Core Curriculum *for* Pediatric Critical Care Nursing

American Association of Critical-Care Nurses

CORE CURRICULUM for PEDIATRIC CRITICAL CARE NURSING

SECOND EDITION

Edited by

MARGARET C. SLOTA, RN, MN

Director, Critical Care Services
Children's Hospital of Pittsburgh
Pittsburgh, Pennsylvania

AMERICAN ASSOCIATION of CRITICAL-CARE NURSES

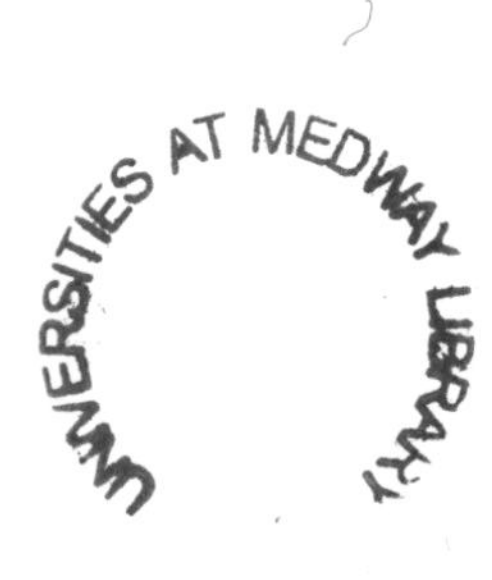

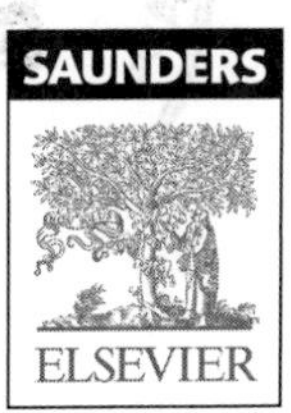

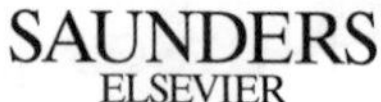

SAUNDERS
ELSEVIER

11830 Westline Industrial Drive
St. Louis, Missouri 63146

CORE CURRICULUM FOR PEDIATRIC CRITICAL CARE NURSING, SECOND EDITION

ISBN-13: 978-1-4160-0157-7
ISBN-10: 1-4160-0157-3

Notice

Knowledge and best practice in this field are constantly changing. As new research and experience broaden our knowledge, changes in practice, treatment and drug therapy may become necessary or appropriate. Readers are advised to check the most current information provided (i) on procedures featured or (ii) by the manufacturer of each product to be administered, to verify the recommended dose or formula, the method and duration of administration, and contraindications. It is the responsibility of the practitioner, relying on their own experience and knowledge of the patient, to make diagnoses, to determine dosages and the best treatment for each individual patient, and to take all appropriate safety precautions. To the fullest extent of the law, neither the Publisher nor the Authors assume any liability for any injury and/or damage to persons or property arising out or related to any use of the material contained in this book.

The Publisher

ISBN-13: 978-1-4160-0157-7
ISBN-10: 1-4160-0157-3

Executive Publisher: Barbara Nelson Cullen
Publishing Services Manager: Deborah L. Vogel
Project Manager: Katherine Hinkebein
Book Designer: Julia Dummit
Marketing Manager: Martin Cronin

Printed in the United States of America

Last digit is the print number: 9 8 7 6 5 4 3 2

With love to my family
George and my children—
Katy, Stephen, Michael, and Christopher

and
My brother David

and in memory of
My parents—Steve and Kathryn
and brother Chuck

All of our work as pediatric critical care nurses is dedicated to the memory of all of the children and families we have cared for—to those for whom our best technology, knowledge, effort, and compassion were not enough for survival and to those children who have gone on with their lives, able to laugh and play again.

Contributors

DEBRA M. BILLS, RN
Transport Team Nurse
Children's Hospital of Pittsburgh
Pittsburgh, Pennsylvania
Multisystem Issues: Septic Shock

NANCY BLAKE, RN, MN, CCRN, CNAA
Director, Critical Care Services
Children's Hospital Los Angeles
Los Angeles, California
Multisystem Issues: Disaster Preparedness

DEBBIE BRINKER, MS, BSN, CCNS, CCRN
Clinical Instructor
Washington State University
Intercollegiate College of Nursing
Spokane, Washington
Hematology and Immunology

LOUISE CALLOW, MSN, BSN, CPNP
Pediatric Nurse Practitioner
Pediatric Cardiovascular Surgery
University of Michigan
Ann Arbor, Michigan
Cardiovascular System

PAULA DICKERSON, RN, BSN
Clinical Documentation Specialist
Burns, Trauma, Ortho, Neurosurgery
Parkland Health and Hospital System
Dallas, Texas
Multisystem Issues: Burns

MICHELLE A. DRAGOTTA, RN, BSN
Transport Nurse
Children's Hospital of Pittsburgh
Pittsburgh, Pennsylvania
Multisystem Issues: Septic Shock

KIMBERLY ANN ETZEL
Professional Staff Nurse
Pediatric Intensive Care Unit
Children's Hospital of Pittsburgh
Pittsburgh, Pennsylvania
Multisystem Issues: Multiple Trauma

MARY D. GORDON, RN, MS, CNS
Adjunct Faculty
University of Texas Medical Branch, School of Nursing;
Burn Clinical Nurse Specialist
Shriners Hospital for Children
Galveston, Texas
Multisystem Issues: Burns

MARY JO C. GRANT, PNP, PHD
Pediatric Critical Care Nurse Practitioner and Researcher
Primary Children's Medical Center
Salt Lake City, Utah
Pulmonary System

MARY JACO, RN, MSN, CNAA
Nursing Director
Inpatient Services
Shriners Hospital for Children
Galveston, Texas
Multisystem Issues: Burns

ANDREA KLINE, RN, MS, PCCNP, CPNP-AC, CCRN
Preceptor for Graduate Nurse Practitioner Students
Rush University
Temple University
Philadelphia, Pennsylvania;
Pediatric Critical Care Nurse Practitioner
Children's Memorial Hospital
Chicago, Illinois
Renal System

BRADLEY A. KUCH, BS, RRT-NPS
Adjunct Instructor, Pediatric Respiratory Care
Indiana University of Pennsylvania
Western Pennsylvania Hospital, School of Respiratory Care;
Transport Therapist
Children's Hospital of Pittsburgh
Pittsburgh, Pennsylvania
Multisystem Issues: Initial Stabilization and Transport

CHRISTINE OWENS LANE, RN, CCRN
Unit Manager III, Burn Intensive Care and Acute Care Units
Parkland Health and Hospital System
Dallas, Texas
Multisystem Issues: Burns

SARAH A. MARTIN, RN, MS, CPNP, PCCNP, CCRN
Advanced Practice Nurse Pediatric Surgery
Children's Memorial Hospital
Chicago, Illinois
Gastrointestinal System

LISA M. MILONOVICH, RN, MSN, PCCNP, CCRN
Pediatric Critical Care Nurse Practitioner
Children's Memorial Center
Dallas, Texas
Renal System

JODI E. MULLEN, MS, RNC, CCRN, CCNS
Clinical Nurse Specialist, Pediatric Intensive Care Unit
Children's Medical Center
Dayton, Ohio
Caring for Critically Ill Children and Their Families

BARBARA MURANTE, BS, MS, ANCC, CPNP
Faculty
University of Rochester, School of Nursing;
Pediatric Nurse Practitioner
Golisano Children's Hospital at Strong
Rochester, New York
Hematology and Immunology

TRACY ANN PASEK, RN, MSN, CCRN
Advanced Practice Nurse, Pediatric Intensive Care Unit
Children's Hospital of Pittsburgh
Pittsburgh, Pennsylvania
Multisystem Issues: Multiple Trauma

MARY FRANCES D. PATE, DSN, RN
Joint Appointment, Assistant Professor
Oregon Health and Science University, School of Nursing;
Clinical Nurse Specialist, Pediatric Intensive Care Unit
Oregon Health and Science University
Portland, Oregon
Caring for Critically Ill Children and Their Families

KATHRYN E. ROBERTS, MSN, RN, CRNP, CCRN
Clinical Nurse Specialist, Pediatric Intensive Care Unit
Children's Hospital of Philadelphia
Philadelphia, Pennsylvania
Hematology and Immunology

SHARI SIMONE, RN, MS, CRNP, FCCM, CCRN
Pediatric Critical Care Nurse Practitioner
Pediatric Intensive Care Unit
University of Maryland Medical System
Baltimore, Maryland
Gastrointestinal System

CAROL A. SINGLETON, RN
Transport Team Manager
Children's Hospital of Pittsburgh
Pittsburgh, Pennsylvania
Multisytem Issues: Initial Stabilization and Transport

ROSE ANN GOULD SOLOWAY, RN, MSED, ABAT
Clinical Toxicologist
National Capital Poison Center
Administrator
American Association of Poison Control Centers
Washington, DC
Multisystem Issues: Toxicology

ELIZABETH C. SUDDABY, RN, MSN
Pediatric Cardiovascular Clinical Nurse Specialist
Inova Fairfax Hospital for Children
Falls Church, Virginia
Cardiovascular System

DEB TEMPLIN
Intermountain Healthcare
Salt Lake City, Utah
Endocrine System

PAULA VERNON-LEVETT, MS, RN, CCRN
Staff Nurse
University of Iowa Hospitals and Clinics
Iowa City, Iowa
Neurologic System

HOLLY F. WEBSTER, MS, PNP
Voluntary Faculty Appointment
University of Utah;
Pediatric Critical Care Nurse Practitioner
Primary Children's Medical Center
Salt Lake City, Utah
Pulmonary System

BARBARA A. WOODRUFF, BS, RRT, CPFT
Transport Respiratory Therapist
Children's Hospital of Pittsburgh
Pittsburgh, Pennsylvania
Multisystem Issues: Septic Shock

Reviewers

SUZANNE E. ANDERSEN, RN, MS, CPNP
Pediatric Critical Care
Children's Hospital of New York Presbyterian
New York, New York

JUDY ASCENZI, RN, MSN
Pediatric Intensive Care Unit
Johns Hopkins Hospital
Baltimore, Maryland

DARLENE NEBEL CANTU, RNC, MSN
St. Luke's Baptist Hospital
San Antonio, Texas

JOSEPH A. CARCILLO, MD
Assistant Professor, Anesthesiology and Critical Care Medicine and Pediatrics
Associate Director, Pediatric Intensive Care Unit
Children's Hospital of Pittsburgh
Pittsburgh, Pennsylvania

JOHN S. COLE, MD, FACEP
University of Pittsburgh Medical Center
Pittsburgh, Pennsylvania

JESSICA STROHM FARBER, MSN, RN
Advanced Practice Specialist
Emergency Medicine and Trauma Center
Children's National Medical Center
Washington, DC

KATE FELMET, MD
Children's Hopital Pittsburgh;
Assistant Professor of Critical Care Medicine
University of Pittsburgh School of Medicine
Pittsburgh, Pennsylvania

MELINDA L. FIEDOR, MD
Clinical Instructor
Department of Critical Care Medicine
Children's Hospital of Pittsburgh
Pittsburgh, Pennsylvania

BARBARA A. GAINES, MD
Director of Trauma
Children's Hospital of Pittsburgh;
Assistant Professor of Surgery
University of Pittsburgh School of Medicine
Pittsburgh, Pennsylvania

SEEMA KHAN, MD
University of Pittsburgh School of Medicine
Children's Hospital of Pittsburgh
Pittsburgh, Pennsylvania

KAREN M. KILIAN, ARNP, CCRN
Pediatric Nurse Practitioner
Children's Hospital and Regional Medical Center
Seattle, Washington

EDWARD P. KRENZELOK, PHARMD, FAACT, DABAT
Director, Pittsburgh Poison Center
Children's Hospital of Pittsburgh;
Professor, Schools of Pharmacy and Medicine
University of Pittsburgh
Pittsburgh, Pennsylvania

AIMEE LYONS
Transport Program Coordinator
Boston Children's Hospital
Boston, Massachusetts

MAUREEN MADDEN, RN, MSN, CCRN, PNP-AC, FCCM
Assistant Professor
UMDNJ–Robert Wood Johnson Medical School
Pediatric Critical Care Nurse Practitioner
Bristol-Myers Squibb Children's Hospital
New Brunswick, New Jersey

H. WILLIAM MCGHEE, PHARMD
Adjunct Clinical Instructor
University of Pittsburgh, School of Pharmacy
Children's Hospital of Pittsburgh
Pittsburgh, Pennsylvania

ELAINE C. MEYER, PHD, RN
Assistant Professor of Psychology
Medical-Surgical Intensive Care Unit
Children's Hospital
Boston, Massachusetts

MICHAEL L. MORITZ, MD
Assistant Professor, Pediatrics
University of Pittsburgh School of Medicine
Pediatric Nephrologist
Children's Hospital of Pittsburgh
Pittsburgh, Pennsylvania

RICHARD ORR, MD, FAAP
Professor, Critical Care Medicine and Pediatrics
University of Pittsburgh School of Medicine
Pittsburgh, Pennsylvania

TRACY PASEK, RN, MSN, CCRN
Advanced Practice Nurse, Pediatric Intensive Care Unit
Children's Hospital of Pittsburgh
Pittsburgh, Pennsylvania

DEVON DRAFFEN PLUMER, CPNP, CCRN
Pediatric Intensive Care Unit/Pediatrics
New Hanover Hospital
Wilmington, NC

RAY PITETTI, MD, MPH
Assistant Professor of Pediatrics
Division of Pediatric Emergency Medicine
Children's Hospital of Pittsburgh
Pittsburgh, Pennsylvania

BONNIE RICE, ARNP, MSN, CCNS
All Children's Hospital
St. Petersburg, Florida

A. KIM RITCHEY, MD
Chief, Pediatric Hematology/Oncology
Children's Hospital of Pittsburgh;
Professor of Pediatrics
University of Pittsburgh School of Medicine
Pittsburgh, Pennsylvania

CAROL G. SCHMITT, BS, PHARMD
Children's Hospital of Pittsburgh
Pittsburgh, Pennsylvania

HARVEY SLATER, MD
Western Pennsylvania Hospital
Pittsburgh, Pennsylvania

DEBORAH J. SOETENGA, RN, MS, CCRN
Children's Hospital of Wisconsin
Milwaukee, Wisconsin

LAUREN SORCE, RN, MSN, CCRN, CPNP
Pediatric Critical Care
Children's Memorial Hospital
Chicago, Illinois

LUCILLE ELIZABETH THOMPSON, RN, MN, CCRN
Advanced Practice Nurse, Cardiac Intensive Care Unit
Children's Hospital of Pittsburgh
Pittsburgh, Pennsylvania

JOYCE WEISHAAR, RN, MSN, CCNS
Children's Memorial Hospital
Chicago, Illinois

Preface

The infants and children cared for in critical care units leave a legacy behind. Beyond the lessons learned from a child's amazing will to survive, the experience of joining the battle for recovery provides knowledge that can never be found in a text. The profession of critical care nursing must continue to grow so that we can meet the demands of this very challenging population, integrating the knowledge and contributions of multiple disciplines and forming a cohesive team of talented caregivers. Although highly skilled and technically competent nursing care has made significant contributions to outcomes, much more is required: compassion shielded by courage; an affirmation to families that although we cannot know their pain, we will always be there for them; persistence blended with realism so that we know when it is time to let go; care focused on not only the children but also their parents, siblings, and extended family who all suffer the consequences; extra caring efforts to make this very difficult period in life a little more endurable; quality monitoring and evidence-based practice that quantifies and ensures the best possible outcomes; and a good, strong sense of humor to help us find the sun in the clouds and the path to tomorrow.

Core Curriculum for Pediatric Critical Care Nursing is intended to serve as a comprehensive reference for nurses caring for critically ill or injured children in any setting. Contributing authors representing pediatric critical care in many geographic regions have created a thorough and relevant source of information that provides a review of a wide variety of conditions. Using a systems approach for easy reference, each chapter includes a review of developmental anatomy and physiology, pathophysiology and defining characteristics of a variety of neonatal and pediatric disorders, clinical assessment, relevant pharmacology, monitoring and diagnostic testing indications, and a multidisciplinary approach to the plan of care. Each pediatric health problem is discussed along the continuum of family-centered care with integration of ethical, legal, and environmental issues. Further clinical integration is achieved with the inclusion of case studies for review in the Appendix. This updated second edition builds on the information presented in the first edition with the addition of two more multisystem issues: initial stabilization and transport of the critically ill neonatal or pediatric patient, and disaster preparedness, focusing on terrorism.

Critical care nurses make a difference in someone's life every single day that they work. My hope is that this book will provide a useful reference to assist in that journey.

Peggy Slota

Acknowledgments

I have learned much from the many children and families I have known and loved over my years in neonatal and pediatric critical care nursing practice. I will always admire and respect the strength and courage of children and families in the face of devastating and unexpected illness and injury. I acknowledge the caring and dedicated health care professionals, including nurses, physicians, respiratory therapists, pharmacists, and all other members of the health care team who play such a vital role in the teamwork required for effective outcomes in a critical care setting. Having worked in five different and challenging pediatric intensive care units, I have developed great admiration for the unparalleled devotion of those who choose this career walk. As an administrator, I have the privilege of hearing and reading praise and gratitude from countless families, who will never forget the staff's efforts to save the life of their beloved child. How wonderful it is to know that their everyday work makes a significant difference in someone's life.

I am very grateful to the contributing authors for their extensive commitment of time and expertise, without which this book would not have been possible, and the thoughtful critiques from the reviewers. I am especially grateful for the thorough and detailed review and suggestions from Lucy Thompson, who went above and beyond in supporting the accuracy and integrity of the work. And truly, the persistent questioning and encouragement from Aunt Ann helped to get the job done. I appreciate the assistance of the editorial staff at Elsevier and the support of my administrative assistant, Vicki Kovac, in fielding numerous communications.

Contents

CHAPTER 1 Caring for Critically Ill Children and Their Families

JODI E. MULLEN AND MARY FRANCES D. PATE

Adam was almost 2 years old and had never been in the hospital. In the weeks before admission, his parents noticed that Adam was holding his head to one side and resisting efforts to straighten it. He was also becoming ataxic. A few days before admission, he experienced emesis and became lethargic. Adam's parents were frightened when they were told that Adam had a malignant brain tumor. Adam was admitted to the pediatric intensive care unit (PICU) after craniotomy for removal of the tumor. He was medically stable and required routine postoperative care. The morning after surgery, Adam was awake and looked around but avoided eye contact. He refused to smile or to pay attention to books or toys. He held his special blanket close to his face. His eyes were huge under the gigantic turban of gauze and tape. With pain medication, he relaxed somewhat but still refused to interact with me.

Adam initially brightened when his mother arrived but showed little interest in her efforts to beguile him. Because Adam was preverbal, it was impossible for him to tell us why he was so unhappy. As his mother and I talked, she told me that Adam was one of four boys. His oldest brother was almost 5 years old, the next boy was 3 years old, and Adam had a twin brother, Noah. Adam's father was at home with the boys until grandparents arrived from another state to help with their care.

I assured Adam's mother that the children were welcome to visit and that I would have the child-life specialist help them understand what to expect before coming into the unit. When the rest of the family arrived, I observed Adam closely. The sight of his father and older brothers elicited a response similar to that of his mother's arrival, but when Adam saw his twin brother, a metamorphosis occurred. When Noah saw Adam, he broke loose from his father's hand and ran to the bed. I suggested that his mother pick up Noah and place him on the bed next to Adam, upon which Adam became a "new man." He sat up straight, looked around the room, and smiled with me and his entire family. Adam's twin had brought Mylar balloons, and within minutes both Adam and Noah were hitting the balloons and laughing out loud. Adam's mother later expressed her feelings to me about the encounter. When she and Adam's father had seen the change in their son, they were able to remain hopeful about their ability to face the future. Their need, at that time, was for their family to be together. Adam's special need was to be with his twin brother. ■

Regardless of the anticipated outcome, admission of a child to the PICU is a highly stressful event for families. Effective pediatric critical care nurses see the child and family as an integral unit that is central to the health care system and are perceptive to the needs of the entire family as they move through the crisis. Nurses who view patients and their families as their partners in care acknowledge both the psychosocial and physical needs of the developing child and family. When guided by the AACN Synergy Model for Patient Care, nursing practice places the patient's and the family's needs as its central or driving force. When nursing competencies are based on these needs, optimal patient outcomes will result (Curley, 2001). By practicing within the Synergy Model for Patient Care, the pediatric critical care nurse can articulate how he or she contributed to the patient's outcomes.

THE SYNERGY MODEL FOR PATIENT CARE

The AACN Synergy Model for Patient Care was initially developed by the AACN Certification Corporation to serve as the foundation for certifying critical care nursing practice (AACN Certification Corporation, 1995).

A. Core Concepts

The following are core concepts of the Synergy Model for Patient Care:

1. **The needs and characteristics** of patients and their families influence and drive the competencies of the nurse.
2. **Synergy occurs** when individuals work together in ways that move them toward a common goal.
3. **An active partnership** between the patient and the nurse will result in optimal outcomes.

B. Patient and Family Characteristics

Every patient and his or her family bring a unique set of characteristics to the care situation. Each characteristic exists along a continuum, and the patient can fluctuate along that continuum as his or her needs evolve over time.

1. **Stability:** The ability to maintain a steady state
2. **Complexity:** The intricate entanglement of two or more systems (body, family, therapies)
3. **Predictability:** A collective characteristic that allows the nurse to anticipate the patient moving along a certain illness trajectory
4. **Resiliency:** Capacity to return to previous level of functioning
5. **Vulnerability:** Susceptibility to stressors that may affect outcomes
6. **Participation in decision making:** Extent to which the patient and family participate in decision making
7. **Participation in care:** Extent to which the patient and family can participate in care.
8. **Resource availability:** Resources (e.g., personal, financial, social) the family brings to the care situation

C. Nurse Competencies

Nursing competencies are driven by the needs of the patient and family. These competencies reflect the integration of nursing knowledge, skills, and experiences that are required to meet the patient's and family's needs and to optimize their outcomes. Each competency has different levels of experience ranging along a continuum from novice to competent to expert practitioner. Although the competencies as a whole reflect the entirety of nursing practice, each competency becomes more or less important depending on the patient's needs at the time.

1. **Clinical judgment:** Clinical reasoning and critical thinking skills
2. **Caring practices:** Creating a therapeutic environment based on the unique needs of the patient and family
3. **Advocacy/moral agency:** Working on another's behalf; resolving ethical concerns
4. **Collaboration:** Working with others in a way that encourages each person's contribution toward the patient's goals

5. **Systems thinking:** Recognizing the interrelationship within and across health care systems
6. **Response to diversity:** Recognizing and incorporating differences into care
7. **Clinical inquiry:** The ongoing questioning and evaluation of practice
8. **Facilitator of learning:** Using oneself to facilitate patient and family learning

D. Outcomes

Optimal outcomes will result when the patient characteristics and nursing competencies are matched. Because the Synergy Model for Patient Care views the patient and family as active participants in the model, the outcomes measured should be patient and family driven. The following are examples of potential outcomes to be measured (Curley, 2001).

1. **Outcomes from a patient perspective**
   - **a.** Functional change
   - **b.** Behavioral change
   - **c.** Trust
   - **d.** Satisfaction
   - **e.** Comfort
   - **f.** Quality of life
2. **Outcomes from a nursing perspective**
   - **a.** Physiologic changes
   - **b.** Presence or absence of complications
   - **c.** Extent to which treatment objectives are obtained
3. **Outcomes from a system perspective**
   - **a.** Costs
   - **b.** Rehospitalization
   - **c.** Resource utilization

The following case study illustrates the use of the Synergy Model for Patient Care in practice.

Duane, a 9-year-old African American male, was diagnosed with asthma at the age of 4. He presented at the emergency department with a 24-hour history of increasing difficulty breathing, wheezing, and cough. Duane had been hospitalized once or twice a year since diagnosis and had been in the PICU on three occasions. Duane had been placed on continuous oxygen and nebulized aerosol therapy and was admitted to the PICU for further observation and care. I had admitted Duane within the past hour and was completing a physical assessment. In addition, I was evaluating Duane from a nursing perspective using the Synergy Model for Patient Care. According to the patient characteristics of the model, Duane could be described as follows.

Stability

Duane was moderately stable. He was currently able to maintain a steady state but had the potential of deteriorating. He was receiving oxygen, aerosol treatments, and intravenous (IV) fluids. He was tachypneic and tachycardic and had moderate work of breathing.

Complexity

Duane's case was mildly complex. Currently only one body system was affected. His family system was relatively uncomplicated; his mother was a single parent, and Duane had two younger siblings, aged 7 and 4 years.

Predictability

Duane's condition was moderately predictable. He was moving along the expected course of his illness. Although he had been in the PICU on three previous occasions, he had not required mechanical ventilation and had always improved as expected once therapies were initiated.

Resiliency

Duane was highly resilient. He had no other underlying conditions that would complicate his situation and had demonstrated previously that he could return to his usual level of functioning.

Vulnerability

Duane had a low level of vulnerability. He was only mildly susceptible to stressors that might affect his outcome. This susceptibility was influenced by his history of asthma, previous medication regimen, and young and relatively healthy physique.

Participation in Decision Making

Duane and his mother had a high level of participation. He was alert and asking questions and had a fairly good understanding of his condition and what would help him get better. His mother was present and asking appropriate questions.

Participation in Care

Duane and his mother had a high level of participation in care. His mother had made care arrangements for her other children so she could remain at the hospital with Duane. I spoke with her about our unit's family-centered care philosophy and invited her to participate as a partner with me in Duane's care.

Resource Availability

Duane and his mother had moderate resource availability. His mother expressed some financial concerns related to recently changing jobs and not yet having health insurance for her family. In addition, the family car had broken down and they were relying on public transportation. She did have an extended family that was supportive of her situation and Duane's medical needs.

By having a holistic picture of Duane and his family's characteristics, I was able to think about what nursing competencies would be an important match for improved patient outcomes. Although all the competencies are important, some would be more valuable in this situation. I would need to rely on strong *clinical judgment* skills to monitor Duane for improvement or worsening of his condition. I would use *caring practices* to create a therapeutic environment for this family, and I would be vigilant to prevent complications from Duane's therapies and the hospitalization itself. I would use *collaboration* skills when working with Duane and his mother and also in determining whom to consult to help with the financial and transportation needs. Finally, I would be a *facilitator of learning* by ensuring that Duane and his mother received additional asthma education.

I discussed outcome goals with Duane and his mother, and we agreed that satisfaction with care, absence of complications, and progressive improvement with discharge from the PICU were important. ■

CHILDHOOD DEVELOPMENT: PSYCHOSOCIAL, EMOTIONAL, COGNITIVE

Knowledge of normal growth and development and the ability to assess the child's developmental level are crucial to working effectively with children and parents in any health care setting. Historically, children were viewed as small adults. Pediatric nurses now conceptualize that using a developmental perspective is the ideal norm. Those who experience children as individuals at a particular level of development find caring for children a rich and rewarding adventure.

The following section describes general childhood development concepts. Individual differences exist, and these stages serve as a general guide for the nurse. Erikson's stages of psychosocial development, Freud's theory of personality development, and Piaget's stages of cognitive development are summarized.

A. Developmental Stages in Infancy (0 to 12 Months)

1. **Psychosocial: Trust versus mistrust**—Infants develop a sense of trust when their basic needs for affection, security, and survival are satisfied. Older infants may fear an unfamiliar person and may not want to be held or approached by a stranger.
2. **Personality: Oral stage**—Sucking provides the major source of enjoyment.
3. **Cognitive: Sensorimotor stage**—Reflexes are gradually replaced with voluntary behaviors. Infants learn to differentiate themselves from others. Infants begin to develop object permanence at 4 to 8 months. Security objects may alleviate anxiety responses in older infants. For instance, infants use their parents as a social reference; that is, by looking at their mother or father, infants determine how to react to new and unfamiliar situations.

B. Developmental Stages of Toddlers (1 to 3 Years)

1. **Psychosocial: Autonomy versus doubt and shame**—Toddlers gradually develop the ability to control their bodies and begin to seek independence. When frustrated or when their need for independence is thwarted, toddlers can express themselves through negativism, temper tantrums, and physical resistance. At times older toddlers are eager to please adults. Toddlers learn through sensorimotor experiences.
2. **Personality: Anal stage**—Toddlers learn bladder and bowel control. They have an egocentric view of life.
3. **Cognitive: Sensorimotor stage matures to preoperational stage**—Toddlers exhibit egocentric development and increased use of language. In addition to early memory development, toddlers develop a sense of time as it relates to their daily routine of meals, naps, and playtime.
4. **Concept of death:** Toddlers view death as a temporary event and may continue to act as though the dead person is still alive (Hockenberry, 2004).

C. Developmental Stages of Preschoolers (3 to 5 Years)

1. **Psychosocial: Initiative versus guilt**—Preschoolers begin to develop the superego and learn right from wrong. They have a strong need to explore the environment. Preschoolers may feel guilt or fear in response to inappropriate thoughts or actions. Many preschoolers are eager to conform to adult expectations.
2. **Personality: Phallic stage**—Preschoolers develop a beginning gender awareness and identify with the parent of the same sex.
3. **Cognitive: Preoperational (2 to 7 years)**—The preschooler's vocabulary increases, and magical thinking is used. Preschoolers communicate through play and have vivid imaginations. They are unable to see anyone else's point of view at this stage of development.
4. **Concept of death:** Death is viewed as temporary. Preschoolers may say that someone is "dead" without any understanding of the finality of death. Preschoolers may fear death as a separation from someone they love, as being injured, or as a punishment for misbehavior (Hockenberry, 2004).

D. Developmental Stages of School-Age Children (6 to 12 Years)

1. **Psychosocial: Industry versus inferiority**—School-age children have a need to develop a sense of achievement and competence and are usually willing and eager to cooperate.

2. **Personality: Latency period**—Development of the superego continues, and school-age children gain a greater understanding about what is right and wrong.
3. **Cognitive: Concrete operational (7 to 11 years)**—School-age children begin to use logic in thought and can consider another person's point of view. Language and problem-solving abilities improve. Rules, rituals, and conformity are important to school-age children because they provide order to their world. They expect others, including parents, to obey the rules and will complain if something seems "unfair" to them.
4. **Concept of death:** Early school-age children still believe death is temporary and may view it as scary or violent (Hockenberry, 2004). Older school-age children understand death as permanent and inevitable (Hockenberry, 2004).

E. Developmental Stages of Adolescents (12 to 18 Years)

1. **Psychosocial: Identity versus role confusion**—Teens are often preoccupied and frequently are dissatisfied with their physical appearance. The adolescent years are a time of emotional struggle for independence as the teen searches for a personal identity.
2. **Personality: Genital stage**—This stage begins at puberty with the development of secondary sex characteristics and sex hormones. Teens display frequent mood swings with emotional lability. Teens often fluctuate between wanting to be with their family and avoiding their family.
3. **Cognitive: Formal operational**—The ability to use abstract thinking begins in the early teens. Logical thinking becomes more developed, although teens may retain some magical thinking as well. For example, they may feel that an illness is a punishment for something they did. Use of verbal communication increases.
4. **Concept of death:** Teens understand death as permanent and inevitable but as something that will occur only in the distant future (Hockenberry, 2004).

DEVELOPMENTALLY APPROPRIATE ASSESSMENT OF CHILDREN

Children usually respond well to honesty, gentleness, and respect. Most children want to please their parents and other adults as well.

A. General Principles for Working with Children

1. **Introduce yourself to the child and family:** Include the child in conversation even if the child does not seem to be responding. Children may not respond verbally but will listen to everything that is said and decide how much comfort or danger the situation holds for them. Assure the child that it is all right to talk or not to talk.
2. **Honesty is vital to establishing a trusting relationship with children:** Be honest with the child if the procedure will hurt. To deny that something will hurt and then deliberately cause pain to a child could destroy the possibility of establishing a trusting, cooperative relationship with that child. Admit that you do not know the answer if the child asks a question you cannot answer. Promise to try to find the answer.
3. **Make eye contact and address the child by name.**
4. **Allow the child to see your hands and any instruments you will use:** If possible, allow the child to touch and examine the instruments because this will tap into his or her curiosity. Most children are cooperative if they know you are not planning a painful procedure.

5. **Allow the child to make choices whenever possible, but avoid giving the child artificial choices:** For example, do not ask permission to measure the child's blood pressure unless you are prepared to respect his or her choice if the child refuses. Simply state what you need to do in a gentle but matter-of-fact manner and do it. Examples of realistic choices include desired popsicle flavor and choice of video game to play.
6. **Allow the parents to participate in the child's care whenever possible:** Some procedures can be accomplished with the child sitting on a parent's lap.
7. **Use a calm, soothing voice.**
8. **Encourage the family to bring the child's favorite articles from home.**
9. **Stoop or bend to communicate at the child's eye level when possible.**

B. Principles for Working with Infants

1. Before touching the infant, assess affect, color, level of consciousness, and respiratory rate and effort because changes can occur in these parameters when the infant is touched. Infants express their distress in physiologic and behavioral ways.
2. When possible, perform the assessment while a parent is holding the infant.
3. Warm the stethoscope and other appropriate instruments before use.
4. Smile and speak softly to the infant before touching and during the examination.
5. Bright objects may be useful as a distraction.
6. Start the examination with the least invasive process, such as listening to breath sounds, and end with more invasive processes, such as examining the ears.

C. Principles for Working with Toddlers

1. Assess affect, color, level of consciousness, and respiratory rate and effort before touching the toddler.
2. Name each body part for the toddler as you examine it.
3. Make the experience fun by drawing faces on tongue blades.
4. The toddler will feel more in control if allowed to sit up and to hold a security item.
5. Allow the toddler to inspect and touch the equipment.
6. Before approaching the toddler, demonstrate the equipment on a doll, a stuffed toy, or the toddler's parent.

D. Principles for Working with Preschoolers

1. In simple terms, explain what you are doing as you progress through the assessment.
2. Praise the preschooler frequently, and make the experience fun.
3. Allow the preschooler to inspect and touch the equipment.
4. Demonstrate the equipment on a doll, a stuffed toy, or the preschooler's parent.
5. Avoid holding your hands behind your back because preschoolers may wonder what you are hiding.
6. Avoid using words or phrases like "cut," "take," "broken," or "put you to sleep."

E. Principles for Working with School-Age Children

1. Speak directly to the school-age child, explaining what you are doing and why.
2. Take time to listen to the school-age child.
3. Allow the child to ask questions. The school-age child can understand simple bodily functions, so incorporate this knowledge into the answers.
4. Accord the child respect, privacy, and dignity.

5. Encourage as much mobility as possible to help reduce stress.
6. As appropriate, allow the child to help with the examination.

F. Principles for Working with Adolescents

1. Respect the adolescent's desire for privacy, and avoid unnecessary physical exposure.
2. Give adolescents the choice of whether or not they want their parents to be present.
3. Explain what you are doing and why.
4. Encourage teens to discuss their concerns, and include them in decision making regarding their health and illness.
5. Teach the adolescent about normal physical and sexual development.
6. Facilitate visits with peers when possible.

G. Principles for Working with Adolescents as Parents

1. Affirm the role of an adolescent parent as "Mom" or "Dad."
2. Discourage grandparents or other relatives from usurping the parent's control.
3. Teach the adolescent parent about normal child development, nutrition, discipline, and care.
4. Assess the parent's level of understanding, and teach without condescension.
5. Direct questions and explanations to the parent even when older relatives are present.
6. Treat the adolescent parent with the same respect given to any parent.

STRESS RESPONSES AND COPING BEHAVIORS

Critical illness and hospitalization in the PICU are stressful experiences for all children. This stress arises not only from the underlying medical condition but also from the PICU environment and experience itself.

A. Physiologic Response to Stress

When a human body is faced with a stressful stimulus, the autonomic nervous system is activated, releasing hormones that control physiologic defense mechanisms. The following are signs of this nervous system activation:

1. Tachycardia, tachypnea, and increased blood pressure
2. Peripheral vasoconstriction with cool extremities
3. Inhibition of the digestive system
4. Inhibition of the immune system
5. Hyperglycemia in older infants or children, hypoglycemia in young infants
6. Dilated pupils
7. Increased level of alertness

B. Response to Psychological Stress and Hospitalization

An important part of the human stress response is what the child thinks or feels about what is happening. As children mature, their perception of stress becomes more important to their overall stress response.

1. **Infants:** Infants respond to stress with crying and increased motor activity. The infant may be experiencing pain or fear or may feel the need to be comforted. Infants may suck on fingers, pacifiers, blankets, or endotracheal tubes to calm themselves and cope with stress. Older infants may avert their gaze or attempt to turn away from an unpleasant experience. In an attempt to calm themselves,

older infants may rock their bodies or use their arms or legs to make rhythmic movements.

Cheyenne is an 11-month-old female who was riding in a car with her 12-year-old brother and her mother. Another car ran a stop sign and collided with Cheyenne's car. Cheyenne and her brother are now hospitalized in the PICU with stable injuries while their mother is being evaluated at another hospital. Cheyenne's father is spending his time going back and forth between both his children's hospital rooms. As Cheyenne's PICU nurse, you notice that every time her father leaves, she screams loudly and cries "Daddy, Daddy" over and over. She reaches her arms toward his direction and searches for him constantly with her eyes. Your attempts to comfort Cheyenne are unsuccessful until she is reunited with her father. ■

2. **Toddlers:** Toddlers may react to stress with increased physical activity, loud crying, or screaming that may continue to the point of exhaustion. The mobile toddler may try to resist a frightening situation physically. This age group is particularly susceptible to distress when separated from parents. Toddlers tend to experience regression when hospitalized. For example, previously toilet-trained toddlers may lose bladder control or revert to thumb sucking. Toddlers are frequently attached to security items and often hold them close to the face.

Twenty-two-month-old Trevor is admitted to the PICU with pneumonia. He is receiving oxygen by face mask, has a pulse-oximeter probe taped to his right index finger, electrocardiographic electrodes on his chest, and an IV catheter in his left hand while his hand is secured to an arm board. Trevor is extremely restless in his crib and keeps getting tangled in the wires and tubing. Additionally, he is left-handed and unable to feed himself because his hand is secured to the arm board. As his mother tries to comfort Trevor, he hits at her with the arm board and cries loudly. The PICU nurse recognizes that this toddler is showing frustration as he tries to maintain his independence despite the medical interventions. ■

3. **Preschoolers:** Hospitalization of preschoolers interrupts and challenges children at a time when they are learning to control their own body and environment. To gain control in at least some area, preschoolers may refuse food and not cooperate with caregivers. Preschoolers continue to hold on to security items. Regression to the toddler stage is common. Preschoolers may project feelings of sadness, anger, or guilt onto others or onto toys and frequently express their feelings about illness through dramatic play. Preschoolers may withdraw from interaction with others if they are angry, sad, or in pain.

Four-year-old Megan needs to have a percutaneously inserted central catheter (PICC) placed for ongoing antibiotic delivery. Recognizing that a child this age has a strong imagination and communicates well through play, the IV therapy nurse brings a doll for Megan to play with. This doll has a PICC taped to her arm, and the nurse guides Megan as she plays with the doll so that she can gain some understanding about the PICC and what it will be like to have the PICC in her own arm. ■

4. **School-age children:** A child of this age will ask questions and try to understand the experience. Fear of a loss of control may lead school-age children to deny fears and act "grown up" even when frightened. School-age children may regress to earlier stages of development and fear bodily mutilation and intrusion. If feeling out of control, school-age children may withdraw from caregivers, refuse to communicate, or use television or sleep as a means of escape. He or she finds comfort in familiar routines, the presence of parents, and contact with siblings.

Brian, who is 8 years old, is recovering in the PICU after having brain surgery to remove a tumor. He is awake and alert. His mother has stated that he likes to put together puzzles. Brian and his mother work on an intricate puzzle all afternoon, and when the puzzle has been completed, Brian shows everyone who comes into the room his "awesome puzzle." The nurse smiles and tells Brian what a great job he has done. In doing so, the nurse is recognizing that a child of this age is developing a sense of achievement and competence. ■

5. **Adolescents:** Teens may deny obvious pain and discomfort, especially if peers are present. If feeling out of control, teens may withdraw and refuse to communicate or cooperate. Teens may regress to an earlier stage and become demanding and clinging with caregivers or parents. The hospitalized teen may experience labile and conflicting emotions, especially about the hospitalization itself and any disruption to body or body image.

Sixteen-year-old Brenda was recently transferred to the PICU because of hemodynamic instability following the administration of several chemotherapeutic agents needed to treat her newly diagnosed leukemia. When she is more stable, Brenda spends time on the telephone with one of her friends. The nurse overhears her crying and talking about how "terrible I'm going to look when I lose my hair! No boys will ever want to talk to me!" The nurse recognizes that adolescents are often preoccupied with their physical appearance and are developing a sense of identity. ■

ISSUES RELATED TO HOSPITALIZATION

A. Fear and Anxiety

Most children experience some fear and anxiety when hospitalized. Fears may be reality based, related to previous procedures or hospitalizations, or the result of magical thinking. Information given to a child by friends or relatives may be incorrect, and the child may inadvertently hear frightening comments made by others. Children in the PICU may witness fear in others and may see or hear things from other bed spaces that cause fear and anxiety.

1. **Age-specific fears related to developmental level**
   - **a.** *Infants:* Separation anxiety and fear of strangers begin at 6 to 7 months of age. Crying and clinging to parents are normal behaviors and generally indicate a healthy parent-child relationship. Older infants frequently resist being separated from parents. When parents leave, infants may exhibit loud and active grief that may continue to the point of exhaustion. Over time, they may become passive and withdrawn if cries do not cause the immediate return of parents or if the separation is prolonged. Infants may accept food and comfort from the nursing staff while avoiding eye contact or other interactions.
   - **b.** *Toddlers* may fear separation from parents, large animals, strangers, "the doctor," changes in their environment, or "shots." Temper tantrums, clinging to parents, attachment to security objects, and regression may be used as means of coping with the fears and perceived threats to security.
   - **c.** *Preschoolers* may fear bodily injury or mutilation, darkness, separation from parents, loss of control, the unknown, death, or "shots." They may regress and act like a toddler or become quiet and withdrawn if feeling out of control. Preschoolers may be able to express anxiety through play and drawing.
   - **d.** *School-age children* may fear bodily injury, loss of control, failure in school, supernatural beings, rejection by others, or death. They may also fear intrusive procedures and being separated from family and friends. Incomplete information and misconceptions about illness, injury, and body function may

exacerbate their fears. For example, they may believe that illness is a punishment for bad behavior. Some school-age children may be reluctant to ask questions and feel that they must act "grown up." Additional explanations may be required by this age group, even if an understanding of information is exhibited.

e. *Adolescents'* fear may revolve around social isolation, loss of control, rejection by peers, the appearance of being different, or helplessness. Teens may use denial or regression despite a fear of appearing younger than they are. They may dramatize events or intellectualize illness or injury.

B. Pain

Children in pain frequently receive too little medication, or they may receive no analgesia at all. Despite an increase in the emphasis on pain management in children over the past several years, some misconceptions about children and pain persist (Table 1-1).

C. Separation from Family and Friends

Support from family and friends is important to children, and the need for support and closeness increases during times of illness. If children are separated from loved ones, long-term effects, such as impaired trust, diminished intellectual and motor functioning, and disturbed behavior, are possible. Preventing separation of the child from his or her family is the standard of care in the PICU (Smith and Martin, 2001). Family-centered care practices ensure the closeness of loved ones as familiar trusted sources of security.

D. Limited Understanding

Misconceptions about illness, treatment, and caregiver motives may result from a child's limited understanding. Magical thinking may lead children to conclude that an illness is punishment for misbehavior. Words such as "cut" or "take" can be misconstrued by children and increase levels of fear. The vivid imagination of childhood supplies answers to any unanswered questions or unexplained situations.

TABLE 1-1
Misconceptions About Pain in Children

Misconceptions	Truth About Pain
Children do not experience pain the same as adults.	"Pain is whatever the experiencing person says it is…" (McCaffrey, 1977) regardless of age.
A child who is not crying is not in pain.	Children express pain in varying ways at different ages.
A child who is asleep is not experiencing any pain.	Some children sleep to try to escape pain, just as adults attempt to do.
Infant nerve pathways are not developed enough to have pain (Schecter, 1989).	Infants may experience harmful physiologic effects from stress responses related to pain (Anand, Phil, and Hickey, 1987).
Children will always tell you if they are in pain.	Children may interpret pain as punishment for misbehavior or believe they are supposed to have pain if nothing is done to relieve it.
Children will become addicted if given narcotics.	Physical dependency is unusual but can occur. These drugs can be weaned just as with adults.
Children always tell the truth about pain.	Children may deny pain to avoid injections. Teens may deny pain in the presence of peers.

E. Loss of Control

Hospitalized children are rarely given choices related to their treatment regimen, which results in little sense of control. Physical restraint can increase the anxiety related to hospitalization and, when at all possible, should be reserved as a measure of last resort. Frequently restraints can be avoided with proper preparation of the child, and therapeutic holding may be used for temporary restraint. Therapeutic holding allows close physical contact with a caregiver or family member during procedures and helps to decrease patient anxiety (Hockenberry, 2003). Allowing choices, when choices are truly present, can assist the child in dealing with feelings of loss of control.

ISSUES RELATED TO CRITICAL CARE UNITS

Ashley was 5 years old and had been admitted to the PICU after she fell from a second- story window while jumping on the bed. She had experienced a traumatic brain injury from the fall and was intubated. She lay unresponsive, sedated, and in a darkened room to decrease stimuli as the rhythmic swoosh of the ventilator breaths continued. Occasionally an alarm or a conversation would break the silence. Another health care provider entered the room to examine her and without a word started turning her side to side as Ashley winced in pain. I gasped, went to the bedside, and stopped any further "assessment." I whispered an apology to Ashley, and as I spoke softly to her, a tear ran down her cheek. ■

A. Sensory Overload

Sensory overload can occur for the child in the PICU because of the around-the-clock activity.

1. **Noise** levels can be high from overhead paging systems, bedrail openings and closings, equipment alarms, pagers not placed in the vibrate mode, telephones, and unchecked voices of families and caregivers (DePaul and Chambers, 1995) (Table 1-2). Recommendations have been made by the World Health Organization

TABLE 1-2
Sound Levels Recorded from Selected Nursing Activities

Activity	dB
Full bottle of formula placed on bedside table	75.3
Storage drawer closed	69.8
Orogastric package opened	71.3
Empty feeding syringe tossed in plastic waste can	55.8
Chair moved across floor	62.0
Running water	54.2
Medication drawer closed	58.9
Medication pump sounding an alarm	57.5
Oxygen disconnected from wall	55.0
Ringing telephone	49.7
Cardiac monitor sounding an alarm at 70% volume	65.8
Cardiac monitor sounding an alarm at 30% volume	55.4

Reproduced with permission from DePaul D, Chambers SE: Environmental noise in the neonatal intensive care unit: implications for nursing practice, *Journal of Perinatal and Neonatal Nursing* 8(4): 71–76, 1995.

and the Environmental Protection Agency stating that hospital noise levels should be no greater than 40 to 45 dB during the day and 35 dB at night (Morrison et al., 2003). Decibel levels no greater than 35 are needed for rest, although noise levels in the PICU have been measured at 55.1 dB with increases as high as 90 dB (Smith and Martin, 2001). Many times the sources of noise, such as monitors and infusion pumps, are located close to the child's head. Hearing loss can result from persistent humming of equipment, especially when these noises are combined with the administration of ototoxic antibiotics (Hockenberry, 2003). Patient annoyance, increased length of stay, intensive care psychosis, and delayed wound healing also have been correlated with excess noise (Morrison et al., 2003).

2. **Constant light** leads to confusion of day and night. Differentiation between day and night is difficult if no windows are available. Lights are frequently bright and directly over the child's head.
3. **Unfamiliar tactile and olfactory stimulation** over which the child has little or no control can be disturbing. Children are unfamiliar with hospital food. Medicinal smells may be powerful and unpleasant.

B. Sensory Deprivation

Although there is an excess of stimulation in most PICUs, there is a lack of the normal types of stimulation beneficial for children. Mealtimes and clothing will most likely change. Important bedtime rituals are changed, especially with unfamiliar blankets, beds, toys, and pajamas. Adults other than parents are directing the child's activities and schedule. Restricted activity leads to feelings of isolation and boredom and interferes with the child's ability to cope with the stress of hospitalization. Physical activity is a method frequently used by children to cope with stress. Sensory deprivation may lead to depression and regression and can interfere with normal development. Children who are intubated also have difficulty communicating. Younger children may fear that they might never be extubated or that they will not be able to speak again (Lebet, 2003).

C. Sleep Deprivation

Children in the PICU may experience sleep deprivation because of repeated caregiver interactions and environmental stimuli (e.g., light, noise) (Slota, 1988) (Table 1-3). Day-night orientation can be lost because children in the PICU sleep less than normal, and often any sleep that is achieved will be interrupted. The physical effects of sleep deprivation may result in immune-system vulnerability, inefficient temperature regulation, and impaired healing of cells and tissues. Anxiety, irritability, confusion, and hallucinations are just a few of the psychological symptoms that may be seen in children experiencing sleep deprivation (Bennett, 2003).

D. Lack of Privacy

Some PICUs are large, open units where patients and families experience "living in public." Open areas allow "strangers" (other visitors and hospital employees) to see the children and their parents. Children may also be aware of procedures and crises that occur at beds close to their own, and the need for close observation sometimes leads to physical exposure of the child.

E. Technology Dependence

The number of technology-dependent patients has increased since the development of mechanical ventilation (Amin and Fitton, 2003). Critically ill, unstable children are the highest priority in the PICU. Chronically ill but stable children who are technology

TABLE 1-3
Causes of Sleep Deprivation in the PICU

Noise levels
Decreased light-dark cycles
Disruption of home sleep rituals
Pain and discomfort
Isolation
Immobilization
Anxiety
Depersonalization
Restraints
Tense atmosphere
Pharmacologic paralysis
REM and NREM suppressant drugs

NREM, non-rapid eye movement (sleep); *REM*, rapid eye movement (sleep).
Reproduced with permission from Slota MC: Implications of sleep deprivation in the pediatric critical care unit, *Focus Crit Care* 15 (3): 35–43, 1988.

dependent may receive less developmental and psychosocial support when the PICU is busy or understaffed. Technology may interfere with parental attachment or lead to the parents' emotional withdrawal from their child. Technology-dependent children may experience long periods of separation from home, school, and friends. Children are aware that alarms are related to them and exhibit fear when any alarm is triggered. Chronic sleep disruption can affect learning, growth, healing, and developmental progress.

DEVELOPMENTALLY APPROPRIATE INTERVENTIONS

A. Pain Management

1. **Assessment of pain:** An accurate assessment of the critically ill or injured child's pain is vital for appropriate pain intervention. The child who states that he or she is in pain should be believed. Family caregivers can provide input about their perception of the child's pain and can also provide a history of the child's experience with pain, what words the child uses to describe pain, and what interventions were previously successful. The pain assessment should be tailored to the child's developmental level and needs (Table 1-4). Other important considerations include the following:
   a. Some children in the PICU may be too ill to display typical pain behaviors because energy is directed toward maintaining physiological stability.
   b. Pain assessment scales are useful to quantify and supplement the nurse's observations.
   c. It may be difficult to distinguish between pain and anxiety. Pain should be considered when the patient's behavior is associated with actual or potential tissue damage or injury. The underlying disease and the presence of lines, tubes, and drains can contribute to the child's pain (American Academy of Pediatrics, 2000).
   d. It is challenging to assess pain adequately in the nonverbal patient (e.g., young child, developmentally delayed patient, sedated or pharmacologically paralyzed patient). The nurse must rely on a myriad of assessment strategies in this situation.

TABLE 1-4
Guidelines for Age-Appropriate Assessment and Nonpharmacologic Management of Pain

Response to pain	Nonpharmacologic pain management (to be combined with appropriate analgesia, as indicated)
NEONATE (0-28 DAYS)*	
BEHAVIORAL INDICATORS OF PAIN Preterm infant may show a less robust response than a term infant Cry (can be high-pitched, tense, or irregular) Facial grimace (eyes tightly closed, brows lowered and drawn together, mouth square-shaped) Increase or decrease in body movements Change in feeding patterns	Swaddling Positioning Developmental care Nonnutritive sucking (e.g., pacifier) Oral administration of sucrose (infants <30 days of age or <44 wk gestation) Music or fetal heart sounds Decrease noxious environmental stimuli
PHYSIOLOGIC INDICATORS OF PAIN Change in vital signs Change in oxygen saturation Vagal tone Palmar sweating	
PAIN ASSESSMENT SCALES Premature Infant Pain Profile (PIPP) (Stevens et al., 1996) CRIES (Krechel and Bildner, 1995) Neonatal Infant Pain Scale (Lawrence et al., 1993) Neonatal Facial Coding System (Grunau et al., 1998)	
INFANT (0-12 MO)	
Response may be blunted by state of arousal, level of consciousness, and severity of illness Cry (can be high-pitched, tense, or irregular) Facial grimace (eyes tightly closed, brows lowered and drawn together, mouth square-shaped) Increased or decreased level of activity, restless, irritable, inconsolable Withdrawal from stimulus (newborns show poorly localized response; older infants localize more and may attempt to pull away) Changes in vital signs Lacrimation	Bundling and rocking Presence of primary caregiver Nonnutritive sucking (e.g., pacifier) Oral administration of sucrose (infants <30 days of age or <44 weeks gestation) Familiar sounds (voices, music, etc.) Security object Distraction with visual stimuli Cutaneous stimulation
PAIN ASSESSMENT SCALES FLACC (Merkel et al., 1997) Nursing Assessment of Pain Intensity (Schade et al., 1996) COMFORT (Ambuel et al., 1992)	
TODDLER (1-3 YR)	
Cries, screams May lie still or rigid Physically attempts to avoid painful stimuli Facial grimace of pain Irritable, sad, uncooperative Touching or guarding site of pain Verbalized expressions ("ow," "ouchie," "it hurts," "stop")	Presence of primary caregiver Rocking, holding, touching Security objects Distraction (e.g., viewmasters, music therapy, books) Controlled breathing (e.g., blowing bubbles)

Continued

TABLE 1-4
Guidelines for Age-Appropriate Assessment and Nonpharmacologic Management of Pain (*cont'd*)

Response to pain	Nonpharmacologic pain management (to be combined with appropriate analgesia, as indicated)
May verbalize where something hurts Unable to describe pain intensity May regress behaviorally	Cutaneous stimulation
PAIN ASSESSMENT SCALES FLACC (Merkel et al., 1997) Nursing Assessment of Pain Intensity (Schade et al., 1996) COMFORT (Ambuel et al., 1992)	
PRESCHOOLER (3-5 YR)	
Cries, screams May demonstrate aggressive behavior Irritable, difficult to comfort Easily frustrated Increasing ability to describe verbally the location and intensity of pain	Presence of primary caregiver Age-appropriate explanations and reassurance Rocking, holding, touching Security objects Distraction (e.g., kaleidoscopes, music therapy, books) Controlled breathing (e.g., blowing bubbles) Cutaneous stimulation
PAIN ASSESSMENT SCALES FLACC (Merkel et al., 1997) Oucher (Beyer and Knott, 1998) Faces Pain Scale (Hicks et al., 2001) Body Outline Tool (Van Cleve and Savedra, 1993) Visual Analogue Scale (Tyler et al., 1993)	
SCHOOL-AGE (6-12 YR)	
May cry less than younger peers May grunt, moan, or sigh Verbalizes protest Describes pain location, intensity, and quality Restless or overly still and quiet Irritable May try to appear brave May clench teeth or fists; body stiffness	Presence of primary caregiver Focused relaxation techniques Distraction (e.g., imagery, music therapy, watching television) Controlled breathing Cutaneous stimulation
PAIN ASSESSMENT SCALES FLACC (Merkel et al., 1997) Oucher (Beyer and Knott, 1998) Faces Pain Scale (Hicks et al., 2001) Body Outline Tool (Van Cleve and Savedra, 1993) Visual Analogue Scale (Tyler et al., 1993) Numeric 1 to 10 Adolescent Pediatric Pain Tool (Savedra et al., 1993) Non-Communicating Children's Pain Checklist (Breau et al., 2000)	
ADOLESCENT (13+ YR)	
Describes pain location, intensity, quality, and duration May clench teeth or fists; body stiffness May grunt, moan, or sigh	Presence of primary caregiver or friends, as desired Focused relaxation techniques

TABLE 1-4
Guidelines for Age-Appropriate Assessment and Nonpharmacologic Management of Pain (*cont'd*)

Response to pain	Nonpharmacologic pain management (to be combined with appropriate analgesia, as indicated)
Restless or overly still and quiet Irritable, moody May be stoic in the presence of peers	Distraction (e.g., imagery, music therapy, watching television) Controlled breathing Cutaneous stimulation
PAIN ASSESSMENT SCALES Oucher (Beyer and Knott, 1998) Faces Pain Scale (Hicks et al., 2001) Body Outline Tool (Van Cleve & Savedra, 1993) Visual Analogue Scale (Tyler et al., 1993) Numeric 1 to 10 Adolescent Pediatric Pain Tool (Savedra et al., 1993) Non-Communicating Children's Pain Checklist (Breau et al., 2000)	

*American Academy of Pediatrics, 2000.
CRIES, Crying Requires increased oxygen administration, Increased vital signs, Expression, Sleeplessness; FLACC, Faces, Legs, Activity, Cry, and Consolability; NFCS, Neonatal Facial Coding System; NIPS, Neonatal Infant Pain Scale.

e. Reassessment of pain should take place at appropriate intervals around nonpharmacologic and pharmacologic interventions to evaluate the adequacy of the interventions. For instance, depending on the route and dosage of a pain medication, reassessment should take place after the onset of action and then at a frequency determined by the duration of action.

2. **Nonpharmacologic management of pain**
   a. Various types of nonpharmacologic measures are useful in the management of children's pain. These techniques work best when combined with appropriate analgesia. (See Table 1-4 for a developmental perspective of nonpharmacologic pain interventions).
   b. When possible, tell the child how long the pain will last, and be sure to tell the child when the procedure ends.
   c. Encourage the child to express feelings of pain. Assure the child that it is all right to cry when something causes pain.
   d. Educate parents about their role in supporting their child who is in pain (Broome, 2000). Ask the parents what comfort measures they have found successful at home.
   e. Distractions such as singing, blowing bubbles, storytelling, reading to a child, music therapy, or watching television may help a child cope with pain.
   f. The use of rhythmic motion is helpful. Infants often like to be patted on the back or bottom. Infants, toddlers, and preschoolers like rocking motions. Holding the child may be comforting at all ages.
   g. Controlled breathing, imagery, and hypnosis can bring about relaxation. These techniques should be practiced before the painful event takes place (Bowden and Greenburg, 2003).
   h. Cutaneous stimulation by means of massage, the application of heat or cold therapy, acupuncture, or acupressure can provide low-level sensory input to reduce the transmission of painful stimuli.

i. Sucking a pacifier may comfort infants experiencing pain. Dipping the pacifier in a 24% sucrose solution may augment pain reduction in preterm and term infants (Stevens and Ohlsson, 2001). Research related to this relatively new therapy is ongoing. Some centers may have inclusion and exclusion criteria to guide the administration of sucrose analgesia. Examples of exclusion criteria might include the risk for necrotizing enterocolitis or unstable glucose levels.

j. Collaborate with child-life specialists, behavioral medicine specialists, and other members of the pain-management team to establish an individualized and comprehensive approach to pain management.

3. **Pharmacologic pain management**

a. *Administration:* The goal of pain-management therapy is to optimize pain relief while minimizing adverse effects (Oakes, 2001). For intermittent dosing, consider the duration of action and anticipate redosing before pain returns. Continuous infusion provides a constant level of analgesia and may be preferable to bolus administration. Administer a bolus dose when the continuous drip is started and each time the infusion rate is increased (Oakes, 2001). Patient-controlled analgesia (PCA) has been used successfully in children as young as 5 years and gives the patient a sense of control over his or her pain. In children younger than 5 years or those who cannot use the PCA system because of developmental delays or neurologic impairment, nurse- or parent-controlled analgesia may be initiated (Berde and Solodiuk, 2003). Some patients in the PICU benefit from epidural analgesia.

b. *Nonopioids* are useful for mild to moderate pain and can frequently be given in combination with opioids for control of more severe pain.

- Acetaminophen is a mild analgesic frequently used for pain and fever in children. It works well for mild pain or when given in combination with an opioid.
- Ibuprofen has anti-inflammatory and analgesic effects with potential for gastrointestinal side effects, platelet aggregation, and bleeding.
- Ketoralac is an anti-inflammatory agent that can be administered via the parenteral route.

c. *Sedatives* can be helpful if the child remains agitated despite receiving appropriate analgesia. Sedatives should not be used in isolation when there is a pain component involved but can work in combination with opioids to control pain more effectively.

- *Benzodiazepines* (i.e., midazolam, lorazepam, and diazepam) provide muscle relaxation, amnesia, and relief of anxiety (Oakes, 2001). When a patient has received a benzodiazepine for an extended period, taper the drug slowly and observe for symptoms of withdrawal such as a state of agitation, confusion, choreoathetoid movements, and ataxia.
- *Ketamine* provides sedation and analgesia. Ketamine raises blood pressure and should not be used in children at risk for increased intracranial pressure. It is a useful drug for children with asthma because of its bronchodilatory effect. Observe for emergence reactions such as excitement, hallucinations, or delirium. Maintain a dark, calm environment if this reaction occurs.
- *Barbiturates* have anticonvulsant and sedative properties. They have a longer half-life and are particularly helpful in patients with acute head injury.
- *Chloral hydrate* can be used to induce sleep and control agitation. Side effects can occur with long-term use because of a buildup of active metabolites.
- *Dexmedetomidine* is an alpha$_2$-adrenergic agonist with sedative and analgesia effects. It is administered via continuous infusion and has minimal effect on

respiration. The patient may need a lower opioid dose when receiving dexmedetomidine (Tobias et al., 2003).

d. *Opioids:* A wide choice of drugs is available to provide relief of moderate to severe pain (Table 1-5). If an opioid is used longer than 4 to 5 days, the child should be weaned from the opioid for a while and observed for withdrawal symptoms (Oakes, 2001). Symptoms may include poor feeding, vomiting, diarrhea, dilated pupils, sweating, nasal congestion, fever, mottling, hallucinations, increased motor tone, and seizures. Because of its longer half-life,

TABLE 1-5
Select Medications Used to Manage Pain and Sedation in the Pediatric Intensive Care Unit (PICU) Patient

Drug	Dose*	Route	Frequency
OPIOIDS			
± Morphine	0.2-0.5 mg/kg/dose Prompt release	PO	Every 4-6 hr as needed
	0.3-0.6 mg/kg/dose Controlled release	PO	Every 12 hr
	0.05-0.2 mg/kg/dose (usual maximum dose: 15 mg/dose)	IV, subcutaneous, IM	Every 2-4 hr as needed
	Neonates (use preservative free formulation)		
	0.01-0.02 mg/kg/hr	IV infusion	Continuous
	Infants/children		
	0.01-0.04 mg/kg/hr	IV infusion	Continuous
Fentanyl	1-4 mcg/kg/dose	IV	Every 1-3 hr
	0.5-5 mcg/kg/hr	IV infusion	Continuous
Meperidine†	0.75-2 mg/kg/dose (maximum dose: 100 mg/dose)	IV, IM, subcutaneous	Every 2-4 hr as needed
± Methadone	0.1 mg/kg/dose initial (maximum dose: 10 mg/dose)	Oral, IM, subcutaneous	Every 4 hr for 2-3 doses, then every 6-12 hr
	Narcotic dependency; 0.05-0.1 mg/kg/dose increase by 0.05 mg/kg/dose until withdrawal controlled		Every 6 hr; after 24-48 hrs the dosing interval can be lengthened to every 12-24 hr during weaning
Codeine	0.5-1 mg/kg/dose (maximum dose: 60 mg/dose)	PO	Every 4-6 hr as needed
NONOPIOIDS			
Acetaminophen	10-15 mg/kg/dose (do not exceed 5 doses in 24 hr)	PO or PR	Every 4-6 hr as needed
NONSTEROIDAL ANTI-INFLAMMATORY			
√ Ibuprofen	4-10 mg/kg/dose (maximum dose: 800 mg/dose)	PO	Every 6-8 hr

Continued

TABLE 1-5
Select Medications Used to Manage Pain and Sedation in the Pediatric Intensive Care Unit (PICU) Patient (*cont'd*)

Drug	Dose*	Route	Frequency
¥ Ketorolac	0.4-1 mg/kg/dose (maximum dose: 30 mg/dose)	IV	Every 6 hr
SEDATIVES			
Lorazepam	0.05-0.1 mg/kg/dose (maximum dose: 2 mg/dose)	IV	Every 4-8 hr
	0.025-0.1 mg/kg/hr (maximum rate: 2 mg/hr)	IV infusion	Continuous
Midazolam	0.05-0.1 mg/kg/dose	IV	Every 1-2 hr
	0.02-0.1 mg/kg/hr	IV infusion	Continuous
Diazepam	0.04-0.3 mg/kg/dose (maximum of 0.6 mg/kg within an 8 hr period if needed)	IV	Every 2-4 hr
Ketamine	0.5-2 mg/kg/dose	IV	Titrate to effect
	5-20 mcg/kg/minute	IV infusion	Continuous
Chloral hydrate	8-25 mg/kg/dose (maximum dose: 500 mg/dose)	PO or PR	Every 8 hr
Dexmedetomidine	0.25-0.5 mcg/kg	IV	Titrate to effect
	0.1-0.7 mcg/kg/hr	IV infusion	Continuous

IM, intramuscular; IV, intravenous; PO, by mouth; PR, by rectum.
From Lexi-Comp Inc., 2004.
Drug dosages may vary based on prescribing practitioner preference, indication for use, and chronicity of the illness. Always check additional references such as the hospital formulary or manufacturer recommendations for dosage and administration guidelines.
*For children weighing <50 kg. Consider maximum recommended dosage in children >50 kg.
+Long-term administration not recommended due to buildup of active metabolites.
±Decrease dose in patients with renal impairment.
¥Do not use in patients with renal impairment.
√Use caution in patients with renal impairment.

methadone is useful as an enteral medication when a child is being weaned from opioids. Help the family understand that opioid dependency is a physiologic phenomenon and that the child is not psychologically addicted. This fact is often not well understood by families and may be a source of anxiety.

4. **Pharmacologic paralysis:** The intubated patient may receive neuromuscular blocking agents to augment other therapies. These medications do not affect the child's state of consciousness or perception of pain. Every child receiving a paralytic should also receive appropriate analgesia and sedation.

B. Communication

The nurse's words, tone of voice, body language, facial expressions, actions, and emotions all convey messages to patients and families. It is important to communicate in a developmentally appropriate manner. Critical care nurses can use communication in a positive way to help children and families as they struggle to cope with the stress of a PICU admission.

1. **Preparation for procedures:** When given the option, most parents will choose to be present with their child during procedures. With proper preparation and

guidance, parents can provide support and comfort to their child. If a parent does not feel able to remain with the child, this decision should be respected. A child-life or play specialist is invaluable in preparing and supporting children for surgery or procedures in a developmentally appropriate manner.

a. *Infancy:* Even infants will learn quickly which cues predict painful events. Awaken infants before any painful procedure so they are not aroused from sleep by pain. Avoid repetitively playing familiar music during procedures such as suctioning or needle sticks so the infant will not associate the music with discomfort or learn to interpret the sounds as a cue to imminent pain.

b. *Toddlers:* Use simple words and phrases to explain the procedure immediately before performing the procedure. Allow the child to handle the equipment when possible. Use restraints only when necessary. Use phrases like "all done" when appropriate so the toddler knows when the procedure is over.

c. *Preschoolers:* Use pictures, puppets, dolls, or toys during explanations or demonstrations, and allow the preschooler to handle them. If time permits, preschoolers may be prepared hours in advance for minor procedures or a few days ahead of time for more serious events. Help preschoolers identify safe times and places when no procedure, vital sign measurement, or other care is planned. Allow preschoolers to keep a security item during procedures. Avoid using confusing phrases such as "put you to sleep" for anesthesia or "move you to the floor" for transfer. The child may interpret these phrases literally.

d. *School-age children:* Use as many choices as possible. Ask the school-age child to explain what was heard to verify understanding of explanations. Allow time for and encourage questions. Depending on the nature of the procedure, school-age children may be prepared weeks before the event. When advanced planning is not possible, allow the school-age child as much time as possible between the explanation and the event. Teach and encourage the use of cognitive-behavioral coping techniques such as imagery and relaxation before the procedure.

e. *Adolescents:* Provide factual explanations of what will happen, and encourage questions. Promote a sense of control by allowing the adolescent to make appropriate choices. Allow teens to choose whether they want to have a parent present. Teach coping techniques such as imagery or relaxation before the procedure. Prepare adolescents as soon as it is known that the procedure or surgery is needed.

2. **Communicating with intubated children:** Children who remember being intubated find the experience of not being able to communicate anxiety producing (Playfor et al., 2000).

Phillip is a 12-year-old male admitted to your PICU with respiratory failure. He is intubated and mechanically ventilated. His arms are restrained to prevent him from dislodging his endotracheal tube. He received some sedating medications and does not remember having the endotracheal tube placed or why he is in your PICU. ■

Strategies for communicating with such a child include the following:

a. Introduce yourself, and orient the child to the place and situation. Speak to the child before and during procedures. Explain what is happening and why the child is in the PICU (i.e., "You were hurt in an accident," "You became very sick," or "You are in the hospital, and you are getting better"). As the child gains awareness, you may need to repeat these explanations.

b. Explain why the child cannot make noise or cry out.

c. Use frequent, gentle touching when you are with the child.

d. Encourage parents to stay with the child, and teach them to assist with appropriate care (i.e., diaper changes, bath, oral hygiene, eye care) if they desire to do so.
e. Allow these children to point to a picture or a word board to express their needs.
f. Teach the child how to summon help if needed (e.g., using a call light).
g. Ask questions that require only a "yes" or "no" answer so the child can shake or nod his or her head or give a thumbs up or down if moving the head is ill advised.
h. Consult a speech or child life therapist as needed for additional augmentative communication devices.

3. **Communication with children who are sedated and pharmacologically paralyzed:** The child receiving sedation and chemical paralysis will retain the ability to hear and may recollect the experience later (Playfor et al., 2000).
   a. Use the child's name, and tell the child what you plan to do even if you think the child might not be able to hear you. Explain noises that the child might hear, such as the monitor alarming or the sounds of the ventilator. Describe things the child might feel, such as vital signs, turning, oral hygiene, suctioning, or bathing.
   b. Touch the child gently, and speak to the child before painful interventions.
   c. Explain to the child why he or she cannot move and that the condition is temporary until the child gets better.
   d. Tell the child that he or she will not be left alone. If the family must leave temporarily, inform the child that the family will return. Family members may record special tapes that can be played in their absence, such as the reading of a favorite story for the child.
   e. Encourage parents to touch, stroke, and talk to the child. Parents may tell the child about things family members are doing, read stories, or sing to the child.
   f. Ask parents what type of music the child prefers, and play this periodically. Before performing any procedures, turn off the music and then explain the procedure. In this way, the child may realize that procedures do not take place while music is playing.
   g. Place a sign in the room that reminds others that the child may hear them, even though he or she is not moving.

C. Interventions for Sleep Deprivation, Sensory Deprivation, and Sensory Overload

1. **Minimize noise levels:** Be aware of the noise level in the PICU, and make attempts to eliminate unnecessary noise. Alarm volumes should be kept just to the level that will alert the nurse to a problem. Monotonous sounds, such as the beep of the QRS, can be turned off if not needed. Limit loud conversation both in and outside patients' rooms, and speak in soft, soothing tones. Use earphones or ear pads to decrease noise exposure for the children even if they are not listening to music. Turn music or headphones off periodically so the child can have quiet periods. Anticipate when infusion pumps are likely to complete their cycle and alarm so they can be responded to quickly.
2. **Maintain a day-night cycle:** Determine the child's usual morning and daytime routines, such as awakening time, mealtime, and playtime. Depending on the child's condition, adhere to these routines when possible. Try to maintain the child's normal bedtime routine, which may include a bath at night, reading a story, or having a security object in bed. Dim lights as much as possible at night, and use indirect lighting around the child. Organize nursing care and that of other caregivers so the child can be undisturbed for at least 90 minutes of sleep. When awakening a child, always offer an explanation before performing any procedures.

For the child who will be in the PICU more than a few days, it can be beneficial to establish a schedule that enhances circadian rhythms when possible. For this schedule to be successful, everyone, including parents, need to follow it as much as possible. Ask parents about their preferences regarding usual home routines. Incorporate this knowledge into the schedule. Initially, the child may be tired and irritable during awake periods and want to sleep. After a few days, however, the child's body will reestablish a circadian rhythm and the irritability and signs of ICU psychosis will diminish. A sample schedule to be used as the child progresses through recovery is outlined in Table 1-6.

D. Facilitation of Play in the PICU

Having an opportunity to play while in the PICU normalizes and humanizes the environment as it allows the child to release tension and express feelings. Play can also provide diversion while giving children the opportunity to exercise control over their hospital experience. The child who is a patient in the PICU presents a different challenge to caregivers interested in providing play opportunities for their patients.

1. Child-life or play specialists can assist in finding appropriate play activities for children at different levels of development.
2. If so desired, parents can bring special toys from home for the child. Children appreciate being surrounded by familiar objects.
3. Caregivers or parents may play for the child who cannot play at all. In some cases, the child can verbally direct the play. Make passive forms of play, such as being read a book, available for these children.
4. Medical play with equipment and supplies can correct misconceptions about the equipment and lessen the anxiety of a procedure (Hockenberry, 2004).

TABLE 1-6
Sample Schedule to Enhance Circadian Rhythms During Hospitalization

Time	Activities
8:00 AM-1:00 PM	Awake Lights on Window blinds open Child out of bed if possible TV on Playtime
1:00 PM-3:00 PM	Nap Lights off TV off Sleep or quiet time
3:00 PM-9:00 PM	Awake Lights on Window blinds open Child out of bed if possible TV on Playtime
9:00 PM-8:00 AM	Asleep Lights off TV off Allow 90 min of uninterrupted sleep when possible by grouping interventions or by delaying interventions that can wait until after the sleep period.

*Schedule adapted as possible during hospitalization and recovery.

5. *Infants* enjoy mobiles, pictures of faces, tapes with soothing music or parent's voices, and soft, cuddly toys. Older infants enjoy toys they can grasp and manipulate. When their use is possible, equipment such as bouncy seats and swings may provide support and enable play.
6. *Toddlers* enjoy books, security objects, and tapes with music, stories, or recorded family voices. Immobility is difficult for the toddler, who may benefit from watching the caregiver play with puppets, cars, or other active toys.
7. *Preschoolers* like to talk and have questions answered. They enjoy water play and having stories read to them. They usually enjoy favorite television shows and will often take part in medical play if given the tools.
8. *School-age children* often enjoy medical play, coloring, books, and crafts. Most enjoy children's movies or television shows. Ask the parents what type of shows the child is allowed to watch at home to avoid conflict related to television. A child of this age may also enjoy playing video or computer games.
9. *Adolescents* enjoy books, magazines, and television. Peer visits and telephone calls, if they can be arranged, are helpful to the teenaged patient. Video or computer games are also an enjoyable distraction.

E. Provision of Psychosocial and Emotional Support for the Child

Samantha and Brooke were 3-year-old and 7-year-old siblings who were unrestrained during a motor-vehicle crash. Both their parents had suffered extensive injuries and were being treated at another hospital. The sisters had serious injuries but were being admitted to the PICU in stable condition. Both were awake and experiencing fear and pain.

Samantha cried as I placed her in the bed and attached electrodes and monitoring equipment to her body. She continually tried to remove her IV catheter. I spoke in soothing tones as I administered pain medication, and I gave her a toy to distract her attention away from the IV. Soon Samantha's grandparents arrived, and I could see Samantha visibly relax when she made reassuring eye contact with a familiar face.

Across the hall, Brooke was very quiet. Because of her injuries, her eyelids were swollen shut. She would not speak but would nod "yes" or "no" when asked a question. I oriented Brooke to the room around her and told her why she was in the hospital, reminding her that nothing was her fault. She nodded "yes" when I asked her if she wanted to listen to the reading of a storybook. I read to her and sat at the side of the bed holding Brooke's hand until her grandfather could come and take my place. ■

1. **Recognize that hospitalized children may experience a range of emotions. Sadness, anxiety, fear, and anger may arise.** These emotions may be a response to being in the hospital, having painful procedures done, having to take medicine, or any number of things that happen in the hospital. Ask about their feelings, and assure them it is all right to feel that way. Some children may be unwilling or unable to express their feelings but sometimes display them by facial expression, crying, withdrawal, or being uncooperative.
2. **Arrange for care by consistent staff members to limit the number of caregivers** each child and family encounter. Having a familiar nurse helps to allay parental anxiety and may make it easier for parents to leave the child's bedside for a time. The nurse who takes time to know the child will become familiar with the child's responses and psychosocial needs. Most children communicate more readily with familiar caregivers. Caregivers who are familiar with a child more easily establish predictable routines.
3. **Some children do not respond verbally but are willing to nod or shake their heads in response** to a "yes" or "no" question or point to a picture on a communication board.

4. **Assure children that they did not get sick because of something they thought or did**. This assumes that the hospitalization is not related to the child's actions or inactions, such as driving without a seatbelt or taking an overdose of medication.
5. **Limit the use of restraints** and remove them whenever someone is able to stay with a child or as soon as the child's condition allows for restraint removal.
6. **Offer hospital and PICU "tours" for both the child and parents** with planned admissions. Identify equipment that will be used with the child. Explain the purposes of the alarms. Assure the parents and the child that the nurses know which alarms require an immediate response and which do not. Introduce the child and parents to at least one nurse or staff member whom they will see when the child is admitted.
7. **If the child chooses, allow him or her to wear personal clothing** as soon as possible. Being able to wear clothing from home, including underwear, socks, and shoes, is comforting for most children.
8. **Respect the child's "space."** Speak when approaching the child. Tell the child what you plan to do before touching the bed or the child.
9. **Explain equipment, medications, and procedures in terms of what the child will experience.** Tell children what they can expect to feel, see, hear, smell, and taste. Run a rhythm strip from the monitor, and give it to the child to take back to school. If the results are normal, tell the child so. Allow the child to hold the electronic thermometer, remove the blood pressure cuff, and remove old tape. Give as much control to the child as is safely possible.
10. **Recognize regression as a normal defense mechanism** in the hospitalized child, and help others, particularly parents, understand the process.
11. **Set reasonable limits that a child can understand.** For example, explain that it is all right to feel angry and cry, but it is not all right to bite or kick people. Do not threaten or shame a child. Positively word phrases, for instance, that you are going to help the child hold still rather than that the child is going to be held down. If parents use threats (e.g., "If you don't hold still, that nurse is going to give you a shot"), explain in a tactful manner, but within the child's hearing, the importance of telling a child the truth and avoiding threats so that the child will trust the caregivers.
12. **Offer whatever comfort the child is willing to accept.** Some children may accept stroking and hugging only in the absence of their parents. Interact with children at their eye level, but do not force eye contact with a child who is avoiding it. Interact with the child in a developmentally supportive manner, which can include being physically close, speaking in a soft voice, and using an empathetic touch.
13. **Suggest that the parents bring in family pictures,** and place them where the child can see them at all times.

PSYCHOSOCIAL NEEDS OF FAMILIES

A. Family Assessment

1. **Sources of stress related to the PICU:** The sight and sound of equipment attached to sick children cause anxiety and fear. Parents often cannot distinguish between alarms that signal life-threatening conditions and those that might indicate something as simple as a completed medication or a false alarm (Board and Ryan-Wenger, 2003). The changes in the appearance of a child and procedures are stressful to parents, especially during the first few days of hospitalization. Later in hospitalization, stress related to the communication and behavior of staff increase

parental stress (Curley and Meyer, 2001). Parents fear that their child is in pain and may fear that the child will die. The presence of other sick, injured, or crying children and their apprehensive parents causes additional stress. Alteration in the parental role occurs as they watch strangers care for their child. This can lead to feelings of loss of control because they do not know how to care for the child themselves. Feelings of inadequacy may result when parents perceive professionals as better able to care for their child. Parents may question their self-image as protector and nurturer of their child as they adjust to a new role as parent to an ill child. Restrictions on visitation and separation from the child can cause additional stress (Board and Ryan-Wenger, 2003).

2. **Needs of parents of children in the PICU** (Curley and Meyer, 2001):
   a. Receiving as much information as possible
   b. Assurance that their child is receiving best possible care
   c. Feeling that there is hope
   d. Vigilance
   e. Being near their child as much as possible
   f. Assistance with physical care
   g. Being recognized as important to the child's recovery
   h. Talking with other parents
   i. Prayer
   j. Resources (e.g., transportation, meals)
3. **Responses to stress and coping behaviors:** Stress reactions for families increase when a child's illness is severe, unexpected, or has an uncertain outcome (Rothstein, 1980).
   a. *Reactions*
      - A shock reaction may occur when parents first see their child in the PICU.
      - Parents might be unable to remember information and might repeat the same question several times.
      - The initial response of parents may be to focus on the equipment and monitors and to be afraid to approach the bed or their child. Parents might want caregiver's "permission" and encouragement to approach the bed and touch their child.
      - Some parents blame themselves or other family members for the child's illness and may show hostility toward caregivers.
      - Parents may assist in their child's care with repetitive tasks such as suctioning their child's mouth or draining urine from the tubing into the bag.
      - Parents may focus on a detail and repeatedly complain if they feel it is not addressed adequately.
      - There may be a delay in approaching the patient's bedside while visually scanning the environment for purposes of orientation to the situation (Lewandowski, 1980).
      - Parents may display signs of withdrawal or passive behaviors, or they may intellectualize the illness (Lewandowski, 1980).
   b. *Support systems*
      - Family members are anyone who is considered important in the child's life (Curley and Meyer, 2001).
      - Family members close to the child may provide emotional support for parents, or they may be an additional source of stress if they are unable to cope with the child's illness or injury.
      - Parents are often more willing to leave the hospital temporarily if a member of their support system remains with their child or if they have grown comfortable with a staff member caring for their child.

- Parents sometimes ask family members of another child in the PICU to "keep an eye on" their child while they leave the hospital for a rest even if a familiar caregiver is providing care for their child.
- Parents may miss and worry about children at home or left in the care of others.

c. *Physical needs*

- If a child's admission to the PICU was unexpected, parents may need assistance with finding a place to rest (if rooming-in accommodations are unavailable), bathe, find clothing, and obtain food.
- If the parents live near the PICU, they may want to go home to rest.
- Some parents are not able to cope with leaving the hospital and will need a place to lie down or a place as close as possible to the PICU.
- Assistance from social services should be obtained if parents do not have enough money for food.
- Parents of critically ill children may forget or decline to eat. Encouraging them to eat and rest will help them to maintain their strength so that they will be able to support and care for their child.

d. *Cultural implications:* The cultural and spiritual identity and perspective of families may influence their understanding, roles, and expectations regarding illness, health care interventions, and end-of-life care.

- Some parents whose first language is not English may be able to speak English but have difficulty understanding what is said because of stress they are experiencing and the unfamiliar medical language. Obtain the assistance of an interpreter when the family is having difficulty understanding. It might be easier for them to ask questions in their own language.
- Be aware that wrist bracelets, ankle bracelets, or objects pinned to the child's clothing may have cultural or spiritual significance for the family. Treat these objects with respect. Consider attaching a patient identification bracelet. Do not remove such objects without parental permission unless absolutely necessary. If objects are pinned to linens, be sure they do not get lost when linens are changed.
- Avoid categorizing or stereotyping members of a cultural group (Society of Pediatric Nurses and American Nurses Association, 2003).

e. *Spiritual considerations*

- Many parents experience guilt and helplessness when a child is ill or injured because they feel they must protect their children from harm of any kind. The illness of a child sometimes causes spiritual distress.
- Some parents express feelings that God caused the child's illness because of a parent's personal sin or fault.
- If the parents are religious, offer to contact a minister, priest, rabbi, or other religious leader. Offer the assistance of hospital chaplains if they are available.
- Assure privacy by closing a door or curtain when parents wish to pray or participate in other religious and spiritual rituals. Some parents believe prayer is more effective when several faith-community members are gathered together and lay their hands on the child. Allowances in visiting policies should be made for this type of visit.
- Assess dietary or treatment restrictions related to religion or culture. These may include rules about some foods or a prohibition against certain treatments, such as a ban on the use of blood products.

f. *Financial concerns:* Critical illness usually causes financial stress. Even parents who have insurance may have additional expenses related to hospitalization, which may include the cost of food, travel, babysitting for other children, or loss of pay. Parents may have to return to jobs earlier than desired. It may be necessary for family, friends, neighbors, and faith communities to assist with financial stressors.

B. Interventions with Families

Multiple studies have been done to identify family needs when a child is critically ill. Families want reassurance, access to the ill child, and information.

1. **Supporting families:** Full partnerships with family members should be developed that impart mutual interdependence and equal status with health care providers. Implementation of the Nursing Mutual Participation Model of Care (Curley and Meyer, 2001) reduces parental stress (Table 1-7). Providing structured education and support to parents has also demonstrated improved outcomes in both mothers and young children. During the COPE (Creating Opportunities for Parent Empowerment) intervention study (Melnyk et al., 2004), mothers of 2- to 7-year-olds admitted unexpectedly to a PICU were educated about young children's emotions and behaviors associated with hospitalization and appropriate parental coping skills and interventions for providing emotional and physical care to their child during and after the hospitalization in the PICU. Mothers who received the COPE program demonstrated improved maternal coping and functional outcomes (less stress, less depression, and fewer PTSD [posttraumatic stress disorder] symptoms) in follow-up assessments compared with the control group

TABLE 1-7
Nursing Mutual Participation Model of Care

ADMISSION
Extend our care to include parents
Acknowledge their importance

DAILY BEDSIDE CONTACT
Enable strategies that provide the parent with system savvy
- Information: teach and clarify
- Anticipatory guidance-illness trajectory
- Provide instrumental resources

Facilitate transition to "parent-to-a-critically-ill-child"
- Enhance parent-child unique connectedness
- Role-model interactions
- Invite participation in nurturing activity
- Provide options during procedures

Communication pattern
- Establish a caring relationship with the parent
How are you doing today?
- Assess parental perception of the child's illness
How does he or she look to you today?
- Determine parental goals, objectives, and expectations
What troubles you most?
- Seek informed suggestions and preferences, and invite participation in care
How can I help you today?

Reproduced with permission from Curley MAQ, Meyer EC: Caring practices: the impact of the critical care experience on the family. In Curley MAQ, Moloney-Harmon PA, editors: *Critical care nursing of infants and children,* 2nd ed. Philadelphia, 2001, W.B. Saunders.

mothers. COPE preschoolers experienced fewer adjustment problems (fewer withdrawal symptoms, fewer negative behavioral symptoms, fewer externalizing behaviors, less reported hyperactivity) at 6- to 12-month assessments following discharge compared with the control group patients.

2. **Communicating with parents**
   a. Make an effort to know the parents' first names so they are not always addressed as "Mom" or "Dad." Ask permission before calling them by their first names.
   b. Make an effort to learn how the parents are coping. Asking whether they were able to sleep or have been able to eat or drink anything demonstrates an interest in their well-being.
   c. Engage the parents as partners in care by asking them how they think the child is doing. Parents often detect subtle changes. Such questions also help the parents feel they are important in the child's care.
   d. Ask about the parents' understanding of their child's condition and whether they have any outstanding questions, worries, or suggestions. After you have responded, explore to ensure that they understood the answers and whether your responses were adequate.
   e. Consider forming a parent support group for the families. Groups can be facilitated by clinical nurse specialists, nurses from the PICU, or social workers. Personally invite each parent of every child in the PICU to the group, and keep all discussions confidential.
   f. Assist the parents with physician contact. Let them know that they may request a joint meeting between the family and staff at any time, or offer to arrange a standing meeting for children anticipated to have a lengthy stay.
3. **Building a relationship of trust:** Parents need to trust the caregivers to feel comfortable enough to leave the bedside. Ask the parents to let you know where they are when they are not in the PICU and how they can be contacted. Agree about when they want to be called. Some parents prefer to be called if any change at all occurs, whether positive or negative. If you have agreed to call the parents when their child asks for them, do so. This will enhance a trusting relationship between the nurse and the parents as well as between the nurse and the child. Consider loaning a pager to the parents so they will know you can easily contact them wherever they are.
4. **Mutual care planning with parents**
   a. Help the family understand which things they can safely touch and which must remain the caregivers' responsibility. Some parents turn off alarms to be helpful. Their point of view may be that they are doing the same thing as the nurse who walks into the room, touches a button, and walks away. Take time to explain the unseen assessment that is performed by the nurse as the alarm is silenced.
   b. Collaborate with the multidisciplinary team (which includes the family) regarding the daily plan for the child. Encourage the family to share their observations about the child, especially any changes they notice. If the plan is to observe the child and not make any changes, let them know that also so that they are not disappointed by a perceived lack of progress.
   c. Assist the parents in gaining as much control as possible by maintaining the parental role. Offer choices as much as possible. For example, when possible, let the parents decide when to give a bath or perform oral hygiene.
   d. Offer to be a gatekeeper for the parents. If parents are being stressed by too many visitors who stay too long, let them know that the staff is willing to place limits on visiting so they do not need to do so.

5. **Caring for parents of chronically ill children**
   a. Children with a chronic illness may experience multiple PICU admissions. When possible, assign nurses who are familiar to the child and family from previous admissions.
   b. Parents may be accustomed to performing many procedures at home and have developed their own ways of doing them. Ask how they perform care at home, and be open to the possibility that the staff can learn from experienced parents. Their expertise and contributions to care should be recognized. Parents will also have the ability to assess their child and provide input into clinical management.
   c. Nurses caring for chronically ill children in the PICU should maintain the child's home routine as much as possible and provide developmentally supportive care.
   d. The multidisciplinary team should convene a discharge-planning session with the family before the child returns home or to another facility to ensure the continuity of care.
6. **Working with siblings of a child in the PICU**
   a. Siblings of critically ill children have special needs. The PICU nurse can help to ensure that family-centered visiting policies are in place and that the PICU environment is such that children feel welcome.
   b. Child-life specialists provide excellent preparation for siblings and help them to know what to expect before they visit in the PICU. Siblings may imagine that a brother or sister is far more seriously ill or injured when they are not allowed to see for themselves. The child-life therapist can assist siblings to communicate feelings they might have difficulty expressing. Formal programs for siblings may also be developed and can decrease behavioral and emotional problems following visitation (Nicholson et al., 1993).
   c. Siblings may fear that they caused the illness or injury by something they said or did. Siblings may also experience signs of stress such as sleep disturbances or changes in behavior.
   d. Parents may need assistance in making decisions regarding care of the child's siblings and whether and when siblings should visit.
   e. Best friends of the child in PICU may have concerns and needs similar to those of the child's siblings (Lewandowski and Frosch, 2003).
7. **Facilitating transfer from the PICU:** Although transfer from the PICU signals the child's improvement and stability, it can engender anxiety and worry about future care.
   a. When their child is transferred, parents may experience anxiety related to the following changes:
      - An unfamiliar unit after becoming accustomed to the PICU
      - Unfamiliar staff members caring for the child
      - Changes in how frequently the child is assessed
      - Discontinuation of frequent monitoring
      - No continuous presence of a nurse at the bedside
   b. Family should be prepared for transfer plans before the event and told of changes to expect. The nurse should assist in understanding that a transfer means the child is now doing better and no longer needs ICU care. If possible, offer a visit to the new unit before transfer, emphasizing the positive aspects of the transfer, such as a more private and quiet environment.
   c. A tour of the new unit and introductions to staff can decrease stress. Care conferences with the family and new unit staff before the transfer and follow-up visits by PICU nurses can facilitate transition.

8. **"Visiting privileges" in the PICU:** To suggest that parents need our permission to be with their child is the antithesis of a system of health care that is driven by the needs of the patient. The primary need of the parents is to be with their child.
   a. Parents should have 24-hour access to their child (Society of Pediatric Nurses and American Nurses Association, 2003).
   b. Parents should be given the option of staying with their child during procedures and tests; studies suggest that families would like to be given the option of and may actually benefit from being present during resuscitation events (Society of Pediatric Nurses and American Nurses Association, 2003).
   c. Extended family and significant individuals who provide caregiving and support should be included in educational and informational processes as desired by the child and family (Society of Pediatric Nurses and American Nurses Association, 2003).
   d. Privacy and confidentiality are important in the PICU but are not barriers to family presence (Ahmann et al., 2003).
   e. Meeting the needs of the children
      - Encourage an open, supportive atmosphere where family members can come and go around the clock to meet their own needs and those of the child.
      - Make exceptions to unit policies based on the child and family's individual needs, especially if a child is dying.

INTERVENTIONS FOR DYING CHILDREN

Nate, a previously healthy 9-month-old, had been admitted to the PICU overnight and diagnosed with bacterial meningitis. His condition had quickly deteriorated, and he required intubation and placement on a mechanical ventilator. Medications were being used to improve his blood pressure, and an arterial catheter and a central venous catheter had been placed. Nate was not responsive and did not seem to be aware of anything taking place around him.

As my shift began, I quickly surveyed the situation in Nate's room. It would be challenging to keep up with the multiple care priorities this patient needed, including ongoing assessments, blood products, antibiotics, and placement of a device to monitor pressure in the brain. In addition, two devastated parents clung to each other in the corner of the room, unable to fathom what unspeakable things were happening to their precious child. I established communication with Nate's parents by introducing myself. Using simple words, I explained what we were doing for Nate and answered what questions his parents could bring themselves to ask. Although I was not aware of it at that moment, I was soon to become the catalyst that would help this family start transitioning from being the "parents of a healthy boy" to the "parents grieving for a lost child."

The extremely high pressure in Nate's brain then confirmed the worst: A child who had been eating cheerios and playing with his 2-year-old brother just yesterday was now neurologically devastated to the point that he would not survive. The critical care team's outcome goals for Nate changed from curing his illness to orchestrating his peaceful and dignified death experience.

I facilitated communication between the pediatric intensivist and the parents. We talked about how they would say goodbye to their son. Our PICU has a strong bereavement philosophy, and our program has many interventions that we offer families during this devastating time. I helped Nate's parents decide what options would be right for themselves and their son. Supported by our research-based policy of family-centered care, loving grandparents, aunts and uncles, a godfather, and the family priest encircled the parents when, for the last time, we placed this child in his mother's arms. At the parents' request, the intensivist and I joined this intimate circle. All eyes were overflowing with tears when the child's godfather said a prayer for the parents and then prayed blessings on the critical care team. ■

A. Pain Management in the Terminally Ill

1. When a child is dying, the focus of care becomes pain relief and promotion of comfort of the child and family. Parents are often more likely to withdraw life support if they perceive their child to be in pain (Meyer et al., 2002). Most parents are keenly sensitive to their child's pain and do not want their child to suffer. Parents place a high priority on the child's perceived degree of pain, and this can influence their decision making regarding withdrawal of life support. In addition, there is a moral imperative to relieve the pain and suffering of dying children.
2. As the child develops a tolerance toward the analgesic used, higher doses of opioids may be required to provide adequate pain relief. High doses of opioids carry the risk of respiratory depression. According to the "principle of double effect," when the intended goal is to relieve pain, it is ethically correct to give whatever dose of analgesic is necessary to relieve pain, even if life is shortened as a secondary effect (Siever, 1994). It is not legal, however, to administer more than is necessary to manage pain or hasten death. Administration of a lethal dose of medication with the intent to cause death as a means of pain relief is not acceptable and is, in fact, active euthanasia (Siever, 1994).
3. Nonpharmacologic means of pain relief are useful in the dying child but should never be used to the exclusion of medications.
4. To provide better control of pain, give analgesics around the clock rather than on an as-needed basis.
5. Fear of tolerance or addiction should not be a consideration in the dying child.
6. Neuromuscular blocking agents do not provide sedation or analgesia for the patient, thereby providing no comfort. Administration of these agents during withdrawal of life support provides no benefit to patients (Truog et al., 2000, 2001).

B. Forgoing Life-Sustaining Medical Treatment

1. Forgoing life-sustaining medical treatment includes decisions to withhold, withdraw, or limit medical treatment.
2. Most ethicists believe there is no difference between withholding medical treatment and withdrawing treatment that has already been in use if the treatment is not beneficial to the patient (American Academy of Pediatrics Committee on Bioethics, 1994).
3. When considering the value of medical treatment in children, the benefits of treatment must be continually weighed against the burdens of treatment placed on the child. For instance, mechanical ventilation may be viewed as life prolonging, whereas noninvasive positive-pressure ventilation may relieve dyspnea and improve the child's time left (American Academy of Pediatrics Committee on Bioethics and Committee on Hospital Care, 2000).
4. In most cases, parents are the appropriate decision makers for children. Ideally, parents and caregivers collaborate in making decisions about limiting or withdrawing treatment. The wishes and desires of conscious, coherent children should be given serious consideration (American Academy of Pediatrics Committee on Bioethics, 1994). Parents not only need to know details, but more importantly they need to know the "bottom line" of the illness and the possibility of survival (Meyer et al., 2002). Parents consider many factors when

deciding whether to withdraw life support for their child, including the quality of life, the likelihood that the child might get better (different from survival), and the amount of pain and suffering, in addition to survival. This is more complex and somewhat different from what the ICU staff may consider. For instance, they may view survivability as the most important factor.

5. A decision to withhold or withdraw any medical treatment applies only to that specific treatment and should not be generalized to other treatments or care.
6. A do-not-resuscitate (DNR) order means only that no life-saving measures will be instituted in the event of a cardiac or respiratory arrest unless other measures have been discussed as well. It does not mean that the child should receive any less or different care compared with the care given to another child. It does not necessarily mean that the child is expected to die soon. A care-and-comfort-only policy is written in positive terms and describes the care that will be given to the child, such as supportive care and pain management. Limitation of treatment may include the decision to not institute any new therapies or to stop specific therapies already in use or both.
7. Any decision to forgo life-sustaining treatment for a child who has been abused should be made using the same process or deliberation criteria used for other critically ill children. Parents or guardians may have a conflict of interest because the perpetrator of the abuse risks having legal charges changed from assault to manslaughter or homicide (American Academy of Pediatrics Committee on Bioethics, 2000).
8. Withdrawal of treatment: Consult parents when planning the time of withdrawal of treatment. There is no urgent need to withdraw support immediately simply because a decision was made. Allow time for parents to gather whatever family members they wish to be with them. Consult multidisciplinary team members, such as a chaplain, child-life therapist, interpreter, and social worker for assistance as appropriate to family needs. Families may want the clergy from their community to be contacted in addition to or instead of the hospital chaplain, or they may not desire either. They may also want the family pediatrician to be involved (Meyer et al., 2002).
9. Acknowledge that parents may be in a stronger agreement with health care providers concerning treatment discontinuation than with family members and friends. This may occur because the health care providers are knowledgeable concerning end-of-life issues and may have been more involved in the decision-making processes. (Meyer et al., 2002)
10. Provide anticipatory guidance to family members related to how treatment will be discontinued and how the child might respond. Allow parents all the time they need to say their good-byes to the child both before and after treatment is withdrawn. Parents may wish to hold the child before and after treatment is withdrawn, especially if death is expected to follow quickly after withdrawal of support. Parents may wish to play specific music for the child, have certain toys or security objects available, or carry out other rituals that have had meaning for them as a family, especially if the child is likely to die when support is withdrawn.
11. Consider discontinuation of monitoring. If the unit has central monitoring capability, consider turning off the monitor in the child's room and continuing monitoring at the central station. Avoid having alarms go off in the child's room if no response to the alarms is planned.
12. Privacy is essential for a family when treatment is withdrawn from a child. Transfer the patient to a private room with less traffic flow, or provide a curtain if no private room is available. Ask parents who, if anyone, they want to have in attendance when life support is withdrawn. Many parents, but not all, wish to be

alone; on the other hand, some fear being alone. Assure parents that if they choose to be alone, assistance will be close by.

C. Caring for the Potential Organ Donor

1. *Brain death* is defined as the irreversible cessation of function of the whole brain, including the brainstem.
2. Critical care staff members are required by law to identify potential organ and tissue donors.
3. Some families see organ donation as a chance to have "something good" come from the death of their child, but other families cannot accept having organs taken from their child related to religious, cultural, or personal convictions (Carnevale, 2003).
4. Early referral to an organ-procurement organization provides assistance of skilled professionals to help both caregivers and parents through the process of organ donation.
5. Uncouple the child's death from the idea of organ donation. Allow the family time to be with the child. Assess the family to determine whether they are acknowledging the child's death to themselves. Note that acknowledgment is not acceptance. If the family is still asking whether there is any chance that the child will recover, they have not acknowledged that the child is dead. Avoid raising the issue of organ donation at the same time the parents are told of the child's death. Allow at least a brief period between these events. If possible, allow some time between raising the issue of organ donation and asking for a decision.
6. It may be difficult for parents to believe a child is dead when the child's chest is still moving and a heart rate is visible on the monitor.
7. Parents may need to ask the same questions repeatedly before they are able to hear and remember what they have been told.
8. Assure the parents that organ donation will not disfigure the child's body, preclude an open casket (Yoder, 1994), or delay funeral arrangements.
9. Offer parents the opportunity to hold the child before the time the organs are removed.
10. Some parents may want to leave the hospital before the child's organs are removed, whereas others may need to see the child again following surgery.
11. Be careful to treat the child who is going to be an organ donor with the same respect and dignity afforded to any child who is still living.
12. In cases of child abuse, federal and state regulations require permission of the parent or guardian for organ donation. If organs are to be donated, the medical examiner or district attorney should be notified so that valuable evidence is not altered or lost during donation (American Academy of Pediatrics Committee on Bioethics, 2000).

D. Caring for the Conscious, Dying Child

Children who are terminally ill frequently know they are going to die even if they have not been told (Wolfe, 2004). Occasionally, families insist that children not be told about their impending death. Whether and how impending death is disclosed to a child can be influenced by the family's religious and cultural heritage, previous experience with death, and other influences. It is important to help the parents realize that the child probably already knows or suspects and may not talk about it simply because he or she senses the parents' avoidance.

1. Ask the family about the child's understanding of death. Explore their thoughts concerning death to help you understand and support them.

2. Encourage parents to discuss the subject with the child and answer the child's questions.
3. Obtain support from clinical-nurse specialists, child-life therapists, psychologists, social services, or chaplains as needed for the family and child.
4. Answer the child's questions openly and honestly.
5. Assure the child that he or she will not be left alone.
6. Allow whatever visitors the child wishes to see.
7. Provide opportunity for a school-age child or adolescent to obtain spiritual guidance as desired, and continue peer relationships as requested (Freyer, 2004).

E. Caring for Bereaved Families

Grief is the cognitive, emotional, physical, psychological, and spiritual response to an overwhelming loss. Grief is frequently described in terms of stages, phases, or symptoms. Although these references are helpful in understanding grief, grief is not a linear process. The bereaved person moves in and out of the phases at various times in the grief process. Symptoms of one phase may overlap with another, and time limits should not be imposed on the individual for completion of this painful process. When a child dies, parental grief is the subjective, individualized response to a hideous loss. The impact is long lasting and life altering.

1. **Lindemann** (1944) described symptomatology that was pathognomonic for grief:
   a. *Somatic distress:* Feelings of tightness in throat or chest, sighing, weakness, shortness of breath
   b. *Preoccupation with the image of the deceased:* Hearing or seeing the person who has died, inability to focus on anything other than loved one who died, emotional distance from others
   c. *Feelings of guilt:* Feeling responsible for the loved one's death, searching for things that could have been done differently, thinking in terms of "if only"
   d. *Hostile reactions:* Feelings and expressions of anger
   e. *Loss of patterns of conduct:* Restlessness and an inability to complete things started
2. **Kübler-Ross** (1969) described the stages of death and dying. As with grief, a person may move in and out of various stages at different times before reaching acceptance:
   a. *Denial:* Shock and disbelief
   b. *Anger:* Angry and hostile reactions expressed
   c. *Bargaining:* Attempts to delay the death
   d. *Depression or despair*
   e. *Acceptance*
3. **Miles and Perry** (1985) identified three phases of parental grief: (1) A state of numbness and shock, (2) a period of intense grief, and (3) a period of reorganization. During the early phase of numbness and shock, parents may use a variety of coping behaviors and display a wide range of emotions.
   a. Some parents may seem to be in a trance and display no emotion at all. They may show concern for others and even try to comfort other family members while expressing little emotion themselves.
   b. Parents can display a wide range of emotions. Many parents will cry. Some express grief loudly with keening and wailing, whereas others cry quietly. Some parents exhibit inappropriate silliness or euphoria. It is a mistake to judge a parent as unaffected or uncaring because of emotional reactions at the time of a death.

c. Although parents are in emotional shock and forget much of what is said to them, paradoxically they often remember verbatim the things that were said to them at the time of their child's death.

d. The psychic numbness protects the person from feeling the full impact of their loss. It protects the mind from a grief that is too horrible to be faced at one time.

4. **Interventions with the family at the time of death**

a. *Be a calm, nonanxious presence.* If you are unable to think of something to say, with family permission, be a silent presence. Being with a family may assist the parents in several ways. Feelings of isolation experienced by the parents may be reduced. Being with the family helps them to know that nothing is being hidden from them. One of the reasons for malpractice suits is that families sometimes feel they are not being told the truth or that information is being hidden. A receptive, nonverbal posture lets people know you are willing to listen if they need to talk. Bereaved family members have described caring people as those who were able to show that they cared by just "being there."

b. *Consider the use of a gentle touch to express caring and concern.* Be sensitive to those who are not comfortable with being touched. This can usually be discerned by stiffening in the person who was touched. Those who respond to touch will frequently grasp your hand or lean toward you as you touch them.

c. *Keep the focus on the family.* Caregivers who feel compelled to share their own losses may be attempting to meet their own needs rather than those of the family.

d. *Provide opportunity to be with the child.* Go into the room with family members. Prepare them for what they will see if they were not there at the time of death. Ask the parents if they prefer some time alone with the child. Remain close by and available to them. Offer parents the chance to hold their child. If death is imminent, be sure they understand their child could die while being held. Offer more than once if they seem to be having difficulty processing information given to them. In some circumstances the parents may ask the nurse to hold their child as he or she dies. Parents may wish to help care for the child's body. Offer the chance to bathe and dress the child or brush the child's hair. Provide a rocking chair if possible for parents to rock their child one last time. Siblings may benefit from being able to say good-bye and need to be reassured that they did not cause the illness and death.

e. *Assist parents to tell siblings* of the child's death. The information given to siblings should be truthful and in terms appropriate to developmental age. Child-life therapists can be helpful with this process. Surviving siblings have had issues with feeling alone or guilty or having concerns for their parents marriage and being compared with the deceased sibling (Carnevale, 2003). Many excellent written resources are available for children to assist them in the grieving process.

f. *Encourage families to seek professional psychosocial support* as needed. It would be impossible to judge who in the family may need professional help following the death of a child. Parents, understandably, might be sensitive if they are deemed to be "coping poorly." Bereavement support groups may also be helpful to families in the aftermath of childhood death.

g. *Call the child by name.* Parents need to know that their child was special to others as well as to them.

h. *Avoid platitudes* such as "Time heals all wounds," "You wouldn't want him or her to live like that," or "You're lucky, it could have been worse." These phrases, although meant to comfort, tend to minimize a person's loss.

i. *Things you can say that are helpful*

- I'm sorry.
- This must be terribly hard for you.
- Is there anyone I can call for you?
- Would you like me to stay with you for a while?

j. *Avoid delaying the onset of grief* by offering the parents tranquilizers or sedatives on a routine basis. Medications may ease the situation for caregivers but only delay the inevitable for the parents. Parents may feel they are being told that their grief is not acceptable.

k. *Offer a remembrance packet to the family.* Keep a camera on the unit and offer to take a picture of the child if the parents wish either before or after the child's death. This may be especially important when an infant dies if the parents have few (if any) pictures. Handprints or footprints can be made easily on a card for the family. Parents may wish to have a lock of hair from the back of the child's head. Ask their permission before cutting the hair. Baptismal certificates or candles can be provided. Handprints or footprints can be easily made in plaster and provide a special keepsake.

l. *Provide factual information, but do not dwell on details that the family has not requested.* Be prepared to answer the same questions more than once.

m. *Allow the family to talk about the child.* Ask questions about the child and listen to the family's answers. Do not be afraid of their tears or your own. Crying is a normal expression of grief for both family and caregivers. There is no need to say, "I didn't mean to remind you"; the parents have not forgotten.

n. *Develop a resource file on the unit* that includes information about grief for families and caregivers, materials to develop a remembrance packet, sympathy cards to be mailed to families, and a list of effective local self-help groups.

o. *A follow-up program is helpful to families.* An index card file system is useful to keep a record of the children who have died. Sympathy cards may be sent to bereaved parents a few weeks following the child's death and again on the first anniversary of the child's death, at Christmas, or any time chosen by the unit staff. Follow-up telephone calls give parents the chance to ask questions and to relate how they are doing. An offer to return to the hospital to visit with physicians or nurses may be helpful for some parents. If an autopsy was done, the parents might have questions and appreciate an opportunity to talk following the autopsy report (Todres et al., 1994).

p. *Consider developing a checklist to guide caregivers at the time of a child's death.* Include those things considered most important on your unit for parents.

5. Staff Support

a. Offer emotional support and assistance to the multidisciplinary team members caring for a child who dies. Allow for the health care providers to "get out of the unit" for a break as necessary.

b. Consider support sessions following a death in the unit. Debriefing sessions may be facilitated by a clinical nurse specialist, child-life therapist, social worker, psychologist, or chaplain.

- Some health care providers may attend the funerals or memorial services for some children for whom they cared. This ritual may assist the caregivers and offer support to the family as well.
- If a child is expected to die, provide a resource person for the nurse who has never cared for a child at the time of death.

REFERENCES

AACN Certification Corporation: Redefining nursing according to patients' and families' needs: an evolving concept. *AACN Clin Issues* 6:153-156, 1995.

Ahmann E, Abraham MR, Johnson BH: *Changing the concept of families as visitors: supporting family presence and participation.* Bethesda, Md., 2003, Institute of Family Centered Care.

Ambuel B et al: Assessing distress in pediatric intensive care environments: the COMFORT scale. *J Pediatr Psychol* 17:95-109, 1992.

American Academy of Pediatrics Committee on Bioethics: Guidelines on forgoing life-sustaining medical treatment. *Pediatrics* 93:532-536, 1994.

American Academy of Pediatrics Committee on Bioethics: Forgoing life-sustaining medical treatment in abused children. *Pediatrics* 106:1151-1153, 2000.

American Academy of Pediatrics Committee on Bioethics and Committee on Hospital Care: palliative care for children. *Pediatrics* 106:351-357, 2000.

Amin RS, Fitton CM: Tracheostomy and home ventilation in children. *Semin Neonatol* 8(2):127-135, 2003.

Anand KJS, Phil D, Hickey PR: Pain and its effects in the human neonate and fetus. *N Engl J Med* 317:1321-1329, 1987.

Bennett M: Sleep and rest in the PICU. *Paediatr Nurs* 15(1):3-6, 2003.

Berde CB, Solodiuk J: Multidisciplinary programs for management of acute and chronic pain in children. In Schechter NL, Berde CG, Yaster M, editors: *Pain in infants, children, and adolescents,* 2nd ed. Philadelphia, 2003, Lippincott Williams & Wilkins.

Beyer JE, Knott CB: Construct validity estimation for African-American and Hispanic versions of the Oucher scale. *J Pediatr Nurs* 13:20-31, 1998.

Board R, Ryan-Wenger N: Stressors and stress symptoms of mothers with children in the PICU. *J Pediatr Nurs* 18(3):195-202, 2003.

Bowden VR, Greenburg CS: *Pediatric nursing procedures.* Philadelphia, 2003, Lippincott, Williams, and Wilkins.

Breau LM et al: Preliminary validation of an observational pain checklist for persons with cognitive impairments and inability to communicate verbally. *Del Med Child Neurol* 42:609-616, 2000.

Broome ME: Helping parents support their child in pain. *Pediatr Nurs* 26:315-317, 2000.

Carnevale FA: The injured family. In Moloney-Harmon PA, Czerwinski SJ, editors: *Nursing care of the pediatric trauma patient.* Philadelphia, 2003, W.B. Saunders.

Curley MAQ: The essence of pediatric critical care nursing. In Curley MAQ, Moloney-Harmon PA, editors: *Critical care nursing of infants and children,* ed 2, Philadelphia, 2001, W.B. Saunders.

Curley MAQ, Meyer EC: Caring practices: the impact of the critical care experience on the family. In Curley MAQ, Moloney-Harmon PA, editors: *Critical care nursing of infants and children,* ed 2, Philadelphia, 2001, W.B. Saunders.

DePaul D, Chambers SE: Environmental noise in the neonatal intensive care unit: implications for nursing practice. *J Perinatol Neonatal Nurs* 8:71-76, 1995.

Freyer DR: Care of the dying adolescent: special considerations. *Pediatrics* 113: 381-388, 2004.

Grunau RE et al: Bedside application of the neonatal facial coding system in pain assessment of premature infants. *Pain* 76:277-286, 1998.

Hicks CL et al: The Faces Pain Scale-Revised: toward a common metric in pediatric pain measurement. *Pain* 93:173-183, 2001.

Hockenberry MJ: *Wong's nursing care of infants and children,* ed 7. St Louis, Mo., 2003, Mosby.

Hockenberry MJ: *Wong's clinical manual of pediatric nursing.* St Louis, Mo., 2004, Mosby.

Kretchel SW, Bildner J: CRIES: a new neonatal postoperative pain measurement score. Initial testing of validity and reliability. *Paediatr Anaesth* 5:51-63, 1995.

Kübler-Ross E: *On death and dying.* New York, 1969, Macmillan.

Lawrence J et al: The development of a tool to assess neonatal pain. *Neonatal Network* 12:59-66, 1993.

Lebet RM: Impact of trauma on growth and development. In Moloney-Harmon PA, Czerwinski SJ, editors: *Nursing care of the pediatric trauma patient.* Philadelphia, 2003, W.B. Saunders.

Lewandowski LA: Stressor and coping styles of parents of children undergoing open heart surgery. *Crit Care Quart* 3:75-84, 1980.

Lewandowski LA, Frosch E: Psychosocial aspects of pediatric trauma. In Moloney-Harmon PA, Czerwinski SJ, editors: *Nursing care of the pediatric trauma patient.* Philadelphia, 2003, W.B. Saunders.

Lexi-Comp, Inc: 2004 Drug information handbook for nursing: pediatric dosage database. Electronic version 1.5.

Lindemann E: Symptomatology and management of acute grief. In Parad JJ, editor: *Crisis intervention: selected readings.* New York, 1944, Family Service Association of America.

McCaffrey M: Pain relief for the child: problem areas and selected nonpharmacological methods. *Pediatr Nurs* 3:11, 1977.

Melnyk BM et al: Creating opportunities for parent empowerment: program effects on the mental health/coping outcomes of critically ill young children and their mothers. *Pediatrics* 113(6):e597-e607, 2004.

Merkel SI et al: The FLACC: a behavioral scale for scoring postoperative pain in young children. *Pediatr Nurs* 23:293-297, 1997.

Meyer EC et al: Parental perspectives on end-of-life care in the pediatric intensive care unit. *Crit Care Med* 30:226-231, 2002.

Miles MS, Perry K: Parental responses to sudden accidental death of a child. *Crit Care Quart* 8:73-84, 1985.

Morrison WE et al: Noise, stress, and annoyance in the pediatric intensive care unit. *Crit Care Med* 31:113-119, 2003.

Nicholson AC et al. Effects of child visitation in adult critical care units: a pilot study. *Heart Lung* 22:36-45, 1993.

Oakes LL: Caring practices: Providing comfort. In Curley MAQ, Moloney-Harmon PA, editors: *Critical care nursing of infants and children,* ed 2, Philadelphia, 2001, W.B. Saunders.

Playfor S, Thomas D, Choonara I: Recollection of children following intensive care. *Arch Dis Child* 83:445-448, 2000.

Rothstein P: Psychological stress in families of children in the pediatric intensive care unit. *Pediatr Clin North Am* 27:613-620, 1980.

Savedra MC et al: Assessment of postoperation pain in children and adolescents using the Adolescent Pediatric Pain Tool. *Nurs Res* 42:5-9, 1993.

Schechter NL: The undertreatment of pain in children: an overview. *Pediatr Clin North Am* 36:781-794, 1989.

Siever BA: Pain management and potentially life-shortening analgesia in the terminally ill child: the ethical implications for pediatric nurses. *J Pediatr Nurs* 9:307-312, 1994.

Slota MC: Implications of sleep deprivation in the pediatric critical care unit. *Focus Crit Care* 15:35-43, 1988.

Smith JB, Martin SA: Caring practice: providing developmentally supportive care. In Curley MAQ, Moloney-Harmon PA, editors: *Critical care nursing of infants and children,* ed 2, Philadelphia, 2001, W.B. Saunders.

Society of Pediatric Nurses and American Nurses Association: In Lewandowski LA, Tesler MD, editors: *Family-centered care: putting it into action.* Washington, DC, 2003, Nursebooks.

Stevens B, Ohlsson A: *Sucrose for analgesia in newborn infants undergoing painful procedures.* Oxford, 2001, The Cochrane Library.

Stevens B et al: The premature infant pain profile: development and initial validation. *Clin J Pain* 12:13-22, 1996.

Tyler DC et al: Toward validation of pain measurement tools for children: a pilot study. *Pain* 52:301-309, 1993.

Tobias JD, Berkenbosch JW, Russo P: Additional experience with dexmedetomidine in pediatric patients. *South Med J* 96:871-875, 2003.

Todres ID, Earle M, Jellinek MS: Enhancing communication. *Pediatr Clin North Am* 41: 1395-1403, 1994.

Truog RD et al: Pharmacologic paralysis and withdrawal of mechanical ventilation at the end of life. *N Engl J Med* 342:508-511, 2000.

Truog RD et al: Recommendations for end-of-life care in the intensive care unit: the ethics committee of the society of critical care medicine. *Crit Care Med* 29:2332-2348, 2001.

Wolfe L: Should parents speak with a dying child about impending death? *N Engl J Med* 351(12):1251-1253, 2004.

Van Cleve LJ, Savedra MC: Pain location: validity and reliability of body outline markings by 4 to 7-year-old children who are hospitalized. *Pediatr Nurs* 19:217-220, 1993.

Yoder L: Comfort and consolation: a nursing perspective on parental bereavement. *Pediatr Nurs* 20:473-477, 1994.

CHAPTER

2 Pulmonary System

MARY JO C. GRANT AND HOLLY F. WEBSTER

DEVELOPMENTAL ANATOMY OF THE RESPIRATORY SYSTEM

A. Embryology of the Lung

1. **Glandular stage: Conception to 16th week**—The lung begins as a bud on the embryonic gut 28 days after conception. These rudimentary solid tubes grow and divide until the 16th week. By the fourth week of gestation, a lung bud branches from the primitive esophagus to form the airways and alveolar spaces. During weeks 7 through 10, the larynx develops (Figure 2-1).
2. **Canalicular stage: 16th to 24th week**—Vascularization of the lung occurs. The first capillaries can be identified in the middle of this phase. Alveolar ducts develop on the terminal bronchioles. Airways are lined with large cuboidal cells filled with glycogen. At about 18 weeks, some of the epithelial cells become alveolar epithelial type II cells, which synthesize pulmonary surfactant. The fetus is potentially viable at the end of the canalicular stage of development (Figure 2-2).
3. **Alveolar stage: 24th week to birth**—Alveolar ducts surrounded by capillaries appear at 26 weeks. Alveoli and alveolar capillaries appear at 30 weeks; columnar cells within the alveolar wall differentiate into type I and type II cells. Type II cells secrete surfactant, which is necessary for sustained inflation of the lung.
4. **The first breath:** The thorax is compressed as it passes through the birth canal, forcing out some of the fetal lung fluid. Chest recoil after the thorax is delivered results in air entry into the lungs. The first inspiratory effort must be large enough to overcome the viscous resistance to movement of the intrapulmonary liquid and overcome the tissue and surface tension. For the first several minutes to 2 hours, expiration is often incomplete, resulting in progressively increasing functional residual capacity (FRC). For infants born by cesarean section, it takes longer to establish FRC.
5. **Prematurity:** The prematurely born infant has a compliant chest cage, making diaphragmatic function inefficient and limiting the ability to generate a large transpulmonary pressure. In a landmark article, Liggins and Howie demonstrated that antenatal corticosteroid therapy administered to women at risk for preterm delivery reduced the incidence of respiratory distress syndrome (RDS) and mortality in their offspring (Liggins and Howie, 1972). Antenatal corticosteroid therapy leads to improvement in neonatal lung function by two mechanisms: enhanced maturational changes in lung architecture and induction of lung enzymes resulting in biochemical maturation (Smolders-de Haas, 1990).

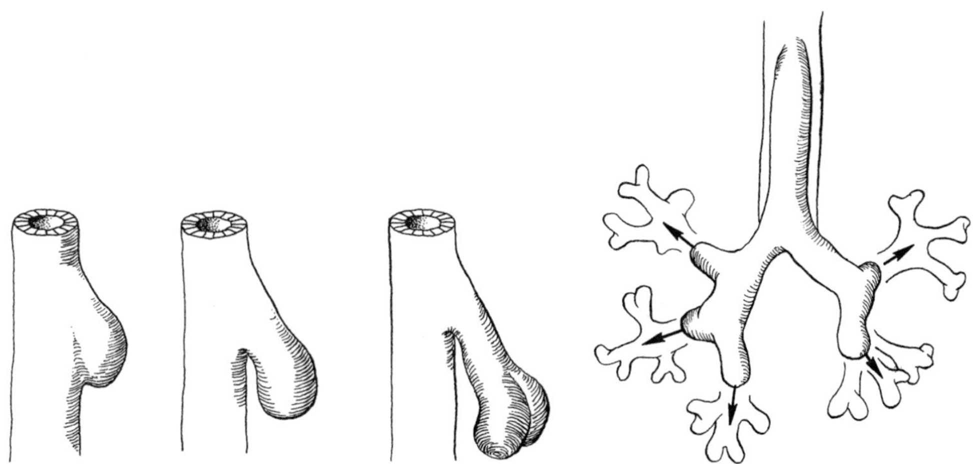

FIGURE 2-1 ■ Embryonic development of the lungs.

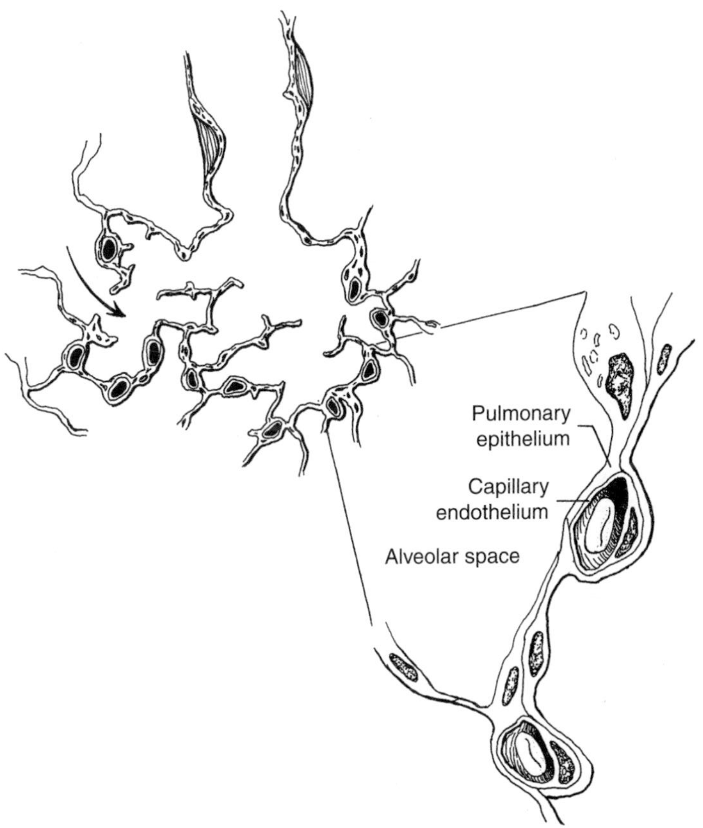

FIGURE 2-2 ■ Epithelial and endothelial development.

B. Postnatal Development (Table 2-1)

1. The **number of airway branches** is fixed at birth, but airway dimensions and alveolar number increase until the child is about 8 years of age. The number of alveoli increases approximately 10-fold, and the air-tissue interface increases to a magnitude 21 times that which exists in the newborn. After birth the number of

TABLE 2-1
Anatomic Differences Between Pediatric and Adult Airways

Anatomic Difference	Clinical Significance
Proportionally larger head	Increases neck flexion and obstruction
Smaller nostrils	Increases airway resistance
Larger tongue	Increases airway resistance
Decreased muscle tone	Increases airway obstruction
Longer and more horizontal epiglottis	Increases airway obstruction
More anterior larynx	Difficult to perfom blind intubation
Cricoid ring is narrowest portion	Inflated cuffed tubes not recommended for routine intubation in children <8 y of age
Shorter trachea	Increases risk of right main stem intubation
Narrower airways	Increases airway resistance

alveoli continues to increase dramatically but ceases by 5 to 8 years of age. The smaller alveolar size of infants predisposes the infant to alveolar collapse; however, alveolar diameter continues to increase until adulthood. Lung volume increases fourfold during the first 12 months of life. Collateral ventilation does not develop until after infancy.

2. The infant chest is **cylindric,** with an anteroposterior (AP) diameter equal to or slightly greater than the transverse diameter. Following birth, growth of the transverse diameter is more rapid. By about 3 years of age, the child has attained the adult chest wall configuration: the transverse diameter is greater than the AP diameter.

C. Upper Airway Development

The upper airway is responsible for warming, humidifying, and filtering air before it reaches the trachea (Figure 2-3).

1. **Nose**
   a. *Embryology:* Nasal cavities begin as widely separated pits on the face of the 4-week-old embryo. At birth the maxillary sinuses are the largest. The ethmoid cells are present and increase in size throughout life. Frontal and sphenoid sinuses do not begin to invade the frontal or sphenoid bones until several years after birth.
   b. Until the age of 6 months, infants are obligatory nose breathers because the elongated epiglottis, positioned high in the pharynx, almost meets the soft palate. However, they are still able to mouth-breathe because blocked nares do not lead to complete upper airway obstruction. By the sixth month, growth and descent of the larynx reduce the amount of obstruction. Nasal breathing doubles the resistance to airflow and proportionately increases the work of breathing (WOB).
2. **Pharynx**
   a. *Embryology:* The oropharyngeal membrane between the foregut and the stomodeum begins to disintegrate to establish continuity between the oral cavity and the pharynx in the 4-week-old embryo.
   b. The *pharynx* is a musculomembranous tube that extends from the base of the skull to the esophageal and laryngeal inlets. The pharynx is the conduit for respiratory gas exchange and vital to the production of speech. The *nasopharynx* is located above the soft palate. The *oropharynx* extends from the soft palate to

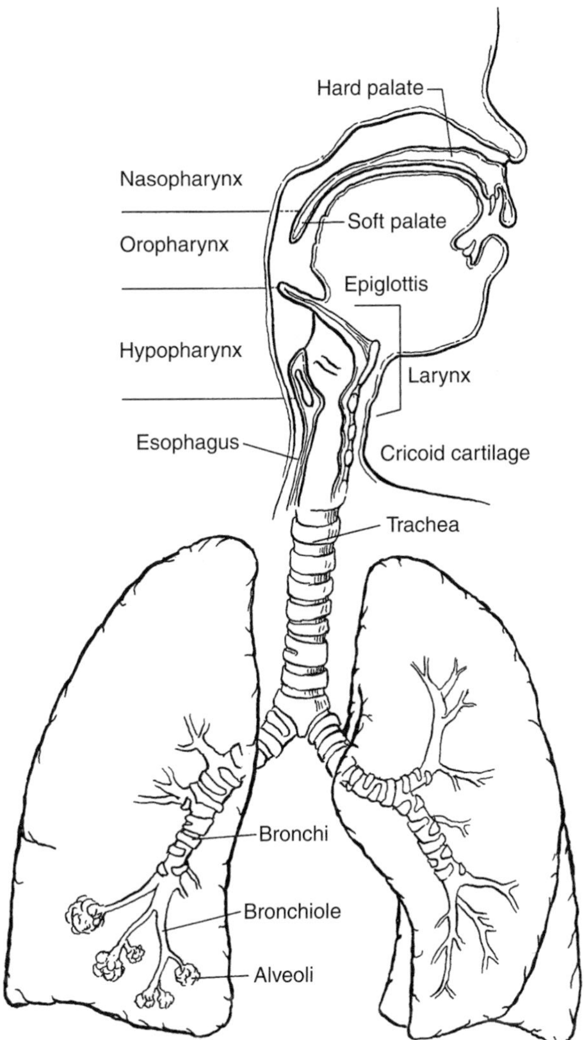

FIGURE 2-3 ■ Airway anatomy.

the level of the hyoid bone. The *hypopharynx* extends from the level of the hyoid bone to the esophageal inlet.

3. **Larynx**
   a. *Embryology:* During the fourth week of embryologic life, the laryngotracheal groove begins as a ridge on the ventral portion of the pharynx. Vocal cords begin to appear in the eighth week. In the newborn infant, the larynx is approximately at the level of the second cervical vertebra. In the adult the larynx is opposite the fifth and sixth cervical vertebrae.
   b. The *larynx* is a funnel-shaped structure that connects the pharynx and trachea. It includes the thyroid cartilage, vocal cords, epiglottis, and the cricoid cartilage. It is important in the production of the cough and protects the airway from aspiration of food during deglutition.
      - Compared with the adult epiglottis, the child's *epiglottis* is longer and more flaccid. The epiglottis in a newborn extends over the larynx at approximately a 45-degree angle. This more anterior and cephalad epiglottis may make intubation of the airway more difficult in the small infant.

- In the infant and small child, the narrowest portion of the airway is the *cricoid cartilage ring*. This is the only point in the larynx in which the walls are completely enclosed in cartilage. In the rest of the trachea, the posterior wall is membranous. Resistance to airflow is inversely proportional to the fourth power of the radius. Thus, swelling from trauma or infection can lead to additional narrowing in this area, producing large increases in airway resistance.
- *Vocal cords* must abduct to allow the exchange of respiratory gases and close to prevent aspiration.

4. Trachea

a. *Embryology:* The trachea begins to develop in the 24-day-old embryo. At 26 to 28 days a series of asymmetric branchings of the primitive lung bud initiate the development of the bronchial tree.

b. The *trachea* is a thin-walled rigid tube characterized by a framework of 16 to 20 cartilages that encircle the trachea, except in its posterior aspect, which is membranous and contains smooth muscle. Because the cricoid cartilage provides a "natural cuff" or narrowing of the airway, an uncuffed endotracheal tube (ETT) is recommended for all children who weigh less than 24 kg (Hazinski et al., 2002).

c. The trachea's nervous, vascular, and lymphatic supplies are independent of those to the lungs.

D. Lower Airway (Lung) Development

1. Lung

a. At birth the lungs weigh about 40 g and double in weight by 6 months. By age 2 years, when most of the alveolarization process is complete, they weigh about 170 g. Normal adult lungs weigh approximately 1000 g.

b. The right lung has three lobes, and the left has two lobes separated by divisions called *fissures* (Figure 2-4), each further subdivided into bronchopulmonary segments. The surface of the lung is covered with the visceral pleura.

2. Conducting airways

a. *Intrapulmonary airways* are divided into three major groups: cartilaginous bronchi, membranous bronchioles, and gas exchange units.
- *Cartilaginous bronchi* are the large airways that include 9 to 12 divisions terminating in bronchi having a diameter of approximately 1 mm.
- *Membranous bronchioles* comprise an additional 12 divisions before ending as terminal bronchioles, the last conducting structure in the lung.

b. The airways are lined with epithelial membrane, which gradually changes from ciliated pseudostratified columnar epithelium in the bronchi to a ciliated cuboidal epithelium near the gas exchange units.

c. In the largest airways a smooth-muscle bundle connects the two ends of the C-shaped cartilage. As the amount of cartilage decreases, the smooth muscle assumes a helical orientation and gradually becomes thinner.

3. Gas exchange units (alveoli)

a. *Alveoli* are complex networks in which gas exchange takes place. Alveoli are lined by two epithelial cell types. Type I cells cover about 90% of the total alveolar surface. These cells are adapted to allow for the rapid exchange of gases. Type II cells constitute the other 10% and secrete surfactant material that lowers surface tension and maintains the patency of alveoli during respiration. Alveoli patency means preventing collapse and allowing the alveoli to maintain a spherical shape for efficient gas exchange.

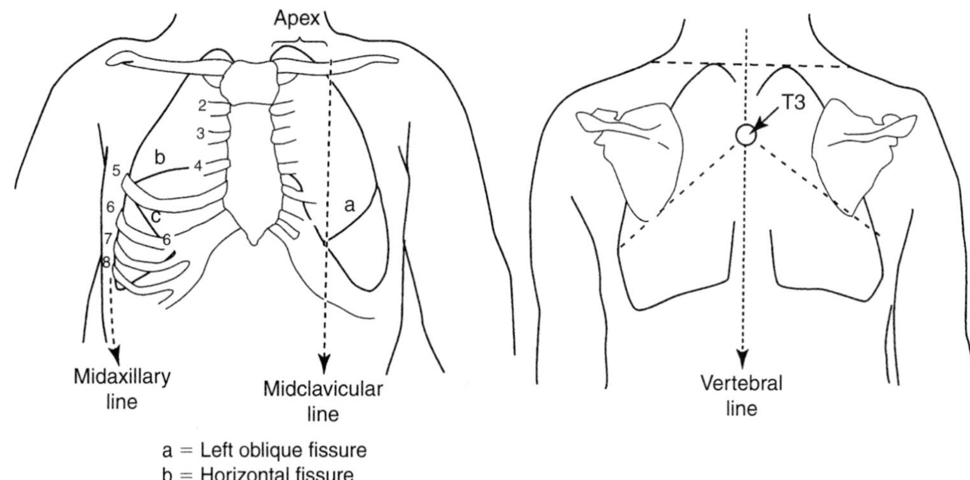

FIGURE 2-4 ■ Anatomic landmarks of the thorax. The lower lobes of both lungs have only small projections on the anterior plane on the x-ray film and can be better visualized on a lateral or posterior x-ray film. The midaxillary line, midclavicular line, vertebral line, and intercostal spaces are frequently used landmarks in describing the location of pulmonary findings. **A**, Anterior view: Left lung is divided into two lobes by the left oblique fissure. The right lung is divided into three lobes by the horizontal fissure with landmarks between the fourth rib medially and the fifth rib laterally. The right oblique fissure is found from the inferior margin (midclavicular line) to the fith lateral rib. **B**, Posterior view: Fissures dividing upper and lower lobes begin at T3, medially, extending in a line inferiorly below the inferior tips of the scapula.

b. Two types of *intercommunicating channels* provide collateral ventilation for the gas exchange units. *Alveolar pores of Kohn* are holes in the alveolar wall that provide channels for gas movement between alveoli. These pores are not present until 6 to 8 years of age. *Canals of Lambert* are accessory channels that connect a small airway to an airspace normally supplied by a different airway.

c. *Gas exchange* involves the movement of gas between the atmosphere and the alveoli and the pulmonary capillary blood. This movement occurs by simple passive diffusion where the gases travel from an area of high to an area of low partial pressure.

E. Thoracic Cavity

1. Diaphragm

a. The *diaphragm* is the principal muscle of inspiration. If the chest wall is stiff, contraction of the diaphragm during inspiration decreases the pressure within the thoracic cavity and increases thoracic volume. This negative intrathoracic pressure in the chest cavity is discussed in detail in concepts of ventilator management. The diaphragm is innervated by the phrenic nerve (third, fourth, and fifth cervical spinal nerves).

b. The *diaphragm* inserts more horizontally in the infant than in the older child or adult.

2. The chest wall: The infant's chest wall is very compliant compared with the rigid chest wall of the older child and adult. In the presence of lung disease, contraction of the diaphragm results in intercostal and sternal retractions rather than in inflation of the lungs. These retractions occur because the intercostal muscles are not strong enough to stabilize the chest against the stronger diaphragm contraction.

F. Pulmonary Circulation

Development closely follows development of the airways and alveoli.

1. **Embryology:** *Preacinar arteries,* which branch along the airways, develop in utero. Muscular arteries end at the level of the terminal bronchiole in the fetus and newborn but gradually extend to the alveolar level during childhood. Prematurely born infants have less well-developed vascular smooth muscle.
2. **Pulmonary blood volume:** The lungs receive the entire cardiac output from the right ventricle if no intracardiac right-to-left shunts are present.
3. **Pulmonary lymphatics:** The lymphatic system is composed of a superficial network in the pleura and the deep network around the bronchi and pulmonary arteries and veins. An increase in the hydrostatic pressure of the pulmonary and systemic circulation can result in effusions by decreasing the rate of pleural fluid absorption. Lymphatics may be disrupted by thoracic surgery or trauma, leading to lymphatic effusions.

DEVELOPMENTAL PHYSIOLOGY OF THE RESPIRATORY SYSTEM

A. Physiologic Function

The primary function of the lung is to deliver oxygen to the body and to remove carbon dioxide. During inspiration, the diaphragm contracts, the chest wall expands, and the volume of the lungs increases. Gas flows from the atmosphere into the lung and oxygen diffuses into the blood at the alveolar-capillary interface. During expiration the diaphragm and the chest wall relax, thoracic volume decreases, intrathoracic pressure increases, and gas flows out of the lung. This process is affected by pulmonary compliance and resistance and by pulmonary vascular pressures and resistance.

1. **Pulmonary compliance and resistance**
   a. *Compliance* is the measure of the distensibility of the lungs influenced by surfactant and elasticity of lung tissue (Figure 2-5).
      - Volume change is produced by a transpulmonary pressure change ($C_L = \Delta V/\Delta P$). For example, if the volume change produced by a given pressure change is small, the lungs are stiff or have decreased compliance.
      - Compliance of the infant chest wall (especially in premature infants) is considerably greater than that of the adult. There is less opposition to lung collapse. Compliance is decreased by pulmonary edema, pneumothorax, pulmonary fibrosis, and atelectasis. Compliance is increased by lobar emphysema.

   b. *Airway resistance* is the driving pressure of air divided by the airflow rate determined by airway diameter. It is directly proportional to flow rate, the length of the airway, and the viscosity of the gas and is inversely proportional to the fourth power of the airway radius *(Poiseuille's law).*
      - The upper airway contributes 70% of the total airway resistance in adults and 50% of total airway resistance in infants. In infants the small peripheral airways may contribute as much as 50% of the total airway resistance compared with less than 20% for the adult.

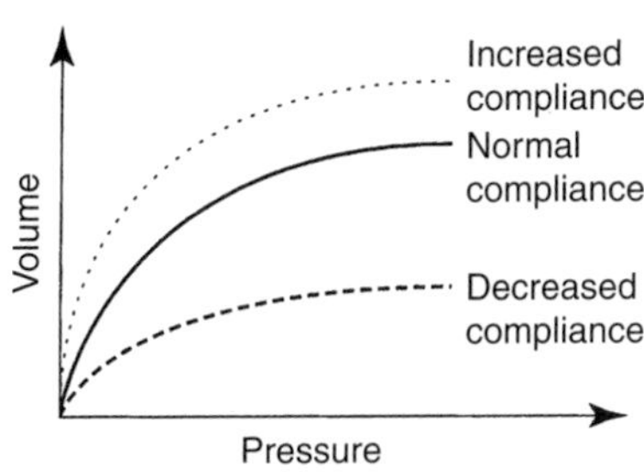

FIGURE 2-5 ■ Compliance curve. Compliance reflects the amount of pressure required to deliver a given volume of air into an enclosed space such as the lung. Increased compliance of a lung unit indicates that less pressure is needed to distend the lung with a given volume. Decreased compliance indicates that more pressure is required to deliver the same volume of air.

- Resistance is increased by asthma, cystic fibrosis, bronchopulmonary dysplasia, bronchiolitis, tracheal stenosis, and increased respiratory secretions. High resistance increases the work of breathing and creates respiratory distress.

2. **Pulmonary vascular pressures and resistance:** See also Fetal Circulation in Chapter 3.
   a. *Changes in pulmonary circulation at birth*
      - The fetus has low pulmonary blood flow from high pulmonary vascular resistance. This high pulmonary vascular resistance is due to hypoxic vasoconstriction, thicker pulmonary musculature, and smaller surface area. At birth there is a decrease in pulmonary vascular resistance associated with ventilation and the effect of oxygen. This drop in pulmonary vascular resistance after birth increases blood flow to lungs, thus facilitating the transition from fetal circulation. In the 6 to 8 weeks following birth, there is a further progressive fall in resistance associated with thinning of the smooth-muscle layer.
      - Pulmonary blood flow is not uniformly distributed throughout the lung. It is gravity dependent related to regional differences in pulmonary vascular pressure and resistance.
   b. *Intravascular pulmonary pressure* is measured by placing a catheter in the pulmonary artery and measuring systolic, diastolic, and mean arterial pressures (MAPs). A balloon-tipped catheter wedged in a pulmonary artery branch approximates the left atrial pressure. Beyond the newborn period, pulmonary artery systolic pressure averages 20 mm Hg, and diastolic pressure is 10 mm Hg with a mean pressure of about 15 mm Hg.
   c. *Ventilation-perfusion matching:* Regional differences in lung perfusion are described by *West's zones of perfusion*. Blood flow is least at the apex and increases at the base of the lung in an upright position (Figure 2-6).
      - Zone I is located in the apexes of an upright adult. Mean pulmonary arterial pressure is less than alveolar pressure.
      - Zone II is located in the midlung field. Pulmonary artery pressure is greater than alveolar pressure, which is greater than pulmonary venous pressure.
      - Zone III is found in the base of the lung of an upright adult. Pulmonary artery and venous pressures are greater than alveolar pressure.
   d. *Pulmonary vascular resistance* is increased by an increase in blood viscosity or a decrease in total cross-sectional area of the resistance vessels related to fewer number of vessels or normal number with narrowing.
      - Increased blood viscosity is most commonly seen as a result of a raised hematocrit from cyanotic heart disease. An increase in hematocrit from 40% to 70% approximately doubles blood viscosity.

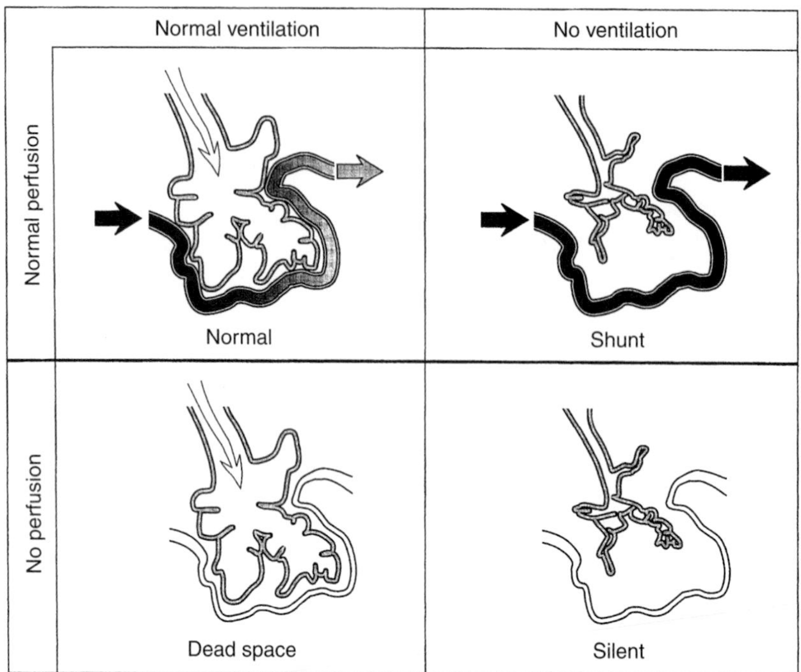

FIGURE 2-6 ■ Ventilation-perfusion relationships.

- A decreased total number of vessels may occur with congenital lung lesions such as hypoplasia or cystic lung changes.
- A decreased luminal diameter with a normal number of vessels is more common. Vasoconstriction can be due to biologically active agents (serotonin, norepinephrine) or alveolar hypoxia and metabolic acidemia. Hypoxic pulmonary vasoconstriction occurs when the lungs are ventilated with hypoxic gas. As a result pulmonary arterial pressure increases almost immediately. This process is reversible with the return to ventilation with normal concentrations of oxygen. Hypoxic pulmonary vasoconstriction shunts blood flow away from hypoxic regions of the lung. This minimizes ventilation-perfusion mismatch and optimizes systemic oxygenation.

3. **Control of breathing**
   a. *Central respiratory centers:* The *medulla* is responsible for the normal rhythm of respiration. The pons contains the apneustic and pneumotaxic centers, which regulate the quality of breathing.
   b. *Peripheral neural reflexes:* Respiratory mechanoreceptors that can affect respiration are located within the upper airways, trachea, and lungs. Impulses are transmitted to the brainstem respiratory centers via the vagus nerve.
   c. *Chemical control of respiration* is mediated by chemosensitive areas in the medulla and through peripheral chemoreceptors (Figure 2-7).
      - When the medulla is perfused with fluid of a low pH or high partial pressure of carbon dioxide in arterial gas ($Paco_2$), it triggers a marked increase in neural discharge. CO_2 freely diffuses from the blood into cerebrospinal fluid (CSF). An increase in $Paco_2$ quickly increases the

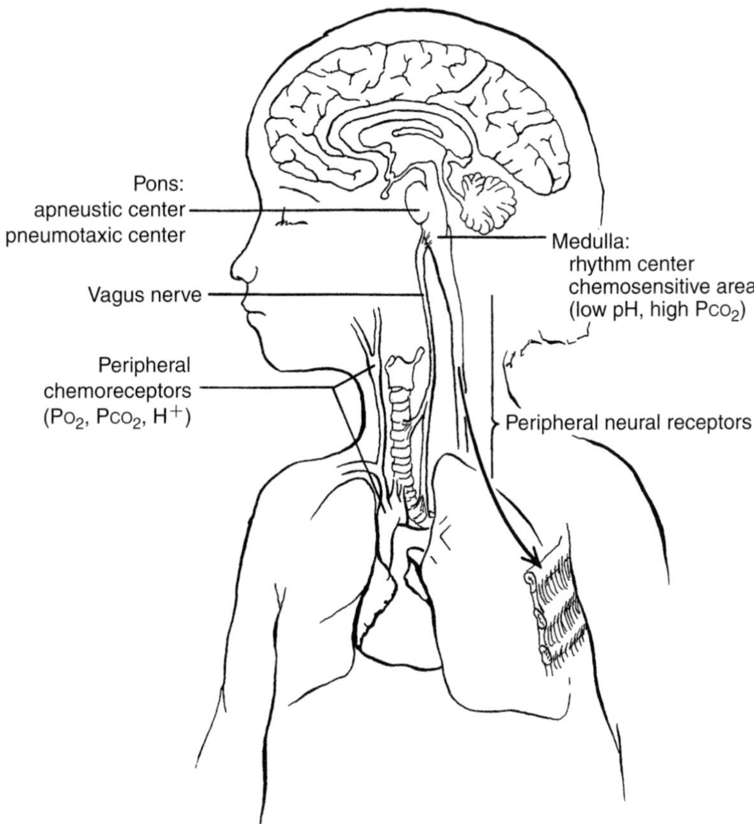

FIGURE 2-7 ■ Chemical control of breathing.

hydrogen ion concentration in the CSF. This occurs as carbon dioxide combines with water to form carbonic acid (H_2CO_3), which then dissociates into bicarbonate and hydrogen ion. The result is a rise in hydrogen ion concentration and a fall in pH, causing respiratory acidosis.

$$CO_2 + H_2O \Leftrightarrow H_2CO_3 \Leftrightarrow H^+ + HCO_3$$

- Peripheral chemoreceptors are located at the carotid bifurcation and the arch of the aorta. They respond to changes in arterial partial pressure of oxygen (Po_2), $Paco_2$, and hydrogen ion concentration.

4. **Mechanics of breathing:** Elastic properties of the lung come from the elastic tissue and collagen that support the lungs' internal structures. Lung compliance changes with age. The thorax of the infant is much more compliant than an adult.
5. **Lung volumes** (Figure 2-8)
   a. *Total lung capacity* (TLC) is the total volume of the gas contained in the lung at maximum inspiration.
   b. *Vital capacity* (V_C) is the maximum volume expired from total lung capacity with maximal expiration.
   c. *Functional residual capacity* (FRC) is the volume of gas remaining in the lungs at the end of a normal expiration.
   d. *Residual volume* is the volume of gas remaining in the lung following a maximal respiratory effort.

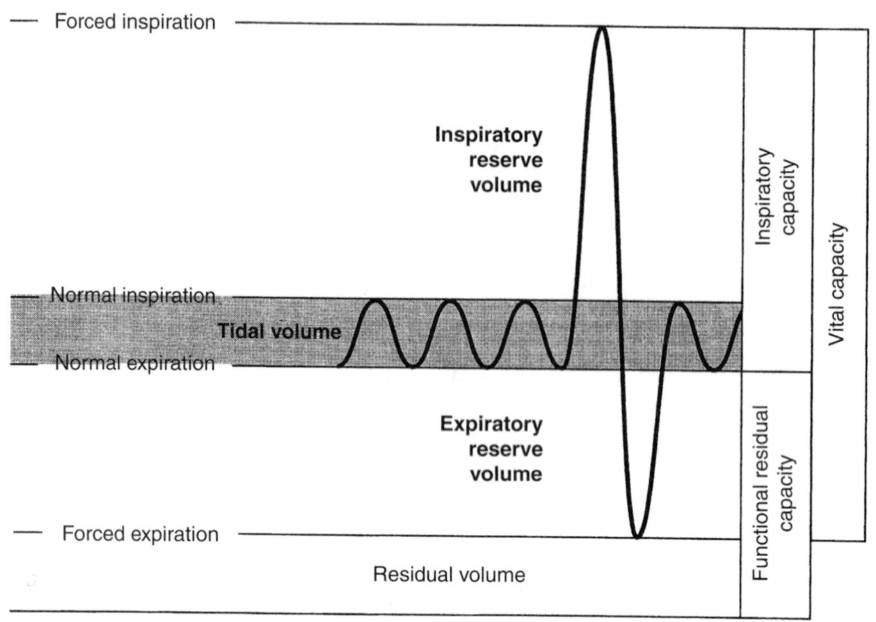

FIGURE 2-8 ■ Lung volumes.

B. Gas Exchange and Transport

Respiratory gas exchange involves the movement of gas from the atmosphere to the alveoli to the pulmonary capillary blood. The alveolar capillary membrane permits the transfer of oxygen and carbon dioxide while restricting the movement of fluid from pulmonary vasculature to alveoli.

1. **Diffusion**
   a. Oxygen diffuses from the alveolus through the alveolar epithelial lining, basement membrane, capillary endothelial lining, plasma, and red blood cell. Blood passing through the lung resides in a pulmonary capillary for only 0.75 second. Diffusion of oxygen depends on a difference (gradient) between alveolar and oxygen tension.
   b. Carbon dioxide diffuses from the red blood cell to the plasma, through the capillary endothelial lining, basement membrane, and alveolar epithelial lining. The pulmonary capillary mean alveolar carbon dioxide gradient is smaller than that of oxygen (i.e., CO_2 diffuses more readily than O_2).
2. **Oxygen transport**
   a. Oxygen is carried in the blood in two forms: in combination with hemoglobin (Hgb) and dissolved in plasma. The arterial oxygen content (CaO_2) describes the total amount of oxygen carried by arterial blood. CaO_2 is represented in the following equation:

$$(\text{Hgb} \times 1.34 \times \text{SaO}_2) + (0.003 \times \text{PaO}_2),$$

   Parameters are defined and other oxygen values are calculated in a similar fashion as in Table 2-2.
   b. Oxyhemoglobin dissociation curve (Figure 2-9)
      - The oxyhemoglobin dissociation curve is an S-shaped curve with Hgb on the Y axis and PaO_2 on the X axis. The release of oxygen to the tissues is directly related to Hgb concentration and the affinity of oxygen for Hgb.

TABLE 2-2
Normal Oxygenation Profile Values

Parameter	Calculation	Norms
CaO_2	$CaO_2 = (Hgb \times 3.4 \times SaO_2) + (PaO_2 \times 0.003)$	20 ml/dl
$C\bar{v}O_2$	$C\bar{v}O_2 = (Hgb \times 3.4 \times S\bar{v}O_2) + (P\bar{v}O_2 \times 0.003)$	15 ml/dl
$a\text{-}\dot{v}DO_2$	$\dot{C}aO_2 = C\bar{v}O_2$	3.5-5 ml/dl
$\dot{D}O_2$	$\dot{D}O_2 = CaO_2 \times CI \times 10$	620 ± 50 ml/min/M^2
$\dot{V}O_2$	$\dot{V}O_2 = (CaO_2 - C\bar{v}O_2) \times CI \times 10$	120-200 ml/min/M^2
O_2ER	$(CaO_2 - C\bar{v}O_2)/CaO_2 \times 100$	25 ± 2%
$S\bar{v}O_2$		75% (60%-80%)

CaO_2, arterial oxygen content; *Hgb*, hemoglobin; *SaO_2*, arterial oxygen saturation; *CI*, cardiac index; *DO_2*, oxygen delivery; *PaO_2*, arterial partial pressure of oxygen; *$C\bar{v}O_2$*, venous oxygen content; *$S\bar{v}O_2$* venous oxygen saturation; *PvO_2*, venous partial pressure of oxygen; *$a\text{-}vDO_2$*, arteriovenous oxygen difference; *VO_2*, oxygen consumption; *O_2ER*, oxygen extraction ratio.

Curley MAQ & Thompson, JE: Oxygenation and ventilation. In Curley MAQ, Moloney-Harmon, PA, eds. *Critical Care Nursing of Infants and Children*, 2nd ed. Philadelphia, 2001, Saunders.

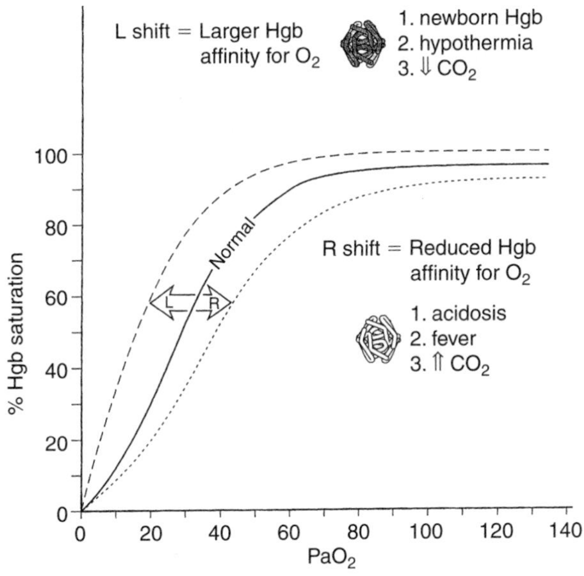

FIGURE 2-9 ■ Oxyhemoglobin dissociation curve. *Hgb*, hemoglobin.

Thus, on the steep portion of the dissociation curve, relatively small changes in PaO_2 cause large changes in oxygen saturation of Hgb.

- A shift to the right, which facilitates the unloading of oxygen from Hgb, is caused by a decrease in pH, an increase in $PaCO_2$, elevated temperature, or an increase in 2,3-diphosphoglycerate (2,3-DPG). 2,3-DPG decreases the affinity of Hgb for oxygen. During hypoxia or anemia, oxygen availability is increased within a matter of hours by an increase in 2, 3-DPG.
- A shift to the left, which increases the binding of oxygen to Hgb, is caused by an increase in pH, a decrease in $PaCO_2$, a decrease in temperature, or a

decrease in 2,3-DPG. Fetal Hgb has decreased 2,3-DPG, shifting the curve to the left of the adult Hgb curve. Thus, at a given PaO_2 and hematocrit, fetal Hgb is more readily saturated than adult blood is. Fetal Hgb also releases oxygen less readily to the tissues than adult Hgb. Fetal Hgb is replaced by adult Hgb within 4 to 6 weeks after birth.

3. **Cellular Respiration**
   All cells depend on a continuous supply of oxygen to support aerobic metabolism. Oxygen delivery data do not provide information about the adequacy of tissue oxygenation. In septic shock, tissue oxygen extraction is altered. To assess tissue oxygen extraction, a true mixed venous blood sample should be obtained from the pulmonary artery.

CLINICAL ASSESSMENT OF PULMONARY FUNCTION

A. History

1. **Prenatal and delivery:** The history should include gestational age and Apgar scores, respiratory distress in the neonatal period (including oxygen requirement and ventilatory assistance), and length of hospital stay.
2. **Childhood history**
   - **a.** Immunizations and tuberculosis tests (verify with records)
   - **b.** Family history of asthma, allergies, or other respiratory illnesses
   - **c.** Wheezing episodes with previous illnesses
   - **d.** Frequency of colds and upper respiratory tract illnesses
   - **e.** Environmental smoke in home
   - **f.** Supervision of child (especially if younger than 5 years) to evaluate the risk of foreign-body aspiration
   - **g.** Recent illnesses of child or family member
   - **h.** Daily medications and medications used to treat respiratory symptoms
3. **Other significant information**
   - **a.** *Chest pain* (rarely of cardiac origin) is described in quality, timing with respiratory phase, duration (continuous or intermittent), and precipitating factors.
   - **b.** *Growth and development:* Failure to gain weight is often the first sign of chronic pulmonary disease. Activity level or milestones may be delayed with chronic pulmonary dysfunction.
   - **c.** *Gastrointestinal (GI) symptoms*
     - Pneumonic processes frequently manifest by generalized abdominal pain in young children.
     - Acute or chronic infection may cause anorexia and occasionally vomiting.
     - Upper airway mucus may impede swallowing and cause gagging, vomiting, or diarrhea in infants and toddlers.
     - Bulky, foul-smelling stools may indicate cystic fibrosis.
     - Gastroesophageal reflux may cause chronic pulmonary aspiration.
   - **d.** *Sleeping habits*
     - Evaluate duration of sleep at night and causes of interruptions. Nighttime coughing is a frequent symptom of asthma or other lower respiratory tract diseases.
     - Note positioning for sleep (e.g., flat or requiring head elevation).
     - If a humidifier is used, note care and maintenance of the humidifier.
     - Note signs of obstructive sleep apnea, such as sleeping propped up on pillows, apnea, orthopnea, and snoring.

B. Physical Examination

1. Inspection

a. *Anatomic landmarks* of the thorax provide a method for describing physical examination findings (see Figure 2-4).

b. *Thoracic inspection*

- Note thoracic contour. A neonate's chest is round with the anterioposterior diameter equal to the transverse diameter. Chest contour is more oval by 2 to 3 years of age. Disproportionate size may be detected by comparing head circumference (occipitofrontal circumference [OFC]) to chest circumference. From birth to 2 years the head and chest circumferences are generally equal. During childhood, chest size is 5 to 7 cm greater than the OFC. Chronic disease may cause enlarged anteroposterior diameter ("barreled-chested," similar to the neonate contour) (Figure 2-10).
- Note any skeletal deformities. Anomalies such as sternal depression (pectus excavatum) or protrusion (pectus carinatum) may cause, or be associated with, respiratory abnormalities by altering pulmonary mechanics. Inspect posterior thoracic structures and the spine. Kyphosis and scoliosis can impair pulmonary mechanics.
- Note symmetry of excursion.

c. *Respiratory effort*

- Rate and rhythm are age related. Respiratory rate is about one fourth of the pulse rate in the normal infant at rest.
- Evaluate the adequacy of thoracic excursion (depth of respiration).
- Note the effort of breathing. Infants and young children breathe principally with the diaphragm related to immature intercostal muscles. Infants in respiratory distress may exhibit nasal flaring, head bobbing, expiratory grunting, or head extension.
- Note the use of accessory muscles. Signs of respiratory insufficiency include suprasternal, substernal, intercostal, and subcostal retractions (Table 2-3).
- Variations in respiratory patterns are also observed with various neurologic abnormalities (Figure 2-11).

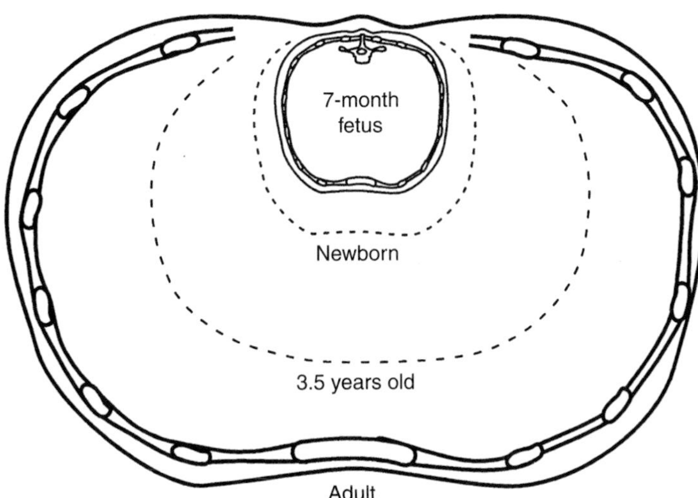

FIGURE 2-10 ■ Thoracic contours by age. Comparison of the anteroposterior diameter and contour of the chest wall according to age.

■ **TABLE 2-3**
■ ■ **Symptoms Associated with Severe Respiratory Insufficiency**

Cyanosis
Nasal flaring
Tachypnea
Quiet, shallow respirations
Tachycardia
Marked retractions
Head bobbing (infants)
Agitation or lethargy
Acidosis
Absent breath sounds
Pulsus paradoxus >20 mm Hg

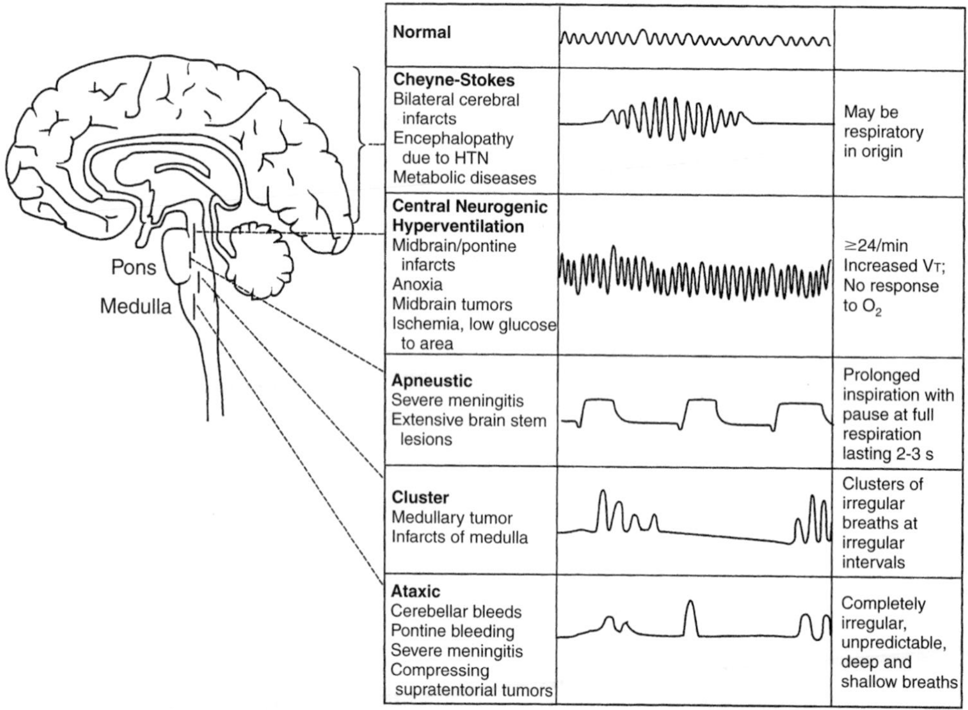

FIGURE 2-11 ■ Variations in respiratory patterns. Breathing patterns as associated with anatomic regions of the brain. Lesions causing global injury tend to cause an orderly progression of respiratory patterns down to the brainstem. Focal lesions may cause a lower central nervous system (CNS) pattern; higher function is otherwise noted on examination. *HTN*, hypertension; V_T, tidal volume.

d. *Note the quality of the voice and breathing,* especially a muffled voice; stridor; expiratory/inspiratory wheezing; and barky, loose, congested, or paroxysmal cough.

e. *Note skin color and appearance.*

- Cyanosis is observed when 3 to 5 g of Hgb becomes desaturated. Conditions that can mask or mimic cyanosis include hypothermia, anemia, or polycythemia. If cyanosis persists with oxygen administration, this may indicate an intracardiac shunt.

- Clubbing of fingertips is an indication of chronic hypoxia. The distal phalanx is flat and broad, causing a "club" appearance.
- Cyanosis is *not* related to increased $Pa{CO_2}$ (hypercarbia). A patient may be well oxygenated with a supplemental flow of oxygen diffusing through the airway but still be significantly hypercarbic and without a cyanotic appearance.

2. **Palpation** is a limited technique in infants, but it is useful in older children.
   a. *Expand the hands bilaterally and symmetrically across the anterior chest wall and then across the posterior chest wall* to evaluate the following:
      - Expansion of the thoracic cage.
      - *Fremitus* is conduction of the child's voice while the child says, for example, "99." Vibrations should be noted at the trachea and upper airway. Decreased sensation is normally observed centrally near large airways; otherwise, it is associated with occlusions. Increased sensation is associated with solid masses (consolidations). In infants, palpation during crying allows a similar evaluation.
      - Palpation of fine vibrations may indicate underlying pleural friction rub.

   b. *Palpate the entire thoracic cage for crepitus,* a coarse, crackly feeling (and sound) of air in the subcutaneous tissue.
   c. *Evaluate the skeletal structure,* especially clavicles with a history of trauma.
   d. *Palpate the tracheal position* (midline); if it is shifted, locate the position of maximal impulse of the heart. A shift in either or both may indicate fluid or air collection or a collapsed lung.
3. **Percussion**
   a. *Percussion* is a technique used to determine the presence of air, fluid, or masses in the underlying lung and to determine anatomic landmarks (such as the upper margin of the liver; Figure 2-12).
   b. *Percuss using the middle finger of one hand flush against the chest wall* in interspaces, noting the quality of sound produced by striking this finger with the middle finger of the other hand.

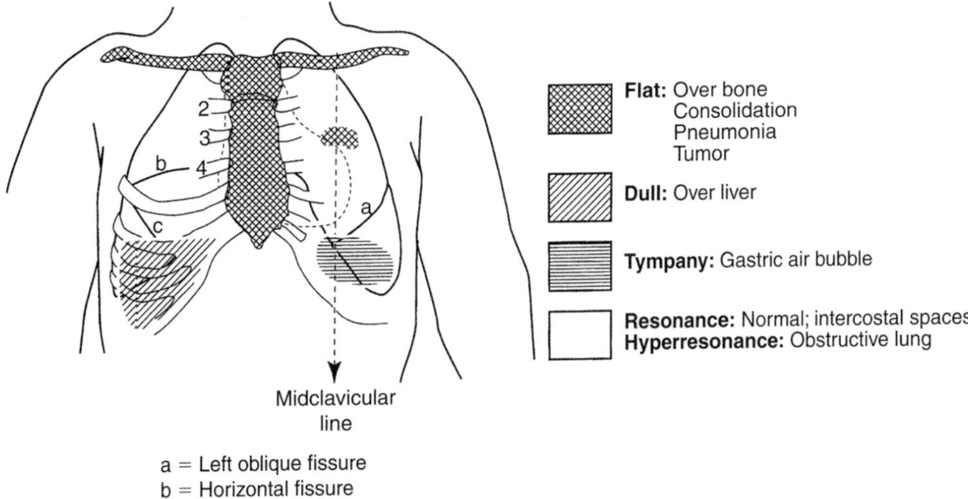

FIGURE 2-12 ■ Percussion of the thorax. Differences in densities are noted to detect the presence of abnormal air, fluid, bones, or mass.

- The right side of the anterior chest: Percussion sounds should be resonant in each intercostal space down to the fifth to sixth intercostal space, where the superior liver margin begins. There the sound changes to a dull quality. Farther down where the lung field ends and liver remains, the percussion note becomes flat.
- The left side of the anterior chest: Percussion of the heart borders can be determined. The superior border is often percussed between the second and third intercostal spaces. The inferior border is at the fourth to sixth intercostal space, and the left border is just lateral to the midclavicular line. At the sixth intercostal space and below, tympany may be observed because of an air-filled stomach.
- Posterior chest: Percuss side to side to identify abnormal densities.

c. *Variations in sounds* define the density of structures:
- Flat: Short, soft; heard over *bone*
- Dull: Medium pitch; duration heard over the liver, spleen, and *mass densities*
- Resonance: Low, loud, and long; heard over an air-filled *lung*
- Hyperresonance: Deep pitched, loud, and prolonged; heard over an *overinflated lung* or air collections such as pneumothorax
- Tympany: High, musical quality, loud; heard over *gas-filled organs such as the stomach*

4. Auscultation

a. *Evaluate the pitch, intensity, quality, and duration of each phase using the diaphragm of the stethoscope.* For small infants, either a small diaphragm or the bell of a stethoscope may enable localization of sounds.

b. *Compare side to side,* starting at the apex and proceeding methodically to the bases. The thin-walled chests of infants create transmitted breath sounds throughout the lung fields. Listen for discreet changes from one location to the next. For emergent situations a quick check under each axilla (rather than the upper lobes of the lungs) allows gross determination of the presence of bilateral aeration.

c. *Quality of pitch: Vesicular breath sounds* (inspiratory [I] > expiratory [E]) are of long inspiration, low pitch, and soft intensity and are heard over most of the lungs. *Bronchial breath sounds* (I < E) have an equal or longer expiratory phase; are high pitched, loud, and blowing; and are heard over the large airways. Bronchial breath sounds are abnormal when heard over the peripheral lung tissue. *Bronchovesicular breath sounds* (I = E) are high-pitched tubular sounds.

d. *Adventitious sounds* are abnormal sounds superimposed on normal breath sounds. Abnormal sounds have classically been defined as rales, rhonchi, and wheezes. However, confusion over definitions has prompted a focus on describing the *quality* and *location* of these sounds to associate them with common causes. Attention should be given to pitch, timing (I or E), location, and whether they clear with cough.
- Fine, high-pitched crackling noises (similar to the sound of rolling hair between fingers) may be heard at end inspiration over peripheral lung fields in pneumonia and pulmonary edema. Medium-pitched crackles are heard in early to mid inspiration with pulmonary edema and diffuse secretions in the bronchioles. These may partially clear with coughing. Upper airway secretions may cause coarse, bubbling (rhonchi) sounds that clear with cough.
- Inflamed pleural surfaces may result in a very fine, low-pitched crackle over the focal areas of the chest during both I and E phases. With cessation of breathing, the crackles are not heard.

- Wheezing results from narrowed airway lumina. Inspiratory wheezing usually results from high obstruction, such as laryngeal edema or foreign bodies. Expiratory wheezing often results from lower obstruction, such as with bronchiolitis, severe asthma, or chronic obstructive lung disease.

e. *Diminished or absent breath sounds* are noted as the focal absence of sounds, with occasional crackling, or as an abnormal quality or abnormal location of normal sounds. This may occur with atelectasis, pneumothorax, or pleural fluid accumulation.

C. Abnormal Physical Examination Findings

1. Stridor (Table 2-4)

a. *Description:* Noisy breathing caused by increased turbulence of airflow through a lumen.

- Inspiratory stridor is related to the inward collapse of structures during inspiration. It is most common with supraglottic or glottic lesions because of the negative pressure generated during inspiration. Inspiratory stridor is common in laryngotracheomalacia and viral croup. Post-extubation endotracheal tube trauma is another possible source of stridor.
- Expiratory stridor is most commonly observed with subglottic lesions.

TABLE 2-4
Evaluation of Stridor

	Supraglottic	Subglottic	Tracheal
Phase of respiration	Inspiratory	Inspiratory or biphasic	Expiratory
Phonation	Muffled	Weak or breathy	Absent or high pitched
Pitch of stridor	Coarse, low pitch	High-pitched, barking or rough cough	
		DIFFERENTIAL DIAGNOSIS FOR UPPER AIRWAY STRIDOR	
Intrinsic lesions		Subglottic stenosis	
		Web laryngocele	
		Tumors such as papillomas	
		Laryngomalacia	
		Tracheomalacia	
		Tracheoesophageal fistula	
Extrinsic lesions		Vascular ring	
		Cyst hygroma	
		Neurologic lesions such as lymphomas	
Infections		Epiglottitis	
		Laryngotracheobronchitis	
		Peritonsillar abscess	
		Bacterial tracheitis	
		Infectious mononucleosis	
Other		Craniofacial abnormalities	
		Trauma	
		Foreign body aspiration	
		Hypertrophic tonsils or adenoids	
		Allergic reactions	
		Corrosive ingestions	

- Fixed lesions (e.g., subglottic stenosis) may cause both inspiratory and expiratory stridor.

b. *Evaluation of the child with stridor includes* nasal patency, the size of tongue and mandible, the quantity of oropharyngeal secretions, the presence of drooling, the quality of phonation, head and neck range of motion, evidence of tooth evulsion or oral trauma, presence of fever or infectious symptoms, neurologic status, and the rate of progression of symptoms.

- Note the position of preference. Infants with laryngomalacia, micrognathia, or macroglossia often have less distress when placed in a prone position. Children with epiglottitis or croup (laryngotracheobronchitis) often position themselves upright; children with moderate obstruction may exhibit forward extension of the head.

2. Cyanosis

a. *Description:* Central or peripheral blue discoloration of skin tissue caused by desaturated Hgb. Cyanosis is usually not appreciated until 3 to 5 g Hgb per deciliter of serum is desaturated, corresponding to an $Sa{O_2}$ of 80% to 85% in a normal child. Cyanosis is *not* caused by an elevated $Pa{CO_2}$. Cyanosis can be caused by other nonpulmonary conditions (Figure 2-13).

- Cyanosis may be masked by anemia, causing a more pallid color, or polycythemia, which may create a more "ruddy" color.

b. *Evaluation of the cyanotic child*

- Oxygen should be administered before proceeding with the evaluation. Note the response to oxygen and the general degree of distress. If distress is moderate or severe, emergency management should be given before proceeding with further evaluation.
- Note whether cyanosis is peripheral (nail beds), central (lip and tongue color), or both.

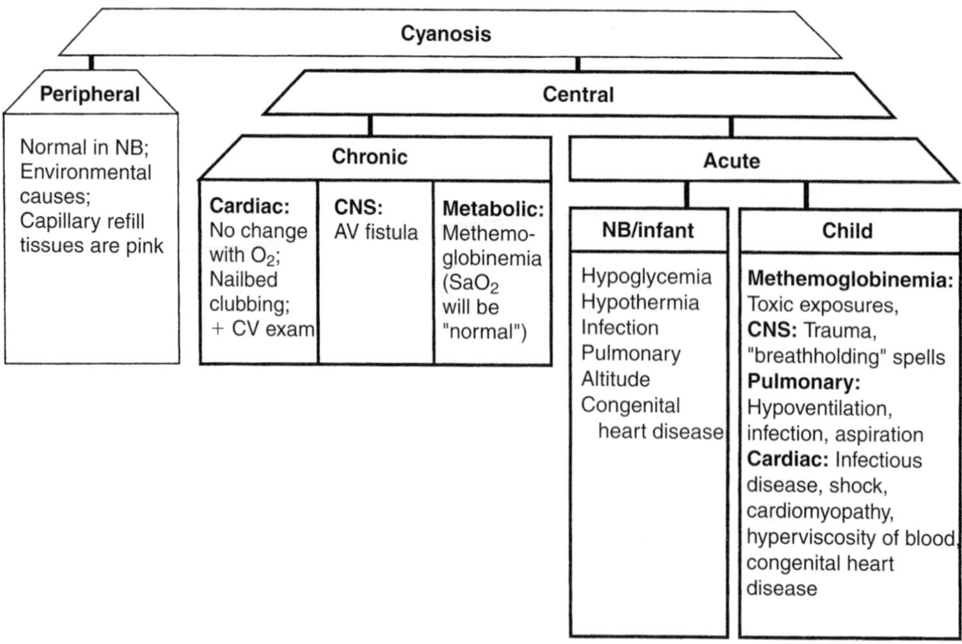

FIGURE 2-13 ■ Etiology of cyanosis. *AV*, arteriovenous; *CNS*, central nervous system; *CV*, cardiovascular; *NB*, newborn.

- Assess pulmonary function to identify upper or lower airway causes, including the presence or absence of stridor, phonation, use of accessory muscles, and general state of alertness and activity level.
- Obtain historical information such as the evolution of the cyanosis (sudden or gradual onset) and associated factors (e.g., illness or decreased environmental temperature).

3. Cough

a. *Description:* A cough is an attempt to clear the airway of particulate matter or may result from general tissue irritation. It is produced by a reflex response in cough receptors, found in ciliated epithelium, or it may be initiated in higher cortical centers.

b. *Evaluation*

- Many causes of cough are age specific (Table 2-5).
- Note historical information such as the presence or absence of infectious disease or exposures.
- Characteristics of the cough may suggest the cause:
  - Loose and productive: Cystic fibrosis, bronchiectasis, asthma
  - Croupy: Viral laryngotracheobronchitis
  - Paroxysmal: Pertussis, mycoplasma, foreign body, chlamydia
  - Brassy: Tracheitis, upper airway drainage, psychogenic
  - Nocturnal: Asthma, sinusitis, gastroesophageal reflux, upper respiratory tract disease
  - During exercise: Asthma, cystic fibrosis, bronchiectasis
  - Loud honking that disappears with sleep: Psychogenic

TABLE 2-5
Common Causes of Cough by Age Groups

Neonates	Infections Chlamydia Viral: Cytomegalovirus, rubella, pertussis Congenital malformations Tracheoesophageal fistula Vascular rings Airway malformations
Infants	Above, plus Infections Viral bronchiolitis Diffuse interstitial pneumonia Gastroesophageal reflux Cystic fibrosis
Preschoolers	Infections in suppurative disease (e.g., cystic fibrosis) Viral infections with or without reactive airway disease Foreign body aspiration Environmental pollutants Gastroesophageal reflux Reactive airway disease
School age/adolescents	Reactive airway disease Mycoplasma pneumoniae infection Cystic fibrosis Cigarette smoking Psychogenic cough tic Pulmonary hemosiderosis

c. *Other associated symptoms:* Examine sputum samples for white blood cells (WBCs) or eosinophils. Note hemoptysis. Poor weight gain, steatorrhea, and cough are strongly suggestive of cystic fibrosis.
d. A *cough* that persists longer than 2 weeks or a cough that causes immediate respiratory distress warrants investigation.

INVASIVE AND NONINVASIVE DIAGNOSTIC STUDIES

A. Diagnostic Approach

1. **Individualization of evaluation:** All sick children are at higher risk for respiratory insufficiency or failure than adults because of the age-related anatomic differences described previously. Monitoring of pulmonary function can be individualized according to the acuity of illness and the age of the child. For a patient with the lowest acuity, clinical examination and serial observations are adequate; but with increasing severity of illness, other monitoring devices should be used. The options for monitoring include continuous observation and clinical examination, oxygen monitoring, CO_2 monitoring, monitoring of pulmonary function, and laboratory and roentgenographic studies.
2. **Immediate assessment and care:** A brief estimation of the severity of distress should be made to determine whether oxygen or airway assistance is needed.

B. Baseline Respiratory Monitoring

1. **Physical examination:** All children suspected of having respiratory distress should have their clothing removed for maximum observation, ensuring that ambient temperature is controlled. Refer to the clinical assessment section for details on physical examination techniques. A quick-look observation should be done with all patients for early recognition of respiratory distress requiring emergency management. This 20-second appraisal should include level of consciousness, color, and respiratory effort.
2. **Diagnostic studies for children in respiratory distress from any cause:**
   a. Complete history and physical examination
   b. Chest x-ray examination
   c. Sinus x-ray examinations (depending on age)
   d. Complete blood count
   e. Tuberculin skin test
   f. Nasopharyngeal swab for respiratory syncytial virus and viral panel and pertussis, if applicable
   g. Diagnostic studies to consider for children in respiratory distress according to symptoms:
      - Bronchoscopy with alveolar lavage
      - Laboratory testing as indicated
      - pH probe testing for suspected gastroesophageal reflux disease (GERD)
      - Pulmonary function testing

C. Laboratory Studies (Table 2-6)

D. Radiologic Procedures for Pulmonary Evaluation

A variety of imaging techniques allow visualization of anatomy, motion dynamics, and identification of abnormalities. Frequently, a patient may require more than one imaging procedure to detail a specific anatomic site.

1. **Chest roentgenography** permits visualization of lung parenchyma (tissue), pulmonary vascular markings, heart silhouette, and bone densities.

TABLE 2-6
Summary of Diagnostic Laboratory Evaluation of Pulmonary Function

Test	Significance
IMMUNOGLOBULINS	Norms are age-related assays. Decreased levels of any immunoglobulin are usually associated with congenital deficiencies and patterns of infections beginning early in life. Altered levels are associated with specific causes as follows.
	INCREASED LEVELS ASSOCIATED WITH
IgA: Deficiency is associated with an increased incidence of mucosal bacterial infections	
IgG: Found in blood, lymph, CSF, pleural fluid, peritoneal fluid, and breast milk; slow response (appears 1 wk after stimulus)	Myeloma Bacterial infections Collagen disorders
IgM: Intravascular; predominant first response to bacterial or viral infection; activates the complement system	Appears early in infectious course but may persist with chronic infection
IgD: Predominant activity on the surface of B cells (involving antibody formation)	Increased with chronic infections
IgE: Found in the serum and triggers release of histamine	Increased with allogenic stimulation (e.g., asthma, associated with allergenic stimulus)
DIFFERENTIAL WHITE BLOOD CELL COUNT Test total WBC <1 y: maximum = 20,000 1–12 y: maximum = 15,000 Segmented neutrophils (PMNs) <12 y = 25–40% ≥12 y = >50%	Infections may cause an elevated or remarkably low (<4000/mm^3) WBC count
Band neutrophils <10%	Increase in bands associated with bacterial infections
Lymphocytes <12 y = >50% ≥12 y = <40% Monocytes 4%–6% Eosinophils 2%–3% Basophils 0.5%	Increased with specific infections such as pertussis, Epstein-Barr virus, hepatitis
PILOCARPINE LONTOPHORESIS (SWEAT CHLORIDE TEST)	
Sodium <70 mEq/L Chloride <60 mEq/L Potassium <60 mEq/L	Higher levels suggest cystic fibrosis
SPUTUM OR TRACHEAL ASPIRATE CULTURES	
Normally should have few if any PMNs and mixed flora Deep tracheal secretions preferred; protected brush specimen technique Evaluate Gram stain for presence of PMNs Endotracheal tubes and tracheostomy tubes become quickly colonized with existing flora, which may be misleading if microbiology results are interpreted independently from other clinical indicators	PMNs: 3–4+ with dominant organism is more likely to be valid indicator of infection than one with <2+ PMNs and multiple organisms

PMNs, polymorphonuclear neutrophils.

2. **Fluoroscopy** provides evaluation of thoracic motion, particularly diaphragm movement, which is essential to the infant, and is especially useful in the evaluation of a paralyzed diaphragm.
3. **Computed tomography (CT) scan** is the visualization of very thin slices of tissue in a predetermined plane of dimension, enabling identification of masses, fluid accumulation, and anatomic definition. A spiral CT may provide better definition.
4. **Magnetic resonance imaging (MRI)** uses an external magnetic field around the patient to cause rotation of cell nuclei. Imaging provides well-defined visualization of soft tissues. No radiation is involved in this procedure.
5. **Ventilation-perfusion scan (V/Q scan)** is obtained by injecting a radioisotope into a peripheral vein and imaging its flow through the pulmonary vessels. The V/Q scan is made following the inhalation of a radioactive gas, which distributes to aerated alveoli. Comparison between *ventilated* areas with *perfused* areas of the lung can be made, looking for "matched" segments. Although many disorders may cause a ventilation-perfusion mismatch, a complete segmental mismatch is a useful clue to the diagnosis of pulmonary embolism.
6. **Pulmonary angiography** involves the introduction of a catheter into a peripheral vein; the catheter is guided to the right side of the heart and to the pulmonary artery trunk. Injection of contrast media with serial radiographic examinations of the pulmonary vascular bed allows definitive recognition of vascular obstruction.

RESPIRATORY MONITORING

A. Oxygen Monitoring

1. **Pulse oximetry**
   a. *Principles of operation:* The device consists of a probe that contains an infrared light source and a photodetector. Both are housed in a wraparound strip so that the light source is aligned to emit light through tissue (such as a nail bed) to the photodetector. Saturated Hgb absorbs little light, whereas desaturated Hgb absorbs a large amount of light. The photodetector measures the amount of light that crosses the tissue and with a microprocessor computes the percentage of saturated Hgb.
   b. *Uses:* The pulse oximeter requires pulsatile tissue to provide accurate measurements. Fingers, palmar wrap (in small infants), toes, and ear clips are used. The microprocessor unit measures pulse rate, and most units have a mechanism to provide a "poor signal" alert or perfusion indicator if the tissue has an inadequate pulse. It provides a stable, accurate measurement over a wide variety of physiologic conditions.
   c. *Limitations:*
      - Poor perfusion (low cardiac output states) may interfere with a stable signal.
      - A major source of error in children is motion artifact, which causes poor tracking of the pulse. New oximeters feature an algorithm to identify both motion artifact and poor perfusion (Barker et al., 1997).
      - With elevated carboxyhemoglobin or methemoglobin levels, the true oxygenated Hgb values are inflated because the pulse oximeter does not distinguish between Hgb saturated with oxygen and other bound molecules.
      - In the neonatal population, where retinopathy is a concern, $Sa{O_2}$ may not provide any margin of safety because the $Pa{O_2}$ can vary widely when oxygen saturations are greater than 90% as the result of factors that alter the oxygen dissociation curve.

- Newborns and children with uncorrected congenital heart disease may have variance in measurements, depending on placement of the oximeter. In cardiac lesions with right-to-left shunting, the right hand or foot is used for preductal measurement and the left hand or foot is used for postductal measurement.

2. **Transcutaneous oxygen monitoring ($Ptco_2$)**
   a. *Principles of operation:* A small, heated probe is placed on the skin surface. Localized heating increases capillary blood flow to the site. Oxygen diffuses across the skin and is measured by a thermistor in the probe.
   b. *Uses:* $Ptco_2$ functions well in infants and has shown good correlation with Pao_2 measurements (DeNicola, 2001). It can reduce the quantity of invasive blood-gas measurements and provide continuous data for patients who are either being weaned or are otherwise labile.
   c. *Limitations:* With increasing skin thickness, the accuracy of measurements diminishes. Poor perfusion and local skin hypoxia can interfere with measurements. The probe requires site change every 4 to 6 hours with a 10- to 15-minute warm-up time (and a blood-gas analysis to verify measurement accuracy). Further, the heated probe may cause blisters in some infants.
3. **Mixed venous oxygen saturation monitoring:**
   a. Many pediatric patients are monitored with pulmonary artery catheters for hemodynamic measurements. One type of catheter includes a fiberoptic tip that measures reflected wavelengths of light from saturated Hgb in the local (pulmonary artery) blood flow.
   b. The mixed venous oxygen saturation (Svo_2) measurement, which is usually between 65% and 80%, is a global indicator of total oxygen consumption (Vo_2).
   c. Either a change in oxygen supply (arterial oxygen saturation) or in oxygen demand (oxygen consumption) will alter this measurement (see Chapter 3 for further information).

B. Carbon Dioxide Monitoring

1. **Transcutaneous carbon dioxide monitoring ($Ptcco_2$) (Meliones, 1996)**
   a. *Principles:* A CO_2 sensor, housed in a small probe, is mounted on the skin surface to measure diffused carbon dioxide with an electrode similar to that found in standard blood-gas machines. Although earlier $Ptcco_2$ electrodes used a local heat to "arterialize" the site, recent studies showed that a predictable linear relationship can be obtained with nonheated electrodes. Typically the $Ptcco_2$ is higher than the $Paco_2$, but the gradient should remain stable.
   b. *Uses:* Consistent correlations have been documented in neonates (Carter, 2001), but less reliability has been demonstrated in older children and adults. After the probe is positioned and the warm-up period is passed, the monitor measurement should be compared with a simultaneous blood-gas measurement to establish the gradient. After this point, blood-gas measurements can be reduced until the next site rotation (usually every 4 hours).
   c. *Limitations:*
      - The sensors appear to be somewhat fragile and prone to discreet alterations, such as inadequate fluid in the sensor. If the gradient between $Ptcco_2$ and $Paco_2$ is unstable, a site change is warranted.
      - Calibration procedures must be exact, necessitating the presence of personnel who are well-trained in the operation of these monitors.
2. **End-tidal carbon dioxide monitoring (E_Tco_2):** The measurement of exhaled carbon dioxide gas provides direct evidence of ventilatory function. An increased carbon dioxide level is an objective parameter for the identification of respiratory failure. This can be measured with or without a waveform.

a. *Principles of operation:* A small device placed in line with the ventilator circuit at the proximal airway measures expired carbon dioxide by mass spectrometry or infrared absorption. Exhaled gas passes through this device, which emits infrared light. A detector measures the light absorption in this sample. The carbon dioxide level is *inversely* proportional to the light absorption.

b. *Uses:* In the normal subject, $Petco_2$ is theoretically within 2 mm of $Paco_2$.
   - Alveolar hypoventilation will lead to an increase in arterial and E_Tco_2, which can be used in patients who are being weaned from mechanical ventilation. E_Tco_2 detection—whether qualitative, quantitative, or continuous—is the most accurate and easily available method to monitor correct ETT position in patients who have adequate tissue perfusion (American College of Emergency Physicians, 2002).
   - An estimation of dead space ventilation can be inferred when $Paco_2$ measurements and E_Tco_2 are compared serially. When the dead space (V_d/V_t) increases, the gradient between $Paco_2$ and E_Tco_2 increases. Conversely, as ventilator adjustments are made in an attempt to improve alveolar ventilation, the gradient should diminish.
   - Exhaled carbon dioxide monitoring should be considered when intubated patients undergo sedation (American Society of Anesthesiologists Task Force, 2002).
   - Carbon dioxide monitoring can be useful in patients with increased intracranial pressure (ICP) or pulmonary hypertension in which the patient's $Paco_2$ needs to be regulated.

c. *Limitations:*
   - The choice of sensor for a child must be guided by the sensitivity for smaller exhaled volumes. Clinically, infants weighing less than 5 kg may not be good candidates for this device, but the final decision should be based on comparative measurements with a blood gas.
   - Additional considerations are the warm-up time required and the calibration process, which requires operator competence for its use.
   - During a cardiac arrest or extubation, the E_Tco_2 measurement acutely disappears.

C. Gastric Mucosal pH Monitoring

1. *Principles of operation*: The gastric mucosa is an early victim of blood flow redistribution. In the normal state, gastric mucosal CO_2 ($Pgco_2$) approximates $Paco_2$. An increase in $Pgco_2$ indicates an imbalance between the production of carbon dioxide metabolism and its removal.
2. *Uses*: In practice, a tonometrics gas-permeable silicone balloon catheter is inserted into the stomach. Carbon dioxide freely equilibrates between the gastric mucosa and the balloon. A sample from the balloon is analyzed automatically with an infrared sensor or blood-gas analyzer for determination of $Pgco_2$. The intramucosal pH value is calculated. Casado-Flores et al. (1998) found that a gastric intramucosal pH value of less than 7.32 at hospital admission and 12 hours after cardiopulmonary bypass was associated with higher rates of mortality and multiorgan failure in children.
3. *Limitations*: Requires placement of a catheter into the stomach.

D. Diagnostic Pulmonary Function Testing

Critically ill children require continuous surveillance of pulmonary function. For those who are not in frank respiratory failure, clinical assessment, including respiratory rate, observation of chest expansion, and use of accessory muscles, provides an estimation of adequacy of minute ventilation. For those in distress, further measurements may be warranted. With children, standard measurements of pulmonary function may not be possible because of lack of patient cooperation.

1. **Spirometry:** In the cooperative child, lung volumes can be estimated with simple flow spirometers. Flow spirometers, which measure exhaled V_T, can provide an *estimation* of vital capacity (V_C) and can be used for trending. In general, 80% of the V_C can be exhaled in 1 second and is called the forced expiratory volume, or FEV_1.
   a. In *obstructive* disease, the patient is unable to breathe out fully and has both decreased V_C and FEV_1.
   b. In *restrictive* disease, in which the lung cannot fully expand, the V_C is low, but FEV_1 is still proportionally normal (i.e., ≥80% of V_C).
   c. In the *weakened patient*, lower volumes may be observed with a faster respiratory rate (Figure 2-14).
2. **Pressure manometers**
   a. Both negative and inspiratory pressure (effort) can be quantified by using a manometer to provide an estimation of muscle condition. A normal school-age child should be able to generate a minimum of about 30 cm H_2O on *inspiration* (called negative inspiratory force, or NIF). An infant may generate an NIF of about 20 cm H_2O, although infant effort is difficult to capture; "crying effort" measurement is sometimes used, however. On *expiration,* a school-age child should be able to generate a pressure of at least +30 cm H_2O.
3. **Measurement of compliance**
   a. *Lung compliance* (C_L) is the measure of the distensibility of the lung and thoracic wall. It is defined as the volume change per unit of pressure change across the lung. This is expressed as $\Delta V/\Delta P$.
   b. *Dynamic compliance* is the relationship of the delivered (tidal) volume to the total pressure required to deliver that volume. Dynamic compliance includes both elastic recoil and airway resistance factors.

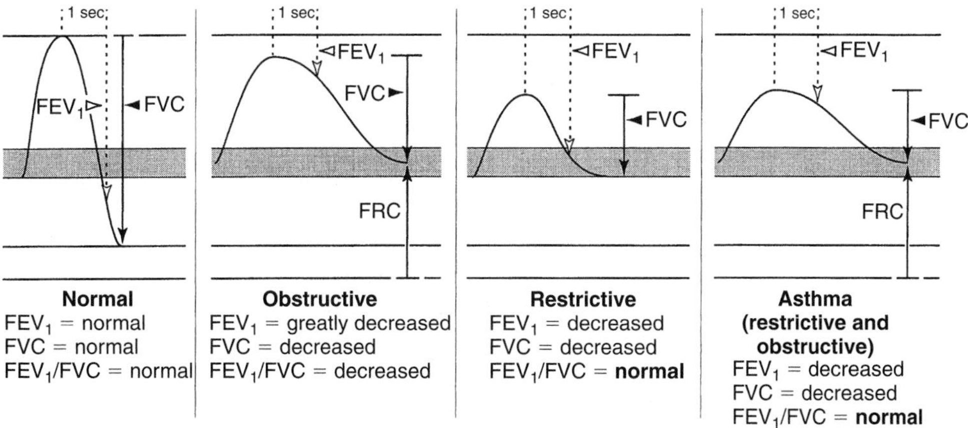

FIGURE 2-14 ■ Normal pulmonary function tests and impact of obstructive and restrictive diseases. Normal pulmonary function measurements. Comparison of pulmonary function measurements in the person with obstructive and restrictive pulmonary disease. The ratio of FEV_1/FVC is greater than 80%. Note that in restrictive disease the ratio is normal, but the separate measurements of FEV_1 and *FVC* are abnormally low. FEV_1, forced expiratory volume in the first second of exhalation; *FRC*, functional residual capacity; *FVC*, forced vital capacity.

c. *Static compliance:* At the end of a breath, gas flow delivery is paused. The friction created by that flow disappears, causing the inspiratory pressure to drop slightly (airway plateau pressure). The $\Delta V/\Delta P$ (*static* pressure) reflects the elastic properties of the lung (or average distensibility of all participating alveoli). Normal range is the same in an infant as in an adult: 60 to 100 mL per centimeter of H_2O. Static compliance decreases with restrictive disease and increases with obstructive disease. Serial monitoring of *static* compliance may facilitate identification of optimal tidal volumes, optimal positive end-expiratory pressure (PEEP), and prediction of weaning readiness.

PULMONARY PHARMACOLOGY

A. General Principles

Pharmacologic management of pulmonary diseases in children requires understanding of both the pharmacokinetics of the various drugs and the disease conditions for which the drugs are prescribed. Most medications have been studied in adult populations, and application to children has often occurred by extrapolation of data. It is beyond the scope of this text to explore these issues, but several ideas merit consideration by the critical care nurse.

1. **Physiologic differences:** Infants and young children have a greater percentage of total body water, predominately extracellular fluid. The total volume of distribution of a drug, depending on solubility, occurs within intracellular, extracellular, and interstitial fluid compartments. In general, drug doses are higher per kilogram of body weight in the infant than in the adolescent or adult.
2. **Enteral absorption:** Gastric acid secretion and motility appear to be developmentally regulated. The rate of gastric emptying in the normal neonate (<10 weeks) is 87 minutes (Blumer, 1992) compared to an adult time of 65 minutes. However, intestinal transit is more rapid in the infant than in the adult. Many medications might not be absorbed as completely as in the older child or adult because of the following factors:
   a. An *acidic pH* favors absorption of acidic medications; likewise, an alkaline pH improves absorption of alkaline compounds.
   b. The *rate of gastric emptying* and intestinal transit affects absorption of medications. Delayed gastric emptying or rapid intestinal motility will decrease absorption. Conditions that can decrease absorption include gastroesophageal reflux, respiratory distress syndrome, and congenital heart disease.
   c. *Gastric or jejunal* feedings may alter bioavailability. Drugs administered through these tubes may bind with proteins in the feedings. Certain drugs that can be monitored by serum assays, such as phenytoin (Dilantin), carbamazepine (Tegretol), or theophylline should be administered in a consistent fashion but preferably through a gastric tube that has been rinsed before administration; feedings should be stopped for a while before and after administration. Adjustment of drug doses (based on serum assay) is reliable only with consistency in the administration of the drugs and when steady-state concentrations have been achieved.
3. **Protein binding:** Binding of drugs to plasma proteins determines the amount of free drug available for body distribution. Although plasma albumin levels reach adult levels soon after birth, differences in the binding properties of infant albumin can influence the dosing of selected medications.
4. **Underlying pathophysiology:** Decreased blood flow to major organs influences absorption, delivery of the drug to targeted site, and elimination. Inflammation

can cause an increase in regionalized blood flow with altered capillary permeability, which can result in abnormally high drug delivery to these regions. Extravascular fluid collections may provide a protein-rich reservoir for drugs, diverting them from their intended distribution site.

5. **Dosing of medications:** The dosing of medication is frequently based on one of two strategies:
   a. *Target concentration:* Drugs used for chronic or chronically intermittent conditions, such as acetaminophen (Tylenol), antibiotics, or theophylline. The basis for this strategy is that serum concentrations for a given drug have defined therapeutic and toxic ranges. These assays are *guidelines* and are not specific to an individual patient. Knowledge of pharmacokinetics is important to the successful use of this strategy.
   b. *Target effect:* A drug is selected with a therapeutic endpoint clearly defined before administration. Dosing is titrated to achieve this effect or until toxic effects are observed. Discontinuation of the drug may be necessary if toxicity occurs or if no therapeutic effect is achieved. Medications frequently administered with this strategy include catecholamines and diuretics. Many of the medications used in a critical care setting are prescribed in this manner.

B. Neuromuscular Blocking Agents (Table 2-7) (Yaster, 1997)

1. **Description:** Muscle relaxants are used in the pediatric intensive care unit (PICU) to facilitate assisted ventilation by intervening within the neuromuscular junction in one of two ways:
   a. *Depolarizing agents* cause a continuous release and subsequent depletion of acetylcholine.
   b. *Nondepolarizing agents* bind the receptor sites of acetylcholine so that synaptic transmission is blocked.
2. **Indications for use**
   a. *Placement of an ETT* requires administration of a neuromuscular blocking agent (NMB) in most instances.
   b. *Control of ventilation* is often needed in patients with severe respiratory disease, increased ICP, cardiac failure, or pulmonary hypertension.
   c. *Reduction of oxygen consumption* from muscle movement can be achieved with the use of an NMB.
3. **Nursing considerations**
   a. The *choice of an NMB* agent depends on the purpose and intended duration of pharmacologic paralysis. All patients who will receive a paralytic drug should be given adequate sedation and analgesia.
   b. *Monitoring* of all children who are given an NMB agent should include electrocardiographic (ECG) monitoring, pulse oximetry (see Respiratory Monitoring), and intermittent peripheral nerve stimulation monitoring. Increased heart rate (increases from baseline) may be caused by pain, fear, or seizures; increased systolic blood pressure may indicate pain or anxiety; and pupil size (dilation) may indicate fear, pain, or other causes of sympathetic stimulation such as seizures.
   c. *Long-term use* of muscle relaxants may mask pain, anxiety, and seizures. Whenever possible, withholding paralytic medications should be scheduled to enable adequate assessment of the patient's awareness and condition. Prolonged use of muscle relaxants has been associated with a myopathy, particularly if steroids are given concurrently (Martin et al., 2001; Marik, 1996). (See Acute Respiratory Failure discussion and Table 2-7 for more information on specific agents.)

TABLE 2-7
Neuromuscular Blocking Agents and Anticholinergic Agents

Drug	Dose/Onset/Duration	Contraindications	Comments
NEUROMUSCULAR BLOCKING AGENTS			
Pancuronium	Dose: 0.02–0.1 mg/kg Onset: 120 s Duration: 45–90 min	Renal failure 60%–90% renal elimination Tricyclic antidepressant use	Vagolytic: Increased heart rate and blood pressure
Vecuronium	Dose: 0.08–0.1 mg/kg Onset: 120 s Duration: 30–90 min	Liver failure	Renal elimination <25%
Atracurium	Dose: 0.3–0.5 mg/kg Onset: 240–420 s Duration: 30–40 min	Asthma Hypotension Need for rapid onset	Hoffman elimination makes it ideal for kidney or liver failure Very slow onset
Succinylcholine	Dose: 1–2 mg/kg Onset: 30–60 s Duration: 3–10 min	Myasthenia gravis Guillain-Barré syndrome Crush, burn, electrical injuries Open globe injury Increased intracranial pressure	Dysrhythmias Fasciculation Potassium efflux Muscle rigidity
Rocuronium	Dose: 0.5–1.2 mg/kg Onset: 30–60 s Duration: 30–60 min	None	Short duration
ANTIMUSCARINIC AND ANTISPASMODIC AGENTS			
Atropine sulfate	Dose: 0.01 mg/kg Minimum: 0.1 mg Onset: 2–4 min Duration: 90 min	Hypersensitivity Narrow-angle glaucoma Tachycardia Thyrotoxicosis Gastrointestinal obstruction Obstructive uropathy	Monitor for muscarinic effect: Bradycardia, salivation, bronchospasm
Glycopyrrolate	Dose to reverse blockade: 0.2 mg IV for each 1 mg of neostigmine or 5 mg of pyridostigmine administered Dose: 0.004–0.01 mg/kg/dose Maximum: 0.1 mg/dose Onset: 10–15 min after IV administration	Narrow-angle glaucoma Acute hemorrhage Tachycardia Hypersensitivity Ulcerative colitis Obstructive uropathy	Reverses neuromuscular blockade and bronchospasm Controls upper airway secretions Children with Down syndrome, spastic paralysis, or brain damage may be hypersensitive

C. Sedatives and Analgesics (Table 2-8) (Yaster, 1997; Siberry, 2003)

1. Benzodiazepines

a. *Description:* Benzodiazepines are believed to cause anterograde amnesia through the inhibition of the neurotransmitter gamma-aminobutyric acid (GABA) in the limbic system. They have little or no effect on retrograde memory and have no analgesic properties.

b. *Indications* include short-term general sedation and amnesia for procedures, long-term use for facilitating compliance with assisted ventilation, and acute therapy for seizure management.

TABLE 2-8
Sedatives and Analgesics

Drug	IV Dose/Onset/Duration	Contraindications	Comments
Propofol	Dose: 0.5–2 mg/kg IV push 50 μg/kg/min infusion Onset: 1–2 min Duration: 5–10 min	Allergies to soybean or eggs Liver failure Disorder of lipid metabolism	Helpful with refractory bronchospasm Caution with hypovolemia or congestive heart failure May ↓ ICP Produces green urine Does not provide analgesia
Thiopental	Dose: 2–5 mg/kg Onset: <30 s Duration: 5–30 min	Hypovolemia or hypotension	Produces general anesthesia and amnesia Decreases ICP and cerebral blood flow Monitor for hypotension
Ketamine	Dose: 0.5–2 mg/kg Onset: <30 s Duration: 10–15 min	Increased ICP Unconsciousness	Analgesic, amnestic, hallucinogen Monitor for emergence delirium and nightmares Bronchodilator used for patients with asthma Prevent emergence reaction with benzodiazepines at the end of the procedure
BENZODIAZEPINES			
Midazolam	Dose: 0.05–0.2 mg/kg Onset: 2–4 min Duration: 20–30 min Maximum dose: 0.2 mg/kg	Severe hypotension CNS depression	Sedative-anxiolytic, anticonvulsant Alternate routes of delivery including oral, rectal, and transmucosal (nasal)
Lorazepam	Dose: 0.05–0.1 mg/kg Onset: 2–4 min Duration: 20–30 min	Severe hypotension CNS depression	4 to 12-hour half-life, may be used by intermittent bolus No active metabolite
Diazepam	Dose: 0.05–0.1 mg/kg Onset: 2–4 min Duration: 20–30 min Maximum dose: 0.6 mg/kg in an 8 h period	Not recommended for use by continuous infusion Severe hypotension CNS depression	Prolonged effect because of long half-life and presence of active metabolites
OPIATES AND ANALGESIC AGENTS			
Fentanyl	Dose: 1–2 mcg/kg Onset: 3–5 min Duration: 0.5–1 h	Severe respiratory depression	Analgesic, mildly sedating
Methadone	Dose: 0.1 mg/kg Onset: 10–20 min Peak effect: 1–2 h Maximum dose: 10 mg per dose		Half-life 15–29 h Used for managing opiate dependence
Morphine	Dose: 0.1–0.2 mg/kg Peak: 20 min Duration: 4–5 h	Respiratory depression Metabolite accumulation in renal failure	May cause histamine release

CNS, central nervous system; *ICP*, intracranial pressure.

c. *Nursing considerations* include the following:
- Benzodiazepines do *not* provide pain relief. In many situations, use of an analgesic in conjunction with sedation should be considered.
- To avoid hypotension, patients should be euvolemic (well hydrated) before administration of a benzodiazepine to avoid hypotension.
- Prolonged administration may result in physical dependence. Withdrawal symptoms, such as anxiety, sweating, agitation, or hallucinations, may occur with abrupt withdrawal.
- Some patients may exhibit a paradoxical response to benzodiazepines, which worsens with escalating doses. If an agitated child is given additional doses and the agitation worsens, consideration of a paradoxical response might prompt discontinuation of the benzodiazepine (Ashton, 1994; Charney et al., 2001).

2. **Morphine-like opioids**

a. *Description:* Opioid receptors are found in the brain and spinal cord. Five receptors have been described, but three—the mu (M), kappa (K), and sigma (S)—are the most clinically recognized targets for opiate binding:
- M: Supraspinal anesthesia. Euphoria, respiratory depression, physical dependence
- K: Spinal anesthesia. Sedation, miosis, and respiratory depression
- S: Central nervous system (CNS) stimulant. Dysphoria, hallucinations, respiratory and vasomotor stimulation
- Most morphine-like narcotics are described as M and K agonists. Other agents work at different receptor sites, such as nalbuphine (Nubain). Nalbuphine is a K and S receptor agonist and M receptor antagonist. Administration of nalbuphine after morphine may "antagonize" or reverse some of the morphine effects because of its antagonistic effects on the M receptor.

b. *Indications* for analgesic medications include procedures, relief of pain from underlying disease, and continuous analgesia for facilitating assisted mechanical ventilation. Opioids are *not* a substitute for an anxiolytic and amnestic agents. Although sedation occurs with opioid administration, the mechanisms do not duplicate those found in conventional sedatives such as benzodiazepines.

c. *Nursing considerations* include the following:
- Some opioids, such as morphine, can cause vasodilatory effects from histamine release. Histamine release is minimal with the synthetic narcotics such as fentanyl. Most opioids, except meperidine, induce a central parasympathetic stimulation and direct depression of the sinoatrial node. All opioids also cause dose-dependent respiratory depression.
- Routes of delivery should be individualized with the goal of using the lowest possible dosing to provide continuous relief without side effects.
- Fentanyl is a synthetic opioid with approximately 100 times the analgesic potency of morphine. This concentrated solution (unless adequately diluted) may increase the risk for chest-wall rigidity especially with rapid, high-dose intravenous (IV) administration, and decreased seizure threshold. These side effects can be seen with all opioids and are not necessarily contraindications for their use. Slower administration and lower dosing can attenuate or prevent these side effects.

3. **Barbiturates**

a. *Description:* Barbiturates are one of the oldest classes of sedative agents in use today. They provide good sedation but are *not* analgesic or amnestic agents. The cardiopulmonary effects are dose dependent and well defined.

Several drugs are available and classified according to the duration of activity. In addition to their sedative effect, barbiturates have potent anticonvulsant properties and can decrease cerebral metabolism, thus affecting ICP.

b. *Indications* include short-term sedation for procedures and long-term sedation for ongoing management of assisted ventilation (rarely), increased ICP, and continuous procedures such as with use of the intra-aortic balloon pump (IABP). Barbiturates are not a substitute for analgesic medications unless the dosing is high enough to produce complete anesthesia.

c. *Nursing considerations* include the following:

- Cardiovascular effects are dose related. With higher doses, venodilation and depressed myocardial function can occur.
- Pulmonary effects are also dose related, with apnea occurring in the mid-dose ranges. Bag, mask, and oxygen should always be at the bedside.
- Most barbiturates are in an alkaline solution and therefore must be administered separately from other medications and IV solutions.

4. Ketamine

a. *Description:* Ketamine is both an analgesic and an amnestic medication. The mechanism of this drug, including S receptor stimulation, is mediated through the sympathetic nervous system causing a brief, immediate release of endogenous catecholamines. A brief increase in heart rate, blood pressure, and general stimulation are observed with administration of lower doses (0.5 to 2 mg/kg). It produces dissociative anesthesia in which the eyes may be open and nystagmus may be noted; even at lower doses, however, it provides intense analgesia and amnesia. Higher doses provide good anesthesia and respiratory depression, but as the patient recovers, the stimulation and dysphoria can reappear.

b. *Indications:* Ketamine has a minimal effect on cardiopulmonary stability at doses less than 2 mg/kg and is a good choice for unstable patients. Bronchodilation occurs (through the release of endogenous catecholamines), which makes ketamine a good agent for patients with bronchospasm. However, ketamine increases cerebral blood flow and ICP and therefore may not be a good agent for patients with altered intracranial compliance.

c. *Nursing considerations* include the following:

- Emergence phenomena are observed more often in older children and adults than in younger children. Previously it was believed that administration of a benzodiazepine at the end of the procedure could decrease or prevent this occurrence. However, more recent data refute this belief; in fact, some children exhibit paradoxical response to benzodiazepines, causing them to be more agitated and dysphoric.
- Although respiratory depression is dose dependent with ketamine administration, even with normal respiratory function, it is unclear whether airway reflexes are completely intact. Therefore bag, mask, oxygen, and suction should be available at the bedside, particularly if any other sedative agents have been given with ketamine.

5. Propofol

a. *Description:* Propofol is a sedative-hypnotic agent administered intravenously, with rapid onset and short duration of action. The effects are dose dependent. Propofol is provided in a lipid emulsion of soybean oil, glycerol, and egg phosphates. It has multiple properties, including bronchodilation and rapid recovery (with minimal posthypnotic obtundation), which make it an attractive agent for deep sedation or anesthetic induction.

b. *Indications* include induction of anesthesia, deep sedation for short procedures, limited sedation for facilitating other patient-care procedures, and relief of bronchospasm refractory to more conventional agents.

c. *Nursing considerations* include the following:
- Before administration, to avoid an allergic reaction, the patient or family should be questioned about possible allergies to eggs or soybeans.
- Propofol may produce hypotension by direct vasodilation.
- Propofol decreases cerebral blood flow and metabolic requirements of the brain, which may be an advantage in some patients.
- Propofol increases central vagal tone and may cause bradycardia. If used with other medications known to cause bradycardia (such as fentanyl or succinylcholine), this effect can be cumulative. Sudden death has been reported with the use of a fentanyl, propofol, succinylcholine sequence (Egan and Brock-Utne, 1991).
- Use of continuous infusions has been discouraged because of the incidence of unexplained metabolic acidosis, bradycardia, and cardiac arrest (Cray et al., 1998; Stricklan and Murray, 1995).
- Isolated reports of neurologic adverse effects, such as myoclonic movements and convulsions, have raised concern for use of propofol as a long-term therapy (Trotter and Serpell, 1992).

D. Remedial Agents

In providing sedation, analgesia, or pharmacologic paralysis for a child, some agents exhibit predictable but unwanted effects that can be prevented or remediated pharmacologically. The following medications may be used to manage the side effects (Table 2-9).

1. **Anticholinergic agents** (atropine-like medications):

a. *Description:* Anticholinergic agents antagonize the actions of acetylcholine, producing a central vagal blockade (tachycardia, increased blood pressure, mitosis) and specific sympathetic effects in target organs.
- Atropine crosses the blood-brain barrier and is known to cause CNS stimulation, whereas synthetic agents such as ipratropium do not cross into brain tissue.
- In addition, the lungs have both cholinergic and adrenergic receptors that regulate bronchomotor tone. An anticholinergic agent is included in the management of the patient with reactive airway disease. (See Asthma discussion.)

b. *Indications* include premedication for procedures or medications known to potentiate bradycardia (such as succinylcholine), reduction of salivary secretions, bronchodilation (not as a first-line agent but as an adjunct), and symptom control while using a beta-blocker agent.

c. *Nursing considerations* include the following:
- Pupil size and responsiveness are altered with atropine administration. This is important to note when a neurologic condition is being monitored.
- Side effects may be bothersome to patients who are awake, including a fast heart rate, dry mouth, and CNS effects (delirium, agitation).
- Atropine does cross the blood-brain barrier and will cause CNS effects such as agitation.

2. **Naloxone (Narcan)**

a. *Description:* Naloxone is an opioid antagonist, which has an affinity for opiate receptors, blocking them from binding to narcotics. Narcotics attached to the

TABLE 2-9
Remedial Agents

Side Effects	Drug	IV Dose Duration	Comments
Bradycardia or Bronchospasm	Atropine	*Bradycardia* Dose: 0.01 mg/kg Minimum: 0.1 mg Maximum: 1 mg *Bronchospasm* Dose: 0.05 mg/kg in 2.5 ml NS q6h MDI* or aerosol	Monitor for muscarinic effect: Bradycardia, salivation, bronchospasm
Pruritus (Epidural opioids)	Naloxone (Narcan)	Continuous infusion 0.001 mg/kg/hr	This dose should not significantly reverse analgesia
	Nalbuphine (Nubain)	0.01 mg/kg IV every 2–3 min	May improve analgesia May cause increased sedation
(Systemic opioids)	Diphenhydramine (Benadryl)	0.5–1 mg/kg IV q6h	Significant sedation may be observed
Respiratory depression			
(Benzodiazepines)	Flumazenil Romazicon	*<20 kg:* 0.01 mg/kg (maximum 0.2 mg) Repeat: 0.005 mg/kg (maximum 0.2 mg) *20–40 kg:* 0.2 mg (maximum 1 mg) Repeat 0.005 mg/kg	Caution in patients with seizure history Does not consistently reverse amnesia Used for reversal of conscious sedation May produce convulsions in patients physically dependent on benzodiazepines
(Opioids)	Naloxone (Narcan)	*Mild oversedation* 0.01 mg/kg; repeat 2–3 min *Opiate intoxication* <20 kg: 0.1 mg/kg >20 kg: 2 mg/dose Repeat 2–3 min until response noted May require repeat doses q20–60 min	May cause abrupt cessation of pain control; sudden awakening with agitation, nausea and vomiting, and headache
Nausea	Metoclopramide (Reglan)	0.1 mg/kg IV q6h	Low incidence of side effects but extrapyramidal symptoms may occur
	Droperidol (Inapsine)	2–12 y: 0.05–0.06 mg/kg/dose q4–6h >12 y: 2.5–5 mg/dose q4h	Can cause dysphoria, severe hypotension, extrapyramidal reaction
	Ondansetron (Zofran)	0.15 mg/kg IV × three doses at 4 h intervals	No sedation; best used prior to anticipated stimulus (e.g., operating room) Low incidence of bronchospasm, seizures, headaches

*Metered dose inhalers.

receptor are displaced. Naloxone is used to reverse the effects of morphine-like drugs. When given intravenously, the duration is 2 to 3 minutes.

b. *Indications* include the diagnosis and treatment of respiratory depression associated with narcotic use and in research for the management of shock.

c. *Nursing considerations* include the following:

- Because of the quick onset of effect with naloxone, the patient may awaken abruptly and may be in pain or exhibit nausea and vomiting.
- Because of the short duration of effect with naloxone, there may be a recurrence of the narcotized state, necessitating repeated dosing or continuous infusion. Therefore the patient requires constant monitoring because the effects of the narcotic may last longer than the effects of naloxone.

3. Flumazenil (Romazicon)

a. *Description:* Romazicon is a reversal agent for the benzodiazepines with a central mechanism of action.

b. *Indications* include the reversal of benzodiazepine-related side effects, especially respiratory depression.

c. *Nursing considerations* include the following:

- Patients should be monitored continuously with airway equipment at the bedside.
- Use flumazenil with caution in patients with a history of seizures, massive overdoses, or concurrent use of tricyclic agents.

4. Other agents: Nausea and pruritis frequently occur with many of the medications discussed in this section. See Table 2-9 for drug recommendations and dosing to manage these problems.

E. Agents That Affect Ventilation-Perfusion Matching

1. Nitric oxide

a. *Description:* Inhaled nitric oxide is a potent vasodilator of pulmonary vasculature. It appears to have no effect on the systemic circulation because it binds to Hgb and is rapidly inactivated. Studies suggest that nitric oxide may effectively reduce mean pulmonary artery pressure and intrapulmonary shunting, allowing reduction of fraction of inspired oxygen (FiO_2) in patients with adult respiratory distress syndrome (ARDS) (Day et al., 1996).

b. *Indications* currently are for patients with worsening oxygenation and known pulmonary hypertension.

c. *Nursing considerations* include the following:

- Nitric oxide is an inhalational gas delivered through the ventilator circuitry at a flow of 10 to 80 parts per million (ppm).
- Methemoglobin levels should be noted on routine blood-gas analysis as methemoglobinemia is a dose-dependent side effect of nitric oxide therapy.
- Nitric oxide should not be abruptly discontinued if used for more than a short time because rebound effects can occur.

2. Surfactant replacement therapy

a. *Description: Surfactant* is a soapy substance secreted by type II pneumatocytes in the alveoi. Its function is to prevent alveolar collapse at end expiration. Premature infants are deficient in surfactant and may develop respiratory distress syndrome (RDS). Surfactant therapy has proven effective in preventing RDS in neonates, shortening ventilator days, decreasing the barotrauma, and decreasing the severity and incidence of chronic lung disease. Until recently, surfactant has not been well studied in other populations. Many supportive studies have since been published that advocate the use of surfactant for viral bronchiolitis, an acute lung injury in which the surfactant may be diminished by the inflammatory process (Lewis and Brackenbury, 2003; Luchetti et al., 2002).

b. *Indications:* Surfactant therapy for premature newborns is well established, and the earlier it is administered, the better. Surfactant therapy for viral bronchiolitis has enough research documentation to suggest that its use is becoming more common. The timing of administration, however, is not clear. The following criteria were used in the study by Luchetti (2002) in patients with viral bronchiolitis:

- Radiographic evidence of air trapping, hyperinflation, and parenchymal disease plus diagnosis by immunofluorescence assay
- $PaO_2/FiO_2 \leqq 150$ and $PaCO_2 \geqq 40$ mm Hg at admission to the ICU
- Ventilation for 12 hours without improvement (a PaO_2 increase of $\geq 30\%$); peak inspiratory pressure (PIP) >35 cm H_2O.

c. *Nursing considerations* include the following:

- The patient should be sedated and paralyzed to avoid a cough reflex during endotracheal administration of surfactant.
- Administration of surfactant to each lung is done as two separate installations with the patient positioned in a lateral position. Between administrations, the patient's side-lying position is altered with the head of the bed up and then down to facilitate distribution of the surfactant in the lung.
- After administration of surfactant, a transient increase in PIP may occur secondary to decreased compliance. A respiratory therapist should be at the bedside with the nurse and remain there until the patient's condition stabilizes.
- Tidal volume should be continuously monitored. As lung compliance improves, the baseline tidal volume may increase if the ventilator is not in a volume-controlled mode. Ideally the tidal volume should be set for 6 to 7 mL/kg.
- Suctioning should be avoided for at least 1 hour after administration unless there is evidence (as on flow loops) of significant airway obstruction.
- Retreatment at 24 hours or longer may be necessary if the PaO_2/FiO_2 ratio is still less than 200 (if oxygenation index is used, a target goal should be established).

3. Sildenafil

a. *Description:* Sildenafil is a phosphodiesterase inhibitor 5 (PDE-5) with selective vasodilatory activity in the lung vasculature. Hypoxia produces a rapid rise in pulmonary artery pressure. Sildenafil inhibits this response to hypoxia.

b. *Indications:* Sildenafil provides an option for the treatment of pulmonary hypertension refractory to more conventional therapies. Sildenafil is thought to impede or possibly reverse the vascular remodeling process that occurs with sustained pulmonary hypertension (Carroll and Dhillon, 2003).

c. *Nursing considerations* include the following:

- Sildenafil is an oral agent, making it an attractive option for treating pulmonary hypertension. Calcium channel blockers, the only other oral agents available, are not effective in more than half of the patients. Nitric oxide must be delivered continually by inhalation, and prostacyclin must be continuously administered parenterally.
- Dosing reported in several studies is 2 mg/kg orally every 6 hours, starting with a test dose of 0.5 mg and increasing upward to achieve effect (Carroll and Dhillon, 2003).

F. Bronchodilators

Direct bronchodilation for reactive airway disease (RAD) can be achieved through anticholinergic blockade, direct smooth-muscle relaxants, or beta-adrenergic stimulation.

1. **β-agonist medications**
   a. *Description:* Dilation of the airways can be achieved through the administration of β-agonist agents, specifically the β_2 receptors, found in the smooth muscle of the airways. Agents such as albuterol or terbutaline exhibit primarily β_2 stimulation.
      - When given as an inhalation agent, albuterol has an onset of action about 3 to 6 minutes after administration, and its effect may last as long as 4 to 6 hours.
      - IV terbutaline may have an immediate effect, depending on initial dosing. A loading dose of 2 to 10 mcg/kg may be given over 5 minutes, followed by a continuous infusion of 0.08 to 0.4 mcg/kg per minute, titrating to effect and toxicity (heart rate, blood pressure). Doses as high as 6 mcg/kg per minute have been used.
      - Epinephrine is the prototype adrenergic agonist, but it stimulates β_1-, β_2-, and α-receptors, thus producing a generalized sympathetic response with earlier toxicity.

   b. *Indications* include the relief of acute bronchospasm and management of RAD exacerbations.

   c. *Nursing considerations* include the following:
      - Adverse side effects are dose related: tachycardia, tremors, headache, nausea, and sleep disturbances.
      - Potassium wasting may occur. Serum potassium should be monitored in anticipation of a decrease in serum potassium levels in patients receiving aerosol treatments more frequently than every 4 hours.

2. **Anti-inflammatory agents**
   a. *Description:* Conditions such as asthma, ARDS, and postextubation stridor are mediated by an inflammatory process triggered by environmental or endogenous stimuli. The host inflammatory mechanisms normally provide protection, but in specific settings the process appears to cause injury. Anti-inflammatories will not provide immediate treatment for bronchospasm; effects are noted 24 to 36 hours after administration of high-dose steroids.

   b. *Indications:* A component of some daily preventative medications for asthma may include nebulized steroids. High-dose steroids are used for acute exacerbations. Steroid treatment for crouplike illnesses and postextubation stridor are commonly used. Corticosteroids (glucocorticoids) are synthetic preparations of the endogenous hormones. They exert general anti-inflammatory effects such as the suppression of hypersensitivity and immune responses and metabolic effects with an influence on lipid, protein, and carbohydrate metabolism and sodium retention.
      - *Dexamethasone* is often prescribed to treat upper airway edema, and more recent data suggest that a single parenteral dose of dexamethasone (0.6 mg/kg) may be useful in aborting an acute RAD episode (Luria et al., 2001).
      - *Methylprednisolone* is a therapy for management and rescue in asthma exacerbation.

   c. *Nursing considerations:* Glucocorticoids interact with many other drugs; therefore, taking the patient's medication history is essential before administering these drugs.

- Many adverse reactions occur in patients receiving steroids, including sodium and water retention, hyperglycemia, hypokalemia, hypertension, and CNS changes ranging from dysphoria to mood disorders.
- Patients receiving long-term therapy are at risk for osteoporosis, ulcers, hyperlipidemia, and increased susceptibility to infection with symptoms that may be suppressed by the steroids.

d. *Nonsteroidal agents:* Nonsteroidal anti-inflammatory agents (NSAIDs) have not proven useful in the treatment of pulmonary disorders. In particular, a subset of patients with RAD may exhibit asthma symptoms from the use of aspirin. In addition, aspirin should not be used in pediatric patients under the age of 18 years because of its clear association with Reye syndrome.

e. *Leukotriene inhibitors:* These agents block or inhibit the synthesis of cysteinyl leukotriene (c-leukotriene), a mediator that causes bronchoconstriction, mucous secretion, increased vascular permeability, and eosinophil migration to the airways. The release of c-leukotriene from mast cells, eosinophils, and basophils appears not to be blocked by steroids (Bisgaard and Nielsen, 2000). These agents do not appear as efficacious as monotherapy, but in combination with inhaled steroids, improved patient baseline function has been noted. Because of the prolonged duration of onset, they are not intended for treatment of an acute episode of asthma.

ACUTE RESPIRATORY FAILURE

A. Definition and Etiology

Acute respiratory failure is inability of the respiratory system to meet the demands of the body for oxygen or provide adequate carbon dioxide elimination, often leading to acidosis. The acute respiratory distress syndrome (formerly called the adult respiratory distress syndrome, or ARDS) is characterized by acute diffuse infiltrative lung lesions with resulting interstitial and alveolar edema, severe hypoxemia, and respiratory failure. The definition of ARDS includes the following components:

1. A ratio of PaO_2 to the $FiO_2 \leq 200$, regardless of the level of PEEP
2. The detection of bilateral pulmonary infiltrates on the frontal chest x-ray
3. Pulmonary artery wedge pressure ≤18 mm Hg or no clinical evidence of elevated left atrial pressure on the basis of the chest radiograph and other clinical data (Bernard et al., 1994)

B. Pathophysiology

Respiratory failure can be related to pulmonary and nonpulmonary causes. The "respiratory pump" includes the nervous system, airways, and respiratory muscles. Respiratory failure can develop as a result of the failure of any component of the respiratory system. The anatomy of the airway of a child differs from that of the adult in many clinically significant ways (See Developmental Anatomy of the Respiratory System). These differences can lead to airway compromise and make airway support more difficult (Figure 2-15).

1. **Pulmonary causes of acute respiratory failure**

   a. *Impaired integrity of lung tissue*

   - Conditions such as atelectasis, pneumonia, bronchiolitis, and ARDS can lead to low V/P.
   - Conditions such as acute lung injury (ALI), alveolar overdistention causing pulmonary injury (Martin, 1995), ARDS, or cyanotic heart disease can cause mismatches between ventilation and perfusion.

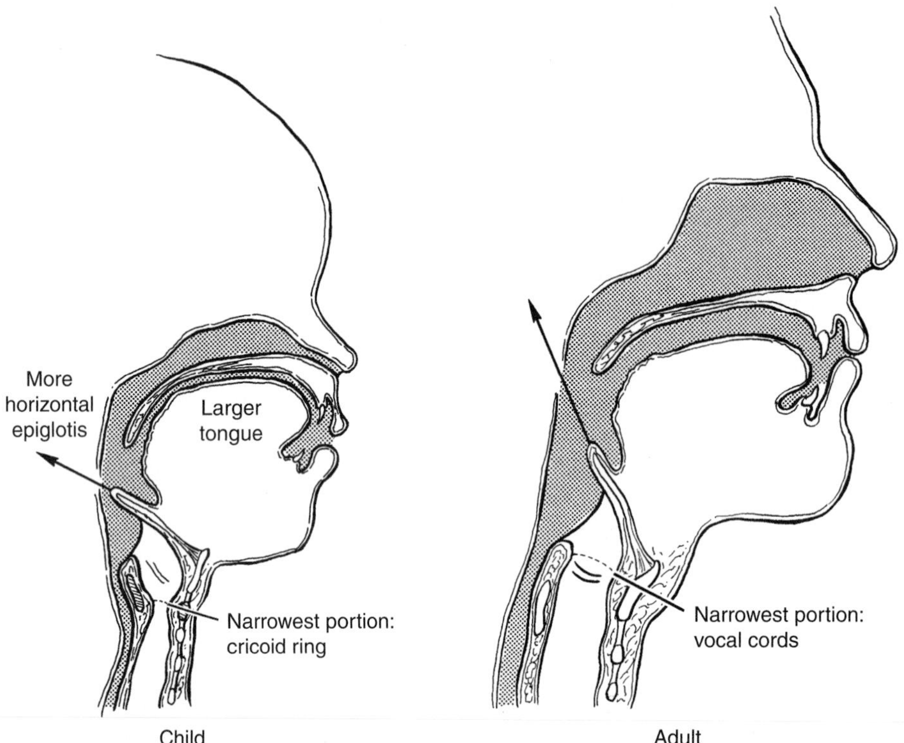

FIGURE 2-15 ■ Anatomic differences between child and adult airways.

- Pulmonary edema results from increased pulmonary extravascular water as a result of increased pulmonary capillary permeability or an increase in pulmonary vascular pressure, which causes impaired gas exchange.

b. *Increased airway resistance*

- Small amounts of edema can significantly reduce airway diameter and increase resistance to airflow and the work of breathing in the infant or child. High compliance makes the child's airway susceptible to dynamic collapse in the presence of airway obstruction.
- Congenital upper-airway anomalies can restrict flow through upper airways. Aspiration of a foreign body may restrict flow by narrowing the airway.

2. Nonpulmonary causes of acute respiratory failure

a. *Respiratory muscle compromise*

- The diaphragm is the primary muscle of inspiration for infants. Movement of the diaphragm is limited, with abdominal distention or poor diaphragmatic function. Diaphragmatic disorders include diaphragmatic hernia, paralysis, and eventration.
- The chest wall is extremely compliant, which can further compromise ventilation and lead to chest-wall retractions.
- Respiratory muscle fatigue leads to hypoventilation, which may progress to hypoxia and acidosis.

b. *Alterations in nervous system control of breathing* include immature CNS function; respiratory depression by narcotics, sedatives, or anesthetics; and CNS disease, such as Guillain-Barré syndrome, head or spinal cord trauma, CNS infection, myasthenia gravis, botulism, or central hypoventilation syndrome.

c. *Upper-airway disorders* include choanal atresia, micrognathia, cystic hygroma, obstruction, and tracheoesophageal fistula.
d. *Cardiovascular and hematologic disorders* include congenital heart disease, anemia, shock, or sepsis.

C. Clinical Presentation

1. **The patient's history** should be evaluated for chronic lung disease and respiratory or nonrespiratory causes of respiratory failure. Evaluate the onset of symptoms, the presence of respiratory distress, fever, activity level, and level of consciousness. Determine home use of respiratory medications.
2. **Physical examination**
   a. Increased work of breathing is related to airway obstruction or alveolar disease and results in tachypnea; nasal flaring; and intercostal, subcostal, and suprasternal inspiratory retractions.
   b. Alterations in respiratory mechanics can be related to alveolar collapse and the loss of lung volume associated with pulmonary edema, pneumonia, or atelectasis. Grunting increases end-expiratory pressure, thereby increasing functional residual capacity. Head bobbing, stridor, and prolonged expiration are additional signs of altered respiratory mechanisms.
   c. Signs of upper-airway obstruction can be related to congenital abnormalities (laryngomalacia, vocal cord paralysis, hemangioma, airway tumor), infections (epiglottitis, croup, bacterial tracheitis), noninfectious upper-airway edema (allergic reaction following intubation and extubation, gastroesophageal reflux), or aspiration of a foreign body. Inspiratory stridor and paradoxical chest movement with sternal and intercostal retractions rather than chest and lung expansion may be seen in upper-airway obstruction.
   d. Lower-airway obstruction can be related to bronchiolitis, asthma, pulmonary edema, or intrathoracic foreign body. Prolonged expiration and wheezing are clinical signs of lower-airway obstruction.
   e. Decreased air entry can be related to hypoventilation, airway obstruction, atelectasis, pneumothorax, hemothorax, pleural effusion, mucous plug, or foreign-body aspiration. Breath sounds are diminished unilaterally or bilaterally.
   f. Perfusion should be evaluated by examining skin color and temperature. Evaluate mucous membranes, nail beds, palms of hands, and soles of feet for cyanosis, which can be caused by hypoxia or poor perfusion.
   g. Changes in the level of consciousness, such as irritability, lethargy, or failure to respond to parents, may be indications of cerebral hypoxia or hypercarbia, which will require immediate intervention.
3. **Diagnostic tests to evaluate for respiratory failure**
   a. *Arterial or capillary blood gas* analysis can assist in the assessment of respiratory failure (Table 2-10).
      - *$Paco_2$* directly reflects the adequacy of alveolar ventilation. Hypercarbia is $Paco_2$ greater than 55 mm Hg.
      - *Oxygenation* is evaluated with the Pao_2. Hypoxemia is an arterial Pao_2 less than 60 mm Hg.
      - *Acid-base balance* is indicated by the pH. *Acidosis* is an arterial pH less than 7.35, and *alkalosis* is an arterial pH greater than 7.45.
   b. *Chest radiographs* are evaluated for areas of consolidation, atelectasis, pneumothorax, effusion, hyperinflation, and edema.
4. **Clinical course:** Determine the cause of the respiratory failure if possible. If spontaneous minute ventilation and oxygenation are effective (as evidenced by

TABLE 2-10
Normal Blood Gas Values

Parameter	Arterial	Mixed Venous	Capillary
pH	7.35-7.45	7.31-7.41	7.35-7.45
Po_2	80-100 mm Hg	35-40 mm Hg	Less than arterial*
O_2 saturation	95%-97%	70%-75%	Less than arterial
Pco_2	35-45 mm Hg	40-50 mm Hg	35-45 mm Hg
HCO_3	22-26 mEq/L	22-26 mEq/L	22-26 mEq/L
Total CO_2 content	20-27 mEq/L	20-27 mEq/L	20-27 mEq/L
Base excess	+2 to −2	+2 to −2	+2 to −2

*Capillary Po_2 is approximately 10 mm Hg less than arterial Po_2 except when decreased tissue perfusion is present, that is, cardiovascular collapse or hypothermia. In these states, capillary samples will not accurately reflect arterial Po_2.
From Powers A: Acid-Base Balance. In Curley MAQ & Moloney-Harmon PA, eds. *Critical Care Nursing of Infants and Children*, 2nd ed. Philadelphia, 2001, Saunders.

good air movement in all lung fields, pulse oximetry saturation ≥90%, and normal mental status), supplemental oxygen can be delivered by cannula or face mask. Intubation or noninvasive positive pressure ventilation (continuous positive airway pressure [CPAP]/bilevel positive airway pressure [BiPAP]) is required if respiratory failure (significant hypoxemia, hypercarbia, acidosis, or altered level of consciousness) is present.

D. Patient Care Management

1. **Prevention** of acute respiratory failure includes general principles of management of the infant or child's airway. Encourage coughing and deep breathing in awake patients. Intervene with frequent position changes. Reduce abdominal distention by nasogastric suction if necessary. Use precautions for known reflux.
2. **Monitoring**
   a. *Noninvasive respiratory monitoring* includes pulse oximetry and E_Tco_2 detectors for intubated patients.
   b. *Invasive respiratory monitoring* includes arterial blood-gas (ABG) analysis and mixed venous oxygen saturation monitoring via pulmonary artery catheter (see Respiratory Monitoring discussion).
3. **Oxygen-delivery systems** provide supplemental oxygen for patients with adequate ventilation (Table 2-11). Bag and mask ventilation is used when a patient's breathing is inadequate. It can be used in conjunction with oropharyngeal or nasopharyngeal airways and allows the administration of PEEP.
   a. *Endotracheal tube (ETT) airways* are indicated for inadequate respiratory effort (drugs, infections, trauma, chest-wall deformities), normal effort but overwhelming demand (bronchiolitis, asthma, pneumonia), inadequate CNS control of ventilation, a need to maintain a patent airway (loss of protective reflexes, obstruction, edema), a need for high PIP, and the anticipated need for mechanical ventilatory support (shock, trauma, increased ICP, status post-cardiopulmonary arrest, or acute respiratory failure).
   b. See Table 2-12 for methods to estimate the size of the ETT and Table 2-13 and Figure 2-16 for intubation equipment.
4. **Medications** such as *neuromuscular blocking agents, anticholinergics* (see Table 2-7), and *sedatives* (see Table 2-8) are often used. See Pulmonary Pharmacology.

TABLE 2-11
Oxygen Delivery Systems

	Indications	FiO_2	Description	Comments
Nasal cannula	Nasal breathing; provide oxygen up to 0.5	0.22–0.5	One prong fits into each anterior naris, maximum oxygen flow 4–5 L/min	Least restrictive, FiO_2 unknown, entrains room air
Head hood	Useful for infant or small child	0.21–0.9	Clear plexiglass box placed over patient's head	Less than 10 kg; requires humidification; flows >10 L/min to flush out carbon dioxide
Simple face mask	Useful for delivering aerosols and oxygen; use with mouth breathing	0.44–0.5	Vinyl, fits over nose and mouth; open ports on side of mask to allow exhalation of carbon dioxide Minimum flow rate: 4 L infant, 5 L child	Entrains room air, child cannot eat or drink; high FiO_2 not attainable; FiO_2 is not correlated with high flow rates
Nonrebreathing mask	Useful for patients who require high FiO_2	0.9–0.95	Vinyl, fits over nose and mouth; reservoir bag attached with one-way gas flow from bag into the mask	No entrainment of room air; oxygen flow determined by patient's minute ventilation
Laryngeal mask airway (LMA)	Used to secure the airway in an unconscious patient	0.21–1	Available in a range of sizes; consists of a tube with a cuffed, masklike projection at the distal end	Introduced into pharynx and advanced until resistance is felt as the tube enters the hypopharynx
Endotracheal tube with mechanical ventilation	Can deliver positive pressure and high FiO_2; does not require patient respiratory drive when used with a ventilator	0.21–1	Sterile, translucent polyvinyl with radiopaque marker; uniform internal diameter; cuffed or uncuffed	Most effective and reliable method of oxygen delivery; can control inspiratory time, PEEP, and tidal volume when used with a ventilator

TABLE 2-12
Methods to Estimate Endotracheal Tube Size

ENDOTRACHEAL TUBE SIZE CALCULATION

$$\text{Internal diameter (mm)} = \frac{16 + \text{age (y)}}{4}$$

MINIMUM DEPTH OF TUBE INSERTION

Size of ETT × 3

TABLE 2-13 Intubation Equipment

Equipment	Types	Comments
Laryngoscope	Miller (Straight) elevates epiglottis MacIntosh (curved)	Size 0–1: Newborns and infants Size 1–4: Children and adults
Endotracheal tube	Uncuffed	Used in those younger than 8–10 y of age to reduce the risk of subglottic edema and stenosis; an uncuffed tube of appropriate size provides a reasonable seal at the cricoid ring
	Cuffed	Used in those older than 10 y of age and when needed to deliver a significant amount of positive pressure; cuff should be inflated with minimal leak to prevent mucosal ischemia
Monitoring equipment	Pulse oximeter ECG Blood pressure cuff	
Oxygen delivery equipment	Bag-valve ventilation device	
Suction	Large bore (14–18F), disposable tracheal suction Yankauer tonsillar suction	
Exhaled or end-tidal CO_2 monitors	Calorimetric or continuous capnography	Recommended to confirm endotracheal tube placement in all patients who weigh > 2 kg and have a perfusing rhythm

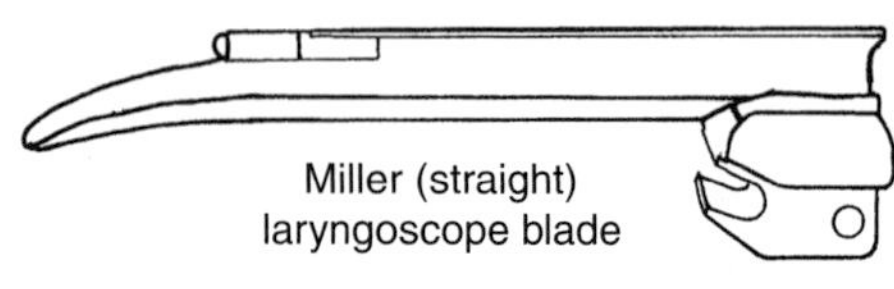

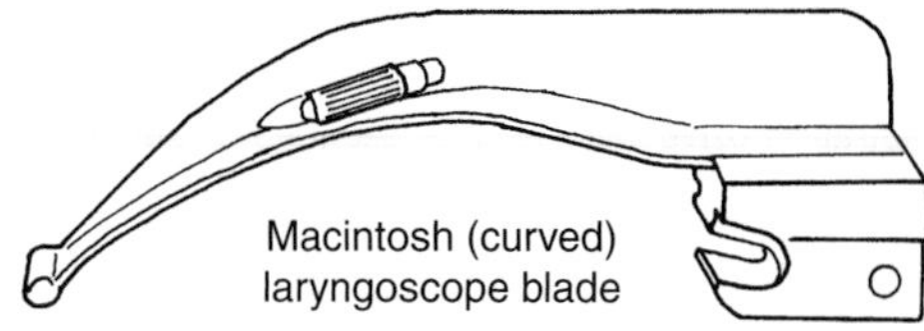

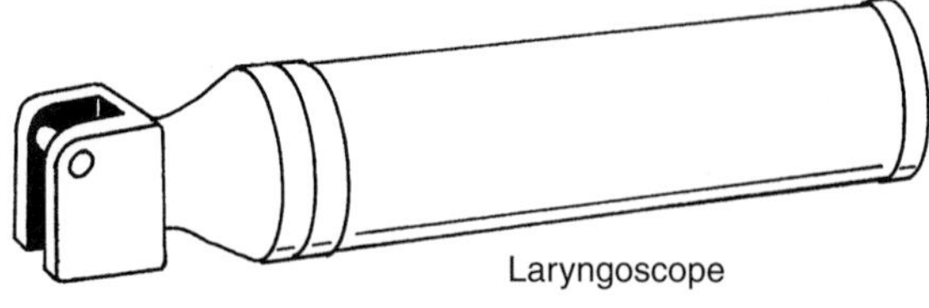

FIGURE 2-16 ■ Intubation equipment.

5. **Rapid-sequence intubation** is used in patients with a "full stomach" when concern about regurgitation and aspiration is present. Cricoid pressure is used to prevent regurgitation of abdominal contents. Bag-valve-mask ventilation of patients is limited to reduce air entry into the stomach.

E. Outcomes

1. **Extubation** is attempted when the indications for intubation have resolved. Excessive sedation is avoided, the oropharynx is suctioned, and the cuff is deflated.
2. **Complications** from endotracheal intubation include airway trauma, such as tracheal laceration or hematoma of the vocal cords, erosions of posterior vocal cords, loss of teeth, aspiration, hypoxemia from prolonged attempts at intubation, ETT obstruction, endobronchial intubation from flexion of the head, esophageal intubation, and dislodgment of the ETT from head and neck extension.
   a. *Postextubation croup* occurs in 1% to 6% of pediatric patients. Most have been intubated longer than 1 hour. Upper-airway obstruction occurs acutely up to 3 hours after extubation. Treatment involves cool humidified oxygen, nebulized racemic epinephrine, or a helium-oxygen gas mixture. Steroids are sometimes beneficial.
   b. *Other postintubation sequelae* include laryngeal webs, laryngeal and tracheal granulomas, tracheal stenosis, vocal cord paralysis, sinus infections, and tracheomegaly.

ACUTE EPIGLOTTITIS

A. Definition and Etiology

1. Acute epiglottitis is a severe life-threatening, rapidly progressive infection of the epiglottis and surrounding area (Figure 2-17).
2. Acute epiglottitis usually occurs in children aged 2 to 6 years but can occur at any age. As many as 6% of children with epiglottitis without an artificial airway die, compared with less than 1% of those with an artificial airway. Before the use of the Hi*B* vaccine, *Haemophilus influenzae* type b was the most commonly identified cause of acute epiglottitis (Adams et al., 1993). The usual cause in the

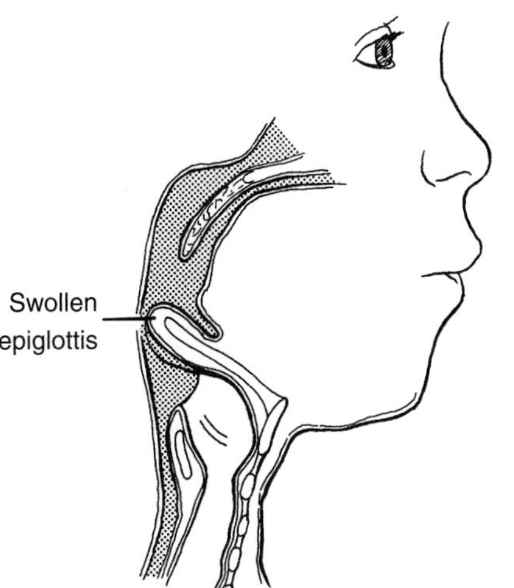

FIGURE 2-17 ■ Swollen epiglottis in acute epiglottitis.

vaccinated child is now *Streptococcus pyogenes, S. pneumoniae,* or *Staphylococcus aureus.*

B. Pathophysiology

1. Thickened epiglottis and aryepiglottic folds lead to narrowing of the airway and turbulent gas flow. Pulmonary edema may occur from an increased transmural pressure gradient from pulmonary vasoconstriction resulting from alveolar hypoxia as well as the negative pleural pressure generated against the airway obstruction.

C. Clinical Presentation

1. **History** usually reveals acute onset of symptoms, including high fever, sore throat, dyspnea, and rapidly progressing respiratory obstruction.
2. **Physical examination**
   a. The term *four Ds and an S* describes the symptoms: dysphagia, drooling, dysphonia, distress, and stridor.
   b. *Presentation* is characterized by an abrupt onset of fever, sore throat, drooling, muffled voice, and hyperextension of the neck. Respiratory distress is usually mild to moderate. Stridor is a late finding and suggests near-complete airway obstruction. The child often attempts to maintain a patent airway by leaning forward while sitting and holding his or her head in a sniffing position.
   c. *Assess* the degree of stridor, color, retractions, air entry, and level of consciousness.
3. **Diagnostic tests**
   a. If *epiglottitis* is suspected, invasive or anxiety-provoking procedures should be avoided. Also avoid direct oral cavity examination because depression of the tongue could force the enlarged epiglottis over the laryngeal opening and agitate the patient.
   b. An *AP radiograph* of the neck may not reveal a swollen epiglottis. A lateral neck radiographic examination, however, is diagnostic and is always indicated in the presence of upper airway lesions.
   c. Obtain *blood cultures* to identify the organism after airway control is established.
4. **Clinical course:** Acute infection usually resolves in 24 to 72 hours with antibiotics; most patients have concomitant bacteremia.
5. **Differential diagnosis:** Distinguish epiglottis from laryngotracheobronchitis by presentation, lateral neck radiographic examination, or direct visualization in the operating room (Table 2-14).

D. Patient Care Management

1. **Prevention:** The HiB vaccine has significantly reduced the incidence of this disease in children and therefore is strongly recommended for infants.
2. **Direct care:** If epiglottitis is strongly suspected, the patient should be taken directly to the operating room for direct laryngoscopy and subsequent intubation. Before endotracheal intubation or tracheotomy is performed, keep the child comfortable and disturb him or her as little as possible. Allow the patient to maintain a comfortable position. Supplemental oxygen can be administered while the child is sitting in a parent's lap. Ceftriaxone, cefotaxime, or a combination of ampicillin and sulbactam should be given parenterally, pending culture and susceptibility reports, because from 10% to 40% of *H. influenzae* type b cases are resistant to ampicillin (Frantz and Rasgon, 1993). Antibiotics should be continued for 7 to 10 days.
3. **Supportive care** includes admission to the PICU for close monitoring. Use sedation and arm restraints or muscle relaxants to prevent self-extubation, and

TABLE 2-14
Diagnostic Features of Infectious Causes of Stridor

	Laryngotracheobronchitis	Epiglottitis	Bacterial Tracheitis
Age range	3 mo–3 y	2–6 y	2–4 y
Etiology	Viral	Bacterial	Bacterial
Pathology	Inflammation of subglottic region, trachea, bronchi, bronchioles	Inflammation of epiglottis, aryepiglottic folds, and surrounding tissue	Acute infectious process in the trachea
Onset	Gradual	Acute	Variable
Signs and symptoms	Hoarseness Barking cough Stridor	High fever Drooling Dysphagia Dysphonia Distress Inspiratory stridor Sniffing position	High fever Inspiratory stridor Drooling May mimic epiglottitis
Diagnosis	History and physical examination	History and physical examination Swollen supraglottis on direct visualization	Thick purulent secretions
Radiographic signs	Subglottic narrowing "Steeple sign"	Increased epiglottic shadow on lateral neck x-ray examination	Subglottic irregularity "Steeple sign" may be present
Treatment	Mist hydration Racemic epinephrine Steroids	Antibiotics Airway management with endotracheal tube	Antibiotics Airway control
Course	Obstructive signs decrease over a period of 3–4 d	Improvement 36–48 h after antibiotics are initiated	Improvement 36–48 h after antibiotics are initiated May require tracheostomy

decrease movement of the ETT in the larynx. Deliver oxygen as necessary. Monitor closely for postobstructive pulmonary edema. Criteria for extubation may include air leak around the artificial airway or direct examination of the epiglottis. Extubation is performed in the PICU or operating room with intubation and emergency tracheostomy equipment available.

4. **Complications:** Intubation has been reported to have fewer complications than tracheostomy. These include self-extubation and obstruction from secretions. Patients who underwent intubation rather than tracheostomy have a shorter period of artificial airway support and hospitalization.

E. Outcome

Given appropriate management of the airway during the initial stabilization, there should be no long-term sequelae for this disease.

ACUTE LARYNGOTRACHEOBRONCHITIS

A. Definition and Etiology

1. **Acute laryngotracheobronchitis (LTB)** is an inflammatory swelling of the submucosa in the subglottic area. *Croup* is a general medical term that refers to this inflammatory process, which results in stridor, cough, and hoarseness.

2. *Croup* usually occurs in children aged 3 months to 5 years, peaking in the second year of life. There is a tendency for LTB to recur in children who have had one episode. LTB can be either viral or bacterial in origin. Viral LTB accounts for 85% of reported cases. The parainfluenza viruses (types 1, 2, and 3) account for about 75% of cases; other viruses associated with this disease include influenza A and B, adenovirus, and respiratory syncytial virus (RSV). Nonviral LTB may result from asthma, angioneurotic edema, foreign-body aspiration, or subglottic stenosis following endotracheal intubation.

B. Pathophysiology

The term *laryngotracheobronchitis* refers to a viral infection of the glottic and subglottic regions. In children the cricoid cartilage makes up the narrowest segment of the upper airway. Swelling and secretions in this subglottic region increase resistance to airflow, leading to respiratory distress (Figure 2-18).

C. Clinical Presentation

1. **History:** Characteristically a gradual onset and symptoms of a preceding upper respiratory tract infection include rhinorrhea, coryza, and low-grade fever. Symptoms vary over several days, with stridor worsening at night.
2. **Physical examination:** Clinical manifestations are produced by subglottic obstruction. Clinical signs of respiratory failure are predictive of severity. The onset of LTB is noted by the development of a barking cough and hoarseness. The patient may also demonstrate inspiratory stridor and thin, copious secretions. The degree of nasal flaring, tracheal tugging, and retraction of the chest muscles depends on the degree of airway resistance. The larynx is nontender on palpation. A low (rather than high) fever helps to differentiate

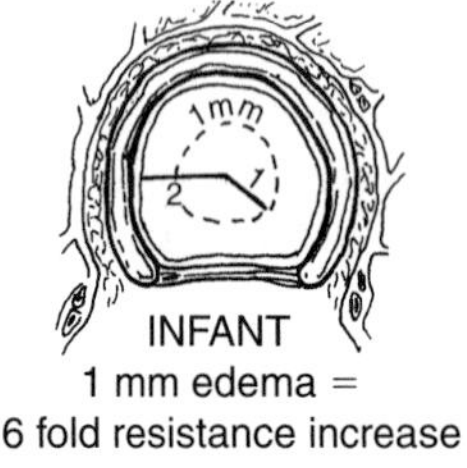

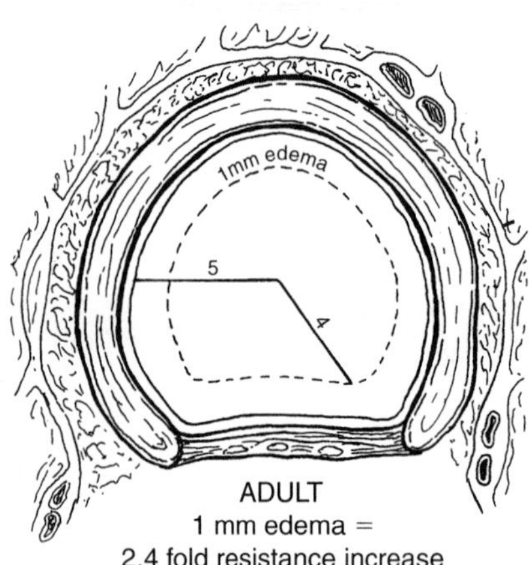

FIGURE 2-18 ■ Airway edema and acute laryngotracheobronchitis.

from bacterial tracheitis and epiglottitis. Normal alveolar gas exchange and low oxygen saturation are seen only when complete airway obstruction is imminent.

3. **Diagnostic tests:** A chest radiograph (AP) demonstrates a funnel-shaped narrowing of the glottis and subglottic airway ("steeple sign"). A lateral radiograph of the neck demonstrates a normal epiglottis. Radiographs should be considered only after airway stabilization.
4. **Clinical course:** Monitor closely for cyanosis, pallor, weakness, or other signs of hypoxemia. Hypoxemia, hypercarbia, tachycardia, and respiratory acidosis may develop if obstruction is severe.
5. **Differential diagnosis:** See Table 2-14 for comparison of LTB, epiglottitis, and bacterial tracheitis.

D. Patient Care Management

1. **Direct care**
   a. Although rare, *intubation* may be necessary for increased WOB, pallor, cyanosis, decreased level of consciousness, worsening hypoxemia or hypercarbia, or respiratory distress unresponsive to treatment. Intubation is necessary if respiratory distress is refractory to medical intervention. Development of an air leak can indicate readiness for extubation.
   b. *Racemic epinephrine* produces topical mucosal vasoconstriction of the precapillary arterioles, thereby reducing mucosal edema. Indications include moderate to severe stridor that does not respond to cool mist. Racemic epinephrine is a 1:1 mixture of the *d*- and *l*-isomers of epinephrine. A dose of 0.25 to 0.75 mL of 2.25% racemic epinephrine in 3 mL of normal saline can be used as often as every 20 minutes (Kristjansson et al., 1994).
   c. After several decades of debate about the effectiveness of *corticosteroids* in viral croup, clear evidence of their benefit has not been established. Most studies have demonstrated the efficacy of dexamethasone used as a single dose of 0.6 mg/kg (Luria et al., 2001).
   d. *Antibiotics* are not indicated.
   e. A *helium-oxygen* gas mixture (30% oxygen plus 70% helium) may be used for severe croup. The lower density provides less turbulent flow than oxygen alone, and it reduces the WOB by decreasing the resistance to turbulent gas flow through a narrowed airway. Preliminary studies with a helium-oxygen mixture (Heliox) have shown similar clinical improvements compared with responses to racemic epinephrine (Weber et al., 2001).
2. **Supportive care**
   a. *Minimize disturbances.* Avoid agitation such as obtaining blood gases.
   b. *Judge severity* using the croup score (Table 2-15). The child should be admitted to the PICU for a croup score of 6 or higher.

TABLE 2-15
Croup Score

Symptom	0	1	2
Stridor	None	Inspiratory	Inspiratory and expiratory
Cough	None	Hoarse	Bark
Air entry	Normal	Decreased	Markedly decreased
Flaring and retractions	None	Flaring and suprasternal	Suprasternal, subcostal, intercostal
Color	Normal	Cyanosis in room air	Cyanosis in 40% oxygen

c. *Provide cool, humidified oxygen* by face mask or through a tube held in front of the patient by the parent. Use humidification and adequate hydration to liquefy secretions. Control fever using antipyretics. Administer IV fluids to ensure adequate hydration. Once epiglottitis and bacterial tracheitis have been ruled out, antibiotic therapy is not needed.
d. *Enteral (transpyloric or gastric) feedings* may be considered in patients with respiratory distress. Transpyloric feeding tubes can be easily placed at the bedside, and tube feedings can be initiated in any patient with moderate respiratory distress or at risk of aspiration (Chellis et al., 1996a, b; Gianotti et al., 1994).

3. **Complications:** Intubation should be performed by a skilled practitioner to limit complications of intubation. ETT size should be 0.5 to 1 mm smaller than that predicted for the patient's age to aid in passing through the narrowed airway and avoid exacerbating subglottic inflammation.

E. Outcome

1. With appropriate management, the mortality for LTB is low.

PNEUMONIA

A. Definition and Etiology

1. Pneumonia is an infection of the lung caused most often by bacteria or viruses.
2. The most likely etiologic agent depends on the age of the patient, how the organism was acquired (community or nosocomial), and the presence of underlying disease. Influenza and RSV are most common in young children. Bacterial and viral causes are found in 44% to 85% of children with community-acquired pneumonia, with more than one pathogen in 25% to 40% (Wubbell et al., 1999). Children fully immunized against *H. influenzae* type b and *S. pneumoniae* are less likely to be infected with these pathogens.
3. Compromised host defenses may predispose a patient to pneumonia, including the following:
   a. *Bypass of nasal defenses* from endotracheal intubation or tracheostomy
   b. *Pulmonary aspiration* from CNS injury or secondary to gastroesophageal reflux or tracheoesophageal fistula.
   c. *Abnormal airway secretion* or mucociliary clearance from infections, bronchopulmonary dysplasia, or cystic fibrosis and in neurologically devastated patients.
   d. *Underlying chronic disease* or poor nutrition.
   e. *Diseases* that alter the immune system.

B. Pathophysiology

1. **Invading organisms** initiate the inflammatory response, which then causes alveolar edema. The edema is a medium for the multiplication of organisms. An inflammatory process of the lungs may involve the interstitial tissue and pleura, leading to lung consolidation, reduced lung compliance, and a decrease in vital capacity and TLC.
2. **Mode of transmission** of the organism is through inspiration of microorganisms, aspiration of oropharyngeal secretions, or systemic circulation. The location of the pneumonia on chest radiograph may help to differentiate the type of pneumonia. The neurologically devastated patient who has poor secretion control is at risk of developing aspiration pneumonia. Generally *lobar pneumonia* involves

one or more lobes of the lung and is observed with bacterial processes. *Bronchopneumonia* involves terminal bronchioles. *Interstitial pneumonia* involves the alveolar walls, producing a hazy, diffuse radiographic pattern characteristic of viral pneumonia.

C. Clinical Presentation

1. **History:** Prodrome may be of a mild upper respiratory tract infection or sudden fever, cough, and chest pain. In infants a prodrome of upper respiratory tract infection and diminished appetite can lead to the abrupt onset of fever, restlessness, and respiratory distress. Examine for etiologic or precipitating factors.
2. **Physical examination:** Shaking chills followed by a high fever, cough, and chest pain may occur, particularly with bacterial pneumonia. Upper respiratory tract symptoms are characterized by stuffy nose, irritability, and poor feeding. Respiratory distress manifests by expiratory grunting, flaring of the nostrils, retractions, tachypnea, and tachycardia. Cyanosis may be present. Abdominal distention may be prominent because of gastric dilation from swallowed air. The liver may seem enlarged because of downward displacement of the diaphragm secondary to hyperinflation of the lungs. Auscultation of the lungs may reveal fine early inspiratory crackles or bronchial breath sounds heard with lobar pneumonia. Infants appear ill with respiratory distress manifesting by grunting, nasal flaring, tachycardia, air hunger, cyanosis, and occasionally apnea (Sectish and Prober, 2004).
3. **Diagnostic tests**
   a. *Chest radiograph:* The chest radiograph confirms the diagnosis of pneumonia and may indicate a complication such as a pleural effusion or empyema. Pneumonia can initially produce a patchy infiltration with fluffy margins. Later a bacterial pneumonia causes more segmental or lobar disease with more homogenous opacification of the involved area of the lung. Aspiration pneumonia usually develops in the portion of the lung that is dependent at the time of aspiration. Bronchopneumonia produces perihilar congestion from inflammation of terminal bronchioles. Pleural effusion may represent empyema, most often associated with bacterial infection.
   b. *Sputum or tracheal secretions* are of limited value and examined only to note the predominant flora and the presence of neutrophils. A tracheal aspirate from a newly intubated patient may be of some diagnostic value. Reliable reagents for the rapid detection of RSV, parainfluenza, influenza, and adenovirus are available.
   c. *Cultures* of blood, pleural fluid, or lung are necessary for definitive diagnosis of a bacterial infection. Results are diagnostic but positive in only 10% to 25% of cases.
   d. *Quantitative bronchoalveolar lavage* (BAL) or *protected brush specimen* may be indicated to reduce some of the diagnostic confusion that may be created by sputum specimen contamination. However, BAL does not always recover the pathogens that produce pneumonia.
   e. *Lung biopsy* may be indicated in the child with severe disease or in the immunosuppressed host. This will provide evaluation of lung tissue and a culture obtained under sterile setting to guide more definitive treatment.
   f. A *serum WBC count* greater than 15,000/mm^3 with a predominance of granulocytes is associated with bacterial pneumonia (Nohynek et al., 1995).
4. **Clinical course**
   a. The clinical course depends on the patient's age, the cause of pneumonia, and the clinical presentation. Occasionally extrapulmonary manifestations of

bacterial pneumonia, such as dehydration and obtundation, result in patient admission to the PICU.

D. Patient Care Management

1. **Prevention**
   a. Immunocompromised patients should receive scheduled trimethoprim-sulfamethoxazole (Septra) as prophylaxis against *Pneumocystis carinii* pneumonia.
2. **Direct care**
   a. Patients are monitored for signs of increasing respiratory distress. A chest radiograph is included in the initial evaluation. ABG levels are monitored at frequent intervals if the pH is low or there is concern of progressive deterioration in respiratory status.
   b. Oxygen delivery should maintain saturations of greater than 90%. Intubate and provide mechanical ventilation for respiratory failure.
3. **Supportive care**
   a. If the patient is dehydrated, a fluid bolus of 10 to 20 mL/kg is administered. Maintenance of hydration can be achieved by IV fluids. If the course is prolonged, enteral feedings are initiated.
   b. Antimicrobials are administered for age group and suspected organism and are continued for 7 to 14 days. Treatment of nosocomial pneumonia involves the use of antimicrobial agents directed at the identified pathogen or, if it is unknown, at the most likely etiologic agent based on the clinical setting and available diagnostic information. Treatment of viral infections is supportive.
4. **Complications**
   a. The complications from bacterial pneumonia stem from lung injury related to the disease process, high oxygen requirement, or complications of mechanical ventilation. Complications such as pleural effusion, empyema, bacteremia, and pericarditis can extend the clinical course of the disease.

BRONCHIOLITIS

A. Definition

Bronchiolitis is an acute inflammatory disease of the lower respiratory tract that results in obstruction of small airways (Figure 2-19).

B. Pathophysiology

1. **Viral replication** in the epithelial cells of the airways results in direct injury of the respiratory epithelium. Abnormal secretions combined with edema of the submucosal layer causes obstruction of the small airways and diffusion impairment. Multiple areas of atelectasis produce ventilation-perfusion mismatching and abnormal gas exchange.
2. **Gas Exchange:** The principal abnormality in gas exchange is hypoxemia. Most infants are able to maintain normocarbia despite ventilation-perfusion mismatch by increasing their respiratory rate. Hypercarbia and respiratory failure develop when the infant becomes fatigued and minute ventilation falls.

C. Etiology

1. **Bronchiolitis** may be caused by a number of viral pathogens, depending on the age of the child, immune function, and seasonal and geographic variables.

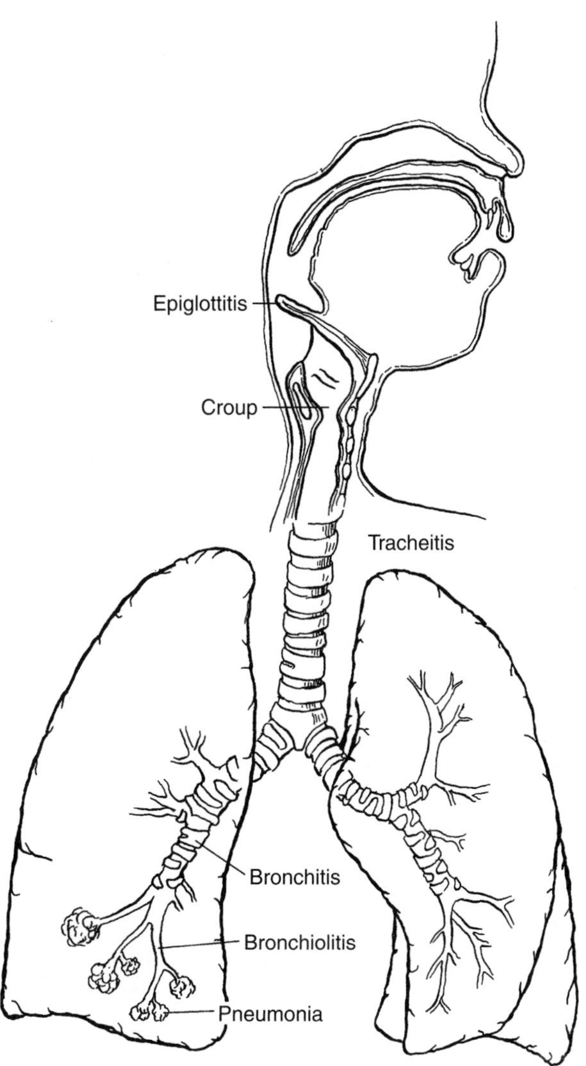

FIGURE 2-19 ■ Anatomic location of respiratory infections.

Influenza, parainfluenza, and RSV are most likely. RSV is the most common pathogen in children younger than 3 years of age (Izurieta et al., 2000).

2. **Peak incidence** occurs during midwinter and early spring and typically affects infants younger than 1 year of age (Izurieta et al., 2000).
3. **Risk factors:** Infants with bronchopulmonary dysplasia, cyanotic congenital heart disease, prematurity, cystic fibrosis, and other chronic illnesses are at risk for severe bronchiolitis.

D. Clinical Presentation

1. **History:** Generally there is a 2- to 5-day history of upper respiratory tract infection with fever and known exposure. Fever is usually present; however, temperatures are generally lower than in bacterial pneumonia.
2. **Physical examination** demonstrates cough, sneezing, rhinorrhea, and respiratory distress with tachypnea, retractions, wheezing, prolonged expiration, rales, and irritability. Infants may also present with poor feeding, low-grade fever, apnea, and cyanosis. Tachypnea is the most consistent clinical

manifestation. Auscultation of the chest may reveal crackles and wheezing throughout the thoracic cavity.

3. **Diagnostic tests:** Diagnosis is based primarily on clinical observations.
   a. *Chest radiography* demonstrates hyperinflation, atelectasis, and peribronchial thickening in 50% of cases. Partial lobar or patchy involvement in multiple areas of the lung or shifting regional infiltrates may be present. Radiographic appearance alone is not diagnostic, and other clinical features must be considered.
   b. *ABG analysis* may show hypoxemia or hypercarbia.
   c. *Pulse oximetry* may demonstrate hypoxemia.
   d. *Reliable reagents* are available for the rapid detection of RSV, parainfluenza, influenza, and adenoviruses. Direct isolation of the virus may be possible through nasopharyngeal washing but may require 5 to 10 days for positive culture results.
   e. *A peripheral serum WBC* count may be useful in differentiating viral from bacterial pneumonia. In viral pneumonia the WBC count is usually not higher than 20,000/mm^3 (Nohynek et al., 1995).
4. **Clinical course:** Viral bronchiolitis generally has a clinical course of 7 to 10 days with peak symptoms at 48 to 72 hours. Severe cases may require mechanical ventilation for apnea, hypoxemia, or respiratory failure.

E. Patient Care Management

1. **Prevention:** Nosocomial spread of viral pathogens can be minimized with good handwashing. Both a humanized murine anti-RSV monoclonal antibody (palivizumab) and RSV intravenous immune globulin (RSV-IVIG) are available for protecting high-risk children against serious complications from RSV infections (IMPACT-RSV Study Group, 1998; Simoes et al., 1998).
2. **Direct care** involves hospitalization if the patient is younger than 6 months of age or has respiratory distress requiring oxygen therapy. Provide oxygen as needed or mechanical ventilation if respiratory failure, hypoxemia, or apnea develops. Nasal CPAP is a reliable alternative to support arterial oxygenation in patients with respiratory failure who are alert and vigorous enough to avoid hypercapnia and respiratory acidosis while breathing spontaneously. Pneumothorax should be considered if sudden deterioration occurs.
3. **Supportive care**
   a. *Fluids and nutritional requirements* are maintained with physiologic maintenance fluids and enteral nutrition if possible. Tube feedings may be considered in infants with tachypnea. Transpyloric feeding tubes can be easily placed at the bedside and initiated in any patient with moderate respiratory distress or at risk of aspiration (Chellis and Sanders, 1996; Gianotti et al, 1994).
   b. *Monitor infants closely* for respiratory failure. Vital signs, sensorium, breathing pattern, and skin color are assessed. Noninvasive measurement includes pulse oximetry and E_TCO_2 for patients using an ETT. Invasive monitoring includes ABG monitoring.
   c. *Medications:* Antibacterial agents are not recommended for the treatment of a viral infection. If bacterial pneumonia cannot be excluded, antibiotics can be started until appropriate culture results are negative. Ganciclovir is an antiviral with significant activity against cytomegalovirus (CMV) in immunosuppressed patients.
4. **Complications** include secondary bacterial infection and ARDS. Up to 30% of patients with known viral infection may have coexisting bacterial pathogens;

deterioration in clinical status could signal the possibility of a bacterial infection (Wubbell et al., 1999).

F. Outcomes

Impaired oxygenation may continue for several weeks after apparent clinical recovery. Studies have shown that between 5% and 50% of children with acute bronchiolitis in infancy develop recurrent wheezing later in life.

ASPIRATION PNEUMONITIS

A. Definition and Etiology

1. Pneumonitis is inflammation caused by pulmonary aspiration of fluids. Aspiration of gastric fluid produces direct injury to the mucosal surface of the respiratory tract. Alveolar damage is followed by an interstitial reaction, causing acute inflammatory and polymorphonuclear cell infiltration of the alveolus. Common aspirates include gastric fluid irritants and hydrocarbons.
2. Any impairment or depression of normal reflexes increases the risk of aspiration, which might be caused by an altered level of consciousness from anesthesia, seizures, toxic ingestion, or neurologic devastation. Altered anatomy or function of the trachea or esophagus may predispose to aspiration of secretions or stomach contents (Table 2-16).

B. Pathophysiology

Initial parenchymal injury occurs from direct epithelial damage. Indirect damage occurs from the generation of toxic radicals, inflammatory cells, and activation of the complement system. Pneumonitis, or inflammation of lung parenchyma, may involve pleura, interstitium, and airways. To be classified as pneumonia, alveolar consolidation must be present.

C. Clinical Presentation

1. **History:** To treat the patient appropriately, it is important to know the nature of the aspirated material. Determine the events surrounding the aspiration episode, such as level of consciousness and feeding history.
2. **Physical examination:** Patients may demonstrate increased cough and fever, acute dyspnea, wheezing, and cyanosis progressing to pulmonary edema. Observe for increased WOB, retractions, and increased respiratory rate. Auscultate for absent breath sounds, crackles, or wheezing in the affected lobes.

TABLE 2-16
Causes of Aspiration Pneumonitis

Altered level of consciousness	Drugs, alcohol, anesthesia, seizures, central nervous system disorders
Altered anatomy of trachea or esophagus	Tracheal or esophageal abnormalities, endotracheal tube, tracheostomy
Altered function of swallow or esophageal motility	Loss of normal reflexes, which prevent aspiration of stomach contents; gastroesophageal reflux, especially when associated with neurologic or anatomic impairment
Inhalation injury	Inhalation of toxic substances such as gastric acids or hydrocarbons

Aspiration of oral secretions manifests with signs similar to acute bacterial pneumonia.

3. **Diagnostic tests**
   a. *Chest radiographic* changes following aspiration are related to irritation, inflammation, and pneumonia. Aspiration pneumonia characteristically produces patchy opacification in the lung bases and perihilar infiltrations. Radiographs may demonstrate slight hyperventilation to diffuse infiltrates or alveolar densities. Infiltrates are most likely to be observed in the right upper lobe in a patient who was supine at the time of aspiration. Chest radiograph changes may worsen over the first 72 hours and then begin to clear. Radiographic abnormalities may persist for 4 to 6 weeks.
   b. *ABG levels* should be evaluated if hypoxemia and hypercarbia is clinically significant.
   c. *Pulse oximetry* gives a continuous measurement of Hgb oxygen saturation.
4. **Clinical course**
   a. *Presentation and management* of aspiration pneumonia depend on the nature and quantity of the aspirated material. The degree of lung injury is dependent on the pH of the aspirated material and the presence of bacteria.
   b. *Materials with an acidotic pH* may produce immediate pulmonary symptoms that worsen over the first 24 hours. Chemical burns increase alveolar capillary membrane permeability with subsequent extravasation of fluid into interstitium and alveoli. Often lung volume decreases, and then ventilation-perfusion mismatch and hypoxia occur. Acidotic fluid produces airway irritation, bronchospasm, peribronchial hemorrhage, and necrosis. *Alkalotic materials* can also cause devastating airway and lung injury.
   c. *Materials with a normal pH* can induce hypoxia or pulmonary edema, but generally there is little necrosis.
   d. *Irritant gases* cause direct injury to the mucosal surface. Epithelial cells become edematous, then necrotic, going through three phases. The *acute phase* is characterized by pulmonary edema, hypoxemia, and respiratory failure. The *delayed phase* is characterized by pulmonary edema, airway obstruction, and superinfection. The *long-term phase* involves reactive airways and interstitial fibrosis.
5. **Differential diagnosis:** Evaluate for foreign-body aspiration. Generally cough, dyspnea, and wheezing are seen with foreign-body aspiration (see Foreign-Body Aspiration discussion). Differentiate between acute bacterial or viral pneumonia by history, chest radiograph, secretions, and tracheal aspirate (if available).

D. Patient Care Management

1. **Prevention**
   a. *An obtunded or tachypneic patient* should not receive oral feedings. Patients with CNS injury, those receiving sedation, or those recovering from intraoperative anesthesia are also at risk.
2. **Direct care**
   a. *Nasogastric feedings* should be monitored closely. Before initiation of feedings, the patient should be assessed for gastric distention and bowel sounds. The volume of gastric aspirate should be checked periodically to ensure adequate emptying of the stomach.
   b. If *gastroesophageal reflux* is suspected, follow reflux precautions. These include small, frequent feedings and raising the head of the bed after feedings.
   c. Consider the use of *transpyloric feedings* if an ETT has been placed or if there is a significant risk of gastroesophageal reflux or poor gastric emptying.

Consideration of gastric versus postpyloric feeding remains controversial (Marik and Zaloga, 2003).

d. *In patient whose stomach is not empty,* rapid-sequence intubation techniques (including cricoid pressure) should be used, and suctioning equipment should be available.

3. Supportive care

a. *High oxygen concentrations,* mechanical ventilation, and high PEEP may be necessary.

b. *Choice of antibiotics* depends on the patient's age and the cause of aspiration. Prophylactic antimicrobials have not been proven beneficial and allow overgrowth of resistant organisms. Antibiotic therapy should be reserved for known or suspected secondary infection.

c. *Reflux aspiration* can often be treated medically through elevation of the head and torso during sleep; antacids; GI motility-enhancing agents; and small, frequent, thickened feedings.

d. *Bethanechol and metoclopramide* are used to increase GI motility and lower esophageal sphincter pressure. Cisapride, cimetidine (Tagamet), and ranitidine can be administered to control gastric pH. Optimal medical therapy may include the addition of a proton-pump inhibitor such as omeprazole or lansoprazole.

e. *Surgical management* by a Nissen fundoplication can be done if medical management fails.

E. Outcomes

Prognosis is generally good. Mild restrictive or obstructive defects such as bronchiectasis (dilation of the bronchi from bronchial wall damage) and reactive airways disease have been observed.

ADULT RESPIRATORY DISTRESS SYNDROME

A. Definition and Etiology

1. **Adult respiratory distress syndrome (ARDS)** is a condition characterized by acute lung injury and noncardiogenic pulmonary edema. It is initiated by a variety of stimuli that trigger the release of systemic inflammatory mediators. These mediators are *not* specific to the lung but in fact may be responsible for a broader spectrum of multiple-organ failure. Therefore the patient with ARDS often exhibits signs of single- or multiple-organ dysfunction as well as symptoms from the initiating insult. ARDS was first recognized in adult war victims, but the pathology has since been observed in children as well.
2. More recently, a less severe form of ARDS, termed **acute lung injury (ALI)** has been proposed as a means of promoting early recognition of lung injury that might have the potential to progress to ARDS. The definition of ALI is Pao_2/Fio_2 less than 300 mm Hg with bilateral infiltrates on chest radiograph, in contrast to ARDS, in which the Pao_2/Fio_2 is less than 200 mm Hg. For simplification of the following section, ARDS will be used to denote the entire spectrum of lung injury.
3. **Etiology** includes the following:

a. *Direct or focal etiologic injuries* include (but are not limited to) gastric aspiration, near-drowning events, toxic inhalation (smoke, oxygen, chlorine, ammonia), pulmonary infection or contusion, pulmonary embolus, foreign-body aspiration, or radiation pneumonitis.

b. *Secondary or systemic injuries* include prolonged hypotension, trauma, sepsis, multiple blood transfusions, ingestions (associated with aspiration), cardiopulmonary bypass, and head injuries.

B. Pathophysiology

1. Mechanisms of ARDS

a. The *final common pathway* observed in ARDS pathology results in increased capillary permeability and pulmonary edema. The hallmark change in pulmonary function is ventilation/perfusion mismatching.

- The host response to a local or systemic insult (such as sepsis or trauma) activates a systemic stress response that causes the release of pro-inflammatory mediators that act on the vascular endothelium.
- The principal mediator of microvascular injury is thought to be the sequestration of neutrophils in the pulmonary vasculature (Figure 2-20). A local injury or an inciting trigger such as endotoxin causes the activation of the complement pathways. The C5a component is thought to be the principal stimulus for neutrophil activation and aggregation in the pulmonary capillary beds.
- Increased fluid and protein leak into the interstitial space, and sloughing of bronchial and alveolar epithelium occurs secondary to the inflammatory process.
- Neutrophils flood the pulmonary capillaries, inducing injury by the release of oxygen radicals and the release of proteolytic enzymes. The oxygen radicals appear to disrupt the alveolar capillary membrane directly. The enzymes not only cause direct injury to the pulmonary vasculature but also generate additional activated complement. Aggregation of neutrophils in the pulmonary vasculature creates a cascade of events that causes the release of cytokines, interleukins, tumor necrosis factor, leukotrienes, and platelet-activating factor, resulting in pulmonary edema and pulmonary vasoconstriction.

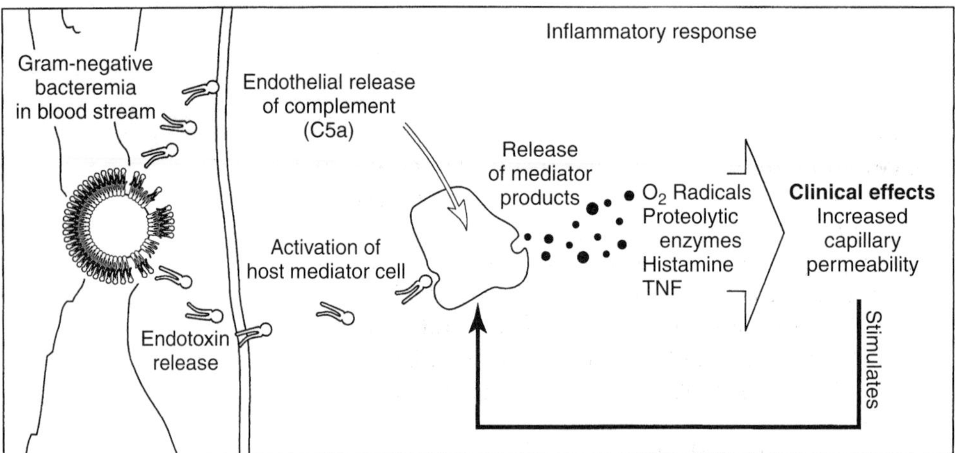

FIGURE 2-20 ■ Mechanisms of inflammatory responses. Pathogenesis of adult respiratory disease syndrome (ARDS): Focal injury or release of an antigenic substance such as endotoxin causes the release of complement and activation of the complement pathway, which stimulates neutrophil aggregation. *TNF*, tumor necrosis factor.

- The influx of protein-rich edema fluid into the alveolus leads to the inactivation of surfactant, causing atelectasis and ventilation-perfusion mismatching (Figure 2-21).

2. **Pulmonary mechanics and dysfunction**
   a. *Pulmonary hypertension* occurs from the action of specific mediators on the pulmonary vasculature, and hypoxemia potentiates this effect because it causes vasoconstriction of the pulmonary vasculature.
   b. *Hypovolemia and increased pulmonary vascular resistance* cause decreased perfusion to alveolar cells, specifically the type II pneumocytes that produce surfactant. The absence of surfactant creates a greater tendency toward alveolar collapse, thus reducing FRC and compliance.
   c. The *lung parenchyma* exhibits an abnormal, heterogeneous pattern, with obstructive air trapping interlaced with atelectatic segments, and infiltrates. The net effect of these parenchymal changes is a significant reduction in FRC and decreased lung compliance. The transpulmonary pressure required to open the lower airways to achieve a specific lung volume is greater than normal.
   d. The *summation* of the inciting injuries to the lung creates a characteristic cascade of effects (Rogers, 1996). Heterogeneous pulmonary parenchymal tissue is created by segmental hypoinflation and hyperinflation. Ventilation-perfusion mismatch (shunting of blood flow to nonventilated areas) is progressive and is aggravated by hypoxemia, which causes vasoconstriction. Positive feedback loops present at various points in the process to sustain the pulmonary dysfunction.

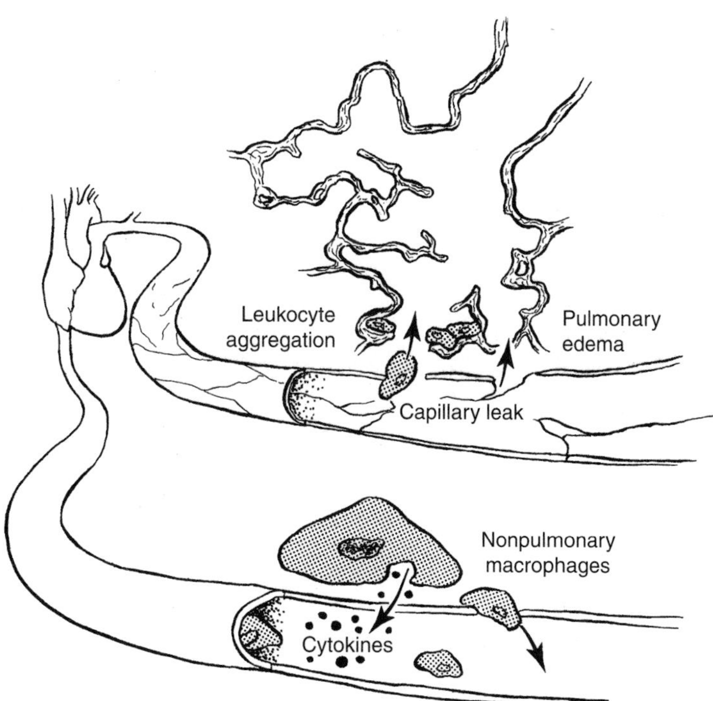

FIGURE 2-21 ■ Mechanism for development of pulmonary edema in adult respiratory disease syndrome (ARDS). The inflammatory response to an inciting injury causes mediator release, which acts on the endothelium of the pulmonary vessels, causing increased permeability.

C. Clinical Presentation

1. **Stage 1 (days 1 to 2):** Symptoms of distress may be subtle, such as mild tachypnea, air hunger or hypoxemia, anxiety, or restlessness.
2. **Stage 2 (days 2 to 3):** Clinical symptoms of distress are clearly apparent and may include cyanosis on room air, tachycardia, increased respiratory effort, and retractions. Parenchymal changes become identifiable on x-ray examination.
3. **Stage 3 (days 3 to 10):** Symptoms change from distress to respiratory failure. Frank respiratory failure occurs, manifested by inability to oxygenate and ventilate, alveolar collapse, desaturation, and fatigue. Clinical signs include diffuse rhonchi or rales, high oxygen requirement, signs of parenchymal consolidation, and a hyperdynamic state. Evidence of multiple-organ failure may occur during this period as well.
4. **Stage 4 (after 10 days):** Stage 3 changes persist with progression of lung restriction. Loculated pneumonia, development of pulmonary fibrosis, and progressive impairment of oxygenation are observed.

D. Diagnosis

1. **Recognition of ARDS** in the early stages requires a high index of suspicion because inciting factors are often nonpulmonary. Presentation always begins with mild tachypnea or dyspnea, for which there are many causes. Conventional criteria for defining ARDS include the following (Zaccardelli and Pattishall, 1996):
   a. *Historical factors* (see etiology)
   b. *Bilateral, diffuse chest radiographic* changes associated with hypoxemia in the absence of cardiomegaly
   c. *Respiratory failure:* (1) Altered oxygenation indices such as PaO_2/FiO_2 ratio less than 200; (2) A-a gradient less than 200; (3) oxygenation index greater than 15; (4) decreased lung compliance; (5) increased intrapulmonary shunt fraction
   d. *Pulmonary artery occlusion pressure* less than 18 mm Hg and the absence of any other signs of cardiac insufficiency

E. Patient Care Management

1. **Goals of therapy**
   a. Ensuring adequate oxygenation and ventilation
2. **Monitoring**
   a. Measuring pulse oximetry, ECG, and ABG and monitoring pulmonary arterial catheter for progressive lung disease requiring high PEEP.
   b. Chest radiographs are used to evaluate disease and to identify evolving pneumothorax or pneumomediastinum. Pneumothorax may cause an acute decompensation or an insidious deterioration of oxygenation.
   c. Monitoring fluid intake and output.
   d. SvO_2 monitoring with a pulmonary artery catheter can be a useful technique for critically ill patients. (See Chapter 3 for more information.)
   e. Continuous clinical evaluation of the patient's response to ventilatory assistance includes observation of chest excursion and patient comfort and auscultation of lung fields to assess the adequacy of aeration and the length of inspiratory and expiratory times.
3. **Patient care management** (Table 2-17)
   a. *Managing the inciting injury* (e.g., aspiration pneumonia or sepsis): Early, aggressive management of hypoxemia and infectious processes is essential. Careful hemodynamic resuscitation is initiated to ensure adequate preload without fluid overload.

TABLE 2-17
Management Principles for ARDS

Early recognition of evolving respiratory insufficiency
Routinely monitor oxygen and chest radiograph
Provide supplemental oxygen; evaluate for risk factors
Determine need for positive airway pressure ventilation
Evaluate low tidal volume, high PEEP ventilator strategies
Avoid oxygen toxicity
Optimize nutrition
Assess for infectious disease

b. *Intubation and mechanical ventilation*

- Indications for intubation and mechanical ventilation include a FiO_2 requirement greater than 60% with a SaO_2 of less than 90% or rapid deterioration with evidence of respiratory fatigue, such as decreased effort, decreased mentation, and increasing $PaCO_2$.
- *Assisted ventilation modalities:* The principal goal is to increase FRC and to minimize potentially traumatic ventilatory (TV) mechanisms. Volume ventilation is a conventional choice for initial management of patients with ARDS. *Initial* ventilator settings may include a tidal volume of 6 to 8 mL/kg with an inspiratory time of 0.5 to 1 second according to body size or age, PEEP of 8 cm H_2O, FiO_2 of 100%, and an adequate inverse ratio ventilation rate to ensure minute ventilation. The ARDS network studies have suggested management with smaller TV mechanisms of 4 to 6 mL/kg using PEEP to achieve oxygenation and allowing CO_2 to increase if needed to keep volumes low and decrease trauma. Some patients require pressure ventilation.
- PEEP is instituted *early* to recruit collapsed alveoli and to increase FRC. After blood-gas evaluation, adjust PEEP to allow the reduction of FiO_2 to the lowest possible setting (<60% is desirable). A gradual increase in PEEP will facilitate alveolar recruitment.
- Pressure control, IRV, and permissive hypercarbia can be used to minimize tidal volume and yet provide adequate mean airway pressure (MAP) and oxygenation.
- Alternative ventilator management may be necessary for refractive disease and may include high-frequency ventilation and extracorporeal membrane oxygenation (ECMO).

c. *Support of optimal oxygen delivery (DO_2):*

- Use of PEEP is the cornerstone of therapy for ARDS, but higher PEEP may in turn compromise cardiac output.
- Preload: Ensure normal preload and support contractility, which may require the use of vasoactive medications. Pharmacologically, contractility can be increased with a β-agonist medication such as epinephrine or dobutamine. A cardiac index greater than 4 L/min/m^2 is often useful as a temporizing measure to improve DO_2 immediately. However, this strategy does not improve long-term outcomes.
- *Maintain an adequate Hgb level* to ensure optimal oxygen-carrying capacity.

d. *Assessment:* Ongoing assessment of intravascular volume with central venous pressure (CVP) measurement and urine output will guide ongoing fluid administration. Placement of a pulmonary artery catheter for monitoring filling pressures and measurement of SVO_2 allows more precise, goal-directed therapy.

e. *Minimize oxygen consumption* (VO_2): Decrease patient activity and anxiety by providing individual comfort measures, frequent explanations and reassurances, and sedation and analgesia. Maintain normal core temperature.

4. **Provide optimal fluid and nutritional support:** The goal of fluid administration is to maintain normal hemodynamics using the CVP for estimation of fluid requirements (CVP of 4-8 mm Hg is usually adequate) and to maintain normal urine output (>1 mL/kg per hour).
   a. *Fluid retention* often occurs because of electrolyte alterations, third spacing, decreased oncotic pressure, or syndrome of inappropriate secretion of antidiuretic hormone (SIADH). Diuretics are often useful, if indicated, in maintaining euvolemia and minimizing extravascular fluid.
   b. *Caloric needs* are best determined by indirect calorimetry. However, a safe estimate of caloric needs is predicted by using the resting energy expenditure (REE) (Sibbery and Iannone, 2002) multiplied by 1.2 for modest stress (e.g., skeletal trauma) or by 1.5 for severe stress (e.g., sepsis) (Trujillo et al., 1999).
   c. *Early use of enteral nutrition* is the preferred method of nutritional supplementation. The most important stimulus for mucosal growth and function is a nutrient supply, even in small quantities. Numerous studies have documented a reduced incidence of sepsis and improved wound healing with early enteral nutrition compared with parenteral nutrition or no nutrition (Romito, 1995). Twenty-five percent of the intestinal mucosa is lymphoid tissue, and as such about 75% of the body's immunologic secreting cells are found in the intestine (Romito, 1995). Altered circulation (from any cause) decreases splanchnic blood flow, leading to gut mucosal damage and a decrease in gastric barrier function, resulting in translocation of endogenous bacteria (generally gram-negative organisms such as *Escherichia coli* (Gianotti et al., 1994). Administration of enteral nutrition can be achieved through a gastric tube or one that is positioned in the jejunum.

      Adverse effects of inappropriate nutritional support sometimes occur. Excessive glucose administration shifts metabolism to lipogenesis, causing increased carbon dioxide production and therefore increasing ventilatory demands. Excessive lipid administration may aggravate hypoxemia.
   d. *Infectious disease surveillance* is important with ARDS patients who are at risk for nosocomial infections. Risk factors include invasive lines, impaired immunity, decreased nutrient supply, antibiotics, histamine blockers, antacids (Ben-Menachem et al., 1996), oral and nasal tubes, and narcotic administration (causing decreased intestinal motility). Surveillance and preventive measures should include the following:
      - Monitoring WBC and temperature pattern daily
      - Observing universal infectious disease precautions, emphasizing strict handwashing by all contacts with patient and restriction of visitors with infectious symptoms
      - Elevating the head of the bed 30 to 45 degrees for all ventilated patients to reduce the incidence of aspiration
      - Decreasing the unnecessary use of antacid regimens in patients with an ETT tube; there is good evidence that an alkaline pH in gastric secretions may foster bacterial growth normally inhibited by acid (Ben-Menachem, 1996; Scolapio, 2002).

- Considering the use of bowel decontamination for prevention of ventilator-associated pneumonia (Scolapio, 2002)

5. **Other therapies for ARDS** that are currently in trials include the following:
   a. *Nitric oxide (NO)* had appeared promising (Day et al., 1996), but more recent data demonstrate that although transient improvement occurs with NO, it does not affect long-term outcomes (Dellinger et al., 1998).
   b. *Liquid ventilation* has improved oxygenation in neonates (Hirschl, 1995); however, results of clinical trials in children and adults are not available at this time.
   c. *Prostaglandin E and prostacylin* interventions have not been shown to be effective in the treatment of ARDS, although trials are continuing (Ware and Mathay, 2000).
   d. *Alveolar surfactant therapy:* In the largest study to date, surfactant therapy was shown to be ineffective in reducing mortality (N = 498) in adult patients (Evans et al., 1996). More recent work has also supported this conclusion (Lewis and Brackenbury, 2003). Ongoing studies are focusing on the timing and drug delivery form of surfactant.

F. Complications and Prognosis

1. **Complications:** The complications observed in ARDS are related to the precipitating illness and to the therapies used to treat it. Barotrauma and recurrent pulmonary air leaks are significant and frequent complications. Secondary infections and multiple-organ failure are significant markers for outcome, with a higher mortality rate observed in patients with failure of two or more major organs.
   a. *Ventilator strategies:* Strategies to reduce morbidity include reducing FiO_2 to less than 60%, using PEEP as the principal intervention for improving oxygenation, and avoiding overdistention by using low tidal volumes of 6 to 8 mL/kg.
   b. *Infection control:* Measures should be implemented early.
2. **Mortality:** The death rate for patients with ARDS is approximately 32% to 45%, compared with 53% to 68% in the 1980s (Ware and Mathay, 2000). Early deaths are usually associated with the severity of the inciting event. Later deaths are usually associated with multiorgan system failure rather than pulmonary disease. Poor outcome is associated with gram-negative sepsis, poor response to PEEP, and underlying malignancy. People who survive ARDS often have a good recovery, with demonstrable improvement in pulmonary function within 3 to 5 months and stable function at 1 year, returning to baseline health in many cases (Aggarwal et al., 2000).

ASTHMA

A. Definition

Asthma is a diffuse, obstructive pulmonary disease characterized by airway inflammation with mucosal edema, thick secretions that cause airway plugging and hyperreactivity of the tracheobronchial tree that results in bronchospasm of the smooth muscle.

B. Pathophysiology

1. **Cellular mediators:** An extrinsic antigen causes immunoglobulin E (IgE) production by plasma cells and lymphoid tissue. IgE binds to mast cells in the

bronchial walls. The mast cells then release several mediators, including histamine and bradykinin. The mediators decrease the intracellular levels of cyclic adenosine monophosphate (cAMP), which causes contraction of smooth muscles and increases the level of guanosine monophosphate (cGMP), which increases the release of these mediators (Figures 2-22 and 2-23).

2. **Neurogenic factors:** Inflammatory mediators are thought to stimulate the vagus nerve (cholinergic stimulation), causing bronchial smooth-muscle constriction and increased production of mucus. β-Adrenergic stimulation, which normally relaxes smooth muscle and decreases vascular permeability, is *inhibited* by the mediators. A relative insensitivity of the β-adrenergic receptors in the smooth muscle may also be responsible for the hyperreactivity observed in this condition.
3. **Pulmonary function:** Airflow obstruction caused by decreased airway caliber causes resistance to inspiratory air entry. Mucus plugging of smaller airways causes air trapping and increased residual lung volumes. The diaphragm assumes a flattened position caused by hyperinflation rather than the dome-shaped position that allows optimal force of contraction. In severe asthma, transpulmonary pressures greater than 50 cm H_2O are not uncommon (Bohn and Kissoon, 2001).

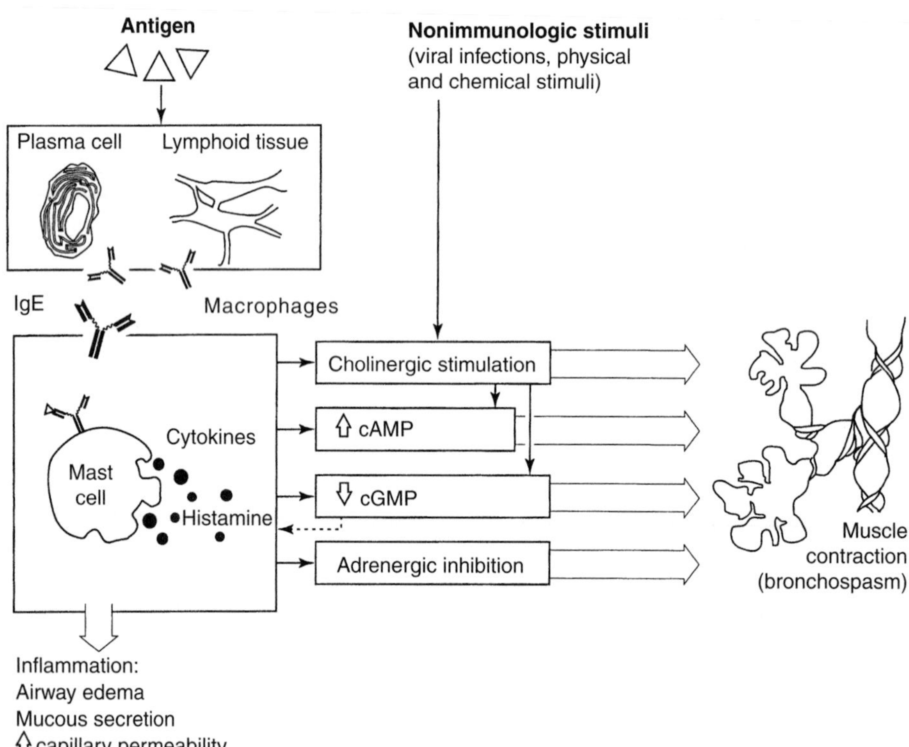

FIGURE 2-22 ■ Mechanisms of bronchoconstriction in asthma. (*1*) Extrinsic antigen causes IgE production by plasma cells and lymphoid tissue. (2) Immunoglobulin E (IgE) binds to mast cells, causing release of mediators. (*3*) Mediators inhibit cyclic adenosine monophosphate (cAMP) production, which normally produces muscle relaxation. Cholinergic stimulation directly inhibits cyclic adenosine monophosphate (cAMP) production.

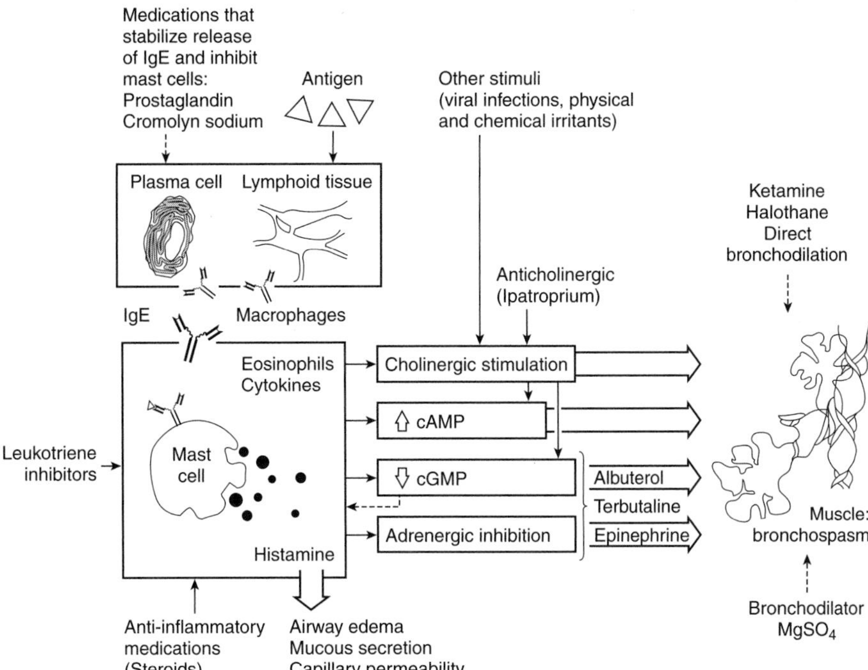

FIGURE 2-23 ■ Pharmacologic management of asthma based on the mechanisms of disease. Medications used for acute exacerbations include steroids to minimize the inflammatory response (causing airway edema and secretions); beta-agonists to enhance bronchodilation; anticholinergic agents to block stimulation, which causes decreased cyclic adenosine monophosphate (cAMP); and direct muscle relaxants, such as ketamine, halothane, and magnesium sulfate. Chronic management of severe asthma includes mast cell stabilizers and leukotriene inhibitors.

4. **Abnormalities of gas exchange in asthma:** Hypoxemia presents early in the course of an asthmatic episode. Copious sticky mucus plugs cause segmental atelectasis, thus creating a V/Q mismatch that is worsened by areas of hyperinflation. The degree of hypoxemia correlates well with the degree of airway obstruction in a symptomatic child (Meliones, 1996). Hyperventilation (with a decreased $Pa{CO_2}$) is observed in the early phases of the episode in response to hypoxemia. As the disease progresses, $Pa{CO_2}$ normalizes or rises above 45 mm Hg with prolongation of expiratory time.

C. Clinical Presentation

1. **Initial appraisal:** The first observation should immediately identify urgent conditions. Symptoms associated with severe respiratory insufficiency in the asthmatic patient requiring *immediate* intervention are summarized in Table 2-18.
2. **History**
   a. *First-time episode*: Use detailed questioning to identify common triggers, including environmental (smoke) and infectious exposures or symptoms (especially respiratory viral symptoms).
   b. *Episodic*: Inquire about previous episodes requiring hospitalization and ventilation, both of which are risk factors for near-fatal asthma episodes. Identify historic triggers, known allergies, and clinical profile of previous episodes. List age of onset and previous outpatient evaluation and treatments.

TABLE 2-18
Clinical Asthma Evaluation Score*

Variables	0	1	2
Pao_2	70–100 mm Hg in room air	≤70 mm Hg in room air	≤70 mm Hg in 40% O_2
Cyanosis	None	In air	In 40% O_2
Inspiratory breath sounds	Normal	Unequal	Decreased to absent
Accessory muscles used	None	Moderate	Maximal
Expiratory wheezing	None	Moderate	Marked
Cerebral function	Normal	Depressed or agitated	Coma

*Clinical asthma score of children with status asthmaticus score ≥5 = impending respiratory failure, score ≥7 = plus $Paco_2$, ≥65 mm Hg = existing respiratory failure.

From Wood DW, Downes JJ, Lecks HL: A clinical scoring system for the diagnosis of respiratory failure, AM J Dis Child 123:227, 1972.

Attempt to determine general, *daily* severity of asthma using criteria from the National Association of Emergency Physicians Asthma Guidelines (NAEP, 1992).

c. *Obtain a complete medication history* both for asthma management and for other medications used at home.
d. *Determine the impact of illness* on the child and the family.
e. *Estimate hydration.* Inquire about all fluids taken during previous 24 hours and voiding frequency.

3. **Physical examination**
   a. *Evaluate respiratory effort.* Patients are typically tachypneic with mild use of accessory muscles *early* in the course. As the episode progresses, a prolonged exhalation time will be observed. End-expiratory wheezing is usually noted early and is associated with lower airway narrowing. With progression, inspiratory (upper-airway narrowing) and expiratory wheezing may be audible. In some children, the wheezing stage may be brief or unappreciated with rapid progression to absent breath sounds segmentally.
   b. *Evaluate cardiovascular status.* Color remains normal in early stages but progresses from pale to cyanotic. Tachycardia is observed early in response to increased WOB and hypoxemia. Increased negative intrapleural pressures reduce cardiac output during inspiration in a spontaneously breathing patient causing a reduction in systolic pressure of greater than 10 mm Hg during inspiration compared with expiration (pulsus paradoxus) secondary to negative intrapleural pressure. Pulsus paradoxus tends to parallel FEV_1 measurements.
   c. *Evaluate ABG levels,* which generally are not used as a definitive marker for treatment options. Clinical judgment of the patient's WOB and level of fatigue are more important information to guide treatment options. However, when they are obtained, the ABG levels in an asthmatic patient follows a predictable course, beginning with a low $Paco_2$ (secondary to hyperventilation) and a pH greater than 7.40. As the condition progresses, the patient is unable to excrete $Paco_2$, efficiently, exhibited by a normal $Paco_2$ and a normal pH. Late in the course, a mixed acidosis occurs; a metabolic acidosis is secondary to increased WOB, causing oxygen consumption to be increased. Hypoxia stimulates pulmonary vasoconstriction, which in turn aggravates the hypoxia. Anaerobic

metabolism is initiated in this phase. A respiratory acidosis, from the inability to excrete $Paco_2$ compounds the magnitude of the acidosis

d. *Evaluate CNS effects.* Level of consciousness is a predictable clinical correlate with severity of disease. Patients who are hypoxic or struggling to maintain normal gas exchange are typically anxious. The use of sympathomimetic medications may further aggravate the anxiety. Respiratory fatigue in this setting results in hypoxemia and elevated $Paco_2$. The patient becomes sleepier and ultimately obtunded.

4. **Summary impression**
   a. *A "quick look" assessment* of a child during an acute episode is conventionally classified as mild, moderate, or severe acuity. With a mild episode, the child's condition can be managed in an outpatient setting. Moderate episodes require hospitalization with close monitoring. Severe episodes require PICU care with intubation equipment at the bedside (Table 2-19, Figure 2-24).
5. **Differential diagnosis of wheezing**
   a. *Bronchiolitis* usually presents with viral upper respiratory tract infection symptoms in children under the age of 2 to 3 years.
   b. *Congestive heart failure* presents with other supportive evidence on physical examination, such as an enlarged liver and heart murmur.
   c. *Foreign-body aspiration* may have unequal breath sounds or a unilateral wheeze; radiologic appearance of foreign body may be observed. The patient often has a history of being well with an abrupt onset of respiratory symptoms.
   d. *Vascular ring* presents with progressive symptoms, usually beginning in the first year of life, and has a typical appearance on esophagography.
   e. *Exposure to irritants* such as smoke or chemicals may cause the child's breath to have a chemical odor. Cold air may also produce mild wheezing.
   f. *Neoplasms* of the airway or chest demonstrate characteristic radiologic findings and, in some cases, concurrent anemia.
   g. *Infectious diseases* such as bronchitis or pneumonia may cause wheezing and are usually identifiable by history of fever, cough, and focal infiltrates on x-ray examination.
   h. *Pulmonary hypertension* or edema may cause wheezing, though of a lower pitch.
   i. *Histrionic behavior* reveals dyspnea disproportionate to the physical examination findings, sometimes causing hyperventilation tetany. Characteristically the pulmonary symptoms are absent during sleep.

D. Diagnostic Evaluation

1. **Laboratory tests**
   a. The *complete blood count* is usually normal but may show evidence of a bacterial process requiring antibiotic treatment.
   b. *Measurement of ABG* may be deferred with mild symptoms; oxygenation should be assessed by pulse oximetry. Although ABG analysis remains the gold standard for evaluation of pulmonary function, close observation of the patient provides essential information about the severity of the illness. The reason for obtaining ABG levels is to measure of $Paco_2$ and pH. Capillary blood gases provide accurate measurements of $Paco_2$ and pH (Harrison et al., 1997) and may be less traumatic to the child than an arterial puncture.
   c. *Fluid and electrolyte* measurements may reflect high fluid loss from the pulmonary system. Slight dehydration, evidenced by high blood urea nitrogen (BUN), may be observed. β-agonist medications increase potassium losses, so serum K^+ should be periodically evaluated.

TABLE 2-19
Classifying Severity of Asthma Exacerbations*

	Mild	Moderate	Severe	Respiratory Arrest Imminent
SYMPTOMS				
Breathlessness	While walking	While talking (infant—softer, shorter cry; difficulty feeding)	While at rest (infant—stops feeding)	
	Can lie down	Prefers sitting	Sits upright	
Talks in	Sentences	Phrases	Words	
Alertness	May be agitated	Usually agitated	Usually agitated	Drowsy or confused
SIGNS				
Respiratory rate	Increased	Increased	Often >30/min	
		Guide to rates of breathing in awake children:		
		Age	*Normal rate*	
		<2 m	<60/min	
		2-12 m	<50/min	
		1-5 y	<40/min	
		6-8 y	<30/min	
Use of accessory muscles; suprasternal retractions	Usually not	Commonly	Usually	Paradoxical thoracoabdominal movement
Wheeze	Moderate, often only end expiratory	Loud; throughout exhalation	Usually loud; throughout inhalation and exhalation	Absence of wheeze
Pulse/minute	<100	100-200	>120	Bradycardia
		Guide to normal pulse rates in children:		
		Age	*Normal rate*	
		2-12 m	<160/min	
		1-2 y	<120/min	
		2-8 y	<110/ min	
Pulsus paradoxus	Absent <10 mm Hg	May be present 10-25 mm Hg	Often present >25 mm Hg (adult); 20-40 mm Hg (child)	Absence may also suggest respiratory muscle fatigue
FUNCTIONAL ASSESSMENT				
PEF % predicted or % personal best	>80%	Approx. 50%-80% or response lasts <2h	<50% predicted or personal best	
PCO_2	<42 mm Hg (test not usually necessary)	<42 mm Hg (test not usually necessary)	≥42 mm Hg: possible respiratory failure	
SaO_2% (on room air) at sea level	>95% (test not usually necessary)	91%-95%	<91%	

*The presence of several parameters, but not necessarily all, indicates the general classification of exacerbation. Many of these parameters have not been systematically studied, so they serve only as general guides.
PEF, peak expiratory flow.

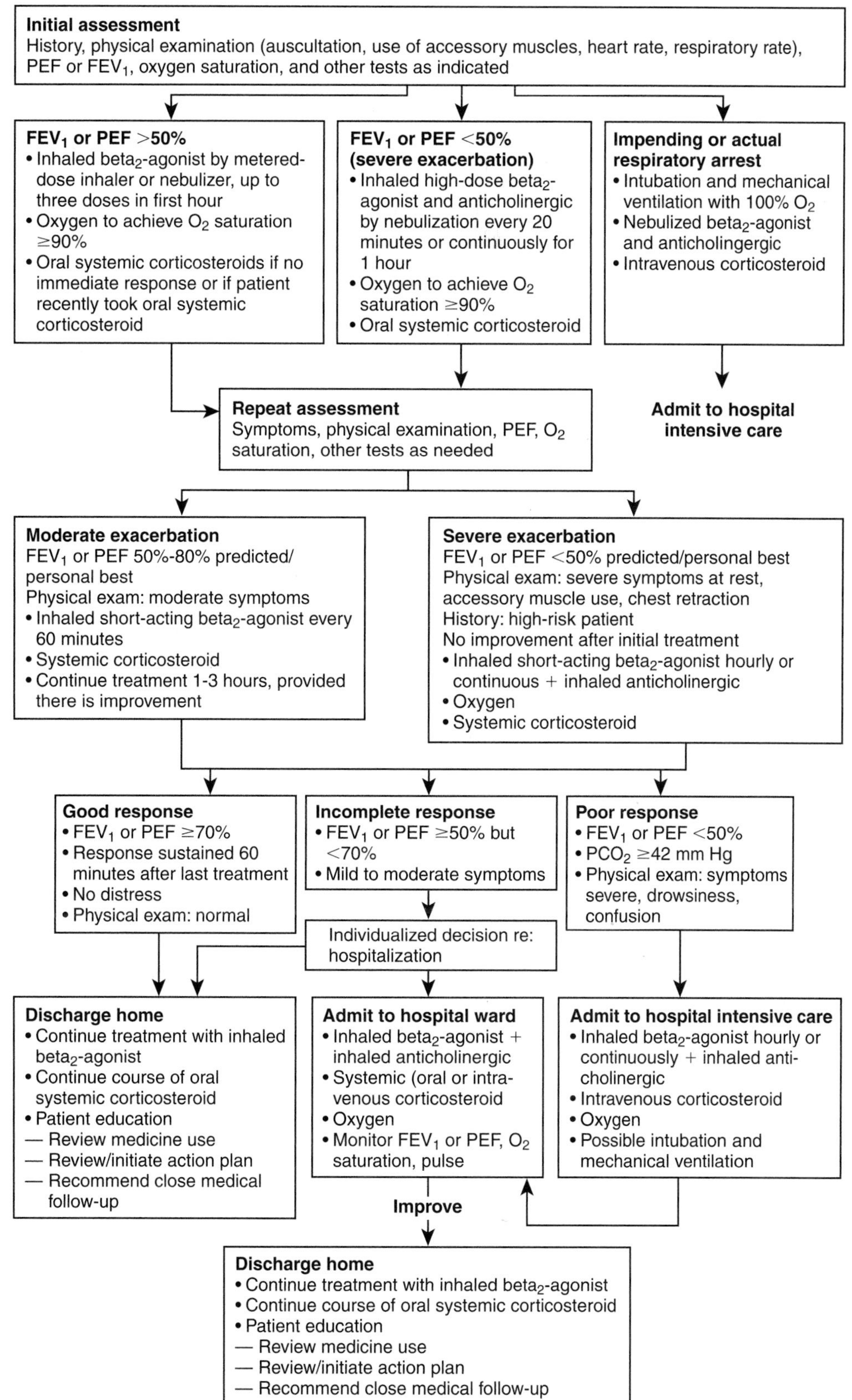

FIGURE 2-24 ■ Management of asthma exacerbations. From National Heart, Lung, and Blood Institute, 2002.

2. **Chest radiographs**
   a. *Chest radiographs* are frequently normal but may reveal a focal infiltrate, hyperinflation, or the presence of a foreign body. Small areas of segmental atelectasis are observed in many patients, which should be differentiated from an infectious infiltrate.
3. **Pulmonary function tests (PFTs) (see Figure 2-14)**
   a. *FEV:* The expiratory volume recorded for an FEV is obtained after a subject inspires maximally and then exhales as hard and as completely as he or she is able. A reduced FEV_1 (the volume of air exhaled in the first second) is observed in subjects with asthma or other obstructive disorders.
   b. *FVC* is the maximal volume that can be exhaled by forceful and complete exhalation after a maximal inspiration. The subject with asthma has a reduced FVC, although not reduced as much as the FEV_1.
   c. *FEV/FVC ratio:* Normally, the ratio is approximately 80%. In an asthmatic patient this ratio is significantly lower.
   d. *Bedside evaluation of pulmonary function* and trend of measurements can be performed on cooperative children with a hand-held spirometer. The peak flow rate is relatively correlated with FEV_1. Trending of the FVC can be a useful method of monitoring clinical progression of obstructive disorders such as asthma.

E. Management of Acute Episodes

1. **Goal of therapy:** The goal is to restore airway patency by reversing the bronchospasm, controlling the inflammatory response, and decreasing secretions. Supportive therapy, including oxygen, ventilation, hydration, correction of metabolic and electrolyte abnormalities, treatment of infections, and management of anxiety, should be provided.
2. **Thorough and continuous assessment:** Continuous observation of the patient is required to enable early recognition of progressive respiratory insufficiency. A brief bedside assessment tool (see Table 2-18) enables swift recognition of risk factors associated with severe episodes and is useful in trending clinical changes. Further, a child old enough to cooperate with a flow spirometer should be evaluated every 1 to 2 hours, trending the measurements.
3. **Medications:** The most frequently used medications to reverse the asthmatic process are directed toward altering intracellular mechanisms that regulate bronchial reactivity and modulate the inflammatory process (see Figure 2-23).
   a. *Sympathomimetics* cause direct bronchodilation by stimulation of β_2-receptors.
   b. *Anticholinergics* block parasympathetic (vagal) receptors found in the pulmonary tree, thus allowing bronchodilation. They also inhibit cGMP metabolism. Anticholinergics are used in conjunction with a B-agonist, not as a sole agent.
   c. *Corticosteroids* blunt the host response to the stimulus by suppressing the immune response and the release of mediators, such as histamine. Clinically this should diminish the secretion of mucus.
   d. *Leukotriene inhibitors* block the action or inhibit synthesis of cysteinyl leukotrienes, which cause bronchoconstriction, secretion of mucus, increased vascular permeability, and eosinophil migration to the airways (Bisgaard and Nielson, 2000; Dworski et al., 1994). A leukotriene antagonist is not first-line therapy for an acute RAD episode because the effects are not noted for a minimum of 24 hours. However, if the child has been taking a leukotriene antagonist before hospital admission, it should be continued during hospitalization.

e. *Aminophylline* is no longer recommended as a first-line treatment of RAD (National Heart, Lung and Blood Institute, 1997). It is considered a weak bronchodilator, but it also has anti-inflammatory properties and ionotropic effects on the respiratory muscles (Bohn and Kissoon, 2001). There is a narrow window between therapeutic effect and toxicity, making it a less attractive agent. In addition, it requires monitoring of blood levels.
f. *Mucolytics* either thin or reduce mucous secretions. This seems intuitively beneficial, but some agents cause drying of airway secretions, which may aggravate airway plugging. Furthermore, many mucolytic agents are also known irritants and may cause bronchospasm. One agent, however, deoxyribonuclease, used in patients with cystic fibrosis, may be useful for breaking up mucous plugs.
g. *Antibiotics* may be used for patients exhibiting clear signs of a bacterial infection (infiltrate on chest radiograph; increased WBC, fever) but are otherwise not indicated.
h. *Magnesium sulfate* is a physiologic calcium antagonist and has a direct effect on calcium uptake in smooth muscle, causing muscle relaxation. Doses of 25 to 50 mg/kg are given IV over 1 to 2 hours. Magnesium levels should be pushed to 3 or 4 mg/dL and monitored every 8 to 12 hours (Ciarollo et al., 2000).
i. *Other pharmacologic modalities* that cause direct bronchodilation include ketamine, halothane, and prostaglandins (Table 2-20).

4. **Intubation and mechanical ventilation**
 a. *Mechanical ventilation* may be required when the following symptoms are exhibited:
 - Decreased respiratory effort with fatigue *or* shallow tachypnea
 - Inability to speak single words
 - Decreased mental status
 - Absence of breath sounds despite respiratory effort, hypercarbia with $Paco_2$ greater than 45, *or* increasing by 5 per hour
 - Hypoxemia with Sao_2 less than 95% refractive to oxygen supplementation (Fio_2 1.00)
 - Pulsus paradoxus greater than 20 mm Hg

 b. *Before intubation* the child should receive 100% Fio_2 by a bag-valve-mask circuit.
 - Clinicians should assume a "full stomach" in all patients and use a rapid-sequence IV induction with cricoid pressure.
 - Premedication with atropine is recommended. Some medications are reported to cause a clinically significant histamine release, which could potentially aggravate bronchial edema. These include morphine, meperidine (Demerol), atracurium, and thiopental (Pentothal). Induction agents may include ketamine, lidocaine (to blunt tracheal reflexes), midazolam (Versed), and propofol. Paralytic agents may include rocuronium, vecuronium, or pancuronium for a rapid-sequence intubation.
 - Asthmatic patients generate large negative intrathoracic pressure while breathing on their own, which increases venous return and augments cardiac output. At the moment positive pressure is initiated, a significant *decrease* in venous return and cardiac output may occur. Anticipatory fluid administration may prevent cardiac decompensation during intubation.

 c. *Modes of ventilation:* Patients usually exhibit thick secretions, mucosal edema, and bronchoconstriction, which cause increased airway resistance. Air trapping is also an important feature when considering ventilatory strategies. Heavy sedation and paralysis may be necessary initially to establish adequate ventilation and oxygenation.

TABLE 2-20
Dosages of Drugs for Asthma Exacerbations in Emergency Medical Care or Hospital

	Dosages		
Medication	**Adult Dose**	**Child Dose***	**Comments**[†]
SHORT-ACTING INHALED BETA$_2$-AGONISTS			
Albuterol			
Nebulizer solution (5.0 mg/ml, 2.5 mg/3 mL, 1.25 mg/3 mL, 0.63 mg/3 mL)	2.5–5 mg every 20 min for 3 doses, then 2.5–10 mg every 1–4 h as needed, or 10–15 mg/h continuously	0.15 mg/kg (minimum dose 2.5 mg) every 20 min for 3 doses, then 0.15–0.3 mg/kg up to 10 mg every 1–4 h as needed, or 0.5 mg/kg/h by continuous nebulization	Only selective beta$_2$-agonists are recommended. For optimal delivery, dilute aerosols to minimum of 3 mL at gas flow of 6–8 L/min.
MDI (90 mcg/puff)	4–8 puffs every 20 min up to 4 h, then every 1–4 h as needed	4–8 puffs every 20 min for 3 doses, then every 1–4 h inhalation maneuver. Use spacer/holding chamber	As effective as nebulized therapy if patient is able to coordinate.
Levalbuterol (R-albuterol)			
Nebulizer solution (0.63 mg/3 mL, 1.25 mg/3 mL)	1.25–2.5 mg every 20 min for 3 doses, then 1.25–5 mg every 1–4 h as needed, or 5–7.5 mg/h continuously	0.075 mg/kg (minimum doses 1.25 mg) every 20 min for 3 doses, then 0.075–0.15 mg/kg up to 5 mg every 1–4 h as needed, or 0.25 mg/kg/h by continuous nebulization	0.63 mg of levalbuterol is equivalent to 1.25 mg of racemic albuterol for both efficacy and side effects.
SYSTEMIC (INJECTED) BETA$_2$-AGONISTS			
Epinephrine 1:1000 (1 mg/mL)	0.3–0.5 mg every 20 min for 3 doses sq	0.01 mg/kg up to 0.3–0.5 mg every 20 min for 3 doses sq	No proven advantage of systemic therapy over aerosol.
Terbutaline (1 mg/mL)	0.25 mg every 20 min for 3 doses sq	0.01 mg/kg every 20 min for 3 doses then every 2–6 h as needed sq	No proven advantage of systemic therapy over aerosol.
ANTICHOLINERGICS			
Ipratropium bromide			
Nebulizer solution (0.25 mg/mL)	0.5 mg every 30 min for 3 doses then every 2–4 h as needed	0.25 mg every 20 min for 3 doses, then every 2–4 h	May mix in same nebulizer with albuterol. Should not be used as first-line therapy; should be added to beta$_2$-agonist therapy.
MDI (18 mcg/puff)	4–8 puffs as needed	4–8 puff as needed	Doses delivered from MDI is low and has not been studied in asthma exacerbations.

TABLE 2-20
Dosages of Drugs for Asthma Exacerbations in Emergency Medical Care or Hospital (*cont'd*)

	Dosages		
Medication	**Adult Dose**	**Child Dose***	**Comments†**
Ipratropium with albuterol			
Nebulizer solution (Each 3 mL vial contains 0.5 mg ipratropium bromide and 2.5 mg albuterol.)	3 mL every 30 min for 3 doses, then every 2–4 h as needed	1.5 mL every 20 min for 3 doses, then every 2–4 h	Contains EDTA to prevent discoloration. This additive does not induce bronchospasm.
SYSTEMIC CORTICOSTEROIDS‡			
Prednisone	120–180 mg/d in 3 or 4 divided doses for 48 h, then	1 mg/kg every 6 h for 48 h then 1–2 mg/kg/d (maximum = 60 mg/d)	For outpatient "burst" use 40–60 mg in single or 2 divided doses for adults
Methylprednisolone	60–80 mg/d until PEF reaches	in 2 divided doses until PEF 70% of predicted	(children: 1–2 mg/kg/d, maximum 60 mg/d) for
Prednisolone	70% of predicted or personal best	or personal best	3-10 d.

Drugs	Dosing/Administration	Comments
OTHER AGENTS		
Ketamine	IV: 1–2 mg/kg per dose	Contraindicated with increased intracranial pressure May cause dysphoria in older children; use benzodiazepine prior to administration
Halothane	Inhalational gas: 0.25–0.5% delivery with oxygen through anesthesia circuit	May cause hypotension
Magnesium sulfate	20–50 mg/kg IV for 20–30 min May repeat q6h	Check Mg levels before redosing Levels >4 mg/dl may cause depressed CNS function, diarrhea, and respiratory depression

Adapted from National Heart, Blood, and Lung Institute National Asthma Education and Prevention Program: *Expert panel report: guidelines for the diagnosis and management of asthma: update 2002.* Washington, DC, 2002, U.S. Government Printing Office.

*Children ≤ 12 years of age

†No advantage has been found for higher dose corticosteroids in severe asthma exacerbations, nor is there any advantage for intravenous administration over oral therapy provided gastrointestinal transit time or absorption is not impaired. The usual regimen is to continue the frequent multiple daily dose until the patient achieves an FEV_1 or PEF of 50% of predicted or personal best and then lower the dose to twice daily. This usually occurs within 48 hours. Therapy following a hospitalization or emergency department visit may last from 3 to 10 days. If patients are then started on inhaled corticosteroids, studies indicate there is no need to taper the systemic corticosteroid dose. If the follow-up systemic corticosteroid therapy is to be given once daily, one study indicates that it may be more clinically effective to give the dose at 3 p.m., with no increase in adrenal suppression. (Beam et al., 1992).

‡Dosages and comments apply to all three corticosteroids.

- Volume-controlled SIMV ventilation has been the preferred mode of ventilation to ensure adequate tidal volumes at the lowest possible inspiratory pressure. Newer ventilators offer a pressure-regulated, volume control mode of ventilation that provides a decelerating flow pattern (high inspiratory flow initially). V_T should be adjusted to allow delivery of approximately 6-8 mL/kg. Exhaled V_T should be monitored to ensure adequate volume delivery.
- Respiratory rate is adjusted to an I:E ratio of 1:2 to 1:4, to ensure adequate exhalation time. Adequacy of exhalation is determined by auscultation. Initial intermittent mandatory rate settings should not be targeted to achieve a normal $Paco_2$. Permissive hypercarbia is an acceptable strategy, to minimize ventilatory manipulations, with the goal to achieve a pH of 7.25 or greater.
- PEEP should be used conservatively, if at all. Asthmatics have very high FRCs because of air trapping. Although minimizing PEEP is the first-line strategy, patients with hypoxemia refractive to all other measures may benefit from cautious increases in PEEP, adjusting the PEEP upward in 1 cm H_2O incremental changes to open atelectatic lung segments.
- After about 24 hours of ventilation, volume or pressure support modes allow patients to use their own respiratory drive but provide assistance with each breath, requiring less sedation and faster weaning.

5. **Monitoring during ventilation:**
   a. An *arterial line* is useful for periodic ABG evaluation. Patient goals for each parameter should be clearly defined by the health care team to ensure continuity and to be able to recognize the earliest opportunity for weaning.
   b. *Continuous noninvasive monitoring* is highly recommended but should not be regarded as a substitute for direct arterial measurements of oxygen and carbon dioxide. Pulse oximetry can be used for monitoring of oxygen saturations, and ventilation can be assessed with an E_Tco_2 or transcutaneous CO_2 monitor. With severe air trapping, E_Tco_2 measurement may be artificially low, in which case, the E_Tco_2 measurements can be used for trending after establishing the arterial-E_Tco_2 gradient.
6. **Indications for weaning:** Often weaning and extubation can be done soon after the underlying pathology is clearly resolving as evidenced by lower peak inspiratory pressures (<30 cm H_2O) and with improved oxygenation. This may be anticipated within 48 hours after institution of steroid therapy in some children. The presence of an ETT in a hyperreactive airway can aggravate the underlying process; accelerated weaning in a pressure support mode will facilitate early extubation.

F. Supportive Care

1. **Hydration:** Patients are often dehydrated from decreased water intake and increased insensible losses. Adequate hydration, evidenced by appropriate urine output (>1 mL/kg per hour), is an important therapeutic goal.
2. **Metabolic acidosis:** Acidosis occurs in most children with moderate disease because of dehydration and hypoxemia. Rehydration of the patient corrects some of the pH abnormalities, but if acidemia continues, sodium bicarbonate administration may be used. Administration of sodium bicarbonate in the absence of adequate ventilation, however, may cause an adverse increase in $Paco_2$ and precipitate respiratory failure. For patients on a ventilator, this is less worrisome if adequate ventilation is ensured. Some researchers report that correction of the acidosis results in an increase in alveolar ventilation (Bohn and Kissoon, 2001; Mansmann et al., 1997).

G. Complications

Complications include secondary bacterial infection, pneumothorax occurring from air trapping and segmental overdistention, sudden airway closure from severe bronchospasm causing respiratory arrest, and chronic illness resulting from malnutrition and medication side effects.

H. Prognosis

1. Acute episodes

a. *Early intervention* with medications and supportive care prevents nearly all episodes from progressing to critical states. About 1% to 7% of asthmatic patients die each year. Early recognition and intervention are key factors toward diminishing mortality.

b. *Individual thresholds* based on FEV or peak flow measurements should be obtained in the history to determine the need for medical intervention, initiation of steroids, and hospitalization.

c. *Risk factors for death:* The cause of death is known to be from asphyxia, not from cardiac arrhythmias as previously thought. The following factors have been identified that may alert the clinician to the patient at risk of impending death (NIH, 2002):

- Previous severe episode requiring hospitalization and intubation
- Three or more emergency department visits for exacerbation in the past year
- Hospitalization or emergency department visit within the past month
- Prior admission to an ICU
- Two or more hospitalizations for asthma in the past year
- Poor compliance with medications or suboptimal treatment of asthma
- Current use of systemic steroids or recent withdrawal from steroid treatment
- Poor perception of dypsnea
- Race: increased risk in African Americans, Hispanics, and young male patients
- Low socioeconomic status
- Illicit drug use
- Urban residence

I. Outcome

The incidence of asthma has increased in the last decade. An estimated 15 million people in the United States have asthma, and children account for about 5 million; 54% of children with RAD report having at least one severe episode in the last year (CDC, 2004). A disproportionate number of people with RAD are African American and poverty-stricken patients. Most asthma-associated deaths occur outside a medical facility. With the current level of understanding about the pathophysiology of asthma and the aggressive interventions that are available, a significant reduction in both morbidity and mortality should be well within reach.

PULMONARY HEMORRHAGE

A. Definition and Etiology

1. **Bleeding** in the lower respiratory tract in children is rare but can be life threatening. *Pulmonary hemosiderosis* is a term to describe persistent or recurrent bleeding.

2. **Causes** of pulmonary hemorrhage include extensive bacterial, fungal, or parasitic infection or chest trauma. Cardiovascular causes include increased pulmonary venous pressure, arteriovenous malformations, or pulmonary emboli. Autoimmune disorders and rare immune-related vascular disease as a cause of pulmonary hemorrhage is generally limited to older children. Swallowed maternal blood may be a cause in the neonate.
3. **Acute, idiopathic pulmonary hemorrhage** in young infants has been found in association with chronic water damage in the children's homes along with the growth of fungi, including *Stachybotrys chartarum* (Dearborn et al., 2002).

B. Pathophysiology

1. Acute, idiopathic pulmonary hemorrhage in young infants has been found in association with chronic water damage in the children's homes along with the growth of fungi, including *Stachybotrys chartarum* (Dearborn et al., 2002).
2. The pathophysiology of pulmonary hemorrhage depends on the etiology. The hemorrhage can be focal from infection, trauma, or foreign bodies or diffuse from abnormalities of alveolar capillaries. The amount of respiratory distress is related to the quantity of blood in the alveoli and airways. After a hemorrhage, macrophages convert the iron of Hgb into hemosiderin, hence the term hemosiderosis (Dearborn, 2004). It takes the macrophage 36 to 48 hours to form hemosiderin.

C. Clinical Presentation

1. **History** includes respiratory distress with or without hemoptysis.
2. **Physical examination**
   a. *Symptoms* are those of recurrent or chronic pulmonary disease and include cough, hemoptysis, dyspnea, wheezing, and occasional cyanosis associated with fatigue and pallor (Dearborn, 2004; Dearborn et al., 2002). The infant or child may vomit large quantities of swallowed blood.
   b. *Respiratory distress* and hypoxia can be severe, requiring immediate endotracheal intubation and ventilation.
3. **Diagnostic tests**
   a. *Acute hemorrhage* is usually accompanied by a drop in hematocrit, an increase in reticulocyte count, and a stool positive for occult blood.
   b. *Diagnosis* is most readily confirmed with the use of Prussian blue staining for hemosiderin within 20% of alveolar macrophages, obtained by BAL or by examination of sputum or gastric aspirates (Dearborn, 2004; Epstein et al., 2001). Angiography is the diagnostic test of choice if a large vessel injury is suspected.
   c. *Culturing of BAL* samples for bacteria, viruses, and fungi helps to exclude infectious processes.
4. **Clinical course**
   a. The clinical course depends on the etiology of the hemorrhage and the extent of bleeding.

D. Patient Care Management

1. **Direct care:** Plasmapheresis has been used successfully during acute massive hemorrhage in Goodpasture syndrome.
2. **Supportive care**: The child is admitted to the PICU for close monitoring; respiratory status and degree of anemia are followed closely. Transpyloric feeding tubes are easily placed at the bedside and tube feedings can be initiated in any patient with moderate respiratory distress or at risk of aspiration (Chellis et al., 1996a, b; Marik and Zaloga, 2003).

3. **Complications** include severe respiratory failure, anemia, and end-organ failure from hypoxia.

E. Outcome

1. **Resolution of pulmonary hemorrhage**

PULMONARY HYPERTENSION

A. Definition and Etiology

1. **Pulmonary hypertension (PHTN)** is defined as a mean pulmonary artery pressure (PAP) of ≥ 25 mm Hg, caused by either increased blood flow or increased resistance to blood flow in the pulmonary vasculature.
   a. An *alternative definition* is a PAP pressure that is greater than one fourth of systemic pressure. If a normal systemic mean blood pressure is 80 mm Hg, the PA pressure should be 20 mm Hg or lower.
   b. PHTN is defined within the context of primary and secondary pulmonary hypertension.
      - *Primary PHTN* is clinically a diagnosis by exclusion. When the evaluation for PHTN has excluded all known causes of PHTN, it is classified as primary.
        - Histologic changes in the vascular wall demonstrate the characteristic hypertrophy or obliteration of the arteriole but without any identifiable reason.
        - In the familial form of primary PHTN, which accounts for approximately 5% of the cases (Thomson et al., 2003), the gene itself has been mapped to chromosone 2q31-32. Mutations in other gene lines have been demonstrated in more than 50% of familial cases; thus the true incidence of "familial" primary PHTN may be greater.
      - *Secondary PHTN* has many identifiable causes, including congenital heart disease, chronic lung disease, and chronic thrombotic disease.

B. Pathophysiology (Figure 2-25)

1. **V/Q mismatching:** Blood is shunted through the lungs to areas of lower pressure (dependent regions), or, if an intracardiac lesion is present, blood is shunted from right to left through the cardiac lesion, resulting in oxygen desaturation.
2. **Pressure, flow, and resistance:** The *pathophysiology* of PHTN can be understood by the equation: $P = F \times R$, where P = pressure, F = flow, and R = resistance. Increased pressure (in the pulmonary arterioles) is caused by either increased flow or increased resistance. *Note:* Increased blood flow may not generate high *pressure* initially until vascular remodeling begins to occur from the sustained stretching of the walls of the blood vessel.
3. **Endothelial dysfunction**
   a. *Endothelium* plays an early role in the evolution of pulmonary vascular disease. Vasoactive substances are produced, metabolized by, or activated by the pulmonary vascular endothelium. Both vasodilating substances and vasoconstricting substances exist in the pulmonary endothelium and are balanced in the normal state.
   b. *Vasodilating substances*, such as prostacyclins and NO, when activated, cause vasodilation.
      - NO is produced by vascular endothelial cells in response to shear stress from the flow of blood.

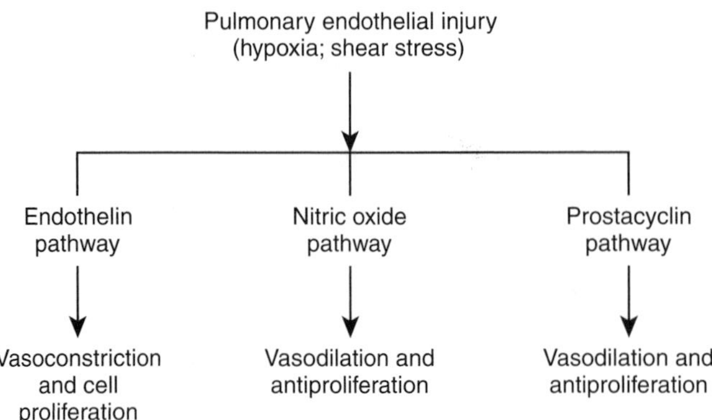

FIGURE 2-25 ■ The genesis of pulmonary artery hypertension (PAH) evolves from the imbalance between those mediators that promote vasodilation/antiproliferation and those that promote vasoconstriction and vascular remodeling. Pharmacologic interventions are directed toward blocking endothelin and promoting both nitric oxide and prostacyclin.

- Prostacylin is also synthesized in the endothelial cell. In addition to vasodilation, prostacyclin inhibits platelet aggregation.
- Oxygen is possibly the most potent vasodilator.

c. *Vasoconstricting substances*: Agents such as endothelin-1 and thromboxane A respond to stimuli to vasoconstrict the pulmonary vasculature.
- Increased levels of both have been found in children with PHTN (Suchomski and Morin, 1998).
- Hypoxia is a potent vasoconstrictor; it normally induces several local factors, which activates endothelin-1 in the vascular cells. In turn, this leads to the production of nitric oxide and vasodilation in the normal subject.
- In patients with PHTN, the enzymes responsible for the synthesis of NO and prostacyclin are decreased, and therefore the hypoxic response is blunted (Giaid, 1993.)
- Finally, adrenergic stimulation causes significant vasoconstriction and is an important point for therapeutic interventions.

4. **Classification of PHTN** (Table 2-21)

a. In 1998 the World Health Organization (WHO, 1998) proposed a new classification with five main categories:
- *Pulmonary arterial hypertension* can be caused by increased pulmonary flow, such as from intracardiac shunts, which causes increased blood flow from the left heart to the right heart and then to the pulmonary arteries. Prolonged shunting eventually causes hypertrophy of the medial wall of the pulmonary arterioles and development of fibrotic lesions.
- *Pulmonary venous hypertension* is caused by increased left ventricular pressure such as with mitral valve disease or left ventricular dysfunction.
- *Pulmonary hypertension associated with chronic respiratory disorders/hypoxemia:* Hypoxia triggers vasoconstriction through endothelial mediators. Blood flow is diverted through or from the lung; when hypoxemia persists for even a few hours, medial smooth muscle, elastin, and collagen proliferate. If corrected at this stage, regression of smooth muscle extension can occur.

TABLE 2-21
Classification of Pulmonary Hypertension

PAH
- IPAH
- FPAH
  - Collagen vascular disease
  - Congenital systemic to pulmonary shunts (repaired or unrepaired)
  - Portal hypertension
  - HIV infection
  - Drugs and toxins
  - Other (glycogen storage disease, gaucher disease, hereditary hemorrhagic telangiectasia, hemoglobinopathies, myeloproliferative disorders, splenectomy)
- Associated with significant venous or capillary involvement
  - Pulmonary veno-occlusive disease
  - Pulmonary capillary hemangiomatosis

Pulmonary venous hypertension
- Left-sided atrial or ventricular heart disease
- Left-sided valvular heart disease

Pulmonary hypertension associated with hypoxemia
- COPD
- Interstitial lung disease
- Sleep-disordered breathing
- Alveolar hypoventilation disorders
- Chronic exposure to high altitude

PH due to chronic thrombotic and/or embolic disease
- Thromboembolic obstruction of proximal pulmonary arteries
- Thromboembolic obstruction of distal pulmonary arteries
- Pulmonary embolism (tumor, parasites, foreign material)

Miscellaneous
- Sarcoidosis, histiocytosis X, lymphangiomatosis, compression of pulmonary vessels (adenopathy, tumor, fibrosing mediastinitis)

PAH, pulmonary artery hypertension; *IPAH*, idiopathic PAH; *FPAH*, familiar PAH; *PH*, pulmonary hypertension; *COPD*, chronic obstructive lung disease

From Rubin LJ: Diagnosis and management of pulmonary artery hypertension: ACCP evidenced-based clinical practice guidelines, *Chest* 126:9S, 2004.

During the period of low pulmonary blood flow, inhibition of pulmonary surfactant production causes alveolar collapse, which increases V/Q mismatching, increasing hypoxia, which then becomes a self-perpetuating cycle.

- *Congestive pulmonary vascular disease:* Pulmonary venous obstruction due to functional or structural abnormalities demands a higher right ventricular work index (RVWI) to generate enough pressure to force blood flow through the obstruction. A low-flow state through the lungs occurs, eventually causing both venous and arteriolar thickening. This is most often seen with congenital heart defects with right outflow-tract stenosis or pulmonary vein hypoplasia.
- *Pulmonary vascular obstruction* is common in pediatric patients. The more common causes include the following:
  - Diaphragmatic hernia (with hypoplastic lung)
  - Arteriovenous malformations
  - Bronchopulmonary dysplasia

- Pulmonary embolism: PEs in children are thought to be uncommon; however, this belief might reflect unrecognized PEs rather than a true low-incidence statistic. Microthrombi are asymptomatic, but with progression, vascular obstruction can create a low-flow state, causing hypoxemia and finally PHTN.

C. Clinical Presentation

1. History

a. *Patients with PHTN* may be asymptomatic, depending on the etiology of the PHTN; however, most children present with syncope, dyspnea on exertion, chest pain, or right-sided heart failure (Haworth, 1998)

b. *Patients with PHTN secondary to congenital heart* disease may present with pulmonary congestion or signs of congestive heart failure.

c. *Patients with a history of lung disease* and persistent hypoxia may be recognized by decreased oxygen saturations (or an oxygen requirement to maintain saturations) and digital dubbing.

d. *Patients or parents* will report varying degrees of activity intolerance, tachypnea, tachycardia, often failure to thrive, and orthopnea.

2. Physical examination

a. *Fatigue and lethargy* increase over time.

b. *Increased respiratory rate* and heart rate are noted.

c. *Lung fields* may or may not reveal rales.

d. *Auscultation* of the heart may reveal a prominent, single S2.

e. *Abdominal examination* may reveal an enlarged liver.

f. *Ambulating patients* will show varying degrees of dyspnea on exertion.

g. *Frank cyanosis* is a late sign of PHTN.

3. Diagnostic evaluations (Gorenflo, 2003)

a. The child who presents with *symptoms suggestive* of pulmonary hypertension should have the following performed:

- ECG: To look for signs of right ventricular hypertrophy or other abnormalities.
- Echocardiography: To look at ventricular function and for the presence of pulmonary or tricuspid insufficiency as well as other structural defects.
- Chest x-ray: Unless an A-V fistula is present or the child is in congestive heart failure, the child with PHTN will frequently have normal chest radiographs.
- Pulmonary function testing
- Computed tomography (CT) scan of the chest: The helical CT scan has been shown to reliably identify emboli if it involves a moderate size embolus or a segment of lung. It is also used for evaluating the presence of parenchymal disease.
- Screening labs: Serology for collagen vascular disease and for coagulation disorder (antithrombin III, protein C and S, lupus anticoagulant, anticardiolipin antibodies, and factor V Leiden).
- Six-minute walking test: A 6-minute walking test to evaluate exercise tolerance is commonly used for establishing a baseline assessment and to evaluate current severity of disease (Garofano and Barst, 2003).
- Pulmonary angiography is considered the gold standard for quantifying the severity of PHTN, for measurement of filling pressures, and calculation of pulmonary vascular resistance. Evaluation of pulmonary reactivity to vasodilators—including calcium channel blockers, NO, and prostacyclin—may also be performed with angiography.

D. Patient Care Management

1. **The goal of therapy** for PHTN is to relax pulmonary vessels and prevent escalation of the vascular remodeling leading to irreversible pulmonary hypertension. Interventions to optimize Do_2 and reduce Vo_2, such as reducing agitation, maintaining a hematocrit above 35% to 40%, and maintaining $Sao_2 >$ 93% are fundamental.
2. **Identifying treatable causes** of PHTN is needed to prevent worsening of PHTN. If PHTN is at an early stage, aggressive measures to remediate PHTN may enhance regression of vascular remodeling.
3. **Direct care**
   a. *Oxygen* by nasal cannula or mask is used to maintain a $Sao_2 \geq 95\%$.
   b. *Pharmacologic interventions* are aimed at altering the balance between vasoconstrictive and vasodilator influences. Vasodilators include the following:
      - NO, which is an endogenous mediator produced in the endothelial cells, may be suppressed. NO administration via inhalation raises cyclic guanosine monophosphate (cGMP) levels, which produces vasodilation. However, administration must be continuous, and long-term outcomes have found that although Sao_2 is raised, no improvement in mortality results (Dent and Fontan, 1999).
      - Prostacyclin is a strong pulmonary vasodilator and may prevent smooth-muscle proliferation in some circumstances as well (Dent and Fontan, 1999). It is available for IV use and as an inhaled aerosol. Recent research (Leuchte et al., 2004) suggests that the combination of a prostacyclin analog and sildenafil together may improve outcomes over either agent alone (Turanlahti et al., 1998).
      - Calcium channel blockers are used for the treatment of primary PHTN in selected patients. Research suggest that there may be an intrinsic abnormality in the membrane mechanisms that regulate intracellular calcium levels in patients with primary PHTN. Thirty percent of patients who respond to NO respond well to calcium channel blockers (Rich and Kaufman, 1991).
      - Sildenafil is a phosphodiesterase inhibitor that might provide new treatment options for PHTN by inhibiting the binding of cGMP thus producing elective vasodilation in the pulmonary arteries (see Pharmacology section).
   c. *Anticoagulation*
      - Anticoagulation is recommended for most patients with PHTN (Dent and Fontan, 1999) secondary to a low-flow vasculature, which is vulnerable to the formation of clots.
4. **Supportive care**
   a. *Early treatment of fever* can minimize cardiopulmonary distress.
   b. *Early treatment of infections,* particularly pneumonia, is important.
   c. *Annual immunizations* for influenza, respiratory syncitial virus, plus one immunization for pneumococcus are recommended.
   d. *Stool softeners,* if indicated, can minimize the risk of cardiac collapse with a valsalva maneuver.
   e. *Prevention and management* of pulmonary hypertensive crisis, including oxygenation, sedation, and a decrease in agitation.

E. Prognosis and Outcomes

Without aggressive management of PHTN, the PA pressures gradually increase, eventually causing irreversible thickening of the medial smooth muscle in the arterioles. *Untreated PHTN* results in rapid development of increased right ventricular pressure and heart failure (cor pulmonale).

Before the availability of prostacyclin, the median survival for childhood PHTN was 10 months (Barst et al., 1996). More recent data report 125 to 150 deaths per year in the United States from PHTN, with a 5-year survival rate of 65%, with prostacyclin management. Sildenafil may be an important adjunct, but the experience using sildenafil is too limited at this time to draw conclusions.

THORACIC TRAUMA

A. Definition and Etiology

1. Trauma results in more deaths among children older than 1 year than all other causes combined. Although most pediatric trauma fatalities result from head injury, thoracic and abdominal injuries are the direct cause of about 20% and 10% of childhood deaths, respectively (Cooper et al., 1994; Furnival, 2001). Knowledge of the manner in which pediatric anatomy, physiology, and injury patterns change with age may expedite the evaluation of the pediatric chest after trauma.
2. Thoracic trauma may be the result of a blunt or penetrating injury. Nationwide more than 85% of pediatric thoracic and abdominal injuries result from blunt mechanisms (Meller et al., 1984; Peterson et al., 1994); however, in adolescents, penetrating trauma has a statistically more prominent role. Rib fractures indicate severe chest trauma, and injury to underlying organs, such as the liver, spleen, and lungs, is likely to be present; but serious intrathoracic injury can also be present in the absence of obvious chest-wall injury. Therefore, intrathoracic injuries must be suspected and ruled out whenever there is a significant history of blunt or penetrating trauma.

B. Pathophysiology

A child's chest wall is extremely compliant, and the mediastinum is mobile. As a result, pulmonary contusions are more common, whereas rib fractures occur less frequently in children than adults (Peterson et al., 1994). Adults may manifest hypotension after a 15% to 20% blood volume loss; however, children may remain compensated with up to a 40% blood loss (Bliss and Silen, 2002).

1. **Rib fractures**
   a. Half of *intrathoracic injuries* in children are not associated with rib fractures. The presence of three or more rib fractures in a child reliably identifies him or her in a subgroup of patients with a significant likelihood of intrathoracic, as well as other organ involvement. In the 0- to 3-year age group presenting with isolate rib fractures, child abuse should be a paramount concern (Bulloch et al., 2000; Cadzow and Armstron, 2000).
   b. *Compared with adults*, first- and second-rib fractures in children do not correlate with the presence of injury to the great vessels; however, great-vessel injury should be ruled out. Thoracic spine fractures should increase the suspicion of great-vessel injury. All patients should be evaluated for the presence of spine injuries.
2. **Pulmonary contusions** result in hemorrhage and edema in the peripheral alveolar interstitium as well as in focal capillary leaks. Blood in the alveoli leads to V/P mismatch. Contusions may be associated with pneumothorax or hemothorax (Figure 2-26). Admission chest radiograph is diagnostic in 85% to 97% of patients (Bliss and Silen, 2002).
3. **Tracheobronchial injuries** from blunt trauma can be difficult to diagnose. Half the deaths from tracheobronchial injury occur within 1 hour after the injury. Generally, tracheobronchial injury is the result of blunt trauma to the neck.

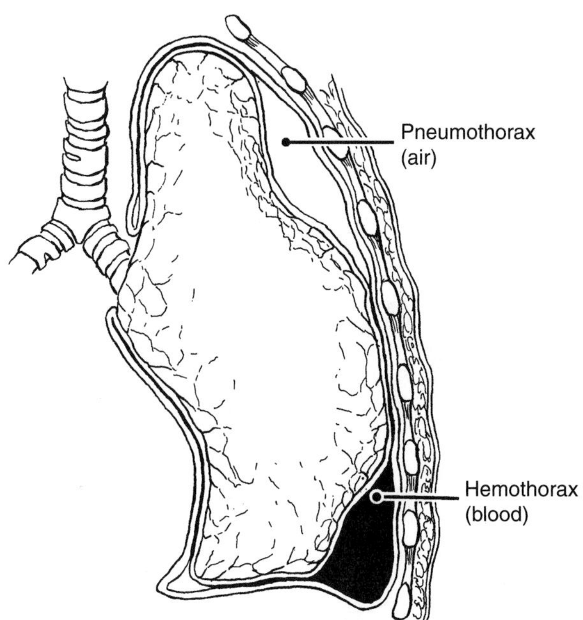

FIGURE 2-26 ■ Pneumothorax and hemothorax.

4. **Pneumothorax and hemothorax** together account for almost half of childhood intrathoracic injuries. Most chest injuries resulting in pneumothorax or hemothorax require only a tube thoracostomy for successful management (see Figure 2-26).
   a. A *tension pneumothorax* produces mediastinal shift with tracheal deviation, which can interfere with central venous return and lead to decreased cardiac output. Tension pneumothorax requires emergency intervention (Figure 2-27).
   b. *Hemothorax* is a blood collection in the pleural cavity (>20 mL/kg). Clinically relevant hemothoraces occur in 14% of children sustaining blunt-force chest injury (Bliss and Silen, 2002). Blood in the thorax is most often asymptomatic unless the volume is large.
5. **Cardiac injuries** generally result from blunt trauma.
   a. *Myocardial contusion* is a cardiac muscle injury secondary to blunt traumatic forces.
   b. *Cardiac tamponade* is a compression of the heart produced by accumulation of blood under pressure in the confined space of the pericardial sac. This results in decreased filling of the heart and decreased cardiac output. Patients present with a narrow pulse pressure, muffled heart sounds, distended neck veins, and shock (Figure 2-28).
   c. *Other cardiac injuries* include valvular dysfunction from papillary muscle or chordae tendineae rupture, cardiac rupture, pericardial effusions, and cardiac dysrhythmia. All cardiac injuries demonstrate signs of decreased cardiac output, such as poor perfusion and poor pulses.
6. **Aortic and great vessel injuries** most commonly involve traumatic aortic disruption in the older adolescent population.

C. Clinical Presentation

1. **History** is important to learn the details of the mechanism of the injury to pinpoint possible sites of injury.

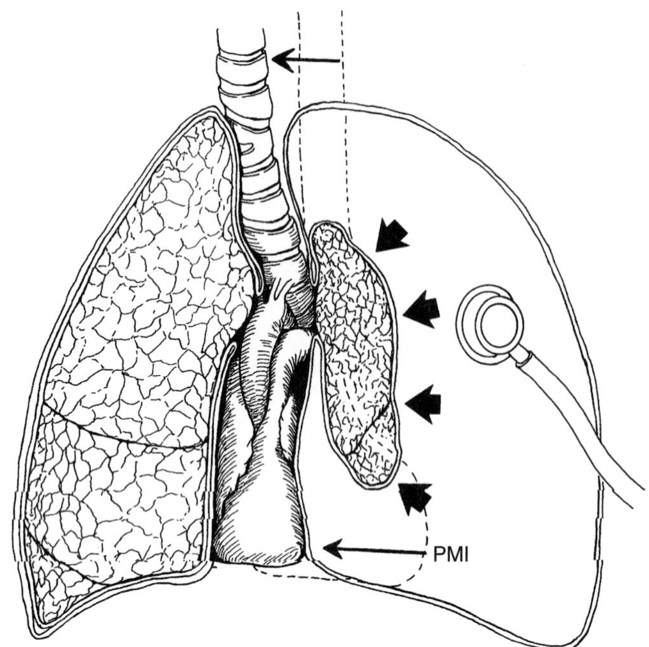

FIGURE 2-27 ■ Tension pneumothorax. *PMI*, point of maximal impulse.

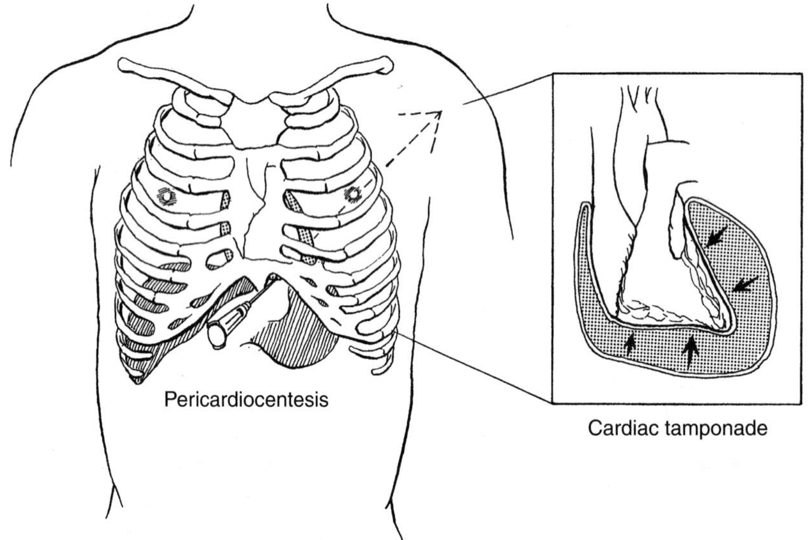

FIGURE 2-28 ■ Cardiac tamponade and pericardiocentesis.

2. **Physical examination**
   a. Children with *significant intrathoracic injuries* may not have suggestive external evidence of these injuries. The primary survey during trauma resuscitation includes a rapid thoracoabdominal examination. Quickly assess airway and breathing. The absence of breath sounds implies the presence of a pneumothorax or hemothorax. However, because of the hyperresonance of the infant's thoracic cavity, breath sounds may be transmitted to the

contralateral side. Observe for chest-wall ecchymosis, bruising, abrasions, sensation of crepitus, point tenderness over a rib, or a displaced trachea.

b. *Tension pneumothorax* causes severe respiratory distress, distended neck veins, contralateral tracheal deviation, and poor systemic perfusion. There may be hyperresonance to percussion, decreased chest expansion, and diminished breath sounds on the side of the injury (see Air-Leak Syndromes discussion).

c. *Hemothorax* manifests with signs similar to those of tension pneumothorax. Tachycardia and hypotension may result from decreased venous return to the heart.

d. In *tracheobronchial injury*, small tears may present with subcutaneous emphysema, dyspnea, sternal tenderness, and hemoptysis. Complete transection presents with severe respiratory distress and failure.

e. *Rib fractures* may cause palpable crepitus, rib deformity, and asymmetric chest-wall movement. Pain leads to splinting of the thorax with impaired ventilation.

f. *Aortic and great vessel injuries* should be suspected if the patient develops midscapular back pain, unexplained hypotension, upper extremity hypertension, bilateral femoral pulse deficits, large initial chest-tube output, sternal fracture, or widened mediastinum demonstrated by radiographic examination of the chest.

3. Diagnostic tests

a. *Radiographic evaluation* of the chest is standard in thoracic trauma cases (Table 2-22).

b. *ABG monitoring* is used to evaluate for hypoxia, hypercarbia, and respiratory acidosis.

c. *CT scan* may be a useful adjunct in the evaluation and management of blunt chest trauma.

d. *Bronchoscopy* is used to confirm the diagnosis of rupture of the trachea or bronchus.

e. *Angiography* is the diagnostic test of choice if large-vessel injury is suspected.

TABLE 2-22
Radiographic Evaluation of the Chest on Trauma

Hemothorax	Fluid assumes a dependent position Complete opacification of the hemothorax with accumulation of pleural fluid The trachea and mediastinum may be shifted away A lateral decubitus view may help confirm the presence of free pleural fluid
Pneumothorax	Presents with unilateral hyperlucency
Tension pneumothorax	Underlying lung will collapse Trachea and mediastinum will be shifted away from the side of the pneumothorax
Rib fractures	Rib and thoracic spine fractures are evaluated Excludes other chest and upper abdominal injuries
Cardiac tamponade, aortic, and great vessel injuries	High mediastinal width–to–chest width ratio Blurring of the aortic knob Tracheal deviation Widened peritracheal stripes Increased heart size with tamponade

f. *ECG* can be used to evaluate for ischemic changes, premature atrial or ventricular contractions, and other arrhythmias that occur with myocardial contusion.
g. *Other diagnostic tests* for myocardial trauma include serum creatinine kinase, CK-MB isoenzyme, radionuclide angiography, and echocardiography.

D. Patient Care Management

1. **Direct care** involves assessment and establishment of an airway, breathing, and circulation and correction of life-threatening injuries.
   a. *Needle decompression* is required for tension pneumothorax (Figure 2-29).
   b. *With hemothorax* the chest tube is placed more posterior if possible. Ideally the fourth to fifth intercostal space along the midaxillary line is used. This presents little danger to the thoracic nerve and little risk to the liver or spleen. If blood from the chest tube is bright red, the source may be intercostal vessels or the internal thoracic artery. In penetrating injuries, the source may be a disruption of the aorta or a hole in the heart, which is generally is followed by rapid decompensation and death if early intervention is not accomplished. Thoracotomy is indicated when the thoracostomy tube output is more than 2 to 3 mL/kg per hour or greater than 20% of the blood volume.
   c. *Myocardial contusion* requires an adequate airway and oxygenation, continuous cardiac monitoring, and serial cardiac isoenzymes or Tropinin Ic levels. Lidocaine infusion may be necessary for dysrhythmias causing hemodynamic compromise.
   d. *Cardiac tamponade* requires establishment of an airway, breathing, and circulation. Pericardiocentesis is performed, and blood is then aspirated from the pericardium (see Figure 2-28). Thoracotomy is indicated for ongoing hemorrhage to drain the pericardium and repair the bleeding site.
   e. *Tracheobronchial injury* requires intubation to ensure adequate oxygenation and ventilation and a chest tube for evacuation of air. Surgical intervention is necessary to overcome a large air leak.
   f. *Rib fractures* may necessitate supplemental oxygen and good pulmonary toilet. Avoid atelectasis and pneumonia by providing analgesia and encouraging deep breathing.
2. **Supportive care:** Continue with chest tube evacuation of air or blood as long as necessary. Provide rigorous pulmonary toilet to prevent atelectasis (postural drainage, cough). If the patient is receiving mechanical ventilation, provide frequent suctioning and monitor peak inspiratory pressures. Use antibiotics only for a confirmed infection. Provide oxygen as necessary.
3. **Complications** include sudden hypotension after the chest tube is placed and the complications of chest tube placement as defined earlier.

E. Outcomes

Most pediatric trauma-related mortality occurs before admission to the hospital, whether in the field or in the emergency department. Initial stabilization of the pediatric trauma victim includes rapid cardiopulmonary assessment, basic airway maneuvers, vascular access skills, and cardiopulmonary stabilization.

FOREIGN-BODY ASPIRATION

A. Definition and Etiology

Foreign-body aspiration is an important cause of accidental death in infants and children. Toddlers younger than 3 years of age account for 60% to 80% of foreign-

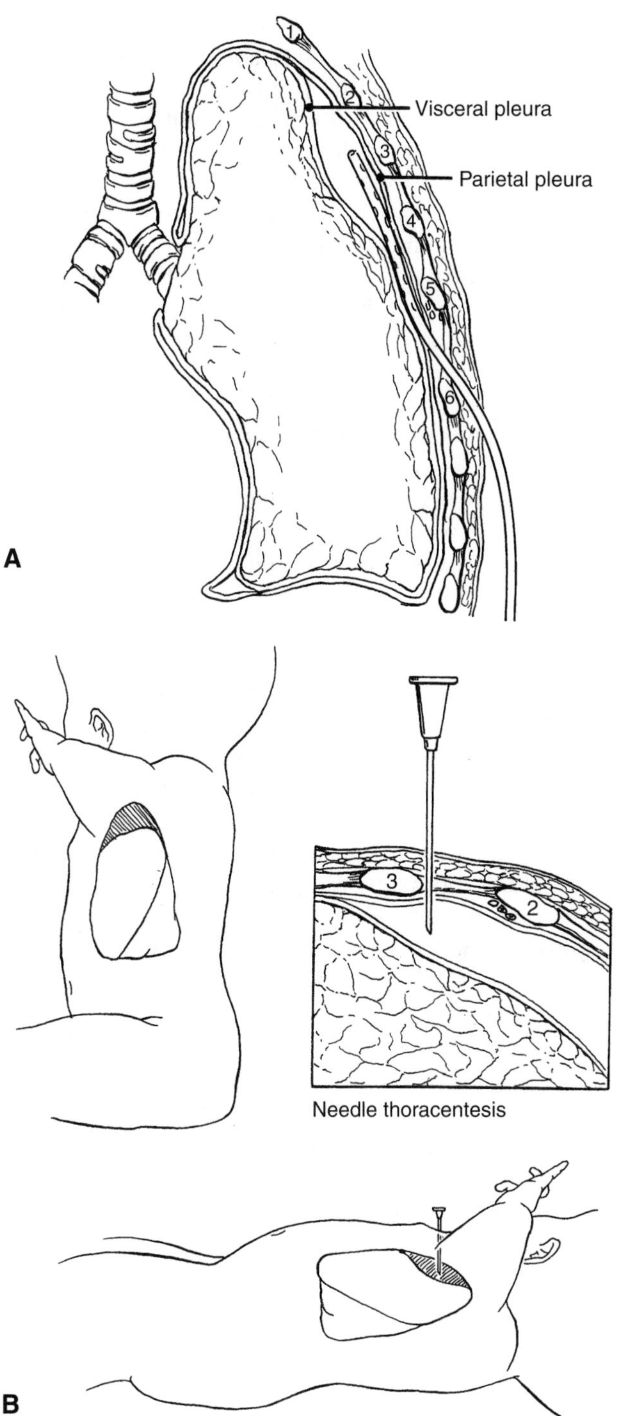

FIGURE 2-29 ■ **A,** Chest tube placement. **B,** Needle thoracentesis location between second and third rib.

body aspirations. Beginning at age 8 to 10 months, the curious infant has developed thumb-forefinger grasp, enabling placement of objects into the mouth, and has learned to crawl. By 1 to 2 years of age, the toddler is climbing. The foreign body is usually organic; nuts are the most common. Other small items frequently found in the environment of a child pose a risk for occluding the airway.

B. Pathophysiology

The severity of lung disease and rapidity of presentation depend on the type of object aspirated and the amount of airway obstruction produced. Fewer than 5% of inhaled foreign bodies are found in the more distal portions of the tracheobronchial tree. Most lodge in a main stem or lobar bronchus. Laryngeal foreign bodies are more common in infants younger than 1 year of age. There are three stages of symptoms resulting from aspiration. The initial event associated with violent paroxysms of coughing, choking and gagging. This is followed by an asymptomatic interval when the foreign body becomes lodged and the immediate irritating symptoms subside. In the third stage, obstruction, erosion, or infection develops.

C. Clinical Presentation

1. **History:** Fewer than 40% of patients give a clear history of an aspirated foreign body. The initial episode is frequently associated with choking and coughing. Often symptoms subside, and the child presents at a later time with diverse symptoms, such as coughing, wheezing, recurrent or protracted pneumonia, and fever. The right bronchus is more often the site of the foreign body than the left bronchus, but the airway might be blocked anywhere from the posterior pharynx to the bronchus (Figure 2-30).
2. **Physical examination:** Examination findings may be normal or reveal nonspecific signs, such as decreased air entry, wheezing, rhonchi, or inspiratory stridor. Patients with laryngeal foreign bodies have stridor, dyspnea, cyanosis, cough, and voice change. Total airway obstruction can occur. Patients with bronchial foreign bodies present with cough, asymmetric breath sounds, wheezing, dyspnea, and fever.
3. **Diagnostic tests:** Chest radiographs may show metallic or radiopaque objects. A single foreign body lodged in a single bronchus may present with obstructive emphysema. Chest radiographs may be normal in as many as 38% of cases. A chest radiograph may demonstrate atelectasis, infiltrate, or hyperinflation; however, it is not a reliable indicator of foreign-body aspiration. Inspiratory and

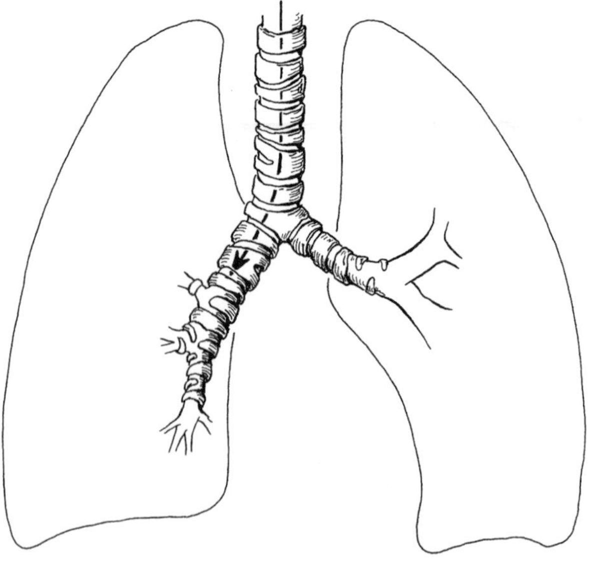

FIGURE 2-30 ■ Anatomy of mainstem bronchus.

expiratory radiographs can be evaluated for ball-valve bronchial obstruction. Soft-tissue lateral neck x-ray films are used to evaluate for the presence of laryngeal foreign bodies (Nova et al., 1998). Direct laryngoscopy is used to confirm foreign body aspiration.

4. **Clinical course** depends on the degree of obstruction, location of the foreign body, nature of the object, and availability of equipment or personnel.
   a. *For life-threatening airway* obstruction follow basic life support emergency measures for the choking child as outlined in the following section. Emergent rigid bronchoscopy should be performed if these maneuvers are unsuccessful.
   b. *Before removal* of the foreign body, a quiet environment should be provided and vital signs and respiratory distress must be watched carefully. Monitor for changes in the heart rate, respiratory rate, increased retractions, pallor, or cyanosis.
   c. *Following removal,* respiratory effort should continue to be monitored, observing for signs of airway obstruction from edema at the site where the foreign body was removed.

D. Patient Care Management

1. **Prevention**
   a. Parents should be *instructed* to limit the availability of nuts, jewelry, small objects, latex balloons, popcorn, and hot dogs to children younger than 3 years.
   b. *Poison control* phone numbers should be readily available in the child's home. The American Academy of Pediatrics is no longer recommending ipecac administration to children.
2. **Emergency care:** Follow Pediatric Advanced Life Support recommendations (Hazinski et al., 2002). If the child still has adequate air exchange and an effective cough, no attempt should be made to dislodge the foreign body before definitive management with a bronchoscopy. If the child has inadequate air exchange, administer five back blows followed by five chest thrusts for a child younger than 1 year or the Heimlich maneuver for the older child. Oxygen should be supplied by face mask.
3. **Respiratory care**
   a. *Monitor* closely for signs of deterioration such as changes in heart rate, respiratory rate, increase in severity of sternal retractions, or increased oxygen requirement.
   b. *Immediate removal* of the foreign body is the most effective intervention for acute aspiration. Laryngoscopy or rigid bronchoscopy may be performed for direct visualization of the airway and removal of the foreign body. Rigid bronchoscopy is performed while the child receives general anesthesia.
4. **Supportive care**
   a. *Administer oxygen* as indicated.
   b. *Infection* can develop in the area of the lung distal to the obstruction and usually resolves rapidly once the foreign body is removed. Antibiotic therapy should be used if a culture of respiratory secretions shows infection.

E. Outcome

Pronounced local inflammation or granulation may be seen in the airway with long-standing foreign bodies. If the foreign body is not readily removed, obstruction from edema, erosion with infection, perforation, and hemorrhage may develop. Generally the outcome is good if appropriate and timely management is provided.

AIR-LEAK SYNDROMES

A. Definitions and Etiology

1. **Pneumothorax** is a collection of air in the pleural space (see Figure 2-26).
2. **Etiology** includes the following:
   a. *Postoperative patients* may have air leaks related to pleural space disruption during surgery, allowing air accumulation or inadequate air drainage by the chest drainage system.
   b. *Air leaks* can occur during chest tube removal, as a complication of mechanical ventilation, or as a complication of respiratory disease.
   c. *Upper airway trauma* can cause severe tracheobronchial disruption after high-energy impact injuries. Injuries range from irregular tears to complete transection.
   d. *Thoracic trauma* (see Thoracic Trauma and Multiple Trauma discussions) may be blunt or penetrating. A penetrating chest wound allows free, bidirectional flow of air between the affected hemithorax and the surrounding atmosphere.

B. Clinical Presentation

1. **History:** Determine the presence of any of the previously mentioned causes. Because of the increased compliance of the child's chest wall, tracheobronchial injury may occur without the suggestive chest wall injuries seen in the adult patient.
2. **Physical examination**
   a. *Pneumothorax* presents with decreased intensity or a change in the pitch of breath sounds over the involved area, increased PIP (in the child receiving mechanical ventilation), tachypnea, increased respiratory effort demonstrated by the presence of retractions, or a sudden change in color to pale or cyanotic. Referred breath sounds may be heard over the area of the pneumothorax in the infant. Decreased breath sounds are noted over the affected area in the older child.
   b. *Tension pneumothorax* may present with agitation, hypotension from obstruction of venous return to the heart, severe hypoxemia, unilateral chest-wall movement, decreased breath sounds on the affected side, and cardiorespiratory distress. Heart sounds may be shifted away from the pneumothorax. Tracheal deviation and mediastinal shift is away from the side of the pneumothorax. Respiratory failure, distended neck veins, and cyanosis can progress to circulatory collapse (see Figure 2-27).
   c. *Tracheobronchial injury* may present with subcutaneous emphysema, dyspnea, sternal tenderness, and hemoptysis. Subcutaneous emphysema is noted when gas tracks along the peribronchial and perivascular tissues to the mediastinum and then up into the neck.
   d. *Open pneumothorax* (sucking chest wound) results from a penetrating chest wound. Paradoxical shifting of the mediastinum to the contralateral side can occur with each spontaneous breath (flail chest). Severe respiratory distress with hypoxia is often seen.
3. **Diagnostic tests**
   a. *Chest radiographs* of pneumothorax demonstrate no pulmonary vascular markings present from the air-tissue interface in the pleural cavity. A

pneumothorax is seen as a uniformly translucent area without lung markings. Free pleural air accumulates in the nondependent portions of the chest. A cross-table lateral radiograph may be necessary to detect intrapleural gas in supine patients. This is particularly important in those with noncompliant lungs that do not readily collapse. Multiple broken ribs are generally noted in flail chest. With a tension pneumothorax, the diaphragm is flattened and the heart and trachea deviate to the nonaffected side.

b. *Chest radiographs of tracheobronchial injury* demonstrate subcutaneous emphysema, pneumomediastinum, pneumothorax, and air surrounding the bronchus.

c. *Diagnostic bronchoscopy* is necessary to confirm the location and the extent of the disruption in tracheobronchial injury.

d. *Transillumination* of the chest may enable detection of pneumothorax in newborns and premature infants.

4. Clinical course depends on the size of pneumothorax and the presence or absence of tension.

C. Patient Care Management

1. Prevention: Care must be taken to avoid reentry of air during chest tube removal. Use ventilatory strategies to minimize barotrauma during mechanical ventilation. Set high-pressure alarms on the ventilator to 10 to 15 cm H_2O above PIPs. Avoid excessive peak pressures when manually bagging a patient by monitoring with a pressure manometer.

2. Direct care

a. *Pneumothorax* should be treated with placement of a chest tube in the fifth intercostal space just lateral to the nipple at the point between the anterior and midaxillary line. After placement, the chest tube is connected to a water seal and suction system. Multiple tubes may be required, depending on the location of air or blood. An emergency needle thoracentesis may be performed if the patient is experiencing significant hemodynamic or respiratory compromise. Needle thoracentesis may be accomplished through the insertion of a 14-gauge needle at the second intercostal space on the midclavicular line, just above the third rib. The catheter may be left in place with a stopcock; some recommend venting to room air until a chest tube is inserted (see Figure 2-29).

b. *Treatment for an open pneumothorax* (flail chest) consists of positive pressure ventilation and covering the wound with an occlusive dressing followed by insertion of a chest tube.

c. *Tension pneumothorax* requires prompt evacuation by needle thoracentesis or a chest tube.

3. Supportive care: Evaluate for the effectiveness of chest tube placement by auscultation and chest radiography. Monitor the function of the chest tube drainage system by observing the quantity of air that is evacuated. Monitor the patient for signs of reaccumulation, such as tachypnea, hypoxia, or increased respiratory effort. Assess for evidence of erythema or drainage when changing the chest tube dressing. Remove the chest tube when evidence of the air leak has disappeared (i.e., there is no air movement through the water seal chamber of chest tube) and risk of further barotrauma is negligible.

D. Outcome

Complications of a chest tube placement include hemorrhage, hemothorax, direct bronchial or parenchymal lung injury, infection, and nerve injury.

CHRONIC LUNG DISEASE OR BRONCHOPULMONARY DYSPLASIA

A. Definition

1. **The classic form**
   a. *Bronchopulmonary dysplasia* (BPD), before the surfactant era, was chronic lung disease (CLD) following a prolonged period of mechanical ventilation with high FiO_2 use, oxygen dependency persisting beyond 36 weeks' corrected gestational age, and abnormal chest radiographs. *BPD* is now defined as the *severe* form of CLD as a natural consequence of prolonged mechanical ventilation or oxygen toxicity causing direct airway damage. Chronic fibrotic changes in the lung architecture are noted on histologic evaluation.
2. **Chronic lung disease**
   a. *CLD is the "new BPD"* (post-surfactant era). It evolves as a milder (although persistent) lung disease; with the use of antenatal steroids, surfactant, new ventilator strategies, and survival of smaller premature infants, the clinical evolution of CLD is more commonly seen today than BPD.
   b. *The definition of CLD*, as with BPD, is lung injury often following a course of mechanical ventilation with an oxygen dependency persisting beyond 36 weeks' corrected gestational age and abnormal chest radiographs. However, CLD typically evolves in a different and sometimes in a more insidious fashion.
3. **Abnormal inflammatory responses**
   a. *The commonality between CLD and BPD* is an abnormal pulmonary inflammatory response that becomes self-perpetuating; however, the triggers and the early management of each differ.
   b. *Early use of antenatal steroids*, surfactant, and CPAP has diminished the early inflammatory responses in neonates with respiratory distress; thus, the milder CLD has become more prevalent.

B. Etiology

Formerly (before surfactant), BPD was more commonly associated with respiratory distress syndrome (RDS) of the neonate; now BPD is more often related to meconium aspiration, persistent fetal circulation, and congenital conditions requiring surgical intervention. CLD is more commonly associated with extreme prematurity, sepsis, and patent ductus arteriosus (PDA). Risk factors for the development of BPD include birth before 32 weeks' gestational age, birth weight less than 1000 g, male gender, and white race. RDS appears in a much milder form secondary to the use of surfactant and antenatal steroids. Contributing factors include high concentrations of oxygen and positive pressure ventilation with substantial damage to the airways evolving to more severe lung disease: BPD (Coalson, 2003).

C. Pathophysiology

1. **BPD** is characterized by the following (Banacalari, 2002):
   a. *Prolonged intubation* that results in reduced mucociliary function and increased dead space, the presence of a PDA, persistent fetal circulation with increased pulmonary vascular resistance, and barotrauma leading to over-distention and remodeling.
   b. *Oxygen toxicity*, which may result in capillary proliferation, stromal edema, and interstitial fibrosis; increased airway resistance resulting in both

overinflation and atelectasis; and an abnormal inflammatory response, which perpetuates the disease. Dilated lymphatics, interstitial pulmonary edema, and increased accumulation of fluids are observed in infants with BPD.

2. **CLD** is characterized by the following (Gomella, 2004):
   a. A *defective pattern of alveolarization* and pulmonary vascular dysgenesis, an interference with septation of alveoli with less fibrosis (than seen with BPD) and fewer and larger alveoli are observed. Fewer pulmonary capillaries combined with fewer alveoli cause a reduction in gas-exchange surface area.
   b. *Hypoxemia* results from the subsequent V/Q mismatch. Chronic hypoxemia may cause increased pulmonary vascular resistance, pulmonary hypertension, right ventricular hypertrophy, and cor pulmonale (see Pulmonary Hypertension).

D. Clinical Presentation

1. **Signs and symptoms** include tachypnea, retractions, failure to thrive, increase in ventilatory requirements or inability to wean, hypoxia, hypercapnia, respiratory acidosis, crackling, wheezing, and bronchospasm.
2. **Increased intrathoracic pressure** may cause SIADH, causing fluid and sodium retention.
3. **Pulmonary hypertension** may evolve to right ventricular failure, tachycardia, hepatomegaly, periorbital edema, with a prominent S_2 or a gallop rhythm.
4. **"BPD spells"** result in irritability, agitation, duskiness, hypercarbia, hypoxemia, and increased respiratory effort. These episodes may be related to bronchospasm or bronchomalacia.
5. **Hypertension** is observed in 40% of these patients secondary to increased renin activity and catecholamine secretion (Gomella, 2004).

E. Invasive and Noninvasive Diagnostic Tests

1. **ABG** may reveal hypoxemia, hypercarbia, and compensated respiratory acidosis.
2. **ECG** findings may reveal right ventricular hypertrophy resulting from the increased pulmonary vascular resistance, which causes increased right ventricular afterload and right axis deviation. This is less common with CLD.
3. **Chest radiograph**
   a. The chest radiograph may demonstrate scattered linear infiltrates, atelectasis, and patch areas of hyperinflation, increased interstitial markings, and cardiomegaly.
   b. With CLD, a more homogeneous pattern of hyperinflation is noted; PE may also be observed with increased interstitial markings.
4. **Pulmonary function studies** may reveal low forced expiratory rates, decreased FRC, increased minute ventilation, increased work of breathing, high airway resistance, low dynamic compliance, and higher oxygen consumption.
5. **Echocardiogram** is used for estimation of pulmonary hypertension and assessment of right ventricular hypertrophy.
6. **Cardiac catheterization** or pulmonary artery catheterization may be performed (rarely) in children with increasing pulmonary hypertension and failure to thrive to further elucidate the extent of pulmonary hypertension.

F. Patient Care Management

1. **Maintain adequate oxygenation and ventilation.** Maintenance of a patent airway and thorough pulmonary toilet is essential.

a. *Early use of continuous positive airway pressure* may prevent or attenuate the need for invasive mechanical ventilation.

b. *Supplemental oxygen therapy* is useful in reducing hypoxemia, decreasing required minute ventilation, stimulating pulmonary vasodilation, avoiding cardiovascular and pulmonary vascular complications, and possibly enhancing growth.
   - Oxygen requirements vary depending on activity level; continuous pulse oximetry or transcutaneous oxygen monitoring is essential.
   - The oxygen saturations ($Sa{O_2}$) should be targeted for 92% to 95% or, if pulmonary hypertension is prominent, targeted to 95% to 97% or greater (Nievas and Chernick, 2002).
   - If an infant's oxygen requirement increases, consider GERD, aspiration, congenital heart disease, or a new pneumonia.
   - If patient is on low-flow oxygen, an infant should have a 10-minute trial off oxygen every 2 to 3 weeks. If $Sa{O_2}$ is 92% or greater, the patient can be off oxygen while awake (Nievas and Chernick, 2002). The same procedure for weaning oxygen while an infant is sleeping is monitored for 2 to 3 weeks.
   - Assessment of the infant's breathing-room air should include noting growth patterns; if the patient stops growing, oxygen therapy may be reinstituted.
   - Weaning from ventilation may be prolonged in some infants and should be done slowly (see Mechanical Ventilation section).

c. *Tracheostomy or home ventilation* may be required in some patients, but many infants with CLD will require supplemental oxygen only.

2. **Pharmacologic interventions**

a. *Bronchodilators* assist in reducing airway obstruction caused by bronchospasm. Beta-adrenergic agonists such as albuterol are not uniformly successful. The airway obstruction, especially with BPD, is caused by metaplasia and mucous plugging of the distal airways and not necessarily by bronchospasm.
   - A trial of nebulized aerosols is warranted for acute desaturation episodes; if the patient is on a ventilator, flow loops should be evaluated before and after the aerosol to document the reversibility of airway obstruction.
   - Up to 50% of infants with CLD have tracheomalacia (Doull, 1997) and would deteriorate from a beta-agonist because of airway collapse.
   - Side effects are related to the adrenergic stimulation and include tachycardia, tremors, and GI disturbances.

b. *Inhaled anticholinergics* are also used to treat bronchospasm and may be useful for bronchomalacia, in which a paradoxical response to beta$_2$-agonists may be seen. Increased dynamic compliance and decreased respiratory effort have been described after administration of nebulized ipratropium bromide.

c. *Methylxanthines* (currently less commonly used), such as theophylline or aminophylline, decrease airway resistance, promote diuresis, stimulate the CNS respiratory center, provide anti-inflammatory action, and increases diaphragmatic contractility. Toxicity (extreme tachycardia, tremors, seizures) is the principal reason for the decreasing use of these agents. In addition they may also decrease esophageal sphincter tone, potentially resulting in GERD. Many factors, including other drugs, affect metabolism and clearance; therefore serum levels should be monitored.

d. *Anti-inflammatory therapy,* such as steroid administration, may not prevent development of BPD/CLD but may acutely improve pulmonary function. Aerosolized steroids have been shown to increase compliance and decrease resistance after 3 weeks of therapy.

- Steroids appear to have little, if any, effect on long-term morbidity and mortality, or health care costs (Nievas and Chernick, 2002). Significant complications from steroids include masking of infection, hypertension, growth failure, glucose instability, and adrenal suppression (Schimmer and Parker, 2001).

e. *Diuretic therapy* is often used to aid in the improvement of pulmonary function and decreased respiratory effort through the reduction of excessive fluids, secondary to SIADH, or iatrogenic administration.
- The efficacy of long-term diuretic use is unproven (Nievas and Chernick, 2002).
- Furosemide and bumetanide are more potent than other diuretics, but both may cause a rapid onset of metabolic alkalosis secondary to chloride excretion, which may cause secondary hypoventilation, renal calculi, and rickets with long-term use. Some investigators (Nievas and Chernick, 2002) recommend a target pH of 7.30 to 7.35, which may require the use of other agents to decrease bicarbonate (e.g., acetazolamide [Diamox]) or increase chloride. In some cases it may be necessary to use alternative diuretics.
- Thiazide diuretics do not affect calcium excretion in the same way as loop diuretics and may be useful for long-term therapy.

3. Prevention

a. *Prevention of infections* with immunizations, including influenza vaccine, pneumoccal vaccine, seasonal administration of palivizumab, and a humanized respiratory syncytial virus monoclonal antibody (IMPACT-RSV Study Group, 1998) are essential for children with CLD. *Promote hygiene measures* with the family, focusing on strict handwashing, avoidance of close contact with the child's face, and enforcing distancing from the child if an obvious infection is noted in the people around the child.

4. Promote normal growth and development

a. *Adequate nutrition* is essential in the recovery of lung function, which often occurs during the first year. Some infants with BPD/LCD may need 170-200 kcals/kg/day (Spitzer, 1995).

b. *Malnourishment* related to chronic respiratory distress and repeated hospitalizations is a common problem in infants with chronic lung disease.

c. *Increased work of breathing* necessitates a higher basal caloric requirement and increased oxygen consumption. Calories should not be withheld because of the possibility of fluid overload. If necessary, diuretics can be adjusted.

d. *Oxygen consumption* ideally is measured with a metabolic cart to provide accurate caloric requirement calculations. Otherwise daily weights on the same scale and same conditions provide an estimation of basal metabolic requirements.

e. *The enteral route* is preferred for feedings. Because fluids are often restricted, infant formulas can be modified to increase caloric content, but the high osmotic load of high-calorie formula may cause diarrhea in some infants. Complicating factors in providing adequate nutrition include the following:
- GERD
- Poor suck and swallow or oral aversion
- Decreased mesenteric flow, a risk factor for necrotizing enterocolitis
- Defective vitamin A kinetics or limited capability to absorb fat (more recently studied by Nievas and Chernick, 2002)

f. *Early speech therapy* is essential for infants who demonstrate an oral aversion or to prevent oral aversion.

5. **Continued assessment**
   a. An *increase in the WOB,* lethargy, increased carbon dioxide level, and a decrease in the arterial oxygen level require immediate attention. The development of respiratory *acidosis* in an infant may require a form of ventilatory assistance.
   b. *Increasing pulmonary vascular resistance* (pulmonary hypertensive crisis) can precipitate right ventricular failure. Distinguishing between a pulmonary alteration and a change in pulmonary vascular resistance requires a pulmonary artery catheter, echocardiogram, or cardiac catheterization. The management for increased PVR is oxygen, pharmacologic treatment or NO (see Pulmonary Hypertension).

G. Complications and Long-Term Outcomes

1. **Respiratory bronchioles and alveoli** continue to increase in number, and size correlates with linear growth; therefore, infants tend to improve with normal growth. Significant improvement can occur during the first 2 years of life with good nutrition and freedom from infections.
2. **BPD/CLD** is characterized by exacerbations and remissions. Children with lung disease have significant respiratory morbidity after discharge (Bhandari and Bhandari, 2003). Frequent hospitalizations of children with BPD/CLD in the year after discharge are most often related to viral respiratory illnesses, with RSV the most frequent etiology. Risk factors for a viral respiratory illness include the following:
   a. *Concurrent cardiac disease*
   b. *Presence of siblings* or other children in the house
   c. *Smoking* in the home
   d. *Supplemental oxygen therapy or other inhaled irritants*
   e. *Poor hygiene* (especially handwashing)
3. **Long-term outcome** studies indicate improvement in the first year of life; however, abnormalities of the small airways often persist, and airway hyperresponsiveness has been reported in long-term survivors (Bhandari and Bhandari, 2003). *Neurodevelopmental* problems in children with severe BPD have also been demonstrated (e.g., learning difficulties, behavior disorders, deficits in motor skills) (Majnemer et al., 2000). However, those complications may be related to the overall neonatal course. Early assessment and intervention for developmental delays and movement disorders are strongly recommended.

PHYSIOLOGIC PRINCIPLES OF MECHANICAL VENTILATION

A. Objectives of Mechanical Ventilation

1. **Improve pulmonary gas exchange.**
2. **Relieve respiratory distress** by relieving upper and lower airway obstruction, reducing oxygen consumption, and relieving respiratory fatigue.
3. **Manage pulmonary mechanics** by normalizing and maintaining the distribution of lung volume and providing pulmonary toilet.
4. **Provide airway protection** in patients with decreased level of consciousness or with neuromuscular disorders.
5. **Provide general support** for hemodynamically unstable patients.

B. Physiologic Principles

1. **Pulmonary function** (Table 2-23)
   a. *Tidal volume (V_T):* Volume of air inspired with each inspiratory effort. The normal V_T in a spontaneously breathing patient is 4 to 7 mL/kg. The calculated tidal volume is the product of inspiratory time and flow rate: $V_T = T_I \times \text{Flow}$
   b. *Minute ventilation (V_E):* Total volume of gas inspired over a period of one minute; V_E is the product of respiratory rate and tidal volume: $V_E = RR \times V_T$
   c. *Alveolar ventilation (V_A):* Volume of air available for gas exchange in the alveoli that accounts for the presence of dead space: $V_A = (V_T - V_D) \times RR$
   d. *Dead-space ventilation (V_D):* Volume of gas occupying airway lumina that does not participate in gas exchange. Normally V_D is approximately 2 cc/kg. Therefore, approximately one third of the V_T.
   e. *Functional residual capacity (FRC):* Volume of gas in the lungs at end-expiration that maintains alveolar distention: FRC ~30 mL/kg
   f. *Vital capacity (V_C):* Volume of gas measured after a forced (maximal) expiration following maximal inspiration: V_C = 40–50 mL/kg
2. **Relationship of pressure (P), flow (F), and resistance (R)** is expressed by the equation: $P = F \times R$
   a. *Pressure:* The driving pressure to transfer flow to the alveoli is directly proportional to flow and resistance; that is, if either flow or resistance increases, pressure will increase.
   b. *Resistance:* Resistance is a force that impedes the flow of gas. It is inversely proportional to the diameter of the airway. Factors that increase resistance should be minimized, such as appropriate size and length of the ET tube and ventilator circuit, treatment of airway edema, and secretions.
   c. *Inspiratory flow*: Appropriate flow rates through an oxygen delivery system or ventilator must provide adequate minute ventilation under a variety of clinical conditions.
3. **Compliance (C_L)**
   a. *Compliance* is the relationship between volume and pressure within a closed space. A change in either volume or pressure will alter compliance:

TABLE 2-23
Pulmonary Function

Respiratory frequency (RR)	=	Infant: 30–40 bpm Child: 20–30 bpm
Inspiratory time	=	Infant: 0.4–0.6 s Child: 0.6–1 s
Inspiratory flow	=	Infant: 2–3 L/min Child: 8–15 L/min
Tidal volume (V_T)	=	$\frac{\text{Inspiratory Time} \times \text{Flow Rate}}{RR}$
Minute ventilation ($\dot{V}_E$)	=	$V_T \times RR$
Physiologic dead space (V_{DS})	=	2 ml/kg (40–50% of V_T)
Alveolar ventilation (V_A)	=	$(V_T - V_{DS}) \times RR$
Functional residual capacity (FRC)	=	30 ml/kg
Vital capacity (VC)	=	Infant: 33–40 ml/kg Child: 40–50 ml/kg
Total lung capacity (TLC)	=	Infant: 63 ml/kg Child: 70–75 ml/kg

$$\text{Compliance } (C_L) = \Delta\text{Volume} / \Delta\text{Pressure}$$

or

$$C_L = \frac{\text{Tidal volume}}{\text{Plateau pressure}}$$

For example, a patient with severe parenchymal lung disease will have decreased compliance ("stiff lung") requiring a greater amount of inspiratory pressure to maintain the same tidal volume.

b. *Total lung compliance* is the summation of chest wall compliance and lung compliance.
c. *Lung compliance* is determined by the elasticity of lung tissue and the presence of surfactant in alveoli (which prevents alveolar collapse).
d. *Chest-wall compliance* is determined by the contour of the thoracic cage, the structural integrity of the thorax and external impedance, such as a distended abdomen.

C. Physiologic Interface Between a Ventilator and a Child

1. **Mean airway pressure (MAP):** MAP is the average airway pressure measured at the proximal airway, from one inspiration to the beginning of the next. MAP directly affects the Pa_{O_2}. It is determined by tidal volume, PIP, flow rate, respiratory rate, and end-expiratory pressure.
2. **Tidal volume (V_T):** Small absolute tidal volumes are observed in infants and small children, necessitating a ventilator that is capable of regulating V_T to as low as 20 mL (for full-term infants). Infants and small children are not capable of increasing V_T spontaneously because of the structural contour of their chest wall and increased compliance. With respiratory distress, the child will instead increase respiratory rate.
3. **Respiratory rate (RR):** The RR observed in children is faster to compensate for the inability to increase V_T and also because of increased metabolic rate. Shorter inspiratory times are observed in children. The spontaneous inspiratory time is determined by lung compliance, airway resistance, and flow rate. A "stiff" lung or narrowed airway may necessitate a longer inspiratory time on the ventilator.
4. **Peak inspiratory pressure (PIP):** The principal determinants of PIP include lung compliance, inspiratory time, airway resistance, and tidal volume. Minimizing PIP is a lung-protective strategy to avoid volutrauma. Normal PIPs in spontaneously breathing newborns are 10 to 12 mm Hg; in older infants and small children, they are approximately 12 to 15 mm Hg. Adolescents and adults are characteristically 20 mm Hg or less.
5. **Inspiratory flow:** Flow patterns and flow rate are more variable from breath to breath in infants and young children. Constant flow is more typical of an adolescent or adult. Appropriate flow rates through an oxygen delivery system or a ventilator must be ensured to provide adequate minute ventilation under a variety of clinical conditions. Additionally, flow patterns can be manipulated on most ventilators to optimize alveolar ventilation and to provide flexibility for the patient. An example is a "decelerating flow" pattern in which a large proportion of the flow is delivered on the initiation of a breath, with the remainder of the flow delivered more slowly, to enhance distribution of oxygen to alveolar units.
6. **Positive end-expiratory pressure (PEEP):** PEEP is a mechanism provided at end-expiration to maintain FRC (Figure 2-31). Some conditions are characterized by decreased FRC (restrictive diseases) in which PEEP is a primary therapeutic intervention to prevent alveolar collapse at end-expiration.
7. **Synchronization:** *The smooth interaction between* the ventilator and the patient is

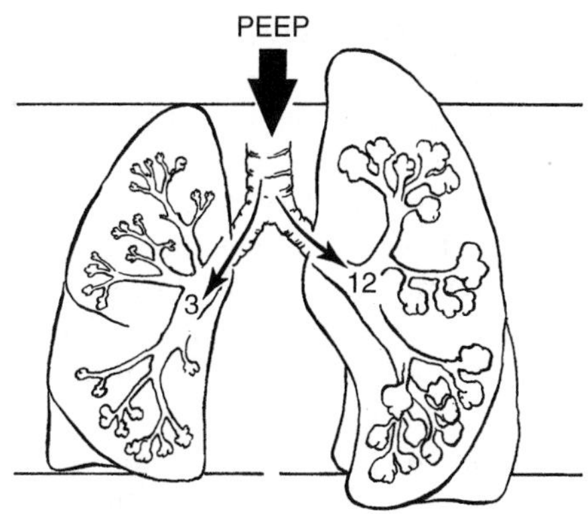

FIGURE 2-31 ■ Effect of positive end-expiratory (PEEP) on functional residual capacity (FRC). In restrictive disease without PEEP, there is increased negative intrapleural pressure at FRC. Alveolar pressures are equal. (Note the left sides of illustration.) With the addition of 12 cm H_2O PEEP, pressure is increased. Alveolar distention is maintained at end expiration. Patients with adult respiratory disease syndrome (ARDS) typically develop patchy atelectasis requiring higher PEEP to maintain FRC.

an important goal. Spontaneous breathing should be maintained and supported whenever feasible. Selection of a ventilation strategy appropriate to the child's physiologic needs and individual comfort should allow good synchronization.

D. Positive-Pressure Ventilation

1. **Positive-pressure ventilators:** Positive-pressure ventilation (PPV) creates a positive pressure at the proximal airway that exceeds alveolar pressure, forcing gas flow to the lungs. The *mode* of ventilation is used as a broad term to describe several phases of PPV. One method for understanding PPV is illustrated in Figure 2-32. The three principal mechanisms are mode, control, and phase variables.
2. **Mode:** A strict definition of mode describes the type of breath (mandatory or spontaneous) that the ventilator allows to the patient as well as how much support the ventilator will give each spontaneous breath.
   a. *Controlled mandatory ventilation:* The ventilator controls every breath with preset parameters. The patient cannot initiate spontaneous breaths.

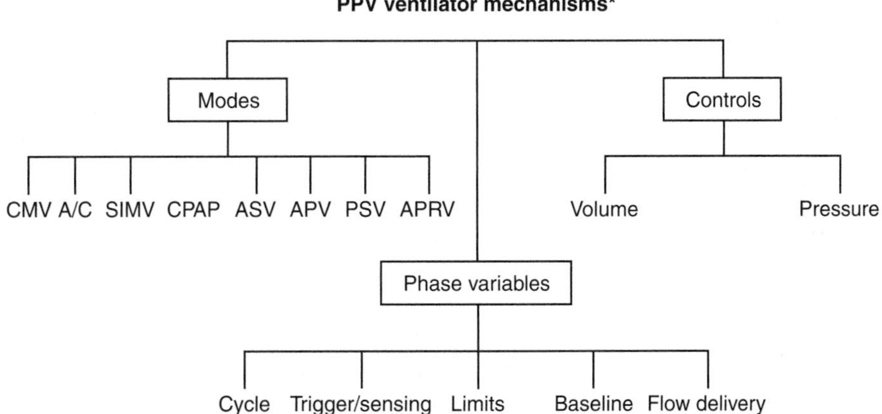

FIGURE 2-32 ■ Mechanics of positive pressure ventilation. *PPV,* positive pressure ventilation; V_T, tidal volume; *PIP,* peak inspiratory pressure; C_L, lung compliance; T_I, inspiratory time; *IMV,* intermittent mandatory ventilation; *PEEP,* positive end-expiratory pressure; *CPAP,* continuous positive airway pressure. *Choose (1) control, (2) mode, and (3) phase variables.

b. *A/C:* Assist/control ventilation. The ventilator breaths are regulated as in controlled mandatory ventilation; however, if the patient initiates a breath, the ventilator will complete the effort with the preset mechanisms. The patient does not exert much work except for the initial effort.
c. *IMV: Intermittent mandatory ventilation.* A preset respiratory rate with other preset limits is delivered to the patient. The patient can breathe spontaneously from the circuit, but the ventilator does not interface with these efforts. If the patient should be midway into a spontaneous breath, when the machine timing initiates a breath, the patient will receive a larger, more uncomfortable breath.
d. *SIMV: Synchronized intermittent mandatory ventilation.* The ventilator has a preset IMV rate and settings. The patient can breathe spontaneously from the circuit. If the patient initiates a breath within the timing window before the next ventilator-timed breath, the ventilator will synchronize its timing with the patient and likewise support the patient.
e. *PSV: Pressure support ventilation* allows the patient to breathe spontaneously, providing pressure/flow support with each effort. The pressure support is predetermined by the clinician. When spontaneous effort is sensed, gas flow is delivered until the airway pressure reaches the preset limit. The higher the pressure, the greater the support for the patient (decreased respiratory work). The patient can continue inspiration with a variable flow rate and variable inspiratory time, whereas the preset airway pressure is sustained. PSV can be used alone or with SIMV facilitating "muscle conditioning."
f. *ASV: Adaptive support ventilation* is similar to *mandatory minute ventilation (MMV)*, in which the minute ventilation is preset based on patient's ideal weight. ASV allows the patient to breathe spontaneously but with a backup RR if the patient becomes apneic. The ventilator compares both the patient's V_T and RR to its internal targets and adjusts either or both to achieve the preset V_E with the lowest possible PIP. MMV, on some ventilators, utilizes a preset IMV rate rather than a backup rate, and the V_T may be determined by the clinician.
g. *APV: Adaptive pressure ventilation* is a form of pressure-regulated volume-control (*PRVC*) mode in which a target V_T is preset, as well as the IMV rate, inspiratory time, and PEEP. In APV, the ventilator monitors lung compliance and airway resistance and continuously adjusts the PIP to deliver the V_T at the lowest possible pressure (thus a variable PIP). Some ventilators do not automatically adjust PIP; instead, it is established by the clinician.
h. *CPAP:* Continuous positive airway pressure is a mode in which the patient is breathing spontaneously, with preset end-expiratory pressure. There is no back-up IMV rate in this mode; PSV can be added for support of patient-initiated breaths.
i. *APRV:* Airway pressure release ventilation is a mode of ventilation that provides a form of pressure control in which the inspiratory time, frequency, PEEP, and PIP are preset, with V_T and V_E variable. It allows spontaneous patient inhalation and exhalation at a preset high CPAP (T-high) for a preset time (e.g. 3 seconds). Periodically the CPAP/PEEP is released for 1 to 2 seconds to allow greater exhalation and therefore CO_2 removal (T-low).

3. **Controls: The control variable regulates inspiration.**
   a. *Pressure control:* The PIP is regulated throughout the inspiratory cycle. It may be set above the patient's PIP to ensure that patient does not exceed the desired PIP, or it may be set to *limit* the patient's PIP at a lower level (Figure 2-33). The V_T volume is determined by the difference between the PIP and PEEP, or delta P

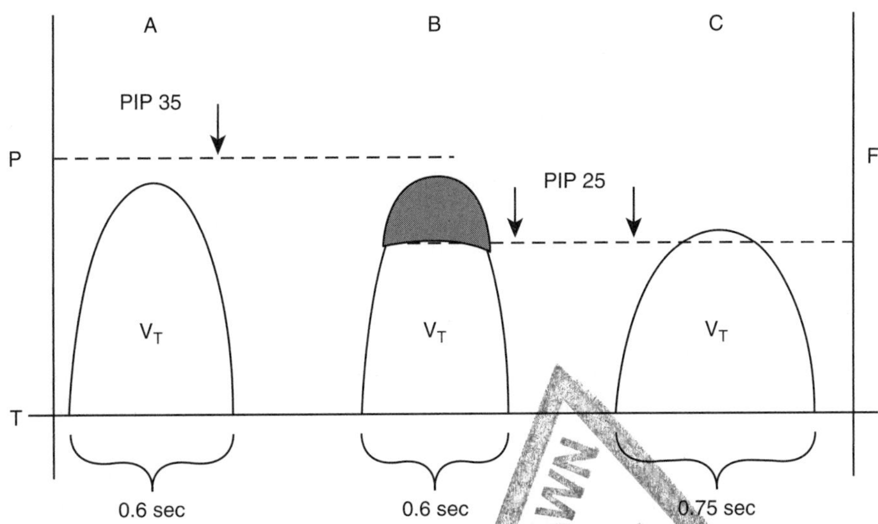

FIGURE 2-33 ■ The relationship between V_T, PIP, flow, and T_I. V_T is a function of flow and T_I and is represented by the area under the curve (**A**). If F and T_I are kept constant, pressure limiting a breath will result in decreased V_T (**B** is shown in black). In order to maintain a constant tidal volume when a pressure limit is set, either the T_I must be increased or the flow rate must be increased (**C**).

(ΔP). A target V_T is established first by setting the desired PEEP, then setting the PIP at a level that allows the desired V_T. This is a lung-protective strategy to minimize high peak pressures while ensuring an adequate V_T. It is commonly used in patients with decreased C_L (stiff lungs). The disadvantage is that, as compliance changes, V_T will be altered. With improving compliance at the same PIP, V_T will increase with the risk of volutrauma.

b. *Volume control:* The V_T is assured throughout inspiration, with variable PIP. A preset inspiratory time and flow rate, plus IMV, PEEP, and PSV, are clinician determined; the flow rate, or I time, is variable, regulated by the patient's lung compliance. PIP is variable according to lung compliance. The disadvantage of this control is that a high PIP may be generated, either acutely (because of airway resistance) or more insidiously, as lung compliance diminishes, with a potential for barotrauma. A high-PIP alarm is set, usually 5 to 10 mm Hg higher than the patient's PIP.

4. Phase variables: These variables are the mechanisms that can be selected to match individual patient needs to achieve an optimal ventilation strategy and synchronization.

a. *Cycle*: The cycling mechanism determines the end of inspiration. The choices are volume-, time-, or flow-cycled ventilation. Currently, pressure-cycled ventilation is rarely used. If a patient is in time-cycled ventilation, inspiration will last only as long as the preset inspiration time (T_I). T_I is one factor of V_T (the other being flow rate). Therefore the time-cycled mode is a type of volume-controlled ventilation.

b. *Trigger and sensing mechanism*: The **trigger** is the mechanism that *initiates* inspiration. The trigger may be a preset IMV rate or patient-initiated breath, which is detected by either a flow or pressure sensor. The **sensing** mechanisms allow the patient to trigger the ventilator. *Pressure sensors* are activated when the patient generates a preset level of negative pressure in the circuit as the patient initiates inspiration. *Flow sensors* are activated when the patient initiates inspiration, displacing a preset level of flow from the circuit. *Placement* of these sensors and their *sensitivity* are important with the goal of minimizing the WOB. Ideally a sensor is positioned at the proximal airway and the flow is accessible at the proximal airway rather than from the ventilator port. A flow sensor generally requires less patient effort than a pressure sensor, and therefore it is preferable for most infants and children.

c. *Flow delivery*: The **rate** of flow during inspiration determines distribution of gas in the lungs. The **availability** of flow determines the ease with which the patient can access flow. The **pattern** of flow delivery—fast, gradual, or slow—will influence patient comfort and synchronization as well as distribution of gas flow in the lungs.

- Continuous circuit flow provides immediate access to flow with minimal patient effort; demand flow requires the patient to inspire the volume of air within the entire inspiratory limb of the circuit before the gas is actually delivered to the patient. The latter imposes a greater WOB and is less desirable for infants and small pediatric patients.
- Fast flow delivery in the initial portion of inspiration is often useful for patients who have noncompliant lung disease or a mixed state in which there is both overdistention and collapse. This flow pattern is described as decelerating flow.

d. *Limits*: Mechanisms that regulate inspiration to provide safety mechanisms. High pressure, time, and flow limits are set, depending on the selected strategies for individual ventilation.

e. *Baseline variables*: Variables that regulate the expiratory phase. PEEP is used to maintain FRC. In children with tracheomalacia, PEEP also appears to "stent" open the airways, which may have a natural tendency to collapse at end expiration.

E. Selection of Ventilation Variables

1. **The choice of mechanisms** is guided by the respiratory compliance of the patient, the ability to breathe spontaneously, and predicted clinical course of the underlying disease.
2. **Preservation of spontaneous breathing efforts** should be maintained whenever possible. The ventilator should have the capability of both allowing spontaneous breathing and providing supported breaths in synchrony with the patient's effort. Examples of ventilator settings for various pathophysiologic conditions are provided in Table 2-24.

F. Alternative Ventilation Strategies (Venkataraman and Orr, 1998)

1. **Inverse-ratio ventilation (IRV)**

a. *Conventional modes* of ventilation use inspiratory:expiratory (I:E) time ratios of typically 1:2 to 1:4. With IRV, the ratio is reversed. The I:E is greater than 1:1 and often 2:1 or more. Lengthening the inspiratory time allows more time for distribution of gas throughout the lungs. The usual sequence of changes that evolves to IRV is a gradual lengthening of the inspiratory time to a point when inspiration is greater than expiration. Lengthening the inspiratory time can cause increased V_T as well as increased PIP, which must be monitored. The $Paco_2$ may eventually rise with the shorter exhalation time, but permissive hypercapnia is frequently tolerated.

TABLE 2-24
Expected Ventilator Requirements Associated with Pathophysiologic Conditions

Conditions	Patient Requirements	Ventilator Settings (Example)
UPPER AIRWAY OBSTRUCTION		
Infectious disease (e.g., epiglotitis)	Normal V_T/PIP Normal FiO_2	Mode: SIMV, APV, CPAP, ASV/MMV, PSV
Facial abnormalities Tracheomalacia	Spontaneous breathing, requires little ventilation unless sedated	Control: Volume Variables: PEEP 3-4 Flow access-continuous
DECREASED LUNG COMPLIANCE		
Surfactant deficiency RDS ARDS Pneumonitis Fibrosis Pulmonary edema Excessive PEEP	Ensure adequate V_T and normal FRC Monitor exhaled V_T and MAP Guard against overdistention (too much V_T) May require patient paralysis or heavy sedation Severe disease or complications (e.g., air leak syndrome): Faster rates, lower V_T, permissive hypercarbia	Mode: SIMV, APV +/–, AC Control: Volume or pressure Variables: PEEP 6-15+ cm H20 Long inspiratory time Vt 6-8 ml/kg
NEUROMUSCULAR DISORDERS (USUALLY WITH NORMAL COMPLIANCE)		
Spinal muscular atrophy Guillian-Barré syndrome Spinal cord injury CNS alterations Sedation Altered consciousness Central apnea	Normal V_T, low to normal PIPs Normal PaO_2/low FiO_2 Spontaneous breathing with support is preferable when possible Monitor exhaled V_T on PSV breaths	Mode: SIMV with PSV, APV, MMV Control: Volume Variables: PEEP 3-4 Vt 5-6 ml/kg Normal I:E Flow sensor

ARDS, adult respiratory distress syndrome; *FRC*, functional residual capacity; *IMV*, intermittent mandatory ventilation; *MAP*, mean airway pressure; *PEEP*, positive end-expiratory pressure; *PIP*, peak inspiratory pressure; *PSV*, pressure support ventilation; *RDS*, respiratory distress syndrome; *SIMV*, synchronized IMV; *APV*, adaptive pressure ventilation; *AC*, assist control; *ASV/MMV*, adaptive support ventilation/minimum minute ventilation.

b. *IRV* is employed when the usual strategies for enhancing oxygenation have failed. IRV is thought to allow MAP and V_T to be maintained at relatively lower levels without increasing PEEP, provided air trapping does not occur. Patients almost always require sedation and paralysis when receiving ventilation in this mode.

2. High-frequency ventilation

a. Historically, *high-frequency ventilation* (HFV) has been used to provide an alternative to patients for whom conventional ventilation is failing. In more recent years, HFV has been used earlier in the course of illness for specific reasons, including ventilation of low-birth-weight infants, prevention of barotrauma with severe restrictive lung disease, treatment for bronchopleural fistulas, airway disruptions, and severe pulmonary interstitial edema with markedly reduced C_L. With HFV, the shearing effect of repetitive opening and closing of alveoli, from PIP to PEEP (ΔP), is minimized compared with conventional ventilation. The two most commonly used are high-frequency oscillation ventilation (HFOV) and high-frequency jet ventilation (HFJV).

- HFOV: This ventilator uses a piston pump to drive a volume of gas into the lungs at a frequency of 60 to 3600 per minute (1-60 Hz). Exhalation is *active* (generated by the piston motion), unlike other high-frequency ventilators. Not only does this facilitate CO_2 removal, but it diminishes the potential for volume-stacking (inadvertent PEEP/MAP). The delivered V_T is less than or equal to the anatomic deadspace (V_D).
  - A *conventional ETT* is used with this ventilator, making the transition from a conventional ventilator to HFOV somewhat easier than with other high-frequency ventilators.
  - *Adequate lung inflation* at the start of this ventilatory technique is essential to avoid extensive microatelectasis. The MAP is initially set approximately 3 to 5 mm Hg higher than the patient's MAP on the conventional ventilator. After stabilization, the MAP can then be weaned.
  - *Four Mechanisms* of HFOV are MAP, power amplitude (ΔP), the frequency in hertz (Hz), and inspiratory time (T_I).
    (i) MAP determines lung expansion and FRC and is the principal mechanism for regulating oxygenation. An estimation of adequate lung volume can be made from a chest radiograph, in which the lung fields should be expanded to 8 to 10 ribs. Greater expansion than this may overly distend the lung, increasing resistance to gas delivery. Lower MAPs may cause microatelectasis to develop.
    (ii) The *power amplitude* (ΔP) regulates the "tidal volume." This mechanism determines the amplitude (or change in position) of the piston. Increasing amplitude will increase V_T to a point at which the V_T actually begins to diminish secondary to inadequate inspiratory time. With experience, a "gestalt" impression of chest "bounce" provides a quick estimate of appropriate ΔP, which may range from 30 to 80.
    (iii) *Frequency* measured in Hertz is similar to the IMV rate on a conventional ventilator, but it also directly influences tidal volume. The "optimal" hertz set point is that which facilitates CO_2 removal (in conjunction with ΔP). Delivered V_T will *decrease* at a threshold (individual) level. An increasing CO_2 can indicate that either the hertz is too high or the ΔP is too low.
    (iv) *Inspiratory time:* If inspiratory and expiratory time constants are equal, then the inspiratory time theoretically would be set at 50% (I:E = 1:1). However, the time constants are rarely equal, and an inspiratory time of 50% will cause air trapping with this form of ventilation. Conventionally, a 33% I time is used.
  - Determining initial HFOV settings:
    (i) MAP should be determined first, generally set 3 to 5 times higher than the MAP on the patient's conventional ventilator.
    (ii) Amplitude selection, estimated from the ΔP of the conventional ventilator, is a safe place to start. If CO_2 retention occurs, the amplitude can be increased, assuming MAP is optimized. The goal is to look for a "plateau" with ABGs to determine the optimal MAP and optimal amplitude.
    (iii) Frequency: Neonates generally require 10 to 15 Hz; infants, 8 to 10 Hz; young preschool age children, 6 to 8 Hz; and older children, 4 to 6 Hz. It is prudent to start on the lower end of the range to avoid air trapping (volume stacking).

(iv) Inspiratory time: Manufacturer recommendations suggest a 33% inspiratory time (66% expiratory time), altering only if all other maneuvers to improve ventilation fail. Volume stacking can occur with shorter expiratory times, which might be first noted with a MAP measurement that is drifting higher than the setting.

- HFJV: *HFJV* is a technique of ventilation that delivers a burst of gas from a high-pressure source at supraphysiologic frequencies, with a rate of 60 to 600 pulses per minute. The burst is delivered through a port of a specialized ETT, providing a V_T that is approximately equal to V_D (±2 mL/kg). Exhalation is *passive* around the jet cannula into the continuous flow circuit of the tandem ventilator. *HFJV* is used in tandem with a conventional ventilator to provide gas flow for entrainment. The V_T is both the burst of gas and the gas entrained from a tandem conventional ventilator at a set peak airway pressure. Disadvantages of HFJV are air trapping causing hypercarbia and overdistention and concern for reintubation in an emergency with the specialized endotracheal tube.
    - *Inspiratory driving pressure* provides the primary mechanism for regulating V_T delivery. The driving pressure range is 0 to 50 psi.
    - A *valve device* on the expiratory limb of the circuit provides PEEP.
    - *Respiratory rate* is regulated by a valve that creates timed flow interruption. The rate is adjusted to between 60 and 150 breaths per minute.
    - *Inspiratory time* is set as a percent of the total respiratory cycle, from 10% to 50%. Inspiratory times greater than 40% generally will not allow adequate expiratory time.

3. ECMO

a. *ECMO* uses a cardiopulmonary bypass machine, which provides an alternative method for gas exchange or cardiovascular support in patients for whom conventional therapy has failed.

b. *Candidates for ECMO:* Patients for whom ventilation strategies are failing or who are in severe cardiac failure refractive to standard therapy are candidates for ECMO. ECMO therapy is applied only to patients with potentially resolvable single-organ failure and potential for good neurologic outcome. Criteria for respiratory patients vary among hospitals but may include the following:

- Oxygenation index greater than 40 with maximal conventional therapy, which predicts 77% mortality
- Alveolar-arterial gradient (A-aDO_2) greater than 580 mm Hg with PIPs above 40, together defining a 81% mortality rate in children
- Static compliance less than 0.5 mL/cm H_2O/kg (Curley and Thompson, 2001)

c. *Contraindications for ECMO* include the following:

- Irreversible conditions
- Previous head bleeds in neonates
- Pulmonary hemorrhage
- Contraindication to heparinization

d. *Application*: The success with ECMO in neonates for respiratory failure has been well established. ECMO support for respiratory failure has not been as successful in pediatric patients as in neonates for reasons that remain unclear (Green et al., 1996).

- *Cardiac bypass*: Cannulation of a major artery and vein is used for both cardiac and pulmonary failure; the blood is diverted from the vein (usually the subclavian or femoral), through the membrane oxygenator, and back to the artery (often the carotid artery in an infant).

- *Pulmonary bypass:* Two major veins are cannulated to divert blood to the oxygenator and returned to the right atrium. This requires good cardiac function to maintain normal cardiac output. Veno-veno bypass is preferred, when possible, to avoid arterial vascular injury or compromise.
- See Chapter 3 for more information.

4. **Negative-pressure ventilation (NPV)**
   a. *Negative pressure ventilators* are used for patients with either neuromuscular disease or central apnea. The patient must have patent airway, and the structural qualities of the lung must be normal. NPV generates lung expansion with a ventilator that uses negative pressure, rather than positive pressure, using a device that surrounds the chest. The operating mechanism mimics a spontaneously breathing patient.
      - *Devices*: The historical model is an "iron lung" tank ventilator, used in the mid-twentieth century for polio patients. More recent devices include the "shell" device, called a *cuirasse,* which surrounds only the thorax like a clam shell. The difficulty is in obtaining a tight seal, requiring some precision in sizing. Another device, called a "raincoat," is aptly named and functions in the same manner as the shell.
      - *Principle of operation:* With the thorax enclosed in a shell or tank, negative pressure is created inside the shell, creating a "vacuum" pressure. The thoracic cage expands outward with this vacuum effect, thus increasing lung volume (and therefore decreasing alveolar pressure). A pressure gradient now exists between the mouth (atmospheric pressure) and the lung (subatmospheric pressure), causing air to fill the lungs. The ventilator is preset to release the negative pressure (an IMV rate), allowing the natural recoil of the lungs to allow exhalation.
      - *Limitations:* The seal of the tank or shell must be very tight. Dilation of the great vessels is exaggerated, diminishing cardiac output. NPV is cumbersome if the child requires 24-hour-a-day ventilation.
      - *Nursing care issues:* Children who need 24-hour-a-day NPV may be at risk for aspiration. Gastric jejunal tubes are indicated for enteral feedings. Hypothermia may also occur because of convective cooling from air being pulled through the collar. Skin integrity may be compromised. Finally, anxiety and claustrophobia may occur.
      - NPV is a method that can avoid a tracheostomy and perhaps is best suited for patients who do not require full time ventilation, such as those with night apnea (Ondine's curse).
5. **Noninvasive positive-pressure ventilation (NPPV)**
   a. *NPPV* provides positive pressure support through a nasal mask or nasal prongs without the use of an ETT, which is more invasive. A simple positive-pressure ventilator is used to deliver CPAP and or BIPAP.
   b. *Indications for NPPV:* Patients with acute respiratory failure may avoid intubation with early use of NPPV. Airway reflexes should be intact. NPPV may also facilitate earlier extubation in some patients as a bridge from intubation to spontaneous breathing. Patients with neuromuscular syndromes and apnea syndromes are also potential candidates for NPPV. All patients should have a normal respiratory drive.
   c. *Principle of operation:* NPPV is a pressure-controlled mode with continuous flow. For simple CPAP or expiratory pressure (EPAP), a baseline expiratory pressure is set as on a conventional ventilator. The patient breathes spontaneously, with the expiratory pressure maintaining FRC. BiPAP provides both inspiratory

pressure support (IPAP) and EPAP. The patient can breathe spontaneously; when the BiPAP ventilator senses patient effort, it delivers flow to achieve the higher pressure until patient demand ceases. A backup IMV rate can be set as well.

d. *Clinical considerations:* Patients must have normal airway secretions and adequate cough and gag reflexes and must demonstrate a sustained effort to breathe spontaneously. Complications include unrecognized ventilatory insufficiency, skin breakdown, aspiration, and gastric distention. Gastric feedings are determined individually; infants and smaller children may be safer with jejunal feedings than with gastric feedings, although more recent research has found no difference in rates of aspiration between nasogastric and jejunal feedings (Marik and Zaloga, 2003).

PATIENT CARE MANAGEMENT AND MONITORING OF THE CHILD ON MECHANICAL VENTILATION

A. Patient Care Management

1. **Airway management**: The goal is to maintain position and patency of the ETT. Retaping of the ETT should always be done with immediate availability of a skilled clinician who can reintubate the patient if necessary. A bag-mask circuit and suction should always be maintained at the bedside. If erosion of the lip, gumline, or tongue occurs, frequent repositioning of the tube is necessary. Some devices are available that can secure the tube in a midline position without pressure on any surface.
2. **Suctioning** the ETT should be performed per hospital standards and when there is evidence of increased airway secretions. Lightly sedated patients may indicate this by coughing. Increased PIP may be noted, and auscultation of the lungs may reveal upper airway rhonchi.
   - **a.** Always preoxygenate the patient before suctioning.
   - **b.** The suction catheter should be an appropriate size to allow ease of insertion. Insertion distance should be known and documented to avoid suctioning below the tip of the ETT.
   - **c.** Sterile technique is important to avoid contamination and possible ventilator-associated pneumonia. In-line suction catheters work well for most patients, particularly those patients with high MAPs, to avoid excessive volume loss (derecruitment).
   - **d.** Routine instillation of normal saline should not be necessary if the humidification is adequate. Tenacious secretions, however, occasionally require instillation (0.5-2 mL); after administration, allow several ventilator breaths to disperse the fluid or provide bag-valve assistance. Chronically tenacious secretions may also respond to deoxyribonuclease (DNAse), an agent commonly used with patients who have cystic fibrosis to break up sticky secretions.
3. **Assessment** of the child receiving mechanical ventilation (See Clinical Assessment discussion on page 52 for detailed information.)
   - **a.** *General observations:* Observe the comfort of the child, the synchrony between patient and ventilator, chest excursion, color and perfusion, and level of consciousness.
   - **b.** *Auscultation*: Note the symmetry of breath sounds; recall that the thin chest walls of infants transmit breath sounds to the opposite side. Evaluate the

quality of breath sounds, noting adventitious sounds, wheezing, or diminished aeration. Absent or severely diminished aeration over one entire lung is an urgent finding, reflecting either a pneumothorax, lung collapse, bronchial obstruction, malpositioned ETT, or a consolidation. Observe chest excursion and expansion (appropriate to the size of the child); observe from the foot of the bed to best appreciate asymmetry in chest expansion.

c. *Note the WOB.* Oxygen consumption (V_{O_2}) is greatly increased with increased WOB.

d. *Insertion distance of the ETT* should be verified and documented at frequent intervals.

e. *Note the volume and quality of secretions.* Ventilator-associated pneumonia (VAP) is a leading cause of nosocomial infection; a change in the quality of the secretions, especially in the presence of a fever, should prompt further investigation.

f. *Evaluate* for the presence of an air leak around the ETT; ideally an air leak will be present at a PIP of 25 mm Hg or less.

g. *Palpation:* Note the presence of crepitus, inspiratory crackles, or bony abnormalities. Note any points of tenderness.

B. Monitoring of the Child During Mechanical Ventilation

1. **Arterial blood gases (ABGs)**
   a. The conventional approach to verifying adequate oxygenation and ventilation is by periodic sampling of arterial blood with the goal of achieving normal blood gas values. However, capillary blood sampling provides reliable measurements of pH and Pa_{CO_2} (Harrison et al., 1997), and pulse oximetry has demonstrated reliability for monitoring of oxygenation.
   b. *Permissive hypercarbia* is a strategy for guiding ventilator manipulations that allows hypercarbia to exist with normal oxygenation, pH greater than 7.25, Pa_{CO_2} 45 to 80 mm Hg, and no evidence of cerebral dysfunction. The benefit of permissive hypercarbia is that it facilitates lower V_T ventilation, thereby minimizing the incidence of ALI (Hickling et al., 1994; Martin, 1995).
   c. *Pulse oximetry* should be used continuously. The oximetry probe should be routinely changed every 2 to 4 hours or by institution protocol to avoid burns.
2. **E_TCO_2 monitors:** E_TCO_2 monitors are useful for infants and children for trending, weaning, and monitoring hyperventilation therapy. They are also essential for quick recognition of ETT dislodgement.
3. **Transcutaneous CO_2 monitoring** (see earlier discussion)
4. **Alarms:** Ensure activation of ECG monitoring alarms. Appropriate ventilator alarms should be used according to the modes used.
5. **Serial chest radiographs:** Radiographs are important to verify ETT position and to evaluate pulmonary processes. The decision for x-ray examinations should be determined by the individual needs of each patient.
6. **Monitoring of neuromuscular blockade:** "Twitch monitoring" with a cutaneous nerve stimulator is used for patients who receive a neuromuscular blocker to assess the level of paralysis. It is performed every 6 to 8 hours to ensure that the minimum amount of medication is used (Murray et al., 1995). Alternatively, discontinuing the paralytic agent every 12 to 24 hours to assess for return of neurofunction may be used ("drug holiday"). The incidence of myopathy in patients who have been paralyzed, particularly those who are concurrently receiving steroids, is significant and should be considered on a daily basis (Martin et al., 2001).

7. **Monitoring ventilator parameters**
   a. Monitor V_T continuously; deviations of greater than 10% should be reported to the therapist for remediation.
   b. Monitor *PIPs* if in a volume-controlled mode; increasing PIP may indicate airway secretions or worsening lung compliance. Uncontrolled PIPs put the patient at risk for barotraumas.
   c. Monitor *PEEP* and observe for the presence of "auto-PEEP," which occurs with breath stacking or patient-ventilator asynchrony.
   d. Monitor patient *efforts to breathe*: How much pressure support does the patient require? Is the chest excursion adequate with the pressure support? Is the patient able to access flow to initiate a breath (sensitivity)? If in a spontaneous mode are the patient's V_T and RR adequate to meet minute ventilation requirements?
   e. *Ventilator graphics* can provide a visual assessment of the patient's pulmonary dynamics and patient-ventilator interface. Overdistention, auto-PEEP, change in C_L, and airway obstruction can be observed on these waveforms (Figure 2-34).

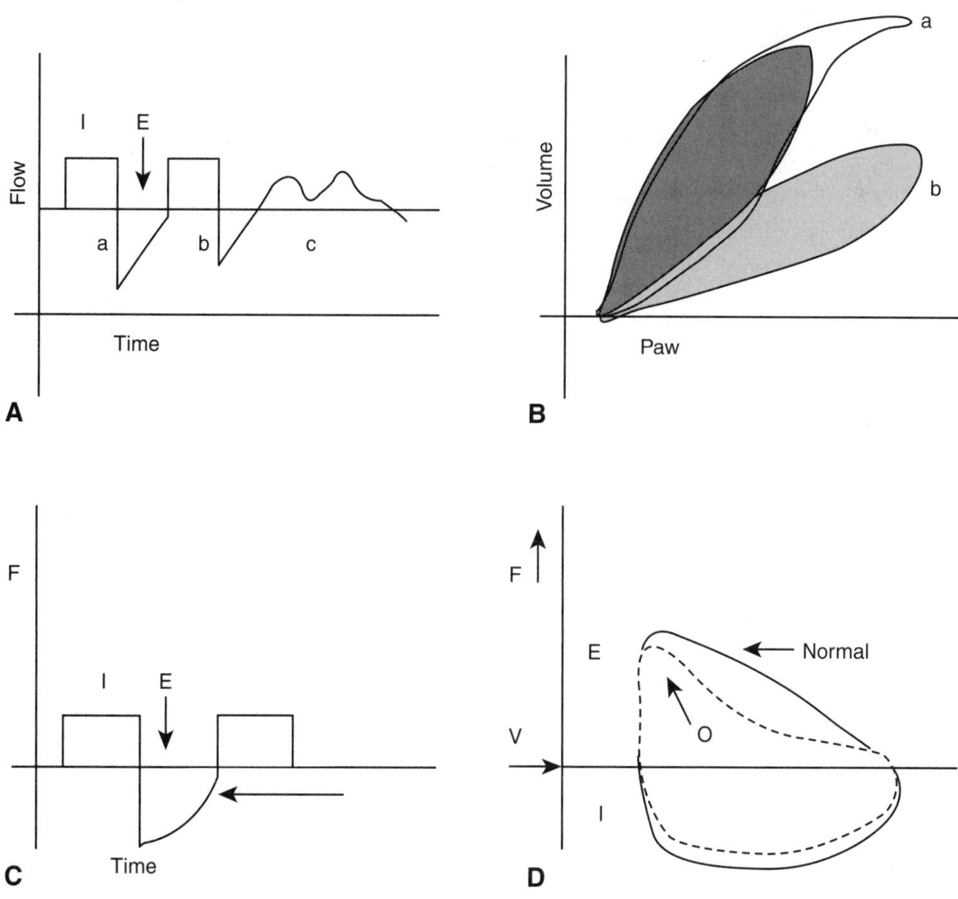

FIGURE 2-34 ■ Ventilator graphics. *PAW,* pulmonary airway pressure; *I,* inspiration; *E,* expiration. **A,** Normal flow-time (a) loop returns to baseline with normal contour; (b) patient dysynchrony. **B,** Volume-pressure loop (gray); (a) overdistention; (b) decreased compliance. **C,** Flow-time loop with auto-positive end-expiratory pressure (PEEP)/airway trapping; inspiration begins before expiration curve returns to baseline. **D,** Flow-volume loop with normal contour and obstruction (dotted line).

C. Supportive Care of the Child on Mechanical Ventilation

1. **Equipment function**
   a. The nurse should be knowledgeable about the mode of ventilation, the ventilator control, and phase variables selected.
   b. Alarm activation and both temperature and humidity of the ventilator should be noted. The temperature should range between 35 and 37 degrees centigrade.
2. **Fluids and electrolytes**
   a. Fluid retention may occur because of underlying disease or SIADH secondary to PPV.
   b. Calculation of input and output of fluid is essential for all patients. Fluid restriction may be used in some settings, but urine output should still be maintained at greater than 1 mL/kg per hour and hemodynamic stability ensured.
   c. Daily weights are valuable in evaluating fluid therapy and should be performed in all patients. Bed scales facilitate this task.
   d. Metabolic alterations affect electrolytes and pH. Permissive hypercarbia causes bicarbonate retention and chloride excretion.
3. **Nutrition**
   a. Early nutrition should be initiated for all patients. Enteral feedings are preferred and can be infused by a nasojejunal tube, even in the presence of hypoactive bowel sounds (Chellis et al., 1996a, b).
   b. Formal nutrition screening should be done early and serially. Indirect calorimetry is the optimal assessment tool, when available, but is usually unnecessary.
   c. Restriction of carbohydrates to less than 30% of metabolic needs may be necessary for patients with ventilatory insufficiency. Excess carbohydrate loads produce excess CO_2 (respiratory quotient [RQ] ≥ 1), thus increasing ventilatory work to remove the CO_2. Difficulty in weaning from a ventilator is attributable to this in some cases.
4. **Skin care:** Patient repositioning is done as often as tolerated at a minimum of every 2 hours. When feasible, the prone position offers significant benefit for lung aeration as well (Curley et al., 2004; Erhard, 1995) by improving ventilation/perfusion matching, although early results of a multicenter trial do not demonstrate a difference in outcomes (Personal communication, Curley). Use dermal protection on pressure points. High-risk patients, especially those who do not tolerate turning, may require pressure reduction or relief from specialized mattresses. Careful inspection of all pressure points should be documented at least every 8 hours.
5. **Mobilization of pulmonary secretions**
   a. Adequate humidification should be ensured, with proper temperature regulation. Low temperatures may cause secretions to become thick and sticky. High and low temperatures may affect the patient's core body temperature.
   b. Assess the patient for airway secretions and suction as indicated. Maintain sterile technique for suctioning. Use of chest physiotherapy either by manual technique or by the vibrating vest technique may be useful.
6. **Sedation and pain management**
   a. Sedation is frequently needed for optimal ventilator management and for patient comfort. However, noninvasive measures should always be offered first, including the presence of parents, a favorite blanket or toy, ear plugs to block out noise (especially with high-frequency ventilators), and darkening the room.

   b. Assess the patient's need for pain medication: The presence of an ETT, suctioning, and ventilator breaths is uncomfortable at the least and often painful.
   c. Conventional pharmacologic therapy usually includes a benzodiazepine or a narcotic. The choice in medications is determined individually.
   d. Children who are paralyzed, pharmacologically or otherwise, must have both sedation and pain medication. Monitor for increased pupil size, tachycardia, or increased blood pressure to determine the adequacy of sedation and pain management.

7. **Psychological needs of the child and family**
   a. Communication barriers and sometimes a diminished level of consciousness alter the child's expressive language and family relationships. Strategies for minimizing barriers include picture boards for preschoolers, picture or alphabet boards for school-age children, or predetermined hand signals. A dry-erase board is appreciated by children old enough to write messages.
   b. Provide sedation as needed for comfort but also provide environmental relief through family presence, family voices on tape, or stories or music on cassettes.
   c. Establish a night-day routine for the patient as early as possible. Include the family in this plan and, optimally, post the plan on the patient's door or at the bedside.
   d. Balance the needs for patient safety with developmental needs. Restraints are usually necessary but can be removed when there is supervision.

D. Strategies for Weaning from Ventilation

1. **Indications for readiness:** Many strategies have been proposed, but currently there is no one documented method for ensuring a successful weaning-to-extubation process. The following criteria are goals to achieve before extubation is actually considered:
   - Hemodynamic stability
   - $Sa{O_2}$ greater than 90% with an $Fi{O_2}$ of 0.4 or less
   - PEEP 5 cm H_2O or lower
   - Adequacy of respiratory muscles to sustain spontaneous ventilation (V_T ≥5 mL/kg)
   - $Pa{CO_2}$ in a range acceptable for the patient
   - Presence of an adequate gag and cough reflex
   - Adequate level of consciousness
   - Adequate respiratory effort, with a negative inspiratory force (NIF) greater than -20 to -25 cm H_2O on serial measurements
   - Pain control is adequate without excessive sedation
2. **Weaning techniques:**
   a. *Before weaning,* parameters to be monitored for each patient should be clearly identified. They may include $Sa{O_2}$, $Pa{CO_2}$, respiratory rate, V_T, and general effort and color. *All* patients should have ECG monitoring and pulse oximetry during this process. There are numerous strategies, but the more commonly employed techniques include the following:
   b. *Spontaneous trials* may occur with SIMV or PSV with a CPAP of 3 to 4 cm H_2O to maintain baseline FRC.
      - Trials of spontaneous breathing without PSV support may be used to verify readiness to extubate or as a method of improving muscle endurance. To assess for readiness to extubate, often a 1- to 2-hour trial is desirable, observing WOB, V_T, and aeration. Spontaneous trials may be also used for

"muscle conditioning" in which planned trials of a stated duration, several times a day, are performed, noting patient tolerance during each. With each successive trial, the time is gradually increased while observing effort, exhaled V_T, and when applicable, ABGs. Patient should be allowed a 6- to 8-hour period (nighttime may be optimal) for full recovery.

- PSV + spontaneous trials provide enough support to overcome the resistance of the ETT; PSV is weaned, by 1 to 2 every 4 to 8 hours, as tolerated, observing trends in exhaled V_T and respiratory rate as support is withdrawn. PSV spontaneous trials can be approached similarly to that with SIMV (when IMV rate is weaned to zero). Again, careful observation of the patient, including spontaneous V_T, WOB, and adequacy of aeration is required. Depending on ETT size, the reccommended *minimum* level of PSV (Randolph et al., 2002) is as follows:

ETT Size	PSV
3.0-3.5	10
4.0-4.5	8
>5.0	6

Be aware that, with reduction in PSV, fatigue or atelectasis may not be apparent for 3 to 6 hours or more.

  ◦ SIMV with PSV weaning: Weaning from this mode can be accomplished either by first weaning the PSV to the recommended minimum, and then weaning the IMV rate or vice versa. The rate of IMV changes and subsequent weaning of PSV should be guided by an individualized plan and assessment criteria. The temptation to accelerate the weaning process in patients who have been intubated for more than a few days may result in atelectasis or a collapsed lung, thereby delaying the entire process.

E. Complications of Mechanical Ventilation

1. **Causes of acute deterioration** in an intubated child can be evaluated using the mnemonic **DOPE:** dislodgement, obstruction, pneumothorax (or other air leaks), equipment failure.
2. **Complications from longer-term ventilation**
   a. *Oxygen toxicity:* Patients receiving greater than 50% FiO_2 for prolonged periods of time may develop parenchymal changes from oxygen exposure (Durbin and Wallace, 1993). Oxygen should be treated as a medication with strict adherence to prescription guidelines. Continuous monitoring of FiO_2 is strongly recommended. The lowest acceptable SaO_2 measurement for the child should be clearly established while FiO_2 is maintained at the lowest possible level.
   b. *Acute lung injury (ALI):* Alveolar overdistention is responsible for the development of pulmonary injury (Martin, 1995). Cyclic opening and closing of lung units with large volumes cause injury by "shearing" forces. Exhaled V_T volumes should be continuously monitored and documented every 1 to 2 hours. Parameters for "acceptable" exhaled volumes should be established for each patient. If the patient is not pressure limited, PIP should be noted; if PIP increases, it is indicative of airway secretions or changes in lung compliance.
   c. *Barotrauma* has been reported to occur in 13% (N = 100) of patients with ARDS who are receiving mechanical ventilation (Schnapp et al., 1995). High PIPs or distending pressures or sudden changes in either may cause alveolar rupture.

Continuous observation of lung volumes and pressures is required to minimize the occurrence of this complication.

d. *Atelectasis* occurs from nonuniform distribution of V_T, inadequate V_T, and adsorption atelectasis. Patient positioning may affect the site of atelectasis. Patient repositioning (including head elevation) should be done every 1 to 2 hours. The prone position is useful for lower lobe aeration and should be used when feasible (Erhard, 1995).

e. *Pneumonia:* VAP is recognized as a significant cause of morbidity in the PICU:

- ETT becomes quickly colonized with bacteria, most commonly gram-negative organisms, thus providing entry to the lungs.
- Aspiration is a constant risk. The presence of an ETT does *not* guarantee protection for patients. A nasogastric tube is usually recommended for drainage. Current research questions the practice of the routine use of gastric acid neutralization by such agents as histamine-2 blockers. It is thought that alkaline gastric secretions impose a greater risk for nosocomial pneumonia than acidic (Apte et al., 1992).
- The head of the bed should be elevated 30 degrees in all ventilated patients.
- The complete blood count with differential and temperature surveillance should be evaluated while the ETT is in place. When a *new* ETT is placed in a patient with a pneumonic process, tracheal aspirate specimens for Gram stain and culture can be useful. However, the specimens should be interpreted in conjunction with clinical factors, types of organisms, and evidence of inflammatory cell infiltration.
- Decreased cardiac output caused by compression of the great vessels secondary to elevated intrathoracic pressures (especially high levels of PEEP) is a potential problem. This can be remediated with adequate volume (preload) expansion.
- A central vascular line for monitoring CVP or pulmonary pressures is often essential in hemodynamically unstable patients.
- SIADH may occur because of stimulation of thoracic receptors, causing third spacing or fluid retention. Hourly urine output measurements and serial serum sodium and protein measurements allow early detection.
- *Complications from intubation* include postextubation edema, tracheal ulcerations, vocal cord injury, granulomas or polyp formation, sinusitis, and airway obstruction resulting from a plugged ETT or bronchospasm.
- Evidence for the use of dexamethasone before extubation continues to be perceived as controversial. However, one recent meta-analysis of six studies supports the use of dexamethasone prior to intubation (Markovitz and Randolph, 2002).
- Helium and oxygen admixture (Heliox) is an intervention for airway disease that has had notable success in children. Helium is a lighter atom than oxygen and therefore the transfer of helium provides more laminar flow; it acts as a carrier of oxygen lower into the respiratory tract.
- All newly extubated children should be positioned upright with humidified air or oxygen. No sedative agents should be administered. Be cautious with deep tracheal suctioning because it might stimulate laryngospasm.
- Pharmacologic management of the patient receiving mechanical ventilation is usually required; if the patient has been on narcotic or benzodiazepine therapy for longer than 5 to 7 days, withdrawal symptoms may occur with abrupt discontinuation.

LUNG TRANSPLANTATION

A. Definition and Etiology

Lung transplant is defined as surgical replacement of one or both lungs or a heart-lung bloc using donor organs for end-stage parenchymal or vascular lung disease. Of the more than 17,500 lung transplants reported to the International Society for Heart and Lung Transplantation Registry as of 2001, more than 1200 pediatric lung and heart-lung transplants have been performed. Since 1996, when 80 transplants were performed that year, the average number of transplants has declined to 50 to 60 per year. Children have undergone heart-lung, double-lung, sequential bilateral single-lung, and single-lung transplantation. The most common procedure today is the sequential bilateral single-lung transplant (Table 2-25).

B. Pathophysiology

1. **Recipient candidates** for lung transplantation have end-stage parenchymal or vascular lung disease with significant impact on activities of daily living.
2. **Candidates with primary PHTN** may have signs of right ventricular failure (increased CVP, hepatomegaly, jugular venous distention, periorbital edema, and pulmonary effusion) and systemic or suprasystemic pulmonary artery pressures.
3. **Candidates with congenital heart disease**, Eisenmenger syndrome, or pulmonary A-V malformation may demonstrate profound cyanosis, clubbing, polycythemia, and hypoxemia exceeding the child's normal values.
4. **Candidates with abnormal airway function** have PFT results (FEV_1, FVC, and forced expiratory flow rates) less than 30% of normal values for age, height, and weight, indicating severe obstructive disease (Armitage et al., 1993).

TABLE 2-25
Indications for Lung Transplantation

Airway diseases
Cystic fibrosis
Chronic bronchitis
Emphysema
Bronchiectasis
Pulmonary hypertension
Primary
Secondary (related to other heart or lung disease)
Interstitial lung diseases
Pulmonary fibrosis
Idiopathic pulmonary fibrosis
Desquamative interstitial pneumonitis
Arteriovenous malformation
Graft-versus-host disease
Congenital heart disease, often with Eisenmenger's syndrome
Cardiomyopathy with elevated pulmonary vascular resistance
Retransplantation related to chronic rejection
Rheumatoid lung
Proteus syndrome

Data from Armitage JM et al: Pediatric lung transplantation: expanding indications: 1985-1993, *J Heart Lung Transplant* 12 (6; pt 2): S246-S254, 1993.

C. Candidate Evaluation

1. **Candidates selected for single-lung transplantation** require normal heart function or reversible right ventricular dysfunction and absence of pulmonary infection.
2. **Candidates for double-lung transplantation** require normal heart function or reversible right ventricular dysfunction but may have some infectious processes present. Both heart and lungs must be transplanted in children with a complex, nonrepairable cardiac defect or inadequate cardiac function in addition to end-stage pulmonary disease. Previous thoracotomy or sternotomy is not an absolute contraindication to transplantation.
3. **Patients with cystic fibrosis** are difficult to evaluate because the course of their disease process will wax and wane. Dependence on supplementary oxygen or an FEV_1 below 40% may indicate the need to begin evaluation for transplantation (Sweet, 2003). The presence of *Pseudomonas cepacia* in the airway or sinuses is usually a contraindication to transplantation, but this is dependent on sputum cultures and sensitivity of the *P. cepacia*.
4. **Invasive and noninvasive diagnostic studies** for transplant evaluation may include the following:
   a. *Chest x-ray examination*
   b. *ECG*
   c. *Transthoracic or transesophageal echocardiogram or both*
   d. *Multiple unit gated acquisition (MUGA) scan* or gated pool study of cardiac function
   e. *Pulmonary function studies*
   f. *ABGs* (in some centers)
   g. *Exercise study with pulse oximetry* (6-minute walk or bicycle test or none if high risk)
   h. *Quantitative V/Q scan*
   i. *Blood chemistry and hematology studies*, including viral serology, PRA (percent reactive antibody), and tissue typing if the PRA is greater than 20%. Tissue typing is done at the time of transplantation.

D. Donor Evaluation

1. **Criteria for acceptance of donor lungs** are continuing to evolve. The opportunity for clinical assessment of the cadaveric donor is helpful in discerning the quality of the lungs for transplantation.
2. **Desirable criteria for donor lungs** include the following:
   a. *A clear chest radiograph*
   b. *Arterial oxygen tension of 400 mm Hg on 100% oxygen*
   c. *Negative results from sputum cultures and Gram stain*
   d. *Direct visualization of the lungs through bronchoscopy at the time of procurement*
   e. *Viral serology of the donor*
   f. *Administration of IV antibiotics and steroids and aerosolized gentamicin*
3. **Relative contraindications** to lung procurement include pulmonary infection (moderate yeast in sputum cultures is an absolute contraindication), pulmonary contusions, chest tubes, tracheostomies, and evidence of significant aspiration.

E. Patient Care Management

1. **Provide and monitor immunosuppression:** Cyclosporine or tacrolimus is initiated in the postoperative period. In addition, patients receive another immunosuppressive agent, such as azathioprine, and steroids.

2. **Monitor and treat rejection:** Bronchoscopy with bronchoalveolar lavage (BAL) and transbronchial biopsy is performed on a regular basis (at least 2 and 4 weeks after transplantation) to assess graft acceptance. BAL specimens are studied for total cell count with differential, microbiologic assays and immunologically with a donor-specific lymphocyte test. Standardized histologic criteria are used for grading rejection; grade A0-A4. Acute rejection grade A2 and above is usually treated with high-dose steroids. Persistent rejection may be treated with a T-cell preparation such as OKT3 or Atgam. Other interventions may include total lymphoidal irradiation or mycophenolate.
3. **Monitor for infection and provide infection prophylaxis:**
   a. *Preoperative evaluations* include titers from the donor and recipient to evaluate hepatitis A, B, C, and D viruses, herpesvirus, Epstein-Barr virus, HIV, toxoplasma, and CMV.
   b. *Serologic follow-up* is performed on patients who have negative results at the time of transplant. Skin testing for tuberculosis and anergy is routine.
   c. *Sputum cultures* are obtained on a routine basis from candidates with cystic fibrosis to guide prophylaxis.
   d. During the perioperative period, *antibiotic coverage* is planned to cover bacterial sensitivities from the donor culture and adjusted if necessary based on surveillance cultures.
   e. *Routine postoperative care* includes thorough pulmonary toilet using strict aseptic technique. Good handwashing should be emphasized, along with assurance of compliance from all health care providers and family members.
   f. *Ventilator tubing* and other invasive tubing are changed regularly.
   g. *Children are monitored*, and cultures are obtained to screen for signs of infection, including: fever or temperature instability, increasing quantity or a change in the nature of the pulmonary secretions, increasing respiratory distress, worsening ABGs, leukocytosis or leukopenia, and radiographic changes.
4. **Monitor systemic perfusion parameters.**
5. **Monitor nutritional status.** Monitor intake, output, and weight and calculate caloric requirements. Nutritional consults should be sought for patients with previous malnourishment (e.g., patients with cystic fibrosis). Provide an enteral or parenteral diet as ordered. Monitor the child's wound healing.

F. Complications of Lung Transplantation

1. **The most serious and frequently occurring complications** in children include rejection, infection, and posttransplantation lymphoproliferative disease (PTLD) (Table 2-26).
   a. Most patients have one to two episodes of *acute cellular rejection* in the first 3 months following transplantation, but this rejection is unrelated to the primary immunosuppressant used.
   b. *Chronic rejection* is characterized by obliterative bronchiolitis (OB), which occurs most commonly 1 to 3 years after transplantation but can occur as early as 6 months; 50% of lung-transplant patients will have OB at 5 years after transplant, and 40% of these patients die.
   c. *Risk factors for the development of OB* include acute rejection grade A2 or greater and prolonged ischemic time (Sweet, 2000).
   d. *Most infections* that cause death in the noncystic fibrosis transplant recipient are related to viral and fungal infections. Severe bacterial infection is common in cystic fibrosis. All CMV-positive or mismatched recipients routinely receive IV ganciclovir (DHPG) for a minimum of 4 weeks after transplantation. Oral

TABLE 2-26
Complications of Lung Transplantation

Postoperative period
Ischemia of the anastomosis site
Bleeding
Infection
Systemic hypertension
Phrenic nerve paresis
First 3 months
Hypertension
Rejection
Infection
First year
Viral infection
Rejection
Hypertension
After first year
Viral infection
Rejection
Posttransplant lymphoproliferative disease (PTLD)

acyclovir has demonstrated poor absorption in pediatric pharmacokinetic studies and has not been shown to be advantageous in most instances. Only CMV-negative blood products are used for transplant recipients. Besides its threat as an infectious process, CMV also increases the risk of subsequent rejection related to upregulation of the immune system.

2. **Pediatric organ recipients** are at increased risk for PTLD, especially when the transplanted organ has significant amounts of donor-derived lymphatic tissue, such as in lung and small bowel transplantations (Armitage et al., 1995).
   a. *Patients who test negative for Epstein-Barr virus* before transplantation and receive donor organs that test positive for Epstein-Barr virus have the greatest risk for PTLD.
   b. Most often *infection* occurs in the lung of a recipient and will occur within the first year after transplantation. In some cases, associated infections will occur.
3. **Children with cystic fibrosis** are an ever-increasing percentage of transplant recipients but are high risk and pose several challenges. Their airways are often colonized with organisms that are resistant to antibiotics or difficult to treat. They are often malnourished, have had long-term IV or enteral catheters, and often have chronic sinusitis and osteoporosis.
4. **Complications** can occur from the sutured airways for the following reasons:
   a. *Systemic arterial revascularization* is not directly reestablished.
   b. *Donor airways* are dependent on collaterals from the pulmonary circulation until revascularization occurs from ingrowth of surrounding tissues.
   c. *Ischemia* surrounding the anastomosis site has been a problem for some patients, especially those with frequent rejection and infection episodes. Collateral flow to the bronchial level is greater than that to the pericarinal trachea. Hence bibronchial anastomosis has been more successful. Heart-lung recipients are protected somewhat after transplantation because less interruption of potential collateral channels occurs with transplantation of the heart-lung bloc and surrounding tissues.

G. Survival and Mortality

1. **Results of lung transplantation** in children have been promising. Since experimentation with lung grafting in adults occurred first, pediatric patients have benefited from the experience. In pediatric patients (as opposed to adults), primary nonfunction of the graft because of preservation injury has been rare. One-year survival rates have been reported by the International Society for Heart and Lung Transplantation registry to be about 80%-90%; 3-year reported survival is 60%-70% depending on age.
2. Lower survival rates at 1 year have been reported for patients with cystic fibrosis compared with survival rates in children with congenital heart disease. Infection poses the highest risk for patients with cystic fibrosis.

REFERENCES

Adams WG, Deaver KA, Cochi SL, et al: Decline in childhood *Hamophilus influenzae* type b (BiB) in the HiB vaccine era. *JAMA* 269:221-226, 1993.

Aggarwal AN, Gupta D, Behera D, et al: Analysis of static pulmonary mechanics helps to identify functional defects in survivors of acute respiratory distress syndrome. *Crit Care Med* 28:3480-3483, 2000.

American College of Emergency Physicians: Clinical Policies Committee. *Ann Emerg Med* 40(5):551-552, 2002.

American Society of Anesthesiologists Task Force on Sedation and Analgesia by Non-Anesthesiologists. CO_2 *Anesthesiology* 96(4):1004-1017, 2002.

Armitage JM, Kurland G, Michaels M et al.: Critical issues in pediatric lung transplantation. *J Thorac Cardiovasc Surg*. 109(1): 60-65, 1995.

Ashton H: Guidelines for the rational use of benzodiazepines: when and what to use. *Drugs* 48(1):25-40, 1994.

Banacalari EH: Neonatal chronic lung disease. In Fanaroff A, Martin RF. *Neonatal perinatal medicine,* ed 7, St Louis, 2002, Mosby.

Barker H, Fanconi S, Baeckert P et al: The effects of motion on performance of oximetry in volunteers. *Anesthesia* 86:101-108, 1997.

Barst RJ, Ivy D, Dingemanse J et al: Pharmacokinetics, safety and efficacy of bosentan in pediatric patients with pulmonary arterial hypertension. *Clin Pharmacol Ther* 73:372-382, 2003.

Barst RJ, Rubin LJ, Long WA et al: A comparison of continuous intravenous epoprostenol with conventional therapy for primary pulmonary hypertension. *N Engl J Med* 334:296-301, 1996.

Ben-Menachem T, McCarthy B, Fogel R: Prophylaxis for stress-related GI hemorrhage: a cost effective analysis. *Crit Care Med* 24(2):338-343, 1996.

Bernard GR, Artigas A, Brigham KL et al: The American-European Consensus Conference on ARDS: definitions, mechanisms, relevant outcomes, and clinical trial coordination. *Am J Respir Crit Care Med* 149:818-824, 1994.

Bhandari A, Bhandari V: Pathogenesis, pathology and pathophysiology of pulmonary sequelae of bronchopulmonary dysplasia in premature infants. *Frontiers in Bioscience* 1(8):e370-e380, 2003.

Bisgaard H, Nielsen KG: Bronchoprotection with a leukotriene receptor antagonist in asthmatic preschool children. *Am J Respir Crit Care Med* 161:1-4, 2000.

Bliss D, Silen M: Pediatric thoracic trauma. *Crit Care Med* 30 (11 Suppl):S4009-4015, 2002.

Blumer JL: Principles of drug disposition in the critically ill child. In Fuhrman B, Zimmerman J, eds. *Pediatric Critical Care*. St Louis, Mo, 1992, Mosby.

Bohn D, Kissoon N: Acute asthma. *Pediatr Crit Care Med* 2(2):151-163, 2001.

Briones TL, Press SV: New ventilatory techniques. *Crit Care Nurse* 12(4):51-58, 1992.

Broide DH: Researchers find clues to which asthmatics are likely to experience near-fatal or fatal attacks. *CHEST 2002*. 68th Annual Scientific Assembly of the American College of Chest Physicians.

Bulloch B, Schubert CJ, Brophy PD et al: Cause and clinical characteristics of rib fractures in infants. *Pediatrics* 105:48-53, 2000.

Cadzow SP, Armstron ML: Rib fractures in infants: red alert! *J Paediatr Child Health* 36:322-326, 2000.

Carroll W, Dhillon R: Sildenafil as a treatment for pulmonary hypertension. *Arch Dis Child* 88(9):827-828, 2003.

Carter BG, Wiwczaruk D, Hochmann M et al: Performance of transcutaneous PCO_2 and pulse oximetry monitors in newborns and infants after cardiac surgery. *Anaesth Intens Care* 29(3):260-265, 2001.

Casado-Flores J, Mora E, Perez-Corral F et al: Prognostic value of gastric intramucosal pH in critically ill children. *Crit Care Med* 26:1123-1127, 1998.

Centers for Disease Control and Prevention (CDC) National Center for Health Statistics: *Health, United States, 2004.* U.S. Department of Health and Human Services, Hyattsville, MD, 2004.

Charney DS, Mihic SJ, Harris RA: Hypnotics and sedatives. In Hardman JG, Limbird, LE, editors: *The pharmacologic basis of therapeutics,* ed 10, New York, 2001, McGraw-Hill.

Chellis MJ, Sanders S: Bedside placement of nasojejunal feeding tubes in the pediatric intensive care unit. *JPEN J Parenter Enteral Nutr* 20(1):88-90, 1996b.

Chellis MJ, Sanders S: Early enteral feeding in PICU. *JPEN J Parenter Enteral Nutr* 20(1):71-73, 1996a.

Ciarallo L, Brousseau D, Reinert S: Higher-dose intravenous magnesium therapy for children with moderate to severe acute asthma. *Arch Pediatr Adolesc Med* 154: 979-983, 2000.

Coalson JJ: Pathology of the new bronchopulmonary dysplasia. *Semin Neonatol* 8(1): 73-81, 2003.

Cooper A, Barlow B, DiScala C et al: Mortality and truncal injury: the pediatric perspective. *J Pediatr Surg* 29:33-38, 1994.

Cray SH, Robinson BH, Cox P: Lactic academia and bradyarrhythmias in children sedated with propofol. *Crit Care Med* 26:2087-2093, 1998.

Curley MAQ, Thompson JE: Oxygenation and ventilation. In Curley MAQ, Moloney-Harmon PA, editors: *Critical care nursing of infants and children,* ed 2, Philadelphia, 2001, W. B. Saunders.

Day RW, Guarin M, Lynch J: Inhaled NO in children with severe lung disease: results of acute and prolonged therapy with 2 concentrations. *Crit Care Med* 24(2): 215-221, 1996.

Dearborn DG, Smith PG, Dahms BB et al: Clinical profile of thirty infants with acute pulmonary hemorrhage in Cleveland. *Pediatrics* 110:627-637, 2002.

Dearborn DG: Pulmonary hemosiderosis. In Behrman RE, Kliegman RM, Eenson HB, editors: *Nelson: textbook of pediatrics,* ed 17, Philadelphia, 2004, W. B. Saunders.

Dellinger RP, Zimmerman JL, Taylor RW et al: Effects of nitric oxide in patients with acute respiratory distress syndrome: results of a randomized phase II trial. *Crit Care Med* 26:15-23, 1998.

DeNicola LK: Noninvasive monitoring in the pediatric intensive care unit. *Pediatr Clin North Am* 48(3):573-588, 2001.

Dent C, Fontan J: Long-term therapy for pulmonary hypertension in children. *Current Opinions in Pediatrics* 11(3):2218-2122, 1999.

Doull IJM, Mok Q, Tasker RC: Tracheomalacia in preterm infants with chronic lung disease. Archives of Diseases of Children. *Fetal Neonatal Ed* 76:F203-205, 1997.

Dworski R, FitzGerald GA, Oates JA: Effect of oral prednisone on airway inflammatory mediators in atopic asthma. *Am J Respir Crit Care Med* 149:953-959, 1994.

Egan TD, Brock-Utne JG: Asystole and anesthesia induction with a fentanyl, propofol, and succinylcholine sequence. *Anesth Analg* 73:818-820, 1991.

Epstein CE, Elidemir O, Colasurdo GN et al: Time course of hemosiderin production by alveolar macrophages in a murine model. *Chest* 120:2013-2020, 2001.

Erhard M: The effect of patient position on arterial O_2 sat. *Crit Care Nurse* 10(10):31-36, 1995.

Evans DA, Wilmott RW, Whitset JA: Surfactant replacement therapy for acute respiratory distress syndrome in children. *Pediatric Pulmonology*, 21(5):328-336, 1996.

Fadler JC, Arnold JH, Nichols DG, et al: Acute respiratory distress syndrome. In Rogers M, editor: *Textbook of pediatric intensive care,* ed 3, Baltimore, 1996, Williams & Wilkins.

Frantz TD, Rasgon BM: Acute epiglottitis: changing epidemiologic patterns. *Otolaryngol Head Neck Surg* 109:457-460, 1993.

Furnival RA: Controversies in pediatric thoracic and abdominal trauma. *Clin Pediatr Emerg Med* 2(1);48-62, 2001.

Garofano RP, Barst RJ: Exercise testing in children with primary pulmonary hypertension. *Pediatric Cardiol* 20:61-64, 1999.

Giaid A, Yanagisawa M, Langleben D et al: Expression of endothelin-1 in the lungs of patients with pulmonary hypertension. *N Engl J Med* 328:175-176, 1993.

Gianotti L, Alexander JW, Nelson JL et al: Role of early enteral feeding and acute starvation post-burn bacterial translocation and host defense: prospective randomized trials. *Crit Care Med* 22:265-272, 1994.

Gorenflo M, Mathias N et al: Pulmonary hypertension in infancy and childhood. *Cardiology in the Young* 13: 219-227, 2003.

Gormella TL: *Neonatology: management, procedures, on-call problems, diseases and drugs*. New York, 2004, McGraw-Hill.

Grant MJC, Curley MAQ: Pulmonary critical care problems. In Curley MAQ, Moloney-Harmon PA, editors: *Critical care nursing of infants and children,* ed 2, Philadelphia, 2001, W. B. Saunders.

Green TP, Timmons OD et al: The impact of ECMO on survival in pediatric patients with acute respiratory failure. *Crit Care Med* 24(2):323-329, 1996.

Harrison AM, Lynch JM, Dean JM et al: Comparison of capillary and arterial blood gases in critically ill pediatric patients. *Crit Care Med* 25(11):1904-1908, 1997.

Haworth S: Primary pulmonary hypertension in childhood. *Arch Dis Child* 79:452-455, 1998.

Hazinski MF, Zaritzky AL et al: *Pediatric advanced life support provider manual.* Dallas, 2002, American Heart Association.

Hickling K, Walsh J, et al: Low mortality rate in adult RDS using low volume, pressure-limited ventilation with permissive hypercapnia: a prospective study. *Crit Care Med* 22(10):1568-1578, 1994.

Hirschl: Liquid ventilation improves pulmonary function, gas exchange and lung injury in a model of respiratory failure. *Ann Surg* 221:79-88, 1995.

The IMPACT-RSV Study Group: palivizumab, a humanized respiratory syncytial virus monoclonal antibody, reduces hospitalization from respiratory syncytial virus infection in high-risk infants. *Pediatrics* 102:531-537, 1998.

Izurieta HS, Thompson WW, Kramarz P, et al: Influenza and the rates of hospitalization for respiratory disease among infants and young children. *N Engl J Med* 342:232-239, 2000.

Jobe AJ: The new BPD: an arrest of lung development. *Pediatr Res* 46:641-643, 1999.

Kristjansson S, Berg-Kelly K, Winso E: Inhalation of racemic adrenaline in the treatment of mild and moderately severe croup: clinical symptom score and oxygen saturation measurements for evaluation of treatment effects. *Acta Pediatr* 83:1156, 1994.

Leuchte, HH, Schwaiblmair M, Baumgartner RA et al: Hemodynamic response to sildenafil, nitric oxide, and iloprost in primary pulmonary hypertension. *Chest* 125:580-586, 2004.

Lewis JF, Brackenbury A: Role of exogenous surfactant in acute lung injury. *Crit Care Med* 31(4):S324-S327, 2003.

Liggins GC, Howie RN: A controlled trial of antepartum glucocorticoid treatment for prevention of the respiratory distress syndrome in premature infants. *Pediatrics* 50:515, 1972.

Luchetti M, Ferrero F, Gallini C: Multicenter, randomized controlled study of porcine surfactant in severe respiratory syncytial virus-induced respiratory failure. *Pediatr Crit Care Med* 3(3)261-268, 2002.

Luria JW, Gonzalez-del-Rey JA, DiBiulio GA et al: Effectiveness of oral or nebulized dexamethasone for children with mild croup. *Pediatr Adolesc Med* 155:1340, 2001.

Majnemer A, Riley P, Shevell M et al: Severe bronchopulmonary dysplasia increases risk for later neurological and motor sequelae in preterm survivors. *Dev Med Child Neurol* 42(1):53-60, 2000.

Mansmann H: Management of status asthmaticus in childhood. In Gershwin NE, Hakpin GM, eds. *Bronchial asthma.* New Jersey, 1994, Human Press.

Marik PE, Zaloga GP: Gastric versus post-pyloric feeding: as systematic review. *Crit Care Med* 7(3), R46-R51, 2003.

Markovitz BP, Randolph AG: Corticosteroids for prevention of reintubation and post-extubation stridor in pediatric patients: a meta-analysis. *Pediat Crit Care* 3:223-226, 2002.

Martin L: New approaches to ventilation in infants and children. *Curr Opin Pediatr* 7:250-261, 1995.

Martin L, Bratton SL, Quint P et al: Prospective documentation of sedative, analgesic, and neuromuscular blocking agent use in infants and children in the intensive care unit: a multicenter perspective. *Pediatr Crit Care Med* 2(3):205-210, 2001.

Martin L, Bratton S, Walker L: Principles and practice of respiratory support and mechanical ventilation. In Rogers MC, editor: *Textbook of pediatric intensive care*. Baltimore, 1996, Williams & Wilkins.

Meliones JN, Wilson BG, Cheifetz IM et al: Respiratory monitoring. In Rogers M, editor: *Textbook of pediatric intensive care*, ed 3, Baltimore, Md, 1996, Williams & Wilkins.

Meller JL, Little AG, Shermeta DW: Thoracic trauma in children. *Pediatrics* 74:813-819, 1984.

National Association of Emergency Physicians (NAEP): Asthma guidelines (June 1991, NIH). *Pediatr Ann* 21(9):545-553, 1992.

National Heart, Lung, and Blood Institute: *Guidelines for the diagnosis and management of asthma, Expert Panel report 2*. National Institute of Health Publication No. 97-4051. Washington, DC, 1997, U.S. Government Printing Office.

Nation Heart, Lung, and Blood Institute National Asthma Education and Prevention Program: *Expert panel report: guidelines for the diagnosis and management of asthma, update 2002*. Washington, DC, 2004, U.S. Government Printing Office.

Nievas FF, Chernick V: Bronchopulmonary dysplasia update. *Clin Pediatr* 41(2)77-85, 2002.

Nohynek H, Valkeila E, Leinonen M et al: Erythrocyte sedimentation rate, white blood cell count and serum C-reactive protein in assessing etiologic diagnosis of acute lower respiratory infections in children. *Pediatr Infect Dis J* 14:484-490, 1995.

Nova A, Muntz H, Clary R: Utility of conventional radiography in pediatric airway foreign bodies. *Ann Otol Rhinol Laryngol* 107:834-38, 1998.

Optiz CF, Wensel R, Bettmann M et al: Assessment of the vasodilator response in primary pulmonary hypertension: comparing prostacyclin and iloprost administered by either infusion or inhalation. *Eur Heart J* 24:356-365, 2003.

Oudiz RJ: Pulmonary hypertension. From emedicine April 13, 2004. Website: http://www.emedicine.com/MED/topic 1962.htm.

Peterson RJ, Tepas JJ, Edwards FH, et al: Pediatric and adult thoracic trauma: age-related impact on presentation and outcome. *Ann Thorac Surg* 1994;58:14-18.

Powers A: Acid-base balance. In Curley MAQ, Moloney-Harmon PA, editors: *Critical care nursing of infants and children*, ed 2, Philadelphia, 2001, W. B. Saunders.

Randolph AG, Wypij D, Venkataraman ST et al: Effect of mechanical ventilation weaning protocols on respiratory outcomes in infants and children. *JAMA* 288(20); 2561-2568, 2002.

Rich S, Kaufman E: High-dose titration of calcium channel blocking agents for primary pulmonary hypertension; guidelines for short-term drug testing. *J Am Coll Cardiol* 18:1323-1327, 1991.

Romito RA: Early administration of enteral nutrients in critically ill patients. *AACN Clin Issues Crit Care* 6(2):242, 1995.

Rubin LJ: Diagnosis and management of pulmonary artery hypertension: ACCP evidence-based clinical practice guidelines. *Chest* 126:9S, 2004.

Schimmer BP, Parker KL: Adrenocorticotropic hormone; adrenocortical steroids and their synthetic analogs; inhibitors of the synthesis and actions of adrenocortical hormones. In Hardman JG, Limbird LE, editors: *The pharmacological basis of therapeutics*. ed 10, New York, 2001, McGraw-Hill.

Schnapp L, Chin DP et al: Frequency and importance of barotrauma in 100 patients with ALL. *Crit Care Med* 23(2):272-278, 1995.

Scolapio JS: Methods for decreasing the risk of aspiration pneumonia in critically ill patients. *JPEN* 26(6S):S58-S61.

Siberry GK, Iannone R, editors: *The Harriet Lane handbook*, ed 15, St Louis, 2003, Mosby.

Sectish, TC, Prober CG: Pneumonia. In Behrman, RE, Kliegman RM, Jenson HB, editors: *Nelson: textbook of pediatrics*, ed 17, Philadelphia, 2004, W. B. Saunders.

Simoes EA, Sondheimer HM, Top FH Jr et al: Respiratory syncytial virus immune globulin for prophylaxis against respiratory syncytial virus disease in infants and children with congenital heart disease. The Cardiac Study Group. *J Pediatr* 133: 492-499, 1998.

Smolders-de Haas H, Neuvel J, Schmand B et al. Physical development and medical history of children who were treated antenatally with corticosteroids to prevent respiratory distress syndrome: a 10- to 12-year follow-up. *Pediatrics* Jul;86(1): 65-70, 1990.

Spitzer AR: Neonatal respiratory care. In Dentzker D, Marini J, Dakow E, editors: *Comprehensive respiratory care.* Philadelphia, 1995, W. B. Saunders.

Stricklan RA, Murray MJ: Fatal metabolic acidosis in a pediatric patient receiving an infusion of propofol in the intensive care unit: is there a relationship? *Crit Care Med* 23:405-409, 1995.

Suchomski S, Morin F: Pulmonary vascular disease after the immediate newborn period. In Fuhrman B, Zimmerman J, editors: *Pediatric critical care,* ed 2, St Louis, 1998, Mosby.

Sweet S: Lung transplantation: outcomes and risk factors. In Tejan A, Fine R, Harmon W, editors: *Pediatric solid organ transplantation.* Copenhagen, 2000, Munskgaard; pp. 491-502.

Sweet S: Pediatric lung transplantation: update 2003. *Pediatr Clin North Am* 50(6): 1393-1417, 2003.

Thomson, J, Machado, R et al: Sporadic pulmonary hypertension is associated with germline mutations of the gene encoding BMPR-II, a receptor member of the TGF-beta family. *J Med Genet* 37: 219-227, 2003.

Trotter C, Serpell MG: Neurological sequelae in children after prolonged propofol infusions. *Anesthesia.* 47:340-342, 1992.

Trujillo E, Robinson M, Jacobs D: Nutritional assessment in the critically ill. *Crit Care Nurs* 19:67-78, 1999.

Turanlahti, M, Laitinen, P, Sarna S et al: Nitric oxide, oxygen and prostacyclin in children with pulmonary hypertension. *Heart* 79:169-174, 1998.

Venkataraman S, Orr RA: Mechanical ventilation and respiratory care. In Fuhrman B, Zimmerman J, eds. *Pediatric critical care,* St Louis, 1998, Mosby.

Ware LB, Mathay MA: The acute respiratory distress syndrome. *N Engl J Med* 342: 1334-1349, 2000.

Weber JE, Chudnofsky CR, Younger JG et al: A randomized comparison of helium-oxygen mixture (Heliox) and racemic epinephrine for the treatment of moderate to severe croup. *Pediatrics.* 107:E96, 2001.

World Health Organization: Executive summary from the World Symposium on Primary Pulmonary Hypertension. 1998. Website available at: http://www.who.int/ncd/cvd/pph.html. Site verified May 15, 2004.

Wubbell L, Muniz L, Ahmed A et al: Etiology and treatment of community-acquired pneumonia in ambulatory children. *Pediatr Infect Dis J* 18:98-104, 1999.

Yaster M: General anesthetics. In Yaster M, Krane EJ, Kaplan RF et al, editors: *Pediatric pain management and sedation.* St Louis, 1997, Mosby.

Zaccardelli DS, Pattishall EN: Clinical diagnosis criteria of the acute respiratory distress syndrome in the ICU. *Crit Care Med* 24(2):247-251, 1996.

CHAPTER

3 Cardiovascular System

LOUISE CALLOW AND ELIZABETH C. SUDDABY

DEVELOPMENTAL ANATOMY AND PHYSIOLOGY

A. Embryologic Development of the Heart

1. **Formation of the heart tube: Days 15 to 23**
   a. The heart is the first functioning organ in the embryo. Although the heart begins as an elongated tube controlled by brain growth, on days 21 through 23, the endothelial tubes fuse to form a single endocardial tube, and the heart begins to beat from a focus in the sinus venosus.
   b. *Cellular units of the developing heart*
      - Central nucleus
      - Sarcoplasm: Intracellular proteinaceous fluid
      - Sarcolemma: The single cell
      - Fiber: Composed of many fibrils, each surrounded by a sarcotubular system
      - Sarcotubular system: A membranous continuation of sarcolemma. The T tubules function to transmit action potential rapidly from sarcolemma to all fibrils in the muscle. Sarcoplasmic reticulum houses calcium ions. Action potentials in the T tubules cause the release of calcium from reticulum, resulting in a contraction.
      - Contractile unit: Sarcomere (muscle fiber composed of fibrils). Each fibril is divided into filaments, and each filament is made up of contractile proteins. Contractile proteins consist of actin, myosin, troponin, and tropomyosin. Myosin forms the thick filaments. Actin, troponin, and tropomyosin form the thin filaments.
2. **Formation of the heart loop: Days 23 to 28 (Figure 3-1)**
   a. The initial straight tube now loops to the right.
   b. The region of tube proximal to the fold becomes the embryonic ventricle.
   c. The atrioventricular (AV) junction moves to the left side of the pericardial cavity.
   d. Cardiac muscle in a mature heart differs from skeletal muscle. It has more mitochondria and can provide more adenosine triphosphate (ATP) and energy for repetitive action. Fibers are connected to each other by intercalated discs that form a lattice arrangement called a *functional syncytium*. When one fiber is depolarized, the action potential spreads along the syncytium to all other fibers, stimulating them also, and the whole syncytium contracts ("all-or-none" response).
   e. Structure of the cardiac wall in the fully developed heart
      - The *pericardium* is a fibroserous membranous sac that encloses the heart. The *fibrous pericardium* is the outermost layer; the *serous pericardium* is composed of the parietal layer; and the *visceral layer* forms the outer surface of the heart.

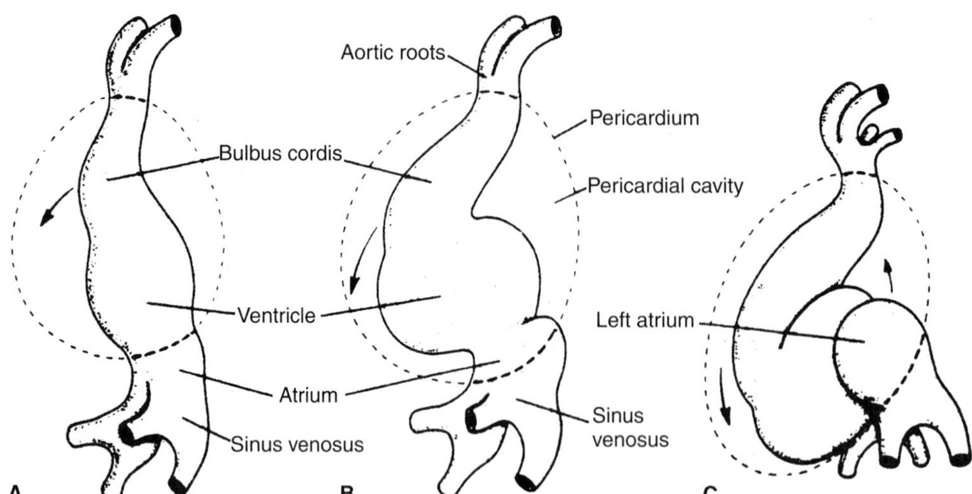

FIGURE 3-1 ■ Cardiac looping to the right as seen from the left side. **A,** At 8 somites; **B,** at 11 somites; **C,** at 16 somites. Dashed line indicates the parietal pericardium. The atrium gradually assumes an intrapericardial position. (Reprinted with permission from Adams FH, Emmanoulides GC, Riemenschneider TA: *Moss' heart disease in infants, children, and adolescents,* ed 4. Baltimore, 1989, Williams & Wilkins.)

- The *epicardium* is the visceral layer of the serous pericardium.
- The *myocardium* is the muscular portion of the heart.
- The *endocardium* is the inner membranous surface of the heart, lining the chambers of the heart.
- *Papillary muscles* arise from endocardial and myocardial surfaces of the ventricles and attach to chordae tendineae. *Chordae tendineae* are the tendinous attachments of the tricuspid and mitral valves, which prevent eversion of the valves during systole.

3. **Formation of embryonic ventricles: Days 22 to 35 (Figure 3-2)**
   - **a.** After looping, the cardiac tube develops expansions that become chambers, and true circulation begins.
   - **b.** The common atrium divides as two tubes fuse.
   - **c.** Endocardial cushions form from cardiac jelly swelling and later divide to create mitral and tricuspid valves.
   - **d.** Ventricles dilate as cardiac output increases by augmented stroke volume (SV).
   - **e.** Trabeculations of the right ventricle form.
   - **f.** The truncoconal portion of the heart moves to lie over the atria.
4. **Formation of cardiac septa: Days 27 to 45**
   - **a.** Active fusion of the cushions or passive expansion of cardiac chambers occurs. Endocardial cushions divide the AV canal into the mitral and tricuspid valves. Conotruncal cushions divide the truncus arteriosus into the aorta and the pulmolnary artery (PA). The septum divides the atria.
   - **b.** Expansion of the trabeculated tissue causes the septum primum to form first, followed by the septum secundum.
   - **c.** The atrial septum forms by the endocardial cushions' fusion of opposing atrial walls.
   - **d.** Pulmonary veins incorporate into the posterior wall of the left atrium.
   - **e.** The septum secundum closes with a remaining perforation called the *foramen ovale.*

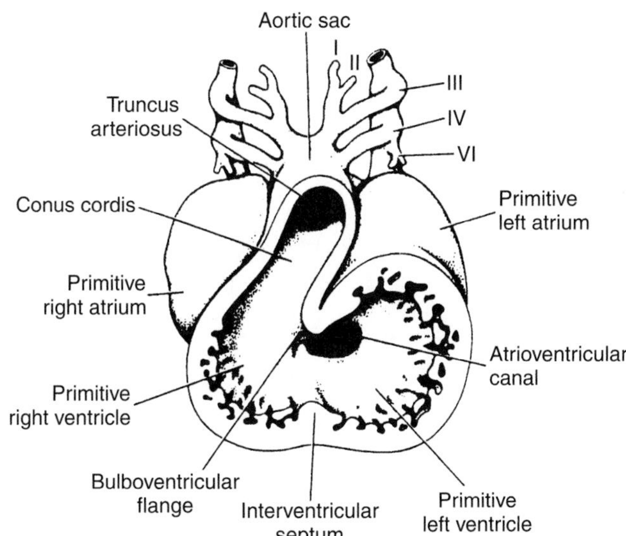

FIGURE 3-2 ■ The primitive atria and ventricles are formed and circulation begins.

(Reprinted with permission from Adams FH, Emmanoulides GC, Riemenschneider TA. *Moss' heart disease in infants, children, and adolescents,* ed 4. Baltimore, 1989, Williams & Wilkins.)

f. While the medial walls of the expanding ventricles fuse, forming the major portion of the ventricular septum, an extension of the endocardial cushions and the truncal conus create the membranous septum.

g. Chambers of the fully developed heart

- The *atria* are thin-walled, low pressure chambers. The right and left atria act as reservoirs of blood for their respective ventricles. Seventy percent of blood flows passively from the atria into the ventricles during early ventricular diastole (protodiastole). The right atrium (RA) receives systemic venous blood via the superior vena cava (SVC), inferior vena cava (IVC), and coronary sinus. The left atrium (LA) receives oxygenated blood returning from the lungs via the four pulmonary veins.
- The *ventricles* are the "pumps" of the heart. The right ventricle (RV), a low-pressure system, contracts (systole) and propels desaturated blood into the pulmonary circulation via the PA, the only artery in the body that carries desaturated blood. The left ventricle (LV), a high-pressure system, ejects blood into the systemic circulation via the aorta.

5. Division of the truncus arteriosus: Days 32 to 33—Outflow tracts divide by fusion of the conotruncal cushions, and spiraling follows the course of cushion development. The conotruncus terminates at the truncoaortic sac, forming six pairs of aortic arches.

6. Formation of cardiac valves: Days 34 to 36

a. The *AV valves* are formed from the endocardial cushion. The mitral valve initially has four cusps; but two cusps grow larger, and papillary muscles fuse into two leaflets (anterior and posterior). The tricuspid valve forms largely from the conus septum, as do the papillary muscles and chordae tendineae. The semilunar valves form at the interface of the truncal cushions and the aorticopulmonary septum.

b. *Cardiac valves in the fully developed heart* (Figure 3-3)

- *AV valves:* The mitral valve is located between the left atrium and LV, and the tricuspid valve is between the right atrium and RV. The mitral valve is bicuspid, and the tricuspid valve consists of three leaflets (anterior, posterior, and septal). The AV valves allow unidirectional blood flow from the atria to the ventricles during ventricular diastole and prevent

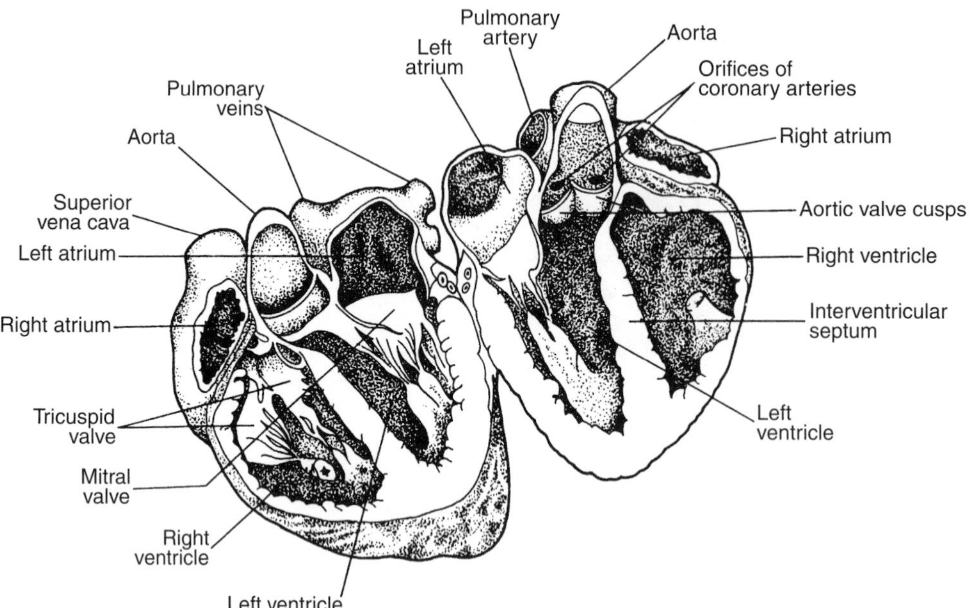

FIGURE 3-3 ■ Illustration of fully developed intracardiac anatomy, valves, great vessels, and pulmonary veins.
(Reprinted with permission from Katz AM: *Physiology of the heart*. New York, NY, 1992, Raven Press.)

retrograde flow during ventricular systole. With ventricular diastole, the papillary muscles relax, the ventricular pressure falls below the atrial pressure, and the valve leaflets open. With increased ventricular pressure and systole, the valve leaflets close completely. Valve closure produces a sound that constitutes the first heart sound, S_1, consisting of a mitral valve and a tricuspid valve component (M_1, T_1). M_1 is the initial and major component of S_1.

- *Semilunar valves:* The pulmonary valve is between the RV and PA and consists of an annulus, three commissures, and three cusps. The aortic valve is situated between the LV and aorta and consists of three valve cusps whose base attaches to a valve annulus. The valves allow unidirectional blood flow from the respective ventricle to arterial outflow tract during ventricular systole and prevent retrograde blood flow during ventricular diastole. Opening occurs when the ventricle contracts, the pressure is greater than the arterial outflow tract, and the valve opens. After ventricular systole, pressure in the arterial outflow tract exceeds pressure in the ventricle, and retrograde blood flow causes valve closure. Valve closure produces a sound that constitutes the second heart sound, S_2, consisting of an aortic and pulmonic component (A_2, P_2). A_2 is the initial and major component of S_2.

7. **Formation of the great veins: Weeks 4 to 7**—Great vein formation is the most variable aspect of cardiac development. Development begins with three pairs of major veins: the cardinal, vitelline, and umbilical veins, which originate in the chorionic villi and return oxygenated blood to the embryo. The right vitelline vein becomes the posthepatic inferior vena cava (IVC). The superior vena cava (SVC) is formed by the right common cardinal vein and proximal right anterior cardinal vein.

8. **Genetic signals to embryonic development**
   a. As more is known about the human genome, gene control of cardiac embryonic events is unfolding and constantly changing, with much more yet to be learned. Genetic control of heart development includes a cascade of signaling molecules that trigger myocardial transcription factors. The transcription factors cause cardiac-specific proteins to be formed. These proteins regulate the growth of muscle types and looping effector genes, resulting in the formation of the normal heart.
   b. Key *signaling molecules* include bone morphogenic proteins (BMPs) and fibroblast growth factors (FGF). BMPs control cell division, cell death, cell migration, and differentiation. FGF signals proteins that cause angiogenesis (blood vessel formation).
   c. Key *transcription factors* include the following:
      - NKX2.5 transcription factor, which is cardiac specific and expressed throughout the heart from the earliest stages and controls differentiation from embryo to cardioblast.
      - Endothelin 1 and other factors, which differentiate cardioblasts into purkinje-type cells.
      - Myocyte-enhancing transcription factor 2 (MEF2) and GATA transcription factors, which cause the cardioblasts to form into the heart tube
   d. *Cardiac specific proteins* that result from transcription factor production control the development of the cardiac chambers.
      - Ventricular differentiation is controlled by MEF2C and Irx4 gene.
      - Formation of the valves by Smad-6 and NF-ATC transcription factors, calcineurin, and transforming growth factor β (TGF-β).
      - Ventricular differences (right from left) are controlled by d-Hand for the right and NKX2.5 stimulation of e-Hand for the left.
      - Ufd1 activates d-Hand and Neuropilin 1, which activate migration of neural crest cells to form the conotruncus, aorta, and aortic arch.
      - PAX 3 gene signals growth of the aortic outflow tract; Forkhead transcription factor Mfh 1 signals growth of the transverse arch. Gridlock gene signals growth in the area of the coarctation, and FAP2b signals the area of the ductus arteriosus.
9. **Systemic vasculature in the fully developed heart**
   a. *Systemic vessels* supply tissues with oxygen and nutrients and remove metabolic wastes. The diameter of the vessels (especially the arterioles) and viscosity of the blood create systemic vascular resistance (SVR). Tissue perfusion is controlled via local chemical reactions and nerves that dilate or constrict blood vessels.
   b. *Major components of systemic vasculature*
      - *Arteries* are a high-pressure circuit composed of strong, compliant, elastic-walled vessels carrying blood from the heart to the capillary beds. Elastic fibers within the arterial wall enable the wall to stretch during systole and recoil during diastole.
      - *Arterioles* are the major vessels controlling SVR and arterial pressure. Arterioles are controlled by the autonomic nervous system and by autoregulation. They contain smooth muscle innervated by sympathetic α-adrenergic nerve fibers. Stimulation causes constriction of the vessels, and decreased adrenergic discharge dilates the vessels controlling blood distribution to various capillary beds. Arterioles may give rise to metarterioles (precapillaries) or give rise directly to capillaries where regulation of flow is through constriction or dilation.

- The *capillary system* allows the exchange of oxygen and carbon dioxide and solutes between blood and tissues and permits fluid volume transfer between plasma and interstitium. Capillary filtration is related to hydrostatic and osmotic pressures across membranes. Increased hydrostatic pressure leads to movement of fluid from vessel to interstitium via osmosis. Greater capillary osmotic pressure leads to fluid movement from interstitium into vessels. Capillaries lack smooth muscle. Diameter changes are passive because of precapillary and postcapillary resistance. Because of their narrow lumens, capillaries can withstand high internal pressures without rupturing. Laplace's law states that the tension in the wall of the vessel necessary to balance the distending pressure is lessened as the radius of the blood vessel decreases. Diffusion is the most important process in moving substrates and wastes between blood and tissues via the capillary system.
- The *venous system* stores approximately 65% of the total volume of blood in the circulatory system. Venules receive blood from capillaries and serve as collecting channels and capacitance (storage) vessels. Veins are capacitance vessels that conduct blood to the heart within a low-pressure system surrounded by skeletal muscles. When muscles contract, they compress veins, moving blood toward the heart. Valves in veins prevent retrograde blood flow. Under normal conditions the venous pump keeps the venous pressure in the lower extremities at 25 mm Hg or less. Gravity has profound effects on the erect, immobile individual. Pressure can rise to 90 mm Hg in the lower extremities, which results in swelling and a decrease in blood volume because of leakage of fluid from the circulatory system into the interstitium.

10. Coronary vasculature in the fully developed heart (Figure 3-4)

a. *Arteries* branch off the base of the aorta, supplying blood to the conduction system and myocardium.

b. The *right coronary artery (RCA)* supplies the sinoatrial (SA) node (55% of hearts), the AV node (90% of hearts), the RA and RV muscles, and the inferoposterior wall of the LV. Eighty percent of the time a branch of the RCA called the *posterior descending artery* is the terminal portion of the RCA,

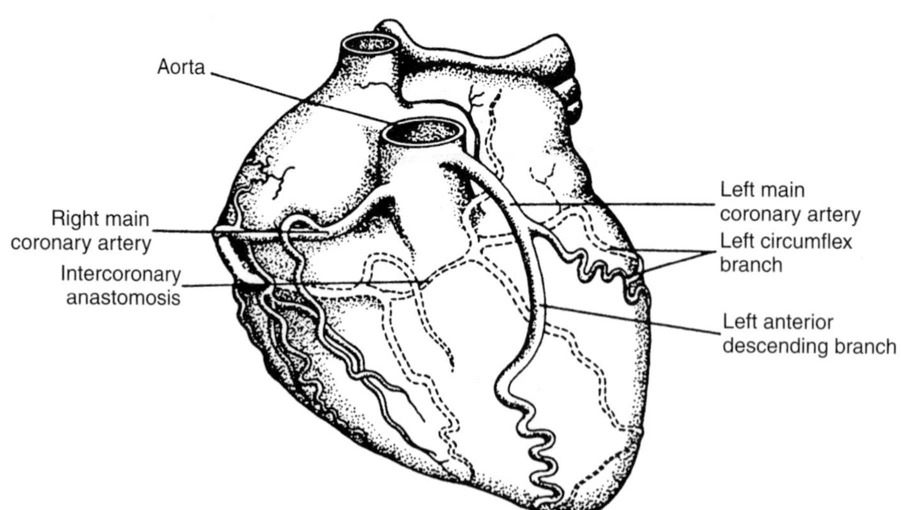

FIGURE 3-4 ■ Location of coronary arteries and branching from aortic root. (Reprinted with permission from Katz AM: *Physiology of the heart.* New York, 1992, Raven Press.)

resulting in a right dominant coronary system. Located in the posterior interventricular groove, it supplies the RV, LV, and the posterior part of the interventricular septum. The RCA gives off a posterior lateral branch that descends from the lateral side of the heart to the apex. It supplies the anteroposterior surface of the RV.

c. The *left coronary artery (LCA)* branches into the left anterior descending artery (LAD), which supplies the anterior part of the interventricular septum, the anterior wall of the LV, the right bundle branch (RBB), and the anterosuperior division of the left bundle branch (LBB).

d. The *circumflex artery,* also branching off from the LCA (into major branches of the circumflex artery and one or more obtuse marginal branches [OMBs]), supplies the AV node (10% of hearts), the SA node (45% of hearts), and the posterior surface of the LV via the OMBs.

e. *Veins* return desaturated blood to the heart. They consist of the great cardiac veins, the small cardiac veins (both drain into the coronary sinus, which drains into the RA), and the thebesian veins (which drain blood into the RA through the atrial wall).

B. Embryonic, Neonatal, and Pediatric Cardiovascular Physiology

1. Fetal circulation (Figure 3-5)

a. Gas exchange occurs in the placenta.

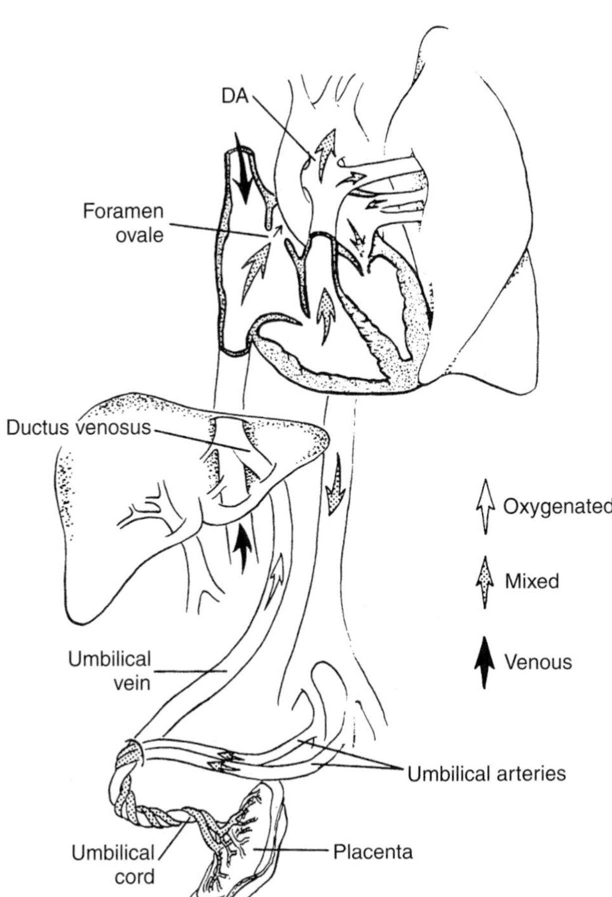

FIGURE 3-5 ■ Fetal circulation with oxygenated placental blood entering umbilical veins, shunting through the ductus venosus, and entering the right side of the heart. Mixed venous blood shunts through the foramen ovale and ductus arteriosus, eventually returning to the aorta and placenta via the umbilical artery. *DA,* ductus arteriosus. (Illustration by Marilou Kundemueller. Reprinted with permission from Hazinski MF: *Nursing care of the critically ill child,* ed 2. St. Louis, 1992, Mosby.)

b. Umbilical venous blood (most highly saturated) returns via the umbilical vein from the placenta and accounts for 42% of fetal cardiac output. From the umbilical vein, about half the fetal blood flows through the ductus venosus to the IVC, and the other half enters the hepatic portal system.
c. There is a preferential flow of more highly saturated blood through the foramen ovale into the LA and LV to the ascending aorta and to the brain and myocardium.
d. The SVC flow is directed to the tricuspid valve and the RV, along with coronary sinus blood. Blood flows from the RV to the pulmonary trunk, and about 8% of RV output perfuses the PA. The rest of the RV output flows through the ductus arteriosus to the aorta. Parallel circulation exists in the fetus: the RV pressure equals the LV pressure.
e. Vascular pressure reflects streaming with RA pressure greater than LA pressure, PA pressure greater than the aortic pressure, and the umbilical vein pressure higher than that of the IVC.
f. The fetal myocardium is less compliant because of the lower ratio of contractile to noncontractile fibers (30% in fetus; 60% in adult).

2. **Transitional circulation (Figure 3-6)**
   a. Interruption of the umbilical cord creates increased SVR and decreased IVC return to the heart. The primary change in circulation after birth is a shift from gas exchange in the placenta to the lungs.
   b. Pulmonary vascular resistance (PVR) rapidly decreases in the first 12 to 24 hours of life, and pulmonary blood flow increases. The reduction to normal PVR occurs slowly over 14 to 21 days.
   c. The ductus arteriosus constricts primarily in response to increased arterial PO_2 but may be influenced by the loss of placental prostaglandin. The ductus arteriosus in the mature infant is functionally closed 12 to 24 hours after birth

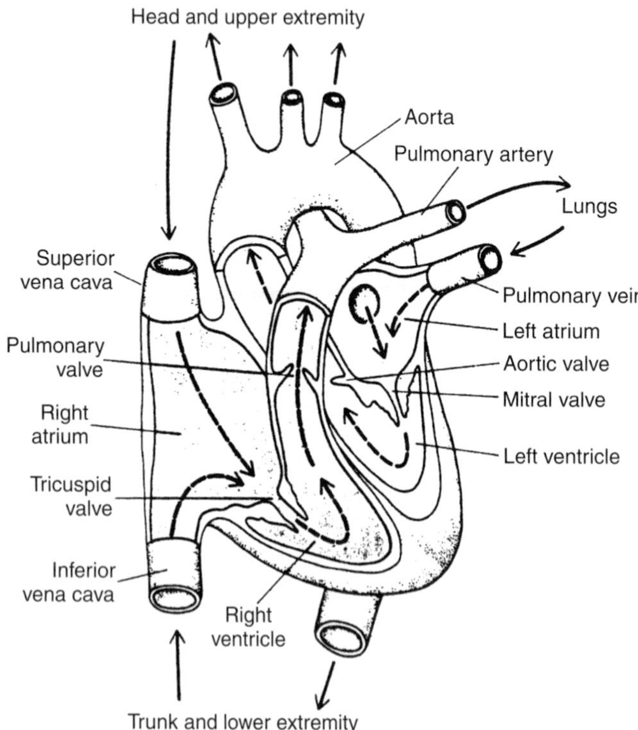

FIGURE 3-6 ■ Structure of the heart and course of normal blood flow through the cardiac chambers. (Reprinted with permission from Guyton AC: *Human physiology and mechanisms of disease.* Philadelphia, 1987, W. B. Saunders.)

but can be reversed with prostaglandin E_1 (PGE_1). Anatomic closure from fibrosis usually occurs within 2 weeks. The RV ejects all blood into the pulmonary circulation when the ductus arteriosus closes and the PVR decreases. The foramen ovale closes as a result of increased LA pressure from increased pulmonary blood return. The ductus venosus closes soon after birth.

d. Rapid loss of the low resistance placental circuit increases the SVR and LV pressure, and LV and RV outputs equalize.

3. Neonatal and pediatric circulation

a. The neonatal myocardium functions at near maximum cardiac output. There is a relatively fixed SV in the first weeks. The larger ratio of noncontractile to contractile muscle fibers disappears after about 1 week.

b. The neonatal myocardium responds to stress by a combination of hyperplasia and hypertrophy. Increased heart rate (HR) produces little change in cardiac output because of a high resting HR; but, because the neonatal myocardium operates high on its cardiac output curve and SV is limited, the cardiac output can be increased by increasing HR more than by increasing contractility. Increased afterload will result in a drop in cardiac output.

c. *Peripheral blood vessel physiology*

- *Local control mechanisms:* The ability of the tissues to control their own blood flow is known as *autoregulation.* Two major hypotheses exist:
  - *Myogenic response hypothesis:* As pressure rises, vessels stretch, stimulating the contraction of smooth muscles *(feedback mechanism).* As tension decreases, smooth muscles relax.
  - *Metabolic hypothesis:* Because of the normal metabolic activity of the tissues, carbon dioxide, potassium, lactate, prostaglandins, and phosphates accumulate and cause vasodilation, which increases the blood flow to the area to flush these waste products away.
  - There may be a delicate balance between these two mechanisms: Myogenic response → vasoconstriction → decrease in blood supply → local increase in metabolites → vasodilation → wastes removed.
- *Autonomic regulation of vessels*
  - *Sympathetic nervous system* fibers secrete norepinephrine at nerve endings, producing vasoconstriction. In arterioles this mechanism helps regulate blood flow and arterial pressure. In veins this mechanism helps to vary the amount of blood stored. (Venoconstriction causes an increase in venous return to the heart.)
  - *Parasympathetic nervous system* fibers secrete acetylcholine at nerve endings (cholinergic effect), producing vasodilation.
- *Stretch receptors:* Baroreceptors (pressoreceptors)
  - Receptor sites are located in the aortic arch, carotid sinus, venae cavae, pulmonary arteries, and atria. Sensitive to arterial pressures, the receptor sites are activated by elevated blood pressure (BP) or increased blood volume, resulting in stretching of the arterial walls. The impulse is transmitted from the aortic arch and the carotid sinus to the medulla. Sympathetic action is inhibited, and the vagal reflex dominates, resulting in decreased HR and contractility, dilation of the systemic vasculature, and normalized BP.
  - In response to decreased BP, the vagal tone decreases and the sympathetic system becomes dominant, resulting in increased HR and contractility and arterial and venous constriction and BP elevated to near normal.
- The *vasomotor center in the medulla* (also called *cardioaccelerator center* or *cardiac center*) consists of the vasoconstrictor and vasodepressor areas.

- Stimulation of the vasoconstrictor area causes increased HR, SV, and cardiac output and, ultimately, increased arterial BP. Venoconstriction, which decreases stores of blood in the venous system, increases venous return and increases SV.
- Inhibition of the vasoconstrictor area stimulates the vasodepressor area, which causes vasodilation. An increase in storage of blood in the venous capacitance system occurs, thereby decreasing SV, cardiac output and arterial BP.
- The vasomotor center works with stretch receptors and chemoreceptors located in the carotid sinus and aortic arch. A rise in BP stimulates the carotid sinus, which inhibits the vasoconstrictor area. This induces vasodilation via stimulation of the vasodepressor area. A fall in oxygen saturation, a rise in carbon dioxide, or a fall in pH stimulates chemoreceptors, which then stimulate the vasoconstrictor center and cause a rise in arterial BP.

3. **Neurohormonal control of the fully developed heart**

a. *Autonomic nervous system*

- Sympathetic stimulation initiates the release of norepinephrine. α-Adrenergic fiber stimulation results in arteriolar vasoconstriction. β-Adrenergic (β_1) fiber stimulation increases SA node discharge (thereby increasing the HR [positive chronotropy]), increases the force of myocardial contraction (positive inotropy), and accelerates AV conduction time (positive dromotropism).
- Parasympathetic stimulation initiates the release of acetylcholine, which stimulates the action of the right vagus (affecting the SA node) and the left vagus nerves (affecting AV nodal conduction tissue). The rate of SA node discharge is decreased and slows the HR (negative chronotropy). It may slow conduction through AV tissue *(negative dromotropism).*

b. *Natriuetric peptides* produced by the atria, ventricles, and brain act as regulators of extravascular fluid volume and BP through control of sodium and water by countering the effects of the renin-angiotensin-aldosterone system.

- *Atrial natriuetic peptide* (ANP) is produced by the atria in response to atrial wall tension from increased intravascular volume. Levels in blood vary significantly with changes in position, exercise, and pacing. ANP reduces sympathetic tone, increases venous capacitance, and shifts intravascular fluid to the extravascular space by increased vascular endothelial permeability. A natural diuresis reduces the extravascular volume by directly affecting the renin-angiotensin-aldosterone receptors in the kidney. ANP reduces peripheral vascular resistance and lowers BP. It lowers the activation of vagal blockers, thus suppressing the reflex tachycardia and vasoconstriction that goes with reduced preload.
- *Brain natriuretic peptide* (BNP) is produced by the ventricles in response to ventricular wall tension and volume expansion. Its effects are similar to those of ANP, producing natriuresis, diuresis, and vasodilation and counteracting the effects of the renin-angiotensin-aldosterone system. BNP also appears to prevent myocardial fibrosis, vascular smooth-muscle cell proliferation, and thrombosis. BNP levels in blood are more stable than ANP. Both ANP and BNP levels rise rapidly after birth in response to increased LV volume and pressure during transition to extrauterine life. Then levels drop to normal within 2 weeks of life. Sex-related differences are noted after puberty (greater in females).
- *C- type natriuretic peptide* is produced mostly by the central nervous system, kidneys, and vascular endothelial cells.

c. *Chemoreceptors* are located in the carotid and aortic bodies and are sensitive to changes in PO_2, PCO_2, and pH. They affect HR and respiratory rate via stimulation of the vasomotor center in the medulla.
d. *Stretch receptors* respond to pressure and volume changes. Stretch receptors located in the atria, large veins, and PA produce the Bainbridge reflex. An increase in venous return stretches the receptors. Afferent nerve impulses transmit to the vasomotor center in the medulla. The medulla increases efferent impulses, increasing HR and cardiac output and enabling the heart to pump out all the blood returned to it.
e. *Respiratory reflex:* Inspiration decreases intrathoracic pressure, increasing venous return to the heart. Inspiration stimulates stretch receptors in the lungs and thorax. Impulses from the stretch receptors inhibit the vasomotor center in the medulla. This inhibition decreases vagal tone, causing an increase in the HR, which allows the heart to pump out the extra blood. This reflex results in "sinus arrhythmia," which may occur in a normal heart.

4. **Variables** that affect the ventricular function of the heart include the following:
   a. *Cardiac output* = SV × HR. *The cardiac index* is used in children because of the variation in cardiac output by body size. Cardiac index is equal to cardiac output divided by body surface area (BSA).
   b. *Stroke volume* is affected by preload, afterload, and contractility.
      - *Preload* is the resting force in the myocardium, which is determined by volume in the ventricles at the end of diastole (left ventricular end-diastolic volume [LVEDV] reflected by left ventricular end-diastolic pressure [LVEDP]). Preload can be related to such variables as volume of blood returned from veins, stretch, and fiber length. An increase in preload stretches myocardial muscle fibers, causing more forceful subsequent ventricular contractions, increasing stroke volume and cardiac output. An increase in preload is accomplished by increasing the volume returning to the ventricles (Figure 3-7). The *Frank-Starling law* states that there is a direct relationship between the volume of blood in the heart at the end of diastole and the force of contraction during the next systole. The preload or ventricular filling pressure reflects the initial sarcomere length, which influences the development of myocardial force. Muscle fibers may reach a point of stretch beyond which contraction is no longer enhanced and stroke volume decreases. Increased preload may be related to mitral insufficiency, aortic insufficiency, ventricular septal defect, atrial septal defect, patent ductus arteriosus, fluid overload, and vasoconstrictors. Decreased preload may be related to mitral stenosis, hypovolemia, and vasodilators.
      - *Afterload* is the initial resistance that must be overcome by the ventricles to open the semilunar valves and propel blood into the systemic and pulmonary circulatory system.
        - Afterload is clinically measured as SVR and PVR (also called *peripheral vascular resistance*).

$$\text{SVR} = (\text{mean arterial pressure [MAP]} - \text{central venous pressure [CVP]})/\text{systemic blood flow}$$

Systemic blood flow is a value measured in resistance units. This number times 80 converts into dynes per second per square centimeter.

$$\text{Normal SVR} = 900 - 1400\ \text{dynes/s/cm}^2$$

- Factors that increase afterload include fixed anatomic obstruction, peripheral arterial vasoconstriction, hypertension, pulmonary hypertension, polycythemia, and vasoconstrictors. Excessive afterload increases

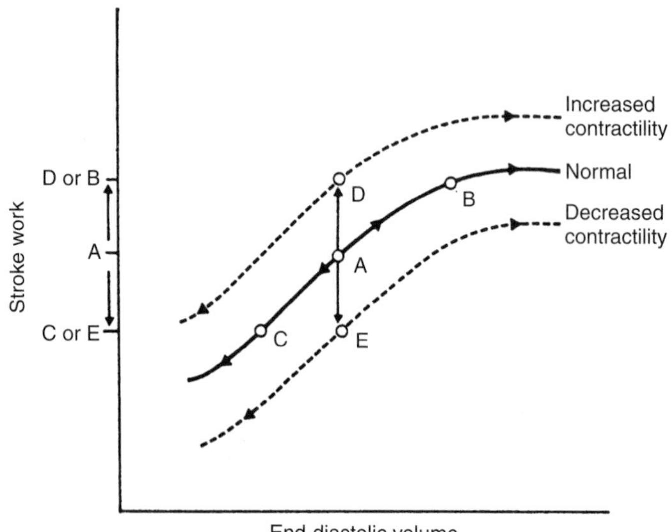

FIGURE 3-7 ■ The work of the heart varies with changing end-diastolic volume according to the Frank-Starling relationship. The work of the heart can also be varied by changes in contractility. The *solid curve (CAB)* describes normal myocardial contractility, and point *A* represents the basal state. Changes in cardiac work that result from alterations in venous return shift the work of the heart along this normal curve. Cardiac work can be increased from *A* to *B* by enhanced venous return and decreased from *A* to *C* by a reduction in venous return. The work of the heart can also be changed by modifications in myocardial contractility. A positive inotropic agent can increase cardiac work from *A* to *D*, even with constant end-diastolic volume. Cardiac work can be decreased from *A* to *E* by a negative inotropic agent without change in end-diastolic volume.
(Reprinted with permission from Katz AM: *Physiology of the heart.* New York, 1992, Raven Press Publishers.)

LV or RV stroke work, increases myocardial oxygen demands, and may result in LV or RV failure. Factors that decrease ventricular afterload include vasodilators and sepsis.

- *Contractility* is the strength and efficiency of contraction (force generated). Positive inotropic drugs, sympathetic stimulation, and hypercalcemia can act to increase the contractile state of the myocardium. Factors that can decrease contractility of the myocardium include negative inotropic drugs; hypoxia; hypercapnia; intrinsic depression attributable in part to long-standing congestive heart failure (CHF); parasympathetic stimulation; metabolic acidosis, hypocalcemia, hypoglycemia, hypomagnesemia, hyponatremia, and hyperkalemia; condition of the myocardium; and intrinsic myocardial disease.

c. *Arterial pressure*

- Factors that can affect arterial BP include cardiac output, HR, SVR, arterial elasticity, blood volume, blood viscosity, age, BSA, exercise, and anxiety.
- *Pulse pressure* is a function of stroke volume and arterial capacitance. This difference between systolic and diastolic BP is expressed in millimeters of mercury ($P_s - P_d$).
- *MAP* is the average pressure in the aorta based on the volume of blood in the arterial system and the elastic properties of the arterial walls.

$$\text{MAP} = \text{systolic BP} + (2 \times \text{diastolic BP}) / 3$$

- *Regulation of arterial pressure:* The renin-angiotensin-aldosterone system involves renin, a protease secreted by the kidney that converts angiotensin I to angiotensin II. Release of renin from the kidney is stimulated by stretch receptors in juxtaglomerular cells that are sensitive to changes in BP. Decreased BP, a rise in sympathetic output, or a fall in sodium concentration results in increased renin secretion. Increased BP results in decreased renin secretion. Angiotensin II is the most potent vasoconstrictor known, producing arteriolar constriction and an increase in systolic and diastolic pressures.
- Other mechanisms include capillary fluid shift mechanisms, local control mechanisms, and the renal-fluid volume process. With a rise in arterial pressure, the kidneys excrete more fluid, causing a reduction in extracellular fluid and blood volume; this reduces circulating blood volume and cardiac output, leading to normalization of arterial pressure. With a fall in arterial pressure, the kidneys retain fluid, causing increased intravascular volume and cardiac output that may result in normalization of arterial pressure.

ANATOMY OF THE CARDIAC CONDUCTION SYSTEM (FIGURE 3-8)

A. Sinoatrial Node (SA Node)

The sinoatrial node is the pacemaker of the heart because it possesses the fastest inherent rate of automaticity (spontaneous generation of impulses.)

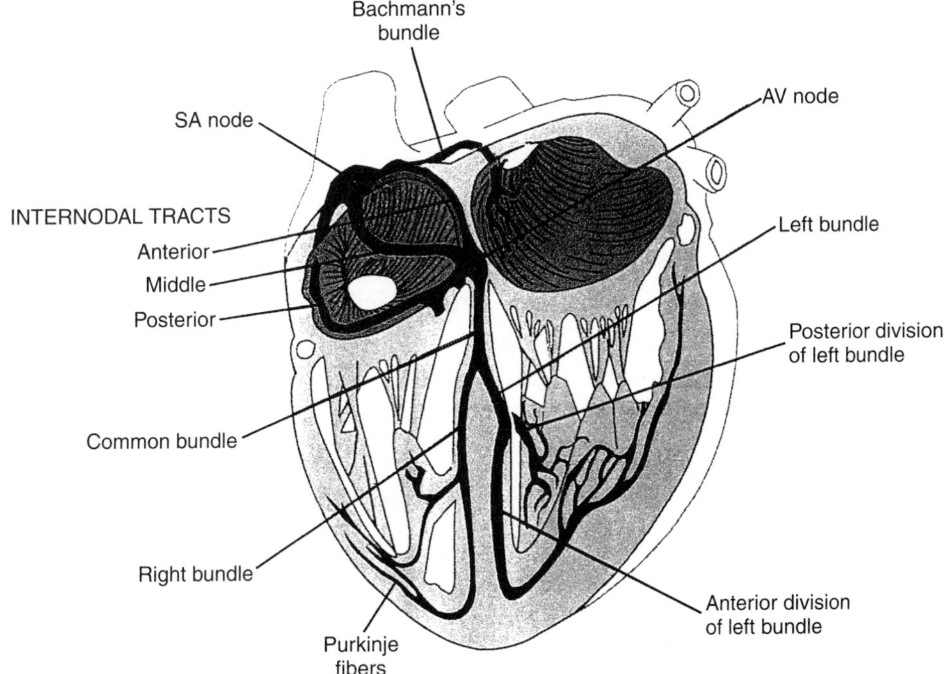

FIGURE 3-8 ■ Cardiac conduction system.
(From Alspach JG: *Core curriculum for critical care nursing,* ed 5. Philadelphia, 1998, W. B. Saunders.)

B. Internodal Atrial Pathways

Internodal atrial pathways, which consist of the anterior tract (Bachmann's), middle tract (Wenckebach's), and posterior tract (Thorel's), conduct impulses from the SA node through the right atrium to the AV node.

C. Bachmann's Bundle

Bachmann's bundle conducts impulses from the SA node to the left atrium.

D. Atrioventricular Node

The AV node (AV junction) delays impulse transmission between atria and ventricles, allowing time for ventricular filling following atrial contraction and before ventricular systole. The AV node controls the number of impulses (if the atrial rate becomes excessive) reaching the ventricles, thereby having some control over HR.

E. Bundle of His

The bundle of His is composed of thick fibers arising from the AV node that travel over the crest of the ventricular septum on its right side to the bundle-branch system.

F. Bundle-Branch System

The bundle-branch system is composed of pathways that arise from the bundle of His. The **right bundle branch (RBB)** is a direct continuation of the bundle of His that transmits impulses down the right side of the interventricular septum toward the RV myocardium. The bundle divides into three parts (anterior, lateral, and posterior), dividing further to become parts of the Purkinje system. The **left bundle branch (LBB)** separates into the left posterior fascicle (which transmits impulses over the posterior and inferior endocardial surfaces of the LV) and the left anterior fascicle (which transmits impulses to the anterior and superior endocardial surfaces of the LV).

G. Purkinje System

The Purkinje system arises from the distal portion of the bundle branches and transmits impulses into the subendocardial layers of both ventricles. It provides for depolarization (from endocardium to epicardium) followed by ventricular contraction and ejection of blood from the ventricles.

ELECTROPHYSIOLOGY

A. Myocardial Conduction System Properties

1. **Automaticity:** Ability to generate impulse spontaneously
2. **Rhythmicity:** Regularity of impulse generation
3. **Conductivity:** Ability to transmit impulses
4. **Excitability:** Ability to respond to stimulation

B. Excitation-Contractile Process of Cardiac Muscle

1. **The sodium and unbound calcium ion concentrations** are greater outside the cell, and the potassium ion concentration is greater inside the cell. The resting membrane potential (RMP) for myocardial muscle fibers is –80 to –90 mV.
2. **Depolarization** can result from chemical, electrical, or mechanical stimulation. The stimulus reduces the RMP to a less negative value (depolarization). The threshold potential is the voltage level where an action potential is produced. For all cardiac tissue except the SA and AV nodes, the threshold potential is –60 to –70 mV. For the SA and AV nodes, the threshold potential is –30 to –40 mV.

Reaching the threshold causes changes in the membrane. The permeability of the cell membrane is altered, opening specialized channels in the membrane, which permits the passage of sodium and calcium ions into the cell. The action potential (AP) is the graphic representation of this change (Figure 3-9).

3. **The AP produced during depolarization** is transmitted to the interior of the cell via T tubules, which transmit the AP to all myofibrils. Calcium is stored in the lateral sacs of the sarcoplasmic reticulum and is released during the AP. Calcium enters the interior of the cell, causing an interaction between actin and myosin filaments through a complex interaction with enzymes. Actin filaments move progressively inward on myosin filaments as successive electrochemical interactions take place (interdigitation). The result is shortening of sarcomeres and then of muscle fibers and thus myocardial contraction. Relaxation of muscle fibers occurs when free calcium is pumped back into the sarcoplasmic reticulum.
4. **"Gate" theory:** Fast channels of the membrane specific for sodium may be controlled by the following:
   - **a.** The *activation gate* opens the fast channels as the RMP becomes less negative, allowing a rapid influx of sodium into the cell, which causes depolarization (phase 0 of the AP).
   - **b.** The *deactivation gate* closes the channels impeding the influx of sodium into the cell. Closure of the gates is complete by *phase 1.*
5. **A return to the RMP** results from an inward current of calcium and potassium ions that diffuse out of the cell.
   - **a.** *Phase 2,* the plateau phase, occurs as calcium flows in and potassium flows out.
   - **b.** *Phase 3,* the rapid depolarization phase, occurs as the calcium channels close and potassium rapidly moves out of the cell.
   - **c.** *Phase 4,* the resting phase, of the sodium-potassium pump regulates the concentration of cations in the cell. This pump, found in the cell membrane, actively pumps excess sodium out of the cell and pumps in the potassium.

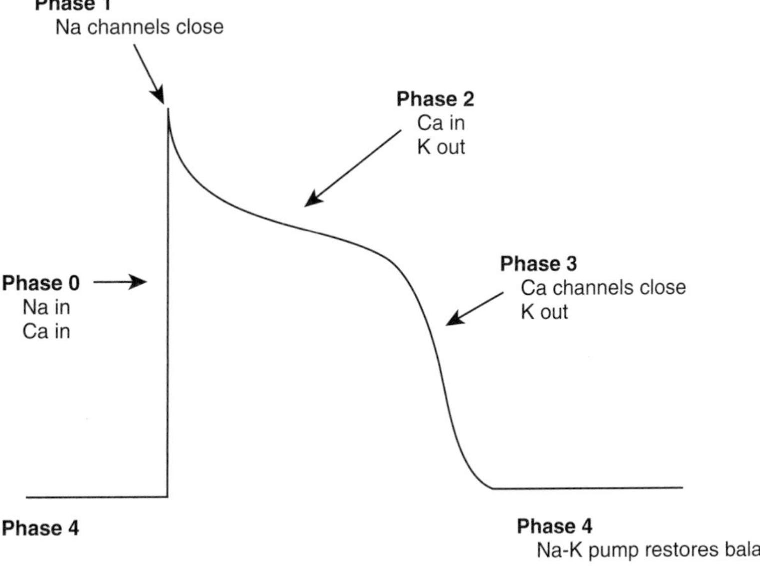

FIGURE 3-9 ■ Action potential.

6. Unlike other cells of the heart that require another stimulus to depolarize them once they have been repolarized, **the SA and AV nodes** spontaneously depolarize (generate impulses) in phase 4. This spontaneous depolarization is due to the steady influx of sodium and the efflux of potassium ions, raising the nodal tissues back to the threshold potential and initiating an AP. This phenomenon is known as *automaticity*.

C. Refractoriness of Heart Muscle

1. **Absolute refractory period** encompasses phases 0, 1, 2, and part of 3 of the APs. During this period of time, the cell cannot respond to another stimulus and produce an AP.
2. **Relative refractory period** (the latter part of phase 3) is a period when a strong stimulus can cause depolarization.
3. **Supernormal period** occurs at the end of phase 3. During this time a very weak stimulus that would not normally elicit an AP can evoke a response and cause depolarization.
4. **Vulnerable period** is the point at the very beginning of the relative refractory period. A stimulus at this time (which corresponds to the peak of the T wave on the ECG) can result in myocardial electrical chaos.

D. Physiologic Response to Depolarization and Repolarization

1. **Electrical depolarization of the atria** is represented by the P wave on the ECG. Following atrial depolarization, the pressure in the atria rises higher than the diastolic pressure in the ventricles, forcing blood from the atria into the resting ventricles.
2. **Electrical depolarization of the ventricles** occurs, producing the QRS complex on the ECG. Isometric or isovolumetric contraction is the first phase of ventricular contraction (systole). Ventricular pressure rises while ventricular volume remains stable because the semilunar valves have not yet opened. The increased pressure in the ventricles closes the AV valves. As ventricular pressure exceeds great vessel pressure, the semilunar valves open. Blood from the ventricles is rapidly ejected into the great vessels. As the outflow of blood from the ventricles decreases, the pressure in the ventricles also decreases, falling below the pressure in the great vessels. This causes a back flow of blood from the great vessels to the ventricles, which closes the semilunar valves. The dicrotic notch on the arterial pressure tracing represents closure of the aortic valve.
3. **Repolarization of the ventricles** occurs during mechanical systole and produces the T wave on the ECG.
4. **Isometric or isovolumetric relaxation** occurs when ventricular pressure falls rapidly following semilunar valve closure. Intraventricular volume remains static before the AV valves open. A "v" wave is produced on the atrial pressure curve during isometric relaxation related to blood flow into the atria from the pulmonic and systemic circuits. As ventricular pressure remains lower than atrial pressure, the AV valves open to initiate the rapid-filling phase.

CLINICAL ASSESSMENT OF CARDIOVASCULAR FUNCTION

A. History

1. **Chief complaint** is the patient's or parents' description of why they are seeking help.

2. **History of present illness:** Determine the onset, description, course, and duration. Evaluate exacerbations and remissions of signs and symptoms, including the following:
   a. *Feeding pattern:* Duration, frequency, associated distress, volume taken, stopping to rest or breathe during eating, caloric supplementation required (earliest sign of CHF)
   b. *Fatigue:* While feeding or playing
   c. *Edema:* Orbital, sacral
   d. *Diaphoresis:* Location, degree
   e. *Dyspnea, tachypnea:* With or without activity
   f. *Cyanosis:* Oxygen saturation with or without activity; skin color
   g. *Squatting:* Frequent in children with cyanotic lesions when repairs are delayed or undiagnosed
   h. *Growth:* Graph against normal limits for height and weight. With CHF, weight will fall below normal limits before height does.
   i. *Frequency of infections*
   j. *Syncope:* Prodrome, with or without dizziness, time of occurrence
   k. *Palpitations:* With or without chest pain
3. **Past history and family history** include all previous illnesses, injuries, and family history of similar disease (i.e., history of congenital heart disease [CHD], not coronary artery disease).
   a. *Prenatal and perinatal history, including in vitro fertilization*
   b. *Family history* should include evaluation of inheritance risk of single gene, chromosomal disorders, or multifactoral syndromes associated with CHD (Tables 3-1, 3-2, and 3-3).
      - Environmental factors include drug teratogens, external radiation exposure, maternal systemic diseases, and infectious exposure of the fetus (Table 3-4).
      - There is a slightly higher risk (2.5% to 16%) of CHD if one parent or sibling has CHD.
4. **Psychosocial history** includes the use of illicit drugs or alcohol during pregnancy or by the child, daily living patterns, relationships with significant others, recreational habits, educational level of the child and parents, and developmental level of the child.
5. The **medication history** should include all medications prescribed or obtained over the counter, including herbal remedies, dosages, and reason for use.

B. Physical Examination

1. **Inspection**
   a. *General appearance:* Note size for age (height and weight graphed against normal limits), activity level, level of consciousness, and physical characteristics of chromosomal defects (genetic phenotypes, i.e., Down syndrome).
   b. *Assess skin and mucous membranes.*
      - Note pallor, cyanosis, or mottling. Skin color is influenced by vasoconstriction. Cyanosis is evident if saturation is less than 85%, which is equivalent to 5 g of reduced hemoglobin per 100 mL of blood. The degree of visible cyanosis is dependent on total hemoglobin and its saturation. Respiratory cyanosis decreases with crying (improved respiratory effort) and oxygen. In cardiac disease, cyanosis increases with crying (increased resistance to pulmonary blood flow and shunting) and remains unchanged with oxygen administration. *Acrocyanosis* (cyanosis of the extremities) is normal in the newborn with vasomotor instability. Note the distribution of

TABLE 3-1
Single Gene Defects Associated with Congenital Heart Disease

Name/Locus	Gene Defect	Phenotype	CV
Marfan's—15q21	Defect for fibrillin, alters growth factor β binding sites, 80 mutations found	Skeletal: tall stature, arachnodactyl, scoliosis, Ocular: retinal detachments Neonatal: valves	Progressive dilation of Ao root with catastrophic aortic dissection, AI, MVP
Holt-Oram—12q24	Defect of transcription factor TBX5	Malformed thumb, hypoplasia of thenar eminence, radial aplasia	80% ASD; also VSD, AVC; conduction abnormalities
Familial ASD—12q?	Defect of transcription factor NKX2.5		ASD and conduction abnormalities; also TOF, DORV, Ebstein's, muscular VSD
Char Syndrome—6q12-21	Defect of transcription factor AP-2b, role in neural crest differentiation	Facial: short philtrum, duck bill lips, ptosis, low-set ears Skeletal: abnormal 5th digit	PDA
Duchenne's MD—Xp21	Mutation of dystrophin gene	Skeletal and smooth-muscle weakness	Dilated cardiomyopathy
Barth Syndrome—Xq28		Immunologic: cyclic neutropenia Renal: organic aciduria Somatic: skeletal myopathy, growth failure	Dilated cardiomyopathy
Alagille's—20p12	Mutation of JAG1, codes for cell surface receptor, results in arteriohepatic dysplasia	Hepatic: liver dysfunction, decreased number of bile ducts Other: eye, skeletal, kidney	67% diffuse peripheral PA stenosis, hypoplasia of pulmonary vascular tree TOF, Pa, coarct, ASD, PDA, VSD
Noonan's—12q24.1	Mutation of PTPN11 gene, encodes nonreceptor protein tyrosine phosphatase SHP2	Skeletal: short stature, shield chest, webbed neck, peripheral edema Face: hypertelorism, downward slant eye, rotated ears low-set posteriorly Head: deafness, delays, 25% MR Hematologic: factor XI deficiency, platelet dysfunction, Von Willebrand's disease	80% heart disease; 40% valvar PS not responsive to balloon dilation; 15% partial AVC; 10% hypertrophic cardiomyopathy; 9% coarctation; also ASD, PDA, mitral valve defects, TOF
Wolff-Parkinson-White—7q34-36	Mutation of gamma-2 regulatory subunit of AMP-activated protein kinase (PRKAG2)		Short PR interval, prolonged QRS, Slurred upstroke of R wave (delta wave) Prone to SVT

AI, aortic insufficiency; *ASD*, atrial septal defect; *AVC*, atrioventricular canal defect; *DORV*, double outlet right ventricle; *MVP*, mitral valve prolapse; *PA*, pulmonary artery; *Pa*, pulmonary atresia; *PDA*, patent ductus arteriosus; *PS*, pulmonary stenosis; *SVT*, supraventricular tachycardia; *TOF*, tetralogy of Fallot; *VSD*, ventricular septal defect

■ TABLE 3-2
■ ■ Chromosomal Defects Associated with Congenital Heart Disease

Name/Locus	Gene Defect	Phenotype	CV
Williams—7q11.23	Monosomy of allele for elastin gene	Face: elfin faces, stellate pattern to iris Behavior: cocktail party personality Mental: developmental delay with language skills preserved	Supravalvar AS Supravalvar PS Renal artery stenosis
Down-21	Trisomy of 21	Face: flattened profile, epicanthal folds, upslanting palpebral fissures, excess nuchal skin, simian crease Mental: MR, hypotonia GI: duodenal atresia, hirshsprung's, imperforate anus 15% hypothyroidism	40% heart disease 45% AVC 35% VSD 8% ASD 5% TOF with or without AVC
Patau-13	Trisomy 13	Head: microcephaly, sloping forehead, cleft lip and palate Seizures, cerebral malformations Overlapping fingers with postaxial polydactyly Severe MR	80% heart disease VSD, ASD, PDA, PS coarctation, dextrocardia
Edwards-18	Trisomy 18	Head: microcephaly, prominent occiput, narrow forehead, cleft lip and palate, low-set ears IUGR, single umbilical artery Extremities: clenched hands with overlapping digits, rocker bottom feet	90% heart disease VSD, ASD, PDA, PS, TOF, bicuspid Ao valve, TGA, coarct, polyvalvar thickening
Turner's—45X		Skeletal: short stature, broad chest with widely spaced nipples, peripheral edema Excess nuchal skin, ovarian dysgenesis Mental: normal intelligence	23% heart disease 50% bicuspid Ao valve 33% coarctation also AS, PAPVR, VSD, ASD 25% multiple cardiac anomalies

Continued

TABLE 3-2
Chromosomal Defects Associated with Congenital Heart Disease (*cont'd*)

Name/Locus	Gene Defect	Phenotype	CV
DiGeorge, velocardiofacial catch 22—22q11	Contiguous gene syndrome with 25 genes in deleted region	Face: cleft palate, high-arching palate, Neck: aplasia/hypoplasia of parathyroids, thymus Learning disabilities, renal anomalies, growth delay, psychiatric disorders	75% conotruncal defects 25-30%truncus arteriosus 25-40% IAA 20% TOF 25% R aortic arch
Cat eye syndrome—22p	Tetrasomy of 22p	Facial: coloboma of iris, down staring palpebral fissures, periauricular tags/pits	TAPVR LSVC

AS, aortic stenosis; *ASD*, atrial septal defect; *AVC*, atrioventricular canal defect; *Coarct*, coarctation of the aorta; *IAA*, interrupted aortic arch; *LSVC*, left superior vena cava, *PAPVR*, partial anomalous pulmonary venous return; *PDA*, patent ductus arteriosus; *PS*, pulmonary stenosis; *TAPVR*, total anomalous pulmonary venous return; *TGA*, transposition of the great arteries; *TOF*, tetralogy of Fallot

TABLE 3-3
Multifactorial Inheritance Syndromes Associated with Congenital Heart Disease

Name/Locus	Gene Defect	Phenotype	CV
Heterotaxy Syndrome	Mutation of Xq26.2 Mutation of ZIC3 gene	Situs ambiguous Asplenia-polysplenia syndrome Lung lobation altered Malrotation	Dextrocardia Other, usually complex heart defects
Jervell-Lange-Nielsen—	Mutation of K^+ ion channel gene	Congenital deafness from ion flow deficit in stria	Prolonged QT, syncope, sudden death
Romano-Ward	Six mutations 11p15.5 defect in encoding K^+ ion channel for phase 3 repolarization 7q35 defect in encoding Ca activated K^+ channel 3p21 Na channel defect 4q25 ? calcium-calmodulin kinase defect		Prolonged QT, syncope, sudden death
Familial hypertrophic	Defect of sarcomeric proteins at 1q3, 19p12.2q13.2, 11p11, 7q3, 3p21, 12q23, 15q14, 14q1		Asymmetric left ventricular hypertrophy with acute obstruction or ventricular arrhythmias

TABLE 3-4
Fetal Environmental and Systemic Exposures Associated with Cardiac Anomalies

Exposure	Cardiac Anomaly
Thalidomide	Truncus, TOF, VSD, PDA
Fetal alcohol	VSD, ASD, TOF
Amphetamines	VSD, PDA, ASD, TGV
Trimethadione	VSD, TOF
Anticonvulsants	PS, AS, Coarct, PDA, TGV, TOF, HLHS
Sex hormones	VSD, TGV, TOF
Lithium	Ebstein's anomaly, tricuspid atresia, ASD
Retinoic acid	TOF, TGV, DORV, truncus, VSD
Rubella	PDA, PS, AS, Coarct, VSD, ASD
Mumps	Endocardial fibroelastosis
Coxsackie	Myocarditis
HIV	Dilated cardiomyopathy
CMV	Myocarditis, fetal heart block
Parvovirus B19	Myocarditis, nonimmune hydrops fetalis with high output heart failure
Diabetes	TGV, VSD, hypertrophic cardiomyopathy
Lupus erythematosus	Congenital complete heart block
Phenylketonuria	TOF, VSD, ASD
Thyroid dysfunction	SVT, cardiomyopathy
Friedreich's ataxia	CHB, PVC's, cardiomyopathy

AS, aortic stenosis; *ASD*, atrial septal defect; *Coarct*, coarctation of the aorta; *DORV*, double outlet right ventricle, *HLHS*, hypoplastic left heart syndrome; *PDA*, patent ductus arteriosus; *PS*, pulmonary stenosis; *PVC*, premature ventricular contraction; *TGV*, transposition of the great vessels; *TOF*, tetralogy of Fallot; *Truncus*, truncus arteriosus; *VSD*, ventricular septal defect

cyanosis over the body. *Peripheral* cyanosis (extremities, perioral [around the mouth]) may represent hypothermia or decreased flow, whereas central cyanosis (inside mucous membranes) indicates reduced hemoglobin saturation. *Chronic* cyanosis stimulates erythropoiesis and polycythemia, which cause increased blood viscosity and an increased risk of spontaneous cerebrovascular accidents, brain abscess, thrombocytopenia with short platelet survival, reduced platelet aggregation with hemorrhagic abnormalities (which may cause operative bleeding), and vascular sheer stress producing increased PVR, even in the face of decreased pulmonary blood flow.

- Note temperature. Skin temperature is influenced by the environment, but it assists in describing the level of decreased perfusion (i.e., cold to knee, cold to midthigh).
- Note edema, which is more common in periorbital and sacral areas of infants.
- Note the presence of diaphoresis.

c. *Observe the extremities.*

- Note clubbing of nail beds indicated by a flattened angle of the nail base to 180 or more degrees (normal is about 160 degrees). Clubbing develops after decreased oxygen saturation persists more than 6 months (Figure 3-10).
- Compare both sides for equal growth, particularly length, in children requiring multiple catheterization procedures.

d. *Observe the chest and precordium* for visible pulsations; active precordium (heaves, thrusts over the precordium noted in volume overload such as left-to-

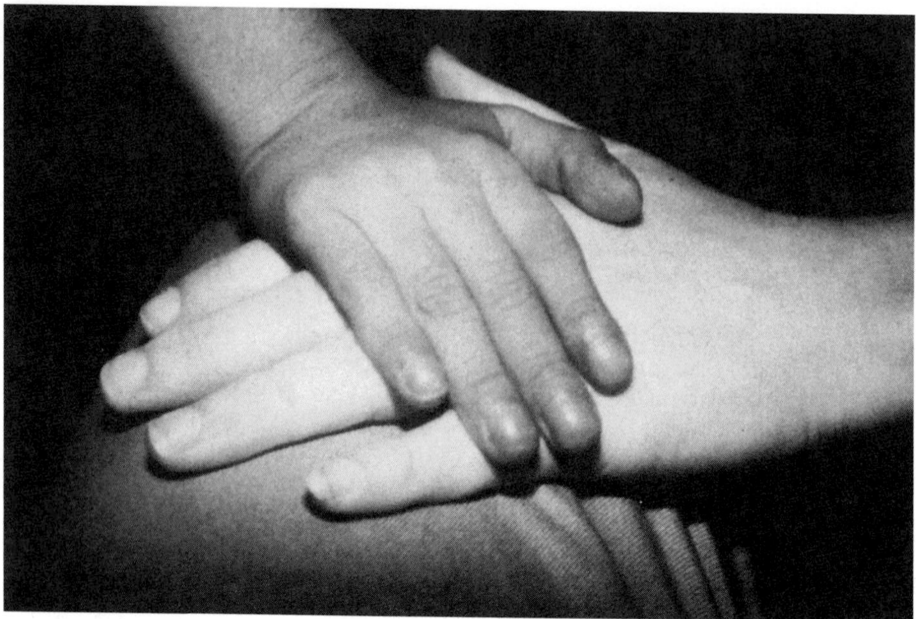

FIGURE 3-10 ■ Example of child's clubbed fingers in contrast to normal fingers. (Courtesy of Elizabeth C. Suddaby.)

right shunts or aortic or mitral insufficiency); shape, contour, and symmetry of the chest; breathing pattern; Harrison's groove in older children; and visible point of maximal intensity of cardiac impulse (point of maximal impulse [PMI]).

e. *Observe the neck for jugular venous distention.*

2. **Palpation**

a. *Precordium*

- Note the PMI, normally found at the fifth left intercostal space (LICS), medial to the midclavicular line after 7 years or at the fourth LICS before 7 years. Lateral displacement of the PMI away from the left sternal border (LSB) indicates elevated diaphragm or left ventricular hypertrophy (LVH). Medial displacement toward the sternum indicates right ventricular hypertrophy (RVH) or an abnormally small LV.
- Seven areas should be palpated (Figure 3-11), including the supraclavicular, aortic, pulmonary, tricuspid, mitral, epigastric, and ectopic areas.
- *Thrills:* Use the ball portion of the palm of the hand to palpate murmurs (feels like a vibration or a cat purring).
  - In the aortic area, thrills indicate aortic stenosis.
  - In the pulmonic area with radiation to the left side of the neck, thrills indicate pulmonic stenosis.
  - In the apical area during systole, this finding indicates mitral regurgitation and during diastole, mitral stenosis.
  - Suprasternal notch may indicate aortic stenosis, pulmonic stenosis, or PDA.
  - Intercostal spaces (ICSs) indicate coarctation of the aorta with collateral circulation.
  - At the mid to lower left sternal border, VSD is indicated.
- *Lifts* are pulsations noted under the palm of the hand. Pulsation in the pulmonic area indicates mitral stenosis or hypertension. Lifts in the tricuspid area may indicate ventricular septal defect (VSD), elevated RV

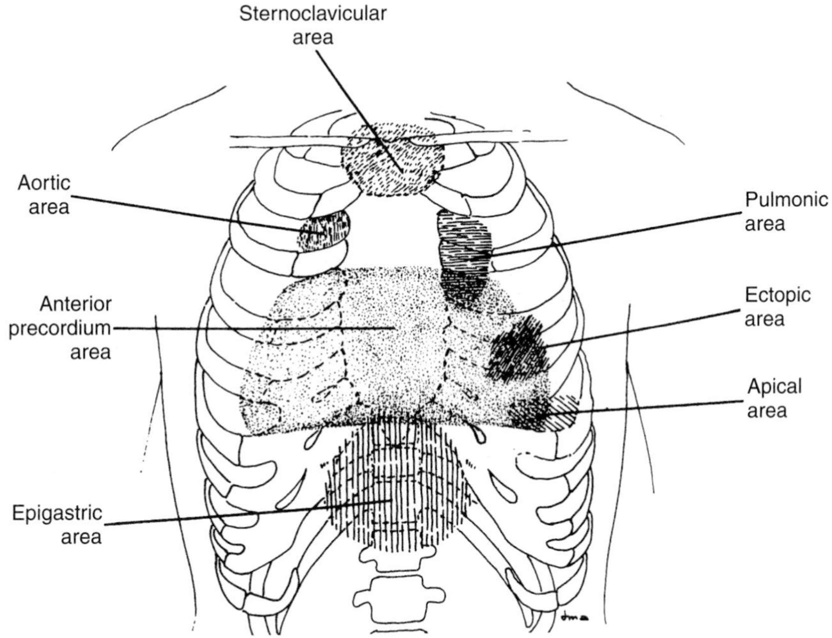

FIGURE 3-11 ■ Seven areas to be examined.
(Reprinted with permission from Alexander MM, Brown MS: *Pediatric history taking and physical diagnosis for nurses.* St. Louis, 1979, Mosby.)

pressure, pulmonary stenosis, pulmonary hypertension, or atrial septal defect (ASD).

- *Friction rubs* are similar to the sensation of rubbing two pieces of material together.

b. *Peripheral pulses* are rated on a scale of 0 to 4, with 0 = absent; 1+ = palpable but thready, easily obliterated; 2+ = normal; 3+ = full; 4+ = full and bounding.

- Common arterial sites for palpation include the carotid, brachial, radial, femoral, popliteal, dorsalis pedis, and posterior tibialis.
- Obtain simultaneous assessments of upper- and lower-extremity pulses to evaluate for coarctation of aorta.
- Strong, bounding pulses are found in PDA, aortic regurgitation, AV fistulas, and truncus arteriosus. Waterhammer pulses may be found with aortic insufficiency or a PDA secondary to low diastolic pressure. Delayed, weak pulses are found in cardiac tamponade, aortic stenosis, mitral stenosis, CHF, shock, and hypoplastic left heart syndrome (HLHS). Pulsus alternans (alternating pulse waves, every other beat weaker than preceding beat) indicates a weak heart muscle as seen in severe hypertension or LV failure.

c. *Capillary filling time* is evaluated by compressing the extremity with moderate pressure and noting the time required for the blanched area to reperfuse. Normal time is less than 3 seconds with the extremity at the level of the heart.

d. The *liver* is palpated starting in the lower abdomen and pressing upward at the right costal margin until the liver edge is palpated. The liver edge of an infant is normally 3 cm below the costal margin. The liver edge of a 1-year-old is at 2 cm below; the liver edge of a 4- to 5-year-old child is at 1 cm below. By adolescence the edge is either not palpable or is at the costal margin.

3. **Auscultation**
   a. *HR and rhythm*
   b. *BP:* Use a cuff bladder that is at least two thirds the circumference and two thirds the length of the extremity. Obtain four extremity BP readings during the initial assessment to rule out coarctation of the aorta. Thigh pressure is equal to upper extremity pressure until a child is 1 year old; after that, the thigh pressure may be higher. Upper-extremity pressures are higher in coarctation. Note the pulse pressure. Low diastolic pressure increases pulse pressure and may indicate PDA or aortic regurgitation. Decreased pulse pressure may indicate aortic stenosis or cardiac tamponade. *Pulsus paradoxus* is an exaggeration of the normal physiologic response to inspiration. Usually on inspiration there is a fall of less than 10 mm Hg in arterial systolic pressure. In pulsus paradoxus the drop exceeds 10 mm Hg during normal inspiratory effort. It can also be found in pericardial effusion, pericardial tamponade, or significant asthma.
   c. *Heart sounds*
      - S_1 represents closure of the mitral and tricuspid valves and the beginning of systole. The mitral component of S_1 is loudest at the apex. The tricuspid component of S_1 is loudest at the fifth ICS to the left of the sternum. S_1 is louder than S_2 at the apex. S_1 is increased in intensity from mitral stenosis, anemia, fever, exercise, and hyperthyroidism; S_1 is decreased in intensity from first-degree AV block, mitral regurgitation, shock, cardiomyopathy, hypothyroidism, and left bundle-branch block (LBBB). A split S_1 denotes separation of mitral and tricuspid sounds and is normally heard in the tricuspid area. If audible at the anterior axillary line, it is more likely an aortic ejection click.
      - S_2 represents closure of the aortic and pulmonic valves at the beginning of diastole. The aortic component of S_2 is loudest at the second RICS. The pulmonic component of S_2 is loudest at the second LICS. S_2 is heard best in the aortic and pulmonic areas. Increased intensity may be normal or may indicate hypertension or coarctation. Decreased intensity (best heard in the aortic area) indicates aortic stenosis. Decreased intensity (best heard in the pulmonic area) indicates pulmonic stenosis or tricuspid atresia. A split S_2 (best heard in the pulmonic area during inspiration) is physiologically related to the increased venous return to the RV, thus delaying closure of the pulmonary valve, and may be normal. A fixed split of S_2 represents delayed closure of the pulmonic valve from increased pulmonary blood flow through the RV as in ASD and total anomalous pulmonary venous return (TAPVR). A widely split S_2 may occur with delayed activation of the RV from right bundle branch block (RBBB), LV pacing, or ectopic beats. A single S_2 may be heard in tetralogy of Fallot, pulmonary atresia or stenosis, and transposition of the great vessels (TGV).
   d. *Extra heart sounds*
      - S_3 is caused by the rapid entry of blood into the ventricles. S_3 is best heard at the apex with the bell and may be heard in normal children. S_3 sounds like "Ken-tuc-ky." A loud S_3 or ventricular gallop is a pathologic finding caused by resistance to ventricular filling related to increased volume load or decreased compliance. It occurs in mitral regurgitation, CHF, tricuspid insufficiency, left-to-right shunts, and anemia.
      - S_4 is produced by atrial contraction, is best heard at the apex, and is almost never heard in normal children. It sounds like "Ten-nes-see." It can indicate aortic stenosis, pulmonic stenosis, hypertension, heart failure, and anemia.

e. *Murmurs* are heard because of turbulent flow through an abnormal opening or obstructed area. The following are evaluated:

- *Timing: Systolic murmurs* are heard between S_1 and S_2 (early, mid, or late). Holosystolic murmurs are heard throughout systole. Midsystolic ejection murmurs start after S_1 and end before S_2, usually with a crescendo-decrescendo sound. *Diastolic murmurs* are heard following S_2 (early, mid, or late).
- *Intensity* is based on a scale:
  - Barely audible (not heard in all positions)
  - Just easily audible (not heard in all positions)
  - Heard well in all positions
  - Heard well, a palpable thrill
  - Louder, can be heard with stethoscope partly off chest
  - Heard with stethoscope off chest
- *Location*
  - Apical area (with some extension up to the pulmonic area): Murmurs of mitral insufficiency or stenosis, subaortic stenosis, aortic insufficiency, aortic ejection click of aortic stenosis, and click or late systolic murmur of mitral valve prolapse.
  - Tricuspid area (with some extension up to the pulmonic area): Murmurs of tricuspid insufficiency or stenosis, pulmonary insufficiency, VSD, and aortic insufficiency.
  - Aortic area: Murmurs of aortic stenosis or insufficiency.
  - Pulmonic area: Murmurs of pulmonary stenosis or insufficiency, ASD, pulmonary ejection click, and PDA.
- *Radiation* to other areas of chest, back
- *Pitch:* High pitch is heard with the diaphragm, and low pitch is heard with the bell.
- *Quality* is described as blowing, rumbling, harsh, or musical.

INVASIVE AND NONINVASIVE DIAGNOSTIC STUDIES

A. Laboratory Studies

Laboratory studies to be ordered may include electrolytes, complete blood count (CBC), lipid profile, calcium (total and ionized), magnesium, BNP levels, lactate levels, and a clotting profile (prothrombin time, partial thromboplastin time, thrombin time, bleeding time, and platelet count).

B. Pulse Oximetry

Pulse oximetry uses changes in infrared light to evaluate the level of saturated hemoglobin, providing an indirect measurement of oxygen saturation (normal 96% to 100%). Pulse oximetry can be used to evaluate or trend cyanosis or to assess tolerance of procedures (suctioning, sedation).

C. Chest Radiographic Examination

1. **Heart size** is evaluated by estimation of the cardiothoracic ratio, which is determined by the largest dimension of the heart compared with the widest intercostal diameter of the chest. The normal size is 50%. A large thymus in infants may be mistaken for cardiomegaly.
2. **Cardiac borders** are evaluated on an anterioposterior film (Figure 3-12). The right border indicates the right atrium. The left lower border indicates the LV; the

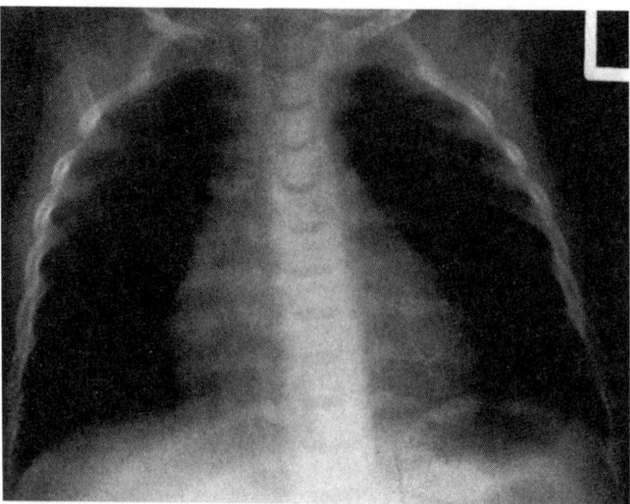

FIGURE 3-12 ■ Heart borders as seen on anterioposterior chest x-ray film.
(Courtesy of Children's National Medical Center.)

left atrium blends into the ventricular shadow unless it is significantly enlarged. The first convexity above the apex is the PA. The second convexity above the apex is the aortic arch. Specific defects can be identified from abnormal borders. A boot-shaped heart can indicate tetralogy of Fallot related to RVH with apex upturned. A convex shoulder of the aorta is seen in transposition of the great arteries (looks like an egg with a narrow superior mediastinum).

3. **Pulmonary vascularity:** Increased pulmonary vascularity is indicated by arteries that appear enlarged and extend into the lateral third of the lung field as seen in ASD, VSD, PDA, TAPVR, truncus, transposition, and AV canal (Figure 3-13). Decreased pulmonary vascularity is noted when the hilum appears small, lung fields are empty and devoid of vessels, and the x-ray image appears black. This may be noted in tetralogy of Fallot, tricuspid atresia, Ebstein anomaly, severe pulmonary hypertension, and transposition with pulmonary stenosis (Figure 3-14).

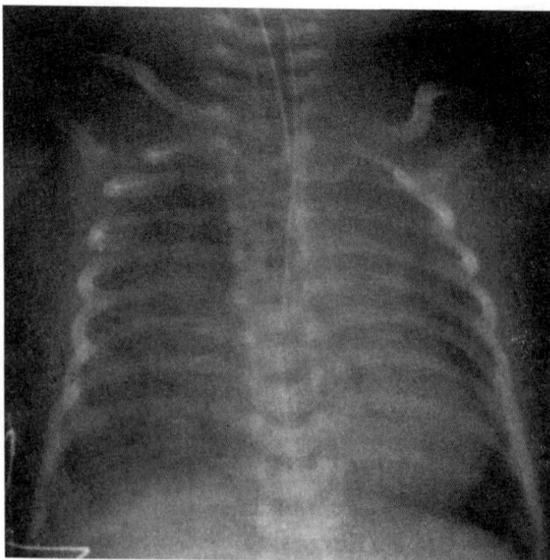

FIGURE 3-13 ■ Chest x-ray film with evidence of increased pulmonary vascularity.
(Courtesy of Children's National Medical Center.)

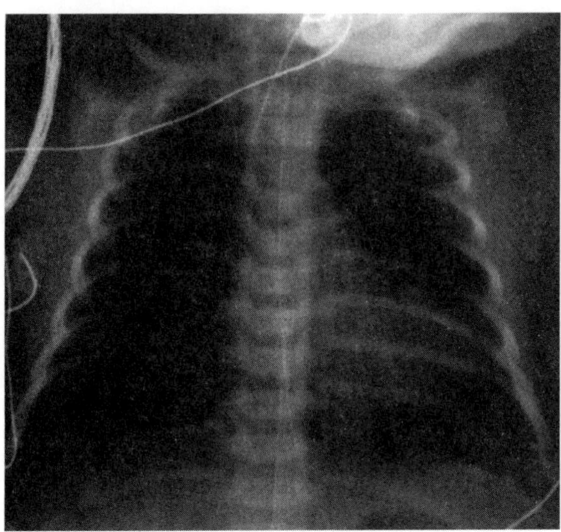

FIGURE 3-14 ■ Chest x-ray film with evidence of decreased pulmonary vascularity.
(Courtesy of Children's National Medical Center.)

D. Electrocardiogram (ECG)

1. The **purpose of ECG** is to measure the electrical activity of the heart by measuring the difference in electrical potential between two points on the body. The recording is used to measure intervals, direction, and amplitudes.
2. **ECG paper** (Figure 3-15)
   a. *Horizontal lines* are a measurement of time. Each small block equals 0.04 second, and each larger dark block equals 0.2 second, with use of standard paper speed of 25 mm/s.

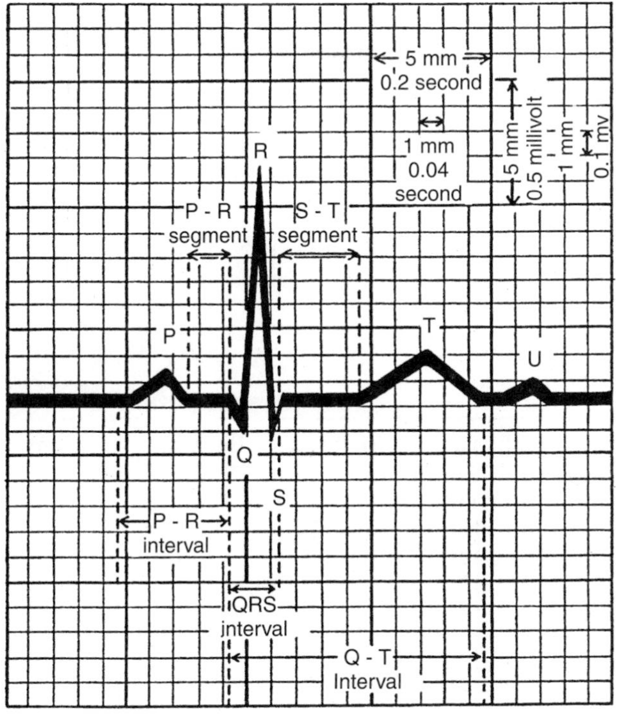

FIGURE 3-15 ■ Electrocardiographic paper and waveforms.
(Reprinted with permission from Sanderson RG, Kurth CL: *The cardiac patient: a comprehensive approach,* ed 2. Philadelphia, 1983, W. B. Saunders, p. 129.)

b. *Vertical lines* represent a measurement of voltage with each small block equal to 0.1 mV or 1 mm and each larger block equal to 0.5 mV or 5 mm (if gain of ECG is set to standard of 1 mV = 10 mm).

3. **ECG waves and intervals** (see Figure 3-15)
   a. The *P wave* represents atrial depolarization. It is measured from the beginning of the P wave to the end of the wave when it returns to the baseline. Usually it is less than 0.08 second. The normal amplitude is less than 2.5 mm (3 mm in the neonate), and it is usually gently rounded with all waves having the same appearance. Right atrial enlargement is noted by tall, peaked P waves greater than 2.5 mm. Left atrial enlargement demonstrates a wide, notched P wave.
   b. The *PR interval* represents atrial depolarization and conduction through the AV node. It is measured from the beginning of the P wave to the beginning of the QRS complex. The normal PR interval is 0.12 to 0.20 second (shorter in younger children with faster HRs). A prolonged PR interval is an indication of first-degree heart block (Table 3-5).
   c. The *QRS interval* represents ventricular depolarization. It is measured from the beginning of the QRS to the end of the QRS. Normal duration is 0.06 to 0.10 second. Prolonged QRS duration may indicate interventricular conduction delay. Although commonly called the QRS complex, the first initial downward deflection is labeled *Q*, the first upward deflection is labeled *R*, the first downward deflection after the R wave is labeled *S*, and any other deflections are labeled with an accent to indicate "prime," such as rSR′. The size of the wave is indicated by a capital or small letter; waves over 5 mm are in capitals.
   d. The *T wave* represents ventricular repolarization and should be in the same direction as the QRS complex. The T wave may change configuration with hypokalemia (flattened) or hyperkalemia (peaked).
   e. The *ST segment* represents ventricular repolarization. It is measured from the end of the QRS to the beginning of the T wave. The ST segment should not vary more than 1 mm from the baseline. Elevations may indicate ischemia and inflammation. Depression may indicate strain or ischemia.
   f. The *QT interval* represents summation of depolarization and repolarization and varies with the HR. It is measured from the beginning of the QRS to the end of the T wave. The QT interval must be corrected for HR. The normal is less than 0.45 second.
   g. The *12-lead ECG* in children should include a recording of V_3r or V_4r, or both. These leads are placed on the right side of the chest in the same positions as the V_3 and V_4 leads are placed on the left side of the chest. The purpose of the

TABLE 3-5
Maximal PR Intervals

	HR (bpm)	HR (bpm)	HR (bpm)	HR (bpm)	HR (bpm)	HR (bpm)
Age	<71	71–90	91–110	111–130	131–150	151
1 mo	0.11	0.11	0.11	0.11		
1–9 mo	0.14	0.13	0.12	0.11		
10–24 mo	0.14		0.10			
3–5 y	0.16	0.16	0.13			
6–13 y	0.18		0.16	0.16		

From Biller JA, Yeager AM: *The Harriet Lane handbook*, 9th ed. Chicago, 1981, Year Book Medical Publishers Inc

V_3r and V_4r leads is to provide an opportunity for analysis of the strong right-sided forces in young children.

4. **ECG analysis**
   a. *Rate* is calculated by counting specific wave patterns during a determined time, such as 6 seconds. An alternative method (used if the rate is regular with no RR variation) is to estimate the rate by noting the position of one wave on a dark line and then noting the next time the wave falls on a dark line. It is essential to remember the six consecutive numbers: 300, 150, 100, 75, 60, and 50. If it is one large block, the rate is 300 per minute; two large blocks equal 150 per minute; and so on. The rate can also be determined in regular rhythm by dividing 1500 by the number of small blocks between complexes. The rate should be determined for both the atrial rhythm (the P wave) and the ventricular rhythm (QRS rate).
   b. *Rhythm* is considered regular if the RR interval and PP interval have less than a three-small-block variation. Note if the rhythm is regularly irregular.
   c. *P-wave relationship to QRS* should be a consistent 1:1 ratio.
   d. *PR interval* should be normal for age and HR.
   e. *QRS interval* should be less than or equal to 0.10 second and have a normal configuration.
   f. *QT interval* (corrected) and *ST segment* are evaluated.

E. Holter Monitoring

Holter monitoring provides a 24-hour record of ECG activity. It is used to document arrhythmias at rest and stress as well as the frequency of occurrence in leads II and V_5. Patients and parents use a diary to record activity.

F. Exercise Stress Testing

1. **Purpose** is to evaluate ECG and simultaneous clinical response to specific stimuli. Exercise stress testing is used to evaluate myocardial oxygen supply and demand, evaluate or provoke arrhythmias, evaluate BP response to exercise, assess aerobic power and "functional" status (or level of conditioning), and evaluate chest pain or syncope.
2. **Technique:** A cycle or treadmill with ECG, BP, oxygen consumption, and cardiac output by rebreathing trend recordings are used. $\dot{V}O_2$ measurements may or may not be included because of the equipment required, technical capabilities, and the ability of the child to wear or tolerate the equipment.
3. **Normal response to dynamic exercise:** HR, cardiac output, and $\dot{V}O_2$ increase. Systolic BP increases with the intensity of the workload, but diastolic BP may remain unchanged. Mean BP rises mildly. Stroke volume increases with work, particularly from rest to moderate effort.
4. **Contraindications to testing** include *acute illnesses* such as myocarditis, pericarditis, asthma, thrombophlebitis, and febrile illness or *chronic illnesses* such as CHF and thyroid, renal, and hepatic dysfunction (relative contraindication depending on patient condition). Special care is required in aortic stenosis, cardiomegaly, hypertension, hypoxemia, anemia, heart blocks, or uncontrolled arrhythmias.
5. **Complications of exercise stress testing** include arrhythmias (supraventricular tachycardia [SVT], ventricular tachycardia [VT], premature ventricular contractions [PVCs]), hypotension, and syncope.

G. Autonomic Testing

Autonomic testing is used to evaluate vasomotor syncope.

1. **Technique:** Place invasive lines and then test the patient in specific positions (flat, then 60 to 80 degrees) and after drug administration (i.e., isoproterenol, propranolol).
2. **Complications** include arrhythmias (asystole, bradycardia), hypotension, and collapse.

H. Echocardiography (ECHO)

1. **Purpose** is to visualize cardiac structures and measure function.
2. **Technique**
   a. *ECHO* uses sound waves to measure the density of tissue and elastic properties of the heart.
   b. *M-mode ECHO* gives a graph of lines for each surface seen by probe with space between surfaces. It allows the most accurate measurement of the dimensions of structures.
   c. *Two-dimensional ECHO* provides a flat picture of structures and is used to identify congenital abnormalities. The *orientation* varies with locations of the probe. The parasternal view reveals left-sided structures, including the left atrium, mitral valve, LV, and aortic valve. The apical view shows all four chambers of the heart (most similar to drawings of the heart) (Figure 3-16). The subcostal view demonstrates the right ventricular outflow tract (RVOT), the RA, and the RV. The suprasternal view shows the aortic arch.
   d. *Three-dimensional ECHO* provides more detailed views of specific structures, allowing measurement of borders and clearer definition of structural anatomy, and measurement of atrial and ventricular volumes, particularly if configuration is not usual.
   e. *Doppler ECHO* measures the velocity of blood flow and is useful to assess the pressure gradient across a valve.

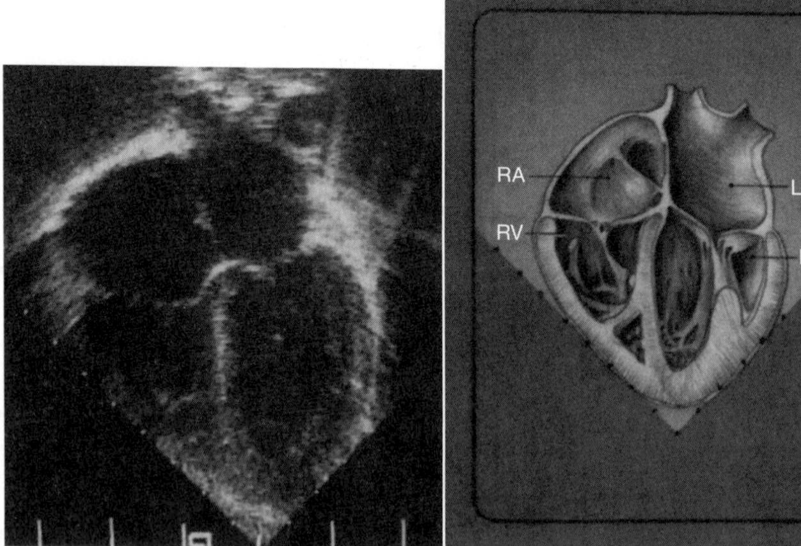

FIGURE 3-16 ■ Echocardiographic image **(A)** and diagram **(B)** of apical four-chamber view of cardiac structures. *LA,* left atrium; *LV,* left ventricle; *RA,* right atrium; *RV,* right ventricle.

(Reprinted with permission from Snider AR, Serwer GA: *Echocardiography in pediatric heart disease.* St. Louis, 1990, Mosby.)

f. *Transesophageal ECHO* is used to look at atrial structures (specifically for clots), to look for endocarditis, and to assess the adequacy of surgical repair during the intraoperative period. It requires placing the ECHO probe orally into the esophagus. To prevent gagging, sedating the patient might be required.

g. *Contrast ECHO* uses the forceful injection of dextrose and water, saline, or blood into a peripheral or central vein to produce microcavitation, which appears as a cloud of "bubbles" inside cardiac structures visualized by ECHO. Contrast ECHO is used to detect intracardiac right-to-left shunts, identify flow patterns, and validate structures.

I. Cardiac Catheterization

1. **Purpose** is to evaluate and measure pressures, saturations, and cardiac output and to outline anatomy with dye. Cardiac catheterization is also used as a treatment modality for specific cardiac or vascular defects.
2. **Technique**
   a. *Pretesting includes an ECHO, ECG, and CBC.* The child receives nothing by mouth (NPO) 4 to 6 hours before the procedure. Blood should be available, depending on the child's age and the procedure planned. Premedication with sedative, analgesic, or amnestic medications is recommended. Non-pharmacologic techniques that are effective in reducing anxiety and promoting comfort include guided imagery, muscle relaxation techniques, and biofeedback.
   b. The *catheter* is placed in the venous or arterial access and advanced into the heart to obtain oxygen saturation samples, make cardiac chamber pressure measurements (Figure 3-17), and inject radiopaque dye at selected locations.
   c. *Contrast agents* have a high sodium concentration and are iodine based. Hypertonic solution may result in changes in cellular membrane potentials, producing stimulation that results in heat sensation, pain, and movement. Isotonic agents are available at a higher cost and result in less hypocalcemia. They are useful in low cardiac output states, renal failure, or reactions to iodinated compounds. Risks of contrast include volume loss (with hypertonic solutions), lower BP from vasodilation, allergic reactions, and decreased

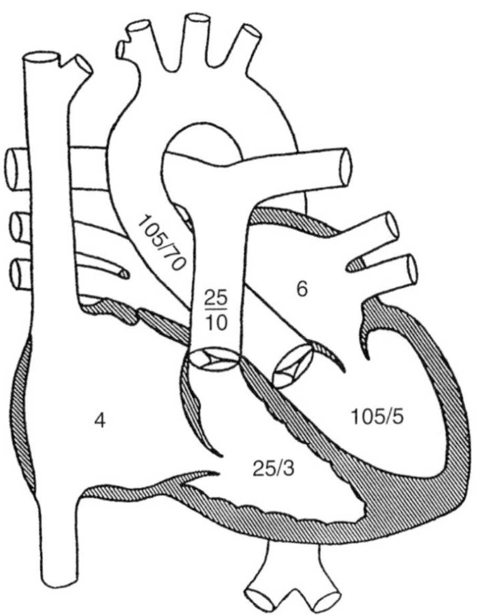

FIGURE 3-17 ■ Normal hemodynamic measurements (mm Hg) found during cardiac catheterization. Numbers *4* and *6* are mean pressures.

contractility; the risks are lower with the use of low ionic or isotonic contrast agents.

d. *Angiography:* The right ventriculogram shows the RV size and structure, RV outflow tract, tricuspid regurgitation, PA anatomy, and pulmonary venous return to the left side of the heart. The left ventriculogram shows the LV size, function, structure, and outflow tract, and left-to-right shunting patterns. The aortogram shows the aortic arch structure, aortic regurgitation, and coronary anatomy. Selective coronary angiography demonstrates coronary blood supply.

e. *Cardiac output* (CO) is measured by the Fick or thermodilution method.
   - CO = SV × HR
   - CI = CO/BSA in m^2; normal is 2.5 to 4 L/min/m^2

3. **Treatment modalities**

a. *Balloon dilation* of valves includes the pulmonary, aortic, mitral, and tricuspid valves. Balloon dilation of vessels has been used with peripheral systemic arteries, native aorta or recoarctation of the aorta, the PA and branches, and pulmonary veins.

b. *Placement of occluding coils* embolizes an abnormal arterial supply or occludes a PDA.

c. *Devices* such as vascular stents, ASD closure devices, VSD closure devices, and PDA occluders are placed.

d. *Other treatments* include balloon atrial or blade atrial septostomy and foreign body removal.

4. **Complications** include arrhythmias from catheter manipulation; arterial and venous thrombosis (and emboli); perforation of atria, ventricles, or vessels; allergic reactions to dye; shock; acidosis; hypotension (from heart failure, stress in a critically ill child, blood loss, or hypoventilation); and death.

J. Electrophysiologic Studies

1. **Purpose** is to evaluate the location and characteristics of abnormal rhythms and the medical therapies to treat them.
2. **Technique:** Pretesting includes an ECHO, ECG, and CBC. The child may also require an exercise stress test, Holter monitoring, and signal-averaged ECG. The patient is NPO 4 to 6 hours before the procedure. Premedication with a sedative, analgesic, or amnestic agent is required. Anesthesia and intubation may be used if an extended period of sedation is anticipated. Special precautions similar to those used in surgery are implemented to protect pressure points (occiput, elbows). A large sheath is placed for threading of marked catheters to identify the location of abnormal electrical tissue of the heart. Multiple catheters are positioned near the high right atrium, coronary sinus, bundle of His, RV, and LV. Pacing through these catheters evaluates conduction intervals as well as stimulates extrasystoles to determine sources of arrhythmias.
3. **Treatment modality:** Specific abnormal rhythms (such as SVT, VT) are initiated to test therapeutic medications. Radiofrequency or cyroablation can be used to eliminate abnormal conduction pathways or areas that generate ectopic beats.
4. **Complications** (in addition to those related to cardiac catheterization) include uncontrollable arrhythmias, which may result in cardiac arrest and death, varying degrees of conduction disorders, and a higher risk of intracardiac clotting when multiple catheters are used.

K. Nuclear Medicine Testing

1. **Perfusion studies** use specific radionuclear materials to evaluate cardiac perfusion. *Thallium-201* detects ischemia (not coronary obstruction) in the

myocardium and can be used at rest or with exercise. *Technetium 99m* detects necrotic tissue or infarcted myocardium.

2. **Multiple unit gated acquisition (MUGA)** uses radionuclear materials to obtain images restricted to specific times during the cardiac cycle (gating) such as end systole and end diastole. Data from hundreds of beats are stored in the computer to obtain adequate intensity. MUGA is used to assess ejection fraction and LV wall-motion abnormalities.
3. **Magnetic resonance imaging (MRI)** uses atomic nuclei subjected to an external magnetic field and stimulated by radio waves to send out energy in the form of radio waves that can be recorded and converted into a map of tissue. MRI is useful in determining structures (Figure 3-18) and in evaluating tissue health based on different image densities. MRI requires patients to remain perfectly still; in children this may require sedation. MRI cannot be applied in patients with magnetizable material in their bodies (i.e., pacemakers or artificial valves) or electromechanically activated devices.
4. **Magnetic resonance angiography (MRA)** uses MRI technology to evaluate blood flow through vascular structures. It is used to create clearer definition of structure and flow.

CARDIOVASCULAR MONITORING AND INSTRUMENTATION

A. Cardiac Monitoring

1. **Indications:** Continuous ECG monitoring is useful for rapid identification and response to rhythm changes. Continual monitoring is required in known arrhythmias and anomalies, the cardiac surgery postoperative period, and drug overdoses. Modified chest lead (MCL)-1 or limb leads (such as leads I, II, III, AVR, AVF) are often used for monitoring.

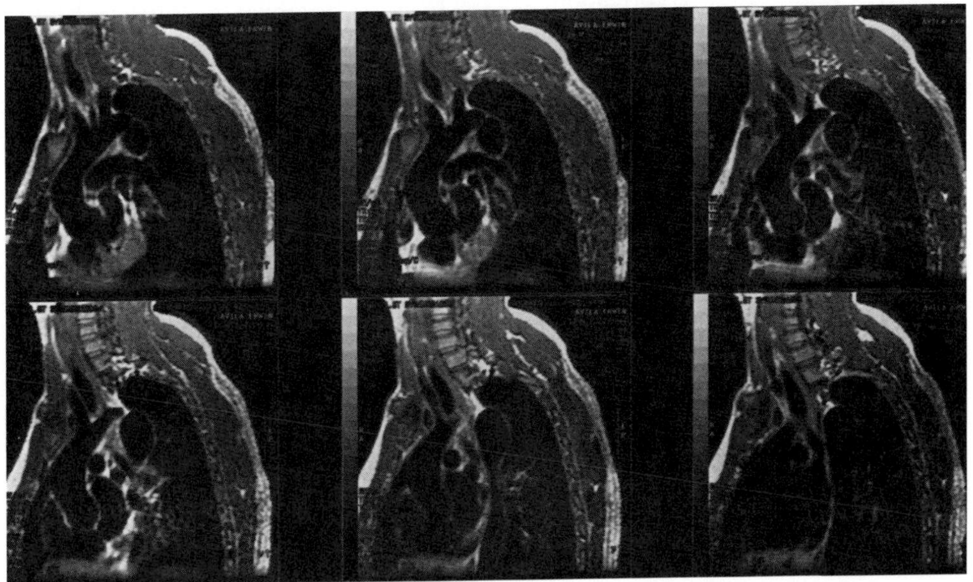

FIGURE 3-18 ■ Magnetic resonance imaging showing a coarctation of the aorta. (Courtesy of Children's National Medical Center.)

2. **MCL 1**
   a. *Lead placement* (Figure 3-19)
      - Ground lead: Right shoulder midclavicular
      - Negative lead: Left shoulder midclavicular
      - Positive lead: Fourth ICS, right sternal border

   b. *MCL-1 allows detection* of arrhythmias, bundle branch block (BBB), and differentiation of aberrancy. MCL-1 typical pattern is negative, similar to V_1.
3. **Monitoring rules**
   a. *Assess the impact of rhythm* on the patient first through assessment of perfusion and BP to determine whether the arrhythmia affects cardiac output.
   b. *The hierarchy providing the most accurate information:* 12-lead ECG where all leads are simultaneously recorded with standardized amplitude size, then recording on monitor paper, then evaluation of monitor screen.
   c. *Consider* the progression and pattern of arrhythmias, impact of surgery on the conduction system, ST segment changes, and usual rhythms with the use of specific drugs.

B. Hemodynamic Monitoring

1. **Arterial pressure monitoring**
   a. *Indications* include situations where a continuous BP reading is desirable, frequent blood sampling is required, or vasoactive medications are in use.
   b. *Insertion sites* can be percutaneous or cut down. The radial site is frequently used. The dorsalis pedis; posterior tibialis; femoral, temporal, and axillary arteries are alternative sites. The Allen test is used to assess ulnar patency or perfusion prior to insertion in the radial site. The Allen test consists of occluding both the radial and ulnar arteries until the patient's fingers and palm blanch and then releasing only the ulnar artery supply to determine whether the alternative blood supply to the hand is adequate if the catheter or clot occludes the radial artery.
   c. *Monitoring equipment required* includes nondistensible tubing, heparinized infusion fluid, and a transducer.
   d. The *phlebostatic axis* corresponds to the RA (Figure 3-20). The fourth ICS at the midaxillary line is used for zeroing.

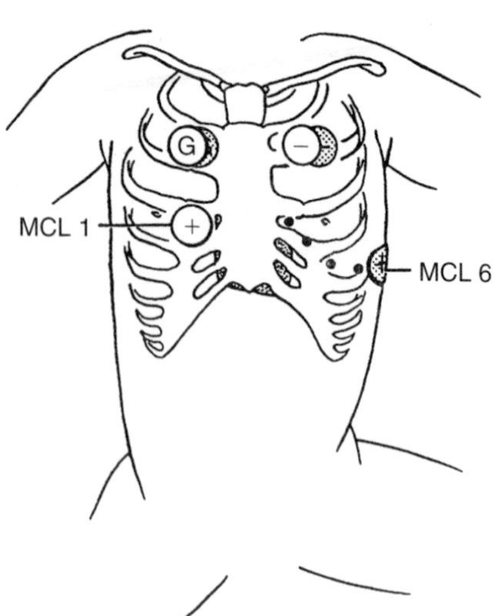

FIGURE 3-19 ■ Modified chest lead *(MCL)*-1 and MCL 6 lead positions. MCLs are useful in identifying aberrant rhythms and bundle branch blocks. *G*, ground lead.

(Reprinted with permission from Hazinski MF: *Nursing care of the critically ill child.* St. Louis, 1992, Mosby-Year Book.)

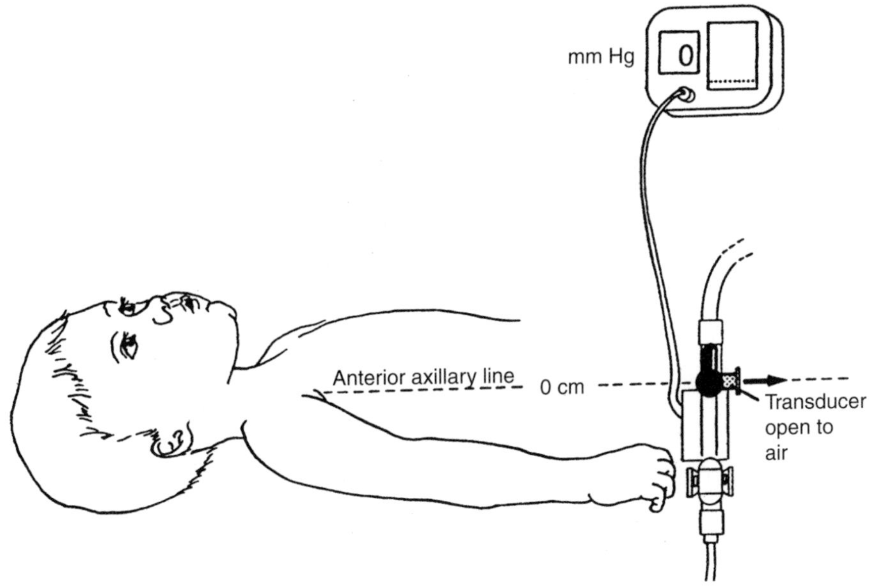

FIGURE 3-20 ■ Diagram of position of phlebostatic axis.
(Modified and reprinted with permission from Hazinski MF: *Nursing care of the*

e. *Waveforms* (Figure 3-21): A normal waveform has a clear dicrotic notch. Fling is related to an unstable catheter. A dampened waveform can be related to occlusion by a clot, absorption by air bubble, a kink, nonpulsatile flow (such as with ECMO), or a loose connection. Absence of a waveform can be related to a displaced or clotted line, nonperfusing rhythm, equipment malfunction, or spasm.

f. *Complications* include hemorrhage, ischemia, hematoma, arterial spasm, infection, and inaccurate readings.

2. **Central venous pressure (CVP) monitoring**

   a. *Indications* include assessment of blood volume and RV function and infusion of large- volume, hypertonic solutions.

   b. *Insertion sites* used include the internal jugular, external jugular, femoral, and subclavian veins, and transthoracic into the RA.

   c. *Monitoring equipment* includes nondistensible tubing, infusion fluid, transducer, and ECG monitor during placement. Choices involved in the selection of the catheter include nonthrombogenic material, the number of lumens, the size of the catheter in relation to blood vessels, and the length of the catheter.

   d. *Normal waveform components* (Figure 3-22) include the *a wave,* which reflects mechanical atrial systole; *x descent,* which reflects the decrease in RA volume during relaxation; *c wave,* which reflects the increase in RA pressure from closure of the tricuspid valve; *v wave,* which reflects mechanical atrial diastole; *y descent,* which reflects emptying of the right atrium into the RV.

   e. *Abnormal readings*
      - High: RV, LV, or biventricular failure; tricuspid regurgitation; tricuspid stenosis; pulmonary hypertension; hypervolemia; cardiac tamponade
      - Low: Hypovolemia, increased contractility

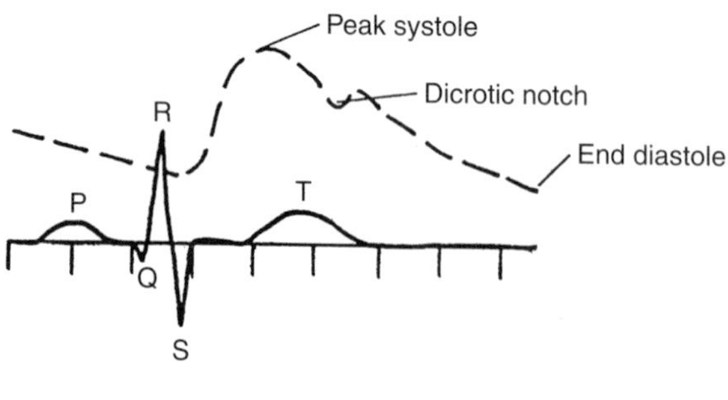

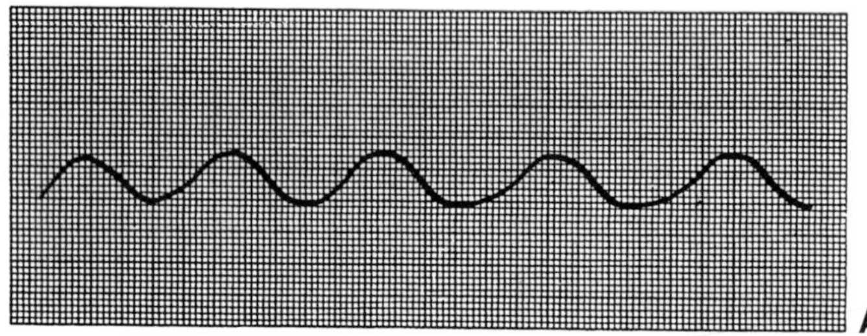

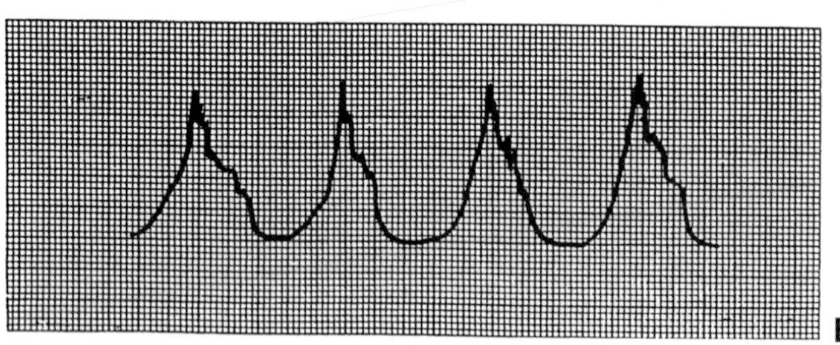

FIGURE 3-21 ■ Diagram of arterial waveform (dotted line) in relation of cardiac cycle by electrocardiography. **A,** Dampened waveform. **B,** Waveform affected by "fling."
(Reprinted with permission from Hazinski MF: *Nursing care of the critically ill child.* St. Louis, 1992, Mosby.)

f. *Complications* include arrhythmias, pneumothorax, infection, air embolism or thromboembolism, hemorrhage, vessel perforation or thrombosis, poor venous return, and inaccurate readings.

3. **Pulmonary artery (PA) and pulmonary artery wedge pressure (PAWP) monitoring**
   a. *PA monitoring* is indicated for use in the diagnosis of cardiopulmonary failure, management of shock, evaluation of abnormal PVR, and measurement of cardiac output.
   b. *Insertion sites* are percutaneous, cut-down, or transthoracic at the time of surgery. The PA can be accessed through the femoral, internal jugular, or subclavian veins.
   c. *Monitoring equipment* requirements are the same as for CVP, with two pressure lines for the CVP and PA ports. Cardiac emergency drugs should be available because of the risk of ventricular arrhythmias from the catheter tip touching the RV wall during passage of the catheter. A defibrillator should be available because of the risk of ventricular arrhythmias deteriorating into a rhythm that requires cardioversion or defibrillation.
   d. *Normal waveform* (see Figure 3-22) *components* include the *a wave,* which reflects LA systole; the *x descent,* which reflects decreased LA volume; the *c*

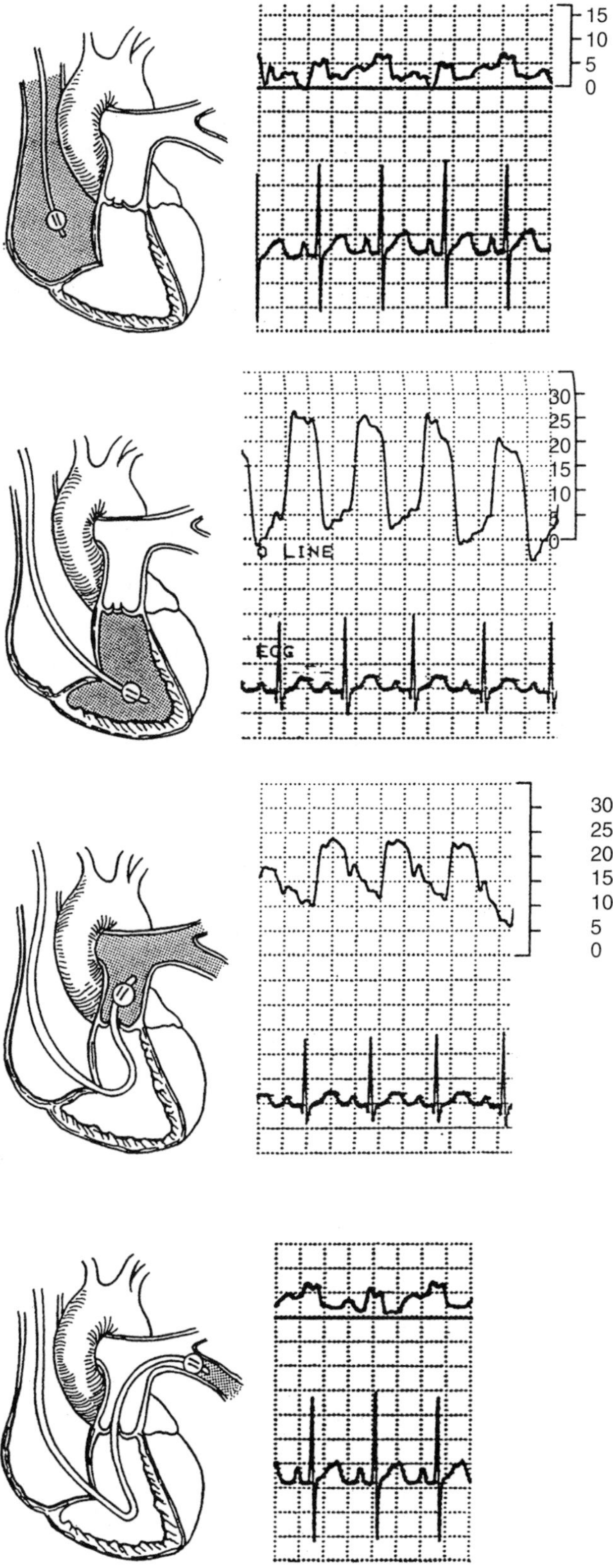

FIGURE 3-22 ■ Catheter positions and waveforms for monitoring the pulmonary artery.

(Reprinted with permission from Hazinski MF: *Nursing care of the critically ill child*. St. Louis, 1992, Mosby.)

wave, which reflects closure of the mitral valve; the *v wave,* which reflects LA filling (diastole); and the *y descent,* which reflects opening of the mitral valve.

e. *Pressure readings*
- RA pressure is the same as CVP. RV pressure is normally 20 to 30/0 to 5 mm Hg, with a mean of 2 to 6 mm Hg. High pressure is related to pulmonary hypertension, pulmonary stenosis, VSD, RV failure, constrictive pericarditis, cardiac tamponade, and chronic LV failure.
- PA pressure is normally 20 to 30/6 to 10 mm Hg, with a mean of less than 20 mm Hg. High pressure is from increased PVR resulting from vascular disease, pulmonary parenchymal disease, mitral stenosis, LV failure, or pulmonary vascular changes from increased pulmonary blood flow.
- Pulmonary capillary wedge pressure (PCWP) is usually 4 to 12 mm Hg. High pressure is related to LV failure, mitral stenosis, mitral regurgitation, cardiac tamponade, hypervolemia, or constrictive pericarditis. Low pressure is related to hypovolemia or vasodilation. PA diastolic pressure reading may be used to avoid risks associated with balloon inflation.

f. *Complications* include arrhythmias, pulmonary infarction, PA rupture, pulmonary embolism, balloon rupture, knotting of catheter, hemorrhage, and infection.

4. Left atrial monitoring is indicated for direct measurement of LA filling pressure, to measure LVEDP, or for indirect measure of LV compliance. *Monitoring equipment* may include air filter, nondistensible tubing, transducer, and infusion to maintain line patency *only*. *Waveform* is illustrated in Figure 3-23.

5. Hemodynamic calculations

a. *CO* = SV × HR; the area under the curve is measured for the change in blood temperature (thermodilution technique).

b. *CI* = CO/BSA; enter height and weight to calculate BSA; normal: 2.5 to 4 L/min/m^2

c. *PVR* = mean PA pressure − PAWP (or LA pressure)/CI × 80; normal: 37 to 250 dynes/s/cm^2 or 0.5 to 3 Wood units

d. *SVR* = MAP − CVP/CI × 80; normal: 900 to 1400 dynes/sec/cm^2 or 11 to 17.5 Wood units

C. Svo_2 Monitoring

1. Indications include the assessment of oxygen supply-demand balance, monitoring of tissue oxygenation, management of shock states, and evaluation of parallel circulation in patients with a single ventricle.

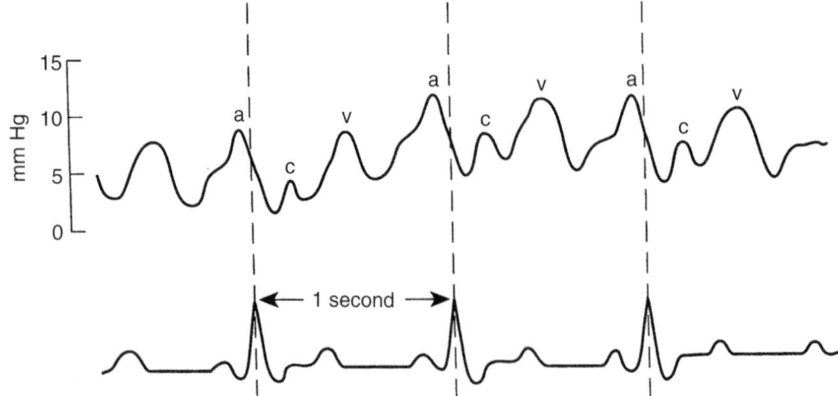

FIGURE 3-23 ■ Left atrial catheter waveform. (Courtesy of Hewlett-Packard Company.)

2. **Physiologic basis:** Oxygen content (CaO_2) is determined by PaO_2, SaO_2, and hemoglobin. Oxygen delivery (DaO_2) is determined by CaO_2, cardiac output, and tissue demand. Hemodynamic monitoring determines the cardiac output, and blood gas analysis can provide CaO_2. Oxygen consumption (VO_2) indirectly reflects tissue demand: $CaO_2 - PvO_2 = VO_2$.
3. **Monitoring mechanism:** The PA catheter with a fiberoptic tip uses light to reflect off blood saturation (the same concept as pulse oximetry). It is floated into place like a PA line, or it is directly placed through the chest wall during surgery. The PA line is used for intermittent analysis of PvO_2.
4. **Interpretation**
   a. Values are influenced by the hemoglobin level. Anemia, cyanide toxicity, and increased hemoglobin affinity impair tissue extraction of oxygen and affect SvO_2 accuracy. Cardiac output, PaO_2, SaO_2, and VO_2 also influence values. If other factors are stable, SvO_2 can be used to estimate changes in cardiac output and states of increased oxygen demand or activities that threaten oxygen delivery.
   b. *Normal* SvO_2 ranges from 60% to 80%. *Low* SvO_2 can indicate low cardiac output or increased demand (that the body cannot meet) such as fever, infection, shivering, burns, or suctioning. *High* SvO_2 can indicate low metabolic rate from anesthesia, use of paralytics, β blockade, hypothermia or high-output cardiac failure from sepsis (in which maldistribution of blood flow allows peripheral shunting in capillary beds and a defect in cellular oxygen utilization.) Right to left intracardiac shunting can raise SvO_2.
   c. *Continuous monitoring* can be used to assess the patient's tolerance of procedures that increase VO_2.

PHARMACOLOGY

A. Inotropic Agents

1. **Mechanism of action:** Inotropic agents work through α- and β-adrenergic receptors on cells. The α_1 receptors cause blood vessels to vasoconstrict. β_1 receptors innervate cardiac muscle and increase AV conduction, HR, and contractility. β_2 receptors innervate vascular smooth muscle in the lungs, and stimulation results in bronchodilation. β_2 receptors also cause arterial vasodilation. In addition, phosphodiesterase inhibitors improve contractility through the cyclic adenosine monophosphate (cAMP) system without any interaction of the α and β receptors.
2. **Milrinone lactate (Primacor)**
   a. *Action*: Improves cardiac contractility and decreases PVR and SVR by inhibiting phosphodiesterase cyclic AMP (cAMP)
   b. *Uses*: Ventricular failure, CHF, pulmonary hypertension
   c. *Side effects*: Hypotension, atrial and ventricular ectopy
   d. *Pharmacokinetics*: Peak action in 2 minutes, half-life of 2 to 3 hours, eliminated unchanged in urine
   e. *Interactions*: Incompatible with furosemide, procainamide
   f. *Nursing implications*: Assess cardiac function, vascular tone, ECG monitoring for arrhythmias, monitor renal function closely
   g. *Dose*: Load 50 mcg/kg over 10 minutes, then infuse 0.2 to 0.75 mcg/kg per minute
3. **Dobutamine (Dobutrex)**
   a. *Action:* Increases contractility, coronary blood flow, and HR by acting on β_1-adrenergic receptors of the heart
   b. *Uses:* To improve cardiac output

c. *Side effects:* Tachyarrhythmias, hypertension
d. *Pharmacokinetics:* Onset 1 to 10 minutes; duration 2 to 3 minutes
e. *Interactions:* Monoamine oxidase inhibitor (MAOI); incompatible in alkaline solutions, $NaHCO_3$
f. *Nursing implications:* Frequent vital signs, ECG monitoring
g. *Dose:* 5 to 20 mcg/kg per minute

4. **Dopamine (Intropin)**
   a. *Action:* Acts on α-adrenergic receptors to constrict blood vessels and thus increase cardiac output at high doses (greater than 15 mcg/kg/min); also selective vasodilation of renal and mesenteric vessels at low doses (less than 5 mcg/kg/min); dose-specific response
   b. *Uses:* Shock, hypotension, improve perfusion
   c. *Side effects:* Arrhythmias, tachycardia, hypertension, slough of extravasation, decreased renal perfusion (high doses), and increased PVR
   d. *Pharmacokinetics:* Onset 5 minutes, duration less than 10 minutes; metabolized in liver, excreted in urine as metabolites
   e. *Interactions:* Hypertensive crisis with MAOI; incompatible with alkaline solutions, $NaHCO_3$
   f. *Nursing implications:* Frequent vital signs, ECG monitoring, volume expanders for hypovolemia; careful monitoring of intravenous (IV) site (preferable to administer centrally)
   g. *Dose:* 1 to 20 mcg/kg per minute
5. **Epinephrine**
   a. *Action:* Catecholamine, which affects both α- (at higher doses) and β-adrenergic receptors on cardiovascular tissue; low dose (0.01 to 0.02 mcg/kg per minute) can cause vasodilation via β_2; higher dose can cause vasoconstriction; bronchodilation is caused through stimulation of α and β receptors
   b. *Uses:* Cardiac arrest, hypotension, acute asthmatic attacks, bronchospasm, severely low cardiac output, and anaphylaxis
   c. *Side effects:* Arrhythmias, cerebral hemorrhage if BP is increased significantly, dyspnea, hyperglycemia; increased doses may cause severe vasoconstriction with decreased perfusion
   d. *Pharmacokinetics:* Onset: 1 minute; half-life: 2 minutes
   e. *Interactions:* Hypertensive crisis with MAOI
   f. *Nursing implications:* Assess perfusion; frequent vital signs; evaluate injection site for tissue sloughing (extravasation is a major concern at high doses; central delivery is preferable); incompatible with sodium bicarbonate or alkaline solutions
   g. *Dose:* 0.05 to 1 mcg/kg per minute for continuous infusion
6. **Isoproterenol (Isuprel)** α_1 and β_2 agonist
   a. *Action:* Catecholamine, which increases levels of cAMP causing smooth muscle relaxation, bronchodilation, and pulmonary vasodilation, which increases HR and contractility
   b. *Uses:* Bronchospasm, heart block, bradyarrhythmias, shock, reactive airway disease
   c. *Side effects:* Tachyarrhythmias, ischemic ECG changes, hyperglycemia, decreased diastolic BP, increased myocardial oxygen consumption
   d. *Pharmacokinetics:* Metabolized in liver, lungs, gastrointestinal tract; half-life: 2.5 to 5 minutes
   e. *Nursing implications:* Check for tissue sloughing at IV site, evaluate the therapeutic effect, ECG monitoring, 12-lead ECG before initiation
   f. *Dose:* 0.05 to 2 mcg/kg per minute

7. **Norepinephrine bitartrate (Levophed)**
   a. *Action:* Catecholamine, which affects both α- and β-adrenergic receptors in cardiovascular tissue, causing constriction of blood vessels, increased contractility of the heart, and increased coronary blood flow
   b. *Uses:* Hypotension
   c. *Side effects:* Tachyarrhythmias; tissue slough with extravasation; increases right and left ventricular afterload
   d. *Pharmacokinetics:* Onset 1 to 2 minutes; limited duration; crosses placenta.
   e. *Interactions:* Hypertensive crisis with MAOI, ineffective in alkaline solution, $NaHCO_3$
   f. *Nursing implications:* Frequent vital signs, ECG monitoring, volume expanders for hypotension, evaluation of ventricular function
   g. *Dose:* Children—Initial dose is 0.05 to 0.1 mcg/kg per minute; maximum dose is 1 to 2 mcg/kg per minute
8. **Vasopressin**
   a. *Action*: Endogenous hormone that acts to mediate systemic vasoconstriction and reabsorption of water in the renal tubules
   b. *Uses:* To increase blood flow to the heart and brain during severe hypotension
   c. *Side effects:* Hypertension, bradycardia, water intoxication, venous thrombus
   d. *Pharmacokinetics*: Potential for excretion in breast milk; onset in less than 1 minute; half-life is 10 to 25 minutes
   e. *Interactions:* Decreased effect with lithium, epinephrine, heparin
   f. *Nursing implications:* Severe tissue necrosis with infiltration, monitor BP and urine output, fluid balance
   g. *Dose:* 0.0003 to 0.002 units/kg per minute continuous infusion for severe hypotension
9. **Phenylephrine hydrochloride (Neosynephrine)**
   a. *Action*: α_1 adrenergic stimulator, which elevates blood pressure via arteriolar vasoconstriction, affects SVR greater than it affects PVR. As blood pressure is raised, baroreceptors trigger vagal stimulation to decrease heart rate
   b. *Uses:* Hypercyanotic spells seen in tetralogy of Fallot, SVT, severe hypotension
   c. *Side effects*: Hypertension, bradycardia
   d. *Pharmacokinetics:* Metabolized by liver; half-life, 2.5 hours; IV route onset, immediately; IV route duration, 15 to 20 minutes
   e. *Interactions:* Potentiates actions of MAOIs
   f. *Nursing implications*: Monitor vital signs; use large veins because extravasation causes severe necrosis
   g. *Dose:* Children—IV bolus, 5 to 20 mcg/kg per dose; IV infusion, 0.1 to 0.5 mcg/kg per minute titrated to desired effect
10. **Digoxin (Lanoxin): Cardiac glycoside**
   a. *Action:* Inhibits the sodium-potassium ATPase pump, providing calcium for contractile proteins of cardiac muscle
   b. *Uses:* Ventricular failure, tachyarrhythmias
   c. *Side effects:* Arrhythmias, AV block, hypotension, blurred vision, or yellow-green halos
   d. *Pharmacokinetics:* IV, onset in 5 to 30 minutes, 1 to 5 hours' duration; half-life, 1.5 days
   e. *Interactions:* Multiple
   f. *Nursing implications:* Assess apical pulse before administration; dose adjustment is required in renal impairment; adjust dose with concomitant use of other antiarrhythmics (e.g., amiodorone or procainamide). Follow PR

interval for prolongation (note pacemaker); assess potassium level; evaluate therapeutic response; teach family signs of toxicity; digoxin immune Fab (Digibind) is the antidote

g. *Dose:* Age dependent—seek specific reference; 15 to 30 mcg/kg total digitalizing dose (TDD) divided with half in first dose, one fourth in next two doses, every 8 hours for TDD over 24 hours; maintenance: 10 mcg/kg daily administered orally divided twice daily; 5 to 7 mcg/kg daily, divided twice daily for IV maintenance

B. Antiarrhythmics

1. **Mechanism of action:** Classified according to the effect on cardiac action potential
   a. *Class I:* Act by depressing the fast inward sodium current across the cell membrane, thus slowing the conduction and lengthening the refractory period
   b. *Class II:* Competitive β-adrenergic blockers that reduce sympathetic excitation of the heart
   c. *Class III:* Act on the potassium channels on the cell membrane in phases 2 and 3 of the action potential, resulting in uniform lengthening of the action potential duration
   d. *Class IV:* Selectively depresses myocardial slow calcium channels in the SA and AV nodes
2. **Adenosine (Adenocard)**
   a. *Action:* Slows conduction through the AV node, depresses SA node automaticity
   b. *Uses:* To convert SVT, produce AV block to unmask atrial flutter
   c. *Side effects:* Minimal due to the rapidity of action; can see a period of sinus arrest on administration; short-term conduction blocks or hypotension
   d. *Pharmacokinetics:* Action in 10 seconds; metabolized in the blood
   e. *Interactions:* Theophylline decreases the activity
   f. *Nursing implications:* IV push as rapidly as possible, followed by a rapid flush; documentation of the rhythm
   g. *Dose:* 0.05 mg/kg per dose; double and repeat every 2 minutes to a maximum dose of 0.25 mg/kg; maximum single dose is 12 mg
3. **Atropine**
   a. *Action:* An anticholinergic agent that blocks acetylcholine at parasympathetic receptor sites, thus blocking vagal stimulation of the heart
   b. *Uses:* Bradycardia
   c. *Side effects:* Urinary retention, headache, dizziness, coma, hypotension, suppression of lactation, tachycardia
   d. *Pharmacokinetics:* Peak 2 to 4 minutes, half-life is 2 to 3 hours; excreted by the kidneys, crosses placenta, excreted in breast milk; minimal dosage required to prevent reflex bradycardia
   e. *Interactions:* Incompatible with most drugs
   f. *Nursing implications:* Document response, ECG monitoring
   g. *Dose:* 0.02 mg/kg per dose; minimum dose, 0.1 mg; maximum single dose in children, 0.5 mg; maximum total dose, 1 mg; maximum single dose in adolescents, 1 mg; maximum total dose for adolescents, 2 mg
4. **Lidocaine (Class I)**
   a. *Action:* Increases electrical stimulation threshold of ventricles, which stabilizes cardiac membrane
   b. *Uses:* Ventricular tachycardia, digoxin toxicity
   c. *Side effects:* Hypotension, bradycardia, heart block, respiratory depression, cardiovascular collapse

d. *Pharmacokinetics:* Onset 2 minutes, duration 20 minutes; metabolized in liver, excreted in urine, crosses placenta
e. *Nursing implications:* ECG monitoring with measurement of PR and QRS duration
f. *Dose:* 1 mg/kg per dose bolus, 20 to 50 mcg/kg per minute infusion

5. **Procainamide (Pronestyl) (Class I)**
   a. *Action:* Depresses excitability of cardiac muscle and slows conduction in the atrium, bundle of His, and ventricles
   b. *Uses:* PVCs, atrial fibrillation, junctional ectopic tachycardia (JET), SVT and VT
   c. *Side effects:* Heart block, cardiovascular collapse, arrest, bone marrow suppression
   d. *Pharmacokinetics:* Monitor levels of drug and metabolites
   e. *Nursing implications:* ECG monitoring, follow PR and QRS duration, observe for PVCs, BP monitoring
   f. *Dose:* Children—3 to 6 mg/kg per dose over 5 to 10 minutes loading dose; then 20 to 80 mcg/kg per minute as continuous infusion; maximum dose, 2 g over 24 hours
6. **Propafenone (Rythmol) (Class I)**
   a. *Action:* Decreases spontaneous automaticity by stabilizing myocardial membranes
   b. *Uses:* Ventricular arrhythmias, atrial tachycardias including reentrant arrhythmias
   c. *Side effects*: Complete heart block, blurred vision, dizziness, taste alterations
   d. *Pharmacokinetics*: Peak action, 3 to 4 hours; half-life, 5-8 hours; protein bound, metabolized in liver, excreted in urine as metabolites, crosses placenta, and excreted in breast milk
   e. *Interactions*: Increases levels of digoxin, warfarin; toxicity induced by amiodorone; phenobarbital decreases levels
   f. *Nursing implications*: ECG monitoring with measurement of QRS duration; monitor for digoxin toxicity or bleeding
   g. *Dose:* IV: 0.1 to 0.2 mg/kg loading dose, then 4 to 8 mcg/kg per minute, PO 3mg/kg every 8 hours; no elixir formulation available
7. **Propranolol (Inderal) (Class II)**
   a. *Action:* Nonselective β-blocker with negative inotropic, chronotropic, and dromotropic activity
   b. *Uses:* SVT, migraine, hypertension
   c. *Side effects:* Laryngospasm, bone marrow suppression, bradycardia, hypotension, bronchospasm
   d. *Pharmacokinetics:* Onset, 2 minutes; peak, 15 minutes; duration, 3 to 6 hours; metabolized in liver; crosses placenta and blood-brain barrier; excreted in breast milk
   e. *Interactions:* AV block with digoxin, calcium channel blockers; less effective with cimetidine
   f. *Nursing implications:* Monitor ECG and BP; follow liver enzymes
   g. *Dose:* IV, 0.01 to 0.1 mg/kg per dose over 10 minutes; maximum dose, 1 mg (infants), 3 mg (children)
8. **Atenolol (Tenormin) (Class II)**
   a. *Action:* Blocks β_1 adrenergic receptors
   b. *Uses:* Hypertension, tachyarrhythmias
   c. *Side effects:* Sinus bradycardia, hypotension, bronchospasm
   d. *Pharmacokinetics*: Oral peak, 2 to 4 hours; half-life, 6 to 8 hours; duration, 24 hours; IV peak, 5 minutes; no hepatic metabolism

e. *Interactions:* Anticholinergics such as atropine can increase drug absorption, and nonsteroidal anti-inflammatory drugs (NSAIDs) may decrease drug activity
f. *Nursing implications*: Monitor HR, assess breath sounds
g. *Dose:* 1 to 2 mg/kg per dose once daily; maximum 2 mg/kg per day; do not exceed 100 mg daily

9. **Esmolol hydrochloride (Brevibloc) (Class II)**
a. *Action:* Short-acting β-adrenergic antagonist by competitive binding of receptor sites
b. *Uses:* SVT, postoperative hypertension
c. *Side effects*: Hypotension, bronchospasm, bradycardia
d. *Pharmacokinetics*: Onset, less than 5 minutes; peak, 10 to 20 minutes; half-life, 10 minutes
e. *Interactions:* Incompatible with procainamide, furosemide, warfarin
f. *Nursing implications*: Monitor ECG and BP
g. *Dose:* Children—50 mcg/kg per minute infusion; range, 1 to 300 mcg/kg per minute

10. **Sotalol (Betapace) (Classes II and III)**
a. *Action:* Slows HR and decreases AV node conduction by blocking β-adrenergic activity and increasing AV node refractory time by affecting K^+ channels
b. *Uses:* Ventricular arrhythmias, difficult-to-control atrial arrhythmias
c. *Side effects*: Torsade de pointes, polymorphic VT, bradycardia, dyspnea, fatigue, dizziness
d. *Pharmacokinetics:* Peak action, 2 to 3 hours; half-life, 8 to 12 hours; absorption affected by food, especially milk products; crosses placenta; excreted in breast milk
e. *Interactions:* Antagonizes beta agonists
f. *Nursing implications*: ECG monitoring, particularly as initiate therapy; measure QT interval; assess for bronchospasm; prepare to treat torsade de pointes with magnesium
g. *Dose*: Children—Oral, 2mg/kg per day divided every 8 hours; increase by increments of 1 to 2 mg/kg per day to a maximum of 8 mg/kg daily

11. **Amiodarone hydrochloride (Cordarone) (Class III)**
a. *Action:* Prolongs action potential and refractory period of myocardial tissue by blocking cellular potassium channels as well as having sodium and calcium channel blocking effects; decreases β adrenergic receptors producing β blockade
b. *Uses:* Supraventricular and ventricular arrhythmias, JET, atrial fibrillation or flutter
c. *Side effects:* Hepatic toxicity, pulmonary fibrosis, fatal gasping syndrome, hypothyroidism or hyperthyroidism, corneal microdeposits, hypotension, photosensitivity, blue skin pigmentation with exposure to sunlight
d. *Pharmacokinetics*: Oral dosing onset 2 to 3 days to 3 weeks; half-life, 3 to 10 days up to 30 to 60 days; IV dosing onset is within hours; metabolized in the liver; stored in fatty tissues
e. *Interactions:* Increases digoxin, warfarin, phenytoin, cyclosporin levels; incompatible with $NaHCO_3$, heparin, cefazolin; use with class I antiarrhythmics prolongs QT
f. *Nursing implications:* ECG monitoring with measurement of PR and QRS durations; monitor BP if using IV infusion; monitor for signs and symptoms of adverse effects; educate on the need for long-term monitoring of side effects; use of sunblock, clothing, and dark glasses advised

   g. *Dose*: Children—IV load (limited data available); 5 mg/kg per dose, followed by a maintenance dose infusion of 5 to 15 mcg/kg per minute; PO load, 10 to 15 mg/kg daily for 5 to 14 days and then maintenance of 5 mg/kg daily reduced to 2 to 5 mg/kg daily; pediatric advanced life support (PALS) dosing 5 mg/kg IV or intraosseous (IO) rapid bolus.

12. **Verapamil (Isoptin) (Class IV)**
   a. *Action:* Inhibits calcium ion influx across the cell membrane, producing a slowing of SA and AV node conduction
   b. *Uses:* Arrhythmias
   c. *Side effects:* CHF, bradycardia, hypotension
   d. *Pharmacokinetics:* IV: Onset, 1 to 3 minutes; peak, 1 to 5 minutes; duration, 10 to 20 minutes; metabolized by liver, excreted in urine
   e. *Nursing implications:* Monitor ECG and BP; evaluate therapeutic response; use in children younger than 1 year contraindicated because of the high incidence of cardiovascular collapse. Keep calcium chloride ready; administer for vascular collapse.
   f. *Dose:* Children 1 to 16 years—Initial dose, 0.1 to 0.3 mg/kg over 2 to 3 minutes; maximum, 5 mg per dose; may repeat dose once in 30 minutes; maximum for second dose, 10 mg per dose

13. **Diltiazem (Cardizem) (Class IV)**
   a. *Action:* Calcium channel blocker inhibits slow channel influx in myocardial and arterial smooth muscle, resulting in decreased action potential excitation
   b. *Uses:* Atrial arrhythmias
   c. *Side effects*: Bradycardia, heart block, headache
   d. *Pharmacokinetics:* Oral peak, 2 to 3 hours; sustained release, 6 to 12 hours; half-life, 4 to 8 hours; IV peak, 5 minutes; half-life, 2 hours; metabolized in liver, excreted in breast milk
   e. *Interactions*: Incompatible with furosemide; additive effect with digoxin; increased digoxin levels; cimetidine increases diltiazem levels
   f. *Nursing implications*: Monitor ECG and BP; give oral doses before meals and bedtime
   g. *Dose:* Children—IV, 0.25 mg/kg per dose bolus over 2 minutes (may be repeated at 0.35 mg/kg per dose after 15 minutes) with infusion of 0.1 to 0.2 mg/kg per hour

C. Antihypertensives

1. **Captopril (Capoten)**
   a. *Action:* Renin-angiotensin antagonist, which selectively suppresses renin-angiotensin-aldosterone system; inhibits angiotensin-converting enzyme (ACE), resulting in arterial and venous dilation
   b. *Uses:* Hypertension, afterload reduction
   c. *Side effects:* Acute reversible renal failure, neutropenia, bronchospasm, hypotension, cough
   d. *Pharmacokinetics:* Peak, 1 hour; duration, 2 to 6 hours; metabolized by liver, crosses placenta, excreted in breast milk
   e. *Interactions:* Increased hypotension with diuretics, adrenergic blockers; use with potassium-sparing diuretics may cause hyperkalemia
   f. *Nursing implications:* Follow CBC, BP, renal studies, potassium level
   g. *Dose:* Neonate, 0.05 to 0.1 mg/kg per dose every 8 to 24 hours; can titrate up to 0.5 mg/kg per dose; infant and child, 0.5 to 1 mg/kg per dose, maximum, 6 mg/kg daily

2. **Enalapril maleate (Vasotec)**
   a. *Action*: ACE that inhibits angiotensin II, which decreases vasopressor action and aldosterone secretion, thereby decreasing peripheral vascular resistance, affecting both preload and afterload.
   b. *Uses:* Afterload reduction, hypertension
   c. *Side effects:* Hypotension, headache, dizziness, renal failure, hyperkalemia, cough
   d. *Pharmacokinetics*: Oral onset, 1 hour; peak, 4 to 8 hours; IV onset, 15 minutes; peak, 4 hours; crosses placenta
   e. *Interactions*: Indomethacin and other NSAIDs decrease activity; may increase digoxin and lithium levels; use with potassium-sparing diuretics may cause hyperkalemia
   f. *Nursing implications*: Monitor BP before and after doses; have volume expansion available for hypotension; follow potassium levels.
   g. *Dose*: Neonate—PO, 0.04 mg/kg per dose every 24 hours; 0.1 mg/kg every 24 hours; child PO, 0.1 mg/kg daily divided and titrated up to 0.5 mg/kg daily; IV, 5 to 10 mcg/kg per dose every 8 to 24 hours
3. **Diazoxide (Hyperstat)**
   a. *Action:* Vasodilates arteriolar smooth muscle
   b. *Uses:* Hypertensive crisis
   c. *Side effects:* Hypotension, SVT, rebound hypertension
   d. *Pharmacokinetics:* Onset 1 to 2 minutes, peak 5 minutes, duration 3 to 12 hours; crosses blood-brain barrier and placenta
   e. *Interactions:* Increases effect of warfarin (Coumadin), hyperglycemia with diuretics
   f. *Nursing implications:* Frequent vital signs (q5min); give over 30 seconds or less; keep patient recumbent
   g. *Dose:* IV: 2 to 5 mg/kg per dose (maximum: 100 mg); may repeat in 30 minutes or 1 mg/kg per dose every 5 to 15 minutes; titrate to BP
4. **Hydralazine (Apresoline)**
   a. *Action:* Decreases BP through vasodilation of arteriolar smooth muscle
   b. *Uses:* Hypertension
   c. *Side effects:* Shock, bone marrow suppression, hypotension
   d. *Pharmacokinetics:* IV onset, 20 to 30 minutes; duration, 2 to 6 hours; PO onset, 20 to 30 minutes; peak, 1 hour; duration, 2 to 4 hours
   e. *Nursing implications:* Frequent vital signs, volume expanders available
   f. *Dose:* Children—IV, 0.1 to 0.2 mg/kg every 4 to 6 hours; do not exceed 20 mg per dose; PO, 0.75 to 1 mg/kg daily in two to four divided doses
5. **Nifedipine (Procardia)**
   a. *Action:* Inhibits calcium influx across cell membrane during cardiac depolarization, dilates peripheral arteries
   b. *Uses:* Systemic or pulmonary hypertension
   c. *Side effects:* CHF, myocardial ischemia, hypotension
   d. *Pharmacokinetics:* Onset, 20 minutes; peak, 30 minutes to 6 hours
   e. *Interactions:* Cimetidine, ciprofloxaxin, erythromycin increase levels; quinidine levels are decreased with concomitant administration
   f. *Nursing implications:* To provide a safe environment until the patient's condition is stable on this drug; monitor BP; difficult to administer in young children because it is available only as a sublingual capsule that might require aspiration to obtain the appropriate dose or use a long-acting delayed-onset tablet
   g. *Dose:* Children—0.25 to 0.5 mg/kg per dose; maximum, 10 mg per dose

6. **Nitroglycerin**
   a. *Action:* Direct vasodilator; dose-related effect on peripheral vasculature
   b. *Uses:* To decrease preload (venous dilator at 1 to 2 mcg/kg per minute) and afterload (arterial vasodilator with decreased SVR at 3 to 5 mcg/kg per minute); selective for coronary circulation
   c. *Side effects:* Hypotension with collapse, headache, flushing, nausea; contraindicated if allergic to nitrates
   d. *Pharmacokinetics:* Onset is immediate
   e. *Nursing implications:* Requires nonpolyvinyl chloride tubing; volume expansion available (relative hypovolemia); note therapeutic effect
   f. *Dose:* Children—0.25 to 3 mcg/kg per minute; usual maximum dose, 5 mcg/kg per minute
7. **Nitroprusside (Nipride)**
   a. *Action:* Directly relaxes arteriolar and venous smooth muscle causing decreased preload and afterload (decreased PVR, SVR, PCWP, MAP, and venous pressure); increases cardiac output by decreasing afterload
   b. *Uses:* Pulmonary or systemic hypertension, afterload reduction
   c. *Side effects:* Hypotension with collapse, coma, cyanide toxicity, ventilation/perfusion mismatch
   d. *Pharmacokinetics:* Onset, 1 to 2 minutes; duration, 1 to 10 minutes; half-life thiocyanate, 2 to 7 days
   e. *Nursing implications:* Protect from light; mix only in dextrose; monitor cyanide and thiocyanate levels and blood pressure
   f. *Dose:* 0.5 to 4 mcg/kg per minute; maximum dose, 10 mcg/kg per minute
8. **See also esmolol and atenolol.**

D. Other Treatments

1. **Carvedilol (Coreg)**
   a. *Action*: α_1- and β-adrenergic blocking agent that reduces BP with peripheral vasodilation
   b. *Uses:* CHF
   c. *Side effects:* Dizziness, bronchospasm, bradycardia
   d. *Pharmacokinetics:* Peak effect, 7 to 14 days; half-life, 8 hours; protein bound, metabolized in liver
   e. *Interactions:* Rifampin decreases drug levels; cimetadine increases levels; carvedilol may increase digoxin levels or mask tachycardia from hypoglycemia caused by insulin
   f. *Nursing implications*: Monitor liver function, monitor for effectiveness as seen by signs and symptoms of CHF
   g. *Dose:* Approved for use in adults; PO 3.125 mg every 12 hours, up to 25 mg every 12 hours
2. **Prostaglandin E_1 (alpostadil, prostin)**
   a. *Action:* Vasodilation with relaxation of smooth muscles
   b. *Uses:* To maintain the patency of ductus arteriosus in infants with ductal-dependent congenital heart disease, pulmonary vasodilator
   c. *Side Effects*: Apnea occurs in 10%, fever, flushing, hypotension
   d. *Pharmacokinetics:* Onset, 15 minutes to 3 hours; half-life, 5 to 10 minutes; metabolized in lungs; excreted through kidneys
   e. *Interactions:* Potentiates effects of warfarin
   f. *Nursing implications:* Evaluate effectiveness by increased blood oxygenation, increased pH, increased BP, return of pulses (depending on the type of congenital heart lesion); monitor ECG, RR, BP, temperature

g. *Dose*: 0.03 to 0.1 mcg/kg per minute of infusion; may start at higher doses and titrate down once ductus is fully open

ADVANCED CARDIAC LIFE SUPPORT

A. Cardiopulmonary Failure

1. **Assess pulmonary and cardiovascular function,** its effect on target organs, and the potential for impending arrest. Cardiac arrest in children is most often the result of respiratory failure as opposed to primary cardiac arrest. Therefore it is essential to recognize and intervene immediately for signs of respiratory distress.
2. **Etiology of respiratory failure:** Respiratory failure is related to inadequate elimination of carbon dioxide or inadequate oxygenation due to intrinsic lung disease or inadequate respiratory effort. (See Chapter 2 for in-depth discussion of respiratory failure.)
3. **Assessment of respiratory failure:** Symptoms include increased respiratory rate or effort, diminished breath sounds, diminished level of consciousness or response to pain, poor skeletal muscle tone, and cyanosis.
   a. *Respiratory rate* may be tachypneic, apneic, or bradypneic. *Tachypnea* is usually the first symptom of increased work of breathing resulting from airway obstruction, pulmonary parenchymal disease, or chest wall disorder. In the presence of nonpulmonary disease, tachypnea without distress usually results in a normal pH. *Bradypnea* results from fatigue, hypothermia, and central nervous system (CNS) depression. Minute ventilation may be low.
   b. *Respiratory mechanics* evaluate *increased work of breathing* as recognized by retractions, flaring, and see-saw breathing.
      - *Stridor* is related to upper-airway obstruction from the supraglottic space to the lower trachea. Causes include congenital abnormalities, vocal cord paralysis, tumor, infections, or aspiration of a foreign body.
      - *Prolonged expiration and wheezing* can be due to bronchial or bronchiolar obstruction caused by bronchiolitis or reactive airway disease.
      - *Grunting* is due to premature glottic closure accompanying active chest-wall contraction during early expiration. Infants grunt to increase airway pressure (autoPEEP) to preserve or increase functional residual capacity. Grunting can be caused by pulmonary edema, pneumonia, atelectasis, and adult respiratory distress syndrome.
   c. *Air entry* is evaluated by chest expansion and auscultation of breath sounds.
      - *Asymmetry* of chest movement during expansion or decreased expansion results from inadequate effort, airway obstruction, atelectasis, pneumothorax, hemothorax, pleural effusions, mucous plug, or foreign-body aspiration.
      - *Breath sounds* should be equal and heard bilaterally. Evaluate both intensity and pitch over all lung fields. Change in pitch may suggest atelectasis, pneumothorax, or effusion.
   d. *Cyanosis* is an inconsistent and unreliable sign of distress. It may occur early in polycythemic infants or late in anemic children.
4. **Assessment of circulation:** Symptoms of circulatory failure include tachycardia, diminished pulses, slow capillary refill, cool or cold extremities, diminished level of consciousness or response to pain, and low BP.
   a. *HR* may be tachycardic as the body attempts to compensate or bradycardic during final common pathway for cardiopulmonary failure.

b. *Perfusion* can be assessed with capillary filling time, temperature of extremities, and palpation of pulses. Diminished circulation can be determined before the loss of adequate BP.
c. *BP* will fall when compensation for shock can no longer be maintained. It is the determining factor between compensated and uncompensated shock.

B. Cardiopulmonary Interventions

1. **Airway and ventilation**
   a. The *goal* is to anticipate and recognize problems that are not dependent on diagnosis of the problem. In recognized distress, immediately provide humidified oxygen in high concentrations.
   b. *Maintain a patent airway* through positioning and suctioning when necessary. Oropharyngeal airways are useful for airway patency in the unconscious child but may stimulate vomiting in a conscious child. Nasopharyngeal airways are better tolerated by conscious patients. The length of the airway should be approximately the same as the measurement from the tip of the nose to the tragus of the ear.
   c. *A bag-valve-mask device* is exceptionally useful. The face mask should provide an airtight seal on the face and extend from the bridge of the nose to the cleft of the chin, avoiding compression of the eyes. The mask is held in place with a one-hand head tilt–chin-lift maneuver using the E-C technique. (Thumb and forefingers form a C to seal the mask to the face while the fingers form an E to lift the jaw, pulling the face up to the mask.) Avoid hyperextension of the neck to prevent airway obstruction. Use a bag-valve device equipped with an oxygen reservoir to deliver the highest oxygen concentration possible. A pressure-limited pop-off valve is available but must be able to be occluded during resuscitation.
   d. *Endotracheal airways* are necessary for prolonged use or to achieve adequate ventilation when other methods fail. Cuffed tubes are usually used only in children older than 8 years, although they may be placed in younger children. Placement may be evaluated by symmetric chest movement, equal breath sounds, end tidal CO_2, or chest x-ray. Other assessments include the absence of breath sounds over the stomach, condensation in the endotracheal tube during expiration, skin color, and oxygen saturation.
2. **Circulatory support and vascular access**
   a. *Chest compressions* are performed when the cardiac rhythm is less than 60 beats per minute (bpm) in infants or the child has signs of poor perfusion (unable to produce a palpable pulse and BP). Compressions are delivered over the lower half of the sternum with the child placed on a rigid surface. The rate is 100 per minute at a depth of one third to one half of the child's chest. One hand is used to deliver compressions in children 1 to 8 years of age, and two hands are used for children over 8 years of age.
   b. *Automatic electrical defibrillation (AED)* is used to deliver rapid shocks in the prehospital setting in the face of ventricular defibrillation. AED-VF algorithms have not been fully established in children, but reports indicate that AEDs can detect VF in children but might not correctly distinguish VT, SVT, or VF in infants. Current AEDs deliver adult energy doses at 200 joules and are recommended for children 8 years of age and older or weighing more than 25 kg. Pediatric adaptor cables are available that deliver 50 joules and are recommended for children younger than 8 years or weighing less than 25 kg.
   c. *Electrical defibrillation* is required when ventricular fibrillation or pulseless ventricular tachycardia is present. Ideally paddles should be of a size to be in

complete contact with the chest without touching each other. The pediatric paddles should be used for infants who weight less than 10 kg or who are younger than 1 year. Front-to-back positioning may be helpful. Use of pregelled electrode pads instead of paddles may ease placement issues. The American Heart Association recommends a starting dose of 2 J per kilogram of body weight. This can be doubled to 4 J/kg and repeated (twice) if it is ineffective. Use of a biphasic defibrillator may be effective with lower doses. If the child is still unresponsive, epinephrine or antiarrhythmics or both and correction of acidosis should be tried to convert fine fibrillation to coarse fibrillation.

d. *IO vascular access* (Figure 3-24) is an alternative temporary measure for resuscitation only. It is safe and effective for medications and fluids in children. Access is successful if the needle is placed in the bone marrow, as evidenced by lack of resistance after the needle passes through the bony cortex; the needle stands upright without support; it can aspirate bone marrow; and free flow of infusion occurs. Location of IO placement can include distal tibia, anterior superior iliac spine, distal radius, distal ulna or sternum.

e. *Central venous vascular access* is essential to provide for faster volume/blood/ medication administration, thereby promoting rapid onset of action and higher peaks of drug levels. The largest and most easily accessible vein is the preferred site. Central cannulation permits infusion of larger volumes of fluid and more direct infusion of medications. Recommended sites include the femoral, internal, or external jugular or subclavian veins.

f. *Until vascular access is achieved,* lipid-soluble medications should be given via the endotracheal route. These include lidocaine, epinephrine, atropine, and naloxone. Medications should be diluted in up to 5 mL of saline before instillation and injected deeply into the tracheobronchial tree, followed by five manual ventilations.

g. *Arterial vascular access* permits direct BP measurement and easy blood sampling for oxygen and acid-base analysis. The radial, femoral, posterior tibialis, and dorsalis pedis arteries are often cannulated. The Allen test should be performed to ensure the adequacy of collateral circulation from the ulnar

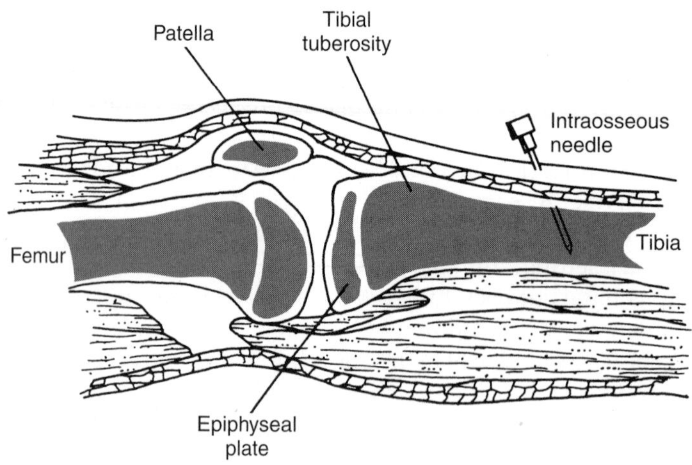

FIGURE 3-24 ■ Intraosseous access.
(From Barkin RM, Rosen P: *Emergency pediatrics,* ed 3. St. Louis, 1990, Mosby.)

artery before cannulation of the radial artery. Placement of arterial access may not be of highest priority during acute resuscitation, but it occurs during postarrest stabilization.

3. **Pharmacologic support**
   a. *General guidelines in acute situations:* Medications are preferably given via central venous access. Oxygen should be given in all arrest situations, in hypoxemia, or respiratory distress. Delivery should be in the highest concentration possible. Oxygen should not be withheld even if the measured arterial oxygen tension is high because tissue delivery may be severely compromised.
   b. *Fluid resuscitation*: Isotonic crystalloid is utilized to expand circulating blood volume in shock and is the key to preventing the progression of refractory shock or cardiac arrest. Hypovolemia is the most common cause of shock in children and can result from diarrhea, vomiting, diabetic ketoacidosis, fluid losses from burns or trauma, and distributive forms of shock with third spacing of fluid. Consider fluid resuscitation in all forms of shock.
   c. *Medications* (see Pharmacology section): Epinephrine is used for hemodynamic instability, bradyarrhythmias, and inotropic support and may be helpful in converting fine fibrillation to coarse fibrillation following unsuccessful electrical defibrillation. Dopamine or norepinephrine may be adjuncts for hypotension. Vasopressin can be an alternative for epinephrine in refractory shock but has not yet met the criteria of evidence for recommendation in PALS guidelines. Other medications to be considered include glucose because limited stores of glycogen may be rapidly depleted; calcium chloride is indicated in hypocalcemia, hyperkalemia, hypermagnesemia, and calcium channel blocker overdose; sodium bicarbonate is indicated for severe metabolic acidosis, hyperkalemia, hypermagnesemia, tricyclic antidepressant poisoning, or sodium channel–blocker poisoning.
   d. A*rrhythmia therapy* recommended in the PALS algorhithms include antiarrhythmic medications such as epinephrine, atropine, adenosine, amiodorone, procainamide, and lidocaine (see Pharmacology section) and defibrillation, synchronized cardioversion, vagal manuevers, and transcutaneous pacing (see Arrhythmias and Myocardial Conduction System Defects).

C. Neonatal Resuscitation

1. **Environment** should protect against excessive heat loss and provide a method to maintain the neonate's body temperature during resuscitation.
2. **Airway and breathing interventions:** The neck should be only slightly extended; the head should be maintained in the sniffing position. Ensure a patent airway by suctioning first the mouth and then the nares when necessary. Respiratory effort and rate should be evaluated immediately. Stimulation for maintenance of respiratory effort should not be done more than twice before further methods of respiratory support (intubation) are used. Indications for ventilation include apnea, HR less than 100 bpm, and persistent central cyanosis in maximal oxygen environment.
3. **Cardiovascular support:** *Bradycardia* (HR <100 bpm) requires respiratory support. Chest compressions should be done if the HR is less than 60 bpm or 60 to 80 bpm but not increasing with adequate ventilation. Compressions can be accomplished using both thumbs side by side on the sternum or two fingers placed one fingerbreadth below the nipple line. The depth of compressions is one third to one half the depth of the chest at a compression rate of at least 100 bpm (120 bpm in neonates) accompanied by ventilation at a rate of 40 breaths per minute.

D. Postresuscitation Care

1. **Continue to assess and support** cardiopulmonary function while maintaining airway patency and administration of humidified oxygen. Delivery of oxygen is titrated by arterial blood gas measurement. Maintain effective breathing and continuously evaluate ventilation. Assess peripheral circulation while adding continuous ECG monitoring, BP recording, and evaluation of end-organ perfusion and level of consciousness.
2. **Serial neurologic examinations** should be performed frequently to evaluate for intracranial hypertension, seizures, or focal findings.
3. **Multiple venous access ports** should be secured for ongoing administration of medications and volume requirements.
4. **Decompression of the stomach** via nasogastric tube improves ventilation and prevents aspiration.
5. **Monitor exposure and environment**, including the child's core temperature.
6. **Investigate underlying causes** for the arrest or respiratory compromise.

E. Parental Presence

1. **Parents** should be notified as soon as possible after the onset of resuscitation and should be provided with support during the process (such as clinical nurse specialists, social workers, or chaplains).
2. **Most family members** report the desire to be present during attempted resuscitation.
3. **Parents or family members** may not ask to be present during the final moments of a child's life, so health care providers need to offer the opportunity.
4. **Presence during resuscitation** may assist families in adjusting to death with less anxiety and depression and more constructive grief behavior related to witnessing the efforts made to keep the child alive.
5. **Surveys of health care providers** find that family members are not disruptive and help staff to view the child in more humane terms.
6. **Survivors of resuscitation** express satisfaction that family members were present.
7. **Development of a hospital protocol** is suggested to establish how to support family members during resuscitation with a facilitator to prepare the family for what they will see and remain with the family to answer questions and provide comfort.

EXTRACORPOREAL LIFE SUPPORT

A. Indications for Cardiac Extracorporeal Life Support

1. **Postcardiotomy low cardiac output syndrome** from arrhythmias, hypovolemic shock, myocardial injury, electrolyte imbalance, or cardiac stun.
2. **Persistent low cardiac output:** From *congenital heart disease,* such as obstructions to blood flow (i.e., aortic stenosis, critical coarctation of the aorta) causing LV dysfunction and failure; anomalous coronary arteries (rare) leading to myocardial ischemia; *cardiomyopathy* with ventricular dysfunction from multiple causes; *inflammatory diseases* such as myocarditis and Kawasaki syndrome; and intractable *arrhythmias.*
3. **Systemic illness:** *Septic shock* results in the release of the myocardial depressant factor related to the endotoxin load. *Metabolic abnormalities* can cause cardiac dysfunction related to hypoglycemia, acidosis, and hypocalcemia. *Toxins* such as doxorubicin (Adriamycin; used in the treatment of cancer), snake bites, antiarrhythmics, and heavy metals (iron) can affect cardiac function.

B. Cardiac Assist Devices (Table 3-6)

1. Extracorporeal membrane oxygenation (ECMO)

a. *ECMO* is a method of gas exchange that provides prolonged cardiopulmonary bypass with membrane oxygenation. The native lungs are not required to participate in gas exchange and can rest with minimal ventilation.

b. *Cannulation* can occur emergently through the carotid, jugular, or femoral arteries or as postcardiotomy support in the operating room. Venoarterial ECMO drains blood from the internal jugular vein in most cases. Blood flows through a circuit composed of a pump, oxygenator, heat exchanger, and power source or backup power source using gravity drainage and a roller-head pump to return blood to the arterial system.

c. *ECMO* is the most commonly used support in children with cardiovascular dysfunction after cardiotomy. Most of these patients have low cardiac output syndrome or severe pulmonary vascular reactivity. ECMO has been used as a bridge to transplantation in other children with myocarditis or cardiomyopathy. The duration of ECMO support is usually shorter in children with cardiac failure than in children with respiratory failure.

d. *Children requiring ECMO* support in the operating room or immediately afterward have increased mortality.

e. *Bleeding, infection, and vascular injuries* are major serious complications.

TABLE 3-6
Cardiac Assist Devices Available for Children

Type	Patient Size	Technical Features	Type of Support	Pediatric Applications
ECMO	2 kg and up	Extracorporeal, requires ACT 180-220, may need left heart venting	Nonpulsatile heart and lung support	Suitable for all ages and weights
Centrifugal pump (Biomedicus)	2 kg and up	Extracorporeal, requires ACT 160-200	Nonpulsatile left, right, or bivad support	Suitable for all ages and weights
Pneumatic pump (Thoratec)	17 kg and up	Paracorporeal, requires ACT 140-160, allows ambulation, higher risk of neurologic events	Pulsatile left, right, or bivad support	Suitable for older children, adolescents
Pneumatic pump (Berlin heart)	3 kg and up	Paracorporeal with choice of 10, 25, 30, or 50 mL stroke volumes, requires ACT 140-160 initially, allows ambulation	Pulsatile left, right, or bivad support	Suitable for all ages and weights
IABP	3 kg and up	Transfemoral or transaortic insertion of balloon, requires ACT 140-160 seconds, timing technically challenging	Nonpulsatile counterpulsation provides left heart support	Suitable for all ages and weights

ACT, activated clotting time; *Bivad*, biventricular assist device

2. **Ventricular assist devices (VADs)**
   a. *VADs* pull blood from the atrium or ventricle and return it to the aorta or PA to provide support for patients with cardiac failure.
   b. *Centrifigal pumps* use a rotating head to suck blood into and force blood out of the pump in a nonpulsatile fashion. Pneumatic pumps use air to force a polyurethane membrane to push blood through the device, providing pulsatile flow to the organs. Both provide cardiac rest off of inotropic support. Biventricular support can be provided with two devices placed (right and left).
   c. *One type of VAD* is not available for all children because of the variable cardiac output required by children. Adult VADs with large stroke volume and low HRs may increase the risk of neurologic complications. VADs require anticoagulation but less than ECMO and with less blood trauma. Risks include bleeding, infection, circuit disruption, and pump malfunction.
   d. *Improved cardiac function* is assessed by the return of pulsatile waveforms on arterial tracing and ECHO evidence of recovery of ventricular function.
3. **Intra-aortic balloon pump (IABP)**
   a. *IABP* uses a balloon-inflated counterpulsation to displace blood volume during diastole, creating increased blood flow and oxygen delivery to the coronary and peripheral circulation. Deflation occurs just before systole, creating a negative aortic pressure, which improves ventricular ejection by decreasing the ventricular afterload.
   b. *Children* require a pediatric balloon (2.5 to 20 mL inflation volumes on 4.5 to 7 French catheter) to provide 40% to 60% of stroke volume. Counterpulsation is timed to the ECG or arterial wave (arrhythmia control is vital) with inflation just before the dicrotic notch or deflation at the onset of the R wave. Timing off a radial arterial line may require adjustments for delays between aortic and radial events. Timing can also be checked using ECHO.
   c. *Balloon placement* is in the descending thoracic aorta between the left subclavian and mesenteric arteries.
   d. *Rapid diffusion of helium* at high HRs requires manual filling of the balloon every 1 to 2 hours.
   e. *Disadvantages* include the need for surgical femoral access, technical knowledge required for optimum timing, elasticity of the aorta in children (which may diminish the effectiveness of the pumping), and anticoagulation.

C. Nursing Care Required for Cardiac Assist

❖ *Decreased cardiac output* related to myocardial dysfunction requiring cardiac assist or RV failure requiring biventricular support
   a. *Outcome measures:* Adequate cardiac output as evidenced by required assist device flow rates, MAP, urine output, peripheral perfusion, and CNS function.
   b. *Nursing actions* include hemodynamic monitoring, assessment of cardiac output to end-organs, monitoring of assist device flow rates, evaluation of volume status and replacement as ordered, assessment for cardiac tamponade, titration of inotropic agents and vasodilators, and monitoring of trends in CVP and PA pressures.

❖ *Bleeding* related to blood component traumatization, surgical dissection, anticoagulation, abnormal liver function due to venous congestion, or disconnection of assist devices
   a. *Outcome measures:* Normalization of blood clotting factors; maintenance of adequate hemoglobin levels

b. *Nursing actions* include the measurement of blood losses from chest tubes, urine, stool, gastrointestinal tract, and dressings; evaluation of hematology profile including the CBC, prothrombin time, partial thromboplastin time, activated clotting time (ACT), fibrinogen, and fibrin split products; replacement of clotting factors; and safety measures such as keeping clamps at the bedside.

❖ Risk for injury from thrombi formation
a. *Outcome measures:* No evidence of thrombi
b. *Nursing actions* include observation of pump head and tubing interfaces, anticoagulation, administration, and monitoring of ACTs.

❖ *Risk for infection* related to invasive device connections, invasive monitoring lines, or depressed immune response
a. *Outcome measures:* Absence of infection as evidenced by absence of redness or drainage, normothermia, and normal white blood cell (WBC) count.
b. *Nursing actions* include assessment for signs and symptoms of infection, strict aseptic technique, surveillance cultures, and prophylactic antibiotic administration.

❖ *Multiorgan system dysfunction* related to low cardiac output state or nonpulsatile flow assist device
a. *Outcome measures:* Normal function of all organ systems resulting in normal arterial blood gases, LFTs, urine output, creatinine, blood urea nitrogen, and mental state.
b. *Nursing actions* to support other organ systems include ventilation and airway support, hemofiltration, nutrition, skin care, and mobility.

❖ *Psychosocial nursing diagnoses* include sensory alteration, pain control, anxiety or fear, sleep pattern disturbance, powerlessness, alienation, disturbance in self-concept and body image, knowledge deficit, and loss of parenting role
a. *Outcome measures:* Normal sleep, ability to express feelings and cope
b. *Nursing actions* include use of support systems, dark quiet environment at night, schedules, family visitation, rest periods, medications, open communication, answering questions, preparation for procedures, and family participation in care.

CONGESTIVE HEART FAILURE

A. Definition

Congestive heart failure is a condition in which the heart is unable to provide adequate cardiac output or regional blood flow to meet the circulatory and metabolic requirements of the body resulting from structural abnormalities that place pressure or volume loads on the heart muscle or from intrinsic myocardial dysfunction.

B. Pathophysiology

1. **Hemodynamics resulting in cardiac failure:** Inadequate emptying of venous reservoirs (backward failure) and reduced ejection of blood (forward failure).
2. **Mechanisms of cardiac reserve** include increased HR and increased stroke volume, increased oxygen extraction, redistribution of blood flow, cardiac dilation, anaerobic metabolism, and cardiac hypertrophy.
3. **Systemic compensatory response** in response to inadequate cardiac output includes the following:
   a. *Salt and water retention* augments preload, causing pulmonary congestion and edema, and results in increased contractility from stretching of the muscle tissue.

b. *Vasoconstriction* helps to maintain BP for adequate perfusion but also increases afterload and myocardial energy and oxygen consumption.
c. *Sympathetic stimulation* increases HR, stroke volume, and energy consumption. Chronic stimulation leads to desensitization.
d. *cAMP* release results in calcium uptake to increase contractility, overloading the system that pumps calcium out of cell during diastole with decreased relaxation. Overload results in transient depolarizations, causing arrhythmias.
e. *Hypertrophy of the cardiac muscle* increases the number of cells to share the workload. Capillary deficit leads to energy and oxygen starvation and myocyte necrosis. Necrosis leads to fibroblast and collagen deposition within the thinned dilated heart. Rapid growth causes variable gene expression of myocardial proteins. Preferential synthesis of "slow" myosin allows increased filling but decreased contractility. Change in the proteins that regulate the calcium channels in the sarcoplasmic reticulum results in rhythm problems.
f. *Desensitization of β-adrenergic receptors* decreases energy use and the functioning number of receptor molecules (downregulation), which decreases contractility.

C. Etiology (Multifactorial)

1. **Obstruction of forward flow** can result from defects such as mitral or aortic stenosis or coarctation of the aorta.
2. **Overload can be due to shunting** (i.e., VSD, AV canal).
3. **Muscular underdevelopment** may occur, such as in HLHS or single ventricle.
4. **Decreased contractility** may result from ischemia, inflammation, or fibrosis.
5. **Arrhythmias** can cause a failure to empty adequately or failure to contract (e.g., bradycardia, conduction disorders).

D. Clinical Signs and Symptoms

1. **Sympathetic stimulation** results in increased HR, increased arrhythmias, peripheral vasoconstriction, mottled and cool skin, and diaphoresis.
2. The **renin-angiotensin-aldosterone mechanism** promotes sodium and water retention, oliguria, peripheral edema, and weight gain (fluid only).
3. **Systemic venous engorgement** is characterized by increased liver size (hepatomegaly), jugular venous distention, peripheral or periorbital edema, ascites, pleural effusion, or a combination of these signs.
4. **Pulmonary venous engorgement** results in tachypnea, rales, wheezing that does not clear until the heart failure is treated, increased respiratory effort, retractions, nasal flaring, pulmonary edema, and central cyanosis.
5. **Low cardiac output** is indicated by irritability, fatigue or lethargy, poor or prolonged feeding with a weak suck, change in responsiveness, poor weight gain, tachycardia, a gallop rhythm, diaphoresis, oliguria, pallor, peripheral cyanosis, decreased capillary refill, pulsus alternans, and pulsus paradoxus.
6. **Redistribution of blood flow** is related to vasoconstricting and vasodilating effects of neurohormonal agents such as norepinephrine, renin-angiotensin-aldosterone, vasopressin, ANP, BNP, dopamine, and paracrine agents. Although protective for the heart and brain, redistributed flow may result in impairment of other organ systems. Long-term redistribution of flow may result in organ impairment (e.g., decreased gut perfusion may result in paralytic ileus; decreased hepatic perfusion results in decreased metabolic function and clotting abnormalities; reduced skin or peripheral perfusion may result in necrotic changes; skeletal muscle may atrophy; and decreased glomerular filtration rate can result in acute tubular necrosis).

E. Diagnostic Studies

1. **History and physical examination** are consistent with the preceding clinical presentation.
2. **Chest x-ray examination** is useful for recognition of cardiomegaly, increased pulmonary vascular markings, pleural effusion, and congestion.
3. **ECG** will determine associated conduction disorders or arrhythmias.
4. **ECHO** establishes the presence or absence of structural defects or pericardial effusion and evaluates contractility.
5. **PA catheter placement** can help determine cardiac index and evaluate management.
6. **Cardiac catheterization** is used to evaluate structural defects, quantify cardiac output, and to evaluate cause.
7. **SVO_2 measurements** provide information about changes in cardiac output and tissue (myocardial) oxygen requirements.
8. **Laboratory studies** diagnose dilutional changes in serum sodium and hemoglobin, anemia, hypoglycemia in infants, digoxin levels, and abnormal results from LFTs related to hepatic venous congestion. BNP levels greater than 650 fmol/mL by enzyme immunoassay are helpful and correlate with ejection fraction.

F. Nursing Diagnoses

- ❖ Alteration in cardiac output related to inadequate tissue perfusion and inadequate nutrition to tissues
- ❖ Alteration in breathing patterns
- ❖ Alteration in fluid and electrolyte balance
- ❖ Activity intolerance
- ❖ Potential for injury from medication therapy

G. Goals and Patient Outcomes

1. Establish hemodynamic stability and optimize cardiac output.
2. Establish positive nutritional state.
3. Maintain optimal level of activity.
4. Prevent medication complications.

H. Patient Management

1. **Improve cardiac output**
   a. Provide *supportive therapy* to increase oxygen supply (supplemental oxygen, semi-Fowler position, bronchodilators) or decrease oxygen demand (normothermia, reduce activity, digoxin therapy, sedation, enteral feedings to decrease energy required for eating, increased caloric intake, and mechanical ventilation).
   b. *Pharmacologic therapy: Vasodilators and inotropic agents* alter the determinants of cardiac output (preload, afterload, contractility, and HR). *Digoxin* improves contractility but increases myocardial oxygen demand and arrhythmogenicity. *Phosphodiesterase inhibitors* provide a positive inotropic effect (nonadrenergically mediated) plus afterload reduction. *β blockers* act to counter sympathetic stimulation.
2. **Control fluid status** through assessment of edema, weight, and breath sounds. Fluid and sodium restrictions may be used. Measure electrolyte levels for elevated sodium and low potassium levels.
   a. *Pharmacologic therapy*: *Diuretics* include *loop diuretics,* which block sodium and chloride reabsorption in the ascending limb of the loop of Henle; *furosemide*

and ethacrynic acid, which inhibit sodium chloride transport in the ascending loop of Henle and in the proximal and distal tubule; *chlorothiazide and hydrochlorothiazide,* which inhibit reabsorption of sodium in the distal tubule and loop of Henle and inhibit water reabsorption in the cortical diluting segment; *metolazone, which* inhibits sodium reabsorption at the cortical-diluting site and in the proximal convoluted tubule; *spironolactone,* which is an aldosterone antagonist that interacts with ACE inhibitors to augment natriuresis.

b. *Complications* include electrolyte imbalances, ototoxicity, and elevated values in renal function studies.

3. **Patient and family education** should include teaching about diet, medications, and signs and symptoms of CHF.
4. **Mechanical and surgical interventions**
   a. *Cardiac assist devices* are not a cure but provide a bridge to recovery or transplantation in patients with CHF and cardiogenic shock.
   b. For *CHF related to correctable congenital defects,* surgery is performed after optimal medical management.

SHOCK

A. Definition

A complex syndrome of decreased tissue perfusion resulting in an inadequate supply of oxygen and nutrients to body cells

B. Etiology and Pathophysiology

1. **Low-flow shock**
   a. *Hypovolemic shock:* Decreased intravascular volume causes decreased venous return, decreased ventricular filling, decreased stroke volume, and decreased cardiac output with decreased blood flow to tissues. *Causes* include blood loss related to trauma, surgery, gastrointestinal tract bleeding, and intracranial hemorrhage; plasma loss from capillary fluid shifts in sepsis, thermal injury, anaphylactic reaction, burns, or nephrotic syndrome; and water loss from vomiting and diarrhea, diuretic administration, or diabetes insipidus.
   b. *Cardiogenic shock* is the inability of the cardiac muscle to pump adequately to meet the metabolic demands of the tissues. Decreased stroke volume results in reduced cardiac output with inadequate blood flow to the tissues. Decreased coronary perfusion and myocardial ischemia lead to further ventricular dysfunction. *Causes* include ischemic injury, arrhythmias, surgical damage and edema, inflammatory injury, obstruction of outflow, and systemic or pulmonary shunting.
2. **Maldistributive shock:** Abnormal distribution of blood volume is evidenced by decreased systemic vascular resistance and shunting of blood past capillary beds.
   a. *Septic shock* (see Chapter 9)
   b. *Anaphylactic shock:* The release of immunoglobulin E (IgE), histamine, serotonin, bradykinin, and prostaglandins in response to anaphylactic reaction. Mediators cause vasodilation and capillary leak.
   c. *Neurogenic:* Massive vasodilation from the loss of sympathetic vasomotor tone caused by pharmacologic blockade or traumatic damage to sympathetic nervous system.
3. **Compensatory mechanisms:** See Table 3-7 for compensatory mechanisms to the lack of oxygen delivery and metabolism to tissues.

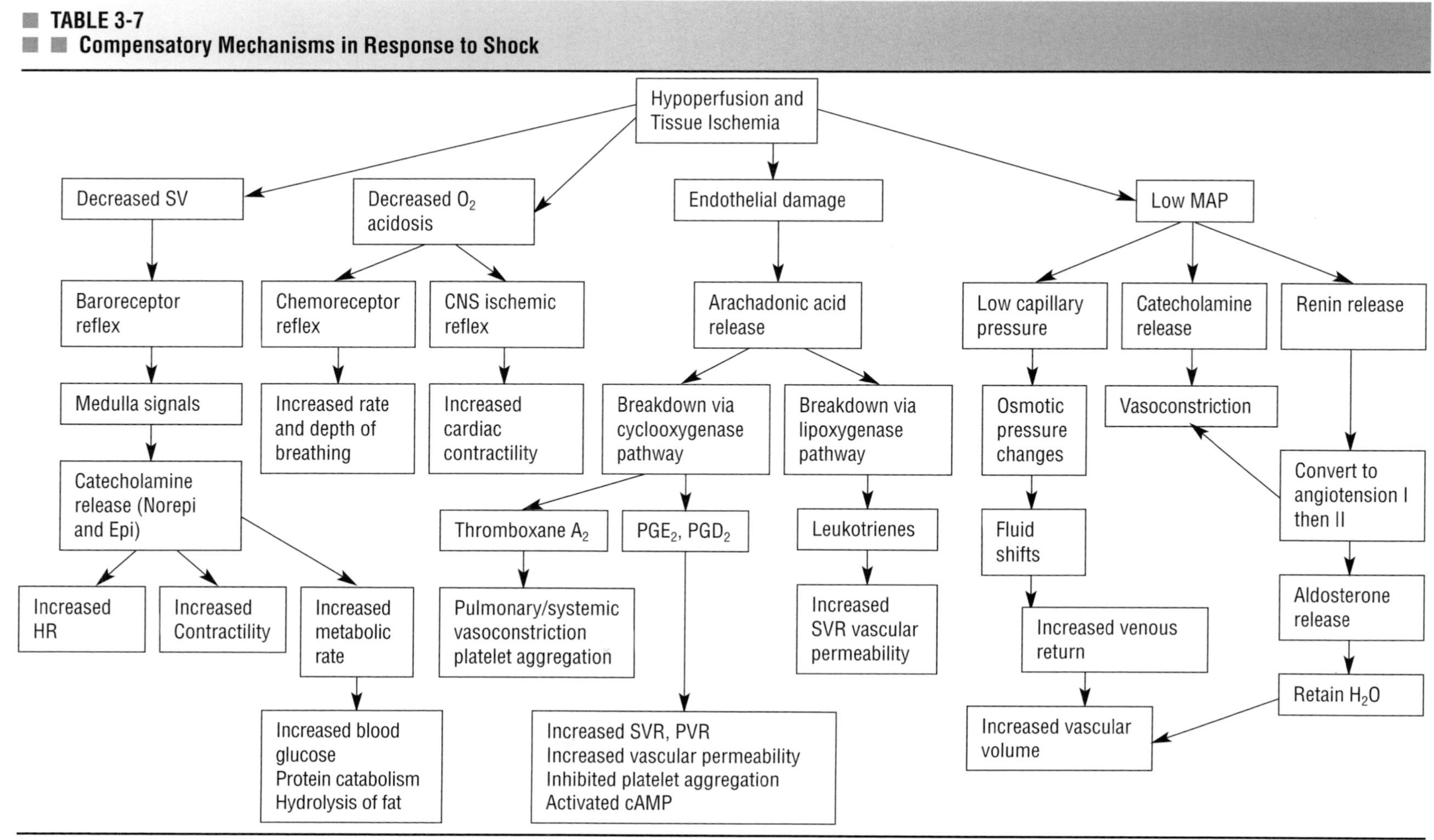
TABLE 3-7
Compensatory Mechanisms in Response to Shock
Hypoperfusion and Tissue Ischemia
Decreased SV
Baroreceptor reflex
Medulla signals
Catecholamine release (Norepi and Epi)
Increased HR
Increased Contractility
Increased metabolic rate
Increased blood glucose
Protein catabolism
Hydrolysis of fat
Decreased O_2 acidosis
Chemoreceptor reflex
Increased rate and depth of breathing
CNS ischemic reflex
Increased cardiac contractility
Endothelial damage
Arachadonic acid release
Breakdown via cyclooxygenase pathway
Thromboxane A_2
Pulmonary/systemic vasoconstriction platelet aggregation
PGE_2, PGD_2
Increased SVR, PVR
Increased vascular permeability
Inhibited platelet aggregation
Activated cAMP
Breakdown via lipoxygenase pathway
Leukotrienes
Increased SVR vascular permeability
Low MAP
Low capillary pressure
Osmotic pressure changes
Fluid shifts
Increased venous return
Increased vascular volume
Catecholamine release
Vasoconstriction
Renin release
Convert to angiotension I then II
Aldosterone release
Retain H_2O

C. Signs and Symptoms

1. **Compensated phase** occurs in response to a deficiency in oxygen and delivery, resulting in anaerobic metabolism and lactic acid production. Vasoconstriction results in cool, pale, or mottled skin with delayed capillary filling time, diminished peripheral pulses, and narrow pulse pressure. Diaphoresis results in clammy, moist skin. Urine output decreases. Poor skin turgor, dry mucous membranes, and sunken fontanelles are noted if dehydration is present. HR and contractility increase with a rise in CVP and PAWP in cardiogenic and a drop in CVP and PAWP in hypovolemic shock. Pulmonary vascular and systemic vascular resistance are elevated and cardiac index decreases. Increased rate and depth of breathing result in respiratory alkalosis. Decreased level of consciousness is indicated by atypical response to parents, restlessness, confusion, and lethargy. Pupils may dilate. Infants may demonstrate a weak cry and poor suck.
2. **Uncompensated phase** of shock, in which compensatory mechanisms fail, leads to multisystem organ failure. The loss of autoregulation in microcirculation increases capillary permeability, leading to third spacing and decreased venous return. Low CVP, BP, and PCWP occur. Coronary perfusion suffers, resulting in ischemic changes on the ECG. Mental status deteriorates, and acute renal failure occurs. Gastrointestinal tract ischemia allows translocation of gram-negative bacteria across damaged mucosa into the circulation, resulting in bowel edema, ulceration, and sepsis. Liver ischemia results in elevated bilirubin and liver enzymes, and jaundice and abnormal clotting/coagulopathy. Alveolar ischemia causes decreased surfactant production, leading to alveoli collapse, atelectasis, and decreased compliance. Ischemia to the distal extremities occurs, with necrosis and ulceration of toes and fingers.
3. **Refractory phase:** Irreversible injury occurs. Bradycardia and profound hypotension occur with no response to potent vasopressors.

D. Diagnostic Tools

1. **Chest radiographic examination** demonstrates cardiomegaly and pulmonary congestion.
2. **ECHO** evaluates the presence of structural disease, systolic function, valvular structure, systolic time intervals, and ejection fraction, specifically noting hypokinetic areas of the myocardium.
3. **Laboratory studies:** Arterial blood gases are used to determine hypoxia and respiratory or metabolic acidosis. Electrolytes diagnose hyponatremia, hyperkalemia, hypoglycemia, and hypocalcemia. Renal and hepatic function studies determine organ function. Lactate levels are used to determine the degree of tissue perfusion. Level greater than 2 mmol/L is indicative of shock.
4. **PA catheterization** measures pressures and cardiac output and evaluates shunting; it allows continuous mixed venous O_2 saturation monitoring.

E. Nursing Diagnoses

- Alteration in tissue perfusion
- Alteration in cardiac output
- Alteration in breathing patterns
- Impaired gas exchange
- Alteration in fluid and electrolyte balance
- Fluid volume deficit
- Potential for infection

F. Goals and Patient Outcomes

1. To reestablish hemodynamic stability
2. To establish adequate ventilation and oxygenation
3. To increase cardiac function by reducing the workload and by improving the efficiency of the heart
4. To provide adequate nutrition and metabolic state
5. To prevent any complications that result from shock

G. Patient Management

1. **Correct the primary cause** of shock.
2. **Evaluate cardiovascular function** via an arterial line for continuous BP monitoring, CVP monitoring to assess preload, a PA catheter to assess therapy, Svo_2 monitoring, and perfusion assessment, which includes assessment of BP, skin color, temperature, capillary refill, and perfusion to organs.
3. **Support cardiovascular function.**
   a. *Optimize preload* with fluid resuscitation (20 mL/kg boluses) until responsive.
   b. *Optimize contractility* with inotropic agents, vasodilators, cardiac rest, and mechanical support when necessary (see Extracorporeal Life Support and Cardiac Assist Devices).
   c. *IV access* is obtained with large-bore catheters in major vessels. In shock, an IO line can be used to infuse large volumes, blood, and drugs in children when IV access cannot be obtained in a timely manner.
4. **Support organ function:** Mechanical ventilation provides cardiopulmonary support. Renal support may require diuretics, continuous AV or venous-venous hemofiltration (CAVH/CVVH), plasmapheresis, or hemodialysis. Prevent any further injury through an assessment of organ systems affected by the redistribution of blood flow.
5. **Provide adequate nutrition** through enteral or parenteral nutrition.

H. Complications

Complications such as renal failure, hepatic failure, sepsis, disseminated intravascular coagulation (DIC), or death may occur.

ARRHYTHMIAS AND MYOCARDIAL CONDUCTION SYSTEM DEFECTS

A. Definition

Arrhythmia is an abnormality in the rate, regularity, or site of origin of a cardiac impulse. A disturbance in the conduction of that impulse prevents the normal sequence of activation of the atria and ventricles.

B. Pathophysiology

1. **Reentry mechanism** is the cause of most SVT and ventricular tachyarrhythmias. Excitation is able to travel via two routes; in reentry it travels down one route and returns up the second route. This implies two discrete pathways and enough delay on one pathway to allow time for a refractory period and recovery. With reentry, rhythm will be regular with an abrupt onset and cessation.
   a. *Orthodromic* describes the path traveling down the AV node to the ventricles and returning retrograde up the accessory tissue (occurs in 90%).

b. *Antidromic* describes the path traveling down the accessory tissue and returning retrograde up through the AV node (occurs in 10%).

2. **Abnormal automaticity** is a derangement of the action potential of cardiac cells, allowing them to reach their threshold voltage prematurely, usually occurring from injured or abnormal cells. With abnormal automaticity, there is variation in rate influenced by sympathetic tone with a gradual warm-up and cool-down of tachycardias. There is an atypical response to antiarrhythmic medications.
3. **Triggered activity** is small oscillations in the cell membrane voltage during repolarization, causing the cell to reach threshold potential.

C. Etiology

Factors that may precipitate arrhythmias include the following:

1. *Cellular milieu*: Hypoxia, hypotension, electrolyte, or metabolic abnormalities
2. *Disease states*: CHD, pulmonary hypertension, diseases of the CNS, sepsis, myocarditis, acute rheumatic fever, or endocrine or metabolic disease
3. *Cardiac procedures* such as cardiac catheterization or catheter placement
4. *Cardiac surgery* with damage to conduction from mechanical manipulation, medication or anesthetics, cannulation from cardiopulmonary bypass, transient conduction system injury from edema, inflammation, ischemia, sutures near the conduction pathway, hemodynamic changes, electrolyte shifts, and medication interactions
5. *Congenital* conduction abnormalities such as congenital complete heart block, Wolff-Parkinson-White syndrome, prolonged QT

D. Supraventricular Arrhythmias (Figure 3-25)

1. **Sinus arrhythmia:** Physiologic variation in sinus rhythm
   a. *Etiology* is related to respiratory variations (HR increases with inspiration and decreases with expiration). It may be marked in children with airway obstruction, asthma, or increased intracranial pressure and after atrial surgery. This is a normal phenomenon in the fetus and in most children at all ages.

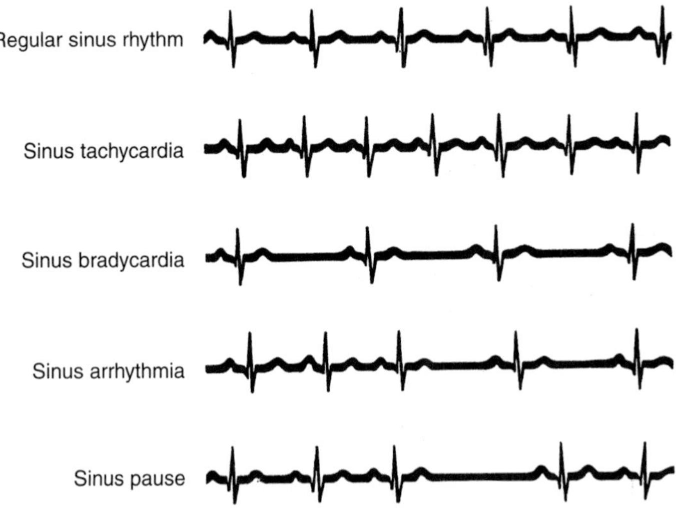

FIGURE 3-25 ■ Normal and abnormal rhythms originating in the sinoatrial node. All rhythms have a P wave in front of each QRS complex with a regular PR interval. (Reprinted with permission from Park MK, Guntheroth WG: *How to read pediatric ECGs*. St. Louis, 1992, Mosby.)

b. *No clinical signs or symptoms* are seen, and the child has a benign, irregular pulse.
c. *ECG findings* include an irregular rhythm; P-P and R-R intervals vary by more than 0.12 second with beat-to-beat variability, upright P waves, one P wave for each QRS complex, and normal PR interval and QRS configuration.
d. *Intervention* is not necessary.

2. **Sinus tachycardia**
   a. *Etiology* is related to increased sympathetic tone, pain, fear, anxiety, anemia, exercise, fever, infection, hypoxemia, shock, CHF, and pulmonary edema.
   b. *History and examination:* History may reveal the underlying causes. The child will have a rapid, regular pulse and may also have palpitations or dyspnea or both or may be asymptomatic.
   c. *ECG findings* include regular rhythm, a higher than normal HR, a P:QRS ratio of 1:1, normal PR interval and QRS configuration, and origin of the rhythm in the SA node. Neonates may have a sinus tachycardia as high as 220 to 250 bpm, overlapping with rates of SVT.
   d. *Interventions* include treating the underlying cause. Digoxin is not effective unless the tachycardia is related to congestive heart failure.
3. **SA node conduction disorders: Pause, block, or arrest**—Brief period of decreased or absent SA node activity
   a. *Etiology of pause, arrest, or block* can be related to hypoxemia, digoxin toxicity, hyperkalemia, increased vagal tone, or cardiac surgery. In addition, myocardial infarction (MI), ischemia, atropine, aspirin toxicity, or infection (myocarditis, rheumatic fever) can be contributing factors.
   b. *History and examination* reveal that the patient is usually unaware of the arrhythmia or may complain of skipped beats. The palpated pulse has a prolonged pause. CHF and decreased cardiac output may develop if the pauses are frequent.
   c. *ECG findings* include a varying or irregular HR, a prolonged pause between QRS complexes, the absence of one or more expected P waves, absent QRS complex unless junctional or ventricular escape beat occurs, and normal QRS duration. In *SA pause,* the pause is less than twice the underlying sinus interval. In *SA block,* the pause is an exact multiple of the underlying sinus interval; the SA node fires but is not conducted. In *SA arrest,* the pause is greater than twice the underlying sinus interval.
   d. *Intervention* includes treatment of the underlying cause, atropine for frequent episodes, or a pacemaker for symptomatic episodes.
4. **Sinus bradycardia:** HR is low for the patient's age and clinical state, but the rhythm is normal.
   a. *Etiology:* The most common cause is hypoxia but causes also include surgical disruption of the SA node, use of digoxin or β-blockers, increased vagal tone, increased intracranial pressure, hypothermia, hypothyroidism, and anorexia.
   b. *History and examination* reveal a slow, regular pulse. In infants, CHF may occur earlier because of the inadequacy of the rate.
   c. *ECG findings* include a P wave before every QRS complex, regular P-P and R-R intervals, normal QRS configuration, normal PR interval, and upright P waves.
   d. *Interventions* include oxygen, bag-mask ventilation to assist breathing if needed, and epinephrine or atropine for symptomatic bradycardia. To determine the exact degree of bradycardia when the patient is asleep and awake, 24-hour ECG monitoring is done. A stress ECG is performed if the patient is older than 5 years to determine the degree of SA node incompetence if the child is asymptomatic.

Transesophageal pacing can test automaticity and sinus node recovery time. Invasive study of the SA node should include the AV node function. If the conduction system is intact, permanent atrial demand pacing can be used.

5. **Sick sinus syndrome (SSS, bradycardia-tachycardia syndrome):** HR varies from rates in excess of 180 bpm to severe bradycardia with long sinus pauses. Arrhythmias may include profound sinus bradycardia, SA exit block, sinus arrest with junctional escape, paroxysmal atrial tachycardia, slow or fast ectopic atrial or nodal rhythm, atrial flutter, or atrial fibrillation.
   a. *Etiology:* Causes include disease or ischemia of the SA node and extensive atrial surgery. It may be of idiopathic origin. SSS may occur following cannulation for cardiopulmonary bypass, hypertrophy of an otherwise anatomically normal heart, fibrosis of areas of the SA node, AV node, or injury to the sinus node artery.
   b. *History and examination:* Patients may experience syncope, seizures, lethargy, poor feeding, seizures, dizziness, exercise intolerance, palpitations, chest pain, or sudden death.
   c. *ECG findings* include an irregular rhythm, variable rate, and P waves that vary in amplitude and morphology.
   d. *Interventions* for symptomatic arrhythmias require a pacemaker for the bradycardia component. Antiarrhythmics are used for the tachycardia component only after pacemaker insertion.
6. **Supraventricular tachycardia (SVT)**
   a. *Etiology:* Most often, SVT is due to a reentry mechanism, but patients can have increased automaticity from hypoxemia, electrolyte imbalance, acid-base abnormalities, myocardial disease, digoxin toxicity, CHD, or rapid firing of a single ectopic focus. Most episodes involve reentry occurring from accessory AV conduction tissue or dual AV node pathways (i.e., AV node reentry).
   b. *History and examination:* Acute SVT often precipitates symptoms of shock and CHF, but older children rarely present in heart failure or shock. They report palpitations, malaise, and a racing heart. SVT can be well tolerated in the neonate; however, prolonged rates in excess of 220 bpm eventually result in CHF.
   c. *ECG findings* include P:QRS ratio of 1:1, a ventricular rate usually greater than 220 bpm in infants and greater than 150 bpm in children, regular P-P and R-R intervals, abrupt onset and termination of rate, normal QRS configuration; P waves may be absent, inverted, or superimposed (Figure 3-26).
   d. *Other findings:* Chronic SVT may be accompanied by evidence of myocardial dysfunction. Electrophysiology studies may reveal automatic ectopic focus located in the atria or bundle of His, concealed AV unidirectional retrograde accessory pathway, or a permanent form of reciprocating junctional tachycardia.
   e. *Interventions* include treatment based on the HR, the mechanism of tachycardia, the degree of myocardial dysfunction, and symptoms.
      - For acute SVT, diving reflex and other vagal maneuvers (rarely effective), pharmacologic treatments (adenosine, propranolol, and verapamil in children older than 1 year), direct current cardioversion, and overdrive pacing can be used in symptomatic children.
      - In chronic SVT, the mechanism of SVT is defined by electrophysiologic catheterization to determine the safety of digoxin use. Vagal maneuvers and pharmacologic treatments (adenosine, verapamil) may be useful. Digoxin improves myocardial performance and slows the HR. Atenolol, propranolol, or amiodorone can be added if digoxin alone is not effective in

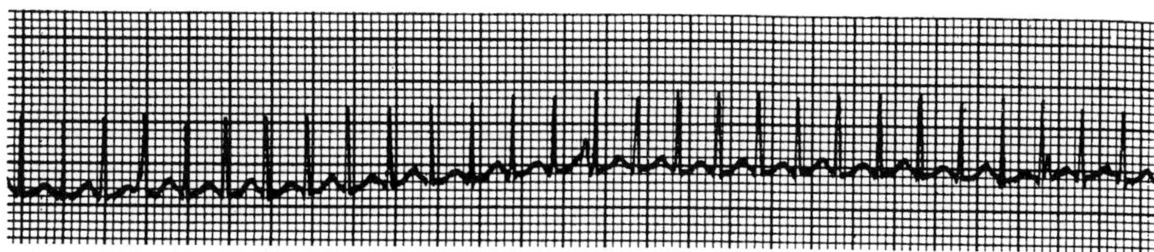

FIGURE 3-26 ■ Electrocardiographic tracing of supraventricular tachycardia with normal QRS complex and regular R-R intervals.

(Reprinted with permission from Park MK, Guntheroth WG. *How to read pediatric ECGs*. St. Louis, 1992, Mosby.)

controlling HR. Radiofrequency or cryoablation may be performed if the SVT is not responsive to medical treatment, the child develops severe side effects, or the child's lifestyle does not allow effective medication regimens. Pacemakers can be used for automatic overdrive or atrial pacing for control of the rate.

7. **Wolff-Parkinson-White syndrome (WPW)**
   a. *Etiology* involves the presence of a congenital accessory connection that conducts electrical activity faster than the AV node. WPW may be an isolated disease or it may be associated with CHD (especially Ebstein anomaly) Pompe disease, and cardiac myopathies. SVT may occur at any age secondary to reentry.
   b. *History and examination:* Frequent tachycardia occurs in infancy with reduced episodes in early childhood and resumption of symptoms at puberty. Symptoms may include palpitations, lethargy, decreased activity tolerance, or, more rarely, syncope, seizures, and sudden death.
   c. *ECG findings:* WPW may be diagnosed by surface ECG or, if it is a concealed pathway, by intracardiac electrophysiology study. ECG features include regular rhythm, frequent episodes of SVT, short PR interval, wide QRS complex, and presence of a delta wave (slurred upstroke of the QRS complex appearance).
   d. *Interventions* include treatment of frequent episodes of SVT or syncope with propranolol or amiodorone, radiofrequency ablation of accessory pathway (especially if not responsive to medical therapy), and avoidance of digoxin in children older than 6 to 12 months.
8. **Junctional tachycardia (nodal; JET)**
   a. *Pathophysiology* involves an accelerated rate originating in the AV node and the loss of atrial kick. This is especially harmful if cardiac output is already compromised by heart disease or cardiac surgery. This type of arrhythmia is common in postoperative patients with cardiac disease and is frequently seen following repair of tetralogy of Fallot.
   b. *ECG findings:* The rate varies from 120 to 200 bpm; QRS complex is usually normal and regular, and an inverted P wave may or may not follow the QRS complex. The child may require an electrophysiologic study to determine the exact origin of the tachycardia.
   c. *Intervention* may be required especially in severely compromised patients. Cooling to a temperature of 35°C, sedation, inotropic support, overdrive pacing when able to capture the rate, paralysis, and medications such as amiodorone or procainamide may be used. Treatment may not be necessary if the rate is within normal limits and cardiac output is adequate.

9. **Atrial flutter**
   a. *Pathophysiology and etiology* are related to a large stretched atria resulting from CHD or acquired heart disease, atrial surgery in neonates, hypoxemia, valvular disease, digoxin toxicity, increased sympathetic tone, or infection.
   b. *History and examination:* Clinical signs and symptoms of heart failure develop if not treated quickly, depending on the ventricular rate. Children may have palpitations, angina, dyspnea, or decreased cardiac output. Symptoms are more pronounced if there is underlying cardiac disease.
   c. *ECG findings* include rapid atrial tachycardia with characteristic flutter waves, normal QRS configuration, atrial rate that is usually 300 bpm and regular (but may go as high as 400 to 450 bpm), ventricular response from 1:1 to various degrees of AV block, sawtooth configuration P waves, and an unidentifiable PR interval. Slower ventricular rates occur if varying degrees of block result in 2:1 or 3:1 flutter (defined as one ventricular contraction in response to every second or third atrial contraction, respectively).
   d. *Intervention* in symptomatic children is direct cardioversion. Rapid overdrive atrial pacing may be useful through transesophageal or transvenous routes. Medications are given to increase AV block, decrease ventricular response rate, and prevent recurrence (digoxin, propranolol, verapamil). Surgical procedures can be used to improve hemodynamics and relieve atrial stretch or for implantation of an automatic atrial antitachycardia pacer.
10. **Atrial fibrillation**
   a. *Pathophysiology and etiology* are related to increased sympathetic tone, hypoxemia, valvular disease, structural heart disease with dilated atria, atrial surgery, digoxin toxicity, disease of the AV node or lower conduction system, or hyperthyroidism (rare in children).
   b. *History and examination:* Clinical signs and symptoms depend on the ventricular response. Children may have palpitations, angina or dyspnea, decreased cardiac output, CHF, ischemia, atrial emboli, and an irregular pulse.
   c. *ECG findings* include a wavy baseline with absent P waves and an "irregularly irregular" ventricular rhythm; a rapid and irregular atrial rate, but with no discernible P waves the rate is unable to be calculated (may be over 350 bpm); an irregular and slower ventricular rate; immeasurable PR interval; and normal QRS configuration.
   d. *Interventions* include digoxin if no WPW is present, propranolol, and cardioversion (in symptomatic patients).

E. Ventricular Arrhythmias (Figure 3-27)

1. Ventricular arrhythmias are rare in otherwise normal hearts, occurring in only 10% of pediatric cardiac arrests, but they are associated with surgical correction of CHD and can occur in newly transplanted hearts. They are also found in myocarditis, cardiomyopathies, idiopathic hypertrophic subaortic stenosis (IHSS), cardiac tumors, metabolic disturbances, drug toxicity, CHD, RV hypertrophy, and QT prolongation. Premature ventricular contractions (PVCs) may be found in utero and in normal children. Sudden death following the repair of CHD or sudden death without known heart disease is most likely due to ventricular arrhythmias.
2. **Ventricular tachycardia (VT)**
   a. *Etiology and pathophysiology* are related to both reentry and enhanced automaticity resulting from intramyocardial tumor, metabolic disturbances, cardiomyopathy, drug ingestion, drug toxicity, long QT syndrome, damage to the His-Purkinje system or myocardium (MI, myocarditis, surgery),

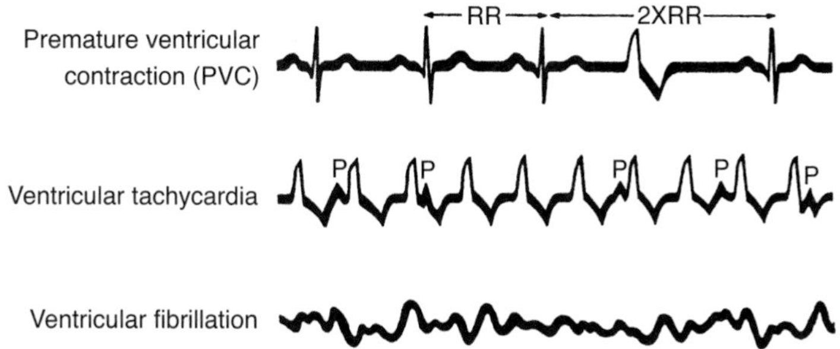

FIGURE 3-27 ■ Ventricular arrhythmias.
(Reprinted with permission from Park MK, Guntheroth WG: *How to read pediatric ECGs*. St. Louis, 1992, Mosby.)

hypoxemia, acidosis, or hypokalemia. Three or more PVCs occurring one after the other are considered VT. This occurrence is uncommon in children who have not undergone intracardiac surgery. In infants younger than 1 year, the QRS complex may not be prolonged. It is more common in children after cardiac surgery, with as many as 18% having nonsustained runs (Hoffman et al., 2002). Torsade de pointes (turning on a point) version may occur from triggered activity.

b. *History and examination:* Patients may experience palpitations, dyspnea, dizziness, anxiety, diaphoresis, angina, decreased level of consciousness, syncope, or decreased BP. VT may be asymptomatic in short bursts, but cardiac output may decrease rapidly with prolonged bursts or short bursts in compromised patients. Rhythm may deteriorate to ventricular fibrillation.

c. *ECG findings* include wide, bizarre, abnormal QRS configuration; a rate usually greater than 100 bpm; P waves not related to the QRS complex; no discernible PR interval; and a sustained or unsustained tachycardia. Diagnosis is confirmed by ECG monitor, surface 12-lead ECG, or intracardiac electrophysiology.

d. *Intervention* for asymptomatic VT in children with normal hearts may not be warranted. Medical treatment for VT associated with abnormal myocardial function includes lidocaine, propranolol, procainamide, or amiodarone. If present, tumors are excised. Radiofrequency ablation is used if reentry VT is demonstrated on electrophysiology study. Cardioversion is indicated for acute events of "perfusing VT," and defibrillation is used for life-threatening events of "nonperfusing VT."

3. Ventricular fibrillation (VF)

a. *Pathophysiology and etiology* include insults to the His-Purkinje system or myocardium, hypoxemia, electrolyte imbalance, hyperkalemia, electrical shock, drugs, prolonged VT, or long QT syndrome.

b. *History and examination:* Clinical signs and symptoms include loss of consciousness; no pulse, respiration, or BP; and possible seizure, cyanosis, and clinical death.

c. *ECG findings* include repetitive series of chaotic ventricular waves varying in size and amplitude; complete absence of characteristic P wave, QRS complex, and T wave; and no measurable HR.

d. *Interventions* include cardiopulmonary resuscitation (CPR) plus defibrillation. VF that is not responsive to three successive defibrillation attempts should be treated with medications. The PALS algorithm includes drug-CPR-shock (repeat).

4. **Long QT syndrome**
   a. *Etiology*: Inherited cardiac ion channel disorder associated with either sodium or potassium channels. It may require the interaction of genes.
   b. *History and examination*: Episodes of syncope or aborted sudden death, family history of sudden death, hearing deficit in 11p15.5 gene disorder. Seizures and palpitations with emotion or exercise (particularly swimming) may also be seen.
   c. *ECG findings*: Prolonged QT interval with corrected QT interval (QT_c) greater than 0.46, abnormal T-wave configuration (notched, biphasic) with ventricular arrythmias including R on T ventricular fibrillation and VT.
   d. *Interventions*: β-blocker medications, demand pacemakers, and internal cardioverter defibrillator placement. Despite therapy there is a continued risk of sudden death.

F. AV Node Conduction Disorders (Figure 3-28)

1. **First-degree AV block**
   a. *Etiology:* Delay in transmission of intra-atrial impulse associated with rheumatic fever, CHD, injury to AV node, certain cardiac drugs, increased vagal tone, surgery, hypoxemia, AV canal defects, Ebstein anomaly, and ischemia of the conduction system.
   b. *History and examination:* Usually there are no clinical signs and symptoms.
   c. *ECG findings* include regular rhythm, P for every QRS complex, regular P-P and R-R intervals, a prolonged PR interval for age and HR (see Table 3-5), a normal QRS configuration, and a constant PR interval.
   d. *Intervention* centers around monitoring because first-degree AV block may progress to second- or third-degree AV block. Treatment is needed only if the cause is drug toxicity.
2. **Second-degree AV block**
   a. *Wenckebach (Mobitz type I)*
      - *Pathophysiology and etiology* are impaired conduction through the AV node and can be found occasionally in normal hearts or after insults to the AV

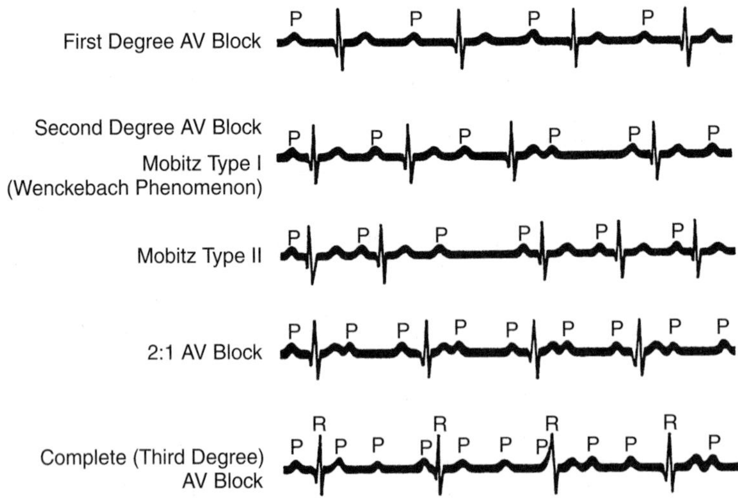

FIGURE 3-28 ■ Disturbances of atrioventricular *(AV)* conduction.
(Reprinted with permission from Park MK, Guntheroth WG: *How to read pediatric ECGs*. St. Louis, 1992, Mosby.)

node, such as inferior MI, hypoxemia, increased vagal tone, and digoxin toxicity.

- *History and examination* usually has no symptoms. If the rate decreases dramatically, cardiac output may decrease. Usually it does not progress.
- *ECG findings* include a regular P-P interval, irregular R-R interval, more P waves than QRS complexes, and a PR interval that progressively increases until a QRS complex is dropped and then the P:QRS relationship resumes.
- *Interventions* include treatment of the underlying cause and observation

b. *Mobitz type II second-degree heart block*

- *Etiology:* This type of block is more serious and is due to a block in the distal AV conduction system near the bundle of His. It is often related to ischemic changes, insults to the AV node, MI, hypoxemia, cardiac drugs, ischemic disease of the conduction system, CHD, and cardiomyopathy.
- *History and examination:* A slower HR may diminish cardiac output. Blocks at the level of the bundle of His may progress suddenly and rapidly to complete the block with significantly lower rates and signs and symptoms of CHF or syncope.
- *ECG criteria* include a regular P-P interval, a slower ventricular response, normal atrial rate, P waves upright and normal, fixed PR interval in the conducted beats, more P waves than QRS complexes, and possibly an abnormal QRS complex.
- *Interventions* include treatment of the underlying cause, close monitoring, and a pacemaker for symptomatic children.

3. Complete AV block (CHB)

a. *Pathophysiology and etiology:* This block is within the AV node, junction, or bundle branches and may be congenital and occur in otherwise structurally normal hearts. Congenital CHB may be diagnosed antenatally and is associated with maternal connective tissue disorders or antinuclear antibodies. Acquired CHB is relatively uncommon in infants and children. It does occur with myopathies, infectious diseases, fibrotic degeneration of the conduction system, CHD, diabetes, collagen disorders or rheumatic fever, surgical interruption of the bundle of His or both bundle branches, and tumors. There is higher risk of mortality if the ventricular rate is less than 55 bpm.

b. *History and examination:* Symptoms include syncope (with lower rates), decreased exercise tolerance, associated ventricular ectopy or standstill, slow HR, and decreased cardiac output. *Examination* usually reveals normal growth and development, but the child may exhibit signs of CHF if the HR is less than 45 bpm during the first year of life. An evaluation for structural disease should be included.

c. *ECG findings* include a regular rhythm, an atrial rate greater than the ventricular rate, regular R-R and P-P intervals, and a variable PR interval. QRS interval will reflect the source of an escape rhythm; for example, a narrow QRS indicates an atrial or junctional origin, whereas a wide QRS may indicate a ventricular origin or a higher origin with aberrant conduction through the ventricles.

d. *Interventions* include an ECG, chest radiographic examination, physical examination, ECHO, and Holter monitor and exercise test every 3 to 5 years beginning at the age of 4 to 5 years. Permanent cardiac pacing is indicated when syncope or heart failure is present, the block is below the bundle of His, in infants with ventricular rates less than 55 bpm, with frequent or complex ventricular arrhythmias, or with moderate to severe exercise intolerance.

G. Bundle Branch Block (BBB)

1. **Pathophysiology and etiology** are related to damage to the bundle branch from fibrotic scarring or ischemia. BBB is common following some forms of surgical repair for congenital heart defects such as VSD or tetralogy of Fallot.
2. **History and examination:** Usually there are no clinical signs and symptoms. If all three bundles are blocked, the child may develop CHB and asystole.
3. **ECG findings** include a QRS width greater than 0.12 second or association with other arrhythmias. Diagnosis of RBBB or LBBB is determined with a 12-lead ECG. To evaluate a BBB from a monitor rhythm strip, find a rabbit-ear configuration (like the letter "M") in V_1 and a broad, wide S wave in V_6 in RBBB; find a broad, wide S wave in V_1; and a tiny R wave with big "S" wave in V_6.
4. **Interventions** include 24-hour ECG monitoring for patients with bifascicular block to assess the development of progressive blocks. Patients are treated with pacing if they are symptomatic.

PACEMAKERS AND INTERNAL CARDIOVERTOR DEFIBRILLATORS FOR TREATMENT OF CONDUCTION DISORDERS

A. Indications for Pacemakers

Pacemakers are used to deliver an electrical impulse (stimulus) to the heart to initiate depolarization and stimulate a cardiac contraction. The most common indications for pacer placement are surgically induced heart block (30%), congenital complete heart block (25%), SSS (15%), other symptomatic bradyarrhythmias, long QT syndrome, and neurocardiogenic syncope. Overdrive pacing may be useful in the termination of accelerated tachyarrhythmias unresponsive to pharmacotherapy. Pacing can provide a reduction in outflow gradient in symptomatic hypertrophic cardiomyopathy.

B. Components of a Pacemaker System

1. The **pulse generator** consists of a battery and programmable circuitry of the pacemaker.
2. **Lead wires** conduct impulses from the pulse generator to the heart. An electrode in contact with the heart delivers the impulse. Most leads are bipolar containing active and ground leads. Unipolar leads use the pacemaker generator itself as the ground pole.
3. **Cable** is used to connect temporary epicardial wires to the pulse generator.

C. Temporary Cardiac Pacemakers

1. **Transvenous catheters** are placed through the femoral or upper extremity veins to the RA or RV using bipolar electrodes. They are most commonly used for congenital CHB or temporary heart block from myocarditis or infection.
2. **Epicardial wires** are placed directly on the RA or RV or both routinely after open heart surgery. Atrial wires exit to the right chest, ventricular wires exit to the left chest. A needle brings the wire through the chest wall, and the needle is broken away to function as the contact pin to a cable that connects to the pulse generator. Wires allow both pacing and the ability to have a direct electrogram from the atrial (or ventricular) chambers.
3. An **esophageal** pacing probe passed via the esophagus paces by the impulse traversing tissue between the electrode and the right atrium. The probe can pace or record an atrial electrogram.

4. **Transthoracic** pacing is accomplished via electrode pads delivering a stimulus through the chest wall. One pad is placed on the anterior chest, and one is placed on the child's back (avoiding the scapula). Noninvasive pacing is not as reliable and requires direct electrical impulses to travel through the chest wall, which is painful. It may be used during resuscitation, until transvenous pacing can be established or as support during anesthesia induction for other pacer placement.

D. Permanent Cardiac Pacemakers

1. **Transvenous (endocardial)** pacing catheters can be threaded through the subclavian or jugular vein to the RA or RV or both. Transvenous pacers are generally used in children who weigh more than 12 kg. Relative contraindications to transvenous pacing include a lack of venous access to the ventricle, intracardiac right to left shunting, elevated pulmonary vascular resistance, or right ventricular dysfunction or fibrosis. Generators are placed in the anterior chest wall (Figure 3-29) or abdominal wall.
2. **Epicardial** leads are placed through a thoracotomy or sternotomy incision on the epicardial surface of the heart using corkscrew coil, fishhook, or suture electrodes. Younger or smaller patients require transthoracic lead placement, as vessel size prohibits transvenous placement. Epicardial leads may be difficult to place in the presence of scar tissue from repeated operations and resultant adhesions. Generators are placed in the anterior chest wall or abdominal wall.

E. Pacemaker Functions

1. **Nomenclature:** The North American Society for Pacing and Electrophysiology (NASPE) and British Pacing and Electrophysiology Group (BPEG) devised a generic code (NBG) used to communicate pacer functions (Table 3-8). The first letter describes chamber paced, the second letter describes chamber sensed, and the third letter describes the mode of response to sensing. In permanent pacers, additional codes include the fourth letter, which indicates the ability of the pacemaker to respond to programming, and the fifth letter, which indicates the ability of the pacer to respond to tachyarrhythmias by burst pacing or shock.
2. **Pacemaker capabilities** include *pacing* (the ability of the pacemaker to deliver an impulse to the heart), *sensing* (the ability to detect intrinsic cardiac activity), and *capture* (the effectiveness of the pacing stimulus to cause contraction). (See Table 3-9 for common pacing modalities.)

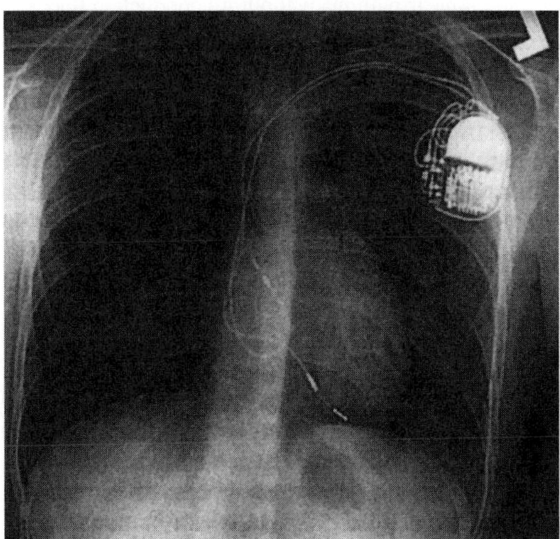

FIGURE 3-29 ■ Standard transvenous lead position in an adolescent.

(Reprinted with permission from Mavroudis C, Backer CL: *Pediatric cardiac surgery*. St. Louis, 1994, Mosby.)

TABLE 3-8
NASPE/BPEG Generic Pacemaker Codes (NBG)

I	II	III	IV	V
Chamber(s) Paced	**Chamber(s) Sensed**	**Response to Sensing**	**Programmable Functions**	**Antitachyarrhthymia Functions**
A = atrium V = ventricle D = dual	0 = none A = atrium V = ventricle D = dual	0 = none I = inhibited T = triggered D = triggered and inhibited	0 = none P = simple programmable M = multiprogrammable C = communicating	0 = none P = pacing S = shock D = dual R = rate modulated

From Craig J, Smith JB, Fineman LD: Tissue perfusion. In Curley MAQ, Moloney-Harmon PA, editors. *Critical care nursing of infants and children*, ed 2. Philadelphia, 2001, W.B. Saunders Company.

TABLE 3-9
Common Pacemaker Modes

Mode	Generator Activity	Indication
AAI-atrial demand	Paces atrium Senses atrium Inhibits pacer if senses atrial activity above set rate	Sinus or high-junctional bradycardias when AV conduction system intact, provides atrial kick
VVI-ventricular demand	Paces ventricle Senses ventricle Inhibits pacer if senses ventricular activity above set rate	Used in emergencies to establish ventricular activity, when AV dissociation present, maintains CO without atrial kick
AOO-atrial asynchronous	Paces atrium Sensing off Triggered to fire at fixed rate	Sinus or high-junctional bradycardias when AV conduction system intact, can trigger atrial arrhythmias, used in emergencies
VOO-ventricular asynchronous	Paces ventricle Sensing off Triggered to fire at fixed rate	Asystole Dangerous as can cause R-on-T with ventricular fibrillation, use DDD or VVI instead
DDD-AV sequential or dual chambered pacing	Paces atrium and ventricle Senses atrium and ventricle Fires only if atrium or ventricle drop below a set rate	Any arrhythmia without AV conduction (blocks) Avoid in atrial fibrillation or flutter as tracks atrial rate Maintains CO with atrial kick

3. **Generator activity modes** (response to sensing)
   a. *Triggered*: Will pace in response to sensing no electrical activity
   b. *Inhibited*: Will not pace in response to sensing electrical activity
   c. *Demand (inhibited and/or triggered) mode:* Allows the pacemaker to sense intrinsic cardiac activity and inhibit pacing when it senses intrinsic activity at a rate equal to or above the set rate. A pacing stimulus is delivered (triggered) when the intrinsic rate is inadequate. Demand pacing avoids complications caused by competition between the child's intrinsic rate and the pacer. AV conduction is required for effective atrial demand pacing. AV conduction is not

required for ventricular demand pacing, but atrial kick is lost. Synchronous AV demand pacing simulates the normal cardiac cycle, but it cannot be used with atrial fibrillation.

   d. *Asynchronous or fixed-rate mode:* Paces at a continuous set rate without sensing or responding to intrinsic cardiac activity. AV conduction is required for an atrial fixed rate pacing mode.
   e. *Rate responsive pacing:* pacemaker rate changes in response to changes in patient parameters
4. **Pacemaker settings**
   a. *Mode*: As described above (see Table 3-9.)
   b. *Rate*: How low the HR must fall to activate pacing and in some cases how high it will track the sinus rate (DDD mode)
   c. *AV interval*: The time between atrial sensing or pacing and ventricular activity (sensing or pacing). Equivalent to PR interval; it is the time to allow atrial contraction and diastolic filling of ventricle.
   d. The *postventricular atrial refractory period (PVARP)* is the time when the atrial lead does not sense or respond to intrinsic atrial activity. It is a protective feature to prevent rapid ventricular pacing to atrial ectopy (PACs, atrial flutter, or fibrillation) and to avoid pacing of retrograde P waves.
   e. *Capture threshold*: The minimum amount of electrical current needed to depolarize the myocardium. It is measured in milliamps (mA). The pacer is usually set at 2 to 3 times the capture threshold to allow for a safety margin.
   f. *Sensing threshold* is the programmed setting for the pacer to recognize intrinsic cardiac activity. It is measured in millivolts (mV). Lowering the millivolts increases sensitivity, whereas raising the millivolts decreases the sensitivity.

F. ECG Evidence of Pacers

1. **Capture:** Depolarization of the atria or ventricle initiated by the pacemaker impulse produces a pacer spike on the ECG. An atrial pacing stimulus is followed by a P wave, and a ventricular pacing stimulus is followed by a QRS complex if the atria and ventricles are captured.
2. **Undersensing** occurs when the pacer fails to identify intrinsic depolarization and paces regardless of the child's rhythm. This can be caused by lead fracture, a lack of connections to the generator, or a low sensitivity setting.
3. **Oversensing** occurs when the pacer detects activity that is not actual cardiac depolarization and inhibits pacing. This can be caused by shivering, chest-wall movement, or ungrounded electrical equipment.
4. **Noncapture** occurs when the pacer fires but fails to cause a myocardial depolarization (no P wave or QRS wave). This can be caused by lead fracture or disconnection, low battery, low-output settings, or high pacing thresholds from edema or scarring at the lead site.

G. Complications of Pacemakers

1. **Insertion** can result in local or systemic infection, pneumothorax, myocardial perforation with transvenous placement, arrhythmias, and hematoma or bleeding.
2. **Component problems** (Table 3-10) or troubleshooting abnormal pacer function.
3. **Bleeding or tamponade** can follow placement of transvenous wires or removal of temporary wires.
4. **Risk of systemic emboli** can occur in children with right-to-left intracardiac shunts with transvenous pacing catheters.
5. **Risk of pulmonary emboli** can occur in children with PA hypertension.

TABLE 3-10
Demonstration of Abnormal Pacemaker Function Related to Undersensing, Oversensing, or Noncapture

	Sample ECG Appearance	Some Possible Clinical Consequences	Some Possible Causes	Corrective Measures
UNDERSENSING Device fails to detect existing cardiac depolarizations, therefore competes with the native rhythm	These native R waves are not detected... ...therefore the pacer emits these unneeded spikes	Competition with a native rhythm Stimulation of dysrhythmias ("R-on-T")	Lead disconnected from pacer or from viable myocardium Sensitivity set too low Lead fracture Low battery	Check connection of lead to pacer Increase sensitivity (turn sensing control to a smaller number) 10 5 15 3 20 1 Sensitivity (mV) Reposition or change lead Change battery
OVERSENSING Device detects noncardiac electrical events and interprets them as cardiac depolarizations, therefore is wrongly inhibited from pacing	Pacing should occur as indicated by the arrows but is inhibited by oversensed non-cardiac electrical noise When the noise ceases, pacing resumes	Pacemaker-dependent patients receive no stimuli from the pacemaker, producing a pause in rhythm and reduction in cardiac output	Electrical potential caused by noncardiac muscle contraction (especially pectorals) is detected and misinterpreted by the device Interference from electrical sources (ungrounded equipment, short circuits) is detected and misinterpreted by the device Sensitivity set too high	Decrease sensitivity (turn sensing control to a larger number) 10 5 15 3 20 1 Sensitivity (mV) Remove all ungrounded electrical equipment or have it evaluated by hospital engineers

TABLE 3-10
Demonstration of Abnormal Pacemaker Function Related to Undersensing, Oversensing, or Noncapture (*cont'd*)

	Sample ECG Appearance	Some Possible Clinical Consequences	Some Possible Causes	Corrective Measures
NONCAPTURE Device emits stimuli that fail to depolarize the myocardium	This dual chamber device paces and captures in the atrium and ventricle for the first two beats. Ventricular capture is then lost; the ventricular pacing spikes are not followed by depolarizations. Fortunately, ventricular escape begins.	Pacemaker-dependent patients receive no stimuli from the pacemaker, producing a pause in rhythm and reduction in cardiac output	Lead disconnected from pacer or from viable myocardium Output set too low in the noncaptured chamber Lead fracture High pacing threshold due to medication or metabolic changes Low battery	Check connection of lead to pacer Increase output in the noncaptured chamber Reposition or change lead Change battery Alter medication regimen, correct metabolic changes

From Witherall CL: Cardiac rhythm control devices, *Crit Care Nurs Clin North Am* 6:95–102, 1994.

H. Automatic Internal Cardiovertor Defibrillator

1. **Indications** for ICD placement include syncope or sudden death episode documented as a ventricular arrhythmia, inducible ventricular arrhythmia by electrophysiology study after undocumented syncope or sudden death episode, drug-refractory VT from long QT syndrome, hypertrophic cardiomyopathy or dilated cardiomyopathy, or repaired congenital heart disease.
2. **Implantation techniques** include both *epicardial* patches, which are sutured to the pericardium (usually for children weighing less than 20 kg), or *transvenous* electrodes.
3. **ICD functions:** The generator is similar to a pacemaker generator and can be programmed to sense, pace, overdrive pace, cardiovert, and defibrillate in response to preset recognition criteria for an arrhythmia (rate, QRS duration, number of beats). The device also has internal memory to allow recording of the rhythm before, during, and after an event that can be downloaded when interrogated with an electromagnetic wand on the pacemaker programmer.

I. Nursing Interventions

1. **For temporary pacers:** Assess the hemodynamic status of the child by his or her vital signs as well as the response to pacing. Evaluate ECG monitoring to determine underlying rhythm, pacing and sensing thresholds, and appropriate capture. Ensure normal electrolytes and acid-base balance. Pacer wires and equipment should be appropriately grounded to prevent accidental electrocution. Also, properly ground all electrical equipment used by the child, including video and electronic games. Dials should be covered to prevent accidental changes in settings when possible. Some pacers do not have covers to protect settings, but they have locking buttons to lock in programmed settings. Note that some models also do not have memory, so that programmed settings are lost if the pacer is switched off. Stabilize the patient's leg if a transvenous electrode is placed in the femoral vein (avoid leg flexion), and observe the catheter site for signs of infection. Patient and family teaching should include indications for pacing and procedures surrounding placement.
2. **For permanent pacers:** Assess the hemodynamic status of the child by his or her vital signs as well as the response to pacing. Evaluate ECG monitoring to determine underlying rhythm, pacing and sensing thresholds, and appropriate capture. Teach the patient and family to assess pacer function. Teach the patient and family to report dizziness, syncope, weakness, fatigue, increased symptoms of CHF, redness, swelling, drainage at the incision site(s), palpitations, unresolved or frequent hiccups, fever, decreased feeding, or irritability. Provide the family with information for medic alert bracelet and transtelephonic pacer checks, and stress the importance of always carrying the pacer identification card with the patient's name; the physician's name, address, and phone number; medications; and the pacer type and settings. If the patient moves out of the area, rapid referral to a new cardiologist is required. Instruct the patient and the family on the appropriate timing to return to normal activity, including school, driving, and exercise (contact sports are to be avoided). Pregnancy generally is well-tolerated, depending on any associated disease.
3. **For ICD:** The function of the device can be determined only in the controlled setting of the electrophysiology laboratory where VT or VF is induced. If an event occurs, record the rhythm and note the response of the ICD. Teach the child and family what action to take when the device fires.

J. Evaluation of Nursing Care

1. The patient is without signs and symptoms of infection.
2. The patient and family verbalize the need for a pacer/ICD and procedure for placement.
3. The patient's ECG demonstrates appropriate sensing and capturing for pacemaker.
4. The patient and family accurately demonstrate the technique for checking pacer function.
5. The patient and family describe the actions to be taken when the ICD fires.

CONGENITAL HEART DISEASE (CHD)

A. Etiologic Aspects of CHD

1. **Cardiovascular diseases** of all types are familial. CHD is 10% attributable to primarily genetic factors, with little environmental influence, and 90% is attributable to genetic and environmental (multifactorial) interactions of equal importance. CHD occurs in 8% to 10% of every 1000 live births.
2. **Genetic factors:** Genetic causes are most likely associated with a syndrome (e.g., Down syndrome). The recurrence risk of the heart lesion is related to the recurrence risk of the chromosomal anomaly. A single mutant gene may cause a syndrome, or others may be related to microdeletions and translocations. It may have dominant inheritance (e.g., IHSS, ASD). With dominance, part of the gene is responsible for the trait. Recessive traits must be present in two copies to permit expression. There are autosomal dominant and recessive forms of conduction defects. With mendelian inheritance, the recurrence risk is high. (See Tables 3-1, 3-2, and 3-3.)
3. **Genetic-environmental interaction:** Multifactorial inheritance is responsible for most CHD. Hereditary predisposition to cardiovascular maldevelopment interacts with an environmental trigger at the vulnerable period of cardiogenesis. Generally the recurrence risk is 1% to 4%. The more common the defect, the more likely it is to recur. Risk increases rapidly with the number of first-degree relatives affected. If two first-degree relatives are affected, the risk recurrence is tripled. If three or more first-degree relatives are affected, the risk is a type C classification with a very high recurrence. Teratogenic exposure in the mother may contribute to the incidence of CHD, although proof is lacking in some cases. Usually the exposure is of short duration. (See Table 3-4.)
4. **Risk to offspring of the affected parent:** Risks are higher for offspring if the mother has CHD.
5. **Child at risk for atherosclerosis as an adult:** There is a 1% incidence of single-gene hyperlipoproteinemia. Most human traits are controlled by more than one gene. Multifactorial inheritance dominates. The single most important risk factor is early onset of coronary disease in a first-degree relative younger than 55 years (heredity, 57% to 63%). Environmental factors such as diet, smoking, and exercise can be manipulated to reduce risk factors.

B. Nursing Diagnoses for Children with CHD

❖ High risk for infection is related to cardiac surgery, invasive lines, and poor perfusion.

1. **Defining characteristics** are temperature above 38.5°C; redness, warmth, and drainage from insertion or incision sites; elevated leukocyte count with increased neutrophils and bands greater than 10%; cloudy urine (leukocytes);

rales and rhonchi present on auscultation of lungs; positive blood or wound culture; chest radiographic examination demonstrating consolidation; temperature and glucose instability; decreased ionized calcium; feeding intolerance; and thrombocytopenia.

2. **Expected outcome:** Patient is free of infection as evidenced by temperature less than 38.5°C, dry wounds that have no redness, normal leukocyte and platelet counts, clear lungs and chest radiographic examination, and tolerance of feedings.
3. **Interventions:** Inspect skin for redness, extreme warmth, or drainage from incisions and peripheral, arterial, and venous lines. Ensure aseptic handling of all IV lines. Administer antibiotics as prescribed. Report elevation in temperature and changes in laboratory data indicative of infectious process (i.e., increased leukocyte count with increased neutrophils). Change IV tubing and dressings as hospital policy dictates. Remove any mucous secretions from the respiratory tract. Encourage deep breathing and coughing, use of incentive spirometer, and blowing bubbles. Assess respiratory status, and monitor for adventitious breath sounds. Assist the patient to change position or change the patient's position every 2 hours. Monitor the hydration status, and administer fluids as ordered. Assess for and provide adequate nutrition. Monitor urine for color, odor, and sediment. Discontinue all catheters, IV lines, and drains as soon as possible. Use body substance precautions. Provide appropriate endocarditis prophylaxis and teach these precautions to the family.
4. **Evaluation of nursing care**
   a. All invasive insertion sites are without signs of infection.
   b. The patient is afebrile.
   c. The patient's lungs are clear to auscultation.
   d. Chest x-ray film is clear without atelectasis or infiltrate.
   e. Leukocytosis and thrombocytopenia are absent.
   f. The patient's skin remains intact with normal turgor.
   g. Incision edges are well approximated without edema, erythema, or exudates.

❖ High risk for knowledge deficit related to diagnosis of congenital heart disease

❖ Ineffective management of therapeutic regimen related to insufficient knowledge of CHF

1. **Defining characteristics** are requests for information; incorrectly relating instructions taught to them; or incorrectly identifying medications, their uses, dosage, time schedule, and side effects. In addition, the patient or family member may incorrectly explain the cardiac diagnosis and therapeutic procedures.
2. **Expected outcomes**
   a. Patient or family member verbalizes understanding of the disease process, causes, treatment regimen, and lifestyle changes that must be taken into account to prevent and control complications.
   b. Patient or family member verbalizes symptoms of complications to be reported.
   c. Patient or family member verbalizes understanding of all medications, their uses, dosage, time of administration, and side effects.
   d. Patient or family member verbalizes understanding of diet regimen and restrictions.
   e. Patient or family member verbalizes impact of growth and development and long-term impact of diagnosis and treatment.
3. **Interventions:** Assess and monitor readiness to learn and support systems and to determine best methods for teaching and learning (i.e., structured, unstructured). Incorporate the patient's family when possible. Individualize the plan. Plan times

for one-to-one interactions with the patient; encourage questions. Teach the patient or family member about the disease process and its ramifications. Provide printed instructions to take home regarding medications; signs and symptoms; activity regimens; dietary restrictions; and what to do if questions, problems, and signs and symptoms arise. Provide video and booklet teaching while the child is hospitalized. Have the patient or family member demonstrate all psychomotor skills necessary for home care when appropriate. Initiate community health and social service consultations as necessary for follow-up care. Stress need for lifelong follow-up care and the impact on growth and development. Assess the family's ability to provide necessary transportation for care.

4. **Evaluation of nursing care**
   a. Patient or family member relates appropriate compliance factors to all nursing and medical regimens.
   b. Patient or family member is able to demonstrate correct procedures regarding home self-care measures.
   c. Patient or family member relates symptoms requiring notification of physician and how to do so.

❖ High risk for altered respiratory function

❖ Dysfunctional ventilatory weaning process

1. **Defining characteristics** are tachypnea, dyspnea, grunting, retractions, and flaring. Arterial blood gases may reflect respiratory alkalosis or acidosis and hypoxemia relative to diagnosis. Bilateral rales and rhonchi, decreased breath sounds, prolonged expiratory phase, and wheezing may occur. Mental status changes such as confusion, restlessness, and irritability may occur. Chest radiographic examination shows pulmonary infiltrates, pulmonary edema, pleural effusions, atelectasis, pneumothorax, or elevated hemidiaphragm. Additional characteristics are pulmonary hypertension, feeding intolerance, lack of appetite, elevated mean and peak airway pressures on ventilator, oversedation or anesthesia with lack of respiratory drive, and paralyzed diaphragm on ECHO or fluoroscopy.
2. **Expected outcomes**
   a. Patient breathes easier, with normal rate, depth of respirations, and work of breathing.
   b. Arterial blood gases are within normal limits for physiology.
   c. Lungs are clear to auscultation, without adventitious lung sounds.
   d. Sensorium is appropriate.
   e. Chest radiographic examination is without effusion, atelectasis, and infiltrates.
   f. Hemodynamic parameters are within normal limits.
3. **Interventions:** Assess the patient for level of consciousness and presence of irritability or restlessness. Maintain a patent airway. Monitor MAP and peak inspiratory pressure (PIP) and minimize PEEP. Expand atelectatic lungs with percussion and postural drainage. Monitor the patient's respiratory status by assessing the lungs for signs of infiltrates and observing the patient's color, respiratory rate, and effort. Institute nursing actions to mobilize secretions (e.g., incentive spirometry, changing positions, chest-wall percussion, postural drainage, delivery of humidified oxygen). Maintain fluid restriction, and administer diuretic therapy. Correct acid-base disturbances as ordered. Assist with placement of and maintain chest tubes as needed. Maintain adequate nutrition and provide medium- or long-chain fatty acid diet for chylous effusion. Use hyperventilation, hyperoxygenation, sedation, paralysis, and pulmonary vasodilators (e.g., nitric oxide) in patients with pulmonary hypertension and avoid noxious stimuli. Assess for signs and symptoms of

pulmonary hypertensive crisis, including hypotension, hypoxemia, bradycardia, and elevated PA pressure (which may proceed to cardiac arrest). Monitor PA pressure, BP, and arterial blood gases. Use a small nasogastric tube in infants because they are obligate nose breathers. Monitoring of the RA and LA pressures will determine transpulmonic gradients.

4. **Evaluation of nursing care**
   a. Patient is hemodynamically stable, and vital signs are within the patient's baseline.
   b. Patient is without pulmonary congestion, effusion, or pulmonary hypertensive crisis.
   c. Lungs are clear to auscultation.
   d. Arterial blood gases are within normal limits for physiology.
   e. Patient is calm or easily soothed.
   f. Patient is able to tolerate diet.

❖ Pain in children related to fear or surgical intervention

1. **Defining characteristics** include description of pain on objective and subjective scoring scale (e.g., Oucher scale), hypertension, tachycardia, crying, grimacing, guarding of incision, tachypnea, grunting, hyperventilation, restlessness, irritability, and poor feeding.
2. **Expected outcomes**
   a. Patient verbalizes comfort level or low pain scale score.
   b. Patient rests comfortably without restlessness, agitation, tachycardia, or hypertension.
3. **Interventions:** Assess factors that decrease pain tolerance, such as age, culture, parental or familial anxiety, child's anxiety, and fear. Determine the child's concept of the cause of pain. Subjectively and objectively assess pain and the response to treatment using accepted pain scoring tools and response to treatment. Prepare the patient and family for procedures. Use anesthesia, sedatives, narcotics, or analgesics as necessary, and provide accurate information to alleviate the patient's or the family's fear of addiction. Provide safe areas and periods of rest using distraction, relaxation, and touch techniques as possible. Reduce or eliminate narcotic side effects (administer stool softeners and antiemetics as needed). Assess the ability for patient-controlled analgesia. Consult with the physician about the use of epidural morphine or narcotic. If at all possible, avoid the use of intramuscularly administered pain medications. Identify coping behaviors, and observe for these to assist the child in coping with pain. Initiate health teaching and referrals, if appropriate.
4. **Evaluation of nursing care**
   a. Patient remains with normal sleep-awake cycles.
   b. Patient's pain is controlled, and hemodynamic parameters are at baseline.

❖ Tissue perfusion, altered cardiopulmonary

1. **Defining characteristics** are hypotension, tachycardia, oliguria, arrhythmias, edema evidenced by a weight gain of more than 30 g per day, irritability, restlessness, failure to thrive, poor weight gain, cool, mottled extremities, delayed capillary refill, decreased peripheral pulses, excessive volume loss through chest drains, acidosis, hypoxemia, presence of extra heart sounds (S_3, S_4), hepatomegaly, splenomegaly, and fever.
2. **Expected outcome**
   a. HR and BP are appropriate for age.
   b. Urine output is 0.5 to 1 mL/kg per hour.
   c. Weight gain is not in excess of 30 g per day.
   d. No arrhythmias or conduction disturbances occur.

e. Warm, perfused extremities with palpable peripheral pulses are noted.
f. The patient has been weaned from all IV inotropic agents and ventilatory support.
g. Volume status is stabilized as evidenced by clear lungs on physical and radiographic examination; intake and output are balanced.
h. Laboratory values reflect balanced electrolytes and acid-base balance.

3. **Interventions**
   a. *Maintain adequate preload:* Monitor CVP and PA and LA pressures, and administer volume infusions as ordered (10 mL/kg bolus). Maintain accurate intake and output; weigh patient daily and record the weight. Administer diuretics as ordered. Monitor signs of tamponade from pericardial effusion or surgical bleeding, such as increased filling pressures, decreased perfusion, oliguria, acidosis, poor peripheral pulses, cool extremities, muffled heart sounds, decreased MAP, and abrupt cessation of chest tube drainage or persistence of bleeding greater than 10% of blood volume per hour for more than 3 hours. Assess coagulation studies and infuse appropriate clotting factors as needed. Monitor for enlarged cardiac silhouette on radiographic examination. Assist with reexploration of the chest in the pedicatric intensive care unit (PICU) if necessary, or return to the operating room. Maintain chest-tube patency.
   b. *Reduce afterload:* Use vasodilators as ordered to improve ventricular ejection or decrease valvular regurgitation, or both. Monitor BP. Monitor the patient's temperature and ensure normothermia.
   c. *Ensure normal cardiac rate and rhythm:* Pace for rate (tachycardia or bradycardia) and AV synchrony or to improve cardiac output. Monitor ECG, and institute appropriate antiarrhythmic medications (monitor drug levels).
   d. *Support myocardial contractility:* Administer positive inotropic drugs. Provide bed rest and rest periods. Observe for changes in level of consciousness, irritability, or restlessness. Obtain arterial and venous oxygen saturations for AV oxygen difference and monitor cardiac output.
   e. *Administer pain medication and sedatives* as ordered.
   f. *Provide nutritional support* using high-calorie formula and nasogastric supplementation to maintain calories for hypermetabolic state. Provide total parenteral nutrition if the patient is unable to tolerate gastric feedings. Consult with nutritional support team as needed.
   g. *Administer oxygen and ventilation support* as needed.
   h. *Assess for decrease in hepatomegaly or splenomegaly* with treatment.
   i. *Monitor laboratory data,* especially electrolytes, arterial blood gases, hematocrit, hemoglobin, and thyroid functions.
   j. *Provide explanations and support* to the patient and family.
   k. *Assess for changes* in level of consciousness, bulging fontanelle, or seizures.
4. **Evaluation of nursing care**
   a. Patient or family member lists symptoms of CHF and actions and side effects of medications.
   b. Patient or family member lists signs and symptoms of tamponade from pericardial effusion and action to take.
   c. Family member relates need for high-calorie formula and is able to provide feedings orally or by nasogastric supplementation.
   d. Patient's HR and BP are age appropriate.
   e. Patient is calm and not irritable.
   f. Cardiac rhythm is normal, without arrhythmia or conduction disturbance.
   g. Blood gases and electrolytes reflect adequate tissue perfusion.

❖ Potential complication: fluid-volume excess

1. **Defining characteristics** are edema (peripheral, facial, periorbital, bulging fontanelle), weight gain in excess of 30 g per day, shiny skin or woody extremities, diaphoresis, shortness of breath, dyspnea, tachypnea, retractions, flaring, grunting, mouth breathing, possible rales, wheezes, prolonged expiratory phase, restlessness, irritability, fatigue, decreased oxygen saturation, dilutional hypovolemia (resulting in a low hematocrit, sodium, potassium, chloride, and albumin), tachycardia with or without arrhythmia, hypertension, hepatomegaly, splenomegaly, ascites, elevated filling pressures (RA, CVP, LA), evidence of pulmonary edema (pleural effusion on chest radiographic examination), and immobility due to illness.
2. **Expected outcomes**
   - **a.** Weight gain is appropriate.
   - **b.** Respiratory functions are normalized, and chest radiographic examination will be clear of edema or effusion.
   - **c.** Vital signs, liver and spleen size, and filling pressures remain at baseline for age and sex.
   - **d.** Laboratory studies reflect a normal volume state.
   - **e.** Patient rests comfortably.
   - **f.** Intake and output are balanced.
   - **g.** No edema is present.
   - **h.** Skin remains intact.
3. **Interventions**
   - **a.** Protect edematous skin from injury. Inspect skin for redness and blanching, breaks in skin, and bony prominence integrity. Reduce the pressure on skin areas by turning the patient at least every 2 hours or by use of a pressure-reduction surface. Provide adequate nutrition.
   - **b.** Accurately record intake and output, and administer medications (albumin, diuretics, electrolyte replacements) as ordered. Maintain fluid restriction by using high-calorie formula. Assess weight daily. Monitor serum electrolytes, albumin, blood urea nitrogen, creatinine, and hematocrit.
   - **c.** Assist with chest radiographic examination and abdominal ultrasound.
   - **d.** Assist with ultrafiltration, peritoneal drain, ascites, peritoneal dialysis, hemofiltration, and hemodialysis.
   - **e.** Assist with placement of chest tubes or thoracentesis for pleural effusion. EMLA cream to chest wall before the procedure may be helpful. Maintain 10 to 15 cm of water suction to chest tubes.
   - **f.** Monitor pulse oximetry and arterial blood gases. Provide oxygen and ventilatory support as needed. Monitor peak and mean ventilatory pressures.
4. **Evaluation of nursing care**
   - **a.** No evidence of skin breakdown is seen.
   - **b.** Chest radiographic examination is free of edema or effusion.
   - **c.** Respiratory effort is normal.
   - **d.** Vital signs are normal for age and sex.
   - **e.** Intake and output are balanced.
   - **f.** Electrolyte values are normal.
   - **g.** Weight gain less than 30 g per day.
   - **h.** Patient or family member correctly states reason for edema and treatment course.

C. Congenital Heart Disease Classifications

1. **Acyanotic lesions** usually are left-to-right shunts. Blood shunts from areas of high to low resistance. These defects generally have symptoms of pulmonary

overcirculation from RV and PA volume and pressure loading, which may result in symptoms of CHF.

2. **Obstructive lesions** produce restrictive blood flow across the stenotic area with hypertensive changes proximal to the obstruction; obstructive lesions may have hypoperfusion states distally.
3. **Cyanotic lesions** usually have obstruction (mechanical [i.e., tricuspid atresia] or anatomic [i.e., total anomalous pulmonary venous return, TAPVR]) to pulmonary blood flow, mandating obligatory right-to-left shunting for blood to enter the pulmonary circulation. This results in intracardiac and/or extracardiac mixing of saturated and desaturated blood and cyanosis. Cyanotic symptoms are related to the degree and number of right-to-left shunts. Cyanosis may also result from anatomically malposed vessels (i.e., transposition of the great vessels [TGV]).

D. Acyanotic Physiology

1. **Expected outcomes**
   a. The patient or a family member will state the need for *lifelong cardiovascular follow-up,* including endocarditis prophylaxis preoperatively and if a shunt is placed.
   b. The patient will have no evidence of hemodynamically significant residual shunt on ECHO or examination.
   c. Operative intervention will occur before irreversible pulmonary vascular obstructive disease (PVOD) or severe ventricular dysfunction occurs.
   d. The patient's symptoms of CHF will resolve, and growth and development will resume on a normal curve.
   e. The patient or a family member can state the signs and symptoms of CHF.
   f. The patient's *exercise tolerance* will be within normal limits for age, or the patient or a family member will state activity limitations if imposed.
   g. The patient is free of *arrhythmia and conduction disturbances,* or the condition will be controlled with medications or with a pacemaker.
   h. Hemodynamic parameters will be normal for age and sex.
2. **PDA:** Persistence of a normal fetal channel connecting the aorta and PA.
   a. *Pathophysiology*
      - In fetal life, the ductus arteriosus permits flow to be diverted away from the high-resistance pulmonary circulation to the descending aorta and the low-resistance placental circulation.
      - Closure of the ductus arteriosus normally occurs from contraction of the medial smooth muscle in the wall of the ductus arteriosus during the first 12 to 24 hours after birth, which is initiated by a rise in the perivascular PO_2 and decreased endogenous prostaglandin. This produces functional closure; however, the ductus may be reopened at this point in response to a strong stimulus such as acidosis, hypoxemia, or prostaglandins. Anatomic closure occurs between 2 and 3 weeks and is produced by fibrosis of the ductal tissue with permanent sealing of the lumen to produce the ligamentum arteriosum. Following anatomic closure, the ductus cannot be reopened.
      - In cases where the ductus fails to close normally, blood shunts from left to right into the PA and lungs. This occurs as the PVR drops and the pressure in the aorta exceeds that of the pulmonary artery. Pulmonary blood flow increases, thus increasing venous return to the LA; LA and LV volume overload and CHF ensue. Over time, the increased flow and pressure on the pulmonary circulation changes the pulmonary vasculature, resulting in PA hypertension and increased PVR. Once these changes have progressed from medial hypertrophy and intimal hyperplasia to fibrosis of the pulmonary

bed, they are irreversible and result in pulmonary hypertension and reversal of the cardiac shunt. Blood is then shunted right to left, causing cyanosis. This reversal of shunt flow resulting from changes in the pulmonary vascular bed from pressure and volume overload is known as *Eisenmenger syndrome.* Once reversal of shunt flow has occurred, surgical closure of the defect is contraindicated. These children may then be candidates for treatment of pulmonary hypertension (prostacyclin infusion) or heart-lung or lung transplant.

- The presence of a large PDA results in a low diastolic pressure. This may adversely affect myocardial function from poor coronary perfusion.

b. *Etiology and incidence:* In preterm infants the response to the vasoconstrictor stimulus of oxygen is not developed, resulting in persistence of the ductus arteriosus. The incidence of PDA in full-term infants accounts for about 5% to 10% of all types of CHD. Failure to close in this population is related to a structural defect in the wall of the ductus. Exposure to rubella during the first trimester of pregnancy is associated with PDA.

c. *Assessment*

- The *presentation* depends on the size and diameter of the ductus; the degree of shunting, which is based on the length and diameter of the ductus; compensatory mechanisms; and the stage of lung development. Full-term neonates have elevated PVR, and therefore shunting is not so pronounced. Premature infants may have severe low cardiac output and require emergency closure to restore adequate diastolic pressure and perfusion of the myocardium as well as other organs. Small PDAs with small shunts rarely produce symptoms, and growth and development are normal. Moderate and large defects produce symptoms of CHF from the left-to-right shunt and LV volume overload.
- *Examination* reveals a machinery-like continuous murmur auscultated at the left upper sternal border. Poor feeding, irritability, tachycardia, tachypnea, and slow weight gain are often present. The pulse pressure is wide, and peripheral pulses may be strong and collapse suddenly because of low diastolic pressure resulting from ductal shunting of blood into the low pressure PA. This is referred to as a *Waterhammer pulse.*

d. *Diagnostic findings*

- *ECG* shows prominent LV forces, LA hypertrophy, and possibly RV hypertrophy.
- *Chest radiographic examination* shows enlargement of the cardiac silhouette with LA and LV enlargement. The MPA segment is prominent. The pulmonary vascular markings are accentuated in moderate to large shunts.
- *ECHO* demonstrates an increased LA diameter. An estimate of the shunt may be made from the left atrium-to-aorta ratio.
- *Cardiac catheterization* is rarely performed. If done, it will demonstrate a step-up in oxygen concentration in the PA. The PA pressure and resistance can also be evaluated and may be elevated in large shunts.

e. *Intervention*

- Medical therapy involves control of CHF with medications or closure of the ductus with indomethacin once normal kidney function and an adequate platelet count are assured.
- Interventional catheterization can be performed to provide closure with intracardiac device in a small- or moderate-sized ductus. Risk of device closure includes residual shunt, embolization of the coil or device, and hemolysis.
- Surgical closure involves division or ligation (or both) of the ductus through a left thoracotomy. Postoperative complications are rare but may include

damage to the recurrent laryngeal nerve, chylous effusion, bleeding, infection, paralyzed phrenic nerve, ligation of the left PA or descending aorta, or tear in the ductus or aorta.

- Use of video assisted thoracoscopic surgery is being introduced at some centers. Risks of this procedure, while low, include injury to the recurrent laryngeal nerve, thoracic duct injury with chylous effusion, prolonged exposure to radiation and residual ductus due to inadequate visualization requiring need to convert to thoracotomy.

3. **Atrial septal defect (ASD):** A defect in the atrial septum from improper embryologic formation of the septal wall (Figure 3-30).
   a. *Classifications*
      - *Sinus venosus:* High in the septum near the junction of the SVC and RA; may be associated with partial anomalous pulmonary venous return.
      - *Ostium secundum:* Most common; region fossa ovalis cordis; may be associated with mitral valve prolapse.
      - *Ostium primum:* Low in septum; may involve defects of one or both AV valves.
      - *Unroofed coronary sinus:* Coronary sinus blood is diverted to the left atrium.

   b. *Pathophysiology:* The defect is created by failure of the endocardial cushion tissue to seal the septum primum (ostium primum defect), failure of the valve of the fossa ovalis cordis to close (patent foramen ovale [PFO]), or failure of closure of the septal fenestration (ostium secundum defect). Defects allow blood to be shunted from the higher-pressure left side of the heart to the lower-pressure right side of the heart, resulting in RV volume and pressure overload with RA and RV dilation. Pulmonary vascular changes occur in 10% to 20% of patients with an ASD. By the third to fourth decade of life, atrial arrhythmias, CHF, and paradoxical embolus become problems. Endocarditis is uncommon.

   c. *Etiology:* Failure of the septum to form in the fetal period results in defects in the atrial septal wall.

   d. *Assessment*
      - Most patients are asymptomatic, but those with large left-to-right shunts may exhibit symptoms of fatigue and dyspnea. Growth retardation is unusual.

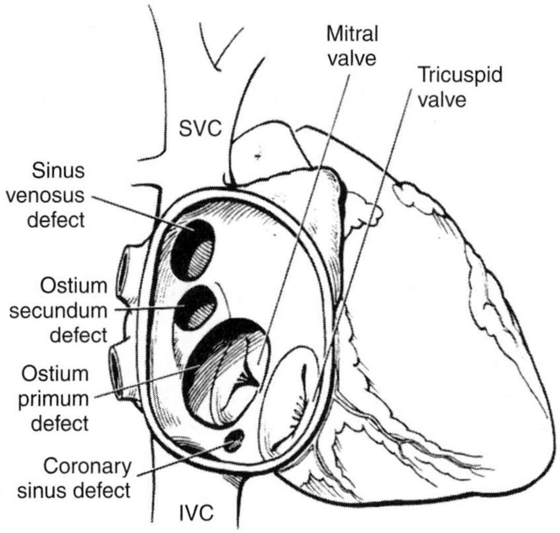

FIGURE 3-30 ■ Atrial septal defect *(ASD). IVC,* inferior vena cava; *SVC,* superior vena cava.
(From Kambam J: Atrial septal defect. In Kambam J, editor: *Cardiac anesthesia for infants and children,* St. Louis, 1994, Mosby.)

- *Examination:* Auscultation may reveal a systolic ejection murmur at the LSB (pulmonary flow murmur); wide, fixed, split S_2; and a diastolic murmur from large-volume flow across the tricuspid valve.

e. *Diagnostic findings*

- *ECG* demonstrates RV and RA hypertrophy, right-axis deviation, RBBB, prolonged PR interval, and possibly evidence of junctional rhythm or a SVT.
- *Chest radiographic examination* may show RVH, RA enlargement, and increased pulmonary vascular markings, but in most cases heart size may be normal.
- *ECHO* confirms the diagnosis in most cases with evidence of RV volume overload, direct visualization of the location and size of defect, and identification of associated defects (most commonly anomalous pulmonary veins or pulmonary stenosis).
- *Cardiac catheterization* is rarely indicated. It demonstrates an increase in oxygen saturation in the RA.

f. *Intervention*

- Many ASDs close spontaneously (up to 85%), but repair of the defect is low risk and is recommended by school age despite presentation to prevent long-term problems with pulmonary disease and arrhythmia. Adult patients undergoing ASD closure may not benefit from complete resolution of symptoms, specifically arrhythmias, but most likely they will have improved quality of life. Closure of a patent foramen ovale/ASD in an adult presenting with paradoxical embolism is indicated to prevent recurrence and avoid risk of lifelong anticoagulation.
- Defects may be closed via a right thoracotomy or through a sternotomy. New techniques of minimally invasive closure of ASD use a small median sternotomy incision with excellent visualization for the surgeon and improved cosmetic results. Surgical repair requires a short period of cardiopulmonary bypass. The defect may be closed directly or patched (Figure 3-31). Postoperative problems specific to this operation include atrial arrhythmia, heart block, residual defect, anemia, phrenic nerve injury, air embolus, patch dehiscence, pericardial effusion/postpericardotomy syndrome, and AV valve regurgitation in ostium primum defects.
- Transcatheter closure of ASD is routinely performed in patients meeting criteria for size and location of the defect (Figure 3-32). The Amplatzer device is approved by the Food and Drug Administration for use in small to medium secundum defects. Risks include incomplete closure, embolization of the device, tricuspid valve injury, and arrhythmia.

4. Ventricular septal defect (VSD): Communication between the right and left ventricles created by an opening in the septal wall.

a. *Classification* (Figure 3-33)

- *Perimembranous* is the most common VSD and is located below the crista supraventricularis adjacent to the tricuspid valve. It may be associated with malalignment of the septum.
- *Infundibular, subpulmonic, subarterial, conal, and supracristal VSDs* are positioned in the RV outflow tract under the pulmonary valve.
- *Inlet VSD* is a common defect located under the AV valve posterior and inferior to the membranous septum.
- *Muscular defects* are located in the muscular septum. If multiple, they are called "Swiss cheese" septum.

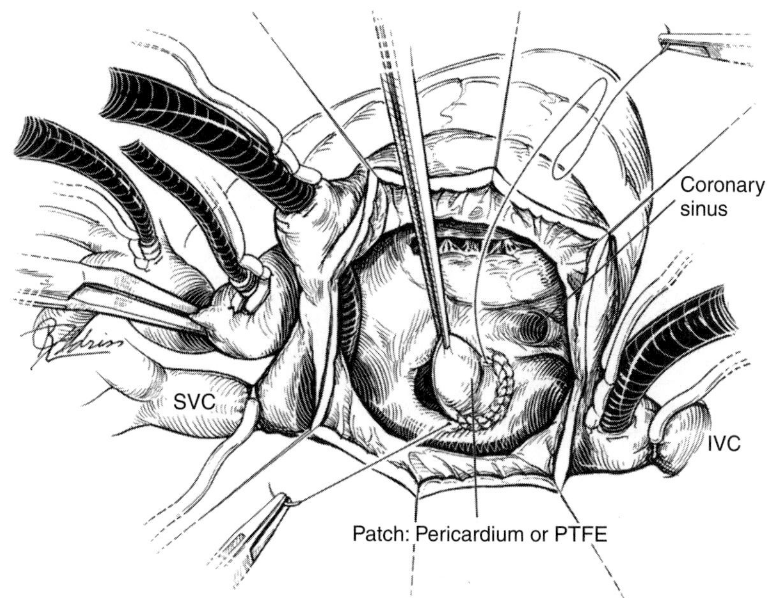

FIGURE 3-31 ■ Closure of an ostium secundum atrial septal defect *(ASD)* with a patch. Cardioplegia has been delivered and the heart arrested. The right atrium has been opened. The ASD is being closed with a patch—usually of autologous pericardium, although polytetrafluoroethylene *(PTFE)* also can be used. *IVC,* inferior vena cava; *SVC,* superior vena cava.

(From Mavroudis C, Backer CL: *Pediatric cardiac surgery,* ed 3. St. Louis, 2003, Mosby.)

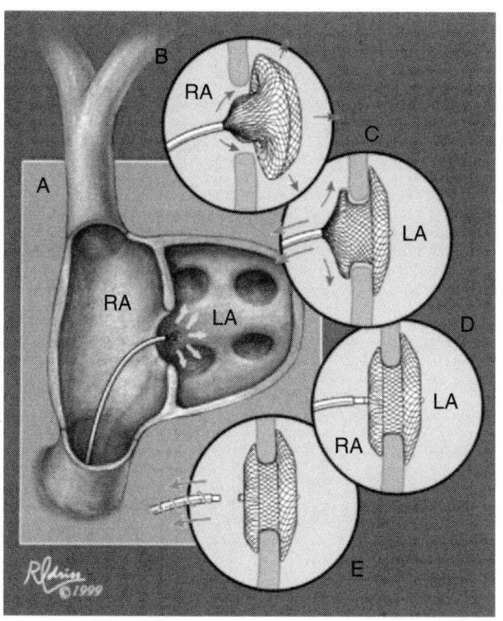

FIGURE 3-32 ■ Implantation of the Amplatzer atrial septal defect *(ASD)* occluder. **A,** The delivery catheter is positioned across the atrial defect. **B,** Left atrial disk *(LA)* with self-centering connecting stalk is delivered. **C,** The device is withdrawn so that the connecting stalk is within the ASD and the left disk is firm against the atrial septum. **D,** Right atrial *(RA)* disk is delivered. **E,** Delivery cable is disconnected; the device can no longer be withdrawn back into the atrium.

(From Mavroudis C, Backer CL: *Pediatric cardiac surgery,* ed 3. St. Louis, 2003, Mosby.)

b. *Pathophysiology*

- Effects of the VSD depend on the size and number of the defects and resistance to flow through the lungs (flow is also affected by the presence of RV outflow tract obstruction). VSDs may present as small defects with

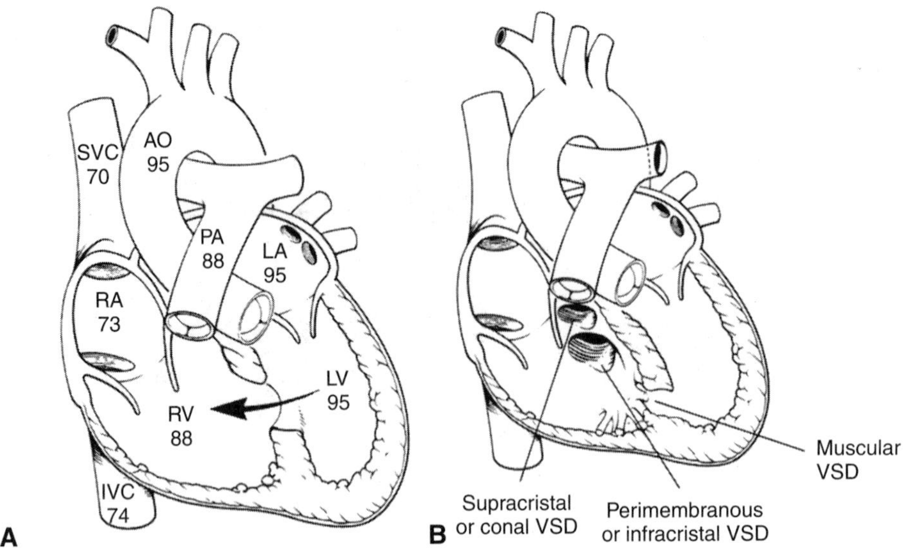

FIGURE 3-33 ■ Ventricular septal defect *(VSD).* **A,** Oxygen saturations within the heart and great vessels are depicted. **B,** Types of VSDs. *IVC,* inferior vena cava; *LA,* left atrium; *LV,* left ventricle; *PA,* pulmonary artery; *RA,* right atrium; *RV,* right ventricle; *SVC,* superior vena cava.

(From Kambam J: Patent ductus arteriosus. In Kambam J, editor: *Cardiac anesthesia for infants and children.* St. Louis, 1994, Mosby.)

normal PVR, moderate defects with variable PVR, or large defects with either mild to moderate or marked elevation of PVR.

- Assess the size of the defect, magnitude of hemodynamic overload, and status of pulmonary vasculature.
- Children are usually asymptomatic until 2 to 4 weeks of age, when PVR drops. The drop in PVR allows shunting from the LV to the RV and creates pulmonary overcirculation. Long-term pulmonary overcirculation causes PA hypertension and vascular changes progressing from medial hypertrophy and intimal hyperplasia to fibrosis and Eisenmenger syndrome (rarely before 1 year of age).

c. *Etiology and incidence:* Defect results from imperfect embryologic formation of the septal wall. VSD is the most common congenital heart defect (20% of all defects) and is slightly more common in girls.

d. *Assessment*

- *Presentation* is dependent on the size of the shunt and PVR.
- *Examination* reveals a holosystolic murmur at the left sternal border (LSB), normal S_1, split and increased S_2, possible S_3, thrill at the LSB, active precordium, and a diastolic rumble at the LSB in large defects. The murmur decreases as PVR increases.

e. *Diagnostic findings*

- *ECG:* Small defects have normal ECG findings. Moderate to large defects have LA enlargement, LVH with or without RVH, left-axis deviation, and BBB.
- *Chest radiographic examination:* Small defects have normal radiographic findings. Moderate to large defects have cardiomegaly, prominent PA segment, and increased pulmonary vascular markings.
- *Echocardiogram* confirms the location, size of defect, associated lesions, and LA and LV dilation. ECHO also quantifies the degree of RV and PA hypertension.

- *Cardiac catheterization* demonstrates an elevated pulmonary-to-systemic flow ratio (Q_p:Q_s), elevated RV and PA pressures, elevated PVR in large defects, and oxygen step-up in the RV and PA.

f. *Interventions*

- Indications for intervention include CHF, PA hypertension, growth failure, or evidence for LV volume overload. Some defects close spontaneously. Medical management is used for control of CHF (see Congestive Heart Failure).
- Surgical palliation with a PA band aims at controlling pulmonary blood flow and protecting the pulmonary vascular bed, mainly for large and multiple muscular VSDs in the lower septum, patients with multiple anomalies, and preterm infants. PA banding via a left thoracotomy decreases the pressure distal to the band to approximately one half the aortic pressure, but it may not restrict flow adequately. Surgery poses the risk of chylothorax, paralyzed hemidiaphragm, and damage to the recurrent laryngeal nerve. Complications include migration of the band, distortion of the vessels, failure to protect the lung vasculature adequately, erosion of the band into the PA, creation of subaortic stenosis from septal hypertrophy, and damage to the pulmonary valve.
- Device closure may be attempted in cases of multple or difficult to reach VSDs, which may require alternative surgical approaches such as ventriculotomy. Device placement avoids ventriculotomy and can be placed in the catheterization laboratory or in the operating room. Disadvantages include peripheral vascular injury from the large venous sheaths, residual shunting, arrhythmia, device migration or embolization, or disruption of papillary muscles.
- For large, hemodynamically important defects, surgical closure is performed at any age to prevent endocarditis and PVOD. A sternotomy and cardiopulmonary bypass is used. Circulatory arrest may be necessary in anatomically difficult lesions or in small patients. Usually defects are closed by a Gore-tex or Dacron patch as opposed to suturing. Complications include systemic hypertension, damage to the aortic valve, heart block, tricuspid insufficiency, residual shunt with low cardiac output, or pulmonary hypertensive crisis. Repair before the patient is 2 years of age usually permits normalization of growth and reversal of any related developmental delays.
- Endocarditis remains a lifelong risk.

5. AVSD (also known as AV canal and endocardial cushion defect): A defect in the atrial and ventricular wall and various degrees of AV valve regurgitation due to deficiency of the endocardial cushion tissue.

a. *Types of AVSD*

- *Balanced:* Ventricles are equal in size
- *Unbalanced:* One ventricle is larger; classified into forms of single ventricular lesions
- *Incomplete:* Separate AV valve orifices (ostium primum defect)
- *Complete:* Common AV valve orifice, usually with five leaflets

b. *Pathophysiology:* AVSD is characterized by a large ASD and VSD and a common AV valve (Figure 3-34). Physiology is similar to ASD and VSD, in which shunting of blood is related to the size of intracardiac septal defects, AV valve competency, PVR, and PA pressure. Usually left-to-right shunting occurs once PVR decreases, causing pulmonary overcirculation, elevation in PA pressure, and eventual rise in PVR from long-standing pressure and

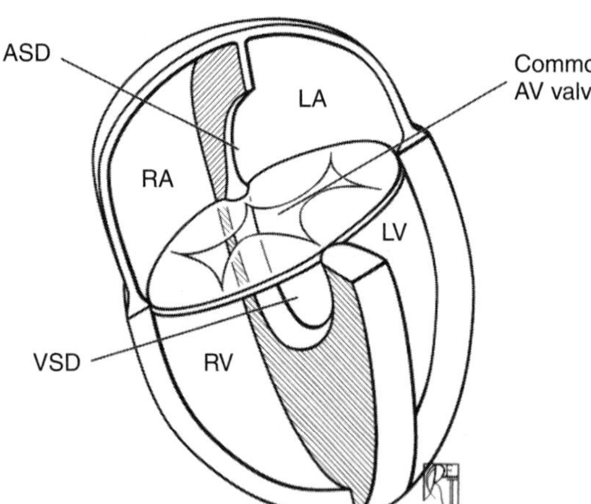

FIGURE 3-34 ■ Anatomy of atrioventricular septal defect *(ASD)*. Complete atrioventricular *(AV)* canal defect.

There is a common AV valve with an ostium primum atrial septal defect *(ASD)* above and a large inlet ventricular septal defect *(VSD)* below. *LA,* left atrium; *LV,* left ventricle; *RA,* right atrium; *RV,* right ventricle.

(From Mavroudis C, Backer CL: *Pediatric cardiac surgery,* ed 3. St. Louis, 2003, Mosby.)

volume overload. A severely regurgitant AV valve leads to early symptoms of CHF and low cardiac output, which may increase PA pressure and PVR and is difficult to treat medically or surgically.

c. *Etiology:* Embryologic deficiency of the endocardial cushion tissue results in ostium primum atrial defect, common AV orifice, inlet VSD, malrotation of the aortic valve, elongation and narrowing of the LV outflow tract, and abnormal attachment of the AV valve to the ventricular septum. AVSD is associated with Down syndrome.

d. *Assessment*

- Symptoms of CHF and pulmonary overcirculation usually occur in early infancy from a large increase in pulmonary blood flow and are associated with elevated PA pressure and complicated by insufficiency of the common AV valve.
- Usually patients are small and undernourished. Oxygen saturation is normal except in the presence of pulmonary vascular disease in older children or accelerated disease in an infant. Desaturation can result from ventilation-perfusion ($\dot{V}\dot{Q}$) mismatch from pulmonary changes secondary to a large left-to-right shunt.
- Examination: Auscultation reveals a systolic ejection murmur at the LSB, mid-diastolic murmur at the lower LSB and apex from AV valve regurgitation, and a split prominent S_2.

e. *Diagnostic findings*

- *ECG* findings are normal sinus rhythm (NSR); prolonged PR interval; RA, LA, or bilateral atrial enlargement; BBB, and left-axis or northwest-axis deviation.
- *Chest radiographic examination* shows an enlarged heart, enlarged RA, prominent PA, and increased pulmonary vascular markings.
- *Echocardiogram* visualizes the VSD and ASD. Both right- and left-sided components of the common AV valve are displaced into the ventricles and are associated with variable deficiency related to the inflow of the ventricular septum. ECHO predicts noninvasive estimates of PA pressure and can quantitate the degree of AV valve regurgitation.
- *Cardiac catheterization* demonstrates an increase in oxygen saturation throughout the right side of the heart; elevated PA pressure and PVR may be present and may or may not be responsive to oxygen.

f. *Intervention*

- Medical treatment of CHF is usually initiated early. Control of the CHF and weight gain are goals of medical management. Elective repair is preferred between 3 to 6 months of age (see Congestive Heart Failure).
- Surgical repair is recommended for any symptomatic infant to prevent early development of pulmonary vascular disease. Surgery involves a sternotomy and cardiopulmonary bypass. One or two patches are used, depending on the preference of the surgeon (Figure 3-35). The VSD is closed and the AV valve is partially anchored to the patch. The atrial component of the patch is partially sewn in place, the AV valve repair is completed, and the atrial defect is closed.
- Complications include heart block, pulmonary hypertensive crisis (rapid fall in BP and HR with concomitant rise in PAP to systemic or suprasystemic levels treated with hyperventilation, hyperoxygenation, pulmonary vasodilators including nitric oxide, sedation, and paralysis), residual shunt, and residual AV valve regurgitation or stenosis.
- Endocarditis remains a lifelong risk.

6. Double-outlet right ventricle (DORV): Origins of both great arteries from a morphologic RV.

a. *Pathophysiology*

- DORV encompasses features of a wide variety of entities including VSD, tetralogy of Fallot, and transposition of the great arteries (Figure 3-36). Both great arteries arise from the RV; usually a VSD is present, and varying degrees of pulmonary stenosis may exist. The great arteries may be in normal position, side by side, in dextroposition or levoposition. The VSD may be subaortic, subpulmonic (Taussig-Bing syndrome), or doubly committed (a large VSD related to both semilunar valves).
- Physiology is based on the degree of pulmonary stenosis and the relationship of the VSD to the PA and aorta. Blood enters the right side of the heart normally. RV output flows to the lowest resistance circuit. Without pulmonary stenosis, blood flow to the lungs is unrestricted and significant pulmonary overcirculation and PVOD occur. If pulmonary stenosis is present, blood may exit to the PA and aorta. The more severe the obstruction, the greater the flow to the aorta.

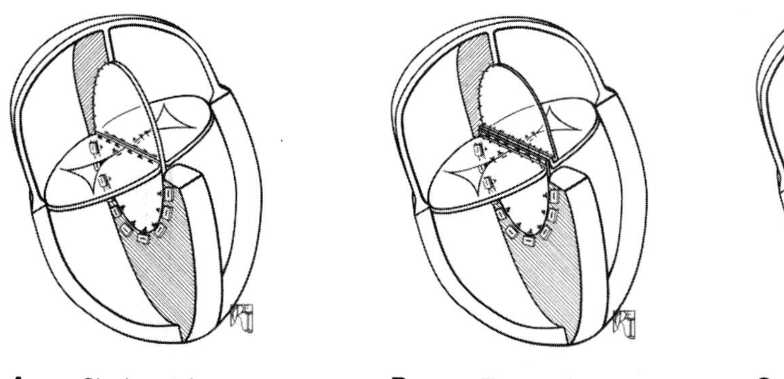

FIGURE 3-35 ■ Schematic three-dimensional reconstruction of the three different surgical techniques: single-patch **(A)**, two-patch **(B)**, and modified single-patch **(C)**. (From Mavroudis C, Backer CL: *Pediatric cardiac surgery*, ed 3. St. Louis, 2003, Mosby.)

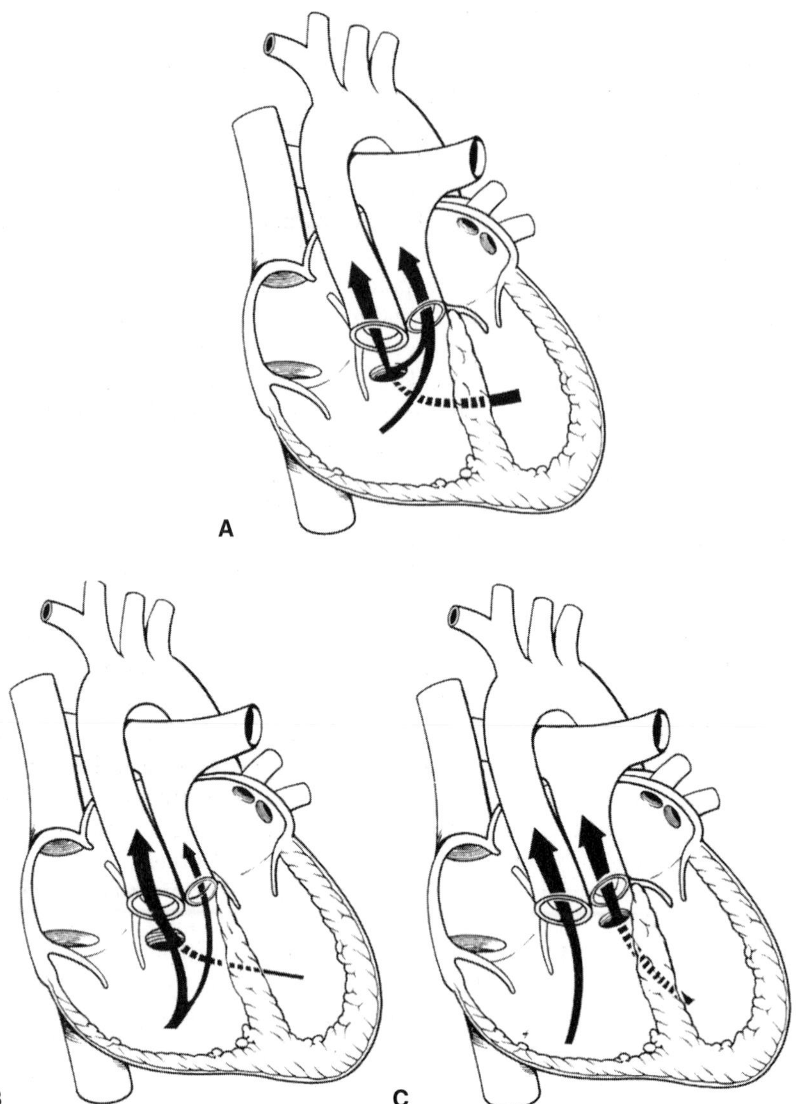

FIGURE 3-36 ■ Double-outlet right ventricle *(DORV)*. There are three major forms of this defect. **A,** DORV with subaortic ventricular septal defect (VSD) without pulmonary stenosis. In this form of DORV, the VSD directs left ventricular outflow into the aorta, with some blood shunting into the pulomonary artery. This defect produces hemodynamics similar to a simple VSD. **B,** DORV with subaortic VSD with pulmonary stenosis. The subaortic VSD directs left ventricular outflow into the aorta. Shunting of right ventricular outflow into the aorta (a right-to-left shunt) will occur if pulmonary stenosis is significant. This defect produces hemodynamics similar to tetralogy of Fallot. **C,** DORV with subpulmonic VSD without pulmonary stenosis. In this form of DORV, the VSD directs left ventricular outflow into the PA and right ventricular outflow to enter the aorta. This produces hemodynamics similar to transposition of the great arteries. (From Hazinski MF: *Manual of pediatric critical care.* St. Louis, 2003, Mosby.)

b. *Etiology and incidence:* DORV is a rare defect (0.09 in 1000 live births) in a spectrum of transposed complexes. DORV is related to failure to achieve conotruncal inversion (rotation) and leftward shift of the conal (aortic or pulmonic) segment of both great vessels from the RV.

c. *Assessment* depends on the anatomic variant.

- Subaortic VSD with pulmonary stenosis is similar to tetralogy of Fallot: Cyanosis, clubbing, exertional dyspnea, polycythemia, RV impulse at LSB, loud systolic ejection murmur, normal S_1, and single S_2.
- Subpulmonic VSD with or without pulmonary stenosis resembles TGV: Cyanosis early, precordial bulge, high-pitched systolic murmur at the upper LSB, and single S_2.
- Subaortic VSD without pulmonary stenosis is similar to a simple VSD: Active precordium, holosystolic murmur at the LSB, and an apical diastolic rumble.

d. *Diagnostic findings*

- *ECG* shows RVH, right-axis deviation, normal to increased LV forces, first-degree AV conduction delay, and RA enlargement.
- *Chest radiographic examination:* With pulmonary stenosis, mild cardiomegaly, absent main PA segment, and decreased pulmonary vascularity occur. Without pulmonary stenosis, cardiomegaly, increased pulmonary vascularity, and prominent main PA segment are seen. With PVOD, "pruning" of the peripheral pulmonary vascular bed occurs.
- *ECHO* displays mitral and semilunar discontinuity, origin of both great vessels from the anterior RV, absence of LV outflow except through the VSD, associated lesions, and accurate position of the VSD.
- *Cardiac catheterization* results are variable, depending on anatomy. It is helpful in quantitating PAP and PVR.

e. *Interventions*

- Intracardiac repair involves closing the VSD via sternotomy utilizing bypass. The goal is complete anatomic repair. Without pulmonary stenosis, early surgery helps to protect the pulmonary vascular bed. Patients may require arterial switch and VSD closure. Alternatively, the anatomy of the VSD and great vessels may best lend itself to intracardiac baffling of the VSD to direct the LV flow into the aorta (Figure 3-37). Neonates may require initial palliation with PA banding for control of CHF while awaiting growth for eventual repair (see Ventricular Septal Defect). Risks associated with VSD closure and arterial switch operation for repair of DORV are the same as each operation (see discussion of VSD and arterial switch operation). Risks associated with intracardiac baffling for repair include residual shunt, low cardiac output/CHF, left ventricular or right ventricular outflow tract obstruction, and heart block, especially if the VSD is enlarged.
- If pulmonary stenosis is associated, the VSD is closed to reestablish LV-aortic continuity. An RV-PA conduit is required to establish RV to PA continuity (Figure 3-38). This conduit will need to be replaced later. If the pulmonary stenosis is mild, it may require only valvotomy or a transannular patch. For infants with a significant degree of pulmonary stenosis, stabilization on prostaglandins followed by palliation with a systemic-to-pulmonary shunt may be necessary, with definitive repair at 6 to 12 months of age. Postoperative complications are the same as those with the Rastelli operation (see Transposition of the Great Arteries).
- Endocarditis is a lifelong risk.

7. Ebstein anomaly: Downward displacement of posterior and septal leaflets of the tricuspid valve with an atrialized portion of the RV.

a. *Pathophysiology*

- Anatomy of the valve is variable, but there is always redundancy of valve tissue and adherence of medial and posterior leaflets to the RV wall. An

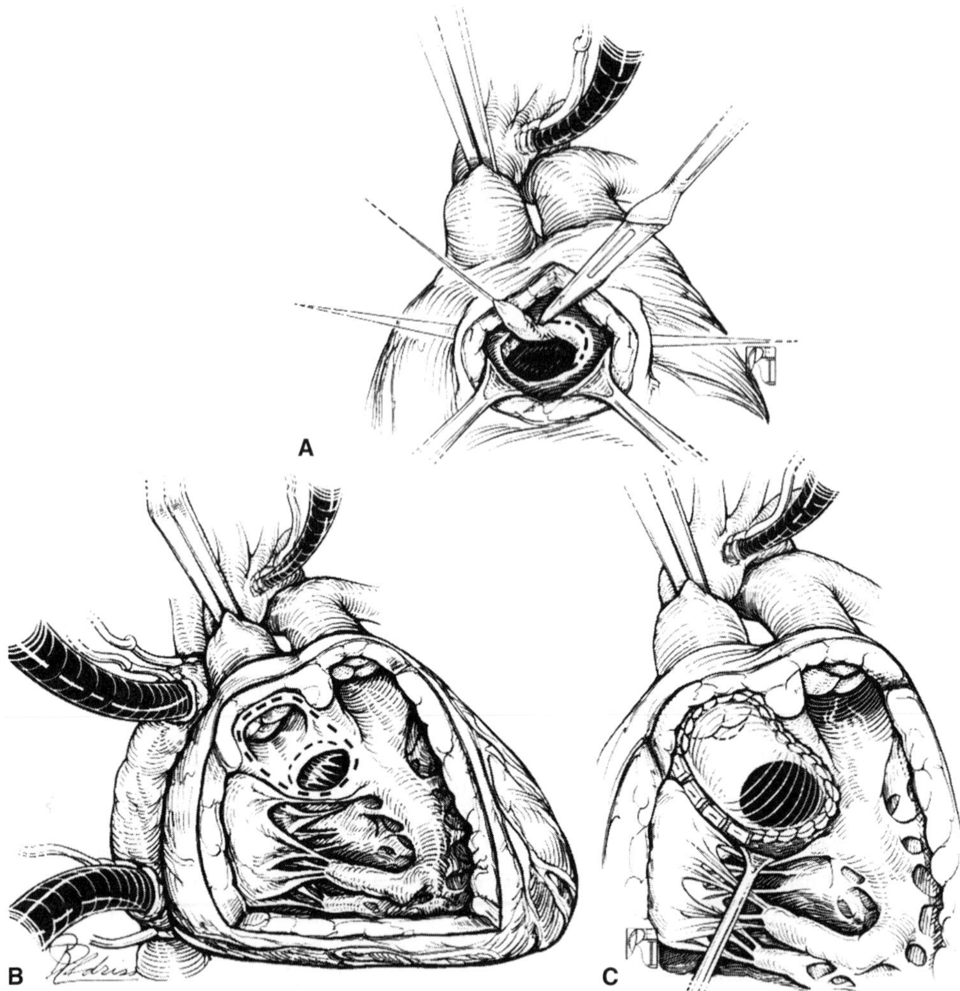

FIGURE 3-37 ■ Intraventricular tunnel repair of double-outlet right ventricle *(DORV)* with subaortic or doubly committed ventral septal defect *(VSD)* without pulmonary stenosis. **A,** If the VSD is restrictive, it is enlarged by resection of the interventricular septum, indicated by inner dashed line. Outer dashed line indicates the portion of the infundibular septum that may require resection to prevent subaortic stenosis. **B,** Enlarging the ventricular septal defect. **C,** Creation of a tunnel connecting the VSD to the aorta.

(From Mavroudis C, Backer CL: *Pediatric cardiac surgery,* ed 3. St. Louis, 2003, Mosby.)

atrialized RV occurs from downward displacement of the tricuspid valve. The RV function is dependent on the amount atrialized (Figure 3-39). It is common to have associated anomalies, including ASD, PFO, VSD, or WPW.

- Physiology depends on the degree of malformation of the tricuspid valve. Mild anomalies may have normal valve function. With severe malformation, cyanosis can occur from right-to-left shunting through the ASD related to massive tricuspid regurgitation and elevated RA pressure. Blood enters the RA normally, but on entering the RV it regurgitates into the RA because of tricuspid insufficiency. In rare circumstances, the tricuspid valve may be

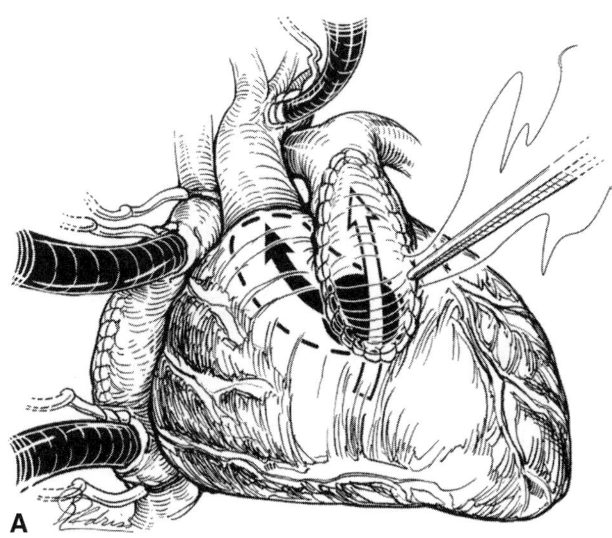

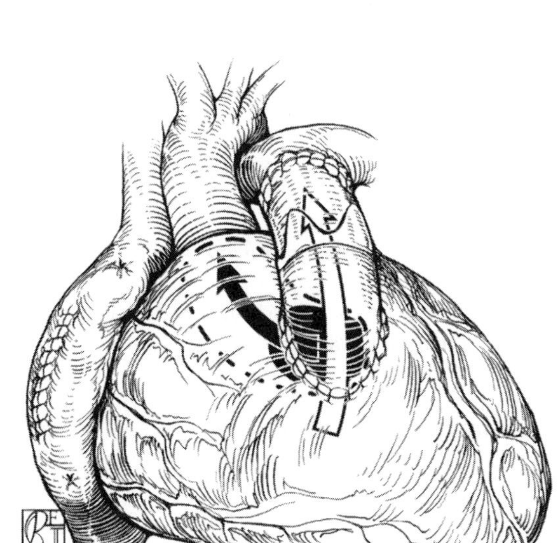

FIGURE 3-38 ■ Reconstruction of the right ventricular outflow tract during repair of double-outlet right ventricle *(DORV)* with subaortic or doubly committed ventral septal defect *(VSD)*. **A,** Patch enlargement of the right ventricular outflow tract with or without transannular extention into the main pulmonary artery *(PA)*. **B,** The use of a valved, extracardiac conduit to establish continuity between the right ventricle and PA.

(From Mavroudis C, Backer CL: *Pediatric cardiac surgery,* ed 3. St. Louis, 2003, Mosby.)

stenotic and cause RA dilation resulting from elevated pressure across the stenotic valve.

- Tricuspid insufficiency in newborns may improve as neonatal elevation of PVR and hence RV hypertension normally regress, thus decreasing cyanosis.

b. *Etiology and incidence:* Ebstein anomaly constitutes 0.5% of CHD cases. The perforations that result in the formation of the chordae tendineae and papillary muscles fail to develop, resulting in tissue redundancy. Unusually high incidence occurs in infants of mothers who are taking lithium.

c. *Assessment*

- History varies based on the degree of tricuspid valve deformity. Cyanosis may be noted in the neonate; the cyanosis disappears over the next few weeks and returns by age 5 to 10 years. Severe tricuspid insufficiency in neonates involves low cardiac output, hepatomegaly, and cyanosis. After infancy, dyspnea on exertion and fatigue may occur. Arrhythmias are common (50%). Growth and development are usually normal.

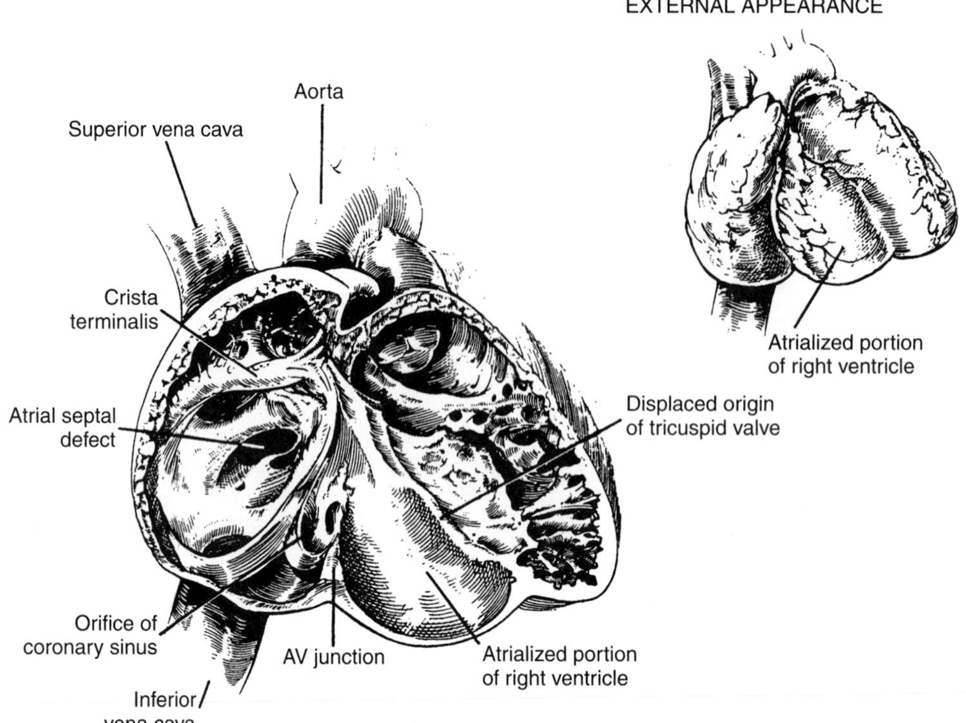

FIGURE 3-39 ■ Ebstein anomaly with displaced tricuspid valve and atrialized portion of the right ventricle.
(Reprinted with permission from Castaneda AR, Jonas RA, Mayer JE, Hanley FL: *Cardiac surgery of the neonate and infant.* Philadelphia, 1994, W. B. Saunders.)

- *Examination* reveals normal cardiac impulse, variable intensity systolic murmur, normal S_1, and possibly a click. If asymptomatic, the S_2 is normal. If symptomatic, the S_2 is diminished or single and an S_3 or S_4 or both may be heard. Hepatomegaly may be present.

d. *Diagnostic findings*

- *ECG* findings are always abnormal and show RBBB, a right-axis deviation, right atrial enlargement, and a prolonged PR interval. WPW may occur (in 5% to 20% of cases).
- *Chest radiographic examination* in the symptomatic infant demonstrates at least moderate, if not massive, cardiomegaly with decreased pulmonary vascular markings (Figure 3-40). Asymptomatic children have normal to slight enlargement of heart size and normal pulmonary vascular markings with RA enlargement of varying degree.
- *ECHO* demonstrates delayed tricuspid valve closure. Valve displacement is present with a sail-like anterior leaflet of the tricuspid valve. Other anatomic findings, specifically RV size or ASD and eccentric coaptation of the tricuspid valve leaflets, can be defined.
- *Cardiac catheterization* is not necessary to delineate anatomy. But arrhythmias are common, so mapping of WPW is warranted. Cardiac catheterization will also demonstrate the portion of the RV that is functioning as the RA.

e. *Interventions*

- No surgery may be required if the degree of tricuspid regurgitation is mild. In moderate or greater TR, tricuspid valvuloplasty with ASD closure or

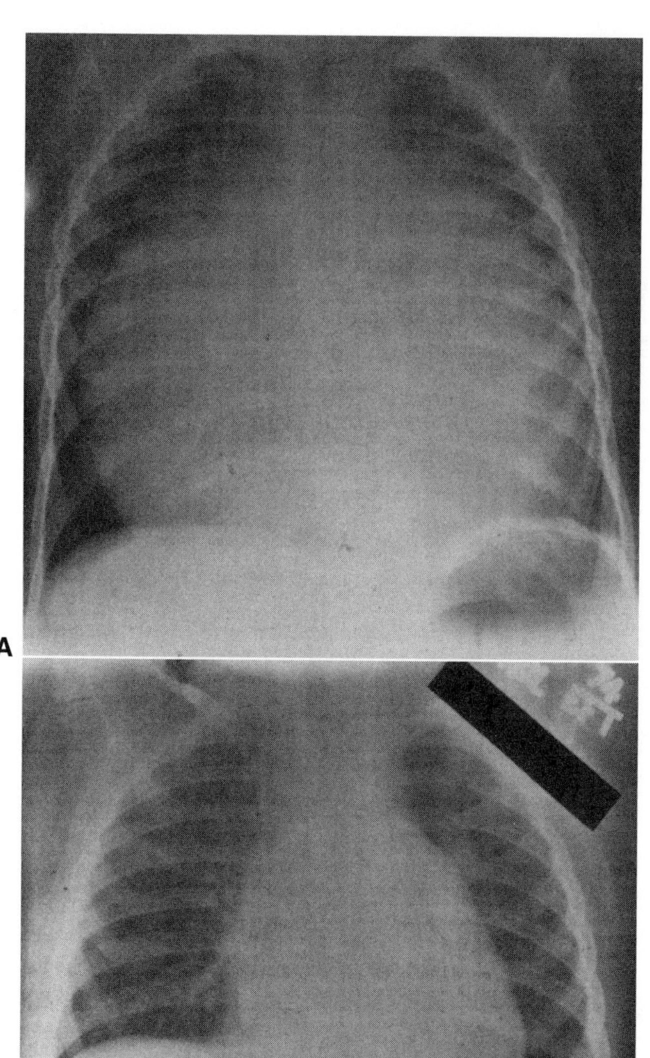

FIGURE 3-40 ■ Chest radiographs of a 2-year-old girl with Ebstein anomaly. **A,** Preoperative (cardiothoracic ratio, 0.96). **B,** Thirteen days after repair (cardiothoracic ratio, 0.55).
(From Danielson GK, Maloney JD, Devloo RAE: Surgical repair of Ebstein's anomaly, *Mayo Clinic Proc* 54:185, 1979).

excision of redundant RA wall may be required to relieve cyanosis, preserve RV function, and prevent paradoxical embolus (Figure 3-41). Valvuloplasty is more effective in older patients. Duran rings may be utilized to stablize a valve repair rather than opting for tricuspid valve replacement. Tricuspid valve replacement is required if valvuloplasty is not effective, usually with plication of the RA.

- For severely symptomatic neonates, prognosis is poor because stabilization of the newborn is difficult. Improvement in oxygenation by manipulation of PVR with nitric oxide, oxygen, and hyperventilation may be helpful. PGE therapy in the absence of severe RV outflow tract obstruction or tricuspid stenosis can be fatal. Tricuspid valve closure to create tricuspid atresia, placement of a systemic-to-pulmonary shunt, and creation of an

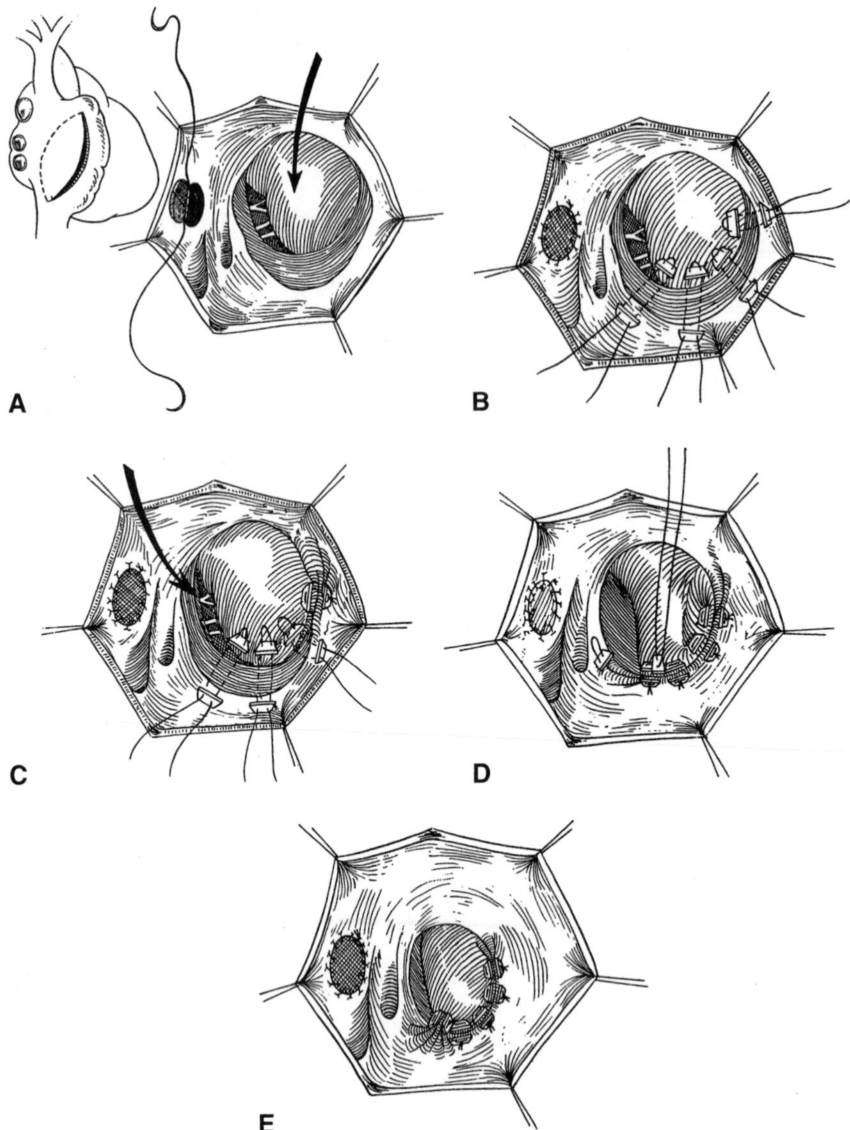

FIGURE 3-41 ■ Diagram of surgical repair of Ebstein anomaly. **A,** *Left:* The right atrium is incised from the atrial appendage to the inferior vena cava. The redundant portion of the right atrium is excised *(dotted line)* so that the final size of the right atrium is normal. *Right:* The atrial septal defect is closed with a patch. The large anterior leaflet is indicated by the arrow. The posterior leaflet is displaced downward from the annulus, and the septal leaflet is hypoplastic and is not visible in this view. **B,** Mattress sutures passed through pledgets of Teflon felt are used to pull the tricuspid annulus and tricuspid valve together. Sutures are placed in the atrialized portion of the right ventricle as shown so that when they are subsequently tied, the atrialized ventricle is plicated and the aneurysmal cavity is obliterated. **C,** The sutures are tied down sequentially. The hypoplastic, markedly displaced deptal leaflet is now visible *(arrow).* **D,** A posterior annuloplasty is performed to narrow the diameter of the tricuspid annulus. The coronary sinus marks the posterior and leftward extent of the annuloplasty, which is terminated there to avoid injury to the conduction system. One or more additional sutures may be required to obliterate the posterior aspect of the annuloplasty repair to render the valve totally competent. The tricuspid annulus at this time will admit two or more fingers in the adult. **E,** Completed repair allowing the anterior leaflet to function as a monocusp valve.

(Modified from Danielson GK, Maloney JD, Devloo RAE: Surgical repair of Ebstein's anomaly, *Mayo Clinic Proc* 54:185, 1979).

ASD is utlized in infants with severe Ebstein anomaly. This is done with cardiopulmonary bypass. These patients will go on to a single-ventricle repair with cavopulmonary shunt and Fontan procedure. Postoperative complications include low cardiac output, RV dysfunction with elevated RV, increased PVR, dysrhythmia, residual tricuspid regurgitation, and persistent pleural effusions.

- Cardiac transplantation for the neonate with severe Ebstein anomaly is another option.
- Ablation (radiofrequency or surgical) of WPW may be required.
- Endocarditis is a lifelong risk.

E. Obstructive Physiology

1. **Expected outcomes**
   - **a.** The patient or a family member will state the need for lifelong cardiovascular follow-up, potential reoperation for valvular regurgitation or stenosis, the need for endocarditis prophylaxis, and activity limitations of the disease state.
   - **b.** The patient or a family member will state the ideal prothrombin time and the side effects of warfarin (Coumadin) where appropriate.
   - **c.** The patient or family member will state action, potential side effects, and complications of all medications.
   - **d.** The patient or a family member will state signs and symptoms of CHF.
   - **e.** The patient's growth and development will be appropriate.
   - **f.** Intervention will occur before development of severe ventricular dysfunction or PVOD.
   - **g.** Systemic hypertension will be controlled to within the 90th percentile for age and sex.
   - **h.** Hemodynamic parameters will be normal for age and sex.
2. **Aortic stenosis:** Malformation of the aortic valve that causes obstruction to ejection of blood from the LV.
   - **a.** *Valvular aortic stenosis:* Obstruction occurs at the valve annulus.
     - *Pathophysiology:* Associated cardiac lesions such as PDA, VSD, or coarctation are common. Valve tissue is thick and rigid with diminished commissural separation of varying degrees, but leaflets are mobile in children. Most often the valve is bicuspid with a single, fused commissure and eccentrically placed orifice. The valve annulus may be hypoplastic (less than 4 to 5 mm). With severe stenosis, the LV develops concentric hypertrophy, decreased LV function, compromised myocardial blood flow, elevated LVEDP, and poststenotic dilation of the ascending aorta. Valvular gradients can give some estimation of the degree of stenosis. This number may be misleading in instances of low cardiac output, where output across the valve is already diminished and the gradient may be falsely low. Estimations of valvular gradients used to determine severity and guide interventional decisions are (1) mild: 5 to 49 mm Hg, (2) moderate: 50 to 75 mm Hg, and (3) severe: greater than 75 mm Hg. Subendocardial or endocardial fibroelastosis may occur in utero if the stenosis is severe and does not regress after repair. Therefore, despite adequate relief of the stenosis, LV function may be permanently compromised. Complications include endocarditis, sudden death, development of valvular insufficiency, and arrhythmias.
     - *Etiology and incidence:* Aortic stenosis occurs more frequently in boys and occurs in about 3% to 6% of congenital heart defects. It may be associated with nonimmunologic hydrops fetalis.

- *Assessment:* Most children are asymptomatic and grow and develop normally. If symptoms occur, they usually involve fatigue, exertional dyspnea, angina pectoris, and syncope with at least moderate aortic stenosis. Severe aortic stenosis has rapid symptoms of CHF and may even have the presentation of HLHS. Examination reveals LV lift, precordial systolic thrill, systolic aortic ejection murmur or ejection click, S_2 delayed or split S_3, and on occasion a diastolic murmur of aortic insufficiency.
- *Diagnostic findings*
  - *ECG* findings may vary with severity but usually include T-wave inversion, deep S wave in V_1, LV strain, LVH, and ST segment depression.
  - *Exercise testing* is used to evaluate BP response and ECG changes with exercise. A fall or a lack of rise in systolic BP suggests the presence of severe obstruction.
  - *Chest radiographic examination* demonstrates normal to minimal enlargement of heart size; rounding of the cardiac apex; LA enlargement if stenosis is severe; pulmonary congestion and enlargement of the PA, RV, and RA; and poststenotic dilation of the ascending aorta.
  - *ECHO* shows diminished systolic valve movement and demonstrates the anatomy of the valve leaflets, an increase in LV wall thickness, transvalvular aortic gradients, end-diastolic dimensions to predict LV peak systolic pressure, and associated cardiac anatomy.
  - *Cardiac catheterization* is more important to establish the site and severity of the stenosis, define associated anomalies, measure cardiac output, and assess valve gradients.
- *Interventions:* Congenital aortic stenosis is a progressive lesion, and most affected children require intervention at least once. The earlier the intervention, the greater the likelihood of further intervention. Intervention is recommended when severe symptoms or LV strain or syncope is present. Stabilization of the neonate with critical aortic stenosis requires prostaglandin therapy.
  - Interventional catheterization or balloon valvuloplasty is successful in opening the valve in most patients, and the results in neonates are similar to those of surgical valvotomy. Arterial access is a problem for the small neonate. Risks include inadequate relief of stenosis, creation of aortic insufficiency, perforation, and acute hemodynamic instability during catheterization.
  - Surgical valvuloplasty carries the same risks as balloon procedures; however, stabilization on cardiopulmonary bypass during the procedure allows time for the ventricle to rest and to resolve acidosis. It also provides a backup in the presence of malignant ventricular arrhythmias with valve manipulation (Figure 3-42).
  - For stenosis (initial or recurrent) in patients with limited annulus size, enlargement of the entire aortic root is required. The Konno procedure with aortic root replacement involves enlarging the LV outflow tract and aortic annulus and incorporating an aortic valve replacement. This is accomplished through a sternotomy on cardiopulmonary bypass (Figure 3-43). Risks of this operation include heart block, myocardial failure and low cardiac output, patch dehiscence of the ventricular patch used to enlarge the septum and aortic root, and perivalvular leak.
  - Some patients require valve replacement for progressive stenosis or insufficiency but have an adequate aortic annulus size. A decision regarding the best valve for that patient's age, lifestyle, sex, and anatomy

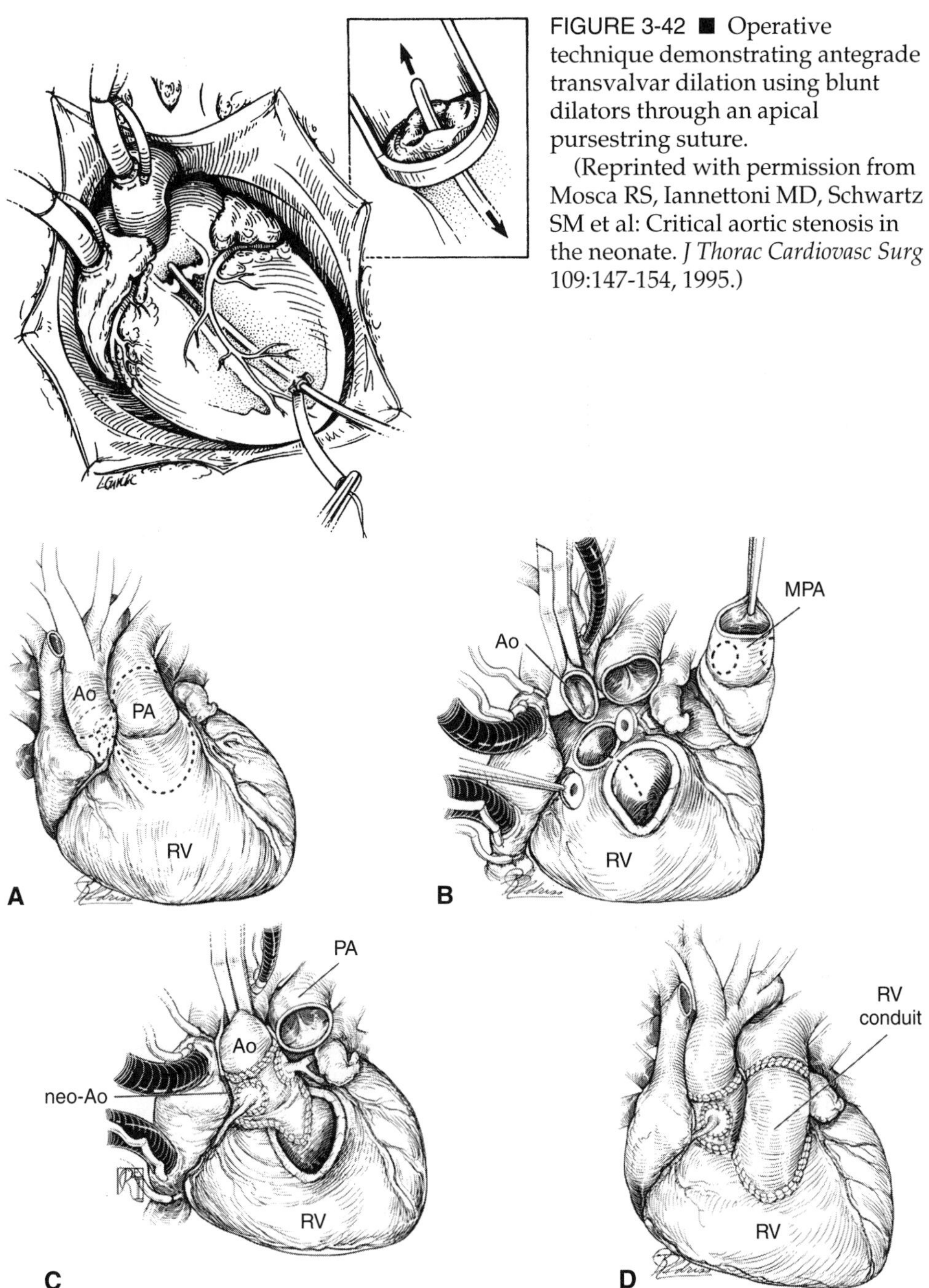

FIGURE 3-42 ■ Operative technique demonstrating antegrade transvalvar dilation using blunt dilators through an apical pursestring suture.

(Reprinted with permission from Mosca RS, Iannettoni MD, Schwartz SM et al: Critical aortic stenosis in the neonate. *J Thorac Cardiovasc Surg* 109:147-154, 1995.)

FIGURE 3-43 ■ **A,** Intended incision and excision boundaries en route to the Ross-Konno procedure. **B,** After aortic cross-clamping, antegrade and retrograde cardioplegic arrest, aortic resention, coronary mobilization, and main pulmonary artery harvest: the interventricular septal incision is noted by the *dotted line.* The pulmonary autograft was harvested, with an extra portion of right ventricle to be used for the ventriculoseptoplasty part of this operation. **C,** The neoaortic left ventricular outflow reconstruction is shown using the pulmonary autograft extension into the interventricular septum. **D,** The completed Ross-Konno procedure is shown after separation from cardiopulmonary bypass. *Ao,* Aorta, aortic; *MPA,* main pulmonary artery; *RV,* right ventricle.

(From Mavroudis C, Backer CL: *Pediatric cardiac surgery,* ed 3. St. Louis, 2003, Mosby.)

is made and replacement performed. In most circumstances these homografts or bioprosthetics require replacement within 5 to 10 years. Prosthetic valves may last 15 to 20 years or longer in older adolsescents or adults. In infants and younger children, the valve will likely require replacement within 5 years.

  - In patients with aortic and pulmonary roots of the same or similar size, a Ross procedure can be performed. This operation involves translocating the native pulmonary valve into the aortic root (autograft) and replacing the pulmonary valve with a homograft. The proposed benefit is that the autograft will grow and not require further replacement. Risks of this operation include bleeding, MI from coronary injury during excision of the pulmonary autograft, aortic regurgitation, and low cardiac output.
- Endocarditis is a lifelong risk.

b. *Discrete subaortic stenosis*
- *Pathophysiology:* Subaortic stenosis includes 8% to 10% of aortic stenosis and occurs more often in boys. It consists of a membranous diaphragm or fibrous ring encircling the LV outflow tract beneath the base of the aortic valve. Progressive aortic regurgitation is found and is an indication for surgery.
- *Assessment*
  - *Examination:* There may be a systolic ejection sound and a diastolic murmur of aortic insufficiency.
  - *ECHO* shows dilation of the aortic root. A fibromuscular ring produces thick echoes from a level near the annular attachment of the anterior mitral leaflet.
- *Intervention:* Surgery is performed through sternotomy on cardiopulmonary bypass. The obstructing membrane or ring is excised along with a small wedge of LV muscle (myomectomy). Myomectomy has been shown to reduce dramatically recurrence of the stenosis. Risks specific to this procedure include aortic insufficiency, mitral valve damage, heart block, and creation of a VSD.
- Endocarditis is a lifelong risk.

c. *Supravalvular aortic stenosis*
- *Pathophysiology:* Congenital narrowing of the ascending aorta may be localized or diffuse, hourglass shaped, membranous type, or hypoplastic type. Coronary arteries are subjected to elevated pressure and may be dilated; the lumin may be narrowed by a thick medial layer. The aortic lumen is constricted, and the distal flow is diminished. It is often associated with Williams syndrome (supravalvular aortic stenosis, PA stenosis, mental retardation, and hypercalcemia in infancy).
- *Assessment:*
  - *History* is similar to valvular aortic stenosis.
  - *Examination* reveals accentuation of aortic closure sound, prominent transmission of a thrill and murmur, narrowing of peripheral pulmonary arteries producing a continuous murmur, and higher BP in the right arm than in the left arm.
  - *ECG* reveals LVH and RVH if peripheral PA stenosis is present.
  - *Chest radiographic examination* rarely shows poststenotic dilation.
  - *Cardiac catheterization* localizes the site of obstruction and degree of hemodynamic alteration. A pressure gradient is found above the aortic valve. Coronary artery problems can be identified, as well as the presence and degree of PA involvement (peripheral pulmonary stenosis).

- *Intervention:* Via sternotomy and cardiopulmonary bypass, an incision is made into the aorta, and a patch is placed to enlarge the area (Figure 3-44). If there is diffuse hypoplasia of the aorta or accompanying PA hypoplasia, transfer of the gradients farther down the aorta or to the PA can occur. Relief of aortic stenosis with significant residual PA stenosis can create suprasystemic PA and RV pressures postoperatively.
- Endocarditis is a lifelong risk.

3. **Hypoplastic left heart syndrome (HLHS):** CHD characterized by various levels of underdevelopment of left heart structures. The left-sided valves may be small or atretic, the LV cavity nonexistent or hypoplastic, and the ascending aorta miniscule to well formed. In all cases of HLHS, the left-sided heart structures fail to form normally and are not large enough to function as systemic ventricles and valves.

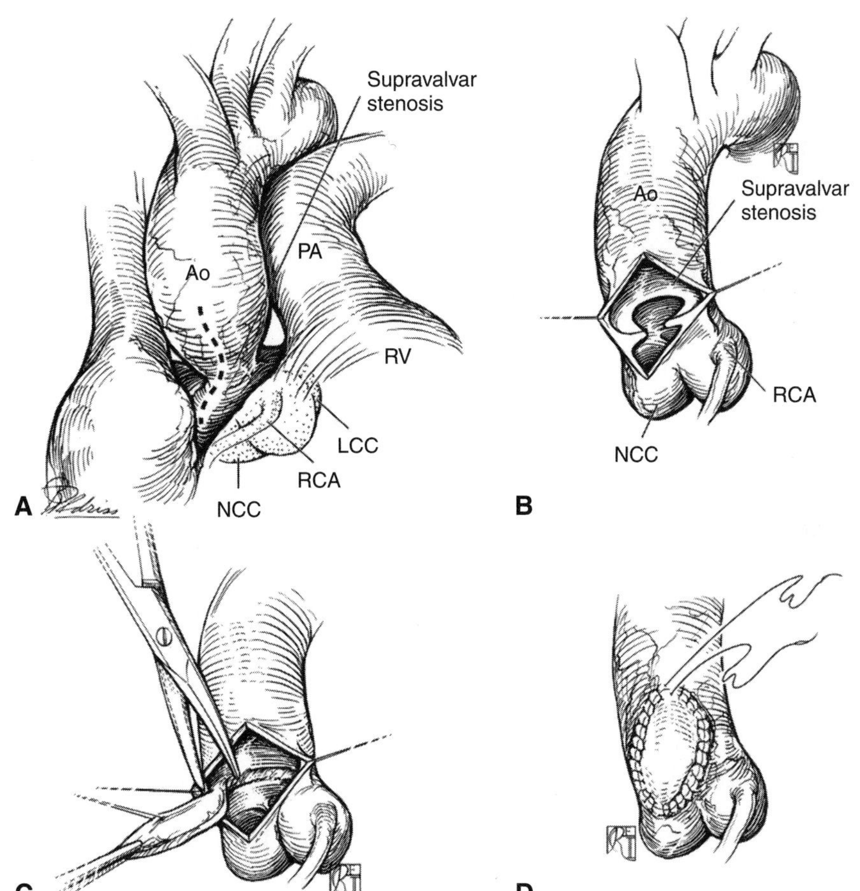

FIGURE 3-44 ■ **A,** Operative conditions showing the proposed incision for repair of supravalvar aortic stenosis by the one-patch technique. **B,** A long incision *(dotted line)* is made in the ascending aorta *(Ao),* which extends through the area of supravalvar stenosis into the noncoronary cusp *(NCC)* of the sinus of Valsalva. **C,** The supravalvar fibrous ring is shown being resected. Care is taken to avoid injury to the orifices of the involved coronary arteries. **D,** The single patch that has augmented the supravalvar area is shown. *LCC,* Left coronary cusp; PA, pulmonary artery; RCA, right coronary artery; RV, right ventricle.

(From Mavroudis C, Backer CL: *Pediatric cardiac surgery,* ed 3. St. Louis, 2003, Mosby.)

a. *Pathophysiology*

- Right-sided structures, the PA, coronary arteries, and lungs are normal, although the RA, RV, and PA may be dilated. Left-sided structures have variable levels of underdevelopment. Mitral valve atresia or stenosis occurs frequently. Aortic atresia or stenosis (annulus ≤5 mm) occurs. Stenotic valves have a small aortic root with leaflets that are thick, dysplastic, and obstructive. LV hypoplasia occurs in varying degrees (volume <20 mL/m^2). There is a non–apex-forming LV (Figure 3-45). The endocardium may be thick or sclerotic. The ascending aorta varies in size but is hypoplastic, usually to the level of the transverse arch (usually 2 to 3 mm). Coarctation is present in 80% of patients.
- Associated lesions are not common with classic HLHS but may include AVSD, TGV, and univentricular heart. A PDA and ASD are essential for survival and are considered part of the complex. Occasionally the ASD is small or restrictive and the newborn presents with obstructed TAPVR.
- Systemic venous blood returns normally to the RA and flows normally out the right side of the heart. Pulmonary venous blood flows across the ASD to the RA because it cannot exit the left side of the heart if mitral atresia is present. Mixing in the RA desaturates the blood. All blood flows across the tricuspid valve to the RV and to the PA. If mitral or aortic stenosis is present, a small amount of forward flow out the LV may occur but not enough to support the cardiac output. Blood flows right to left across the PDA to supply systemic blood flow distally and flows proximally to feed the coronary arteries.

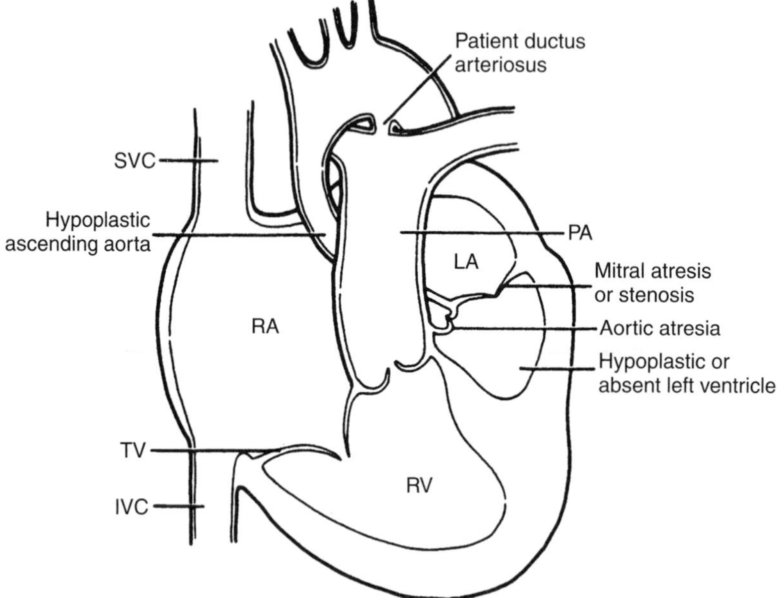

FIGURE 3-45 ■ Hypoplastic left heart syndrome. *IVC,* Inferior vena cava; *LA,* left atrium; *PA,* pulmonary artery; *RA,* right atrium; *RV,* right ventricle; *SVC,* superior vena cava; *TV,* tricuspid valve.

(Reprinted with permission from Callow LB: Current strategies in the nursing care of infants with hypoplastic left-heart syndrome undergoing first-stage palliation with the Norwood operation, *Heart Lung* 20:463-470, 1992.)

b. *Etiology and incidence:* HLHS occurs in 7% of CHD cases or in 0.163/1000 live births. Research suggests an autosomal-recessive transmission. Recurrence risk in siblings is 0.5%; HLHS is more common in boys, and 10% of infants with HLHS have associated extracardiac malformations.

c. *Assessment*

- *History:* Cyanosis is rare at birth; however, as normal involution of the PDA occurs, systemic perfusion is compromised. Symptoms of CHF become evident and, if unrecognized, will progress to vascular collapse. Tachypnea, dyspnea, grunting, cool and poorly perfused extremities, lethargy, and pallor or gray color will be noted.
- *Examination* reveals auscultation of crisp, loud heart sounds; a single S_2; a pulmonary ejection click and an S_3; an enlarged liver; a left precordial bulge; a soft systolic ejection murmur; and variable femoral pulses. There may be no gradient with low cardiac output or an open PDA.

d. *Diagnostic findings*

- *ECG* demonstrates sinus tachycardia, peaked P waves, RA enlargement, RVH, and lack of LV forces and may show ST-T wave changes.
- *Chest radiographic examination:* Levocardia, an enlarged, globular-shaped heart, and variable pulmonary vascular markings (severe pulmonary edema and increased markings if ASD is restrictive) are present.
- *ECHO* is a valuable diagnostic tool that defines all anatomic variants of HLHS: the RV and PA are enlarged; mitral valve leaflets are not visualized; the LV cavity is hypoplastic; the LV is nonapex forming; the aortic root is 5 mm or smaller; and hypoplasia of the aortic arch is present. Anatomy and function of the tricuspid valve are evaluated.
- *Cardiac catheterization* is not required initially unless there is an extreme anatomic variant. It will demonstrate an obligatory left-to-right atrial shunt with increased oxygen saturation in the RA, RV, and PA; aortic saturation equal to PA saturation; RV pressures elevated and equal to or in excess of systemic arterial pressure; PCWP and LA and RA pressures equal except in the presence of obstructive ASD, in which PCWP and LA pressure are greater than RA pressure.

e. *Interventions*

- Ductal patency is maintained while the diagnosis is confirmed and decisions are made for interventions. Treatment options include transplantation (requires maintenance with prostaglandin therapy until a donor is found) or staged surgical reconstruction. Compassionate care (death occurs within 1 week in 95% of cases) is rarely offered but may be considered specifically in certain variations of HLHS or infants with severely obstructed pulmonary veins or ASDs.
- Preoperative stabilization: Balance is maintained between systemic and pulmonary blood flow by manipulating SVR and PVR. If the patient is cyanotic with low pulmonary blood flow, interventions include ensuring patency of the ASD and PDA, hyperventilation, hyperoxygenation, and relief of pulmonary congestion. Pulmonary vasoconstriction and systemic vasodilation are avoided to balance the two circulations, and the hematocrit is maintained at a level between 40 and 55 mL/dL. Pulmonary over-circulation can result in poor cardiac output (hypotension, acidosis) with good oxygenation (PaO_2 usually greater than 45 mm Hg). Nitrogen administration with FiO_2 less than 21% can help to maintain mild metabolic acidosis (pH 7.35) and pulmonary vasoconstriction in the infant with too much pulmonary blood flow. Cardiac output is maintained with

medications and volume. Adequate organ function should be present before surgical intervention.

- *First-stage palliative reconstructive surgery with the Norwood operation* creates an unobstructed RV outflow tract to prevent ventricular hypertrophy and dysfunction and provide good coronary artery flow (Figure 3-46). Pulmonary blood flow is controlled to prevent PVOD via use of a nondistorting shunt to allow growth of the central main PA. A large ASD (atrial septectomy) is created to allow mixing of venous blood return at the atrial level and LA decompression and to avoid elevated PA pressure or PVR. The Norwood operation is aimed at maintaining anatomic and physiologic criteria for an eventual Fontan procedure. The Norwood operation is done via sternotomy with cardiopulmonary bypass. The aortic arch and RV outflow tract are reconstructed using the proximal PA and aorta and homograft augmentation. The incision is carried 10 mm past the insertion of the PDA to ensure that ductal tissue is excised and to reduce or eliminate the risk of postoperative coarctation formation. Careful reconstruction of the proximal PA-aortic anastomosis is completed to avoid torsion and

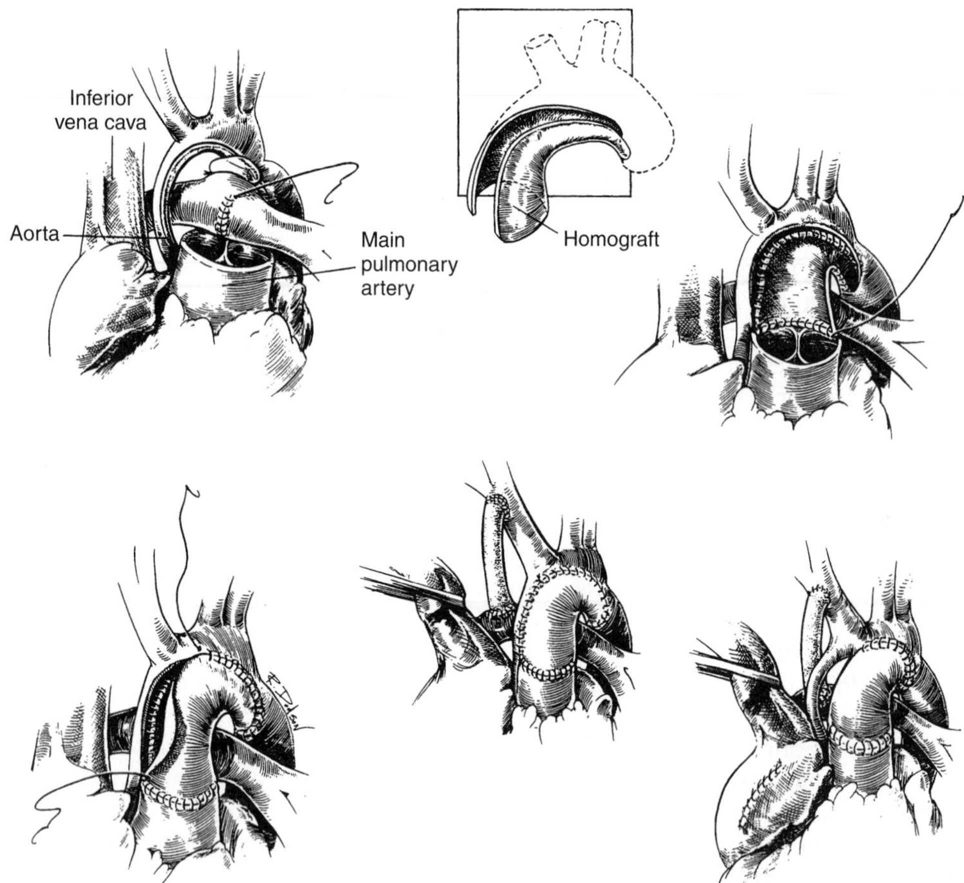

FIGURE 3-46 ■ Surgical reconstruction in hypoplastic left heart syndrome.
Using a homograft patch, the aorta is reconstructed and a systemic-to-pulmonary shunt provides pulmonary flow to the now transected pulmonary artery.
(Reprinted with permission from Castaneda AR, Jonas RA, Mayer JE, Hanley FL: *Cardiac surgery of the neonate and infant*. Philadelphia, 1994, W. B. Saunders.)

obstruction to coronary artery flow. Pulmonary blood flow is created by a systemic-to-pulmonary Gore-tex shunt. An RV to PA conduit may be utilized to supply pulmonary blood flow. The *Sano operation* is believed to increase diastolic BP by eliminating runoff into the PA from the aorta. This would increase coronary artery perfusion and decrease the risk of ischemia to the ventricle. This is considered especially helpful in small or preterm infants and in those with exceptionally small ascending aortas. Manipulation of systemic and pulmonary resistance has questionable effect on pulmonary blood flow in these circumstances. Long-term concerns with this type of conduit include the long-term effects of a ventriculotomy on a single systemic ventricle and the incidence of sudden occlusion and growth of the central and peripheral PAs. Postoperative complications include an unbalanced flow between systemic and pulmonary circulations or severe cardiovascular collapse. The inability to maintain balanced circulation or preoperative obstructed atrial septum may require ECMO for cardiac or pulmonary healing (see Extracorporeal Life Support [ECLS]/Extracorporeal Membrane Oxygenation [ECMO]). The shunt may be occluded temporarily to permit adequate circulation on ECMO. Problems with temporary and reversible elevated PVR and severe hypoxemia may be managed by inhalation of nitric oxide. Low cardiac output may respond to reduction of inhaled oxygen to 21% or subatmospheric oxygen reducing pulmonary blood flow and increasing systemic blood flow. Desired oxygen saturations vary between 70% and 80%, depending on the patient's hemodynamic state. Measurement of Svo_2 and calculation of shunt fractions (Q_p:Q_s) can assist in the manipulation of PVR or SVR. Coupling the Svo_2 with serum lactates provides early warning of inadequate cardiac output and the need for treatment of PVR and SVR based on Svo_2 and shunt fractions.

- *Second-stage palliation: Bidirectional cavopulmonary shunt or hemi-Fontan (3 to 6 months after initial palliation):* Full hemodynamic and anatomic catheterization to assess the size and architecture of the pulmonary arteries, PA pressure, pulmonary blood flow, and RV function is necessary before cavopulmonary shunt (Figure 3-47). The purpose of the cavopulmonary shunt is to provide venous blood flow to the lungs and a stable form of oxygenation, remove volume overload from the RV, protect the RV from hypertrophy, and preserve long-term function. It is performed via sternotomy on cardiopulmonary bypass and may require hypothermic circulatory arrest. If necessary, PA stent or arterioplasty is performed to ensure unobstructed pulmonary blood flow to permit passive flow without excessively high SVC pressures. The pulmonary arteries are repaired as necessary. The SVC is connected end to side with the right or main PA, and flow goes passively from the SVC to the right and left pulmonary arteries by pressure gradient. A bulging fontanelle; high SVC pressure; irritability; low saturations; and edema of the face, neck, and upper extremities (SVC syndrome) are signs of high venous pressure. PVR is optimized, and early heparin use with conversion to aspirin later may prevent PA clots. Any alteration in PVR will affect pulmonary blood flow because there is no ventricular pump to overcome this added resistance. Effusions are treated, diuretics are used to reduce volume overload and improve pulmonary mechanics, and appropriate ventilatory support is given. MAP is maintained in a lower range. Early extubation permits physiologic negative pressure, and spontaneous respiration may reduce MAP. Hematocrit should be maintained greater than or equal to 40%. IVC blood still flows

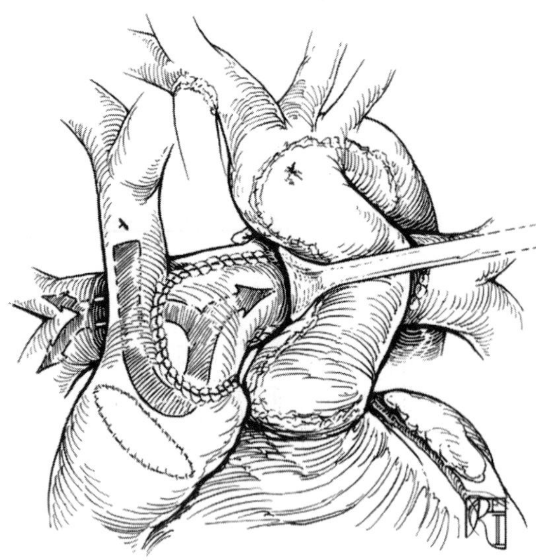

FIGURE 3-47 ■ The completed hemi-Fontan repair.

A polytetrafluorethylene patch is in place to prevent the superior vena caval return from entering the right atrium.

(From Mavroudis C, Backer CL: *Pediatric cardiac surgery*, ed 3. St. Louis, 2003, Mosby.)

through the RV, so complete unloading of the RV volume overload is not accomplished, and mixing of oxygenated and unoxygenated blood occurs with expected saturations of 80% to 85%.

- *Final-stage physiologic palliation: Fontan procedure (also done for tricuspid atresia or single-ventricle hearts of diagnostic categories other than HLHS):* Recommended age is less than or equal to 4 years at operation to prevent ventricular hypertrophy and dysfunction from volume overload and to optimize long-term ventricular function. Full hemodynamic and anatomic catheterization is required before performance of a Fontan procedure to assess for suitability. Criteria for adequate outcomes include good branch PA architecture without stenosis and normal PA pressure, PVR, and ventricular function. Relative criteria include competent AV valve and normal sinus rhythm. The operation is done via sternotomy on cardiopulmonary bypass, possibly with circulatory arrest (Figure 3-48). The systemic venous return is directed to the PA. A lateral tunnel with a 3- to 4-mm fenestration is sewn inside the RA directing IVC flow to the PA. An external IVC-PA conduit is used for systemic or pulmonary venous anatomic aberrations prohibiting previous connections. The goal is to achieve passive flow from the systemic veins to the lungs based on the pressure gradient from the SVC or IVC, to the main PA, to the left and right pulmonary arteries, and to the lungs. Relief of any PA stenosis via arterioplasty or stent placement, or both, is mandatory to prevent a fixed elevation in PVR. Relief of significant AV valve regurgitation is necessary to prevent elevations in atrial pressure transmitted to the lungs.
- Postoperative care may be complicated by ventricular dysfunction, arrhythmias, elevated PVR, and excessive cyanosis from a baffle leak. Observation of the RA-LA gradient may demonstrate a widening gradient with RA hypertension from increased PVR or a narrow gradient but high LA pressure that may signify LV dysfunction. Ideally the RA pressure will be less than 15 mm Hg, with transpulmonary gradient not greater than 10. Ventilation should be optimized with low MAP, and extubation should occur as early as possible. Late complications include thromboembolic events, rhythm disturbances, protein-losing enteropathy, aortopulmonary

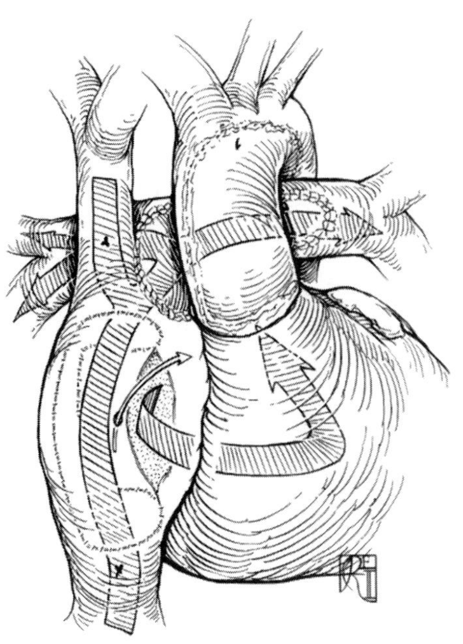

FIGURE 3-48 ■ The completed Fontan procedure showing the systemic venous return from the superior and inferior venae cavae directed to the pulmonary artery.
(From Mavroudis C, Backer CL: *Pediatric cardiac surgery*, ed 3. St. Louis, 2003, Mosby.)

collaterals, pathway obstruction, AV valve regurgitation, and ventricular dysfunction. Neurologic outcomes are encouraging. Resting cardiac output is normal, although at maximal exercise it may be limited. Atrial arrhythmias, primarily sick sinus syndrome and atrial fibrillation or flutter, can occur. Recurrent pleural effusions, hepatic congestion, protein-losing enteropathy, and exercise intolerance may develop. Long-term ventricular failure requires transplantation. Many Fontan procedures are now fenestrated (controlled hole in intra-atrial baffle allowing right-to-left shunting when systemic venous pressures are excessively high). This is believed to decrease the risk to marginal candidates, maintain cardiac output and volume load in the ventricle, and ease transition to passive flow. The right-to-left shunt and cyanosis continue until the fenestration is closed. If performed, fenestration closure is done weeks to months after the initial operation. Initially there is a decrease in cardiac output despite normalization of oxygen saturation in patients with fenestration closure.

- Endocarditis is a lifelong risk.

4. **Coarctation of the aorta:** Narrowing of the aorta causing elevation of pressure proximally and decreased pressure distally
   a. *Pathophysiology:* Classification of coarctation is based on the presence or absence of severe isthmus narrowing and major associated lesions. It is associated frequently with PDA, VSD, aortic stenosis, aortic insufficiency, bicuspid aortic valve, mitral and tricuspid valve anomalies, and DiGeorge syndrome (usually with interrupted arch). Constriction of the aorta occurs most often at the junction of the ductus and aorta just distal to the left subclavian artery–juxtaductal coarctation. The most severe form of coarctation is the interrupted aortic arch, which is a congenital absence of a portion of the aorta. The types of aortic interruption are based on location. ***Type A*** is distal to the left subclavian artery (42%); ***type B*** is distal to the left common carotid artery (53%); and ***type C*** is between the right and left common carotid arteries (4%) (Figure 3-49). Evaluation of coarctation is an ongoing process because the obstruction can worsen over time, resulting in

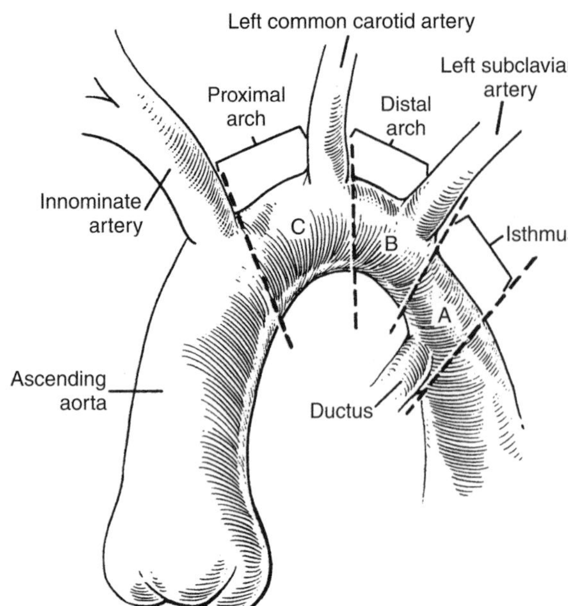

FIGURE 3-49 ■ Depiction of aortic arch in three segments: proximal arch, distal arch, and isthmus. *Ductus,* ductus arteriosus.

(Reprinted with permission from Castaneda AR, Jonas RA, Mayer JE, Hanley FL: *Cardiac surgery of the neonate and infant.* Philadelphia, 1994, W. B. Saunders.)

increased upper-extremity hypertension. Blood exits the LV normally but has varying degrees of difficulty crossing the obstruction. This results in LV hypertension and hypertrophy. In some cases blood cannot cross the constriction. In this case the infant is dependent on right-to-left shunting across the ductus to perfuse the distal aorta and body. As the child grows older, significant aortic collaterals may form to perfuse the aorta distal to the coarctation. Complications of LV failure, long-standing systemic hypertension, stroke, and endocarditis are risks of unrepaired disease.

b. *Etiology and incidence:* Local-area intimal thickening and distortion are found distal to the contraductal shelf. Coarctation occurs in about 8%-10% of CHD and is more common in males.

c. *Assessment*

- *History* depends on the degree of constriction. Neonates with severe obstruction present with severe CHF and cardiovascular collapse and require prostaglandin to maintain ductal patency and reestablish systemic flow until surgical correction. Older children rarely have symptoms but may complain of cramps or pain in calves with exercise.
- *Examination* of the infant reveals a heaving precordium, equally diminished pulses if the ductus is open, and a nonspecific systolic murmur at the LSB. In the child, a BP differential between the upper and lower extremities, systemic hypertension, a short systolic ejection murmur at the LSB, and a continuous murmur if collaterals are present occur.

d. *Diagnostic findings* in the infant and child include the following:

- *ECG:* RVH and LV strain in the infant; increased LV forces and strain in the child.
- *ECHO* defines anatomy, LV function, and associated lesions.
- *Chest radiographic examination* demonstrates cardiomegaly and possibly increased pulmonary vascular markings in the infant; normal heart size, LV prominence, rib notching, and a prominent descending aorta in the child.
- *Cardiac catheterization* determines associated lesions, anatomy of coarctation, gradient across the coarctation unless there is low cardiac

output or a PDA, and descending aortic saturation less than the ascending aortic saturation (from right-to-left shunting at the ductal level).

e. *Intervention:* Interventions depend on age, degree of constriction, ductal dependency, and associated lesions. In the neonate, initial stabilization on prostaglandin and correction of any end-organ failure at diagnostic presentation is required. Medical management is not indicated long term. Short-term stabilization of CHF may be necessary.

- Interventional cardiac catheterization is done primarily for older children or residual coarctation after repair (Figure 3-50). Risks include aneurysm, recurrent coarctation, difficult access in small infants, and inadequate relief. Reduction of collateral vessels following relief of the coarctation by balloon dilation may make operative intervention more hazardous if recoarctation occurs. There is increased risk of paraplegia from low perfusion pressure distal to the aortic cross-clamp during surgery when collateral flow is diminished. Cardiopulmonary bypass may be used to prevent this complication.
- Surgical repair is accomplished via left thoracotomy with one of several methods. Subclavian flap angioplasty, end-to-end anastomosis following resection of the coarcted segment (Figure 3-51), patch aortoplasty (Figure 3-52), and interposition graft are surgical options used. Sternotomy and bypass are

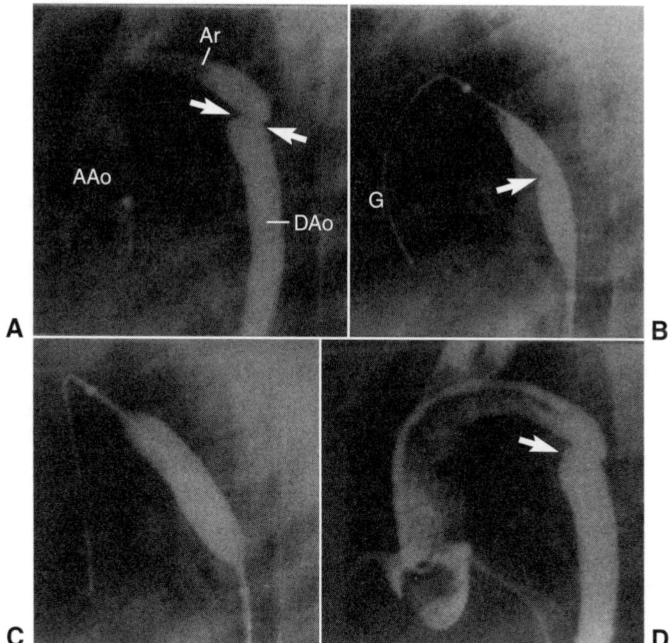

FIGURE 3-50 ■ Balloon angioplasty of recoarctation after surgical repair with subclavian flap. **A,** Predilation aortogram demonstrating the narrowed recoarcted segment *(arrows)*. **B,** Initial balloon inflation with creation of waist from obstructive shelf. **C,** Upon full inflation, the waist is relieved. **D,** Postangioplasty aortogram shows successful dilation of recoarcted segment. Note the irregularity of vessel wall in the dilated area *(arrow)*. *AAo,* Ascending aorta; *Ar,* aortic arch; *G,* guidewire; *Dao,* descending aorta.

(From Zales, VR, Muster AJ: Balloon dilation angioplasty for the management of aortic coarctation. In Mavroudis C, Backer CL, editors: *Cardiac surgery: state of the art reviews, vol* 7. Philadelphia, 1993, Hanley & Belfus, p. 133.)

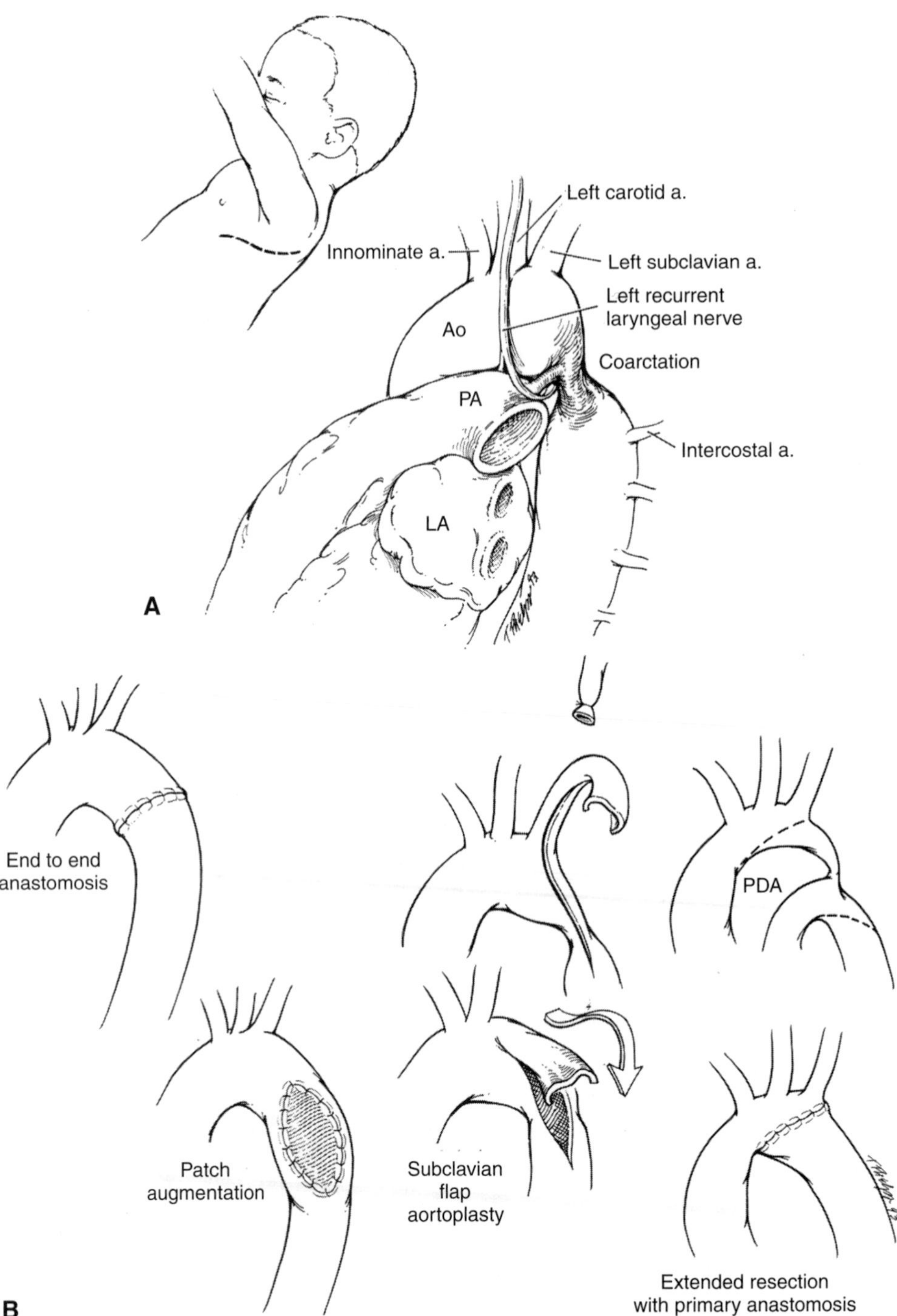

FIGURE 3-51 ■ Surgical approach to coarctation of the aorta *(CoA).* **A,** Placement of a typical surgical incision and surgical anatomy. **B,** Four operative procedures commonly used in repair of CoA; resection of the stenotic segment and end-to-end aortic anastomosis, patch augmentation, subclavian flap aortoplasty, and extended resection with primary anastomosis. *Ao,* Aorta; *PA,* pulmonary artery; *LA,* left atrium; *a.,* artery; *PDA,* patent ductua arteriosus.

(From Nichols DG: *Critical heart disease in infants and children.* St. Louis, 1999, Mosby.)

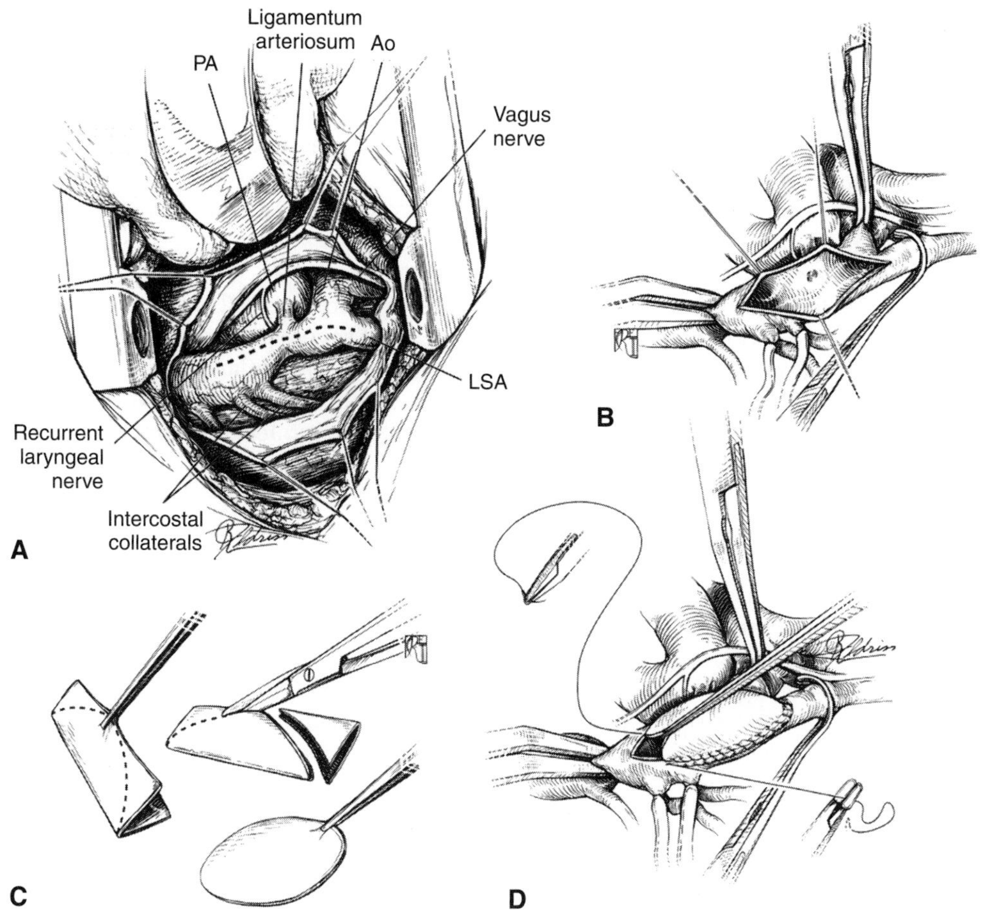

FIGURE 3-52 ■ Patch aortoplasty. **A,** Exposure of the coarctation through a left thoracotomy. Note juxtaductal coarctation and enlarged intercostal collateral arteries. **B,** Clamps have been applied and the aorta opened laterally opposite the site of the ligamentum. Note that intercostal arteries are controlled with small Rumel tourniquets. The coarctation ridge is *not* excised. **C,** An elliptical polytetrafluoroethylene *(PTFE)* patch is fashioned before clamp placement. **D,** The patch is sutured in place so that the PTFE creates a "roof" over the coarctation ridge. *Ao,* Aorta; *LSA,* left subclavian artery; *PA,* pulmonary artery.
(From Mavroudis C, Backer CL: *Pediatric cardiac surgery,* ed 3. St. Louis, 2003, Mosby.)

used if complete arch reconstruction is required or associated lesions are to be repaired (i.e., VSD, subaortic stenosis). Specific postoperative complications include paradoxical hypertension, mesenteric arteritis (feed slowly, await return of bowel sounds), and paralysis (bypass is used if distal aortic pressure is less than 40 mm Hg).

5. **Mitral valve disease or mitral stenosis:** Obstruction of pulmonary venous blood flow from the left atrium to the LV.
   a. *Pathophysiology:* Mitral stenosis is classified by the component of mitral valve that is abnormal. Abnormalities include thick, rolled leaflet margins, abnormal chordae tendineae, papillary muscle hypoplasia, LV endocardial sclerosis, hypoplasia or atresia of the mitral valve, commissure fusion, excessive tissue, parachute mitral valve, or supramitral ring. Left atrial, pulmonary venous, and pulmonary capillary wedge pressures increase relative to resistance to flow

across the mitral valve into the LV. Eventually, mitral stenosis may cause PA hypertension, elevated PVR, and RV dysfunction from PVOD. LV volume load decreases, causing ischemia, fibrosis, and further LV dysfunction and decreased cardiac output.

b. *Etiology:* Mitral stenosis is a variable expression of developmental abnormality involving the LV. Excessive or abnormal deposition of tissue occurs embryologically. Deficiency or excess of endocardial cushion tissue is related.

c. *Assessment*
   - *History:* Timing and type of symptoms of mitral stenosis are based on the degree of obstruction to LV inflow. The most severe presentation (related to ductal closure with systemic hypoperfusion) is similar to the history of HLHS. A history of frequent pulmonary infections, poor weight gain, irritability, tiring with feeding, diaphoresis, tachypnea, chronic cough, and increased work of breathing are noted.
   - *Examination* reveals an active RV impulse with PA hypertension, soft S_1, split S_2, possible S_3 or S_4, and a low-frequency middiastolic murmur at the apex.

d. *Diagnostic findings*
   - *ECG:* LA and RA enlargement or RVH suggest PA hypertension and severe mitral stenosis. Diminished LV forces are noted.
   - *Chest radiographic examination* demonstrates LA enlargement, prominence of pulmonary vascular markings, and right-sided enlargement.
   - *Echocardiogram* shows decreased mitral valve opening, abnormal posterior leaflet motion, LA enlargement, reduced aortic wall motion, and diminished LV dimensions. It defines abnormalities of chordae tendineae and papillary muscles and estimates transvalvular gradients, ASD size, and changes in pulmonary vein inflow patterns.
   - *Cardiac catheterization* reveals mild systemic desaturation and hypoxemia, left-to-right atrial shunt with severe mitral stenosis, elevation of PA pressure, PVR, PCWP, and LA pressure; a diastolic pressure gradient from the LA pressure to the LVEDP; and a transpulmonary gradient if PVOD has developed.

e. *Interventions:* CHF is medically managed. Surgical intervention is considered for elevated PAP and PVR. The success of the operation is related to mitral valve and annulus size, LV size, PVR, PA pressure, and age. Older patients have better results if no PVOD is present. The mitral valve orifice must be opened to allow adequate LV inflow and pulmonary vein drainage. Commissurotomy is done via sternotomy and bypass with excision of excess tissue and membranes. Mitral valve replacement is difficult in infants with small annulus size. Postoperative care is directed at PA hypertension, low cardiac output, arrhythmias, and conduction disturbances.

6. **Congenital mitral insufficiency:** Failure of the valve leaflets to coapt normally, which allows regurgitation of blood into the pulmonary veins

   a. *Pathophysiology:* Congenital mitral insufficiency is associated with or secondary to other cardiac disease, such as single ventricle, AVSD, cardiomyopathy, Kawasaki syndrome, connective tissue disorders, metabolic disorder, and mucocutaneous lymph node disease. Classically, there is mitral valve prolapse. Failure of the valve leaflets to coapt normally allows regurgitation of LV volume into the left atrium and, depending on the severity of mitral valve incompetence, into the pulmonary veins, causing PA hypertension and elevated PVR over time.

b. *Etiology and incidence:* Congenital mitral insufficiency is rare and usually is associated with other defects. As with congenital mitral stenosis, consider an isolated cleft in the mitral valve.

c. *Assessment*

- *History* depends on the severity of insufficiency as with mitral stenosis (see Mitral Stenosis).
- *Examination* reveals diffuse apical impulse, active precordium, soft S_1, S_3, split S_2 in the presence of PA hypertension, high-frequency blowing or harsh holosystolic murmur at the apex, and a low-frequency apical diastolic murmur.

d. *Diagnostic findings*

- *ECG* shows LA enlargement and LVH.
- *Chest radiographic examination* shows an enlarged heart with LA and LV enlargement, increased pulmonary vascular markings, and congestion.
- *ECHO* demonstrates an abnormal valve anatomy, increased LA and LV dimensions, normal to increased LV systolic indexes, insufficiency or overlapping of anterior and posterior leaflets, a break in leaflet echo suggesting a cleft, and regurgitant flow into the LA and pulmonary veins if insufficiency is severe.
- *Cardiac catheterization* reveals elevated PCWP, PA pressure, PVR, LA pressure, LVEDP, LA opacification to a varying degree with LV injection, and a deceptively normal LV ejection fraction because of the ability to eject retrograde to low-pressure atrium.

e. *Interventions:* Treatment may be medical if the child is not in severe CHF. The child must be watched closely for signs of PA hypertension and the development of PVOD. Afterload reduction and diuretics (see Pharmacology) may be used cautiously. Surgical intervention is required in the presence of severe CHF, ventilator dependency or PA hypertension, and vascular changes. Valvuloplasty may be difficult if there is deficient valvular tissue. Prosthetic rings may be used. Cleft or elongated chordae tendineae are repaired. Mitral valve replacement is used as a last resort. Relief of mitral insufficiency producing a competent mitral valve may unmask LV dysfunction.

7. Valvular pulmonary stenosis (valvular PS): Narrowed pulmonary valve causing obstruction to flow from the right ventricle to the pulmonary artery, resulting in RVH (Figure 3-53)

a. *Pathophysiology:* The pulmonary valve is conical or dome-shaped and is formed by fusion of valve leaflets. It may be bicuspid (20% of cases). Thickened and immobile leaflets provide obstruction to RV outflow. The endocardium of the infundibulum may be thick and endocardial fibroelastosis may develop. In severe cases there is tricuspid valve regurgitation and RA dilation. If an ASD or patent foramen ovale is present, right-to-left shunting can occur, resulting in cyanosis of varying degrees. If pulmonary stenosis is severe and significant right-to-left atrial shunting occurs across the ASD, the RV and pulmonary valve may be hypoplastic. Grading of PS severity is based on transvalvular gradients of (1) mild, 25 to 49 mm Hg; (2) moderate, 50 to 75 mm Hg; and (3) severe, greater than 75 mm Hg.

b. *Etiology and incidence:* Pulmonary stenosis results from an embryologic error in the formation of pulmonary leaflets. It occurs in 25% to 30% of children with CHD. Dysplastic pulmonary valve is common in association with Noonan syndrome.

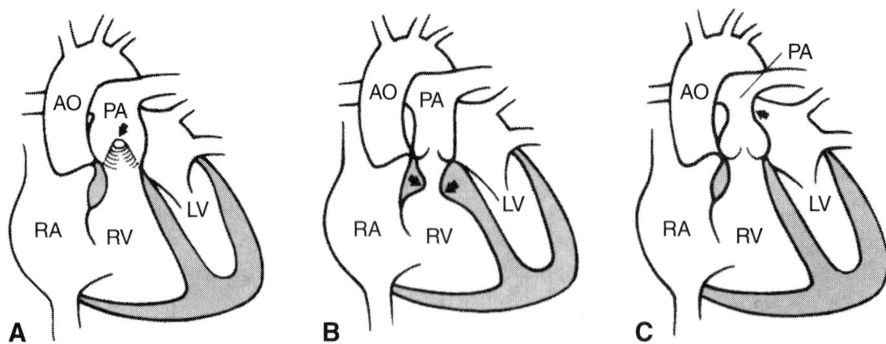

FIGURE 3-53 ■ Anatomic types of pulmonary stenosis *(PS)*. **A,** Valvular stenosis. **B,** Infundibular stenosis. **C,** Supravalvular pulmonary stenosis (or stenosis of the main pulmonary artery [PA]). Abnormalities are indicated by *arrows*. *AO,* aorta; *LV,* left ventricle; *RA,* right atrium; *RV,* right ventricle.
(From Park MK: *Pediatric cardiology for practitioners,* ed 4. St. Louis, 2002, Mosby.)

c. *Assessment*
- *History* may vary from an asymptomatic presentation to mild exertional dyspnea and cyanosis to severe CHF, depending on the degree of pulmonary stenosis. Dyspnea and fatigue with exercise are the most common complaints at first; as stenosis progresses, they occur even at rest. Growth and development are usually normal. The presence of cyanosis from right-to-left atrial shunting indicates moderate pulmonary stenosis.
- *Examination* reveals a normal S_1, pulmonary ejection click, and a diastolic ejection murmur (shorter in milder pulmonary stenosis, longer in severe pulmonary stenosis). The holosystolic murmur of tricuspid insufficiency and soft or absent S_2 are characteristic of severe pulmonary stenosis. In the newborn with severe pulmonary stenosis, S_2 is almost always single.

d. *Diagnostic findings*
- *ECG* is useful to assess the severity of pulmonary stenosis. In mild stenosis, normal RV forces are present. Severe RVH and RA enlargement are present in severe stenosis.
- *Chest radiographic examination* demonstrates a prominent main PA segment, RVH and downward apex, and cardiomegaly in severe pulmonary stenosis only (usually only mild enlargement).
- *ECHO* determines function and anatomy of the pulmonary valve and associated lesions, septal and RVH, prominent valve with restricted systolic motion, poststenotic dilation of the PA, and size of the tricuspid valve and RV (small only in severe pulmonary stenosis). It is also used to quantify the PVR and valve gradient.
- *Cardiac catheterization* is not required for diagnosis, but it excludes other diagnoses or is used to perform interventional therapy. RV pressure is elevated. The valve area and gradient and anatomy are defined. Oxygen saturations are usually normal. Cardiac output is quantified to use in determining the accuracy of the valve gradient.

e. *Interventions:* Intervention is required for moderate or greater pulmonary stenosis. Balloon valvuloplasty is the currently accepted treatment and provides excellent short-term and long-term results. The balloon catheter is inserted across the pulmonary valve and inflated to a size 10% to 20% greater than the annulus (Figure 3-54). Valvuloplasty is not as effective for dysplastic

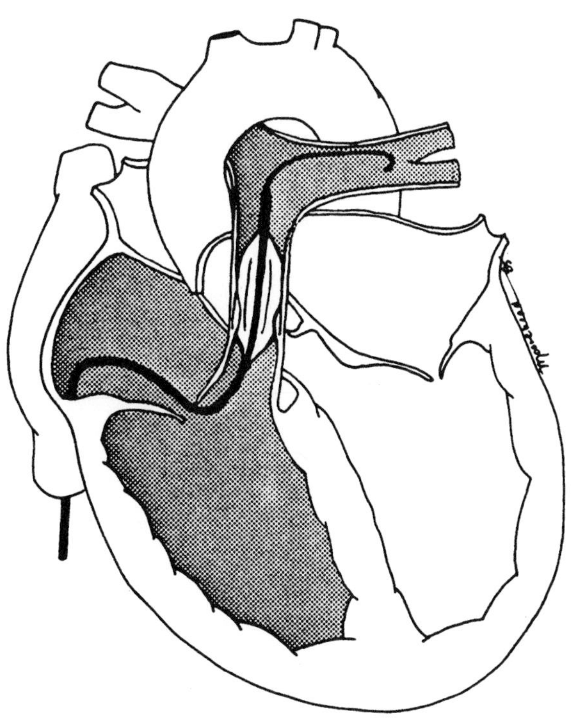

FIGURE 3-54 ■ Illustration of balloon valvuloplasty catheter positioned across the pulmonary valve.

(Reprinted with permission from Adams FH, Emmanoulides GC, Riemenschneider TA: *Moss' heart disease in infants, children, and adolescents,* ed 4. Baltimore, 1989, Williams & Wilkins.)

valves and neonates with critical pulmonary stenosis, although results in this group are improving. Risks include RV perforation, residual stenosis, and creation of insufficiency. Surgical valvotomy (Figure 3-55) may be done in cases where the catheter cannot pass through the pulmonary valve or when associated lesions require surgery. Progressive dilators are inserted through the pulmonary valve via incision in the PA to 1 cm greater than the valve annulus. Surgery requires sternotomy and a short period of cardiopulmonary bypass. Risks include RV failure, creation of pulmonary insufficiency, and inadequate relief of pulmonary stenosis.

f. *Endocarditis* is a lifelong risk.

F. Cyanotic Physiology

1. Expected outcomes

a. The patient or a family member will state activity limitations of disease.

b. The patient or a family member will state signs and symptoms of CHF.

c. The patient or a family member will state actions, side effects, and complications of medications.

d. The patient or a family member will state need for lifelong cardiovascular follow-up and endocarditis prophylaxis.

e. Hematocrit will be greater than 40%, and oxygen saturation will be greater than 70%.

f. The patient's growth and development will be optimized.

g. Arrhythmia or conduction disorders will be absent or controlled by medications or pacemaker.

h. Stenosis or obstruction of prosthetic material will be detected before ventricular dysfunction occurs or PVOD develops.

i. The patient or a family member will state need for staged operative intervention and repeated catheterization.

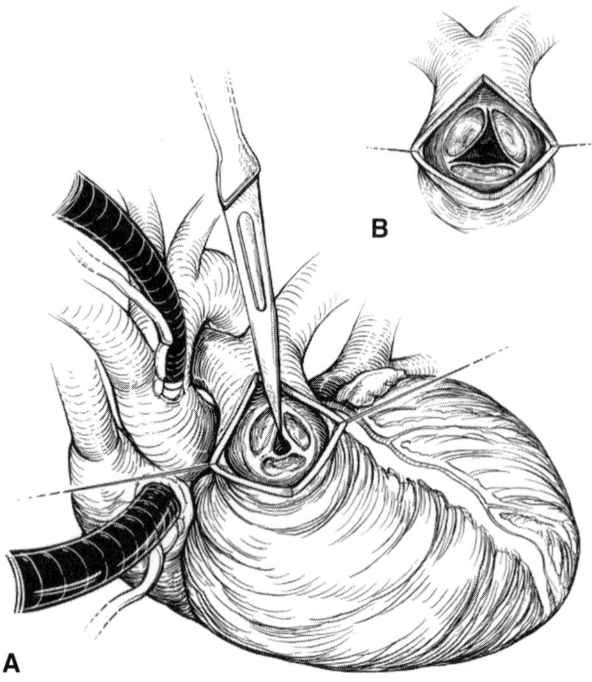

FIGURE 3-55 ■ Technique of pulmonary valvulotomy. **A,** Fused leaflet commissures are incised to the PA wall. **B,** Completed valvulotomy.
(From Mavroudis C, Backer CL: *Pediatric cardiac surgery,* ed 3. St. Louis, 2003, Mosby.)

j. Caloric intake, including nasogastric supplementation, will be maximized for growth.
k. Hemodynamic parameters will be normal for age and sex.

2. **Tetralogy of Fallot:** Combination of congenital heart defects consisting of a VSD and RV outflow tract obstruction.
   a. *Pathophysiology:* Major features of classic description include a nonrestrictive VSD, RVH secondary to outflow obstruction, aortic override, and pulmonary stenosis of varying degrees but progressive in nature because of the anterior deviation of the infundibular septum (subvalvular or infundibular, valvular, and supravalvular) (Figure 3-56). Associated anomalies include coronary artery anomalies, AVSD (newborns will present with CHF and cyanosis), absent pulmonary valve (usually dilated PA with degrees of respiratory compromise from bronchial compression by dilated PA), ASD, or pulmonary atresia.
      - Blood enters the RV normally. RV outflow obstruction causes shunting across the VSD to the aorta, thereby mixing systemic venous and pulmonary venous return. The severity of the pulmonary stenosis determines the severity of the cyanosis. As the aorta handles biventricular cardiac output, it is often dilated. Patients are at risk for endocarditis, RV dysfunction, polycythemia, brain abscess, and stroke from cyanosis.
      - Classic hypoxic episodes are marked by increasing cyanosis, hyperpnea, and irritability progressing to unconsciousness, seizures, or cardiac arrest. Usually they occur early in the day, probably secondary to a spasm of the infundibulum of the outflow tract or a drop in the systemic resistance, increasing right-to-left shunt and decreasing pulmonary blood flow. The murmur disappears as no flow occurs across the narrowed pulmonary outflow tract. Patients are treated with sedation, volume (hematocrit ≥45%), bicarbonate, oxygen, knee-chest position, and intubation and anesthesia if necessary. Morphine sulfate is the drug of choice to relieve agitation. IV

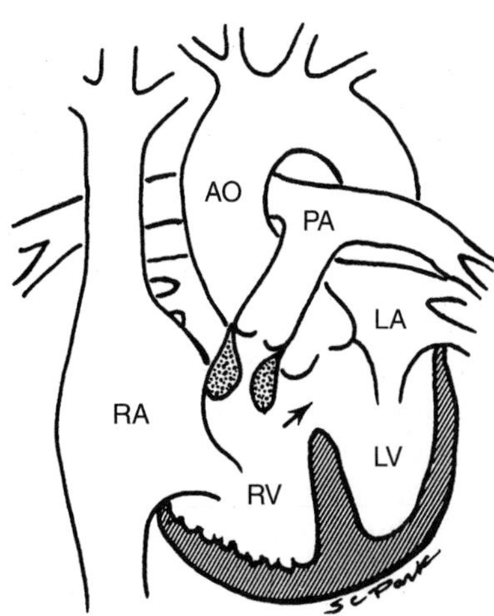

FIGURE 3-56 ■ Anatomy of tetralogy of Fallot with ventral septal defect, pulmonary stenosis, and overriding aorta. *AO*, aorta; *LA*, left atrium; *LV*, left ventricle; *PA*, pulmonary artery; *RA*, right atrium; *RV*, right ventricle.

(Reprinted with permission from Garson AG, Brecker TJ, McNamara DG. *The science and practice of pediatric cardiology.* Philadelphia, 1990, Lea & Febiger.)

propranolol (Inderal) or other beta-blocker may be used to relax the RV infundibulum and decrease the ventricular response to agitation. Phenylephrine (Neo-Synephrine) IV increases the systolic BP and ideally decreases shunting away from the RV outflow tract. Occurrence of spells may indicate a need for earlier repair.

b. *Etiology and incidence:* Tetralogy of Fallot is the most common form of cyanotic CHD and is possibly related to abnormal septation of the conus. The cause is essentially unknown. It occurs slightly more commonly in boys.

c. *Assessment*

- *History* depends on the degree of pulmonary stenosis. If stenosis is severe, neonates are ductal dependent and require immediate surgery. If pulmonary stenosis is not severe, symptoms are mild and include dyspnea on exertion, clubbing, squatting, and cyanosis. Hypercyanotic spells may occur.
- *Examination* reveals a normal cardiac impulse, normal S_1, single S_2, systolic ejection murmur at the LSB (related to pulmonary stenosis), diastolic murmur (with absent pulmonary valve, and a continuous murmur of collaterals or PDA.

d. *Diagnostic findings*

- *ECG* shows right axis deviation, RVH, normal conduction, and rarely ectopy.
- *Chest radiographic examination* demonstrates a boot-shaped heart from absence of the PA segment, normal cardiac silhouette, normal or diminished pulmonary vascular markings, and a right aortic arch (in 25% of cases).
- *ECHO* is the major diagnostic tool for definition of essential morphology, gradients, and identification of associated lesions (anomalous coronary arteries are often difficult to visualize).
- *Cardiac catheterization* may be necessary to adequately detail the RV outflow tract. It will show equal pressures in the right and left ventricles. Coronary arteries are difficult to visualize.

e. *Interventions:* Medical intervention is necessary for hypoxic spells associated with deep cyanosis, hypoxemia, acidosis, or seizures. Maintenance of adequate volume, hematocrit, sedation, oxygenation and knee-chest position are utilized to break spells. Inderal may be useful. The presence of hypercyanotic spells is an indication for surgery. In elective situations, complete repair can be accomplished from newborn period on. Medical management includes prostaglandins in neonates who are ductal dependent for pulmonary blood flow.

- Surgical palliation is provided by a systemic-to-pulmonary shunt (usually a modified Blalock-Taussig shunt with Gore-tex interposition tube between the subclavian artery and ipsilateral PA) via thoracotomy (Figure 3-57). Too large a shunt causes pulmonary overcirculation, symptoms of CHF, and risk of pulmonary vascular disease. Too small a shunt does not relieve cyanosis. Risks of aortopulmonary shunts include chylothorax, damage to phrenic or recurrent laryngeal nerve, infection, PVOD, and distortion of the PA.
- Corrective operation via sternotomy and cardiopulmonary bypass can be performed at any age. It consists of VSD closure (Gore-tex patch) directing LV flow to the aorta, relief of RV outflow tract obstruction, and shunt takedown if one was done previously. Infundibular muscle resection or division of muscle bundles with pulmonary valvotomy or transannular Gore-tex patch results in pulmonary insufficiency. In cases of anomalous coronary arteries or small-branch pulmonary arteries, an RV-PA conduit is used. Risks of operation are low and include heart block, residual pulmonary

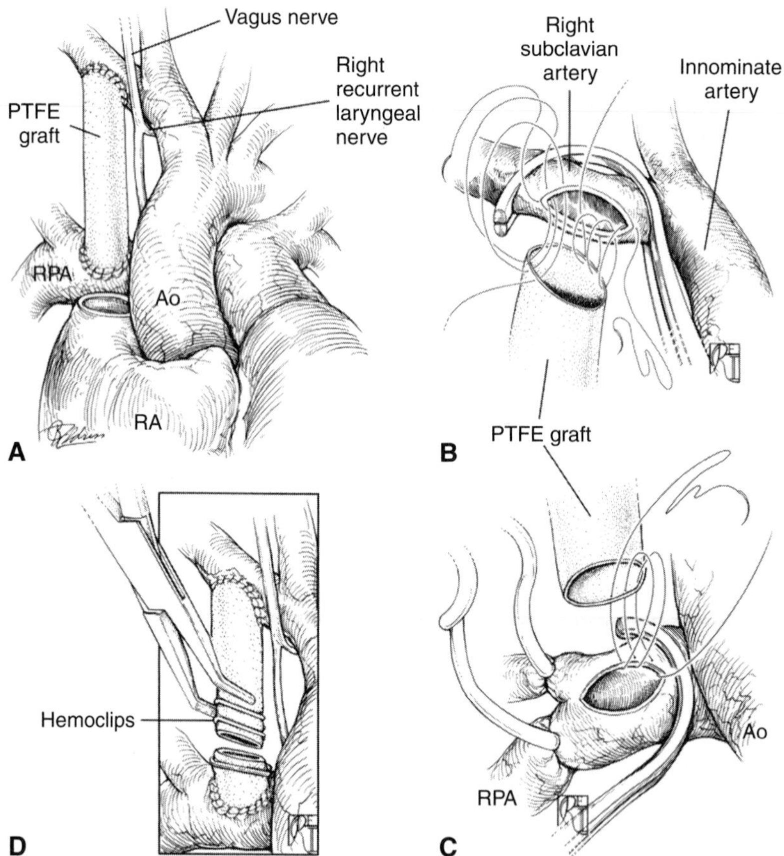

FIGURE 3-57 ■ **A,** Modified Blalock-Taussig shunt using a polytetrafluoroethylene *(PTFE)* graft. **B,** Proximal anastomosis. **C,** Distal anastomosis for modified Blalock-Taussig shunt. **D,** Takedown of a modified Blalock-Taussig shunt with hemoclips and shunt division. *Ao,* Aorta; *RA,* right atrium; *RPA,* right pulmonary artery.
(From Mavroudis C, Backer CL: *Pediatric cardiac surgery,* ed 3. St. Louis, 2003, Mosby.)

stenosis, residual RV outflow tract obstruction, VSD, RV dysfunction, pulmonary insufficiency, or damage to the aortic valve. Late reoperation for PS may be necessary to preserve RV function and exercise tolerance.

- Endocarditis is a lifelong risk.

f. *Pulmonary atresia with a VSD (PA-VSD)* is considered a more extreme form of tetralogy of Fallot. Catheterization is routine at diagnosis to assess the anatomy of the PA, which is extremely variable but frequently is small and nonconfluent. Patients may not be diagnosed until several months of age because collateral flow masks cyanosis. Collaterals are frequently stenotic at either the aortic or pulmonary end. Presentation is usually marked by CHF and failure to thrive by 3 to 6 months, occasional cyanosis, continuous murmurs of collaterals, and single S_2. Chest radiographic examination demonstrates mild to moderate cardiomegaly with no main PA segment and increased pulmonary vascular markings. Results and long-term outcome is based on PA architecture and the state of the pulmonary vascular bed at diagnosis. Often the child requires several surgical interventions. First, the pulmonary arteries are unifocalized, and a RV-PA conduit is placed to promote growth of the proximal and distal PA (Figure 3-58). VSD closure (full repair) is accomplished only in children who have forward RV output and adequately sized pulmonary arteries demonstrated by CHF, increasing saturations, an adequate number of PA segments encorporated into the RVOT, and a predominant left-to-right shunt at catheterization. A postoperative RV:LV pressure ratio of less than 3:4 to 2:3 is necessary to provide good long-term results. An LV/RV pressure ratio greater than 90% generally requires reopening or fenestration of the VSD patch. Reoperation for conduit replacement resulting from conduit stenosis or regurgitation is expected. Complications of operation include residual VSD, PA stenosis, RV hypertension, aortic regurgitation, and arrhythmia, including CHB. Postoperative cardiac

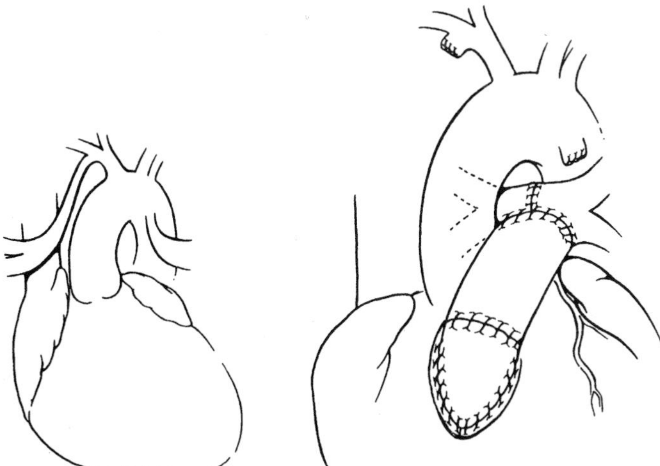

FIGURE 3-58 ■ Technique of complete repair with insertion of homograft conduit after primary unifocalization in patients with complete absence of both interpericardial pulmonary arteries.

(Reprinted with permission from Shanley CJ et al: Primary unifocalization for the absence of interpericardial pulmonary arteries in the neonate, *J Thorac Cardiovasc Surg* 106:237-247, 1993.)

catheterization is not uncommon to assess the PA vasculature and the need for balloon or stenting of stenotic vessels.

g. *Endocarditis* is a lifelong risk.

3. **Transposition of the great arteries (TGA):** TGA is a ventriculoarterial discordance in which the morphologic LV gives rise to the PA and the morphologic RV gives rise to the aorta, creating parallel circulations (Figure 3-59).

a. *Pathophysiology:* Simple TGA is associated with ASD, VSD, and PDA 80% of the time. Parallel circulation exists in that the systemic venous blood enters the right side of the heart normally but exits through the aorta back to the body. Pulmonary venous blood enters the left side of the heart normally but exits through the PA to the lungs. The child requires intracardiac mixing to survive. The degree of cyanosis or acidosis depends on the number, location, and size of intracardiac and extracardiac shunts (ASD, VSD, PDA). Mixing of blood allows systemic saturation of 75% to 90%. LV pressure is maintained at systemic levels for the first 1 to 2 weeks of life. After that, PVR and LV pressure fall. Repair via arterial switch must be done before the fall of LV pressure and mass regression because the LV will have to handle the systemic pressure load. Early development of PVOD in infants with TGA has been found and is an indication for early repair. PVOD is more common if a VSD is present. PVOD can develop as early as 2 weeks of age and occurs in most patients with TGA by 1 year.

- Complications include endocarditis, risk of cyanosis, CHF, and PVOD.

b. *Etiology and incidence:* Although the cause is largely unknown, TGA may be due to a left shift in the pulmonary conus. It is more common in boys of normal birth weight and size. TGA is the most common form of cyanotic CHD to present in the newborn period.

c. *Assessment*

- *History* depends on the degree of shunting. Cyanosis within 24 hours of birth is the most common presentation. If a large VSD is present, the infant may present at 2 weeks of age with CHF.
- *Examination* reveals cyanosis if there is an intact septum; hepatomegaly, tachycardia, tachypnea if with VSD; and clubbing after 6 months. TGA without a VSD reveals a normal S_1, single S_2, continuous murmur of the

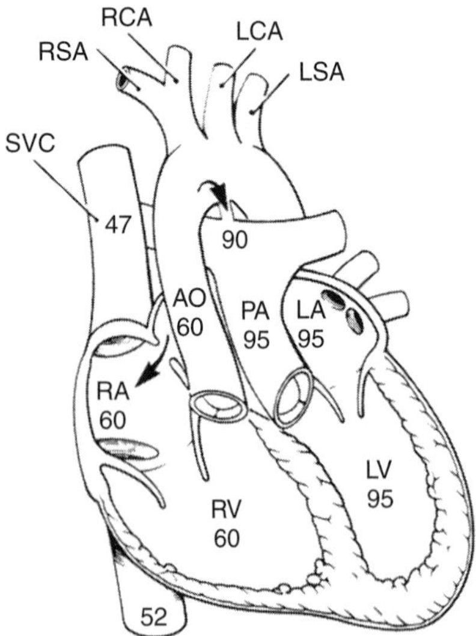

FIGURE 3-59 ■ Transposition of the great arteries. Oxygen saturations in the cardiac chambers and great vessels are depicted with some shunting (mixing) of blood at the atrial level and through a patent ductus arteriosus. *RCA,* Right carotid artery; *LCA,* left carotid artery; *RSA,* right subclavian artery; *LSA,* left subclavian artery; *SVC,* superior vena cava; *AO,* aorta; *PA,* pulmonary artery; *LA,* left atrium; *LV,* left ventricle; *RA,* right atrium; *RV,* right ventricle.

(From Kambam J: Transposition of the great arteries. In Kambam J, editor: *Cardiac anesthesia for infants and children,* St. Louis, 1994, Mosby.)

PDA, and an occasional systolic ejection murmur on auscultation. For TGA with a VSD, auscultation reveals a normal S_1, single S_2, and soft systolic ejection murmur at the LSB.

d. *Diagnostic findings*

- *ECG* shows right-axis deviation, RVH, or biventricular hypertrophy, or findings may be normal for age. In the presence of a VSD, the ECG shows biventricular hypertrophy and a normal QRS axis.
- *Chest radiographic examination* demonstrates an oval-shaped "egg on its side" silhouette, narrow superior mediastinum, and moderate cardiomegaly that may be normal for age. With a VSD, the chest radiographic examination demonstrates moderate cardiomegaly, a narrow superior mediastinum, and increased pulmonary vascular markings.
- *ECHO* plays a dominant role in diagnosis by establishing major anatomic features and anatomic variants, but it might not define the coronary anatomy.
- *Cardiac catheterization* is used mainly for balloon atrial septostomy. It demonstrates increased saturation with shunting, LV outflow obstruction and slight increases in atrial pressure.

e. *Interventions*

- Medical stabilization with prostaglandin therapy is necessary if atrial communication is not sufficient to provide mixing and oxygenation (see Pharmacology). Medications for CHF are used while awaiting operation if there is a large VSD.
- Interventional catheterization is used if the ASD is restrictive or surgery is delayed. Balloon septostomy via catheterization tears the atrial septum. Blalock-Hanlon operation or atrial septectomy via sternotomy on bypass is used to excise the atrial septum surgically, to improve mixing and saturation, and to reduce acidosis.
- Surgical intervention depends on age at presentation, LV pressures, and associated lesions.
  - The *Mustard-Senning operation* (venous switch) redirects venous inflow via intra-atrial baffling, draining the pulmonary veins via the tricuspid valve to the RV to the aorta and the systemic veins, and draining via the mitral valve to the LV and to the PA. The procedure includes closure of the ASD, VSD, and PDA if present. The RV and tricuspid valves remain systemic for life. Complications include early and late atrial arrhythmias, late RV dysfunction and tricuspid regurgitation, venous baffle obstruction, and late development of PVOD.
  - *Arterial switch* (operation of choice) (Figure 3-60) provides anatomic correction involving transection of both great vessels. The pulmonary valve becomes the aortic valve with anastomosis of the distal aorta to the proximal PA and closure of associated shunts. Coronary arteries with a button of PA tissue are transferred to the new aortic root. Criteria for an arterial switch are timing of repair and no fixed pulmonary stenosis, which would become aortic stenosis after the switch. This procedure leaves the LV and mitral valve on the systemic side and avoids a complex intra-atrial baffle, which decreases the risk of significant atrial arrhythmias. Early postoperative problems center on LV dysfunction, low cardiac output, and myocardial ischemia or infarction from kinking or distorting of the coronary arteries during transfer. To date, the most common residual defect has been the development of supravalvular pulmonary stenosis.
- Timing of repair of transposition with VSD is somewhat elective but operation by 2 weeks of age is preferred to avoid CHF and early

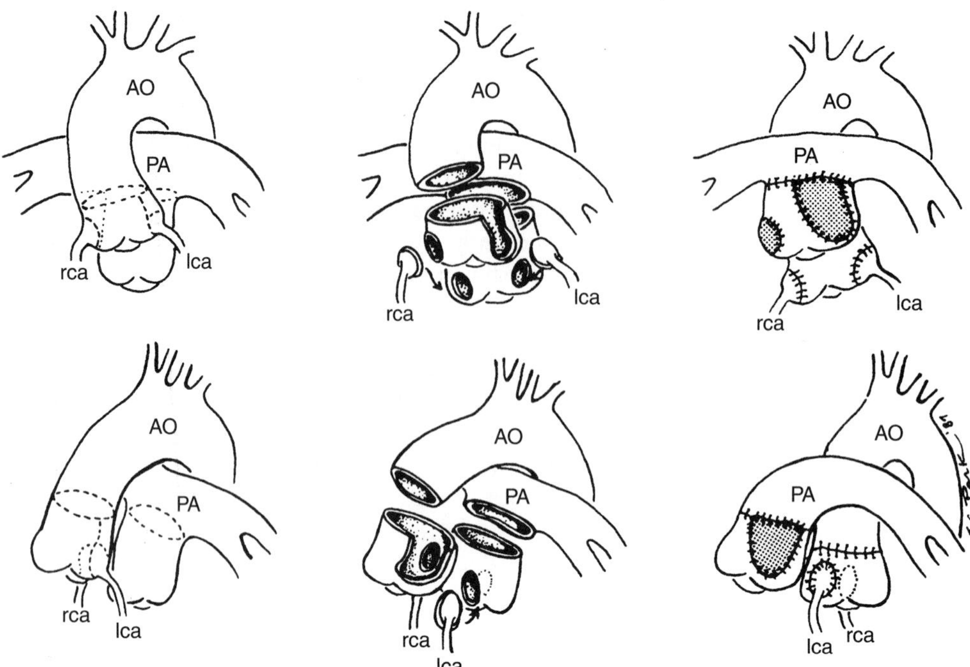

FIGURE 3-60 ■ Arterial switch operation for transposition of the great arteries. Transection of both great vessels followed by anastomosis to the anatomically correct ventricles with coronary transfer. *AO,* aorta; *lca,* left coronary artery; *PA,* pulmonary artery; *rca,* right coronary artery.

(Reprinted with permission from Garson AG, Brecker TJ, McNamara DG: *The science and practice of pediatric cardiology.* Philadelphia, 1990, Lea & Febiger)

development of PVOD. In complex VSD and small patients, a PA band may be used until the infant is older.

- Late diagnosis of transposition with intact ventricular septum can be managed with PA band and placement of a systemic to pulmonary shunt. The shunt overloads the LV with volume and pressure to prepare it to accept systemic pressure workloads following an arterial switch operation. The exact length of time from palliation to arterial switch is still not clear but it has been done as soon as 2 weeks later. Indicators of RV preparation are LV/RV pressure ratio greater than 70%, LV volume/mass normal for age, and LV-wall thickness normal for age.
- Complex TGA includes TGA with VSD and pulmonary stenosis. Palliation with a systemic to pulmonary shunt occurs in the neonatal period. Correction is completed in 6 months to 1 year with the Rastelli operation, which reestablishes LV-aortic continuity (Figure 3-61). The VSD is patched to direct LV flow to the aortic valve, and RV-PA continuity is established with an RV-PA conduit. The size of the VSD and location to the semilunar valves determine the degree of surgical difficulty. If the VSD is small and enlargement is necessary, the risk of postoperative complete heart block increases. Postoperative complications with the Rastelli operation include arrhythmia, VSD patch dehiscence or residual VSD, aortic obstruction, residual pulmonary stenosis, tricuspid insufficiency, and myocardial dysfunction.
- Endocarditis is a lifelong risk.

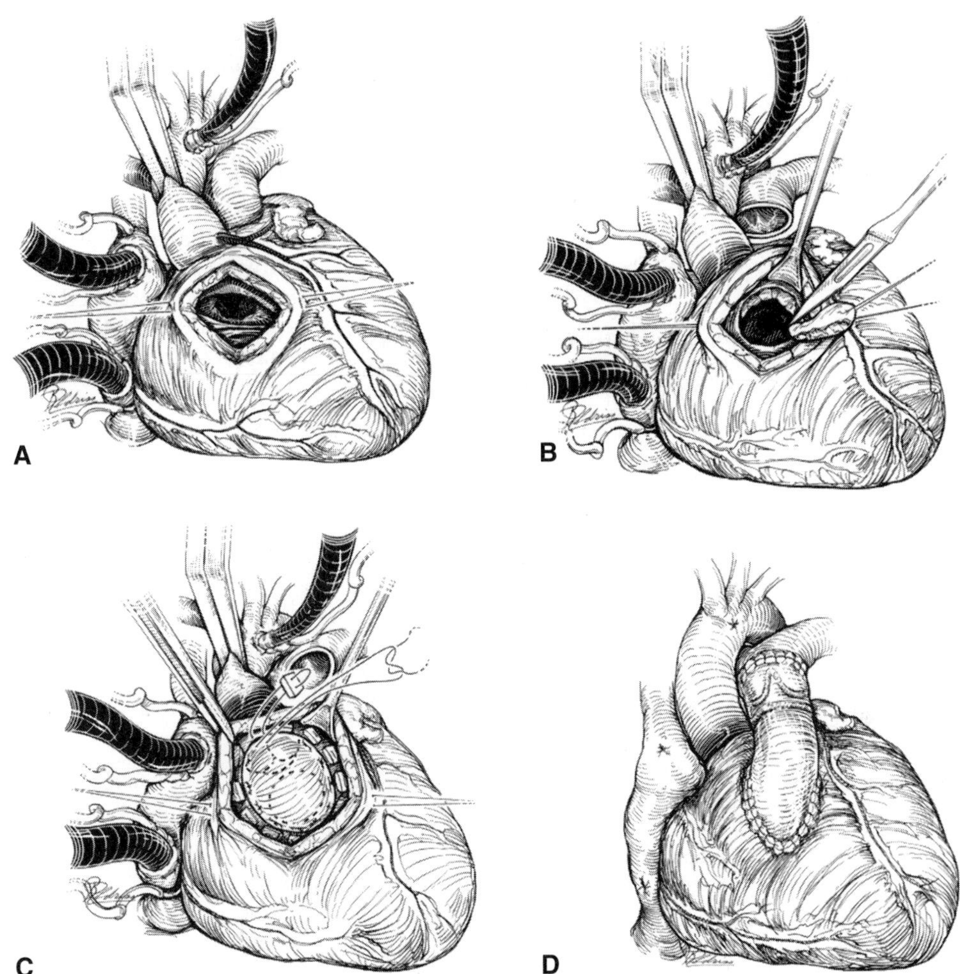

FIGURE 3-61 ■ The Rastelli operation. **A,** A right ventricular incision is made with due regard to the tricuspid valve attachments, the ventricular septal defect anatomy, coronary artery distribution, and intended position of the conduit. **B,** A comprehensive infundibular resection is performed to maximize left ventricular-to-aortic continuity. **C,** The ventricular septal defect is closed with a large patch, creating an ample tunnel to the aorta. The distal pulmonary artery is opened at the most appropriate site for the distal conduit anastomosis. **D,** The valved conduit is in place afer separation from cardiopulmonary bypass.
(From Mavroudis C, Backer CL: *Pediatric cardiac surgery,* ed 3. St. Louis, 2003, Mosby.)

4. **Tricuspid atresia (TAT):** Imperforate tricuspid valve resulting in mandatory right-to-left atrial shunt and eventual single ventricle repair
   a. *Pathophysiology*
      - Agenesis of the tricuspid valve results in no communication between the RA and RV. TAT is associated most often with a small RV, ASD, and an aortopulmonary connection (PDA) (Figure 3-62). Physiology and symptoms depend on the degree of pulmonary stenosis or pulmonary atresia and the presence or absence and size of the VSD. Because blood cannot exit the RV, it is shunted right to left at the atrial level and systemic desaturation occurs. Blood then flows across the left side of the heart to the RV via the VSD and out to the lungs if there is little or no pulmonary stenosis. The result is

Tricuspid Atresia with No Transposition (69% - 83%)

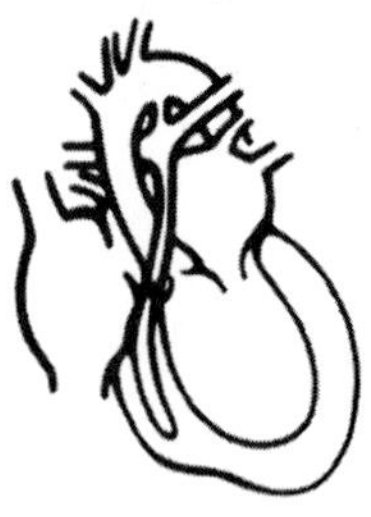

I(a)
Pulmonary atresia

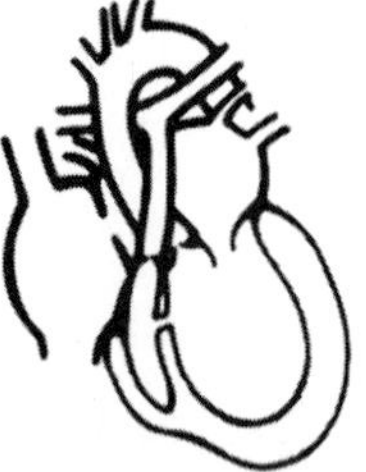

I(b)
Pulmonary hypoplasia, small ventricular septal defect

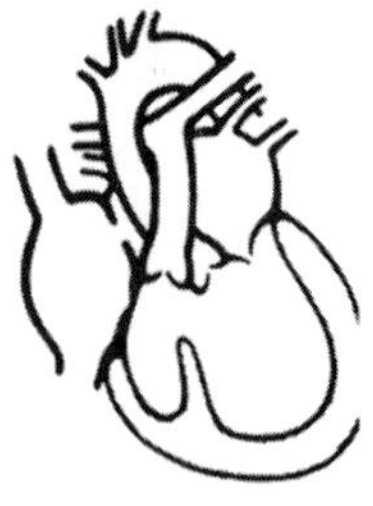

I(c)
No pulmonary hypoplasia, large ventricular septal defect

Tricuspid Atresia with D Transposition (17% - 27%)

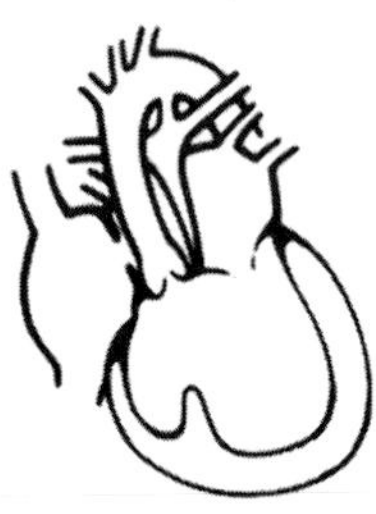

II(a)
Pulmonary atresia

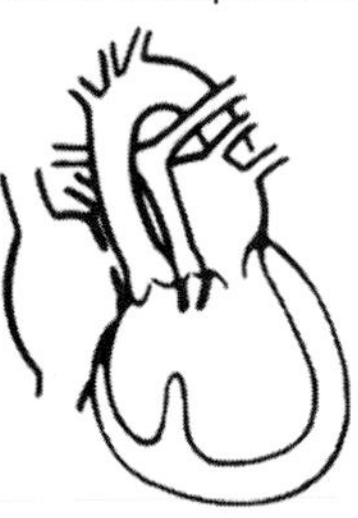

II(b)
Pulmonary or subpulmonary stenosis

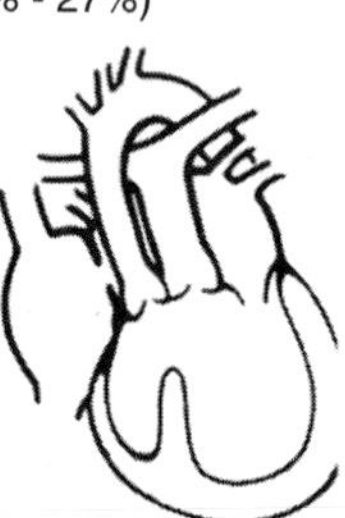

II(c)
Large pulmonary artery

Tricuspid Atresia with L Transposition (3%)

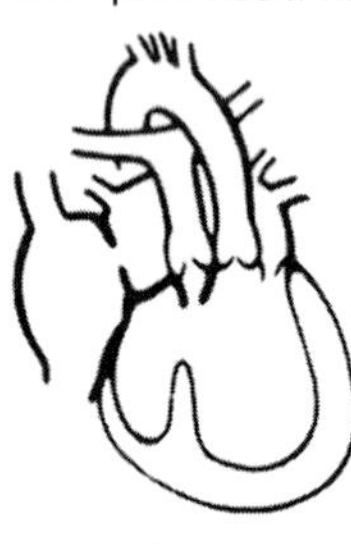

III(a)
Pulmonary or subpulmonary stenosis

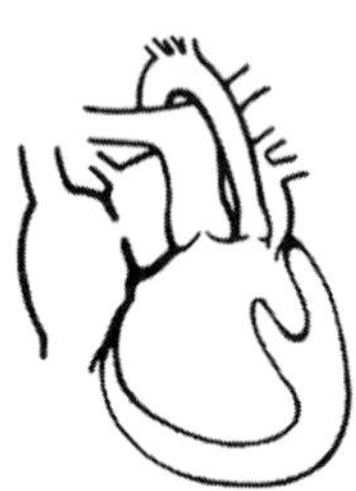

III(b)
Subaortic stenosis

FIGURE 3-62 ■ The anatomic classification of the tricuspid atresia, as suggested by Tandon and Edwards in 1974.

(From Pearl JM, Permut LC, Laks H: Tricuspid atresia. In Bauer AE et al (editors): *Glenn's thoracic and cardiovascular surgery*, ed 6. Stamford, Conn., 1996, Appleton & Lange.)

normal to increased pulmonary blood flow with clinical manifestations of CHF.

- With associated pulmonary stenosis or pulmonary atresia, there will be little or no flow to the PA. These infants usually have small RVs, are cyanotic early, and are ductal dependent for pulmonary blood flow. With VSD, systemic output may be seriously compromised if the VSD is small or restrictive or becomes so early in life.
- In single-ventricle (or univentricle) hearts, both AV valves empty into one ventricle (known as *double inlet*) (Figure 3-63). Ventricles are differentiated based on trabeculations. These lesions, as with TAT, may have normal, increased, or decreased pulmonary blood flow based on the degree of pulmonary stenosis. Clinical manifestations, physical examination,

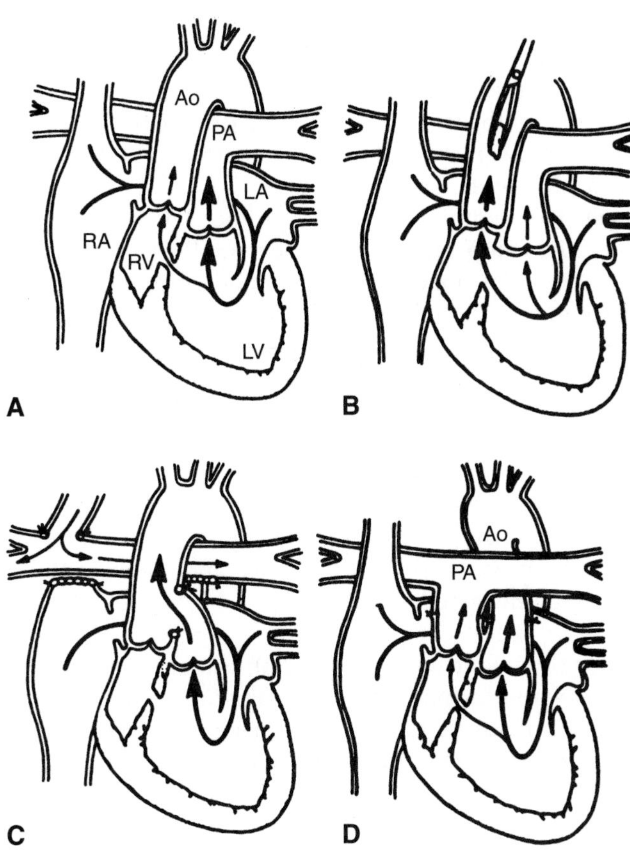

FIGURE 3-63 ■ Methods of treatment of subaortic stenosis in hearts with functional single ventricle. **A,** Anatomy of type IIc tricuspid atresia with significant subaortic stenosis. **B,** Direct resection of myocardium with ventricular septal defect enlargement. **C,** Damus-Kaye-Stancel operation, main pulmonary artery to ascending aortic anastomosis. **D,** Palliative arterial switch operation. *Ao,* Aorta; *LA,* left atrium; RA, right atrium; LV, left ventricle; RV, right ventricle; PA, pulmonary artery.

(From Mavroudis C, Backer CL: *Pediatric cardiac surgery,* ed 3. St. Louis, 2003, Mosby.)

diagnostic findings, and interventions depend on the degree of AV valve regurgitation, extracardiac or intracardiac shunting, and pulmonary obstruction.

b. *Etiology and incidence:* Etiology is agenesis of the tricuspid valve (TAT) or failure of trabecular components of the ventricle to develop (single ventricle). There is no known cause, but TAT may be associated with polyhydramnios or maternal toxemia and has been reported with use of thalidomide. TAT is an uncommon defect (2.7% CHD cases).

c. *Assessment*

- *History* is dependent on the amount of pulmonary blood flow (presence of a VSD, degree of pulmonary stenosis or pulmonary atresia). Early cyanosis is common (50%) and expected (78%) by 1 month because of the obligatory atrial shunt. CHF may occur with VSD and no pulmonary stenosis. Hypoxic spells occur in 16% to 45% of patients younger than 6 months. The risk of complications is from cyanosis, stroke, and brain abscess. Patients with CHF from excessive pulmonary blood flow may develop PVOD. All patients are at risk for endocarditis. Atrial arrhythmias are not uncommon. Delayed growth and development may be seen.
- *Examination* reveals a hyperactive apical impulse, clubbing, left precordial prominence, single S_1 and S_2 (most common unless pulmonary blood flow is increased), systolic ejection murmur at the mid to upper LSB from the pulmonary stenosis, occasional holosystolic murmur at the LSB if a VSD is present, and a continuous murmur of the PDA or collaterals if PVR is normal.

d. Diagnostic findings

- *ECG* shows a superior and leftward QRS axis, RA enlargement, absent or diminished RV forces, and increased LV forces.
- *ECHO* demonstrates absence of the tricuspid valve and diminished RV size. It also defines associated defects, increased LV dimensions, size of the VSD and ASD, and the relationship of the great vessels.
- *Chest radiographic examination* with diminished pulmonary blood flow demonstrates normal to mild cardiomegaly, concave main PA segment, and diminished pulmonary vascular markings. Chest radiographic examination with increased pulmonary blood flow demonstrates gross cardiomegaly and increased pulmonary vascular markings.
- *Cardiac catheterization* is not necessary for first-stage palliation but is necessary before further surgery. On catheterization, the RV is not entered from the RA, and flow of systemic venous blood from the RA to the LA through the ASD results in decreased saturation of the LA blood. The RA pressure is greater than or equal to the LA pressure. It defines the presence of a VSD, collaterals, the relationship of the great vessels, and the degree of pulmonary stenosis. If no pulmonary stenosis is present and there is a VSD, PA pressure and PVR may be elevated.

e. *Interventions*

- Medical interventions for the infant with tricuspid atresia and pulmonary stenosis include initial stabilization with prostaglandin infusion to maintain ductal patency until surgery. Initial treatment for patients with nonrestrictive pulmonary flow involves medical management with the use of CHF medications.
- Initial surgical palliation for those with decreased pulmonary blood flow involves placement of an *aortopulmonary* shunt via thoracotomy. Initial palliation for increased pulmonary blood flow involves ligating the PA and performing an aortopulmonary shunt. A second option is PA banding. The third option is a *Damus-Kaye-Stancel operation* in the cohort of patients with transposed great vessels and a hypoplastic systemic outflow chamber. This operation is similar to a Norwood operation in that a systemic outflow is created by aortic-to-pulmonary (off the LV) anastomosis, ligation of the PA, and creation of a systemic-to-pulmonary shunt.
- Regardless of initial palliation, patients with tricuspid atresia or univentricular hearts will undergo three-stage reconstruction ending with a Fontan (see HLHS). Second-stage palliation will be either a bidirectional Glenn or hemi-Fontan, depending on the venous anatomy and surgeon preference. Fontan operation via lateral tunnel or extracardiac conduit is the final palliation (Figure 3-64). Extracardiac conduits are used especially in patients with univentricular hearts and complex venous anatomy such as heterotaxy to avoid obstruction or compression of venous return.
- Improved survival for the Fontan procedure can be related to younger age at operation, refined surgical technique and staging procedures, and postoperative management. Complex single ventricles, heterotaxy, PA distortion, PAH, or long bypass times during Fontan increase morbidity and mortality. Late complications include thromboembolic events, rhythm disturbances, protein-losing enteropathy, development of aortopulmonary collaterals, Fontan pathway obstruction, AV valve regurgitation, and ventricular dysfunction. Neurologic outcomes are encouraging. Resting cardiac output is normal; however, at maximal exercise, it may be limited.
- Endocarditis is a lifelong risk.

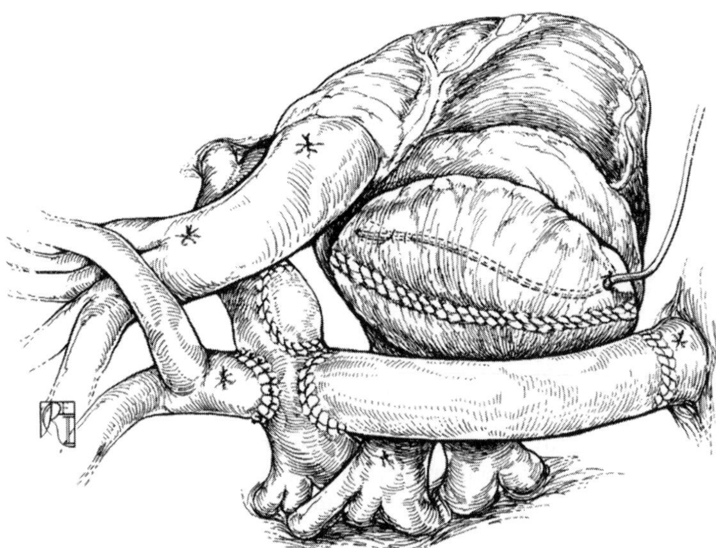

FIGURE 3-64 ■ The total extracardiac conduit type of total cavopulmonary connection. In this instance, a right-sided superior cavopulmonary anastomosis is combined with the interposition of a polytetrafluoroethylene graft conduit between the divided inferior vena cava and the underside of the PA confluence.
(From Mavroudis C, Backer CL: *Pediatric cardiac surgery,* ed 3. St. Louis, 2003, Mosby.)

5. **Truncus arteriosus (TRU):** A single arterial trunk arises from the base of the heart giving rise to pulmonary, systemic, and coronary circulations.
   a. *Pathophysiology*
      - Truncus includes an unrestrictive VSD, a single semilunar valve with possible truncal valve abnormalities, and override of the ventricular septum by the truncal valve. Tricuspid truncal valve occurs in 69% of cases, quadricuspid truncal valve in 22% of cases, and bicuspid truncal valve in 9% of cases. Truncal valve insufficiency is related to thick dysplastic cusps. Truncal valve stenosis is rare.
      - The type of truncus is differentiated by the existence and location of the main pulmonary artery and the PA branches (Figure 3-65). *Type I* has a short main PA segment, which arises from the trunk and then branches into the right and left pulmonary arteries (48%). In *type II* the pulmonary artery arises separately from the trunk but in close proximity to it (29% to 48%). In *type III* the PA arises separately from the trunk and at some distance from it (6% to 10%). In type IV, arteries arising from the descending aorta supply the lungs.
      - Common associated lesions include coarctation and interrupted aortic arch. Coronary artery anomalies may occur. Extracardiac anomalies occur in about 21% to 30% of children and most often include DiGeorge syndrome, bowel malrotation, and hydroureter. Right aortic arch is more commonly associated with truncus arteriosus than with any other congenital heart defect. Complications of this diagnosis include subendocardial ischemia and PVOD early on from the high pressure and volume of pulmonary flow and progressive truncal valve insufficiency.
      - Systemic and pulmonary venous blood returns normally and enters the respective ventricle. Ventricular blood mixes through the VSD and exits the heart through the truncus. Blood then flows to the lungs and body, depending on the respective resistance in the systemic and pulmonary

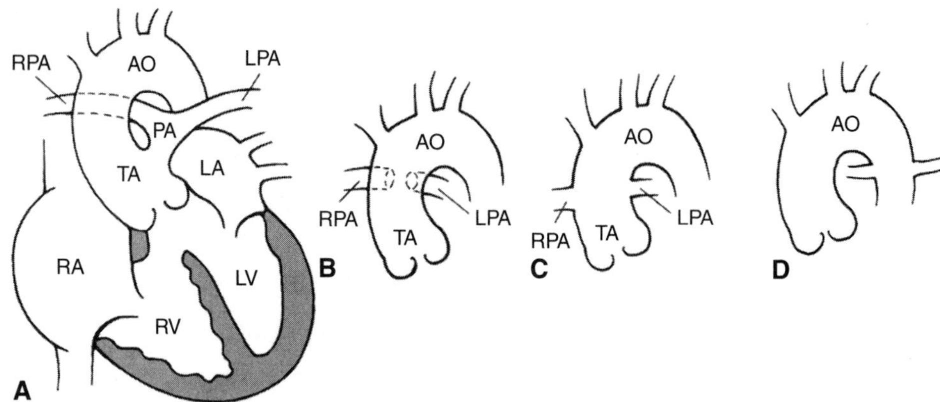

FIGURE 3-65 ■ The anatomic type of persistent truncus arteriosus *(TA)* is determined by the branching patterns of the pulmonary arteries. **A,** In type I, the main pulmonary artery *(PA)* arises from the truncus and then divides into the right *(RPA)* and left PA *(LPA)* branches. **B,** In type II, the pulmonary arteries arise from the posterior aspect of the truncus. **C,** In type III, the pulmonary arteries arise from the lateral aspects of the truncus. **D,** In type IV, or pseudotruncus arteriosus, arteries arising from the descending aorta *(AO)* supply the lungs. *LA,* Left atrium; *LV,* left ventricle; *RA,* right atrium; *RV,* right ventricle.

(From Park MK: *Pediatric cardiology for practitioners,* ed 4. St. Louis, 2002, Mosby.)

circuits. Symptoms appear when the PVR begins to fall around 2 to 4 weeks of life. In the event of severe truncal valve insufficiency (or more rarely stenosis), low cardiac output and cardiac compromise occur almost from birth.

b. *Etiology and incidence:* This accounts for 1% to 4% of all cases of CHD. Conotruncal or truncoarterial separation does not proceed normally. Either a deficiency or an absence of conal (infundibular) septum causes a large VSD.

c. *Assessment*

- *History:* Symptoms of CHF occur when the PVR drops and pulmonary blood flow increases. In infants with associated DiGeorge syndrome, hypocalcemia and hypomagnesemia are frequently noted.
- *Examination* reveals cyanosis only when PVR is increased; this is a concern for eventual repair. Active precordium, normal S_1, loud ejection click, loud and single S_2, and S_3 heard at the apex is common. In addition, a systolic ejection murmur at the LSB and frequently an apical diastolic murmur can be heard. If truncal valve insufficiency exists, a blowing diastolic high-pitched murmur is heard at the LSB.

d. *Diagnostic findings*

- *ECG* shows a normal QRS configuration or minimal right-axis deviation, normal sinus rhythm, biventricular hypertrophy, and left atrial enlargement (LAE).
- *Chest radiographic examination* demonstrates moderate cardiomegaly, increased pulmonary vascular markings, right arch in one third of patients, and dilated truncal root. In the presence of PVOD, enlargement of the PA and a tapering of the distal pulmonary vascular tree occur.
- *ECHO* confirms the diagnosis, and anatomic features are identified. Origin of the pulmonary arteries, VSD location and size, and anatomy of the truncal valve are accomplished. The pressure gradient across the truncal valve and the degree of insufficiency are determined if necessary.

- *Cardiac catheterization* is not necessary except in complex variants. Right and left ventricular pressures are equal, and there is increased oxygen saturation in the PA. PVR may be elevated, and PA pressure is elevated.

e. *Interventions*

- Repair should not be delayed because PVOD develops rapidly. Medical management to control CHF is warranted. Irradiated blood should always be used until DiGeorge syndrome can be ruled out.
- Surgical repair entails sternotomy and cardiopulmonary bypass possibly with deep hypothermic circulatory arrest. The VSD is closed to the truncal valve, creating LV-to-truncal valve continuity (Figure 3-66). The PAs are connected to the distal end of the RV conduit; the conduit is then connected to the RV outflow tract, reestablishing RV-to-PA continuity. Truncal valve insufficiency or stenosis is addressed only if severe. Moderate insufficiency or stenoses often improve when the volume load crossing it is decreased after separation of the circulations. In most neonatal repairs, the ASD or PFO is left open to allow bidirectional shunting until RV compliance improves.
- Complications particular to this operation are conduction disturbances, including heart block, low cardiac output, residual pulmonary stenosis or VSD, PA hypertensive crisis, and progressive truncal valve insufficiency.

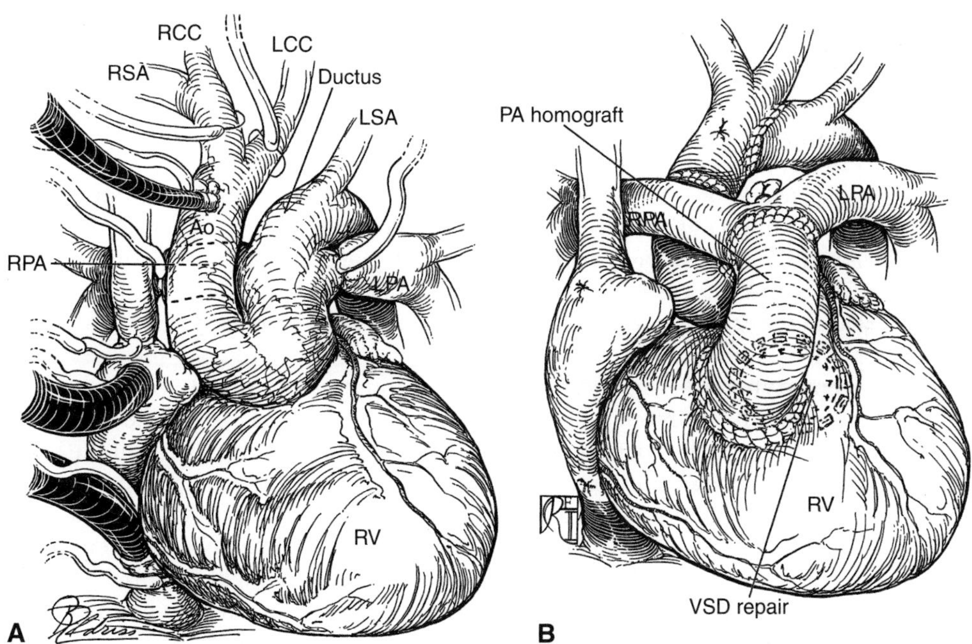

FIGURE 3-66 ■ Diagramatic representation shows a patient with truncus arteriosus and interrupted aortic arch. **A,** Aortobicaval cardiopulmonary bypass is established with bilateral pulmonary artery *(PA)* constriction (enforced snuggers). Lower-extremity flow is accomplished thought the patent ductus arteriosus. **B,** Completed repair of truncus arteriosus with interrupted aortic arch. Direct aortic reconstruction is performed without foreign material. The maneuver of Lecompte facilitates right ventricular-to-PA continuity. *Ao,* Aorta; *LCC,* left common carotid artery; *RCC,* right common carotid artery; *LPA,* left pulmonary artery; *RPA,* right pulmonary artery; *LSA,* left subclavian aratery; *RSA,* right subclavian artery; *PA,* pulmonary artery; *RV,* right ventricle; *VSD,* ventricular septal defect.

(From Mavroudis C, Backer CL: *Pediatric cardiac surgery,* ed 3. St. Louis, 2003, Mosby.)

No increased mortality has been found with repair of interrupted aortic arch and truncus arteriosus. Requirement for truncal valve replacement for severe regurgitation at presentation increases surgical morbidity and mortality. Repair of the valve, even if residual moderate tuncal valve stenosis exists, has had improved results. Pulmonary homograft conduits are currently the preferred material for initial establishment of RV to PA continuity because of the ease of use, improved hemostasis, and improved longevity. Failure of homograft conduits is related to the size of the conduit and the child at implantation, growth of the patient, pulmonary versus aortic homograft, Dacron extension, and extracardiac placement of the valve. Debate continues as to whether the homograft, porcine-valved heterograft, or bovine jugular vein conduit provides the best conduit over time. Branch PA stenosis is not uncommon and requires balloon dilation or patch arterioplasty at reoperation for conduit replacement.

- Endocarditis is a lifelong risk.

6. **Total anomalous pulmonary venous return (TAPVR)** occurs when all four pulmonary veins drain anomalously into the right side of the heart. Partial connection (PAPVR) occurs when one to three pulmonary veins drain anomalously.

   a. *Pathophysiology*

   - Pulmonary veins have no connection to the LA. The LA is often small and noncompliant. The pulmonary veins may empty in various ways to the RA (Figure 3-67). Supracardiac pulmonary veins drain to the left SVC or right SVC via the vertical vein, forming a confluence posterior to the LA (45%). Intracardiac pulmonary veins drain to the IVC via the vertical vein (frequently obstructed at the level of the diaphragm [8%]). Cardiac pulmonary veins drain to the coronary sinus or RA and rarely are obstructed or stenotic (35%). Mixed pulmonary veins drain via a combination of the preceding means (1% to 2%).
   - An ASD is considered part of the complex and is mandatory for survival. One third of cases have other cardiac anomalies such as TAT, TGV, pulmonary atresia, or single ventricle. TAPVR is increased in patients with asplenia and other forms of CHD.
   - Hemodynamics depend on the distribution of mixed venous blood between the pulmonary and systemic circulation, the size of the ASD, and the degree of obstruction. All venous blood enters the right side of the heart and exits the PA. This creates pulmonary overcirculation and hypertension. For survival, blood must enter the LA via the ASD. If the ASD is small, the LV volume will be low and cardiac output will be severely compromised. If the ASD is large and the LA is compliant, LV volume will be appropriate. If the pulmonary veins are obstructed, blood cannot exit the lungs, creating a critical situation of low cardiac output from LV-volume underloading, severe pulmonary congestion from the obstruction, hypoxemia, and acidosis. Increased pulmonary venous pressure is transmitted to the pulmonary vascular bed, and reflex PA vasoconstriction occurs to prevent pulmonary edema. The result is decreased pulmonary blood flow, RA dilation, RVH, and RV failure. Even if the veins are not obstructed, the increased pulmonary flow creates medial hypertrophy and intimal hyperplasia, ending with PVOD by the third to fourth decade of life.

   b. *Etiology*

   - TAPVR is an embryologic error of incorporation of pulmonary veins into the LA.

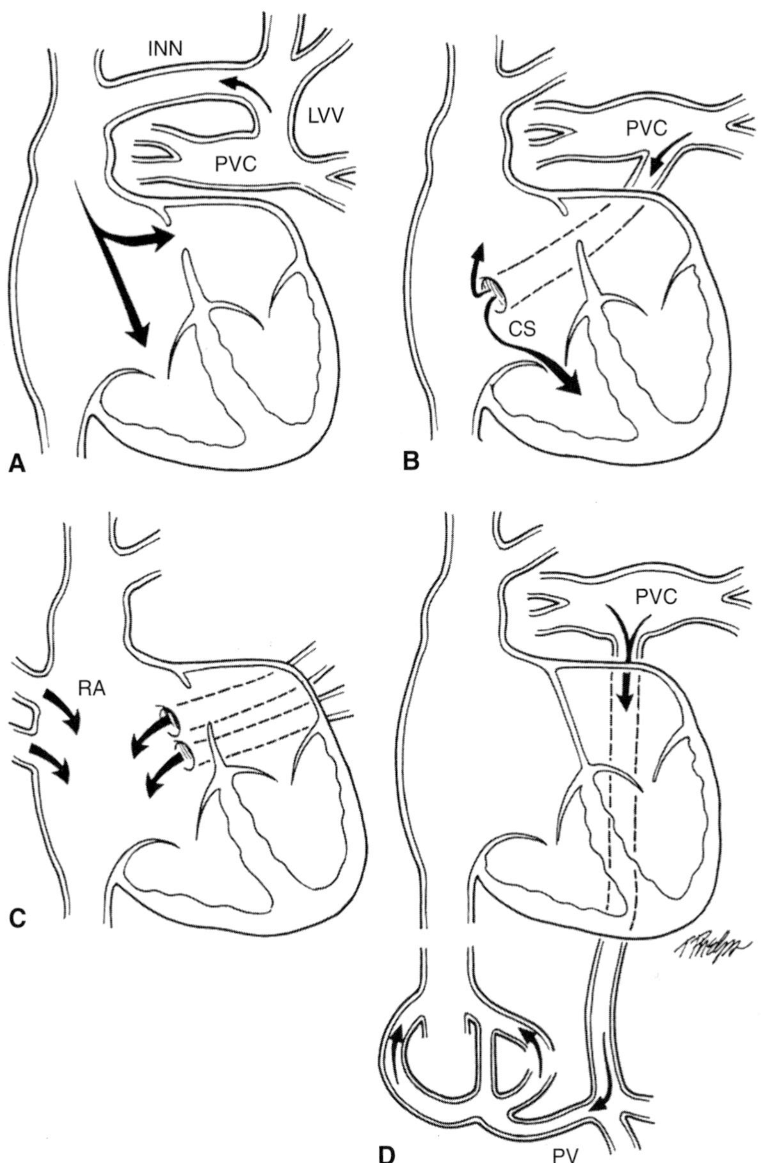

FIGURE 3-67 ■ The four most common anatomic defects in total anomalous pulmonary venous connection *(TAPVC)*. **A,** TAPVC drainage to the innominate vein *(INN)* via a left vertical vein *(LVV)*. **B,** TAPVC from the common pulmonary venous confluence *(PVC)* to the coronary sinus *(CS)*. **C,** TAPVC to the right atrium *(RA)*. **D,** Infradiaphragmatic TAPVC from the common pulmonary venous confluence to the portal vein *(PV)*.
(From Nichols DG et al: *Critical heart disease in infants and children*. St. Louis, 1999, Mosby.)

c. *Assessment*
- *History:* Patients with obstructed veins present with a history of severe respiratory distress, cyanosis, acidosis, and low cardiac output shortly after birth from reduced blood flow to the LV and pulmonary congestion from obstruction of flow through the veins. Patients with unobstructed veins present with CHF after 2 to 4 weeks of life when PVR decreases and shunting increases.

- *Examination:* Children with obstructed veins have marked respiratory distress, cyanosis, dyspnea, tachycardia, tachypnea, RV heave, a systolic ejection click, increased S_1, a fixed and split S_2, low cardiac output, and acidosis. With unobstructed veins, there is an increased and split S_2, an S_3, and a systolic ejection murmur at the upper LSB. Although difficult, the diagnosis of obstructed TAPVR must be differentiated from persistent pulmonary hypertension of the newborn.

d. *Diagnostic findings*

- *ECG* shows RA enlargement, RVH, and right axis deviation (if veins are obstructed).
- *Chest radiographic examination* demonstrates increased pulmonary blood flow, RA and RV dilation, a prominent PA segment, "snowman configuration" of the heart in older infants with supracardiac TAPVR, and cardiomegaly if presentation is with volume overload and CHF.
- *ECHO* confirms the diagnosis and localizes the site of venous drainage. Pulmonary venous obstruction is quantified by Doppler. Associated lesions are defined; RV pressure and PA hypertension are noted; and PA, RA, and RV volume overload are noted.

e. *Interventions*

- Medical treatment for CHF is required for patients with unobstructed veins. In severely obstructed TAPVC, preoperative stabilization with intubation, hyperventilation, hyperoxygenation, and nitric oxide may be needed. ECMO support may be necessary to support cardiac output in the most severe situations until surgical relief of obstruction can be performed.
- Obstructed veins are almost always surgical emergencies. Unobstructed veins are repaired early to prevent PVOD. Surgical repair is aimed at returning pulmonary vein flow to the left side of the heart, eliminating obstruction, closing the ASD, and preventing PVOD. Repair is done via sternotomy on cardiopulmonary bypass using deep hypothermic circulatory arrest. The pulmonary vein confluence is anastomosed to the posterior wall of the LA, or the veins are directed through the ASD by an intra-atrial patch, thereby redirecting pulmonary venous return correctly and closing the ASD.
- Postoperative problems include pulmonary hypertensive crisis, SSS and other atrial arrhythmias, restenosis of the anastomosis, and inability to relieve the stenosis fully. Hyperventilation and nitric oxide and in some cases ECMO may be required postoperatively for pulmonary stabilization. LV compliance is poor, and the LA cannot easily dilate. Slow volume infusion prevents further increase and transmission of elevated pressure to the lungs. Use of inotropic agents may decrease the amount of volume needed to maintain the BP and thereby decrease extracellular water, edema, and elevated LA/PA pressure.
- Long-term prognosis depends on the presence of diffuse pulmonary vein obstruction, the relief of all existing stenosis, any associated cardiac lesions, and the state of the pulmonary vascular bed. About 10% of these children have a second obstruction usually associated with intracardiac or mixed types of veins. Use of sildenafil for treatment of PA hypertension has proven successful over the long term.

7. **Pulmonary atresia with intact ventricular septum (PA/IVS):** Complete obstruction of the RV outflow requiring shunting at the atrial and great vessel level for survival

a. *Pathophysiology*

- The defect is characterized by variable size and function of the RV and tricuspid valve. The RA may be dilated proportional to the degree of tricuspid insufficiency from a lack of RV outflow. An ASD is always present. RV size may be decreased or normal but capable of handling forward cardiac output with relief of obstruction at the pulmonary valve. RV pressure increases relative to the outflow obstruction and can cause tricuspid insufficiency and increased RA pressure. Shunting can occur across the ASD into the LA. Flow into the PA and lungs is maintained by the PDA. The LV manages the total cardiac output.
- Coronary artery anomalies may include fistulous communication between coronary arteries and the RV, which can cause retrograde flow of desaturated blood into the coronary arteries, resulting in ventricular ischemia and even death. Coronary arteries may be stenotic.

b. *Etiology and incidence:* PA/IVS is an uncommon defect (3% of all CHD) that is associated with complex RV lesions. The cause is essentially unknown but may be an interruption of the neural crest cells, or it may be a viral or other infectious agent introduced early in fetal life.

c. *Assessment*

- *History* includes cyanosis evident shortly after birth as the PDA physiologically closes. CHF is uncommon unless the defect is accompanied by tricuspid insufficiency.
- *Examination* reveals an S_1, normal intensity, single S_2, and a continuous murmur of the PDA. When there is significant tricuspid insufficiency, the child may have a holosystolic murmur.

d. *Diagnostic findings*

- *ECG* shows LV predominance and RA enlargement. ST-T wave changes reflect major underlying coronary anomalies when present.
- *Chest radiographic examination* results are normal in most cases (with decreased pulmonary blood flow). Marked cardiomegaly is present with severe tricuspid insufficiency.
- *ECHO* defines an imperforate pulmonary valve, tricuspid valve size and anomalies, and visualization of the ASD and may be able to assess abnormal coronary artery connections.
- *Cardiac catheterization* is essential in full delineation of all anatomic defects. Low systemic venous saturations, decreased LA saturation from right-to-left shunting, and RV pressure are noted. Coronary artery fistulas and stenosis are visualized.

e. *Interventions*

- Ductal patency is mandatory for survival until full diagnostic evaluation and surgical repair are completed.
- All operations are aimed, when possible, at encouraging growth of the tricuspid valve and RV. The surgical approach depends on multiple factors, including predicted RV function and size, the presence of RV-dependent coronary blood flow or coronary artery stenosis, and the size of the tricuspid valve and ASD. The ASD is left open in these infants to provide pressure relief for noncompliant RVs (Figure 3-68). It is closed only after final palliation in patients with a usable RV with good function. For the diminutive RV, small tricuspid valve inlet or for patients with RV-dependent coronary blood flow, initial palliation with a systemic-to-pulmonary shunt and progression to a single ventricle repair with Fontan operation are performed. For patients with moderate RV hypoplasia and

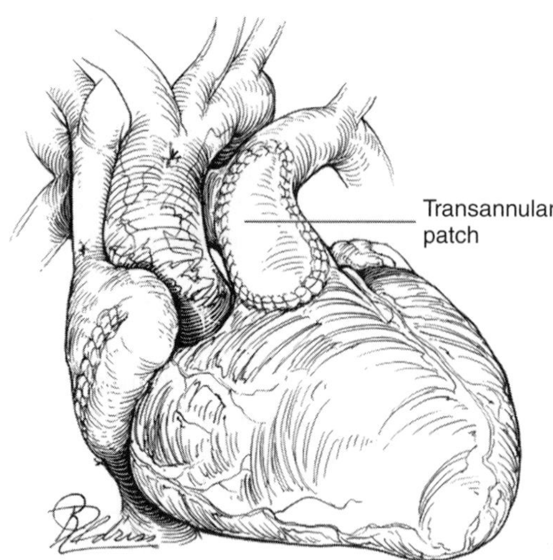

FIGURE 3-68 ■ Appearance of a transannular patch used to enlarge a hypoplastic pulmonary valve annulus and main pulmonary trunk. The patch extends onto the origin of the left pulmonary artery *(PA)*. The proximal extent of the patch on the right ventricular outflow tract should be as short as possible.

(From Mavroudis C, Backer CL: *Pediatric cardiac surgery*, ed 3. St. Louis, 2003, Mosby.)

tricuspid valve annulus who may be able to progress to biventricular repair, a RVOT patch and shunt are performed. Repair with ASD closure alone is feasible if the RV/tricuspid valve can handle the entire forward cardiac output. If not, the $1/2$ ventricle repair with SVC to PA connections and ASD closure may be the best option. In mild RV hypoplasia, the likelihood of a biventricular repair is high. RV to PA continuity is performed using a transannular patch or valvotomy (membranous pulmonary atresia) initially.

- Early and late mortality of this defect remains high, and consensus has yet to be reached regarding optimal patient management. Orthotopic heart transplant is a debatable option in patients with RV dysfunction and coronary artery stenosis or sinusoids.
- Endocarditis remains a lifelong risk.

HYPERTENSIVE CRISIS

A. Definition

An acute, life-threatening elevation in systolic and diastolic BP potentially resulting in end-organ damage or death.

B. Pathophysiology

1. **Normal or abnormal BP** should be determined in infancy. Appropriately sized cuffs are vital for accurate measurements. The American Academy of Pediatrics (AAP) recommends that all children age 3 years and older have their BP measured at least yearly. The AAP Task Force established norms, taking into account race, ethnic group, height, and weight for age. BP varies normally with time of day, physical activity, body position, and emotional state. Hypertension is defined as a BP greater than the 95th percentile for age, sex, and height on at least three different occasions (see Tables 3-11 and 3-12). According to the AAP Task Force, children with elevated BP between the 90th and 95th percentile for age are "at risk" and should be followed more closely.

TABLE 3-11
Blood Pressure at 95th Percentile for Boys (Levels Indicate Hypertension)

Age (years)	Systolic and Diastolic Blood Pressure by Percentile of Height in mm Hg						
	5%	10%	25%	50%	75%	90%	95%
1	98/55	99/55	101/56	102/57	104/58	106/59	106/59
2	101/59	102/59	106/60	106/61	108/62	109/63	110/63
3	106/63	105/63	107/64	109/65	111/66	112/67	113/67
4	106/66	107/67	109/67	111/68	113/69	114/70	115/71
5	108/69	109/70	110/70	112/71	114/72	115/73	116/74
6	109/72	110/72	112/73	114/74	115/75	117/76	117/76
7	110/74	111/74	113/75	115/76	116/77	118/78	119/78
8	111/75	112/76	114/76	116/77	118/78	119/79	120/80
9	113/76	114/77	116/78	117/79	119/80	121/80	121/81
10	114/77	115/78	117/79	119/80	121/80	122/81	123/82
11	116/78	117/79	119/79	121/80	123/81	124/82	125/83
12	119/79	120/79	121/80	123/81	125/82	126/83	127/83
13	121/79	122/80	124/81	126/82	128/83	129/83	130/84
14	124/80	125/81	127/81	128/82	130/83	132/84	132/85
15	127/81	128/82	129/83	131/83	133/84	134/85	135/86
16	129/83	130/83	132/84	134/85	136/86	137/87	138/87
17	132/85	133/85	135/86	136/87	138/88	140/89	140/89

Adapted from Update on the 1987 task force report on high blood pressure in children and adolescents: a working group report from the National High Blood Pressure Education Program, *Pediatrics* 98:653, 1996.

TABLE 3-12
Blood Pressure at 95th Percentile for Girls (Levels Indicate Hypertension)

Age (years)	Systolic and Diastolic Blood Pressure by Percentile of Height in mm Hg						
	5%	10%	25%	50%	75%	90%	95%
1	101/57	102/57	103/57	104/58	105/59	107/60	107/60
2	102/61	103/61	104/62	105/62	107/63	108/64	109/65
3	104/65	104/65	105/65	107/66	108/67	109/67	110/68
4	105/67	106/67	107/68	108/69	109/69	111/70	111/71
5	107/69	107/70	108/70	110/71	111/72	112/72	113/73
6	108/71	109/71	110/72	111/73	112/73	114/74	114/75
7	110/73	110/73	112/73	113/74	114/75	115/76	116/76
8	112/74	112/74	113/75	115/75	116/76	117/77	118/78
9	114/75	114/76	115/76	117/77	118/78	119/78	120/79
10	116/77	116/77	117/77	119/78	120/79	121/80	122/80
11	118/78	118/78	119/79	121/79	122/80	123/81	124/81
12	120/79	120/79	121/80	123/80	124/81	125/82	126/82
13	121/80	122/80	123/81	125/82	126/82	127/83	124/84
14	123/81	124/81	125/82	126/83	128/83	129/84	130/85
15	124/82	125/82	126/83	128/83	129/84	130/85	131/86
16	125/83	126/83	127/83	128/84	130/85	131/86	132/86
17	126/83	126/83	127/83	129/84	130/85	131/86	132/86

Adapted from Update on the 1987 task force report on high blood pressure in children and adolescents: a working group report from the National High Blood Pressure Education Program, *Pediatrics* 98:654, 1996.

2. **Peripheral vascular resistance and cardiac output** determine BP. As total PVR or cardiac output increases, BP rises. PVR is mediated by blood viscosity, arteriolar smooth muscle structure and function, vasoconstrictor substances, renin, angiotensin I, angiotensinogen, vasorelaxants including natriuretic peptides, and the amount of autonomic discharge.
3. Over time, hypertension produces necrosis and inflammation in the arterioles that eventually cause decreased blood flow to end organs.
4. **Uncontrolled hypertension** may induce a sudden rise in BP, which may lead to accelerated or malignant hypertension.
   a. *Accelerated hypertension* is associated with rapid vascular changes and retinal exudates and hemorrhages (rare in infants and young children). Failure to treat accelerated hypertension aggressively will result in malignant hypertension.
   b. *Malignant hypertension* differs minimally from accelerated hypertension in infants. Retinal exudates and hemorrhages, when present, advance to papilledema. Large amounts of renin and angiotensin cause arterial dilation and contraction. This produces turbulent blood flow, which causes microangiopathic hemolytic anemia and intravascular coagulation. The arterial walls swell with fluid, causing fibrinoid necrosis. Hypertensive encephalopathy ensues.
5. Excessive elevation of the BP causes dysfunction of cerebral autoregulation, which in turn causes vasospasms, ischemia, increased capillary pressure and permeability, and cerebral edema and hemorrhage.

C. Etiology

1. **Renal parenchymal disease** (acute glomerulonephritis, chronic pyelonephritis, renal vascular disease, renal secreting tumors, chronic renal failure, polycystic disease, Wilms tumor, hemangiopericytoma) is the most common cause of hypertension. Renal vascular diseases also contribute to the incidence of hypertension, including thromboembolic phenomena related to umbilical artery catheterization or coagulopathy, fibromuscular dysplasia, neurofibromatosis, vasculitis, arteritis, congenital aneurysms, renal vein or artery thrombosis, or segmental hypoplasia (Ash-Upmark kidney).
2. **Neurologic causes** of hypertension from increased intracranial pressure include tumors, Guillain-Barré syndrome, dysautonomia, intraventricular hemorrhage, obstructive hydrocephalus, and porphyria.
3. **Early development of essential hypertension** is associated with familial patterns of hypertension, with genetics accounting for 60% of BP variation. Cardiac risk factors include obesity, elevated lipid levels, and insulin resistance, now called *Syndrome X*.
4. **Other contributing factors** include pheochromocytoma, pituitary tumors, coarctation of the aorta, congenital adrenal hyperplasia, Cushing syndrome, polycythemia, primary aldosteronism, Williams syndrome, and Turner syndrome.

D. Assessment

1. **History** reveals clinical complaints, familial hypertension, etiologic factors, or evidence of complications of hypertension (renal dysfunction, stroke). Diet history may indicate a high sodium intake.
2. **Clinical presentation** of a hypertensive crisis includes decreased femoral pulses (if coarctation is also present), convulsions, mental status changes or focal neurologic changes, dyspnea, headache, restlessness, epistaxis, tachycardia, rales, S_3, S_4, nonspecific signs of uremia, and blurred vision. A bruit may be

auscultated over the femoral area, carotid arteries, abdominal aorta, anterior fontanelle, and anteriorly over the renal vascular area.

3. **Diagnostic findings**
   a. *Laboratory studies*
      - CBC: Anemia is associated with renal disease.
      - Serum blood urea nitrogen, creatinine clearance, and uric acid values are elevated with renal disease.
      - Serum glucose level is elevated in Cushing syndrome, pheochromocytoma, and diabetes, all three of which are potential causes of hypertension.
      - Urinalysis demonstrates proteinuria and hematuria (evidence of renal disease).
      - Serum potassium is used to rule out primary aldosteronism, which causes hypokalemia and hypertension.

   b. *Radiologic findings*
      - Renal arteriography is used to show renal artery stenosis, lesions, and dysplasias as causes of hypertension.
      - IV pyelography may indicate the presence of kidney disease but cannot differentiate the type.
      - Chest radiographic examination may reveal cardiomegaly and pulmonary edema.
      - Computed tomography (CT) scan shows diffuse brain edema in patients with encephalopathy and also demonstrates hemorrhage.

   c. *ECG* may reveal signs of LVH and ischemia.

E. Interventions

1. **Effectiveness and toxicity of drug therapies** vary widely among patients. Therapy is often lifelong when hypertensive crisis occurs in childhood, so doses must be adjusted for growth and maturational changes. Medications include α- and β-blockers, diuretics, vasodilators (including calcium channel inhibitors), and renin-angiotensin inhibitors.
2. **Positive-pressure ventilation** is helpful if pulmonary edema, CHF, and cerebral edema are present.
3. **Reduction of anxiety or pain**, if present, aids in a reduction of BP.
4. **Lifestyle changes** may be required for long-term control and avoidance of future crisis. Diet should be low salt, low cholesterol, and low fat. Exercise programs are prescribed with consideration of limitations of the underlying disease.

F. Nursing Diagnoses

❖ Excessive elevation of systemic BP

1. **Defining characteristic:** Patient exhibits BP greater than the 95th percentile for age, sex, and height.
2. **Expected outcome:** BP will return to normal limits.
3. **Interventions**
   a. *Continually reassure* the patient and family. Maintain a calm, quiet environment.
   b. *Assist* in the insertion of hemodynamic monitoring lines to monitor the patient's response to therapy. Monitor ECG for arrhythmias.
   c. *Administer drugs as ordered:* Monitor response and side effects, and titrate to maintain desired BP level. Goal is to reduce to below the 95th percentile within minutes and to the 85th percentile slowly over hours. Administer diuretics and monitor intake and output.

4. **Evaluation of nursing care**
   a. The patient's BP is within prescribed limits.
   b. ECG demonstrates normal sinus rhythm.

❖ Potential for hypotension secondary to diuretic and antihypertensive drug therapy

1. **Defining characteristics**
   a. BP and urine output are below prescribed limits.
   b. Serum electrolyte levels are abnormal.
   c. The child may exhibit hypovolemic shock symptoms.
2. **Expected outcomes**
   a. BP is within normal limits.
   b. ECG demonstrates normal sinus rhythm.
   c. The child is normovolemic.
3. **Interventions**
   a. Monitor hemodynamic pressures closely. Monitor ECG continuously.
   b. Monitor the patient's response to the drug therapy and report values that reflect hypotension. Titrate or stop antihypertensive drugs when necessary.
   c. Administer fluids to restore volume. Monitor electrolytes for abnormalities.
4. **Evaluation of nursing care**
   a. BP is within prescribed limits.
   b. Hemodynamics reflect adequate filling pressures and cardiac output.
   c. Electrolytes are within normal limits.
   d. ECG demonstrates normal sinus rhythm.

CARDIOMYOPATHY

A. Definition

Cardiomyopathy is a myocardial muscle disease.

B. Pathophysiology

1. **Cardiomyopathy is characterized by changes in the myocardium** that produce myocyte degeneration. Compensation for myocyte loss is hypertrophy with resulting interstitial fibrosis and scarring that decreases contractility. Disorganized alignment of cellular structures leads to ineffective depolarization and contraction. Incidence is 1.13 per 100,000 children per year.
2. **Cardiomyopathies** are classfied as hypertrophic, dilated, and restrictive.
   a. *Hypertrophic* cardiomyopathy is characterized by a thick muscle-bound LV with marked increase in myocardial mass and varying degrees of myocardial fibrosis, a decreased ventricular cavity size, and resistance to LV filling. Frequently there is asymmetric septal hypertrophy and LV posterior-wall hypertrophy. Systolic contraction may produce obstruction of outflow. Diastolic stiffness of the LV impairs filling, producing atrial enlargement. Incidence is 42% of all cardiomyopathies.
   b. *Dilated* cardiomyopathy is characterized by extensive dilation of the ventricles associated with mild to moderate ventricular hypertrophy, reduced stroke volume, low ejection fraction, and low cardiac output resulting from poor contractile force, which leads to increased systolic and diastolic volumes. Stasis of blood can occur within the cardiac chambers. Incidence is 51% of all cardiomyopathies.
   c. *Restrictive* cardiomyopathy is characterized by fibrosis of the ventricle, resulting in minimal contractile movement, poor ventricular compliance, and inadequate filling. Incidence is 3% of all cardiomyopathies.

C. Etiology

1. *Hypertrophic cardiomyopathy (HCM)* has autosomal-dominant transmission in 60% of cases. All mapped genes are genes that encode proteins as part of the sarcomere and are involved in energy production within the cardiac myocyte. There may be a family history of sudden death or HCM. HCM can also be secondary to hypertension caused by obstruction to flow such as aortic stenosis, coarctation, or renal artery stenosis. HCM is associated with specific chromosomal syndromes such as Noonan syndrome.
2. *Dilated cardiomyopathy (DCM)* has multiple identified pathways, including automosomal-dominant, X-linked, autosomal-recessive, and mitochondrial inheritance in 30% to 40% of cases. Mutations of genes result in disease by altering the sarcolemma to sarcomere cytoskeleton within the myocyte. DCM after viral myocarditis may occur from viral damage to these same protein structures. DCM can also occur as a result of ischemic damage as seen in anomalous left coronary artery, metabolic disorders such a hemochromatosis, carnitine deficiency, or glycogen-storage diseases and drug toxicity.
3. *Restrictive cardiomyopathy* is related to endocardial fibroelastosis and hyper-eosinophilic syndrome (infiltration of eosinophils with fibrosis and scarring in leukemia).

D. Signs and Symptoms

1. Children may be asymptomatic until significant disease develops.
2. Most children have an enlarged heart. DCM causes poor contractility; HCM causes supercontractility. With restrictive cardiomyopathy, there is normal systolic function but diminished diastolic function.
3. Low cardiac output results in signs of CHF such as tachypnea, tachycardia, easily fatigued, and diaphoresis at rest. This can progress to poor perfusion, shock, low urine output, and decreased level of consciousness. There may be an LV lift, gallop rhythm, systolic ejection murmur, split S_2, arrhythmias, syncope, thromboembolic events, angina, irritability, cough, and anorexia.

E. Diagnostic Studies

1. **Chest radiographic examination** shows an enlarged heart, normal or increased CT ratio, pulmonary venous engorgement, and interstitial edema and may show pleural effusions.
2. **ECG** shows RBBB, LBBB, conduction delays, arrhythmias, LVH with or without ST depression, and T-wave inversion or other nonspecific T-wave changes as well as possible atrial enlargement.
3. **ECHO** is used to assess contractility and to rule out CHD. It will define ventricular dilation, disproportionate ventricular septal thickening, and possible obstruction of RV or LV outflow tracts and will measure ejection fraction.
4. **Laboratory studies** will rule out metabolic causes and assess viral titers. Brain nateuretic peptide (BNP) may be used to determine the level of heart failure and to trend efficacy of therapy.
5. **Cardiac catheterization** is used to assess cardiac function and obtain endomyocardial biopsy for myocarditis.

F. Nursing Diagnoses

- Alteration in cardiac output due to inadequate tissue perfusion and arrhythmias
- Activity intolerance
- Potential for thrombus formation

G. Goals and Patient Management

1. **Improve and maximize cardiac output and activity level.**
   a. *Pharmacologic therapy*: In HCM, β-adrenergic agonists reduce ventricular workload; calcium channel blockers provide afterload reduction, decrease myocardial contractility, and thereby improve LV diastolic function; diuretics are used judiciously because they may reduce blood volume and increase the risk of obstruction of LV. Inotropic agents are avoided because they may burn out muscle by increasing contractility in an already hypercontractile muscle without increasing underlying coronary supply. In DCM, digoxin and positive inotropic agents (dopamine, dobutamine, milrinone) have been used to improve contractility, but that may be at the cost of earlier lethal heart failure. β blockers are used to counter-regulate sympathetic stimulation. ACE inhibitors have been shown to prolong life.
   b. *Surgical resection* of hypertrophic septal tissue (ventricular septal myotomy) can be used in hypertrophic cardiomyopathy. Resection of the LV outflow tract is used with IHSS.
   c. *Pacing* can change the timing of ventricular responses, producing an asymmetric RV and septal motion away from the area of the LV outflow tract obstruction during contraction (only in HCM).
   d. *Fluid therapy* is aimed at fluid and sodium restriction. Edema, weight, rales, and electrolyte levels are assessed, and diuretics are used.
   e. *Cardiac workload is decreased* through oxygen therapy, intubation or ventilation, rest periods, enteral feedings, and increased caloric intake.
2. **Prevent thrombus formation** with medications (e.g., heparin, aspirin, warfarin, enoxaparin).
3. **Transplantation** is used for end-stage disease. Ventricular assist devices are also utilized as a bridge to transplantation or recovery in patients with cardiomyopathy. Advances in research have enabled certain VADs, such as the Berlin Heart, to be used in very small children.

H. Complications

Complications include arrhythmias, emboli, CHF, and death.

ACUTE INFLAMMATORY DISEASES

A. Definition

Myocardial diseases that produce inflammation of cardiac or vascular tissues including myocarditis, endocarditis, pericarditis, Kawasaki syndrome, and rheumatic heart disease.

B. Myocarditis, Endocarditis, and Pericarditis

1. **Pathophysiology**
   a. *Myocarditis* occurs in focal or diffuse inflammation of cardiac muscle producing temporary or permanent damage to the myocardium. During the acute phase (when the causative organism can be cultured), there is initiation of direct myocardial damage with necrosis of myocardial cells, including specialized tissues such as the conduction system. Cellular infiltration of macrophages and natural killer cells results in disintegration of heart muscle, fibrosis, hypertrophy, chamber dilation, mural thrombi, and release of cytokines, such as tumor necrosis factor, and interferons that block viral

replication while enhancing negative inflammatory effects. The chronic phase is mediated by T cells and natural killer cells that continue to attack the myocardium. The necrotic area of muscle is replaced with scar tissue. Focal hemorrhage, edema, fatty infiltration of the muscle, and fibrosis may also occur. Persistent activation of T-cell presentation of myosin as an antigen and autoantibodies found in genetically at risk indivduals may result in DCM.

b. *Endocarditis* is an inflammation of a valve, endocardium, or endothelium that results from a bacteria or fungus in a child with valvular or structural heart disease or invasive vascular catheter. Turbulent blood flow or disruption of endothelial tissue from line placement results in mural tissue damage with deposition of platelets and fibrin and thrombus formation with entrapment of circulating organisms. Large colonies of bacteria become encased in masses of fibrin-forming vegetations. Vegetations usually occur at the location of jet lesions. In addition, infection may destroy the valve, invade the myocardium to form an abscess, or result in thrombus formation on valves and eventual deformation and valve insufficiency. Portions of the lesions may embolize to other organs, resulting in complement activation and inflammatory responses that may contribute to renal dysfunction.

c. *Pericarditis* is inflammation of the pericardium that can produce effusion fluid (ranges from serous to thick and cheesy exudate) and fibrin deposits within the pericardial sac. As effusion volume increases, cardiac tamponade can occur with a rise in intracardiac pressure, cardiac filling decreases, and cardiac output decreases.

2. Etiology

a. *Myocarditis* can be caused by any pathogen, including bacteria, viruses, and fungi. Most cases are associated with a viral illness (especially RNA type, e.g., coxsackievirus A and B, influenza A and B), a systemic infection, or active endocarditis. Noninfectious myocarditis may be caused by systemic autoimmune diseases (e.g., systemic lupus erythematosus).

b. *Endocarditis* is usually bacterial (especially *Streptococcus viridans, Staphylococcus aureus*) and rarely fungal. It is most likely to affect children with underlying heart disease or intracardiac catheters, especially children with prosthetic valves or those who have undergone surgical interventions (e.g., open heart surgery with foreign patch material, or gastrointestinal tract, genitourinary tract, or dental procedures). Fungal organisms are most likely to be identified in infants or immunocompromised children.

c. *Pericarditis* results from trauma; postcardiotomy; infection (bacterial, viral, fungal, protozoal); toxic reactions from radiation, drugs, or uremia; and collagen diseases.

3. Signs and symptoms

a. *Myocarditis* involves a history of bacterial or viral illness, fever, tachycardia, arrhythmias, signs of CHF, lethargy, chest pain, weakness, myalgia, poor systemic perfusion with shock, systolic murmur, pulsus alternans, or pericardial or pleural friction rub.

b. *Endocarditis* is characterized by new or changing murmurs, fever, chills, sweating, fatigue, malaise, anorexia, headache, splenomegaly, valve insufficiency, CHF, and arthralgia. Systemic emboli may produce pain or compromise in the perfusion of extremities, petechiae, splinter hemorrhages of fingernails, hematuria, cerebral infarct, and renal dysfunction. Osler's nodes, Janeway lesions, and Roth spots rare in children.

c. *Pericarditis* produces precordial chest pain, pericardial friction rub (grating, scratching sound), ST elevation on ECG, signs of cardiac tamponade such as decreased cardiac output and systemic BP, increased intracardiac pressures, and muffled heart sounds from pericardial effusion. In addition, cough, fever, dyspnea, arrhythmias, and pulsus paradoxus (with effusion) may be noted.

4. **Invasive and noninvasive diagnostic studies**
   a. *Chest radiographic examination* demonstrates an enlarged heart when effusion is present.
   b. *ECG* may show ST changes (elevation or depression), inverted T wave, prolonged PR interval, diminished QRS complex and T-wave voltage, or arrhythmias.
   c. *ECHO* is used to size any effusion, locate and visualize vegetations and abscesses, rule out structural problems, measure end-diastolic pressures, and evaluate valve function. A transesophageal view may be used for better visualization.
   d. *Laboratory studies* include cultures (minimum of three blood cultures), WBC (leukocytosis may be present), titers to assess for elevated IgM, cardiac enzyme studies, and sedimentation rate (may be elevated).
   e. *Cardiac catheterization* is used to identify restrictive pericarditis or cardiomyopathy, evaluate the severity of constriction, and obtain an endomyocardial biopsy for histologic grading, culture (rarely positive), and polymerase chain reaction (PCR) analysis of tissue for viral genomes.
   f. *Pericardiocentesis* is a needle aspiration used to obtain pericardial fluid for analysis and culture and to relieve tamponade.
5. **Nursing diagnoses**
   ❖ Alteration in cardiac output
   ❖ Alteration in breathing patterns
   ❖ Alteration in comfort
   ❖ Potential for embolic damage
6. **Goals and desired outcomes**
   a. *Myocarditis*
      • Treat infection.
      • Maximize ventricular function.
      • Provide cardiovascular support.
   b. *Endocarditis*
      • Provide prevention for susceptible patients.
      • Treat infection.
      • Provide cardiovascular support.
      • Treat CHF.
   c. *Pericarditis*
      • Treat infection.
      • Treat inflammation.
      • Drain effusion fluid if hemodynamically significant.
7. **Patient care management**
   a. *Myocarditis:* Provide continuous monitoring (risk of serious arrhythmias and sudden death), bed rest, antibiotics/antivirals, antipyretics, corticosteroids, and intravenous immune serum globulin (IVIG; controversial), treatment of CHF with ACE inhibitors and diuretics to decrease filling pressures and vascular resistance, and β-blockers once stable. Treat shock with inotropes or short-term circulatory support (ECMO or VAD allows for remodeling of heart) as well as antiarrhythmics. Many children recover with no sequelae. Some develop progressive dilation with decreased ventricular function and AV valve insufficiency. In some, the primary manifestation is arrhythmias with sudden death.

b. *Endocarditis* requires appropriate IV antibiotic therapy for 6 weeks, neurologic checks, treatment of CHF, and bed rest. Lesions eventually heal following weeks of treatment, although sequelae from embolization and renal dysfunction from the inflammatory response may result. Therapeutic antibiotic levels and continuing assessment of effective coverage should be maintained even with home IV therapy.

c. *Pericarditis:* Pericardiocentesis is both diagnostic and therapeutic to prevent cardiac tamponade. Antibiotics are prescribed. Anti-inflammatory medications are indicated for pain control and a decrease of effusion volume. Diuretics also decrease effusion volume.

8. **Complications** include CHF, end-stage myocardial damage, tamponade, arrhythmias, valve failure, and microemboli causing infarcts.

C. Rheumatic Fever

1. **Pathophysiology:** Group A β-hemolytic streptococci pharyngitis initiates an autoimmune process in a genetically susceptible host that attacks collagen. Streptococcal and myocardial tissues have similar antigenic determinants, creating antigenic mimicry (antibodies produced for streptococcal infection react with host tissue producing antibody-induced tissue damage).
2. **Incidence:** Rheumatic fever most often occurs in the age group of 6 to 15 years (rare in children younger than 2 years or older than 15 years). The incidence in the United States decreased after the introduction of antibiotics; it remains most common in Third World countries.
3. **Signs and symptoms** include recent pharyngitis or upper respiratory tract infection, new murmur, cardiac enlargement, friction rub or effusion, and CHF. Arthritis occurs in 70% of patients and may be the presenting symptom. Children experience migratory heat, redness, and pain that is greater than the evidence of involvement. CNS involvement is characterized by chorea resulting in grimacing, slurred speech, weakness, and purposeless movements (Sydenham chorea or St. Vitus dance). Skin involvement includes painless, firm subcutaneous nodules (0.5 to 2 cm) over the extensor surfaces of joints, such as elbows, knuckles, knees, ankles, the scalp, and the spine. Erythema marginatum rheumaticum is a rash characterized by pink, raised, small irregular macules that are nonpruritic. It usually appears on the trunk and limbs but not on the face.
4. **Diagnostic studies**

   a. *Laboratory studies* include throat culture (positive for group A streptococci), WBC, sedimentation rate, C-reactive protein, and elevated antistreptolysin O antibody titer.

   b. *ECG* may show a prolonged PR interval indicating first-degree AV block, diffuse ST-T wave changes, or T-wave inversion.

   c. *ECHO* is used to evaluate for myocarditis, decreased contractility, and valvular insufficiency.

   d. *Jones criteria* are used for diagnosis. The patient needs two major or one major and two minor manifestations to have a high probability of rheumatic fever (Table 3-13).
5. **Nursing diagnoses**
   - ❖ Alteration in cardiac output
   - ❖ Alteration in comfort
6. **Goals and desired outcomes**

   a. *Reestablish* and maintain hemodynamic stability.

   b. *Arrest or control* inflammatory processes.

   c. *Treat* infectious processes.

TABLE 3-13
Jones Criteria

Major Manifestations	Minor Manifestations
Carditis	Clinical
Polyarthritis	Previous rheumatic fever
Chorea	Arthralgia
Erythema marginatum rheumaticum	Fever
Subcutaneous nodules	Laboratory
	Sedimentation rate
	C-reactive protein
	Leukocytosis
	Prolonged PR interval

  d. *Optimize* cardiac output.
  e. *Optimize* level of comfort.

7. **Patient care management:** Streptococcal infection is treated with antibiotics. Cardiac workload is decreased with bed rest in a quiet and dark environment, control of arrhythmias, and pain.
8. **Complications** include valvular and myocardial damage.

D. Kawasaki Disease

1. **Pathophysiology:** Microvasculitis of medium-sized muscular arteries. Immunologic activation causes cytokines to make vascular endothelium susceptible to lysis by antibodies. Myocarditis develops within 3 to 4 weeks and is associated with WBC infiltration and edema of the conduction system and myocardial muscle. Occasionally severe valvulitis and coronary artery dilation and aneurysms develop.
2. **Etiology** is unclear. It is more prevalent in children of Japanese ancestry and in children younger than 5 years of age. Seasonal outbreaks in winter and spring occur in geographic clusters.
3. **Signs and symptoms** include high, often spiking, fever (lasting 5 or more days); skin rash; conjunctivitis; injected, fissured lips and erythema of the buccal mucosa; strawberry tongue; cervical lymphadenopathy; and erythema and edema of the hands and feet followed by desquamation 2 to 4 weeks later. Other manifestations have been observed.
4. **Diagnostic studies**
   a. *Laboratory studies* are done to evaluate anemia, leukocytosis, thrombocytosis, elevated erythrocyte sedimentation rate (ESR), elevated serum amylase, liver function, C-reactive protein, pyuria, and proteinuria.
   b. *ECG* shows nonspecific ST-T wave changes, and there may be a prolonged PR interval.
   c. *ECHO* helps in diagnosing coronary aneurysms (may also need arteriography or angiography), pericardial effusions, ventricular dysfunction, and valvular insufficiency. Serial studies are done early and at 6 months.
   d. *Cardiac catheterization* is used to assess coronary aneurysms and stenosis (Figure 3-69).
5. **Nursing diagnoses**
   - ❖ Alteration in cardiac output
   - ❖ Potential for shock related to MI
   - ❖ Alteration in comfort

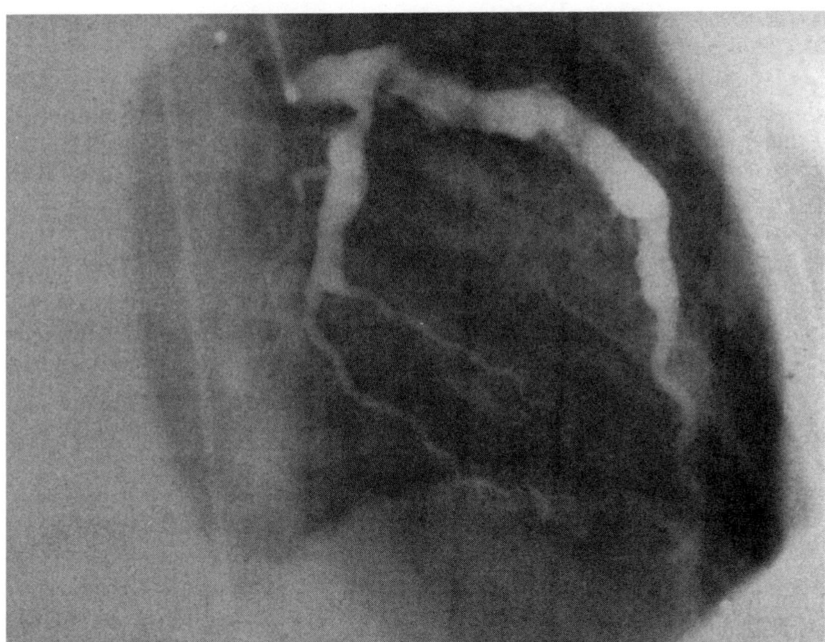

FIGURE 3-69 ■ Cineangiogram photo of aneurysms created by Kawasaki syndrome. (Courtesy of Children's National Medical Center.)

6. **Goals and desired outcomes**
   a. *Reestablish* and maintain hemodynamic stability.
   b. *Arrest* and control inflammatory processes.
   c. *Optimize* cardiac output.
   d. *Prevent* embolic damage and coronary involvement.
   e. *Optimize* level of comfort.
7. **Patient care management**
   a. *Anti-inflammatory agents* reduce inflammation and decrease the incidence of coronary abnormalities. Examples of agents are high-dose aspirin 30 to 100 mg/kg daily divided in 4 doses with IVIG 2 g/kg over 10 to 12 hours. Repeat doses of IVIG or pulse steroids are used if treatment fails (i.e., continued fever).
   b. *Serial ECGs and cardiac isoenzymes* are evaluated on a regular basis. Tissue plasminogen activator (tPA) is used if symptoms of an infarction develop. Coronary artery bypass graft can be used for large aneurysms or significant areas of stenosis.
   c. *Recovery* is usually complete in those who do not develop coronary vasculitis, although second attacks may occur. Regression of aneurysms can occur. The long-term impact of coronary vasculitis on future cardiovascular disease is not known.
8. **Complications** include coronary aneurysms. If an aneurysm is larger than 8 mm in size, there is a higher risk of infarct.

CARDIAC TRANSPLANTATION

A. Definition

Surgical replacement of the heart is used for end-stage, irreversible disease in which no other medical or surgical therapy will be successful.

B. Indications for Transplantation

Indications include end-stage cardiomyopathy, complex CHD not amenable to surgical repair, ischemic damage from anomalous left coronary artery, nonmalignant cardiac tumor not amenable to resection, or life-threatening arrhythmias not responsive to medical and surgical therapy.

C. Clinical Signs and Symptoms

Signs and symptoms are related to the underlying condition (see Cardiomyopathy, Congestive Heart Failure, Congenital Heart Disease).

D. Diagnostic Studies

1. *Cardiac evaluation* includes an ECG and ECHO and cardiac catheterization to assess function and PVR. A PVR greater than 4 Wood units is of concern, and a PVR greater than 8 Wood units is considered a contraindication. Exercise stress testing and Holter monitoring can evaluate for arrhythmias as a sign of myocardial dysfunction.
2. *Other organ system evaluation* includes neurologic examination, liver function studies, and renal function analysis by serum laboratory studies, creatinine clearance testing, and glomerular filtration rate renal scan. Serologies determine exposure to viral illnesses (used as baseline for future exposure as well), and cultures rule out current infection. Because of the risk of superinfection with immunosuppression, current infection is a relative contraindication to transplantation until the infection is appropriately treated.
3. *Immune system* is evaluated with human leukocyte antigen (HLA) testing (HLAs that determine tissue type, used retrospectively to determine degree of matching with donor), the percent of reactive antibody (PRA; antibodies within the blood to other human blood that can produce hyperacute rejection during transplant procedure), and other immune markers used to assess function of immune system cell lines (center specific).
4. *Genetic evaluation* rules out genetic syndromes that might produce disease or prevent optimum outcome from transplantation.
5. It is preferred that all organ systems have normal function to provide the best possible outcome of transplantation. Surgeons may accept relative abnormalities that can be explained by poor cardiac output and are reversible once transplantation occurs. Active malignancy is avoided. Recent pulmonary embolism or infarction is avoided because of the risk of pneumonia after transplantation.
6. *Financial screening interview* is used to determine insurance plan coverage for transplantation, to assess the family's ability to provide long-term medical care, and to assess drug coverage needed to provide expensive long-term immunosuppressive medications.
7. *Psychosocial evaluation* assesses the patient's or family's problems that might prevent positive outcomes of transplantation; identifies problem issues that may need to be addressed during the stress of waiting, transplantation, and long-term care; and considers drug and alcohol history, psychiatric disorders, child abuse and neglect history, and evidence of the family's inability to care for the child.

E. Nursing Diagnoses

- Alteration in cardiac output due to preoperative condition, ischemic heart during early operative recovery, or rejection
- Alteration in immune function
- Risk of infection
- Patient and family knowledge deficit

F. Goals and Patient Outcomes

1. **Establish** hemodynamic stability.
2. **Prevent** cardiac rejection and infection.

G. Patient Management

1. **Evaluate cardiovascular function** as with all postoperative cardiovascular surgery patients. Assess for bradycardia resulting from denervated heart, and prepare for the use of chronotropic agents such as isoproterenol (Isuprel) or pacing to maintain cardiac output. PVCs and short runs of VT may occur in the transplant patient; management is determined by hemodynamic status, frequency of occurrence, and the condition of the donor organ and time involved in transplanting the new heart.
2. **Assess for symptoms of rejection**, including fever, lethargy, malaise, decreased appetite, signs of CHF, decreased ECG voltage, decreased function by ECHO, and grade of rejection by endomyocardial biopsy.
3. **Provide immunosuppressive medications** (see Chapter 8 for further discussion of immunosuppression).
4. **Assess for signs and symptoms of infection.**

H. Complications

Complications include rejection, infection, lymphoproliferative disease, accelerated coronary artery disease, hypertension, renal failure, primary organ failure, and death.

CARDIAC TRAUMA

A. Pathophysiology

The pathophysiology of cardiac trauma depends on the mechanism of injury.

1. **Myocardial contusion** may cause bruising, swelling, muscle dysfunction, internal bleeding, and tamponade.
2. **Major vessel or cardiac rupture** can occur by narrowing the anteroposterior diameter of the chest. This results in rapid compression and expansion of vessel structures, which produce shearing forces, tearing the aorta, SVC, IVC, or atrial appendage leading to sudden massive blood loss with shock or tamponade (Figure 3-70).
3. **Cardiac tamponade** can occur from contusion or penetrating trauma, resulting in blood or fluid accumulation in the pericardial sac. The fluid accumulation impairs ventricular filling.

B. Etiology

1. **Compression** provides a direct blow when the sternum or ribs impact the heart. This can cause septal defects, wall or valve rupture, and coronary artery occlusion. Direct blows can cause fatal arrhythmias.
2. **Acceleration/deceleration injury** may result in avulsion or tears of the aorta, SVC, or IVC.
3. **Changes in intrachamber pressures** from crush of the abdomen produces blow out ruptures.
4. **Punctures** occur from fractured ribs, bullets, or knifes.

C. Signs and Symptoms

1. A high index of suspicion is seen with **rib fractures and other chest trauma**. A pliable thorax decreases the likelihood of rib fractures in children. With fractures of the first or second rib, look for aortic injury.

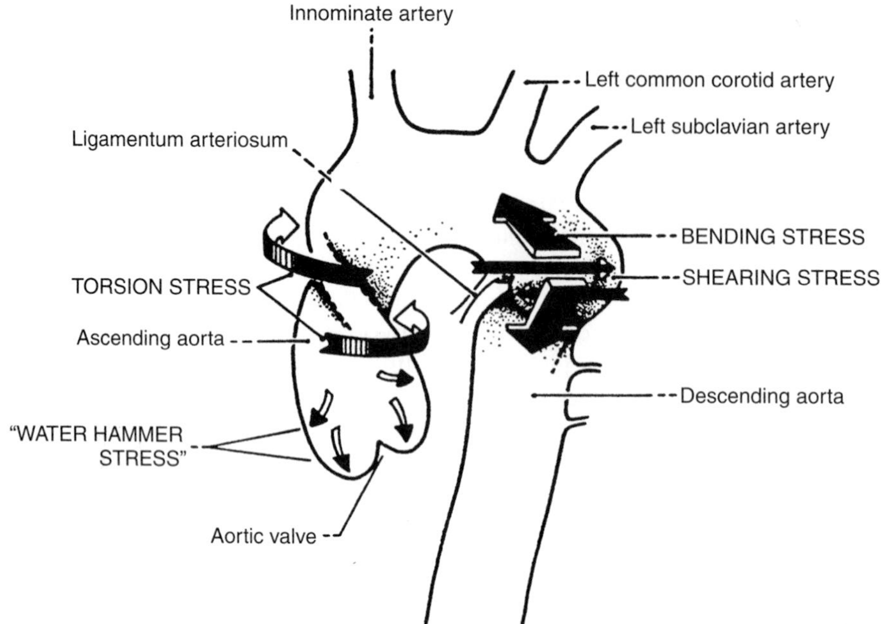

FIGURE 3-70 ■ Diagram of stresses producing trauma to great vessels. (Reprinted with permission from Synbas PN: *Trauma to the heart and great vessels.* Philadelphia, 1978, W.B. Saunders.)

2. **Symptoms of cardiac injury** include widening of the superior mediastinum on chest radiograph, deviation of the nasogastric tube from midline, chest pain, arrhythmias (particularly during transport), bruising on the chest, jugular venous distention, signs of shock, muffled heart sounds, higher BP in arms than legs, and pulsus paradoxus.

D. Diagnostic Studies

1. **Chest radiographic examination** may demonstrate changes in the cardiac shadow.
2. **ECG** is relatively insensitive but may show conduction problems such as RBBB.
3. **Cardiac enzymes** are evaluated. If creatine phosphokinase alone is high, it may be from skeletal muscle trauma. Enzyme levels may rise slowly if there is no period without blood flow.
4. **ECHO** is used to identify tamponade and show differential wall motion. A transesophageal ECHO is used to rule out aortic dissection if the mediastinum is widened.
5. **Aortogram or CT angiogram** defines aortic injuries.
6. **Radionuclide angiography** delineates vascular injuries.
7. **Pericardial tap** relieves the pressure of cardiac tamponade.

E. Nursing Diagnoses

- ❖ Alteration in cardiac output related to hypovolemic shock, inadequate tissue perfusion, arrhythmias, or cardiac tamponade
- ❖ Risk of infection related to emergency thoracotomy

F. Goals and Patient Outcomes

1. Reestablish and maintain hemodynamic stability.

2. Prevent the complications of cardiac tamponade, life-threatening arrhythmias, and infection.

G. Patient Management

1. **Treat shock** (see Shock).
2. **Surgical intervention** may be required, including pericardiocentesis or emergency thoracotomy.
3. **Endovascular stents** are used for aortic rupture if the risk of cardiopulmonary bypass or bleeding is high.
4. **Minimize shear stress** on aortic wall before repair with β-blockers.
5. **Support cardiac recovery** with the use of inotropic agents and afterload reduction.

H. Complications

Complications include exsanguination, cardiac arrest (mortality for traumatic cardiac arrest is very high), arrhythmias, and tamponade. (See also Multiple Trauma in Chapter 9.)

REFERENCES

Adams FH, Emmanoulides GC, Riemenschneider TA: *Moss' heart disease in infants, children, and adolescents,* ed 4, Baltimore, 1989, Williams & Wilkins.

Alexander MM, Brown MS: *Pediatric history taking and physical diagnosis for nurses.* St Louis, 1979, Mosby.

Alspach JG: *Core curriculum for critical care nursing,* ed 5, Philadelphia, 1998, W. B. Saunders.

American Academy of Pediatrics: Revised indications for the use of palivizumab and respiratory syncytial virus immune globulin intravenous for the prevention of respirtory syncytial virus infections. *Pediatrics* 112(6):1442-1452, 2003.

American Heart Association: *Pediatric advanced life support provider manual.* Dallas, 2002, American Heart Association.

Attin M: Electrophysiology study: a comprehensive review. *Am J Crit Care* 10: 260-273, 2001.

Ayoub EM: Acute rheumatic fever. In Allen HD, Clark EB, Gutgesell HB, Driscoll DJ, editors: *Moss and Adams' heart disease in infants, children, and adolescents,* ed 6, Philadelphia, 2001, Lippincott Williams & Wilkins.

Barkin RM, Rosen P: *Emergency pediatrics,* ed 3, St Louis, 1990, Mosby.

Benson DW: Advances in cardiovascular genetics and embryology: role of transcription factors in congenital heart disease. *Curr Opin Pediatr* 12:497-500, 2000.

Biller JA, Yeager AM: *The Harriet Lane handbook,* ed 9, Chicago, 1981, Year Book.

Bliss D, Silen M: Pediatric thoracic trauma. *Crit Care Med* 30(11 suppl):S409-S415, 2002.

Blume ED: Current status of heart transplantation in children: update 2003. *Pediatr Clin North Am* 50:1375-1391, 2003.

Booker PD: Pharmacological support for children with myocardial dysfunction. *Paediatr Anaesth* 12:5-25, 2002.

Boucek MM et al: The registry of the international society for heart and lung transplantation: sixth official pediatric report—2003. *J Heart Lung Transplant* 22(6): 636-652, 2003.

Bove EL: Surgical treatment for hypoplastic left heart syndrome. *Jpn J Thorac Cardiovasc Surg* 47(2):47-56, 1999.

Brogan PA et al: Kawasaki disease: an evidence based approach to diagnosis, treatment, and proposals for future research. *Arch Dis Child.* 86:286-290, 2002.

Brown JW et al: Surgery for aortic stenosis in children: a 40-years experience. *Ann Thorac Surg.* 76:1399-1411, 2003.

Burch M: Heart failure in the young. *Heart* 88:198-202, 2002.

Callow LB: Current stratgies in the nursing care of infants with hypoplastic left-heart syndrome undergoing first-stage palliation with the Norwood operation. *Heart Lung* 20:463-470, 1992.

Castaneda AR, Jonas RA, Mayer JE, Hanley FL: *Cardiac surgery of the neonate and infant.* Philadelphia, 1994, W. B. Saunders.

Charpie JR et al: Serial blood lactate measurements predict early outcome after neonatal repair or palliation for complex congenital heart disease. *J Thorac Cardiovasc Surg* 120(1):73-80, 2000.

Cowie MR, Mendez GF: BNP and congestive heart failure. *Prog Cardiovasc Dis* 44:293-321, 2002.

Craig J, Smith JB, Fineman LD: Tissue perfusion. In Curley MAQ, Moloney-Harmon PA, editors: *Critical care nursing of infants and children*, ed 2, Philadelphia, 2001, W. B. Saunders.

Cremer JT et al: Different approaches for minimally invasive closure of atrial septal defects. *Ann Thorac Surg* 67:1648-1652, 1999.

Danielson GK, Maloney JD, Devloo RAE: Surgical repair of Ebstein's anomaly. *Mayo Clinic Proc* 54:185-192, 1979.

Dearani JA et al: Late follow-up of 1095 patients undergoing operation for complex congenital heart disease utilizing pulmonary ventricle to PA conduits. *Ann Thorac Surg* 75:399-411, 2002.

Dearani JA et al: Surgical patent foramen ovale closure for prevention of paradoxical embolism-related cerebrovascular ischemic events. *Circulation* II:171-175, 1999.

Dichter CH, Curley MAQ: Shock. In Curley MAQ, Moloney-Harmon PA, editors: *Critical care nursing of infants and children*, ed 2. Philadelphia, 2001, W. B. Saunders.

Dorman BH et al: Magnesium supplementation in the prevention of arrhythmias in pediataric patients undergoing surgery for congenital heart defects. *Am Heart J* 139:522-528, 2000.

Duncan BW et al: Mechanical circulatory support in children with cardiac disease. *Ann Thorac Surg*. 73:1670-1677, 2002.

Eades SK: Pharmacotherapy of congenital heart defects. *J Pediatr Pharm Pract* 5(1): 15-34, 2000.

Feldman AM, McNamara D: Myocarditis. *N Engl J Med* 343:1388-1398, 2000.

Ferrieri P et al: Unique features of infective endocarditis in childhood. *Circulation* 105(17):2115-2131, 2002.

Flori HR et al: Transthoracic intracardiac catheters in pediatric patients recovering from congenital heart defect surgery: associated complications and outcomes. *Crit Care Med* 28:2997-3001, 2000.

Garson AG, Brecker TJ, McNamara DG: *The science and practice of pediatric cardiology*. Philadelphia, 1990, Lea & Febiger.

Geiger J et al: Intra-aortic balloon pumps in children: a small-nursing-team approach. *Crit Care Nurs* 17(3):79-86, 1997.

Genizi J et al: Kawasaki disease in very young infants: high prevalence of atypical presentation and coronary arteritis. *Clin Pediatr* 42:263-267, 2003.

Goldmuntz E: The epidemiology and genetics of congenital heart disease. *Clin Perinatol* 28(1):1-10, 2001.

Guyton AC: *Human physiology and mechanisms of disease*. Philadelphia, 1987, W. B. Saunders.

Hanisch D: Pediatric arrythmias. *J Pediatr Nurs* 16:351-362, 2001.

Hazinski MF: *Nursing care of the critically ill child*, ed 2, St Louis, 1992, Mosby-Year Book.

Hazinski MF: *Manual of pediatric critical care*. St Louis, 2003, Mosby.

Hoffman TM et al: The incidence of arrhythmias in a pediatric cardiac intensive care unit. *Pediatr Cardiol* 23:598-604, 2002.

Hoffman TM et al: Postoperative junctional ectopic tachycardia in children: incidence, risk factors, and treatment. *Ann Thorac Surg* 74:1607-1611, 2002.

Hutter PA et al: Twenty-five years' experience with the arterial switch operation. *J Thorac Cardiovasc Surg* 124(4):790-797, 2002.

Jesurum J: SVO_2 monitoring. *Crit Care Nurs* 21:79-83, 2001.

Kambam J: Cardiac anesthesia for infants and children, St Louis, 1994, Mosby.

Karl TR, Horton SB: Options for mechanical support in pediatric patients. In Goldstein DJ, Oz MC, editors: *Cardiac assist devices*. Armonk, NY, 2000, Futura Publishing.

Karmy-Jones R, Hoffer E, Meissner M, Bloch RD: Management of traumatic rupture of the thoracic aorta in pediatric patients. *Ann Thorac Surg* 75:1513-1517, 2003.

Katz AM: *Physiology of the heart*. New York, 1992, Raven Press.

Koch A, Singer H: Normal values of B type natriuretic peptide in infants, children and adolescents. *Heart* 89:875-878, 2003.

LeRoy S et al: Recommendations for preparing children and adolescents for invasive cardiac procedures. *Circulation* 108:2550-2564, 2003.

Lewin MB: The genetic basis of congenital heart disease. *Pediatr Ann* 29(8):469-480, 2000.

Liedel JL et al: Use of vasopressin in refractory hypotension in children with vasodilatory shock: five cases and a review of the literature. *Pediatr Crit Care Med* 3:15-18, 2002.

Linder CM, Suddaby EC, Mowery BD: Parental presence during resuscitation: help or hindrance? *Pediatr Nurs* 30(2), 2004.

Lipshultz SE, Sleeper LA, Towbin JA: The incidence of pediatric cardiomyopathy in two regions of the United States. *N Engl J Med* 348:1647-1655, 2003.

Luikart H: Pediatric cardiac transplantation: management issues. *J Pediatr Nurs* 16(5): 320-331, 2001.

Mann K, Berg RA, Nadkarni V: Beneficial effects of vasopressin in prolonged pediatric cardiac arrest: a case series. *Resuscitation* 52:149-156, 2002.

Marban E: Cardiac channelopathies. *Nature* 415:213-218, 2002.

Marx GR, Sherwood MC: Three-dimensional echocardiography in congenital heart disease: a continunuum of unfulfilled promises? No. A presently clinically applicable technology with an important future? Yes. *Pediatr Cardiol* 23:266-285, 2002.

Mavroudis C, Backer CL: *Pediatric cardiac surgery*, ed 3, Philadelphia, 2003, Mosby.

McElhinney DB et al: Management and outcomes of delayed sternal closure after cardiac surgery in neonates and infants. *Crit Care Med* 28:1180-1184, 2000.

McGahey PR: Family presence during pediatric resuscitation: a focus on staff. *Crit Care Nurse* 22(6):29-34, 2002.

McKee MR: Amiodarone—an "old" drug with new recommendations. *Curr Opin Pediatr* 15:193-199, 2003.

Meghani SH, Becker D: β-blockers: a new therapy in congestive heart failure. *Am J Crit Care* 10:417-427, 2001.

Mir TS et al: Plasma concentrations of aminoterminal pro atrial natriuretic peptide and aminoterminal pro brain natriuretic peptide in healthy neonates: marked and rapid increase after birth. *Pediatrics* 112:896-899, 2003.

Mir TS et al: Plasma concentrations of N-terminal pro-brain natriuretic peptide in control children from the neonatal to adolescent period and in children with congestive heart failure. *Pediatrics* 110(6):e76, 2002.

Mosca RS et al: Critical aortic stenosis in the neonate. *J Thorac Cardiovasc Surg* 109: 147-154, 1995.

Mowery B, Suddaby EC: ECG interpretation: what is different in children? *Pediatr Nurs* 27(3):224-229, 2001.

Nichols DG: *Critical heart disease in infants and children*, St Louis, 1999, Mosby.

Ohye RG et al: The Ross/Konno procedure in neonates and infants: intermediate-term survival and autograft funciton. *Ann Thorac Surg* 72:823-830, 2001.

Okubo M et al: Outcomes of intraoperative device closure of muscular ventricular septal defects. *Ann Thorac Surg* 72:416-423, 2001.

Overt C, et al: Balloon angioplasty of native coarctation: clinical outcomes and predicotra of success. *J Am Coll Cardiol* 35(4): 988-996, 2000.

Park MK: *Pediatric cardiology for practitioners*, ed 4, St Louis, 2002, Mosby.

Park MK, Guntheroth WG: *How to read pediatric ECGs*, St Louis, 1992, Mosby.

Paul S: Understanding advanced concepts in atrioventricular block. *Crit Care Nurs* 21:56-66, 2001.

Pearl JM, Permut LC, Laks H: Tricuspid atresia. In Baue AE et al, editors: *Glenn's thoracic and cardiovascular surgery*, ed 6, Stamford, CT, 1996, Appleton & Lange.

Prahash A, Lynch T: B-type natriuretic peptide: a diagnostic, prognostic, and therapeutic tool in heart failure. *Am J Crit Care* 13(1):46-55, 2004.

Ravishankar C, Tabbutt S, Wernovsky G: Critical care in cardiovascular medicine. *Curr Opin Pediatr* 15:443-453, 2003.

Reinhartz O et al: Multicenter experience with the Thoratec ventricular assist device in children and adolescents. *J Heart Lung Transplant* 20:439-448, 2001.

Rheuban KS: Pericardial diseases. In Allen HD, Clark EB, Gutgesell HP, Driscoll DJ, editors: *Moss and Adams' heart disease in infants, children, and adolescents*, ed 6, Philadelphia, 2001, Lippincott Williams & Wilkins.

Rosero SZ, Akiyama T: Newer indications for permanent pacemakers. *Comp Ther* 26(2):96-102, 2000.

Sanderson RG, Kurth CL: *The cardiac patient: a comprehensive approach*, ed 2, Philadelphia, 1983, W. B. Saunders.

Saulsbury FT: Comparison of high-dose and low-dose aspirin plus intravenous immunoglobulin in the treatment of Kawasaki syndrome. *Clin Pediatr* 41:597-601, 2002.

Schieken RM: Systemic hypertension. In Allen HD, Clark EB, Gutgesell HP, Driscoll DJ, editors: *Moss and Adams' heart disease in infants, children, and adolescents*, ed 6, Philadelphia, 2001, Lippincott Williams & Wilkins.

Seirafi PA et al. Repair of coarctation of the aorta during infancy minimizes the risk of late hypertension. *Ann Thorac Surg* 66:1378-1382, 1998.

Serwer GA, Dorostkar PC, LeRoy SS: Pediatric pacing and defribillator usage. In Ellenbogen KA, Kay GN, Wilkoff BL, editors: *Clinical cardiac pacing and defibrillation*, ed 2, Philadelphia, 2000, W. B. Saunders.

Shaddy RE: Optimizing treatment for chronic congestive heart failure in children. *Crit Care Med* 29 (suppl):S237-S240, 2001.

Shanley CJ et al: Primary unifocalization for the absence of interpericardial pulmonary arteries in the neonate. *J Thorac Cardiovasc Surg* 106:237-247, 1993.

Shillingford AJ, Weiner S: Maternal issues affecting the fetus. *Clin Perinatol* 28(1): 31-70, 2001.

Snider AR, Serwer GA: *Echocardiography in pediatric heart disease*. St Louis, 1990, Mosby.

Snyder M: Pediatric viral myocarditis. *Air Med J* 22(4):6-8, 2003.

Srivastava D, Olson EN: A genetic blueprint for cardiac development. *Nature* 407(9): 221-226, 2000.

Stausmire JM: Temporary epicardial pacing, *Crit Care Nurs* (100110):1-29, 1998.

Stiller B et al: Heart transplantation in children after mechanical circulatory support with pulsatile pneumatic assist device. *J Heart Lung Transplant* 22:1201-1208, 2003.

Suddaby EC: Contemporary thinking in congenital heart disease. *Pediatr Nursing* 27(3):231-237, 2001.

Suddaby EC, Schiller S: Management of chylothorax in children. *Pediatr Nursing* 30(4):290-295, 2004.

Synbas PN: *Trauma to the heart and great vessels*. Philadelphia, 1978, W. B. Saunders.

Takahashi M: Kawasaki syndrome (mucocutaneous lymph node syndrome). In Allen HD, Clark EB, Gutgesell HP, Driscoll DJ, editors: *Moss and Adams' heart disease in infants, children, and adolescents*, ed 6, Philadelphia, 2001, Lippincott Williams & Wilkins.

Towbin JA, Bowles NE: The failing heart. *Nature* 415:227-233, 2002.

Update on the 1987 Task Force Report on High BP in Children and Adolescents: A Working Group Report from the National High BP Education Program. *Pediatrics* 98:649-658, 1996.

Uzark K: Therapeutic cardiac catheterization for congenital heart disease—a new era in pediatric care. *J Pediatr Nurs* 16(5):300-307, 2001.

VanOrden Wallace CJ: Diagnosing and treating pacemaker syndrome. *Crit Care Nurs* 21(1):24-35, 2001.

Vick GW: Recent advances in pediatric cardiovascular MRI. *Curr Opin Pediatr* 15:454-462, 2003.

Vizgirda VM: The genetic basis for cardiac dysrhythmias and the long QT syndrome. *J Cardiovasc Nurs* 13(4):34-45, 1999.

Walsh EP: Clinical approach to diagnosis and acute management of tachycardias in children. In Walsh EP, Triendman JK, editors: *Cardiac arrhythmias in children and young adults with congenital heart disease*. Philadelphia, 2001, Lippincott Williams & Wilkins.

Ware LE: Inhaled nitric oxide in infants and children. *Crit Care Nurs Clin North Am* 14(1):1-6, 2002.

Weber M: Pulsus alternans a case study. *Crit Care Nurs* 23(8):51-54, 2003.

Wedekind CA, Fidler BD: Compatibility of commonly used intravenous infusions in a pediatric intensive care unit. *Crit Care Nurse* 21(4):45-51, 2001.

Wessel DL: Managing low cardiac output syndrome after congenital heart surgery. *Crit Care Med* 29:S220-S230, 2001.

Wiegand DLM: Advances in cardiac surgery: valve repair. *Crit Care Nurse* 23(2):72-91, 2003.

Wilson BA, Shannon MT, Stang CL: *Nurses drug guide 2004*. Upper Saddle River, NJ, 2004, Pearson Prentice Hall.

Windecker S et al: Percutaneous closure of patent foramen ovale in patients with paradoxical embolism. *Circulation* 2: 893-98, 1999.

Witherall CL: Cardiac rhythm control devices. *Crit Care Nurs Clin North Am* 6:95-102, 1994.

Wolfson BJ: Radiologic interpretation of congenital heart disease. *Clin Perinatol* 28:71-89, 2001.

Zales VR, Muster AJ: Balloon dilation angioplasty for the management of aortic coarctation. In Mavroudis C, Backer CL, editors: *Cardiac surgery: state of the art reviews*. Vol 7, Philadelphia, 1993, Hanley & Belfus.

CHAPTER

4 Neurologic System

PAULA VERNON-LEVETT

CENTRAL NERVOUS SYSTEM

A. Developmental Anatomy

1. **Embryogenesis:** The nervous system is one of the first organ systems to develop in the embryo (neurula).
   a. All body tissues are derived from three different *germ cell layers:*
   - ❖ Mesoderm forms future muscle, skeleton, connective tissue, and the cardiovascular and urogenital systems; assists in the early development of neural tissue; and forms notochord, which is incorporated into the future spinal column.
   - ❖ Endoderm forms the future gut and associated organs.
   - ❖ Surface ectoderm forms future skin, nails, epidermis, hair, and mammary glands; the neuroectoderm forms future neural tissue.

   b. *Neurulation* is the process of neural tube formation and development (Figure 4-1).
   - The *neural plate* is the specialized neuroectoderm cells of the embryo that thicken on either side of the neural groove (on the dorsal surface), forming a flat plate with distinct lateral edges present at approximately 20 days' gestation.
   - The neural groove is the anteroposterior groove in the ectoderm that appears at 2½ weeks' gestation. Development proceeds cranially.
   - The neural crest contains the specialized cells that originate from the neural plate but separate from it to form a parallel band extending the length of the neural plate. The neural crest gives rise to the future peripheral nervous system, spinal and autonomic ganglia, and some nonneural tissue (including the meninges). It is present at 3½ weeks' gestation.
   - The neural tube is formed by the lateral edges (folds) of the neural plate that fold and grow medially until they meet and form a tube. The cavity of the neural tube becomes the future ventricular system of the brain and central canal of the spinal cord. It is closed at 4 weeks' gestation.
   - Epidermal (sensory) placodes are composed of 9 or 10 pairs that arise from separate ectoderm thickening in the head region. Together with the neural crest, they give rise to cranial nerves and cranial sensory organs.

   c. *Brain development:* Further specialization of the neural tube forms three distinct swellings (vesicles) at the rostral end of the tube (Figure 4-2).
   - The neural tube forms three bulges (primary brain vesicles) at its cephalic end that develop future parts of the brain (represented at 4 weeks' gestation): prosencephalon (forebrain), mesencephalon (midbrain), and rhombencephalon (hindbrain).
   - Early in the second fetal month, two of the three primary brain vesicles further subdivide to form secondary vesicles. The prosencephalon forms

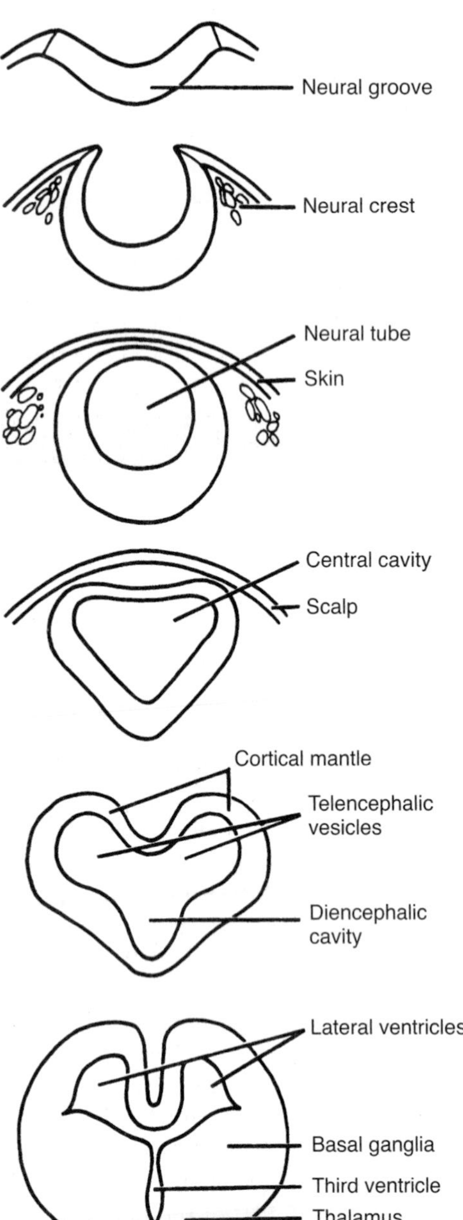

FIGURE 4-1 ■ Cross sections showing early development from neural groove to cerebrum.

(Reprinted with permission from Waxman SG: *Correlative neuroanatomy,* 23rd ed. Stamford, Conn., 1996, Appleton & Lange.)

the telencephalon (future preoptic region and paired cerebral hemispheres of the mature brain) and the diencephalon (future hypothalamus and thalamus of the mature brain). The mesencephalon remains the midbrain (future superior and inferior colliculi; red, reticular, and black nuclei; and cerebral peduncles of the mature brain). The rhombencephalon forms the metencephalon (future pons and cerebellum of the mature brain) and the myelencephalon (future medulla of the mature brain).

- Fissure formation begins in the fourth fetal month with development of the lateral sulcus (of the cerebrum) and the posterolateral sulcus (of the cerebellum). The central sulcus, calcarine sulcus, and parieto-occipital

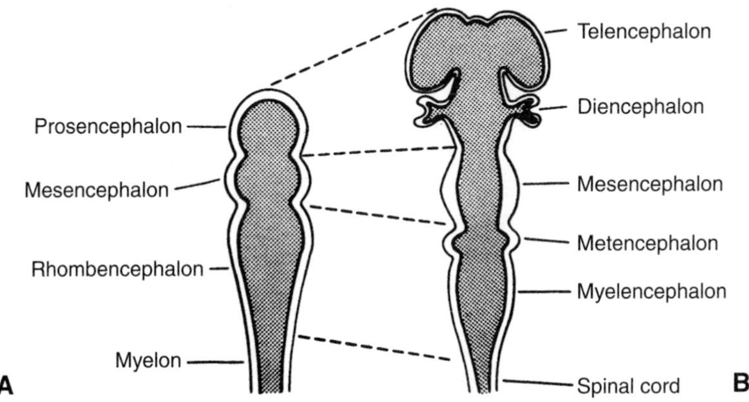

FIGURE 4-2 ■ Subdivisions of the embryonic human brain. **A,** Primary vesicles. **B,** Secondary vesicles.
(Reprinted with permission from Jensen D: *The human nervous system*. New York, 1980, Appleton-Century-Crofts.)

sulcus are visible in the fifth fetal month. All main gyri and sulci are present by the seventh fetal month.
- Myelinization of the brain begins at 10 months' gestation.

d. *Spinal cord development* begins from the caudal portion of the neural tube. The earliest nerve-fiber tracts appear around the second month. Long association tracts appear in the third month. Pyramidal tracts appear in the fifth month. Myelinization begins in the fifth month and is not completed in some tracts for 20 years.

e. *Neural tissue specialization*
- Neural tissue further differentiates into four concentric zones around the central canal that develop into specific areas of the mature brain. The *ventricular* zone is located adjacent to the central canal and is a precursor to neurons and macroglia. The *subventricular* zone generates certain classes of neurons and macroglia and some deep structures of the cerebrum. The *intermediate (mantle)* zone evolves into gray matter. The *marginal* zone has no primary cells of its own but evolves into most of the white matter.
- Sensory components of the central nervous system (CNS) develop from further divisions of the neural tube. The basal plate is the ventral portion of neural tube that contributes to the efferent (motor) system. The alar plate is the dorsal portion of the neural tube that contributes to the afferent (sensory) system.

2. Neuron and associated cells

a. The *neuron* is the functional and anatomic unit of the nervous system (Figure 4-3). The *cell body (soma)* contains the nucleus and gray matter. The *perikaryon (neuroplasm)* is cytoplasm surrounding the nucleus. The perikaryon contains granular, filamentous, and membranous organelles. Two types of neuronal processes include the dendrites and axons.
- Each neuron usually contains several dendrites that conduct impulses toward the cell body (afferent).
- Each neuron only has one axon. A myelin sheath encases some axons (white matter) and increases transmission of impulses. Nodes of Ranvier are anatomic interruptions in the myelin sheath. Axons conduct impulses away from the cell body (efferent).

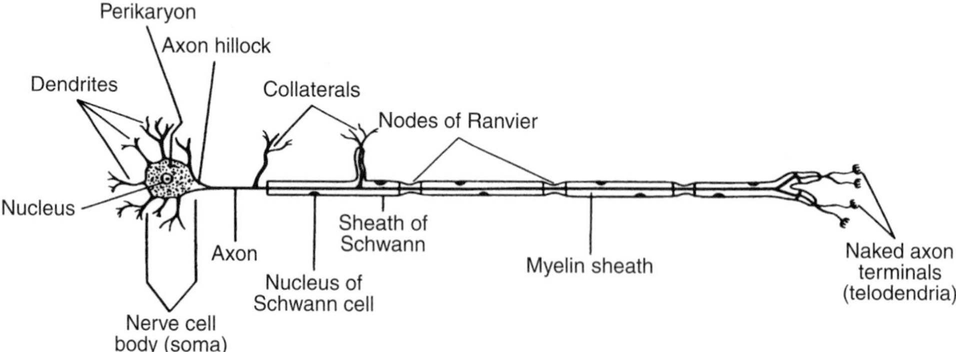

FIGURE 4-3 ■ The principal morphologic features of a peripheral motor neuron. The total length of the fiber has been shortened considerably.
(Reprinted with permission from Jensen D: *The human nervous system*. New York, 1980, Appleton-Century-Crofts.)

- The *synapse* is the site of contact of one neuron with another. The synaptic cleft is the space between the bouton of one neuron and the cell body of another. The *neuromuscular junction* is the termination of nerve fiber in muscle cell, and the neuroglandular junction is the termination of nerve fiber in glandular cell. The *presynaptic* membrane is the cell membrane of the axon at the synapse, and the *postsynaptic* membrane is the cell membrane of the dendrite to cell body, muscle, or glandular cell. The presynaptic vesicle is present in the cytoplasm of the bouton and contains the active neurotransmitter agents.

b. *Neuroglia* are the supporting and nourishing structures of the nervous system. There are four main types: oligodendrocytes (produce myelin), astrocytes (support, bind, and nourish neurons), microglial (phagocytic properties), and ependyma (line the ventricular system and choroid plexus and produce cerebrospinal fluid [CSF]).

3. **Extracerebral structures** (Figure 4-4)
   a. The *scalp* is composed of skin, subcutaneous tissue, galea aponeurotica, and pericranium.

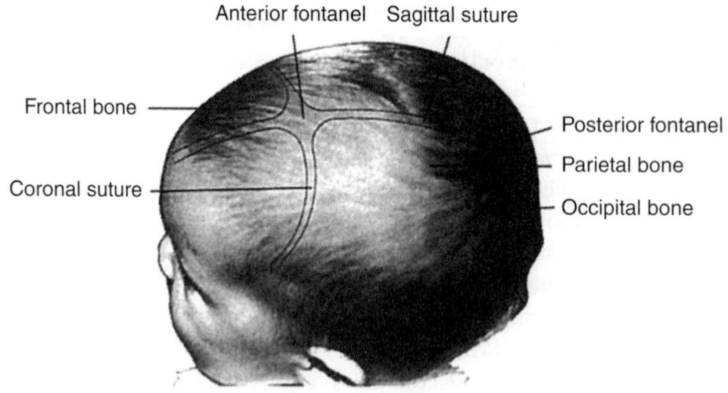

FIGURE 4-4 ■ Cranial sutures and fontanelles in infancy.
(Reprinted with permission from Betz CL, Hunsberger MM, Wright S: *Family-centered nursing care of children*, 2nd ed. Philadelphia, 1994, W. B. Saunders.)

b. The *skull* consists of eight bones: one frontal, two parietal, two temporal, one occipital, one ethmoid, and one sphenoid.

c. The *sutures* are dense, white, fibrous, connective tissue membranes that separate the bones. The sagittal suture separates the two parietal bones on top of the skull. The coronal suture (frontoparietal) connects the frontal and parietal bones transversely. The basilar suture is created by the junction of the basilar surface of the occipital bone with the posterior surface of the sphenoid bone. The lambdoid suture connects the parietal and occipital bones transversely.

d. The *fontanelles* are areas where several sutures join together. The posterior fontanelle is formed by the intersection of the sagittal and lambdoid sutures. Two anterolateral fontanelles are formed by intersection of the frontal, parietal, temporal, and sphenoid bones. The anterior fontanelle is formed by the intersection of the coronal and sagittal sutures. Two posterolateral fontanelles are formed by intersection of the parietal, occipital, and temporal bones. The posterior and anterolateral fontanelles close 2 months after birth. The anterior fontanelle closes between 12 and 18 months. The posterolateral closes at 24 months.

e. *Meninges* are three membranous connective tissue layers that cover the brain. The dura mater is the outermost layer and consists of two layers. The outer periosteum adheres to the inner surface of the skull and vertebrae. The inner layer divides the cerebral hemispheres (falx cerebri), cerebral hemispheres from the cerebellum and brainstem (tentorium cerebelli), and the two cerebellar hemispheres (falx cerebelli). The arachnoid is the middle transparent avascular covering with many fine collagen strands (trabeculae). The pia mater is the inner, delicate, clear membrane that adheres directly to the surface of the brain and spinal cord.

f. *Ventricular system and CSF circulation*

- The ventricles are four interconnecting chambers lined by ependyma. The paired lateral ventricles are contained within the cerebral hemispheres, subdivided into four parts: the anterior horn located in the frontal lobe, the body located in the parietal lobe, the inferior horn located in the temporal lobe, and the occipital horn located in the occipital lobe. The third ventricle is connected to the lateral ventricles via the foramen of Monro and connected to the fourth ventricle via the aqueduct of Sylvius. The fourth ventricle communicates with the third ventricle and subarachnoid space around the brain and spinal cord via three exit points. The foramen of Magendie exits to the cisterna magna (central canal of spinal cord) and the spinal subarachnoid space. The foramina of Luschka exit to the cisterna magna and the subarachnoid space around the brain.
- The choroid plexus is a three-layer membrane consisting of the choroid capillary endothelium, pial cells, and the choroid epithelium. It is located in all four ventricles and parenchyma and is responsible for CSF production.
- CSF is produced by the choroid plexus and, to a lesser degree, by ependymal cells lining the ventricles and spinal cord (Jensen, 1980). The rate of production of CSF varies by age (Swaiman, 1999). Newborns produce approximately 1 mL per hour. Adults produce approximately 30 mL per hour. The total volume of CSF in the ventricular system also varies by age (Swaiman, 1999): newborn, 50 mL; adult, 150 mL.
- Circulation of CSF is detailed in Figure 4-5. From the lateral ventricles, CSF passes to the third ventricle via the foramina of Monro. It travels from the third ventricle to the fourth ventricle via the aqueduct of Sylvius. The combined CSF volume passes through two lateral foramina of Luschka and

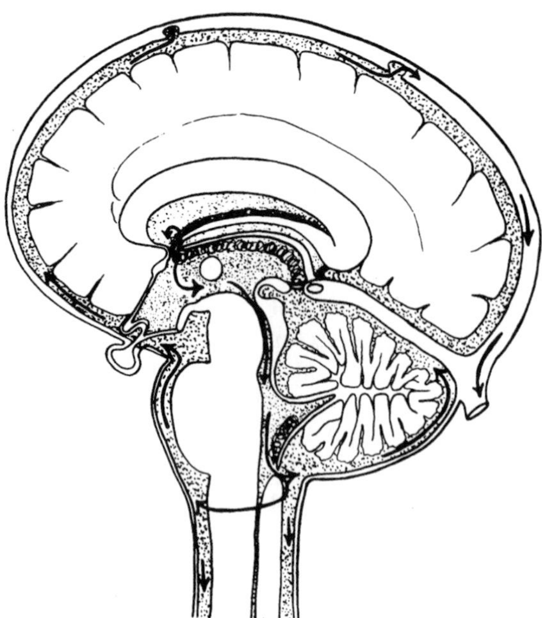

FIGURE 4-5 ■ Schematic representation of cerebrospinal fluid (CSF) circulation.

(Reprinted with permission from Behrman RE, Vaughan VC: *Nelson textbook of pediatrics,* 13th ed. Philadelphia, 1987, W. B. Saunders.)

the medial foramen of Magendie into the cisterna magna. CSF travels upward around the cerebrum via the subarachnoid space and downward around the spinal cord via the spinal subarachnoid space.

- Absorption occurs primarily through the arachnoid villi. Fingerlike projections from the arachnoid layer extending into the superior sagittal sinus function as one-way valves, allowing CSF to exit the sagittal sinus, but the projections prevent blood from entering the subarachnoid space. The rate of absorption depends on CSF pressure (higher pressures result in more absorption to a certain point) and venous pressure (higher venous pressures can impede absorption).
- Characteristics of normal CSF include the following: CSF is clear and odorless, glucose concentration is one half to one third of the serum glucose concentration, protein concentration is 15 to 45 mg/dl (higher in neonates), white blood cells (WBCs) are usually absent (however, a few may be present, especially in neonates), and red blood cells (RBCs) are absent except during traumatic lumbar tap. The opening pressure is dynamic related to the patient's body position and activities. The normal range is 60 to 180 cm H_2O.

4. The **brain** is divided into the cerebrum, diencephalon, brain stem, reticular formation, and the cerebellum.

   a. *Cerebrum (telencephalon)*

   - The *cerebral hemispheres* consist of four lobes (Figure 4-6): The frontal lobes hold the primary motor cortex, Broca's motor speech area (written and spoken language), and personality. The temporal lobes are responsible for reception and interpretation of auditory information, emotional and visceral responses, and retention of recent memory. The parietal lobe is responsible for comprehension of language, orientation of spatial relationships, and initial processing of tactile and proprioceptive information. The occipital lobe is responsible for the reception and interpretation of visual stimuli.
   - *Basal ganglia* are located deep in the cerebral hemispheres and are composed of four nuclei, providing unconscious control of lower motor neurons. The

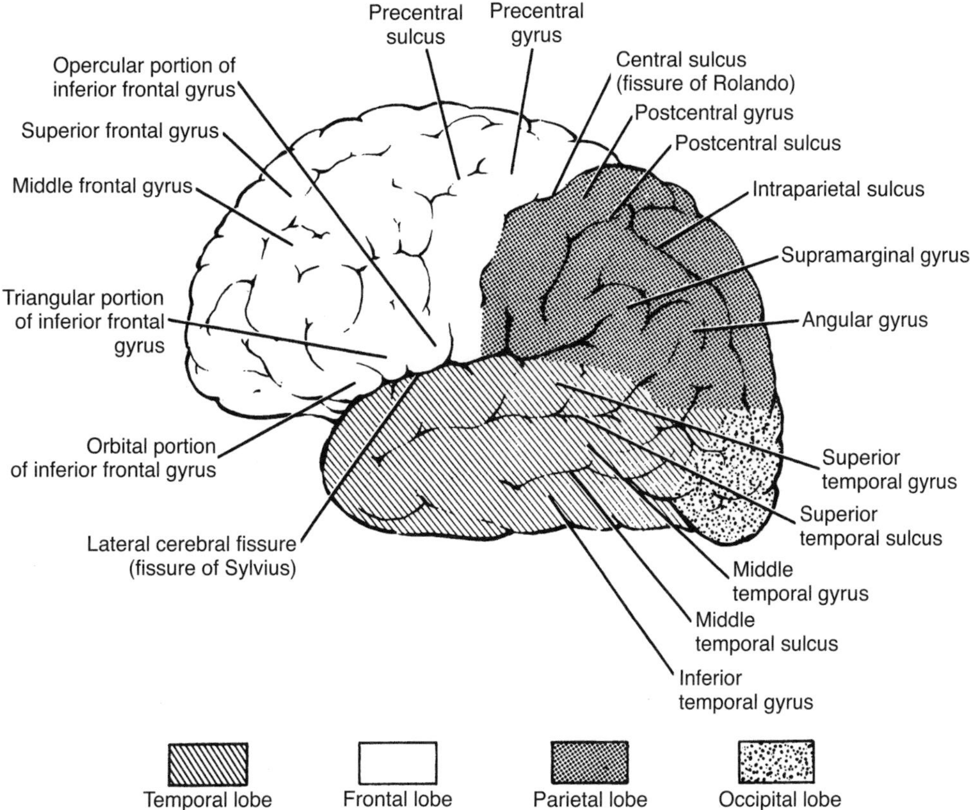

FIGURE 4-6 ■ Lateral view of the left cerebral hemisphere illustrating four lobes: temporal, frontal, parietal, occipital.
(Reprinted with permission from Waxman SG: *Correlative neuroanatomy,* 23rd ed. Stamford, Conn., 1996, Appleton & Lange.)

basal ganglia are processing stations, linking the cerebral cortex to specific thalamic nuclei.

- The *corpus callosum* is the largest commissural tract and is composed of a bundle of transverse nerve fibers connecting the two cerebral hemispheres. It transfers information between cerebral hemispheres and makes up the roof of the lateral ventricles and the third ventricle.
- The *limbic system* denotes several structures, including the limbic lobe, hippocampus and connections, amygdala, septal nuclei, hypothalamus, anterior thalamic nuclei, and portions of the basal ganglia. This system is primarily responsible for affective behavior and autonomic control.

b. The *diencephalon* is the rostral end of the brainstem and is located deep within the cerebrum. Sometimes it is classified as part of the brainstem. Anatomically it is divided into the following:

- The *epithalamus* is a narrow band forming the roof of the diencephalon. The epithalamus's exact function is not well understood, but it is associated with the limbic system, optic reflexes, and reproductive activity.
- The *thalami* are the largest subdivision of the diencephalon. Two egg-shaped masses are located deep in each cerebral hemisphere, and their primary function is to be a relay station for sensory input.

- The *hypothalamus* forms the base of the diencephalon and the floor and inferior lateral walls of the lateral ventricles. The primary function of the hypothalamus is physiologic homeostasis by regulating a number of visceral responses as well as more complex behavioral and emotional responses.
- The *subthalamus* is located lateral to the hypothalamus and is functionally integrated with the pyramidal system (Jensen, 1980).

c. The *brainstem* consists of three continuous structures (Figure 4-7).
   - The *mesencephalon (midbrain)* is located rostral on the brainstem between the diencephalon and metencephalon and is the origin of cranial nerves III and IV. The primary functions of the mesencephalon include serving as a relay center for visual and auditory reflexes and as the center for postural reflexes and the righting reflex (i.e., it maintains the head in an upright position).
   - The *metencephalon (pons)* is located above the medulla and ventral to the cerebellum; it serves as the origin of cranial nerves V, VI, VII, and VIII and contains nerve fibers that form the reticular formation and are continuous with other parts of the brain. The metencephalon also contains the medial longitudinal fasciculus (MLF) composed of efferent fibers. The pons helps to regulate respiration.
   - The *myelencephalon (medulla oblongata)* is continuous with the pons rostrally and the spinal cord caudally and is the origin of cranial nerves IX through

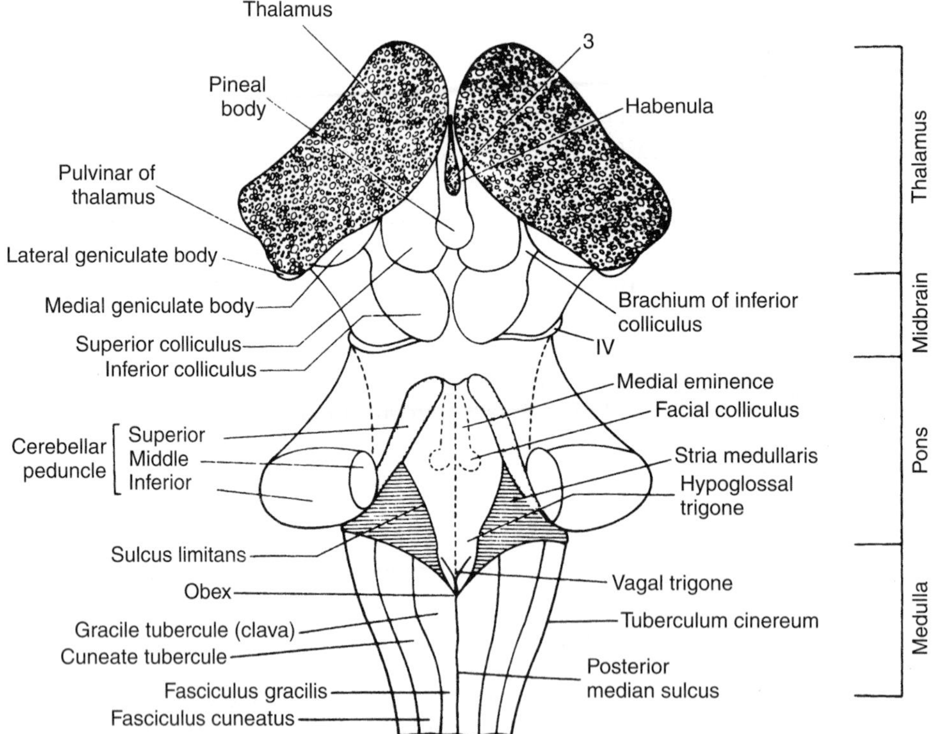

FIGURE 4-7 ■ Gross anatomic features of the brainstem, dorsal aspect. *3*, Third ventricle.

(Reprinted with permission from Jensen D: *The human nervous system*. New York, 1980, Appleton-Century-Crofts.)

XII. Primary functions of the myelencephalon include the primary respiratory and cardiac centers and the vasomotor centers.

d. The *reticular formation* is a diffuse network of neurons located in the brainstem. It begins at the upper end of the spinal cord and extends upward to the hypothalamus and adjacent areas. This formation contains both sensory and motor neurons, nuclei that interact with the extrapyramidal motor control system. The reticular formation is the site of the reticular-activating system (RAS), which assists in regulating awareness (sleep-wake cycles).

e. The *cerebellum* is located superior to the fourth ventricle and contains two lobes. It is connected to the brainstem via three pairs of fiber bundles (cerebellar peduncles). Primary functions of the cerebellum include coordination of voluntary movements, control of muscle tone, and maintenance of equilibrium.

5. Cerebral circulation

a. *Arterial blood* is supplied by two paired vessels, the common carotid arteries and the vertebral arteries.

- The common carotid arteries are located anteriorly; each bifurcates into two vessels. The internal carotid artery enters the cranial cavity and extends to the circle of Willis, where several major vessels meet. The anterior cerebral arteries supply the medial aspect of the cerebral hemispheres and the frontoparietal regions. The middle cerebral artery supplies much of the lateral aspect of the cerebral hemispheres and basal ganglia. The posterior cerebral arteries supply the lateral, medial, and inferior occipital cortex. The posterior communicating arteries connect anterior and posterior circulation.
- The external carotid arteries supply arterial circulation to the extracerebral structures (skin and muscle of the face and scalp).
- The vertebral arteries are located posteriorly; they originate from the subclavian arteries and join to form the basilar artery. Numerous vessels arise from the vertebral and basilar arteries and include the superior cerebellar artery, anterior inferior cerebellar artery, posterior inferior cerebellar artery, meningeal artery, anterior and posterior spinal arteries, and posterior cerebral arteries. Collectively, all the above vessels supply the cerebellum, brainstem, occipital lobe, and inferior and medial surfaces of the temporal lobes.

b. *Venous blood* is supplied by a network composed of valveless, thin-walled cerebral veins. The superficial veins drain the external surfaces of the brain and include the superior cerebral vein, middle cerebral vein, and inferior cerebral vein, which empty into the dural venous sinuses. The deep veins drain internal areas of the brain and include the basal veins, vein of Rosenthal, and the great vein of Galen. All venous drainage empties at the base of the skull via the internal jugular veins.

c. The *blood-brain barrier* is composed of the anatomic structures and physiologic processes that separate the brain and blood compartments. Brain capillaries are characterized by tight junctions among endothelial cells, astrocytes with foot processes that encase capillaries and neurons, and endothelial cells with large numbers of mitochondria (responsible for energy-dependent transport). The blood-brain barrier is believed to be incompletely developed in the preterm neonate (Johnston, 1998). Physiologic properties of the morphologic barrier prevent rapid transport of blood to the brain and maintain a delicate homeostatic balance within the internal brain environment. Chemical barriers restrict some substances, such as large serum-protein molecules and some chemotherapeutic agents. Substances easily transported across the membrane include water, oxygen, carbon dioxide, glucose, and some lipid-soluble substances such as alcohol and anesthetics.

d. The *blood-CSF barrier* is composed of the anatomic structures and physiologic processes that separate the brain and CSF compartments (functionally similar to blood-brain barrier). The morphologic barrier is created by high impermeability of choroid epithelial cells to most substances.

6. **Spinal cord and column**

a. The *spinal column* consists of 33 vertebrae: 7 cervical, 12 thoracic, 4 lumbar, 5 sacral, and 4 or 5 coccygeal segments (Figure 4-8).

b. *Vertebrae:* The cylinder body is located anteriorly and increases in size as it progresses downward. The posterior arch has two pedicles and two laminae.

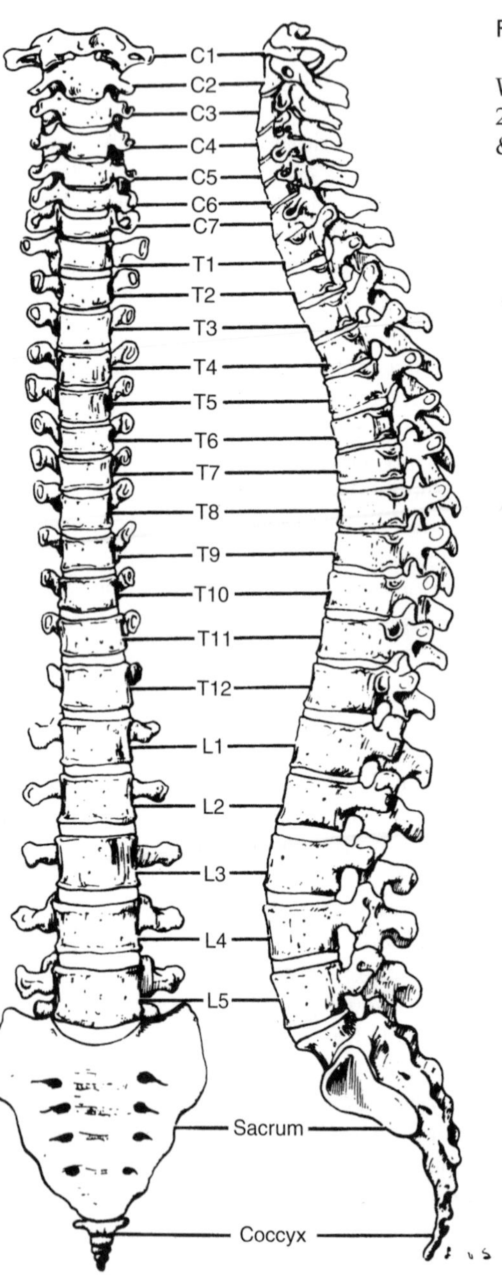

FIGURE 4-8 ■ The vertebral column. (Reprinted with permission from Waxman SG: *Correlative neuroanatomy*, 23rd ed. Stamford, Conn., 1996, Appleton & Lange.)

The pedicles project posterolaterally from the bodies and form part of the transverse foramen. The two laminae are located posteriorly and are thin and relatively long. The spinous processes are formed by fusion of the two laminae and vary in shape, size, and direction, depending on location. The transverse process is located on each side of the arch, providing a lever for muscle attachment. The articular processes (two superior and two inferior) form synovial joints with corresponding processes on adjacent vertebrae. The intervertebral foramina are formed by notches on the superior and inferior borders of the pedicles of the adjacent vertebrae, providing a channel for spinal vessels and nerves. The intervertebral discs are fibrocartilage tissue interposed between adjacent vertebrae consisting of an outer concentric layer of fibrous tissue (annulus fibrosus) and a central spongy pulp (nucleus pulposus). The discs provide an elastic buffer to absorb mechanical shocks.

c. The *spinal cord* is an extension of the medulla oblongata. It extends downward, tapering (conus medullaris), and terminates at the lower border of first lumbar vertebra in the adult and at the third lumbar vertebra in the neonate. The filum terminale is a slender, median, fibrous thread that extends from the conus medullaris to the coccyx.

- Outer coverings are continuous with the corresponding cerebral meninges. The *dura mater* consists of only one layer, does not adhere to vertebrae, and merges with the filum terminale. The spinal cord is suspended from the dura mater via a series of 22 pairs of denticulate ligaments. The epidural space is located between the dura layer and periosteum of the vertebrae. It contains venous plexuses and fat and is the location for injection of anesthetics. The *arachnoid* is nonvascular and extends caudally to the second sacral level, where it merges with the filum terminale. The subarachnoid space contains CSF and blood vessels and surrounds the spinal cord (spinal or lumbar cistern). The *pia mater* is directly attached to the spinal cord, its roots, and the filum terminale and is vascular.
- The inner core of the spinal cord is composed of gray and white matter. Butterfly- or H-shaped *gray matter* consists of cell bodies and unmyelinated fibers. They are anatomically and functionally divided into regions (Figure 4-9). The anterior (ventral) horns contain the neuronal cell bodies of motor neurons supplying the skeletal muscles. The posterior (dorsal) horns contain the neuronal cell bodies involved in sensory input to the spinal cord. The lateral horns contain preganglionic fibers of the ANS.
- *White matter* surrounds the gray matter and consists of myelinated (predominately) and unmyelinated fibers. They are arranged into three pairs of funiculi (columns): posterior, lateral, and anterior. Funiculi are subdivided into bundles of nerve fibers (tracts or fasciculi) that are functionally distinct. Ascending (sensory) pathways transmit sensory information from peripheral receptors to the cerebral and cerebellar cortex and transmit pain, touch, temperature, spatial relationships, vibration, passive movement, and position sense. Descending (motor) pathways contain upper motor neurons, originate from the cerebrum, and descend to the spinal cord (and brainstem). They play a major role in voluntary motor movement. The central canal is lined with ependymal cells, contains CSF, and is continuous with the fourth ventricle in the medulla oblongata. Tracts are of clinical significance (Table 4-1) and are named based on the column in which the tract travels, the origination of cells, and the termination of fibers.

d. The *reflex arc* is an intrinsic neural circuit that, once activated, follows a specific response without conscious control. The *monosynaptic reflex arc* consists of a

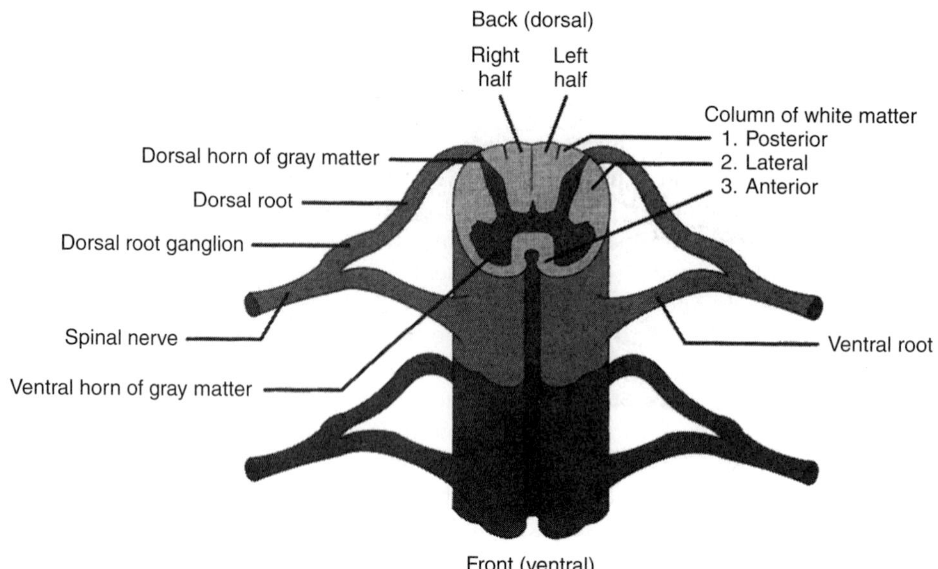

FIGURE 4-9 ■ Cross section of spinal cord.
(Reprinted with permission from Curley MAQ, Moloney-Harmon P: *Critical care nursing of infants and children*. Philadelphia, 2001, W. B. Saunders.)

TABLE 4-1
Common Ascending and Descending Spinal Tracts

Tract Name	Function
ASCENDING (SENSORY)	
Dorsal (posterior) spinocerebellar	Proprioception
Ventral (anterior) spinocerebellar	Proprioception
Lateral spinothalamic	Pain, temperature
Ventral (anterior) spinothalamic	Touch, pressure
DESCENDING (MOTOR)	
Corticospinal (pyramidal tracts)	
Ventral (anterior) corticospinal	Skilled voluntary movements
Lateral corticospinal	Skilled voluntary movements
Rubrospinal	Fine movements, muscle tone
Vestibulospinal	Aid equilibrium, extensor muscle tone
Reticulospinal	Posture, muscle tone
Tectospinal	Mediates optic and auditory reflex movement

From Curley MAQ, Vernon-Levett P: *Critical care nursing of infants and children.* Philadelphia, 2001, WB Saunders.

sensory end-organ (receptor), afferent nerve fibers, one synapse, efferent nerve fibers, and muscle fiber or glandular cell (effector). A classic example is a deep tendon reflex (Figure 4-10). The *polysynaptic reflex arc* consists of a sensory end organ, afferent nerve fibers, multiple interneurons and synapses, efferent nerve fibers, and an effector. A classic example is withdrawal of an extremity from pain stimuli.

7. **Spinal column circulation:** Arterial blood is supplied from branches of vertebral arteries and the radicular arteries derived from segmental vessels (i.e., deep

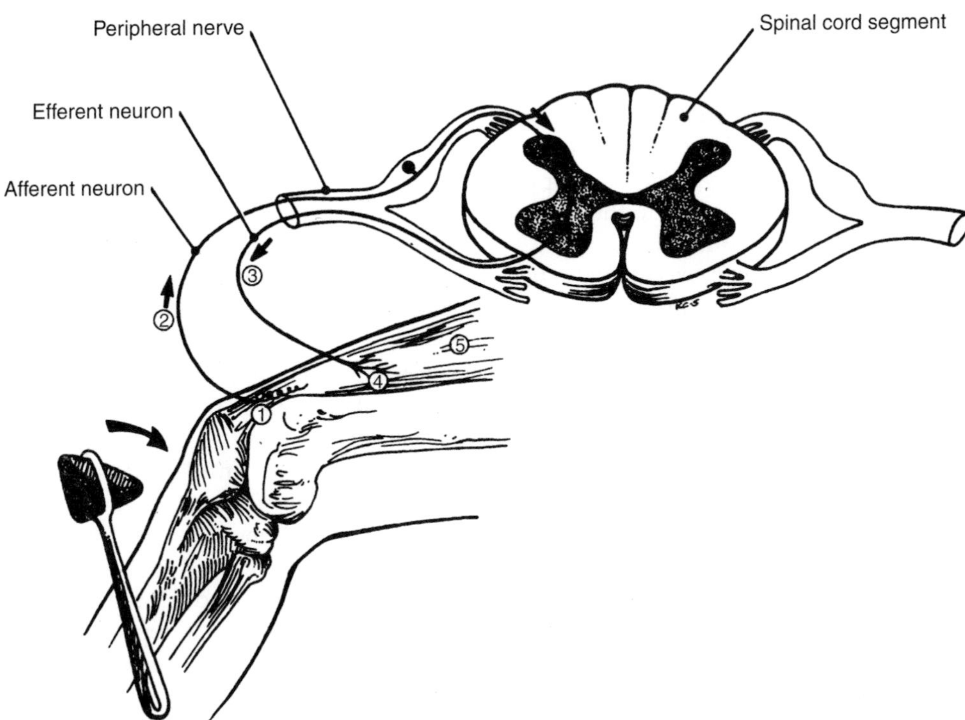

FIGURE 4-10 ■ Simple reflex arc (knee-jerk reflex). *1*, The receptor, the sensory nerve fiber that first picks up the impulse as the hammer strikes the tendon; *2*, the sensory transmitter, the afferent neuron that passes the impulse to the spinal cord; *3*, the motor transmitter, the efferent neuron that passes the impulse to the effector (muscle); *4*, the neuroeffector junction, a specialized endplate of motor nerves; *5*, the effector, a muscle that carries out the actual response (jerking of knee).
(Reprinted with permission from Abels L: *Critical care nursing: a physiologic approach.* St. Louis, 1986, Mosby.)

cervical, intercostal, lumbar, and sacral arteries). The arteries pass through the intervertebral foramina and divide into two branches: the smaller anterior spinal artery and the larger posterior spinal artery. Venous drainage is via the venous plexus and the veins that parallel arteries.

B. Developmental Physiology

1. Impulse conduction

a. During the *resting membrane potential (RMP)* (i.e., not conducting a nerve impulse), the intracellular fluid (neuroplasm) of a neuron has a more negative electrical charge than extracellular fluid. Na^+ and Cl^- are in higher concentrations in extracellular fluid, and K^+ is present in higher concentrations in intracellular fluid. Concentrations are maintained by ionic pumps.

b. As *depolarization* occurs in response to an electrochemical stimulus, the cell membrane becomes more permeable to Na^+. Na^+ enters the cell, and the membrane becomes less negative internally. Initial depolarization must be greater than a certain threshold value for depolarization to continue.

c. The *action potential* is the response of the neuron to depolarization. Impulsive flow of ionic current is produced briefly. After a brief delay, the membrane potential shifts back to negative. Na^+ flow is inactivated, and K^+ permeability increases.

d. *Repolarization* is the reestablishment of negative polarity of the RMP. The cell membrane becomes impermeable to Na^+ and more permeable to K^+. RMP returns to normal via the sodium-potassium pump.
e. The *action potential* is self-propagating and is an all-or-none phenomenon. The impulse travels as a full-blown force or not at all. The action potential in a myelinated nerve fiber is propagated by saltatory conduction, jumping from one node of Ranvier to the next node of Ranvier. Myelin improves conduction of action potentials.
f. The *presynaptic membrane action potential* activates the release of neurotransmitters contained in vesicles. Neurotransmitters diffuse across the synapse, producing a synaptic delay.
g. The *postsynaptic membrane* contains receptors that combine with neurotransmitters to alter the membrane permeability to specific ions. Excitatory neurotransmitters include glutamate, aspartate, and acetylcholine. The receptor responds with increased permeability for Na^+ and K^+, net influx of Na^+, and cell-membrane changes in a depolarizing direction (excitatory postsynaptic potential [EPSP]), and it initiates an action potential. Inhibitory neurotransmitters include glycine and γ-aminobutyric acid (GABA). The receptor responds with an increase in permeability for K^+ and Cl^- but not Na^+, an outward flow of K^+, and cell-membrane potential shifts in a hypopolarizing direction (inhibitory postsynaptic potential [IPSP]), decreases excitability, and inhibits an action potential.

2. **Intracranial pressure (ICP) dynamics**
a. *Modified Monro-Kellie doctrine:* The rigid skull contains three volume compartments: brain tissue (80% to 90%), CSF (5% to 10%), and blood (5% to 10%). If any one or more of the volume compartments increase, there must be a reciprocal change in one or more of the other volume compartments to maintain pressure equilibrium:
b. Intracranial volume = $Vol_{brain} + Vol_{CSF} + Vol_{blood}$
c. *Pressure-volume relationships*
- Normal ICP varies in different age groups and is lowest during infancy (Welch, 1980):
- Newborn: 0.7 – 1.5 mm Hg
- Infants: 1.5 – 6 mm Hg
- Children: 3 – 7.5 mm Hg
- Adult: Less than 10 mm Hg
- The volume-pressure curve represents the relationship between changes in intracranial volume and the resulting ICP (Figure 4-11). Elastance is the change in pressure that occurs with a change in volume ($\Delta P/\Delta V$). Compliance is the inverse relationship of elastance ($\Delta V/\Delta P$). The ICP curve is not linear but a three-phase hyperbolic curve. *Phase 1*, the compensatory phase, is the flat portion of the curve, reflecting good compliance and normal ICP. Temporary increases in ICP are "buffered" by several mechanisms: CSF translocation to the spinal subarachnoid space, venous blood displaced to the extracranial compartment through valveless veins, and decreased production or increased reabsorption of CSF. *Phase 2* is the exponential portion of the curve, representing early decompensation with normal ICP but poor compliance (i.e., slight increases in volume are not tolerated). The critical point when compliance is lost varies and depends on several factors: rate of volumetric change (rapid increases in ICP are not tolerated well), age (younger child has less buffering capacity with acute increases in ICP), and medical interventions. *Phase 3* is the steep portion of

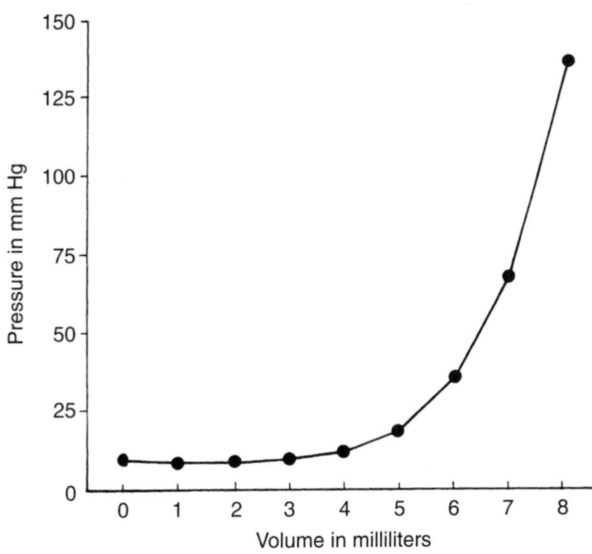

FIGURE 4-11 ■ The relationship between volume and pressure within the intracranial space.

As the volume reaches the point where pressure begins to rise, small increases in volume cause large rises in intracranial pressure.

(Reprinted with permission from Marshall SB, Marshall LF, Vos HR, Chestnut RM: *Neuroscience critical care: pathophysiology and patient management*. Philadelphia, 1990, W. B. Saunders.)

the curve, representing the failure of compensation with increased ICP and poor compliance.

3. **Brain metabolism**
   a. *Oxygen:* Twenty percent of cardiac output is delivered to the brain, although the brain is only 2% of the total body weight. Brain cells require a constant and consistent delivery of oxygen and are dependent on aerobic metabolism. The cerebral metabolic rate of oxygen ($CMRo_2$) is approximately 3 to 3.5 mL/100 g per minute in the adult, but it is not consistent throughout the brain. The exact $CMRo_2$ in the neonate and infant is unknown.
   b. *Glucose:* Glucose stores in the brain are minimal; therefore cells also require a constant and consistent delivery of glucose. Glucose is associated with significant brain cellular processes, including protein synthesis, amino acid metabolism, neurotransmitter release, membrane function, and pH homeostasis. The cerebral metabolic rate of glucose ($CMR_{glucose}$) is 4.5 to 5.5 mg/100 g per minute in the adult. The exact $CMR_{glucose}$ in the neonate and infant is unknown. Hypoglycemia and hyperglycemia can cause neurologic damage (Sieber and Traystman, 1992).
4. **Cerebral blood flow (CBF)**
   a. *Normal CBF* in the brain of the neonate is widely variable and has an unknown lower limit (Altman et al., 1988). The actual delivery of oxygen to the tissues is affected by the percent of circulating fetal hemoglobin. The child's CBF is 105 mL/100 g per minute (Jensen, 1980). Adolescents and adults have a CBF of 55 mL/100 g per minute.
   b. *Determinants of CBF*
      - The smaller the arteriolar radius, the greater the resistance to CBF. The mechanisms that change the caliber of the vessel are cerebral autoregulation and chemical regulation. Autoregulation is a compensatory mechanism that matches CBF to CMR by altering the radius of the cerebral vessels (i.e., vasoconstriction or vasodilation). A constant CBF is maintained when the mean arterial pressure (MAP) is between 50 and 150 mm Hg. The $Paco_2$ (pH) affects the cerebral arteriolar radius: low $Paco_2$ (elevated pH) causes vasoconstriction, and high $Paco_2$ (decreased pH) causes vasodilation. Pao_2, to a lesser extent, affects the cerebral arteriolar radius: Pao_2 less than 50 mm Hg

causes vasodilation, and PaO_2 greater than 50 mm Hg causes vasoconstriction but remains constant. Increased blood viscosity (polycythemia) decreases CBF. The length of the vascular bed is constant at any point in time. Increased length increases resistance to CBF.

- *Cerebral perfusion pressure (CPP)* represents the pressure difference between inflow (arterial) pressure and outflow (venous) pressure across the cerebral vascular bed. Clinically, it is most often calculated by the following equation: CPP = MAP – ICP
- Normal CPP in the neonate is unknown. The child's CPP should be greater than 50 mm Hg, and the adolescent's CPP should be greater than 60 mm Hg.

PERIPHERAL NERVOUS SYSTEM

A. Developmental Anatomy

1. Sensory and motor components

a. *Spinal nerves* are connected to the spinal cord via two roots.

- The *dorsal (posterior) root* carries afferent (sensory) fibers that transmit impulses from sensory receptors in the body to the spinal cord. The fibers supply the innervation for a particular segment of the body called a *dermatome* (Figure 4-12). *Afferent fibers* are subdivided according to their function. General somatic afferent (GSA) fibers transmit impulses from sensors in the extremities and body wall. General visceral afferent (GVA) fibers transmit impulses from sensors in the viscera.
- The *ventral (anterior) root* carries efferent (motor) fibers that transmit impulses from the spinal cord. Efferent fibers are subdivided according to function. General somatic efferent (GSE) fibers innervate voluntary striated muscle. General visceral efferent (GVE) fibers innervate involuntary smooth muscles, cardiac muscle, and glands.
- Fusion of the roots forms 31 spinal nerves: 8 pairs of cervical, 12 pairs of thoracic, 5 pairs of lumbar, 5 pairs of sacral, and 1 coccygeal. Cauda equina (horse's tail) is the long root of lumbar and sacral nerves contained within the spinal cistern (the spinal cord is shorter than the vertebral column). Thoracic, lumbar, and sacral nerves are numbered according to the vertebra just rostral to the foramen through which they pass. Cervical nerves are numbered for the vertebra just caudal to the foramen through which they pass. Fibers are also classified functionally according to conduction velocity.

b. *Cranial nerves* are the peripheral nerves of the brain. Cranial nerve I originates from the cerebrum, and cranial nerves II through XII originate from the brainstem

- *Classification* by type and function is described in Table 4-2.

c. *The ANS*

- Components of the ANS are located in the CNS and the peripheral nervous system. The primary (preganglionic) neuron originates in the CNS. The axon of the primary neuron travels outside the CNS to synapse on a secondary (postganglionic) neuron found in one of the autonomic ganglia. The postganglionic fiber terminates in an organ or structure.
- In the *sympathetic (thoracolumbar) division* (Figure 4-13), preganglionic fibers originate in the intermediolateral cell column of segments T1 through T12. Fibers emerge from the spinal cord through the ventral roots and branch into the white rami communicants. White rami communicants send fibers

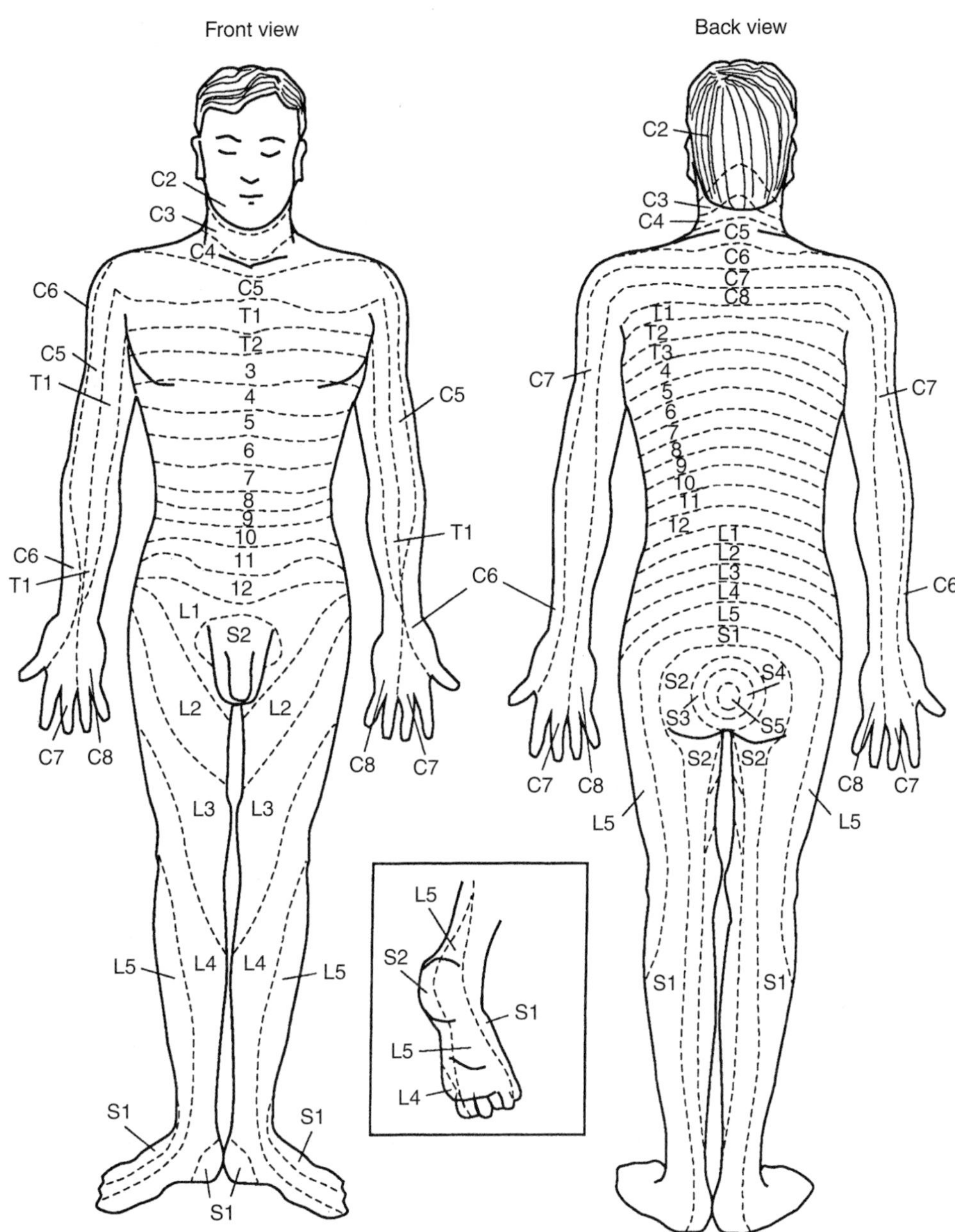

FIGURE 4-12 ■ Dermatomes.
(Reprinted with permission from Cardona VD et al.: *Trauma nursing from resuscitation through rehabilitation,* 2nd ed. Philadelphia, 1994, W. B. Saunders.)

to the paired trunk ganglia (located laterally on each side of the thoracic and lumbar vertebrae), where they synapse with postganglionic fibers. The postganglionic fibers exit the trunk ganglia and innervate different organs and structures. T1 to T5 are to the head and neck; T1 and T2 to the eye; T2 to T6 to the heart and lungs; T6 to L2 to the abdominal viscera; and L1 and L2 are to the urinary, genital, and lower digestive systems.

TABLE 4-2
Classification of Cranial Nerves

Cranial Nerve	Name	Type	Function
I	Olfactory	Sensory	Olfaction
II	Optic	Sensory	Vision
III	Oculomotor	Motor	Pupillary constriction and accommodation, extraocular movements, elevation of upper eyelid
IV	Trochlear	Sensory and motor	Deviation of the eye (inward on adduction, downward on abduction)
V	Trigeminal	Sensory and motor	Muscles of mastication; sensory innervation of the face, nose, and mouth
VI	Abducens	Motor	Lateral deviation of the eye
VII	Facial	Sensory and motor	Muscles of facial expression; sensory components of taste and salivation
VIII	Acoustic	Sensory	Hearing and balance
IX	Glossopharyngeal	Sensory and motor	Motor to pharyngeal region (swallowing); salivation and taste; thermal sensations from posterior tongue, tonsils, and eustachian tubes
X	Vagus	Sensory and motor	Sensory innervation of the larynx and pharynx; motor innervation of the palate and pharynx; and parasympathetic functions
XI	Spinal accessory	Motor	Motor innervation of the sternocleidomastoid muscle and the upper portion of the trapezius muscle (shoulder shrug, turning head)
XII	Hypoglossal	Motor	Movement of the tongue

- In the *parasympathetic (craniosacral) division* (Figure 4-14), preganglionic fibers originate from two areas: brainstem preganglionic fibers (often travel in the cranial nerves, specifically cranial nerves III, VII, IX, and X) and the middle segments of the sacral region. Nerve fibers are distributed exclusively to visceral organs. Most preganglionic fibers have long axons that synapse with a few postganglionic fibers with short axons. The synapse usually occurs in the end organ. The cranial fibers innervate visceral structures, including the head, thoracic cavity, and abdominal cavity. The sacral fibers give rise to the pelvic nerve, which innervates most of the large intestine, pelvic viscera, and genitalia.

B. Essential Physiology

1. **Neural transmission** in the ANS occurs via neurotransmitters. Sympathetic-division preganglionic nerve terminals secrete acetylcholine (cholinergic), postganglionic nerve terminals secrete norepinephrine (adrenergic), and the postganglionic nerve terminals to sweat glands secrete acetylcholine. Parasympathetic division preganglionic nerve terminals secrete acetylcholine, and postganglionic nerve terminals secrete acetylcholine. Acetylcholine is deactivated by cholinesterase. Norepinephrine is deactivated by monoamine oxidase (MAO) and catechol *O*-methyltransferase (COMT).

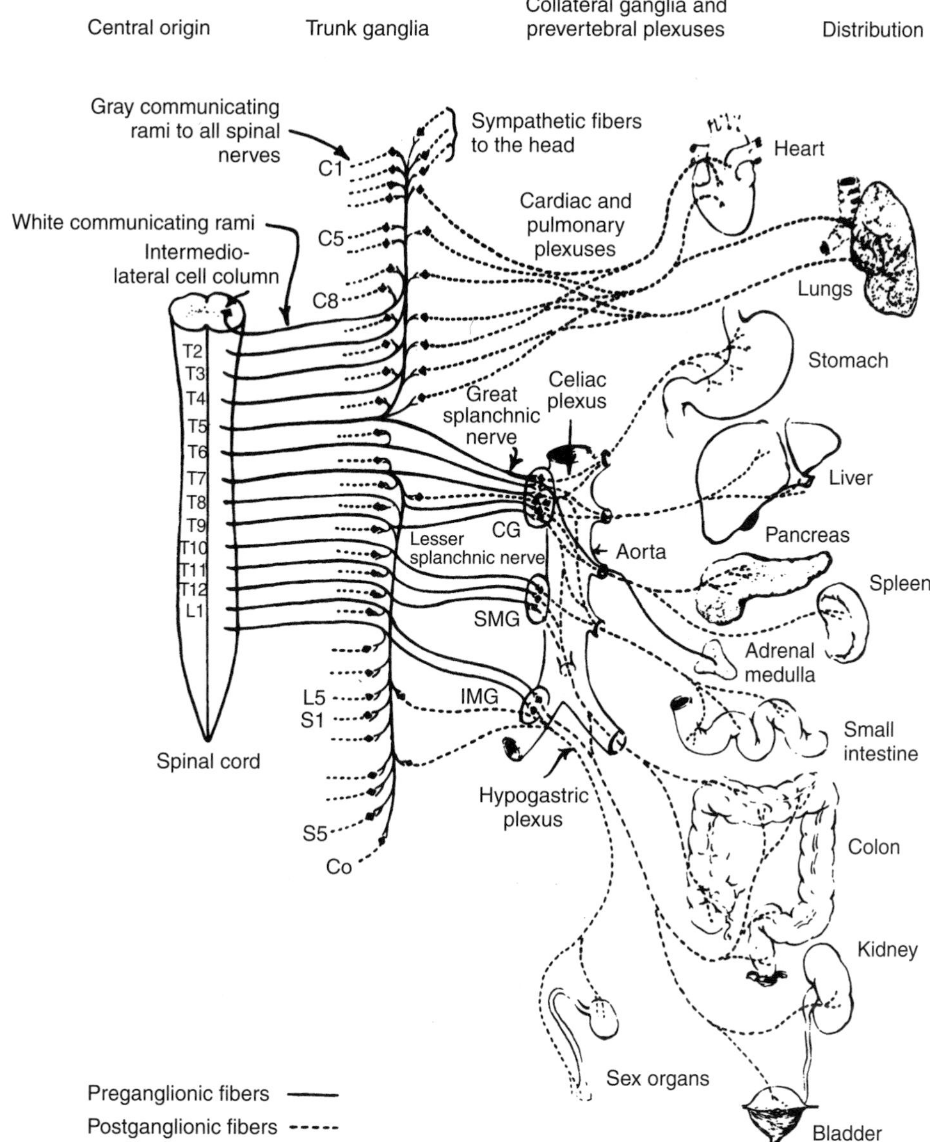

FIGURE 4-13 ■ Sympathetic division of the autonomic nervous system *(left half)*.
CG, celiac ganglion; *SMG*, superior mesenteric ganglion; *IMG*, inferior mesenteric ganglion.
(Reprinted with permission from Waxman SG: *Correlative neuroanatomy*, 23rd ed. East Norwalk, Conn., 1996, Appleton & Lange.)

2. **Systemic effects of ANS innervation** (Table 4-3): The sympathetic division is organized to exert influences over widespread body regions. Stimulation prepares the body for intense muscular activity, such as in the "fight or flight" response. The parasympathetic division is organized to exert influences in localized discrete areas of the body. Stimulation prepares the body primarily for "resting" bodily functions.

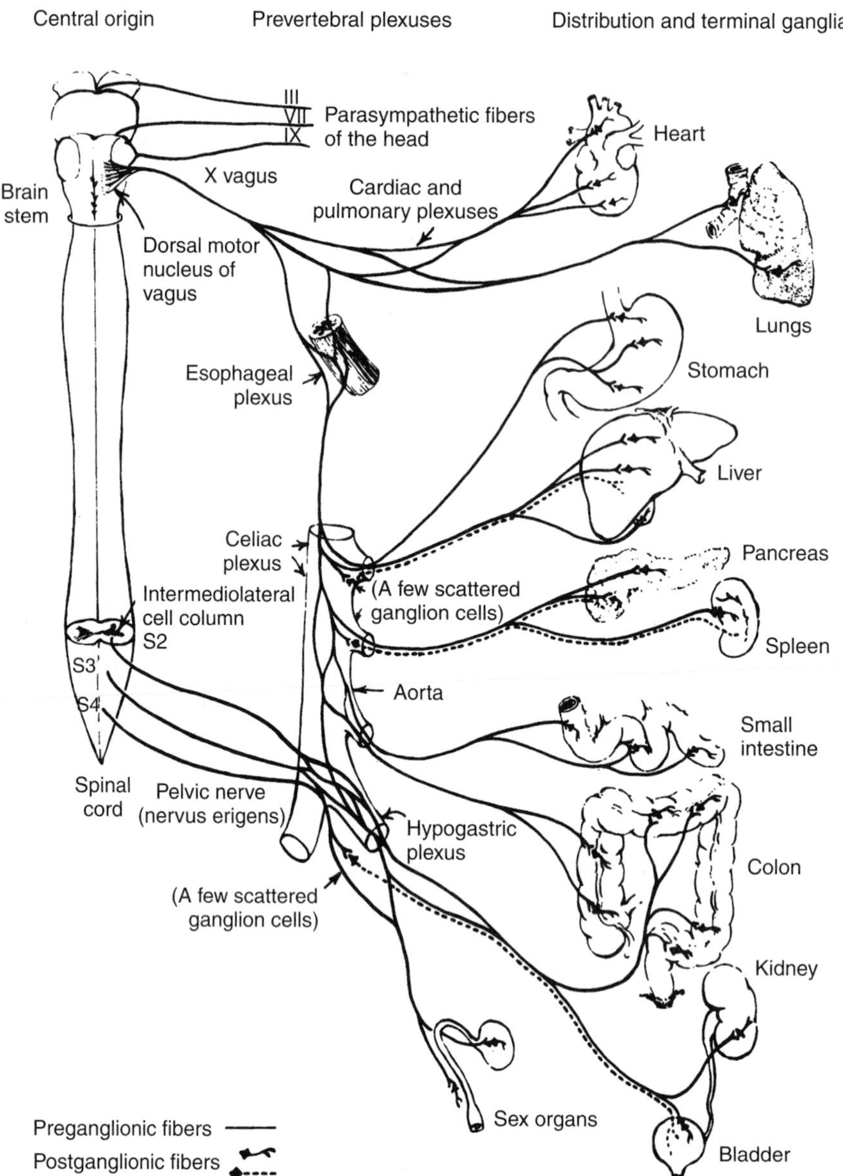

FIGURE 4-14 ■ Parasympathetic division of the autonomic nervous system *(only left half shown)*.
(Reprinted with permission from Waxman SG: *Correlative neuroanatomy*, 23rd ed. East Norwalk, Conn., 1996, Appleton & Lange.)

CLINICAL ASSESSMENT OF NEUROMUSCULAR FUNCTION

The nervous system is incompletely developed at birth and takes several years to mature. Consequently, neurologic assessment of the infant and young child must be individualized to reflect neurodevelopment and temperament of the child.

A. History

1. **Chief complaint:** Use the parents' own words and description, and solicit information from school-age and older children when their condition permits.

TABLE 4-3
Effects of Autonomic Nerve Stimulation

Organ or Structure	Sympathetic (Adrenergic) Effects	Parasympathetic (Cholinergic) Effects	Type of Receptor*
Eye			
Iris: Radial muscle	Contraction; dilates pupil (mydriasis)	Contraction; constricts pupil (miosis)	α
Iris: Circular muscle	—	Contraction; lens thickens, accommodates for near vision (strong effect)	—
Ciliary muscle	Relaxation; lens flattens, accommodates for distant vision (minor effect)	—	β
Smooth muscle: Orbit, upper lid	Contraction	—	—
Heart			
Sinoatrial node	Increased heart rate (tachycardia)	Decreased heart rate (bradycardia); vagal arrest	β
Atria	Increased contractility; conduction velocity	Decreased contractility; some increase in conduction velocity	β
Atrioventricular node, conducting system	Increased conduction velocity	Decreased conduction velocity; atrioventricular block	β
Ventricles	Increased rates of idiopathic pacemakers, contractility, conduction velocity	Decreased contractility (?)	β
Blood vessels			
Cutaneous (skin)	Constriction	Dilatation (minor; doubtful physiologic significance)	α
Buccal mucosa	Dilatation	—	—
Coronary	Dilatation, esp. in vivo; constriction (minor effect)†	Constriction (minor); dilatation (strong)	α, β
Skeletal muscle	Dilatation‡; constriction‡	Dilatation§	α, β
Cerebral	Constriction (minor effects)	Dilatation (minor; doubtful physiologic significance)	α
Pulmonary	Dilatation; constriction (minor effect)	Dilatation (minor; doubtful physiologic significance)	α, β
Abdominal, pelvic viscera	Constriction (strong); dilatation§	—	α, β
External genitalia	Constriction	Dilatation	—
Salivary glands	Constriction	Dilatation	α
Lung			
Bronchial muscle	Dilatation	Constriction	β
Bronchial glands	Inhibition (?)	Stimulation	—
Stomach			
Stomach wall, motility and tone	Decrease or increase (variable response)	Increase or decrease (variable response)	β
Sphincters	Contraction (generally)	Relaxation (generally)	α
Secretion	Inhibition (?)	Stimulation (marked)	—
Intestine			
Motility and tone	Decrease (slight)	Increase (marked)	α, β
Sphincters	Contraction (generally)	Relaxation (generally)	α
Secretion	Inhibition (?)	Stimulation	—

Continued

TABLE 4-3
Effects of Autonomic Nerve Stimulation (*cont'd*)

Organ or Structure	Sympathetic (Adrenergic) Effects	Parasympathetic (Cholinergic) Effects	Type of Receptor*
Gallbladder, ducts	Relaxation	Contraction	—
Urinary bladder			
Detrusor	Relaxation (generally)	Contraction (generally)	β
Trigone, sphincter	Contraction	Relaxation	α
Ureter			
Motility and tone	Increase (generally)	Increase (?)	—
Uterus			
Nonpregnant	Inhibition‖	—	β
Pregnant	Contraction‖	—	α
Sex organs	Ejaculation	Erection	—
Skin			
Pilomotor muscles	Contraction	—	α
Sweat glands	Slight local secretion¶	General secretion (strong response)	α
Splenic capsule	Contraction	—	α
Adrenal medulla	Catecholamine secretion (epinephrine, norepinephrine)	—	—
Pancreas, acini	—	Secretion	α
Liver islets	Glycogenolysis gluconeogenesis	—	β
Salivary glands	Viscous secretion#	Copious, watery secretion	α, β
Lacrimal glands	—	Secretion	—
Nasopharyngeal glands	—	Secretion	—

*These receptor types are based on the response of various tissues to the action of various sympathomimetic amines, i.e., compounds that initiate or mimic sympathetic nerve stimulation. In general, α-receptors are most sensitive to epinephrine and least sensitive to isoproterenol, the effect being excitatory; β-receptors, on the other hand, are most sensitive to isoproterenol and least sensitive to epinephrine, the effect being inhibitory.

†Indirect effects in vivo cause primarily vasodilatation.

‡In vivo, released epinephrine produces a β-receptor response, i.e., vasoconstriction in blood vessels of skeletal muscles and liver. In other abdominal viscera, an a-response, i.e., vasodilatation, is elicited by this catecholamine.

§Sympathetic cholinergic nerves induce vasodilatation in skeletal muscle.

‖Response variable, depending on stage of menstrual cycle and levels of circulating sex hormones (estrogen and progesterone) among other factors. Pregnant and nonpregnant uteri differ in their responses.

¶For example, palms of hands (so-called adrenergic sweating).

#The parotid glands are not innervated by sympathetic nerves.

From Jensen D: *The human nervous system.* New York, 1980, Appleton-Century-Crofts.

2. **Present illness:** Describe onset and development, associated symptoms, and factors that relieve or exacerbate symptoms.
3. **Past history:** Infant and toddler history should summarize antenatal, perinatal, and postnatal courses, including maternal infections, medications taken during pregnancy, Apgar scores, gestational age, and birth complications such as meconium aspiration, seizure activity, or respiratory status (oxygen requirements). History should include a chronologic list of developmental milestones, childhood illnesses, immunization status, significant or chronic illnesses (e.g., seizures, diabetes, head injury), and medications.
4. **Family history:** Some neurologic disorders manifest themselves as disturbances in other body systems; therefore it is important to review the patient's past history.
   a. *Neurologic disorders* may be static or progressive and may be traumatic (acquired) or congenital.
   b. *Endocrine disorders* with neurologic implications include diabetic coma and thyroid disease and hormonal imbalances (growth disorders).
   c. *Cardiovascular disorders* with neurologic implications include cyanotic heart disease (risk for brain infarcts and abscesses) and aneurysms (which may have a higher incidence in families with a known history).
   d. *Congenital disorders* with neurologic implications include neural tube defects and metabolic disorders (e.g., phenylketonuria [PKU], cretinism).
   e. *Genetic disorders* may have a neurologic origin, or they may affect the neurologic system. Most neurodegenerative disorders are transmitted as a recessive gene. Epilepsies and migraine headaches tend to be transmitted as a dominant trait.
   f. *Renal disorders* may produce metabolic imbalances that affect neurologic functioning (e.g., acute renal failure, the increased risk of cerebral edema).
5. **Social history** should include school performance, types of play activities and recreation, substance abuse, and smoking.

B. Physical Examination

1. **General appearance** evaluation includes behavior, dress, speech and conversation, gait, emotional state, and symmetry of body structures.
2. **Skull examination**
   a. *Inspection* (Vernon-Levett, 2001a) of the skull includes occipitofrontal head circumference, shape and symmetry of the head, and transillumination (increased with serous fluid [caput succedaneum] and decreased with blood fluid [cephalhematoma]). Extreme downward rotation of the eyes and paralysis of upward gaze (setting sun sign) is often seen with hydrocephalus.
   b. *Palpation* of the *fontanelles* should occur while the infant is upright and quiet. Fontanelles that remain open beyond the usual period of closure may be related to disorders that abnormally increase the intracranial contents (e.g., tumors, hydrocephalus). The anterior fontanelle is usually 4 to 6 cm at its largest diameter at birth, and the posterior fontanelle is usually 1 to 2 cm at its largest diameter at birth. The anterior fontanelle may be full and tense with increased ICP, crying, vomiting, or coughing in the infant. Pulsations of the anterior fontanelle reflect the peripheral pulse and are normally barely palpable. Palpation of sutures reveals overriding sutures, which are common with vaginal deliveries or present with premature closure of the sutures. Widely separated sutures may suggest hydrocephalus.
   c. *Auscultation* of the skull using a bell stethoscope with the child in an erect position is performed over six areas: the temporal fossae, both globes, and the

reticuloauricular or mastoid regions. In all cases, a transmitted cardiac murmur should be excluded. Bruit (spontaneous) in the young child may be normal, but an abnormal bruit is often loud, harsh, and asymmetric or accompanied by a thrill or both.

d. *Percussion* of the skull is normally dull. A "cracked-pot" sound (Macewen's sign) is heard with separated sutures and increased ICP.

3. Level of consciousness

a. Altered states of consciousness are on a continuum (Plum and Posner, 1982). *Clouding of consciousness* is characterized by reduced wakefulness, confusion, and alternating drowsiness and hyperexcitability. *Delirium* is characterized by disorientation, fear, irritability, visual hallucinations, and agitation. *Obtundation* is characterized by mild to moderate reduction in alertness, reduced interest in the environment, and increased periods of sleep. *Stupor* is indicated by unresponsiveness except to vigorous and repeated stimuli. *Coma* is indicated by no verbal or motor response to environmental stimuli.

b. Mental status may be assessed in children with minimal alteration in consciousness. In infants, assess the quality of the cry, alertness and level of activity, feeding patterns, language development, presence or absence of primitive reflexes, patterns of sleep and wakefulness, and responses to caregivers. In children, assess attention, alertness, orientation, cognition, memory, affect, and perception.

c. Coma scales are used to grade the degree of unresponsiveness by standardized assessments. *Glasgow Coma Scale (GCS)* (Table 4-4) assesses arousibility in relation to three responses: eye opening (arousal state), verbal response (content of consciousness), and motor response (arousal state and content of consciousness). Each response is given the best number for a given response.

TABLE 4-4
Glasgow Coma Scale

Activity	Score*
Verbal response	
None	1
Incomprehensible sounds	2
Inappropriate words	3
Confused	4
Oriented	5
Eye opening	
None	1
To pain	2
To speech	3
Spontaneously	4
Motor response	
None	1
Abnormal extensor	2
Abnormal flexor	3
Withdraws	4
Localizes	5
Obeys	6

*Total score = sum of the score for each of the three components. Score for a fully oriented alert patient = 15. Score for a mute immobile patient with no eye opening = 3.

From Teasdale G, Jennet B: Glasgow Coma Scale, *Lancet* 2:81–83, 1974. © by The Lancet Ltd. 1974.

The sum of the numbers ranges between 3 (least responsive) and 15 (normal). A number of coma scales have been developed to accommodate preverbal children and infants (see Multiple Trauma in Chapter 9). Most scales are scored in similar fashion to the GCS.

4. **Motor function:** Assessment of normal motor development proceeds cephalocaudal and proximodistal.
   a. Assess *primitive reflexes* in infants and toddlers and determine their presence or absence, time of disappearance, and the symmetry of the reflex. The most commonly evaluated reflexes include the following:
      - *Moro:* Elicited by a sudden movement of the body that causes a change in equilibrium. The response is extension and abduction of the upper extremities (fingers fan), followed by flexion and adduction. The reflex appears at between 28 to 32 weeks' gestation and disappears between 3 and 5 months after birth.
      - *Palmar grasp:* Elicited by the examiner placing his or her index finger into the ulnar side of the infant's hand and pressing against the palmar surface. The response is immediate flexion of the infant's fingers around the examiner's finger. The reflex appears at 28 weeks' gestation and disappears between 4 and 6 months after birth.
      - *Parachute:* Elicited by holding the infant in a ventral position. A sudden plunge downward produces extension and abduction of the infant's arms and fingers. The reflex appears at 4 to 9 months after birth and persists throughout life (the response is usually covered up with voluntary movement in older individuals).
      - *Rooting:* Elicited by stroking the perioral skin at the corner of the mouth, moving laterally toward the cheek, upper lip, and lower lip. The infant turns his or her head toward the stimulated side with sucking movements. The reflex appears at 28 weeks' gestation and disappears between 3 and 4 months after birth.
      - *Placing:* Elicited with the infant supported in a vertical position with the dorsum of one foot pressed against a hard surface. The infant's foot will flex and extend, simulating walking. The reflex appears at 35 to 37 weeks' gestation and disappears at 1 to 2 months after birth.
      - *Asymmetric tonic neck response:* Elicited by rotating the infant's head to the side while the infant's chest is maintained in a flat position. The arm and leg extend on the side to which the infant's face is turned, and the opposite arm and leg flex. The reflex appears at birth to 2 months and disappears between 4 and 6 months.

   b. Assess for *developmental milestones* (e.g., sitting, crawling, walking).
   c. If the patient can follow commands, assess *muscle strength and tone, symmetry of movement, and deep-tendon reflexes (DTRs)*. Not all DTRs are present in the infant because of the immaturity of the corticospinal tracts. DTRs are tested based on the segmental level they innervate. The usual reflexes include biceps (segmental levels C5 and C6), brachioradialis (segmental levels C5 and C6), triceps (segmental levels C7 and C8), knee (segmental levels L2, L3, and L4), and ankle (segmental levels S1 and S2). The technique for eliciting DTRs is similar to that used for adults; however, the hammer may be replaced with the examiner's semiflexed index finger. The technique includes positioning the limb so that the muscle is slightly stretched, striking the tendon briskly to create an additional sudden tendon stretch and testing both muscle groups on each side of the body. Reflex responses are usually graded on a scale from 0 (no response) to 4+ (very brisk, hyperactive; may be indicative of disease).

Abnormal findings include very brisk or asymmetric responses or deviations from a previous assessment.

d. *Superficial reflexes* include the Babinski, abdominal, and cremasteric reflexes. The technique for eliciting *Babinski's reflex* includes using a sharp object (thumbnail) to stimulate the plantar surface of the foot. Stimulation begins at the heel and travels along the lateral border of the sole, crossing over the base of the metatarsals to the great toe. A normal response in children younger than 1 to 2 years is immediate dorsiflexion of the great toe and subsequent separation (fanning) of the other toes; this response is abnormal in older children and adults. A normal response beyond the second year is plantar flexion of the toes. The *abdominal reflex* is elicited by lightly but briskly stroking each side of the abdomen, above and below the umbilicus. A normal response is contraction of the abdominal muscles and deviation of the umbilicus toward the stimulus. The reflex may not be present at birth but is consistently present at 6 months of age. A unilateral absent response is abnormal. The *cremasteric reflex* is elicited by lightly but briskly stroking the inner aspect of each of the upper thighs. A normal response is elevation of the testicle on the stimulated side. It may not be present at birth but occurs consistently at approximately 6 months of age. An asymmetric response is abnormal.

e. *Abnormal motor responses* in the comatose patient include *decorticate posturing* (consisting of flexion and adduction of the upper extremities and extension of the lower extremities with plantar flexion representing dysfunction of the cerebral hemispheres or upper part of the brainstem), *decerebrate posturing* (extensor posturing consisting of extension, adduction, and hyperpronation of the upper and lower extremities and plantar flexion representing dysfunction at the pontomesencephalic level), and *flaccidity* (no motor response to external stimuli representing severe dysfunction of the lower brainstem and vital centers for which spinal cord injury and stroke must be ruled out).

f. *All extremities* should be assessed independently. Specific stimuli to solicit a motor response should be documented.

5. **Sensory function**

a. *In infants, sensory testing results are variable* and less reliable than in the older child. Light touch is assessed by stroking an extremity (the normal response is to withdraw the limb). Vibration sense is assessed with a tuning fork over bony areas (the normal response is cessation of movement and often a look of surprise). Proprioception cannot be tested in infants or comatose patients because it requires participation of the patient. Pain sensation is assessed with nail-bed pressure (at the end of examination).

b. *Light touch and superficial pain* are assessed in older children in all four extremities. If abnormalities are noted, a more detailed segmental assessment is done. Proprioception is tested by asking the child to close his or her eyes and move a finger or toe up or down and then asking the child to identify whether the movement is up or down. Pain sensation is tested at the end of the examination by using a pin to test the various dermatomes.

6. **Cerebellar function**

a. *In infants and toddlers, cerebellar function* should be assessed by observing the child during play or usual activities. Abnormal findings include tremors, which are rhythmic alterations in movement and, unlike spontaneous seizures, are usually precipitated by a variety of stimuli (e.g., sudden changes in movement) with no alteration in the level of consciousness. Dysmetria (inability to control the range of movement in muscle action) or gait abnormalities (e.g., wide-based or waddling type of gait) may also be noticed.

b. *Maneuvers to assess older children* include the finger-to-nose test, the heel-shin test, observation of gait, and toe-to-heel walking. The finger-to-nose test is performed while the child stands erect with arms extended at the sides; then the child is asked to touch his or her nose with alternating index fingers. An abnormal finding would be the child completely missing the nose. The heel-shin test is done while the child is in a supine position. The child is asked to place one heel rapidly down the shin from the knee to the ankle and to repeat this movement on the other side. Movements should be coordinated and accurate. The child can also be instructed to touch each finger to the thumb of the same hand in rapid succession. Each hand is tested, and the response should be symmetric. Observation of gait can be made while the child walks toward and then away from the examiner. The child should have good posture and balance. During toe-to-heel walking, the child places the heel of one foot to the toe of the other foot and continues this maneuver for several feet. The child should have good balance.

7. Cranial nerve function: The order and specific nerves to be tested depend on the age and condition of the child. The techniques for the assessment of specific cranial nerves are included in Table 4-5.

8. Fundoscopic examination

a. *Normal findings* include a red reflex that is orange-red and fairly uniform in color, creamy pink optic disc with indented center (physiologic depression) and smooth margins, and veins that are slightly wider than arteries.

b. *Abnormal findings* include papilledema, which is characterized by blurring of the nasal and upper margins of the optic disc. Papilledema is seen with increased ICP in the older child or in the infant with acute, rapid increased ICP. Retinal hemorrhage may occur with subarachnoid hemorrhage, severe diabetes, and shaken-baby syndrome.

9. Vital signs

a. *Respiratory patterns* (Table 4-6): Respirations are the first of the vital signs to change with neurologic dysfunction. Respiratory patterns are more informative than respiratory rate. Patterns may overlap or change, depending on the progression of neurologic dysfunction. (See also Chapter 2.)

- *Cheyne-Stokes respirations* are described as periodic breathing with phases of hyperpnea alternating with apnea. The location of the lesion is bilateral, hemispheric, or diencephalic.
- *Central neurogenic hyperventilation* is sustained rapid and fairly deep hyperpnea. The exact mechanism in the brain (if any) is unknown.
- An *apneustic respiratory pattern* is characterized by a prolonged inspiration with a pause at full inspiration lasting 2 to 3 seconds. This finding represents damage to the brainstem near the level of the fifth cranial nerve nucleus.
- *Ataxic respirations* are a completely irregular breathing pattern with deep and shallow breaths. They are seen in patients with damage to the respiratory centers in the medulla.

b. *Temperature:* Temperature changes are nonspecific in most patients with neurologic dysfunction. Hyperthermia may result from abnormalities of the brain itself or from toxic substances that affect the temperature-regulating centers. Patients at risk for hyperthermia include neonates (due to immature development of thermoregulation centers), children with CNS infections (due to the effects of pyrogens on the hypothalamus), and children with status epilepticus (which might be due to hypothalamic dysfunction as well as to

Text continued on p. 349.

TABLE 4-5
Cranial Nerve Evaluation

Cranial Nerve	Functions	Methods of Testing	Comments
INFANT*			
I	Olfactory Sense of smell	Assess patency of both nostrils. Hold noxious odor near each nostril separately. Observe for generalized body movement or cry.	Unreliable test for infants. Although smell is intact, the immature myelinization prohibits an integrated, voluntary motor response.
II	Optic Vision	Inspect the fundus with an ophthalmoscope. Test visual fields by introducing a brightly colored object into each visual field from behind the infant. In the infant with a pincer grasp, observe the visual acuity used in spotting and picking up crumbs and small objects.	The optic disc is pale, grey, and poorly developed in the infant. The macula (area of central vision) is not fully developed until 4 mo, at which time the infant will notice light contrast and different colors. Infants are capable of binocular fixation at 3 mo and can follow the object for visual field testing.
III	Oculomotor Pupillary constriction, elevation of the upper eyelid, and most of the extraocular movements.	Check pupillary responses: shine light directly into each eye from the side and observe the briskness and completeness of the direct pupillary response. Check the consensual response by shining the light into one eye and observing the response in the other eye. Record the size of the pupil in millimeters (mm). Note the shape and equality of the pupils. Note the infant's spontaneous eye opening and any ptosis. Note the presence of doll's eyes (oculocephalic reflex): turn the head to one side quickly and watch the position of the eyes. A positive response, when the eyes move in the opposite direction as though still gazing in the initial direction, is present with an intact brain stem. Check extraocular movements (cranial nerves III, IV, and IV). Test for accommodation, noting constriction and convergence as a bright object is brought toward the nose.	Early signs of increased ICP include a sluggishly reactive pupil and incomplete constriction. Infants older than the age of 3 mo are able to accommodate for near vision. The setting sun sign (portion of sclera visible between the iris and upper eyelid) can result from hydrocephalus and brain stem irritation. A negative oculocephalic reflex (doll's eyes) can result from a lesion of the midbrain or pons or from a deep coma.

*From Slota MC: Neurological assessment of the infant and toddler, *Crit Care Nurse* 3:87–94, 1983.

TABLE 4-5
Cranial Nerve Evaluation (*cont'd*)

Cranial Nerve	Functions	Methods of Testing	Comments
IV	Trochlear Downward inward movement of the eye	Check the six fields of gaze: hold a bright object 18 in from the infant and move it from the midline into each of the six fields of gaze (upward outward, laterally, and downward outward) for each eye with someone else holding the infant's head steady. Note conjugate movements of the eyes.	Infants should attempt binocular fixation at the age of 3 mo and be able to follow the object smoothly by the age of one year. Nystagmus is normal in premature infants and neonates. Dysconjugate movements after the age of 6 wk can be indicative of blindness.
VI	Abducens Lateral deviation of the eye		
III	Oculomotor All other extraocular movements		
V	Trigeminal Motor: Innervation to the temporal and masseter muscles; responsible for jaw clenching and lateral movement. Sensory: Innervation to the face with three branches: (1) opthalmic, (2) maxillary, and (3) mandibular	Test the strength of the temporal and masseter muscles by assessing the infant's sucking hold on the nipple or finger. Note jaw symmetry while the infant is crying. Test for the rooting reflex by stroking the cheek and watching the infant turn to the stimulated side. Test the corneal reflex with a cotton wisp touched lightly to the cornea only. Note the response of blinking and possible tearing.	Jaw weakness and an impaired suck can be present in infants with trigeminal damage. Infants can blink asymmetrically in response to corneal stimulation. Most infants produce tears by the age of 2 to 3 mo. The sensory component of the corneal reflex is the trigeminal nerve, and the motor component is the facial nerve.
VII	Facial Motor: Innervation to the muscles of the face including the forehead, eyes, and mouth. Sensory: Innervation to the anterior $^{2}/_{3}$ of the tongue where sweet, sour, and salty sensors predominate	Observe facial symmetry during crying and smiling.	While taste is intact at birth, taste testing is not reliable in infants and rarely done. Infants will usually wrinkle their foreheads when crying. Central facial damage will result in paralysis from the eye down, and peripheral damage produces paralysis on the entire side of the face.

Continued

TABLE 4-5
Cranial Nerve Evaluation (*cont'd*)

Cranial Nerve	Functions	Methods of Testing	Comments
VIII	Acoustic Cochlear division: Hearing Vestibular division: Balance	Test acoustic blink reflex by creating a loud noise near infant and noting the blink in response. Create loud noise and note appropriate response for age. Test vestibular branch with doll's eye maneuver (see cranial nerve III) and caloric testing; iced saline is injected into the ear canal with a syringe by the physician after assuring that the tympanic membrane is intact. Note the normal response of nystagmus with the eye jerking away from the irrigated ear.	During the neonatal period, there is a generalized response to noise, usually a cry or Moro reflex. At about 8 to 10 wk, the infant will stop moving to listen to the sound. At about 3 to 4 mo, the infant will turn his head toward the noise. This response is expected by the age of 8 mo at the latest. In coma with an intact brain stem, caloric testing can demonstrate deviation of eyes toward the irrigated ear. With brain stem lesions, there is usually no response.
IX	Glossopharyngeal Sensory: Innervation to the pharynx and taste on the posterior $^1/_3$ of the tongue	Stimulate a gag. Note hoarse or stridorous crying. Observe swallowing with feedings, and note excessive drooling.	Some drooling is normal in infants. The autonomic system is intact at birth, but infants are particularly sensitive to parasympathetic stimulation. For example, the infant can readily demonstrate bradycardia during gagging or suctioning.
X	Vagus Sensory: Innervation to the pharynx and larynx Motor: Innervation to palate and pharynx and parasympathetic functions		
XI	Spinal accessory Motor: Innervation to the sternomastoid muscle and the upper portion of the trapezius muscle	Observe the infant's head movement from side to side.	Damage to the nerve can result in difficulty in turning the head from side to side.
XII	Hypoglossal Motor: Innervation to the tongue	Gently pinch the infant's nostrils to produce reflex opening of the mouth and raising of the tongue. Note tongue asymmetry, deviation, or atrophy. Observe the tongue movements during sucking.	Damage to the nerve can result in paresis, paralysis, deviation, or fasciculations.

TABLE 4-5
Cranial Nerve Evaluation (*cont'd*)

Cranial Nerve	Functions	Methods of Testing	Comments
CHILD[†]			
I	Olfactory Sense of smell	Assure that both nasal passages are patent and unobstructed. Ask child to close eyes and identify smells, testing each nostril separately. Use familiar odors, such as peanut butter, oranges, and chocolate.	Unreliable test results are common in toddlers and young children. Damage to this nerve results in perversion or loss of smell. Unilateral loss of smell can indicate a tumor of the anterior fossa. Temporary or permanent loss of smell can also be related to trauma to the olfactory bulbs or tracts or an upper respiratory tract infection.
II	Optic Vision	Test visual acuity in the younger child by observing recognition of familiar objects or people at a distance. This nerve can be tested with an eye chart (such as a Snellen chart) when children are about 6 to 7 y of age. Test color acuity through recognition of colored objects. Determine visual fields through the confrontation method: (1) seat the child at your eye level approximately 2 to 3 ft away; (2) ask the child to stare at your nose (using a bright sticker on the end of your nose can help); (3) bring a brightly colored object into the child's field of vision from the nasal, lateral, superior, and inferior fields; (4) compare the child's visual fields to your own. Inspect the fundus with an ophthalmoscope for optic atrophy or papilledema.	Damage to this nerve can result in ipsilateral visual impairment. Homonymous hemianopsia can result from spastic hemiplegia. Bilateral (bitemporal) hemianopsia can result from a tumor of the optic chiasm or craniopharyngioma. The confrontation method is a rough evaluation of visual fields. Specialized testing is required for an accurate evaluation. Specific fundoscopic findings in the pediatric patient include: (1) the child's retina is lighter than the adult's, (2) the macula is not fully differentiated, and (3) papilledema is rare in children before complete closure of the fontanelles and sutures.
III	Oculomotor Pupillary constriction, elevation of the upper eyelid, and most of the extraocular movements	Check pupillary responses by shining a light directly into each eye from the side and observing the briskness and completeness of the direct pupillary response. Check the consensual response by shining the light into one eye and observing the briskness in response of the other pupil. Record the size of pupil in	Compression of the parasympathetic nerve fiber on the third cranial nerve allows sympathetic dominance and pupillary dilatation. Since the third nerve is located at the tentorial notch, increases in ICP can result in ipsilateral, contralateral, or bilateral pupillary dilatation. Early signs of increased ICP include

† From Slota MC: Pediatric neurologic assessment, *Crit Care Nurse* 3:106–112, 1983.

Continued

TABLE 4-5
Cranial Nerve Evaluation (*cont'd*)

Cranial Nerve	Functions	Methods of Testing	Comments
		millimeters. Note the shape and equality of the pupils. Note the opening of the upper eyelids and ptosis (drooping). Check the extraocular movements.	a sluggish response to light or incomplete constriction. Other abnormal findings that should be noted include: (1) anisocoria (unequal pupils), (2) bilaterally pinpoint fixed pupils (damage to sympathetic nerves at brain stem), and (3) hippus (rhythmical dilatation and constriction of pupils in response to light).
IV	Trochlear Downward, inward movement of the eye	Check the six fields of gaze by holding a bright object 18 in from the child and moving it from the midline into each of the six fields of gaze for each eye.	Damage to the fourth nerve can cause diplopia (double vision) and altered downward eye movement.
VI	Abducens Lateral deviation of the eye	Ask the child to follow the object with his or her eyes but to keep the head steady. Note conjugate movements of the eyes and absence of nystagmus except in the extreme lateral position.	Damage to the sixth nerve can produce deviation of the head toward the weak muscle to avoid diplopia. Dysconjugate gaze can indicate blindness, and a conjugate horizontal gaze palsy suggests a lesion of the brain stem or cerebral hemisphere. Vertical gaze paralysis suggests brain stem dysfunction, and upward gaze paralysis suggests hydrocephalus or a tumor of the pineal region.
III	Oculomotor All other extraocular movements	Check for accommodation by bringing an object from 18 in out in toward the nose. As the object is brought toward the nose, check for convergence of the eyes and pupillary constriction.	Damage to the third nerve can result in ptosis, outward and downward displacement of the eye, and a large, sluggish pupil (in addition to the changes noted earlier).
V	Trigeminal Motor: Innervation to the temporal and masseter muscles; responsible for clenching and lateral movement of the jaw	Motor: While palpating the temporal and then masseter muscles, ask the child to clench his or her teeth or bite on a safe object. Note the muscle strength. Ask the child to move his or her jaw from side to side and observe the symmetry of jaw movement during laughter, crying, or talking.	Damage to the motor component of the nerve can result in impaired mastication. A unilateral paralysis can cause deviation of the jaw to the affected side when the child opens his or her mouth. Trauma, infections, or tumors can impair facial sensation or produce paroxysmal facial pain.
	Sensory: Innervation to the face with	Sensory: With the child's eyes closed, test the three sensory branches of the nerve by	The sensory component of the corneal reflex is the trigeminal nerve, and the motor component

TABLE 4-5
Cranial Nerve Evaluation (*cont'd*)

Cranial Nerve	Functions	Methods of Testing	Comments
	three branches: ophthalmic, maxillary, and mandibular	using first a cotton wisp and then a sharp object on the forehead, cheeks, and jaw. Substitute the dull end of the object occasionally to test the child's reliability. If abnormal findings are present, evaluate temperature sensation using test tubes filled with hot and cold water. Test the corneal reflex with a cotton wisp touched lightly to the cornea only. Note the response of blinking and some tearing.	is the facial nerve. Use of contact lenses in the older child can diminish or abolish the corneal reflex. If the child in an intensive care setting is being tested frequently for pain sensation, it may be wise to use a sterile needle for testing.
VII	Facial Motor: Innervation to the muscles of the face including the forehead, eyes, and mouth Sensory: Innervation to the anterior $^{2}/_{3}$ of the tongue where sweet, sour, and salty sensors predominate	Motor: Inspect the child's face for asymmetry during rest and while talking or crying. Ask the child to raise eyebrows, make a "mad" face, close eyes very tightly, show teeth, smile, puff out cheeks, and make a "funny" face. In the younger child, watch facial expressions during play. Sensory: Ask the child to hold out his or her tongue. Using an applicator, apply sweet, salty, or sour substances to the child's tongue.	Damage to this nerve can result in facial weakness or paralysis. Central facial damage will result in paralysis from the eye down, while peripheral damage can produce paralysis on the entire side of face. Damage can also result in the loss of taste sensation on the anterior $^{2}/_{3}$ of the tongue. Younger children may not cooperate or be reliable in responding to taste testing.
VIII	Acoustic Cochlear division: Hearing	Cochlear: Check fine hearing by holding a ticking watch 1 or 2 in from one ear while occluding the other ear. Repeat on the opposite side. Check for gross hearing by standing 1 to 2 ft away from the child and whispering something the child will be able to repeat.	Damage to the nerve can result in impaired hearing, tinnitus, vertigo, nystagmus, and unilateral or bilateral deafness. The Rinne and Weber tests can be used for further assessment of this nerve.
	Vestibular division: Balance	Vestibular: Test the vestibular branch with caloric testing. Iced saline (of varying amounts for different ages) is injected into the external ear canal with a syringe. Note the normal response of nystagmus with eye jerking away from the irrigated ear.	Deviation of the eyes toward the irrigated ear can occur in coma with an intact brain stem. Caloric testing usually results in no response in brain stem lesions.

Continued

TABLE 4-5
Cranial Nerve Evaluation (*cont'd*)

Cranial Nerve	Functions	Methods of Testing	Comments
IX	Glossopharyngeal Sensory: Innervation to the pharynx and taste on the posterior $^1/_3$ of tongue	Test the two nerves together by asking the child to say "ah" or yawn. During this action, observe the upward motion of the soft palate and uvula and the upward, inward movement of the posterior pharynx.	Damage to these nerves can result in impaired sensation, dysphagia (difficulty swallowing), dysarthria (difficulty talking), dysphonia, excessive drooling, stridor, and autonomic nervous system changes related to the vagus nerve. Adolescent boys can demonstrate hoarseness and voice changes related to normal puberty.
X	Vagus Sensory: Innervation to the pharynx and larynx Motor: Innervation to the palate and pharynx and parasympathetic functions	Touch the side of the uvula with a tongue blade, and note the upward movement and deviation to the stimulated side. Touch the posterior portion of the tongue with a tongue blade to stimulate a gag reflex. Note any hoarseness, and observe the child's ability to swallow without pain or choking. Note excessive drooling or coughing. Test bitter taste on the posterior $^1/_3$ of the tongue.	
XI	Spinal accessory Motor: Innervation to the sternocleidomastoid muscle and the upper portion of the trapezius muscle	Ask the child to turn his or her head from side to side against the pressure of your hands to test for strength. Note the normal range of motion of approximately 170 degrees. Ask the child to shrug his or her shoulders against the pressure of your hands. You may need to demonstrate this action to younger children.	Damage to this nerve can produce asymmetrical shoulder posture, drooping shoulders, impaired strength in lifting the shoulders, or difficulty in turning the head to either side.
XII	Hypoglossal Motor: Innervation to the tongue	Inspect the younger child's tongue for fasciculations and symmetrical movement. Ask the older child to stick out his or her tongue, and observe for asymmetry, deviation, or atrophy.	Damage to this nerve can result in atrophy, weakness, deviation, or fasciculations of the tongue. Fine, irregular, occasional tremors of the tongue are normal when holding out the tongue.

TABLE 4-6
Common Respiratory Patterns in Comatose Clients

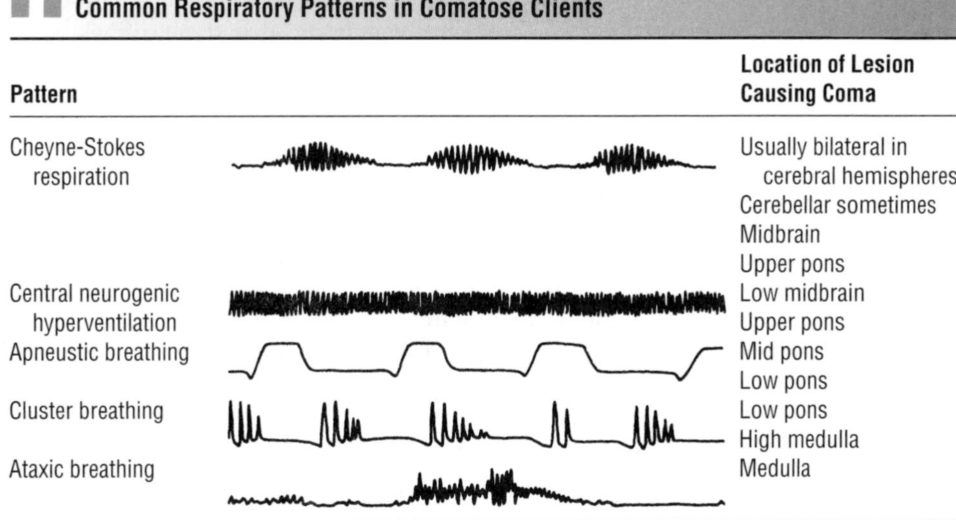

Pattern	Location of Lesion Causing Coma
Cheyne-Stokes respiration	Usually bilateral in cerebral hemispheres Cerebellar sometimes Midbrain Upper pons
Central neurogenic hyperventilation	Low midbrain Upper pons
Apneustic breathing	Mid pons Low pons
Cluster breathing	Low pons High medulla
Ataxic breathing	Medulla

From Ignatavicius D et al.: *Medical-surgical nursing: a nursing process approach*, 2nd ed. Philadelphia, 1995, WB Saunders Co.

increased total-body oxygen consumption). Hypothermia may be seen in neonates (same as the preceding) and in brain death because of loss of hypothalamic function.

c. *Pulse and blood pressure:* Changes in pulse and blood pressure are very late and ominous signs of neurologic dysfunction. *Cushing's reflex* is an increase in systolic pressure greater than diastolic pressure (i.e., widened pulse pressure) and bradycardia. Cardiac dysrhythmias are seen with some traumatic brain injuries (TBIs). Vasodilation with systemic hypotension may be seen with spinal trauma or sympathetic insufficiency (Davis et al., 1992).

C. Determination of Brain Death

1. Most states have adopted guidelines to define death the same way for infants, children, and adults. One of two conditions must exist:
   a. Irreversible cessation of breathing and circulation *or*
   b. Irreversible cessation of whole-brain function (i.e., cortical and brainstem)

2. The difference in brain death determination between children and adults lies not in the legal definition of death but rather in the process of confirming brain death. Several sets of guidelines have been published for the determination of brain death in children. The most widely accepted guidelines are those published by the Ad Hoc Task Force for the Determination of Brain Death in Children (Guidelines, 1987).
   a. *History:* The cause of coma must be known to establish irreversibility. There must be an absence of complicating factors, such as hemodynamic instability, use of sedatives and paralyzing agents, severe hypothermia, or hypoxemia.
   b. To determine brain death the *physical examination* should demonstrate coma, normothermia, normal blood pressure, flaccidity, absence of movement (except for spinal cord reflexes), and absence of brainstem function. Loss of brainstem function is determined by nonreactive midposition or fully dilated pupils; the absence of oculocephalic (doll's eyes) and oculovestibular (cold calorics) reflexes; the absence of movement of bulbar musculature and corneal,

gag, cough, sucking, and rooting reflexes; and the absence of respiratory effort with standardized apnea testing (Jumah et al., 1992; Outwater and Rockoff, 1984). Following disconnection from the ventilator, several conditions must occur: adequate time (5 to 10 minutes) to allow $Paco_2$ to increase to levels sufficient to stimulate respiration, adequate oxygenation, and absence of cardiovascular instability.

c. *Consistent examination techniques* are required throughout the observation period. For infants aged 7 days to 2 months, two examinations and electroencephalograms (EEGs) are performed 48 hours apart. For infants aged 2 months to 1 year, two examinations and EEGs are performed 24 hours apart, or one examination and an initial EEG showing electrocerebral silence (ECS) combined with a radionuclide angiogram showing no CBF is used. In children older than 1 year, two examinations are performed 12 to 24 hours apart. EEG and isotope angiography are optional.

d. *Controversies* (Freeman and Ferry, 1988; Shewmon, 1988): The exact cause of coma is often unknown in the newborn because many hypoxic-ischemic injuries occur in utero. The accuracy of confirmatory tests in the newborn is unknown.

NEURODIAGNOSTIC MONITORING

A. Assessing Anatomic Integrity

1. Radiograph

a. *Description:* Roentgenographic films of skull and spine demonstrate structural deficits only. The radiation penetrates all body tissues and is absorbed to varying degrees, resulting in different shadow intensities.

b. *Clinical use: Skull films* are used to determine fractures, widened sutures, tumors, calcification, and bone erosion. *Spinal films* are used to evaluate the integrity of the vertebral structures, including the vertebral body, disc interspace, lamina, and pedicles. Spinal films are also used to evaluate fractures, dislocations, and degeneration of bone.

c. *Nursing implications:* Immobilize fractures with splints, cervical collars, traction devices, or age-appropriate immobilizers. Provide routine safe-transport care, including the use of appropriate monitoring devices, elevation of side rails, good alignment of affected body structure(s), securing standby emergency equipment, and serial monitoring of neurovascular status. Explain the procedure to older children and parents, including the length of the procedure, purpose of the procedure, sensations and appearance of the environment, and expectations of the child during the procedure (e.g., to remain quiet without body movement).

2. Computed tomography (CT) scan

a. *Description:* CT scans use multiple x-ray beams that pass through the brain at different angles. The beams are picked up by receptors that digitally send the information to a computer. The computer formats the information and displays an image for every section of the brain that is studied. Different anatomic structures of the brain absorb various levels of radiation energy, depending on the tissue density of the structure. CT scan differentiates tissue density relative to water via a computer. Highly dense structures (e.g., bone, fresh blood) appear white, and low-density areas (e.g., air, CSF, fat) appear dark.

b. *Interpretation:* CT scans are interpreted sequentially and systematically. The left side of the brain is displayed on the right of the scan as the viewer faces it.

Each CT scan section is examined for characteristic anatomic landmarks, some requiring measurement. The first image usually begins with a cut through the posterior fossa, followed by sections that advance superiorly. Anatomic structures are viewed in terms of size, location, and symmetry. Figure 4-15 is an example of a CT scan with normal anatomical landmarks. The view is taken above the level of the fourth ventricle and shows the cerebellar hemispheres and the posterior fossa. Sections are then examined for abnormal densities (e.g., blood clots, tumors) and enlarged structures. The basilar cistern is the area of subarachnoid space that surrounds the midbrain. Diffuse brain swelling is recognized on CT scan as a decrease in ventricular size, absence or compression of the basilar cistern, and loss of differentiation between gray and white matter. Visual loss of the third ventricle and loss of sulci indicate an increase in brain bulk (swelling). Asymmetry is almost always an abnormal sign that indicates volume changes between compartments. Figure 4-16 demonstrates four CT scans that show abnormalities.

c. *Clinical use:* Because of cost, speed, and availability, CT scan is used for examination of acute neurologic dysfunction. CT scan is superior to magnetic resonance imaging (MRI) in detecting new blood (especially subarachnoid hemorrhage) and in evaluating cortical bone structures of skull and spine. Contrast-enhanced CT (CECT) is used to detect lesions that cause breakdown of the blood-brain barrier, to visualize blood vessels and well-vascularized lesions, and to rule out cerebral metastases. It is difficult to visualize the posterior fossa because of bone obstruction.

d. *Nursing implications:* Before the procedure, the patient and family should be told that the machine surrounds the body and that clicking and whirring noises may be heard. The procedure is painless, except for a venipuncture if contrast medium is used. The child is required to remain still throughout the procedure; sedation may be required. If contrast medium is used, the patient may experience an unusual sensation during the procedure (e.g., a burning or warm sensation for about 20 to 30 seconds during injection of the contrast medium). The use of contrast media is contraindicated in patients with acute renal failure.

e. *Postprocedure monitoring* includes assessing for an allergic reaction to the contrast medium (e.g., tachycardia, hypotension, fever, chills) and observing the contrast injection site (if used) for bleeding, swelling, redness, and pain.

3. Magnetic resonance imaging

a. *Description:* MRI differentiates tissues by their response to radiofrequency pulses in a magnetic field; lesions have either a high or low signal (in contrast to x-ray density seen with a CT scan).

b. *Clinical use:* MRI is used to identify small infarcts, infections, inflammatory areas, and demyelinating plaques. MRI provides clear sagittal images; therefore it is the procedure of choice for suspected lesions of the spinal cord or cervicomedullary junction. MRI can delineate between tissue structure (e.g., white and gray matter).

- The advantages of MRI compared with CT scan include better definition of normal and pathologic lesions (except those listed previously for CT scan), better three-dimensional information and relationships, demonstration of blood and CSF flow, and evaluation of tumors in the posterior fossa that are normally obstructed by bone artifact in CT imaging.
- Disadvantages of MRI compared with CT scan are the requirement of more time and cooperation from the patient and difficulty in continuously monitoring the patient during the procedure because of the magnetic field;

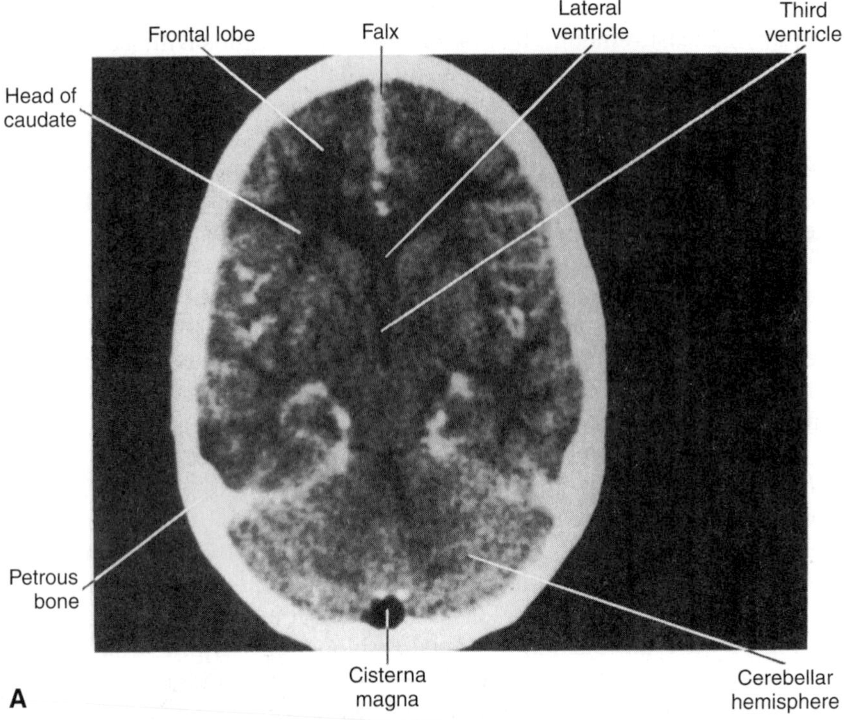

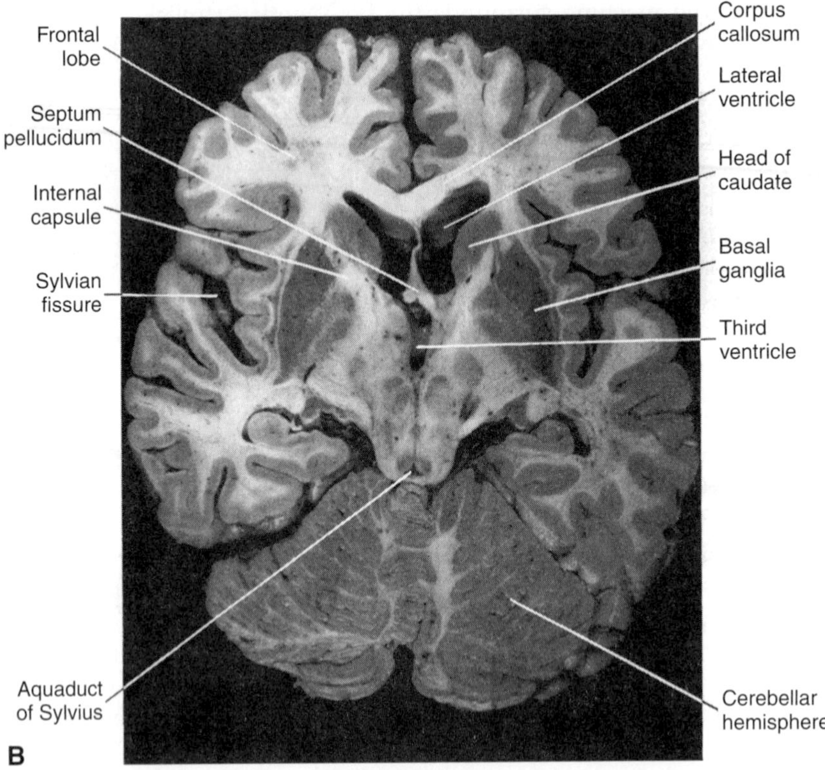

FIGURE 4-15 ■ **A**, Transverse CT scan. **B**, Corresponding anatomical slice including cerebellum, aqueduct of Sylvius, and lateral ventricles.

(From Marshall SB, Marshall LF, Vos HR, Chestnut RM: *Neuroscience critical care: pathophysiology and patient management*. Philadelphia, 1990, Saunders.)

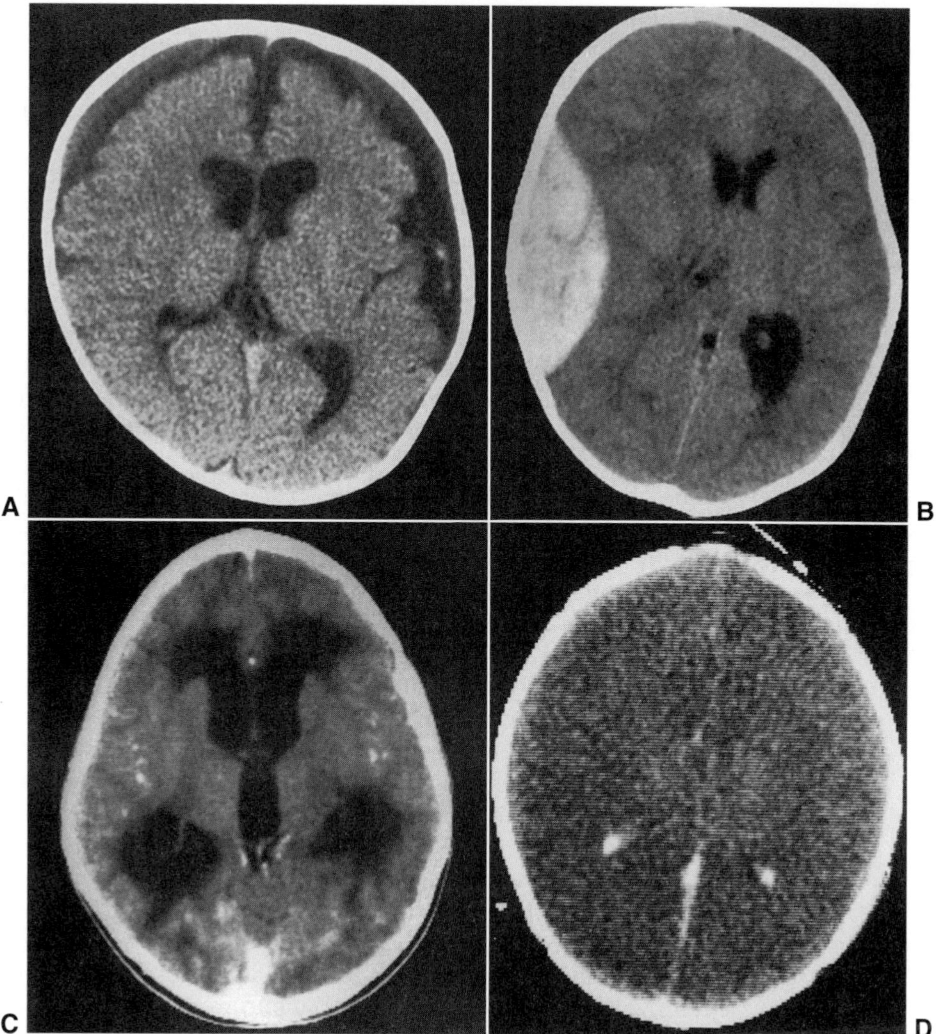

FIGURE 4-16 ■ **A,** Nonenhanced computed tomography (CT) scan of a 9-month-old infant showing bilateral acute and chronic subdural hematoma. Ventricles are mildly enlarged. **B,** CT scan showing a large right-sided epidural hematoma with a characteristic biconvex appearance in a 10-month-old girl. The midline structures are displaced to the left, with effacement of much of the ventricular system on the right, moderate dilatation of the front horns of both lateral ventricles and marked dilatation of the posterior portion of the left lateral ventricle. The basal cisterns are effaced. **C,** CT scan demonstrates enlarged lateral and third ventricles caused by obstruction of the aqueduct of Sylvius by a venous angioma. **D,** CT scan of a severely asphyxiated term newborn at 3 days of age. Note the generalized decreased densities with total loss of gray matter and white matter differentiation.

(From Swaiman KF, Ashwal S: *Pediatric neurology: principles and practice,* 3rd ed. St. Louis, 1999, Mosby.)

however, newer MRI-compatible monitors are becoming increasingly more available. Another disadvantage of MRI is that it is contraindicated in patients with metallic implants (e.g., pacemakers, aneurysm clips).

c. *Nursing implications:* When the patient's condition permits, preprocedural education should include the information that the machine turns around the patient and makes a loud noise much like a washing machine. The procedure is long, and the child must lie still. If a contrast medium is used, an unusual sensation may occur (i.e., a warm rushing sensation for approximately 20 to 30 seconds during injection). The procedure is painless except for venipuncture involving use of contrast medium. All metallic objects must be removed from the patient, parents, and supportive staff who accompany the patient. Inquire about implantable metallic objects (e.g., pacemakers, electronic implants, surgical clips, ferromagnetic items). Sedation is often required for small children. Postprocedure monitoring is the same as for CT scan.

4. Cerebral angiogram

a. *Description:* Intra-arterial injection (usually femoral cannulation) of radiopaque dye is followed by sequential skull radiographs or digital subtraction technique. Cerebral angiogram is used to outline the intracranial and extracranial vessels. A series of radiographs are taken once the arterial system is accessed and contrast dye is injected.

b. *Clinical use:* Since the advent of CT scan and MRI, angiogram use is more restricted. It is usually reserved for confirmation of lesions and identification of vascular occlusions, recanalization, ulceration and dissection of large arteries, and stenosis of small arteries. It is the procedure of choice for aneurysms and arteriovascular malformations and is used to detect CBF alterations.

c. *Nursing implications*

- Preprocedural education should include describing the purpose of the procedure, the length of the procedure (it usually takes several hours), possible sensations the patient may experience during the procedure (e.g., a burning or warm sensation for about 20 to 30 seconds during injection of the contrast medium), and the possible need for sedation and its expected effects. Contrast medium is excreted by the kidneys; patients are encouraged to drink liberally the day before the procedure, or intravenous (IV) fluids may be increased as ordered. Nothing by mouth restrictions before the test usually apply for 12 hours. All jewelry and hair ornaments must be removed.
- Postprocedure monitoring: Patients should avoid movement of the affected extremity to prevent dislodgment of a clot, bleeding, and hematoma formation. Frequently assess the neurovascular status and pressure dressing of a cannulated extremity: usually every 15 minutes for an hour, then every 30 minutes for an hour, and then every hour until the patient is stable. Assess for bleeding, hematoma, or infection at the cannulation site. Restrict activity initially, usually for 12 to 24 hours. Monitor vital signs for indications of shock (e.g., hypotension, diminished pulses, and tachycardia) at the same intervals as the neurovascular assessment. Assess for an allergic reaction to contrast medium (e.g., tachycardia, hypotension, fever, chills). Encourage hydration with sips of water or IV fluids. Maintain intake and output record for 24 hours.

5. Radioisotope scan

a. *Description:* A radioisotope is injected into the circulation, and a brain scanning device detects areas of abnormal uptake of the isotope (occurs with altered blood-brain barrier or highly vascularized area).

b. *Clinical use:* The use of a radioisotope scan has been limited since the development of the CT scan. A radioisotope scan is effective in identifying isodense lesions such as subdural hematoma, blood clots with the same density as adjacent tissue, intracerebral infection, and inflammation. A radioisotope scan is also effective in the evaluation of patients with epilepsy because it can help to identify epileptic foci before excision is done.

c. *Nursing implications:* Preprocedural education includes explaining the purpose for and length of the procedure. A small venipuncture is necessary for isotope injection. Time delay may be necessary for adequate uptake of the isotope. There is a small radiation hazard to the patient and staff; however, the half-life of nuclides is extremely short.

B. Assessing Physiologic Alterations

1. ICP monitoring

a. *Description:* ICP monitoring is a technique in which a catheter is placed directly within the cranium to measure ICP. Less frequently, a transducer is placed indirectly on the anterior fontanelle to measure ICP.

b. *Clinical uses* include assessment for the prevention of herniation and the preservation of cerebral perfusion.

c. *Classification of systems:* Type of transducer

- In *fluid-filled systems,* the compartment that is being monitored is connected to a strain-gauge transducer via a fluid pathway. Fluid-column pulsations are converted into millimeters of mercury. Advantages include the low cost, accuracy (with an intraventricular catheter), and ability to zero and recalibrate after insertion. Disadvantages are that the accuracy depends on the catheter location, artifact is present with movement, the procedure requires transducer leveling with position changes, and the system may become obstructed with tissue, blood, air, or bone.
- *Fiberoptic catheters* have a transducer tip that is non–fluid-filled. A mirrored diaphragm (in the tip of the transducer) moves in response to pressure and is sensed by light fibers. Information is converted into an analog signal and displayed on a pressure monitor. Advantages include the theoretical low risk of infection because of the lack of a fluid column and stopcocks, accurate ICP value, excellent waveform quality with less artifact, placement in brain parenchyma, and the fact that transducer leveling is not required. Disadvantages include a greater cost than with the fluid-filled system, the requirement for dedicated hardware, special handling of the catheter and cable to avoid breakage, inability to rezero after insertion, and inability to drain CSF as a treatment modality unless a catheter is placed in a lateral ventricle.
- A *catheter-tip strain-gauge catheter* is a monitoring system that consists of a miniature strain-gauge pressure sensor positioned at the tip of a 100-cm flexible nylon tube. It is similar to the fiberoptic systems in that several brain locations can be monitored and the microsensor is calibrated before insertion. Unlike the fiberoptic systems, it is housed in flexible nylon tubing that is resistant to breakage and allows for tunneling under the scalp (Vernon-Levett, 2001a).
- An *external fiberoptic transducer* is applied to the anterior fontanelle and measures ICP indirectly. Fontanelle tonometers are used only rarely in infants. Advantages include its noninvasive nature and lack of complications. Disadvantages include the lack of accurate ICP measurements (the amount of external pressure applied to the sensor can alter measurements),

the fact that it may underestimate ICP and may not record acute increases in ICP, additional cost, and that compliance testing and CSF drainage are not possible.

d. *Classification of systems: Anatomic locations* (fluid-filled, fiberoptic, or catheter-tip strain-gauge systems)

- The *intraventricular* location is the gold standard of ICP monitoring. Ventricular monitoring is located deep within the brain and is therefore considered to be more accurate in reflecting whole-brain pressure. The catheter tip is placed in the anterior horn of the lateral ventricle through the nondominant cerebral hemisphere. Waveform quality is excellent. Advantages are that the catheter allows drainage of CSF, is accurate and reliable, permits administration of medications, and permits volume-pressure compliance testing. Disadvantages include the high risk of infection and bleeding, the longer insertion time (collapsed or small ventricles make insertion difficult or prohibitive), and the risk of CSF leakage.
- *Subarachnoid bolts* are inserted into the subarachnoid space via a twist drill hole in the nondominant prefrontal cranium behind the hairline just anterior to the coronal suture. Different types of bolts are available (e.g., Philly bolt, Richmond bolt, Leeds screw). Pediatric bolts are usually shorter and lighter compared with those used in adult bolts. Waveform quality is good initially, but it may dampen with time when using a fluid-filled system. Advantages are that subarachnoid bolts are quick to insert and useful when ventricles are collapsed and access is impossible. Disadvantages are that tissue may occlude the device, CSF leakage may occur, ICP may be underestimated, and the bolt requires the skull to be intact.
- *Subdural catheters* are inserted below the dura mater and above the subarachnoid space in the same manner as the subarachnoid bolt. Used primarily after surgery for evacuation of a clot, the catheter is placed at the operative site (Germon, 1994). Waveform quality is poor and used primarily for trending. Advantages include the low risk of hemorrhage, quick and easy insertion, usefulness when the ventricles are collapsed and access is impossible, and a lower infection risk than with an intraventricular catheter. Disadvantages include the potential underestimation of ICP, the inability to drain CSF, and the requirement of an intact skull.
- *Epidural catheters* are inserted below the skull and above the dura mater. They are considered an indirect measure of ICP. Waveform quality is poor and used primarily for trending. Advantages are that epidural catheters have the least invasive placement (dura mater remains intact) and that it has a low risk of infection, quick and easy insertion, no risk for CSF leakage, and low risk for brain injury. Disadvantages are that epidural catheters provide an indirect measurement that is not as accurate and reliable as measurements made with other catheter systems and that epidural catheters are unable to drain CSF.
- *Intraparenchymal fiberoptic transduced tipped or strain-gauge tipped catheters* are placed directly into the brain tissue (via a bolt or screw device) approximately 1 cm below the subarachnoid space. Waveform quality is good. Advantages include the low risk of infection, quick and easy insertion, and accuracy and reliability. Disadvantages are the same as for all fiberoptic systems.

e. *Nursing implications*

- *Zeroing and calibrating* the fluid-filled systems depend on the manufacturer's recommendations, unit practice, location of the catheter, and the risk of

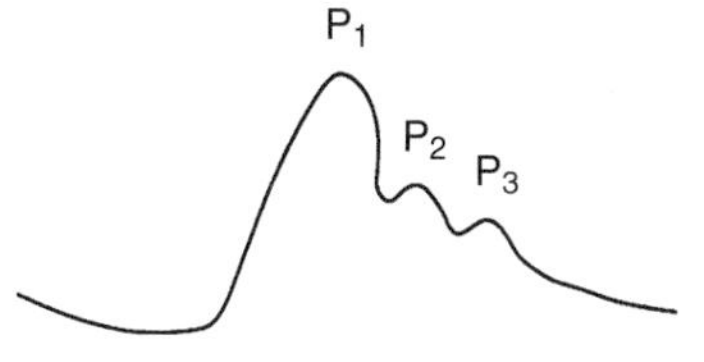

FIGURE 4-17 ■ Components of a normal intracranial pressure waveform.

infection. Because fiberoptic transducers are zeroed before insertion and are factory set, no calibration is required. Fiberoptic transducers may be calibrated with the bedside monitor. The fluid-filled transducer should be *level* at the foramen of Monro (e.g., outer canthus of the eye, tragus of the ear). The level should be changed with every position change. Leveling for fiberoptic systems is not required. The transducer is located at the tip of the catheter.

- *Insertion site care* is basically the same for all systems. Maintain a dry and intact occlusive dressing. Maintain aseptic technique with dressing changes. Notify the physician of any leakage on or around the dressing. Evaluate the insertion site for CSF leakage, bleeding, hematoma, and infection. The diagnosis of meningitis or ventriculitis is made on the basis of positive results from CSF cultures; fever and leukocytosis are less predictive. Local signs of catheter infection include redness, swelling, and drainage at the insertion site.
- *Maintain infection control* by using aseptic technique when handling the system. In fluid-filled systems, minimize the number of connections and stopcocks. Maintain a closed system by covering all entry ports with dead-ender caps. Minimize the number of times the system is entered. Avoid dislodgment or breakage of the system by avoiding tension on the tubing or fiberoptic cables. Tape the tubing to the dressing, clip or pin the cable to the patient, avoid kinking the cable, and use caution when repositioning or transporting the patient. Notify the physician of any loose connections at the insertion site.

f. *Waveform analysis:* The normal ICP waveform (Figure 4-17) resembles the arterial waveform with three descending peaks:

- P_1 (percussion wave) is the first peak that originates from pulsations of the choroid plexus. It is a sharp peak, consistent in amplitude, and the largest of all waves.
- P_2 (rebound or tidal wave) is more variable in shape and amplitude and smaller than the percussion wave and may become larger than the other two waves with decreased intracranial compliance.
- P_3 (dicrotic wave) follows P_1 and P_2 and is the smallest of the three waves. After the dicrotic wave, pressure usually decreases to diastolic baseline.

g. *Abnormal ICP waveforms* (Figure 4-18)

- *A waves* (plateau) are spontaneous, rapid, irregular increases in ICP to 50 to 100 mm Hg lasting 5 to 20 minutes. They are frequently associated with dilated pupil(s), vomiting, abnormal posturing, decreased level of consciousness, widened pulse pressure, dysrhythmias, and decreased respirations. They represent impaired CBF and occur most often with decreases in blood pressure associated with hypovolemia.
- *B waves* are sharp, rhythmic increases in ICP to 50 mm Hg lasting 30 seconds to 2 minutes. B waves are related to respirations. They may precede

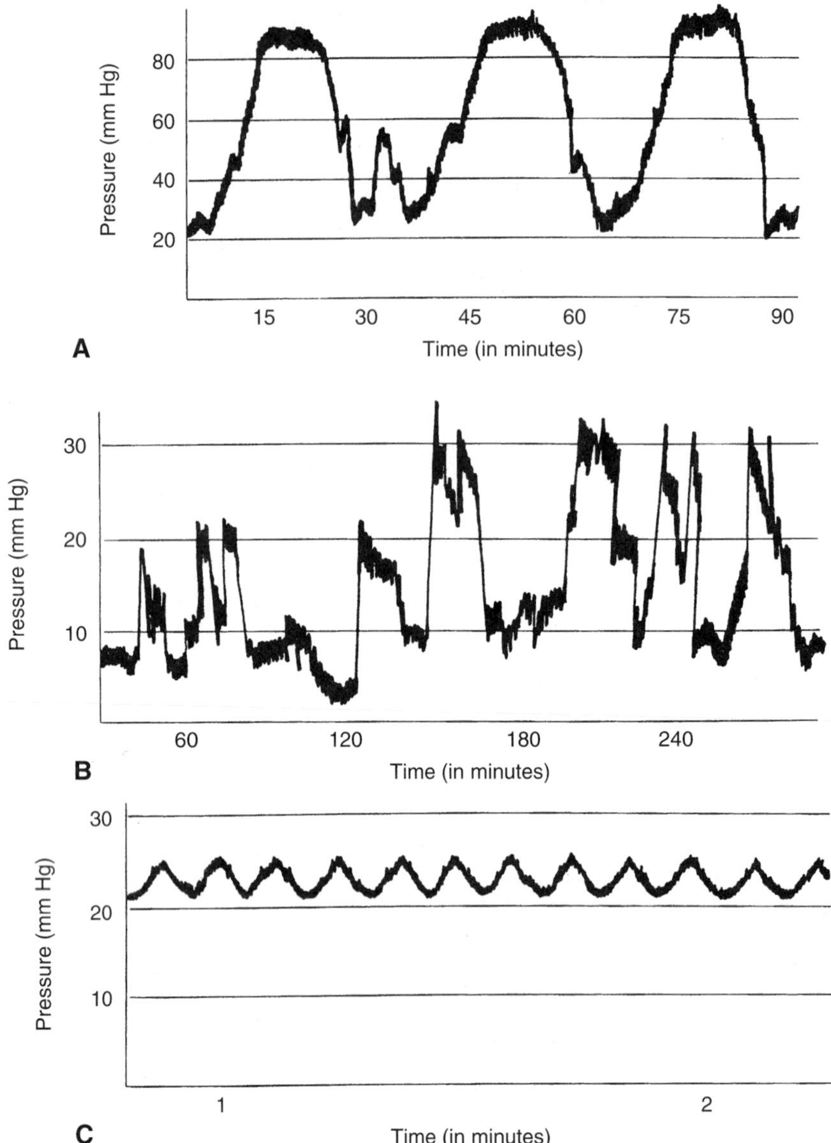

FIGURE 4-18 ■ Abnormal intracranial pressure waveforms. **A,** A or plateau waves. **B,** B waves. **C,** C waves.
(Reprinted with permission from McQuillan KA: Intracranial pressure monitoring: technical imperatives. *AACN Clin Issues Crit Care Nurs* 2(4):632-633, 1991.)

A waves or seizures or occur during a headache, posturing, or decreased level of consciousness.

- *C waves* are small waves that occur every 4 to 8 minutes and result from fluctuations in the systemic pulse and respirations. They are clinically insignificant.

2. **Transcranial Doppler ultrasound**
   a. *Description:* Calculation of mean velocity and direction of CBF is achieved by means of a 2-MHz ultrasound probe held to thin areas of the skull. Velocity signals are displayed as pulsatile waveforms that can be recorded. Transcranial

Doppler ultrasound does not directly measure blood flow, but the velocity signals are directly proportional to blood flow and therefore can accurately measure any change in flow (Unwin et al., 1991).

b. *Clinical uses* are for diagnosis of vasospasm, diagnosis of vessel occlusion, monitoring for cerebral emboli, testing of carbon dioxide and blood pressure vasoreactivity, and detection of changes in ICP (an increase in pulsatility).

c. *Nursing implications:* Ultrasound may be done at the bedside and has no major complications or contraindications. Preprocedural education should include instructing the patient to lie still. Sedation may be required.

3. **Xenon CT scan of CBF**

a. *Description:* The CT technique uses the high density of stable nonradioactive xenon to measure brain tissue buildup of this atom following inhalation of a xenon gas mixture. It is based on the principle that the rate of uptake or clearance of an inert diffusible gas is proportional to blood flow in the tissue. The brain is scanned before, during, and after the procedure, and end-tidal xenon concentration is measured and computer calculated to estimate CBF.

b. *Clinical uses* are for diagnosis of stroke, diagnosis of massive cerebral hypertension, confirmatory test for determination of brain death (i.e., absence of uptake indicates no CBF, which is a definitive diagnosis of brain death), assessment of global hypoxic ischemic injury, and assessment of intracranial trauma.

c. *Nursing implications:* Preprocedural education includes instructing the patient to lie still and inhale a gas mixture. The CT scanner may frighten patients. There are no known risks with the procedure.

4. **Electroencephalograms**

a. *Description:* An EEG records spontaneous electrical activity across the surface of the brain. Activity is characterized by the frequency and voltage of electrical signals. Common EEG abnormalities include the following:
   - Diffuse slowing of background rhythms is a common nonspecific finding seen in patients with diffuse encephalopathies and some structural abnormalities.
   - Focal slowing of parenchyma indicates localized dysfunction.
   - Triphasic waves seen in toxic metabolic encephalopathies consist of generalized synchronous waves occurring in brief runs.
   - Epileptic discharges are associated with seizure disorders.
   - Periodic lateralizing epileptiform discharges (PLED) suggest an acute destructive cerebral lesion.
   - Generalized periodic sharp waves are seen most commonly in patients following cerebral anoxia.

b. *Clinical uses* include the diagnosis of epilepsy, dementia and diffuse encephalopathies, brain lesions, some cerebral infections, and brain death.

c. *Nursing implications:* Preprocedural teaching should include a description of the sensations and setup of scalp leads. Sleep deprivation may be used to precipitate certain types of seizure discharges. It involves keeping the patient awake for all or part of the night before the EEG is to be performed. Depending on specific orders, the patient may be awake or asleep during the EEG. Discontinuation of anticonvulsants may be used before an EEG as an activation technique for seizure discharges. Describe the testing procedures to the child or family. Hyperventilation is an activation technique (i.e., induces seizure discharges) that requires voluntary hyperventilation. Photic stimulation is an activation technique (flashing a light in the eyes at various frequencies). Routine monitoring during the procedure includes observation of seizure activity, observation of other activity, and monitoring of vital functions as dictated by the patient's condition. Accurate documentation of the patient's behaviors and nursing interventions with continuous EEG recording is essential. Shampoo the patient's hair after the procedure.

5. **Evoked potential (EP) studies**
   a. *Description:* EPs measure electrical activity produced by a specific neural structure along a sensory pathway. The measurement is called an *evoked response* (ER). EP electrical activity is generally much slower than spontaneous cortical electrical activity (EEG) and measures minute voltage changes produced in response to a specific stimulus, such as a click, shock or light pattern. EP studies assess the entire sensory pathway from the peripheral sensory organ all the way to the brain cortex. Neural pathways studied are visual (VER), brainstem auditory (BAER), somatosensory (SSER), and multimodality (MMER), depending on the sensory system suspected to be pathologic.
      - VER uses a visual stimulus to the eye, usually a strobe light, which causes an electrical response in the occipital area. The response is recorded with electrodes placed on the scalp overlying the vertex and occipital area.
      - BAER uses a clicking sound applied to either ear to evaluate central auditory pathways of the brainstem.
      - SSER uses a sensory stimulus applied to a specific area of the body. The time it takes the stimulus to travel from the peripheral nerve to the cortex of the brain is measured.
      - MMER uses a combination of the above stimuli to evoke multiple responses from different locations of the brain.

   b. *Clinical uses* are to identify dysfunction in specific sensory pathways. EP studies do not require voluntary patient response and therefore can be used in comatose and nonverbal patients. VER studies are used to detect blindness and eyesight problems in infants. In older patients, it can be used to detect multiple sclerosis, Parkinson disease, occipital lobe tumor, and cerebrovascular accident (CVA). BAER studies are used primarily to detect hearing disorders in infants and may also assist with detection of posterior fossa tumors, CVA of the brainstem or temporal lobe cortex, auditory nerve damage, acoustic nerve neuroma, and demyelinating diseases. SER studies are used to detect spinal cord injuries and monitor spinal cord function during surgery.
   c. *Nursing implications:* Preprocedural education includes teaching the patient what to expect from stimuli. In visual testing, the patient sees a strobe or alternating checkerboard. In auditory testing, the patient hears clicks. In somatosensory testing, the patient feels an electrical current on the skin. The procedure is lengthy. Sedation may be required for agitation or anxiety. After the test, completely remove the gel and glue from the patient's scalp to prevent skin breakdown.

C. Assessing Metabolic Alterations

1. **Jugular venous oxygen saturation (SjO_2) monitoring**
   a. *Description:* SjO_2 monitoring is used to measure the balance between cerebral oxygen delivery and cerebral oxygen consumption. Jugular venous oximetry requires retrograde cannulation of the internal jugular vein. A 16- to 20-gauge introducer is used to thread a 4 French fiberoptic catheter. The catheter is advanced and placed in the jugular venous bulb, where there is the least amount of extracerebral venous contamination (Kidd and Criddle, 2001). The right internal jugular vein is cannulated more often than the left because it is

usually larger and drains a greater proportion of blood from the sagittal sinus. Normal SjO_2 values are maintained at between 60% and 75%. Abnormalities that increase oxygen consumption (e.g., fever or seizures) or that decrease oxygen delivery (e.g., increased ICP, hypotension, hypoxia, hypocapnia, or anemia) can decrease SjO_2. Nonviable brain tissue does not extract oxygen; therefore SjO_2 may be abnormally high (>75%). Two SjO_2 values below 55% are associated with high mortality (Bader, 2003).

b. *Clinical use* is to evaluate and manage patients with cerebral ischemia. SjO_2 monitoring may be used with ICP monitoring and CPP measurements to determine whether a given CPP is sufficient to supply adequate cerebral oxygenation.

- The advantage of SjO_2 monitoring is more accurate identification of cerebral ischemia compared with ICP and CPP monitoring alone.
- Disadvantages include the questionable reliability of low SjO_2 values; verification with blood sampling is required. SjO_2 values represent more global ischemia and are less representative of local ischemia. Because of catheter size, continuous SjO_2 monitoring is not suitable for infants and small children, usually those younger than 8 years or who weigh less than 30 kg; the catheter may impede venous drainage or cause obstruction of the internal jugular vein (Bader, 2003).

c. *Nursing implications*

- Verify low levels of SjO_2: Check the light intensity indicator on the monitor, send a blood sample for laboratory measurement, reposition the patient's head and neck, and flush the catheter with 2 to 3 mL of normal saline (Kidd and Criddle, 2001).
- Recognize SjO_2 desaturation (below 50%) and identify possible causes: Low SaO_2 (below 90%), increased oxygen consumption, hypercarbia, hypotension, increased ICP, and anemia (see section on Multidisciplinary Management of alteration in cerebral tissue perfusion).
- Anticipate potential complications from catheter cannulation: Hematoma formation, catheter sepsis, venous thrombosis, and local infection.
- Calibrate the oximetry catheter at regular intervals (usually every 8 to 12 hours) with venous blood gas analysis.
- Avoid excessive flushing of catheter and medication administration through the catheter.

2. Brain-tissue oxygen monitoring $PbtO_2$

a. *Description:* Brain-tissue oxygen ($PbtO_2$) monitoring is a newer technique to evaluate brain-tissue oxygenation and, in some cases, brain temperature. A $PbtO_2$ catheter is inserted through a cranial bolt deep into the white matter of the brain. Precise normal $PbtO_2$ values are not known but are believed to range between 20 and 35 mm Hg, depending on the monitoring system used (Bader, 2003; Littlejohns et al., 2003). A lower critical $PbtO_2$ threshold has not been established in children. A $PbtO_2$ less than 5 mm Hg is associated with high mortality (Bader, 2003).

b. *Clinical use* is to identify patients at risk for cerebral ischemia and evaluate the effectiveness of interventions that alter cerebral oxygenation (e.g., TBI, systemic arterial hypertension [SAH], ischemia, intraoperative monitoring). It is most accurate when used as complementary monitoring with SjO_2 catheters (Gopinath et al., 1999).

c. *Nursing implications:* Maintain infection control with sterile dressings over the insertion site. Assess and document $PbtO_2$ values in response to changes in clinical status and in response to clinical interventions.

3. **Lumbar puncture and CSF analysis**
   a. *Description:* Lumbar puncture is the most frequently performed neurologic diagnostic test to assess CSF composition. Lumbar puncture is performed by inserting a needle into the spinal subarachnoid space distal to the spinal cord (between L3 and L4 or L4 and L5 vertebral interspace).
   b. *Clinical use* is to measure CSF pressure, analyze CSF, inject or remove substances, and deliver spinal anesthesia.
   c. *Nursing implications:* Preprocedural education includes a description of the sensations. Local anesthetic is used requiring a small needle insertion at the site of the lumbar puncture. A topical anesthetic, prilocaine-lidocaine (a eutectic mixture of local anesthetics, or EMLA) can be used, but it requires application a minimum of 30 minutes before the procedure. Burning may be felt for a few seconds at the infiltration site. A side-lying position is used most often with the child's knees flexed to the chest. The child is held in place with the back close to the edge of the examining table. The nurse should avoid placing any weight on the child. An alternative position for infants to distend the dural sac slightly, and therefore ease insertion, is the sitting position. The infant's buttocks are placed at the edge of the table, and the infant's neck and hips are flexed and stabilized. After the procedure, assess the insertion site for bleeding, infection, leak, hematoma, and swelling. Potential complications include brainstem herniation with elevated ICP at the time of the test; hematoma; infection; headache; radiculopathy; and spinal, epidural, or subarachnoid bleeding.

INTRACRANIAL DEVICES

A. External Ventricular Drainage

1. **Description:** External ventricular drainage (EVD) is a temporary straight Silastic catheter placed in the lateral ventricle (usually on the right) through a burr hole. The catheter is externalized through the ventriculostomy site or from a secondary incision after being tunneled under the scalp. It may be attached to an ICP monitoring catheter (Figure 4-19), or it may function just as a drainage system. The distal end of the catheter is connected to a simple extraventricular drain.
2. **Indications** include intermittent drainage of CSF for acute intracranial hypertension, ventricular shunt malfunction, or acute hydrocephalus following intracranial hemorrhage.
3. **Potential complications** include infection, hemorrhage, collapse of ventricles, leakage of fluid, leakage of air into the ventricular system, and seizures.
4. **Nursing implications**
   a. *Several EVD systems* are available but have similar components, including a drip chamber, collection bag, and drainage-pressure scale.
   b. *Specific orders* are obtained from the physician for care. With the foramen of Monro or lateral ventricles used as the zero reference point, the drip chamber is moved up or down to adjust the amount of CSF drainage. Anatomic location of the zero reference point is usually the external auditory meatus. The height of the drip chamber is usually 27 cm above the reference point. In this position CSF automatically drains when the ICP is greater than 20 mm Hg (1 mm Hg is equal to 1.36 cm H_2O). Specific times when the tubing should be clamped (e.g., too much CSF drainage, during transport, during vigorous activity) or unclamped (e.g., signs and symptoms of increased ICP) and the level of head elevation are ordered by the physician.

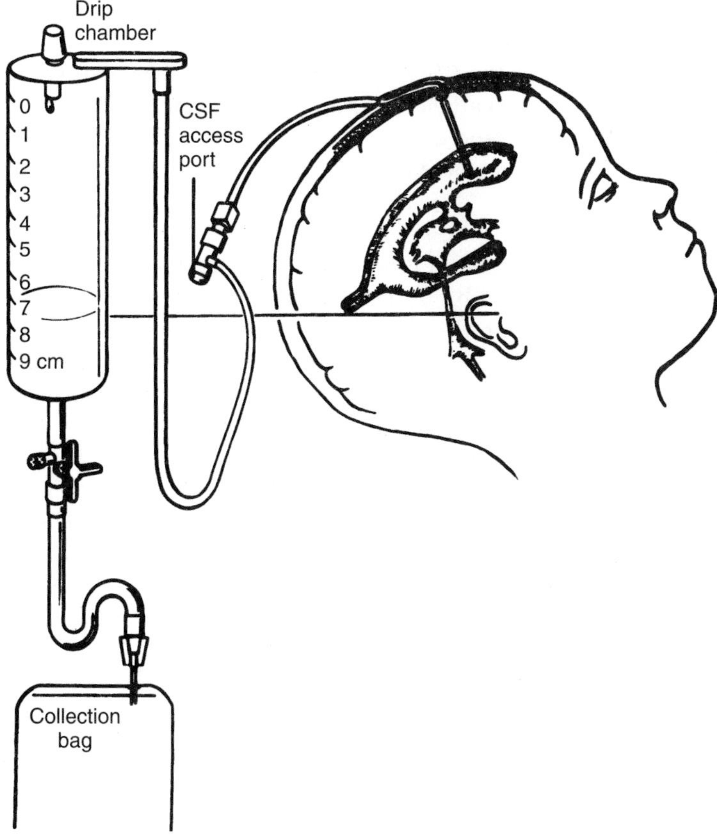

FIGURE 4-19 ■ Intraventricular intracranial pressure monitor with drainage system. *CSF,* cerebrospinal fluid.
(Reprinted with permission from Fuhrman BP, Zimmerman JJ: *Pediatr crit care.* St Louis, 1992, Mosby-Year Book.)

c. *Nursing responsibilities* include assessing and documenting the amount of CSF drainage. CSF flow is controlled by physician order (i.e., level of the drip chamber), the initial problem, and hydration status. However, normal CSF flow is usually 3 to 5 mL per hour in an infant, 5 to 10 mL per hour in a toddler or child, and 10 to 15 mL per hour in an adolescent. CSF should be clear and colorless. Initially CSF may be blood tinged, but it should become clear in 1 to 2 hours.
   - Assess the system for patency by assessing the ICP waveform if a transducer is being used (i.e., the waveform would be dampened if not patent). Assess for fluctuation of the CSF fluid in the tubing with each heartbeat and respiration (if the system does not have a one-way valve). When the system is not draining, lower the collection cylinder until you see drainage; if the system has an external valve, compress the valve several times with the clamp open. Refer to the specific manufacturer's recommendations.
   - Assess the system for loose connections.
   - Notify the physician for significant changes in the patient's neurologic status or for abrupt cessation or too much drainage of the CSF (i.e., if beyond the initial evacuation period, CSF drainage exceeds the established norms or exceeds the physician's prescribed amount).

- Document the reference level and maintain the drip chamber or drainage bag at the prescribed level.
- Prevent infection of the CSF. Observe the catheter exit site or dressing for drainage. Change the catheter dressing using aseptic technique. Monitor the patient's temperature and other signs of systemic infection (e.g., hypotension, increased WBC count, positive results from blood or CSF cultures).

B. Ventricular Shunt

1. **Description:** A ventricular shunt is an internal catheter system designed to drain the lateral ventricles of CSF by bypassing part of the ventricular system. Many systems are available, but the major components are similar. A ventricular catheter is placed in the anterior horn of the right lateral ventricle. It is inserted through a burr hole, usually in the region of the right parietooccipital area; the left side is avoided because of the location of the speech center. The catheter is tunneled under the skin to minimize infection. A reservoir and pumping device are placed directly under the scalp on the skull bones. The pump contains a one-way valve that is usually pressure regulated. Distal tubing is attached to the valve and may be placed in one of several body cavities. The peritoneum (Figure 4-20) is the most commonly used cavity. The distal catheter is tunneled subcutaneously to the upper quadrant of the abdomen. A small incision is made in the abdomen, and the catheter is guided into the peritoneum, where CSF is absorbed. Extra tubing is coiled in the abdomen to allow for growth. The right atrium is only used if abdominal problems preclude a peritoneal catheter. The distal catheter is

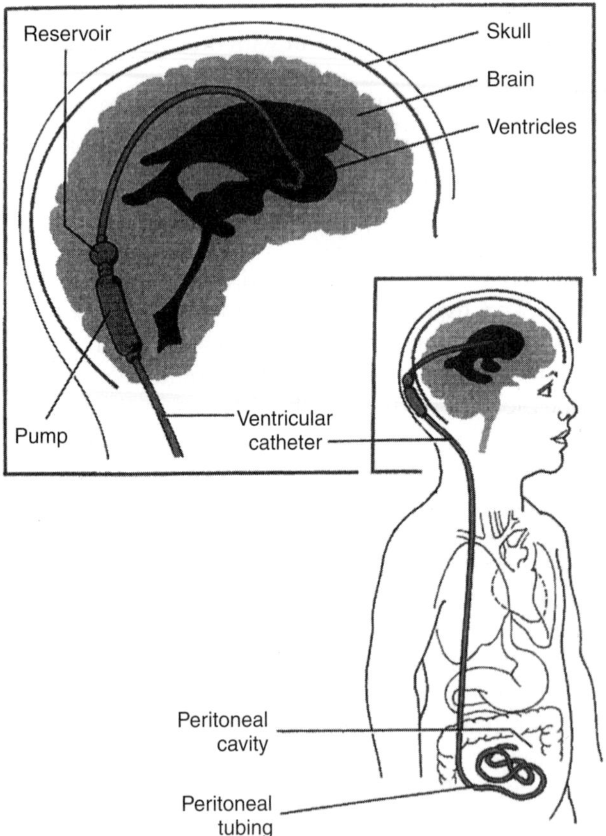

FIGURE 4-20 ■ Placement of a ventriculoperitoneal *(VP)* shunt.

(Reprinted with permission from Betz CL, Hunsberger MM, Wright S: *Family-centered nursing care of children*. 2nd ed. Philadelphia, 1994, W. B. Saunders.)

inserted into the right atrium via passage through the subclavian vein or, less frequently, inserted directly into the right atrium. The pleural cavity is used infrequently: only when the other locations are contraindicated.

2. **Indicated** for hydrocephalus (acute and chronic).
3. **Complications** of the ventriculoperitoneal (VP) shunt include bowel perforation, ascites, and ileus. Complications of the ventriculoatrial (VA) shunt include catheter movement, dysrhythmias, operative risks with more extensive surgery, endocarditis, and congestive heart failure (CHF). Complications of the ventriculopleural shunt include pleural effusion, pulmonary infection, and respiratory compromise.
   a. *All shunting devices* and body cavities that are receptacles are at risk for infection, including ventriculitis, meningitis, and systemic infection.
   b. *Mechanical failure,* although rare, may occur from valves that stick and reservoirs that become obstructed with debris or disconnected from the distal catheter. The distal catheter may become disconnected and migrate to other areas (e.g., right ventricle or pulmonary artery from a VA shunt, perforated intestine from a VP shunt). Obstruction from tissue, clots, and debris may occur in the ventricular tip, valves, reservoir, internal catheters, and distal catheter tip.
   c. *Clinical manifestations* of shunt obstruction and malfunction are similar and generally relate to increased ICP (e.g., a tense and bulging anterior fontanelle, poor feeding, or an increase in head circumference in the infant; headaches, vomiting, or papilledema in the toddler and child).
4. **Nursing interventions**
   a. *Monitor neurologic status.* Rapid evacuation of the ventricles may cause collapse of the ventricles, shearing of small vessels, and intracranial hemorrhage. Obstruction of the system can cause signs and symptoms of increased ICP. Seizures may occur.
   b. *Monitor for signs of infection,* including redness or drainage at the shunt site; hypothermia (more often in the neonate) or hyperthermia; redness, swelling, and tenderness along the subcutaneous tract; and nonspecific signs (e.g., lethargy, irritability, poor feeding, weight loss, pallor).
   c. *Monitor for signs of excessive CSF drainage,* including a sunken fontanelle and increased sodium loss.
   d. *Prevent skin breakdown* by elevating the head of the bed as ordered, positioning the patient on the unaffected side of the skull, or using pressure-reduction devices to protect the skin over the shunt when the patient is lying on the affected side, promoting good nutrition, and turning the patient every 2 hours.
   e. *Monitor for signs of ileus,* including abdominal distention, vomiting, large orogastric residuals (i.e., more than one half of previous hours' intake), and hypoactive or absent bowel sounds.

INTRACRANIAL HYPERTENSION

A. Description

Intracranial hypertension is defined as sustained elevation of ICP above 15 mm Hg. Increased ICP is not a disease state; rather, it is a final common pathway for a number of neurologic pathologies.

B. Incidence

Specific occurrence rates are unknown.

C. Etiology

1. **Neurologic pathologies** that produce increased ICP are broadly classified into (specific pathologies are discussed in later sections) those that increase cerebral blood volume, CSF, or brain tissue.
2. **Cerebral edema** may increase ICP and results from a number of different pathologies. It is defined as an increase in the fluid content of brain tissue. It is not a single entity and occurs in several different forms (Fishman, 1995).
   a. *Cellular (cytotoxic) edema* is characterized by intracellular swelling. It is caused by hypoxia, producing failure of intracellular active transport systems and an increase in intracellular osmoles as water enters rapidly into the cell or acute hypo-osmolality of the plasma that results in water rapidly shifting into cells. This occurs primarily in gray matter.
   b. *Vasogenic edema* is characterized by increased permeability of the capillary endothelium to macromolecules. Large plasma molecules move from the vascular compartment into the extracellular spaces, pulling water with them. Vasogenic edema occurs after vascular injury (e.g., abscess, hemorrhage, infarction, contusion), tumors, or disruption of the blood-brain barrier and accumulation of extracellular fluid.
   c. *Interstitial edema* is characterized by transependymal movement of CSF fluid from the ventricles into the extracellular spaces of brain tissue. It results from increased CSF hydrostatic pressure associated with noncommunicating hydrocephalus. This edema is most prominent in the white matter around ventricles.

D. Pathophysiology

1. Regardless of the cause, when intracranial volume exceeds the buffering capacity of the brain, ICP increases (see Intracranial Pressure Dynamics discussion).
2. Increased ICP causes a number of interrelated pathologic processes resulting in distortion and herniation of brain tissue (Figure 4-21).
   a. *Supratentorial herniation* occurs with an increase in intracranial volume and ICP in the brain structures above the tentorial membrane.
      - *Uncal herniation* is a unilateral displacement of the uncus through the tentorial notch from a large lateral lesion of the middle fossa. Disruption of the parasympathetic fibers to the third cranial nerve causes unilateral pupil dilation on the same side as the lesion and contralateral hemiplegia. Later signs include paralysis of extraocular eye movements; coma; and, if left untreated, death.
      - *Central herniation* is a symmetric downward displacement of the cerebral hemispheres, basal ganglia, diencephalon, and midbrain through the tentorial notch. Early signs include alteration in the level of consciousness, alteration of the respiratory pattern (e.g., yawning, sighs), small reactive pupils, and bilateral Babinski reflexes. Later signs include Cheyne-Stokes breathing, decorticate posturing, oculocephalic reflex, and coma.
      - *Cingulate herniation* is displacement of the cingulate gyrus under the falx cerebri into the opposite hemisphere, causing compression of the internal cerebral vein. There are few signs specific to cingulate herniation. Changes in the patient's mental status and level of consciousness may be the only clues.
   b. *Infratentorial herniation* occurs with an increase in intracranial volume and ICP in the brain structures below the tentorial membrane. Downward displacement of one or both of the cerebellar tonsils occurs through the foramen magnum, and symptoms occur very rapidly (e.g., cardiorespiratory

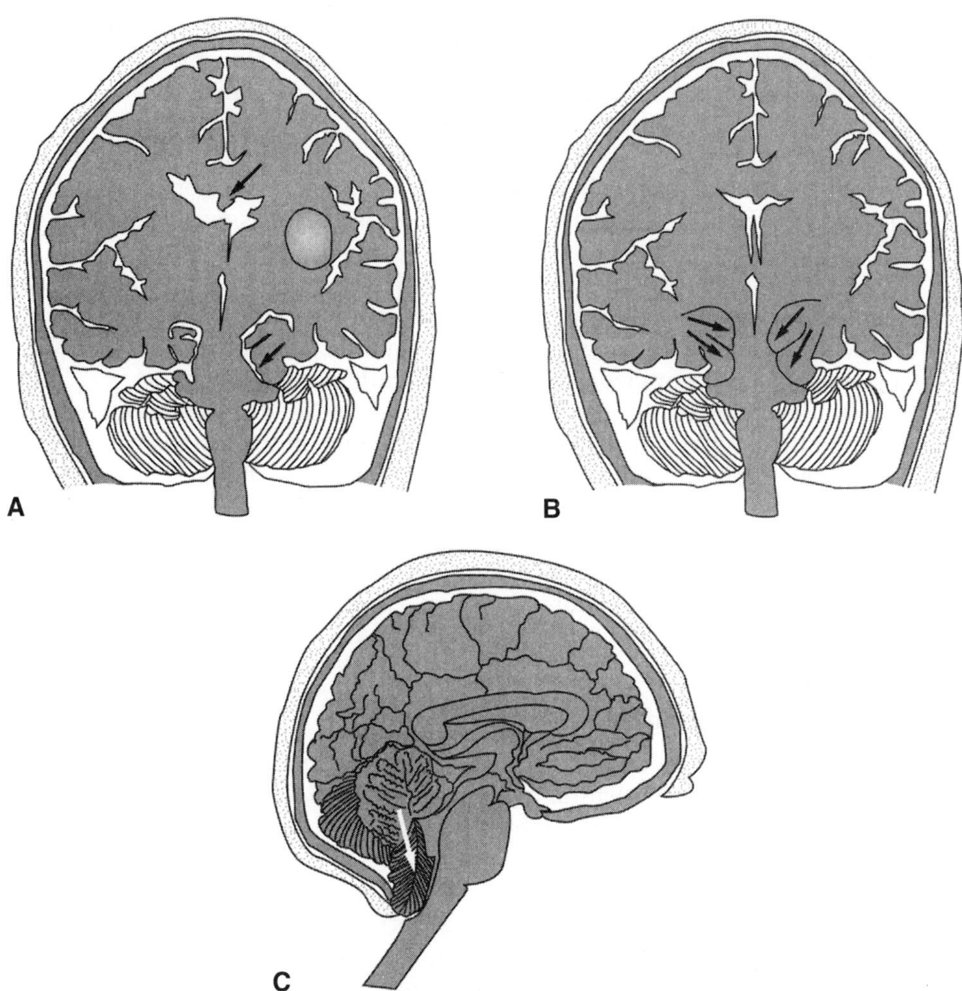

FIGURE 4-21 ■ Herniation syndromes. **A,** Midline shift indicating cingulate herniation. **B,** Protrusion of uncus through the tentorial notch. Downward displacement of supratentorial region through the tentorial notch as seen in central herniation. **C,** Herniation of cerebellar tonsils into the foramen magnum.

(Reprinted with permission from Morrison CAM: Brain herniation syndromes. *Crit Care Nurs* 7(5):35-38, ABC, 1987.)

failure). Upward displacement of the lower brainstem through the tentorial notch can also occur. Clinical signs include developing hydrocephalus and coma. *Midbrain compression* produces downward deviation of the eyes, and *pontine compression* produces small reactive pupils and decerebrate posturing.

3. Increased ICP also results in a reduction in CBF. With loss of cerebral autoregulation, CBF passively follows systemic arterial pressure. Brain ischemia, anoxia, and neuronal cell death occur.

E. Defining Characteristics

Symptoms depend on the age of the child and how rapidly the ICP increases.

1. **Chronic symptoms in infants** are usually nonspecific and include irritability, poor feeding, and lethargy. An abnormal increase in head circumference is

noted; patients in the 95th percentile require further evaluation. The normal rate of head growth in the first year of life is 2 cm per month for 3 months, 1 cm per month for 3 months, and 0.5 cm per month for the remaining 6 months (Jacobson, 1989). The setting sun sign is a classic "sunset" appearance of the eyes (i.e., the sclera are visible above the iris, and the infant is unable to look upward with the head facing forward). Vomiting, a large and full anterior fontanelle, the "cracked-pot" sound when the skull is percussed, and separation of cranial sutures also occur.

2. **Chronic symptoms in children** include headache (local or generalized); vomiting in the absence of nausea, especially on rising in the morning; blurred vision and decreased acuity; altered mental status (e.g., confusion, memory loss, fatigue, irritability); papilledema; and gait disturbances.
3. With **acute changes,** age becomes less a factor in differentiating clinical manifestations. Vital sign changes include a change in the respiratory pattern, progressing from irregular to absent respirations. The systolic pressure increases relative to the diastolic pressure (widened pulse pressure), and the pulse decreases. The pupils are dilated and fixed because of cranial nerve III compression. The patient's level of consciousness progresses from restlessness to unresponsiveness. Motor function progresses from hemiparesis, hemiplegia, or decorticate posturing to flaccid paralysis or decerebrate posturing.

F. Neurodiagnostic Studies

Selection of specific studies depends on the cause of the increased ICP. CT scan and MRI are used to identify structural causes of increased ICP. ICP, Sjo_2, and $Pbto_2$ monitoring are used to detect ICP, cerebral ischemia and evaluate interventions.

G. Medical Management

The cause of increased ICP is identified and corrected (e.g., insert a shunting device for hydrocephalus, excise tumors, and remove extradural hematomas). An ICP catheter is inserted for monitoring ICP, and a ventriculostomy is established for CSF drainage and ICP monitoring. Sjo_2 and $Pbto_2$ monitoring may be used to identify and treat cerebral ischemia. Medications to reduce cerebral swelling (e.g., diuretics, hyperosmolar agents) are administered. Decompressive craniectomy (removal of part of the skull) is used to treat patients with uncontrolled ICP following head trauma (Adelson et al., 2003).

H. Multidisciplinary Management

Alteration in cerebral tissue perfusion related to increased ICP

1. **Expected outcomes**
   a. Maintain a normal ICP range.
   b. Maintain a normal MAP for age.
   c. Maintain CPP in an age-related continuum: 40 to 65 mm Hg (Adelson et al., 2003).
   d. Maintain $Pbto_2$ at greater than 20 mm Hg and Sjo2 greater than 55%.
2. **Nursing assessment:** Perform baseline and serial neurologic assessments. Monitor serum medication levels, urine and serum osmolality, electrolytes, ICP, CPP, Sjo_2, $Pbto_2$, arterial blood gases, end-tidal CO_2 (E_TCO_2), and arterial saturation.
3. **Collaborative interventions to reduce ICP**
   a. *Avoid prophylactic hyperventilation* ($Paco_{2n}$ below 35 mm Hg). Mild hyperventilation ($Paco_2$ 30 to 35 mm Hg) may be considered for intracranial hypertension refractory to all other conventional treatments (Adelson et al.,

2003). Low $Paco_2$ causes the pH to increase (decreased H^+ concentration) and initially decreases cerebral tissue acidosis. Precapillary arterioles constrict in response to decreased H^+ concentration. CBF, cerebral blood volume, and ICP decrease. Prolonged use of hyperventilation may produce abnormally low CBF, especially adjacent to injured tissue, and ischemia may result (Marion et al., 2002). Correlate Sjo_2 and $Pbto_2$ with $ETco_2$ values. Monitor CPP, Sjo_2, and $Pbto_2$ to prevent ischemia.

b. *Maintain neuromuscular blockade* that allows for controlled ventilation and improved cerebral venous outflow. It reduces shivering, posturing, and airway and intrathoracic pressures and also prevents increases in metabolic demand by eliminating skeletal muscle contraction (Adelson et al., 2003).

c. *Maintain oxygenation and normal Pao_2.* Hypoxemia (i.e., Pao_2 below 50 mm Hg) produces vasodilation and an increase in cerebral blood volume. Individualize the endotracheal tube suctioning procedure based on the patient's response. Lidocaine may be given before suctioning to blunt increases in ICP during suctioning. Perform serial respiratory assessments and continuously monitor arterial oxygen saturation.

d. *Promote cerebral venous drainage.* Elevate the head of the bed 30 degrees to promote displacement of venous blood volume to extracranial vessels (Winkelman, 2000). Prevent increased intraabdominal pressure by using stool softeners, decompressing the stomach, and minimizing gastric residuals. Prevent increased intrathoracic pressure by individualizing the use of positive end-expiratory pressure (PEEP) and avoiding chest physiotherapy during periods of poor cerebral compliance. Maintain body alignment (e.g., flexion of the hips, flexion of the neck) to prevent cerebral venous drainage obstruction (Arbour, 1998).

e. *Minimize environmental stimuli* by minimizing noxious procedures, individualizing nursing activities to control ICP, avoiding cluster care, and maintaining effective pain control (Palmer, 2000).

f. *Control cerebral metabolism.* An increase causes elevation of CBF and cerebral blood volume. Treat hyperthermia aggressively with antipyretics and cooling devices. Moderate hypothermia (35 to 35.5°C) may be an option for refractory cerebral hypertension (Abhik et al., 2002; Adelson et al., 2003; Biswas et al., 2002; Tokutomi et al., 2003). Control seizures quickly with anticonvulsants. Barbiturate coma is generally used when all other conventional therapies have been exhausted in hemodynamically stable patients with salvageable head injury (Adelson et al., 2003). An induced barbiturate coma reduces cerebral metabolism and therefore decreases CBF and cerebral blood volume. It is associated with significant negative cardiac effects (e.g., decreased contractility, dysrhythmias, vasodilation, hypotension). Inotropic agents are used concomitantly or are on standby.

g. *Administer hyperosmolar therapy.* Hypertonic saline is effective for lowering cerebral hypertension. It is commonly used as a continuous infusion of 3% saline ranging between 0.1 and 1.0 mL/kg of body weight per hour. The lowest dose needed to maintain the ICP below 20 mm Hg is used. Mannitol (Osmitrol) is a widely used agent that produces an osmotic gradient between the intravascular and extravascular compartments. The net effect is movement of water from the interstitium into the cerebral vasculature, where it can be removed via the kidneys. A secondary effect of mannitol is a compensatory vasoconstriction due to decreased blood viscosity (with intact autoregulation). Dosing guidelines for mannitol range from 0.25 mg/kg to 1.0 mg/kg of body weight. Euvolemia is maintained by fluid replacement. Serum osmolality is monitored and maintained below 320 mOsm/L for mannitol and below 360 mOsm/L for hypertonic saline (Adelson, et al., 2003). Potential complications of mannitol, when used in high doses and at frequent intervals (i.e., creating hyperosmolality), include acute renal failure, possible rebound intracranial swelling (when mannitol diffuses into the extravascular compartment and reverses the osmotic gradient), electrolyte imbalances from increased diuresis via the kidneys, and fluid shifts.

h. *Administer diuretics* that can be used alone or, more frequently, in combination with mannitol. The proposed effects are total-body fluid reduction and decreased CSF production. Monitor fluid and electrolytes. Fluid restriction must be individualized because hypovolemia must be avoided. Frequently monitor serum and urine electrolytes and osmolalities.

i. *Avoid the use of corticosteroids.* The use of steroids in children with severe head injury lowers endogenous cortisol levels and may have an associated increased risk of infection (Adelson et al., 2003).

j. *Promote CSF drainage* by elevating the head of the bed to promote displacement of CSF to the spinal subarachnoid space. Maintain ventricular CSF drainage (see intraventricular devices). Decrease CSF production. Acetazolamide (Diamox) and furosemide (Lasix) transiently decrease ICP by reducing CSF. Long-term success of these medications is unproven (Bruce, 1989; Fishman, 1995).

k. *Avoid hypotension* with fluid resuscitation using crystalloids, colloids, and blood products. When the patient is euvolemic, vasopressors may be used to increase MAP and CPP.

l. *Correct hyponatremia* resulting from the syndrome of inappropriate secretion of antidiuretic hormone (SIADH) (see Chapter 6) or cerebral salt wasting syndrome (CSW). Unlike SIADH, in which free water is retained and hyponatremia results from elevated antidiuretic hormone (ADH), CSW syndrome is associated with increased urine output, increased urine sodium concentration, low serum sodium, normal ADH, and increased atrial natriuretic hormone (ANH). Treatment for CSW syndrome includes fluid and sodium replacement with normal saline (contraindicated in SIADH). The use of fludrocortisone acetate (Florinef) to increase sodium reabsorption by the renal tubules may be an alternative approach (Betjes, 2002).

SEIZURES

A. Definitions

1. A *seizure* is an uncontrolled, time-limited alteration in behavior that results from abnormal electrical discharge from cortical neurons.
2. *Status epilepticus* is a prolonged seizure (usually defined as 30 minutes or longer) or multiple consecutive seizures without regaining consciousness (Scott et al., 1998).
3. *Epilepsy* is a term used to define seizures that are chronic (two or more unprovoked seizures) (Camfield and Camfield, 1999).

B. Incidence

Seizures are the most common neurologic disorder seen in children. Febrile seizures are the most common form of childhood seizures with the peak incidence at 18 months of age (American Academy of Pediatrics, 1996). The overall incidence of epilepsy from birth to 16 years is approximately 40 per 100,000 children per year

(Camfield and Camfield, 1999). Forty-one per 100,000 population have 50 episodes of status epilepticus per year (Pellock, 1999). Seventy-five percent of patients who develop epilepsy do so before 20 years of age. Forty million people are affected worldwide. Males are affected more often than females.

C. Etiology

Except for epilepsy (unprovoked seizures), the most common causes of childhood seizures include fever (non-CNS infection), medication change, chronic neurologic disease, metabolic/toxic disorders, anoxia, CNS infection, and acute trauma. Idiopathic seizures account for a high percentage of seizures in children and are presumed to be genetically determined (Ozuna, 2000). Risk factors include age (it is more common in youth and elderly people), a family history of previous seizure, neurologic disease, head trauma, and neurodevelopmental abnormalities.

D. Classification of Seizures

Classification of seizures varies among experts, but the most widely used system is from *The International Classification of Epileptic Seizures* (Dreifuss, 1989). There are two broad categories of classification:

1. **Partial (focal, local) seizures** include simple partial seizures (consciousness not impaired), complex partial seizures (impairment of consciousness), and partial seizures evolving secondarily to generalized seizures.
2. **Generalized seizures (convulsive or nonconvulsive)** include absence seizures, atypical absence seizures, myoclonic seizures, clonic seizures, tonic seizures, tonic-clonic seizures, and atonic seizures.

E. Pathophysiology

1. In the absence of a compromised CNS, the brain is usually protected from a seizure by compensatory mechanisms. After approximately 20 to 30 minutes, severe alterations in brain function occur. Seizures increase the metabolic demand and CBF requirements of the parts of the cortex with repeated neuronal discharges. Prolonged seizures cause an uncoupling of CBF and metabolic demand, resulting in regional hypoxia, which leads to cell death (Orlowski and Rothner, 1998).
2. **Systemic effects** may also occur and are most often a result of hypoxia (Orlowski and Rothner, 1998). Cardiovascular effects include alterations in heart rate, cardiac arrest, cardiac failure, hypertension, hypotension, and shock. Respiratory effects include apnea, tachypnea, aspiration, respiratory acidosis, and airway obstruction. Renal effects include oliguria, uremia, and acute tubular necrosis. ANS effects include hyperpyrexia, diaphoresis, vomiting, and hypersecretion. Metabolic or biochemical effects include metabolic acidosis, hypoglycemia, hyperkalemia, and elevated creatine phosphokinase (CPK).

F. Defining Characteristics

The defining characteristics vary with the type of seizure. The most common type of seizure requiring admission to the ICU is generalized tonic-clonic (GTC) status epilepticus (formerly known as a grand mal seizure).

1. A **prodromal period** may precede a GTC seizure. The prodrome may occur days to hours before the seizure. Symptoms include headache, irritability, loss of appetite, insomnia, and change in mood. The physiologic basis is unknown.
2. An **aura** may precede a GTC seizure by seconds. It represents an abnormal focal electrical discharge from the brain. Clinical manifestations of aura vary considerably among patients and may include focal motor symptoms such as

finger movement and clonic movement of an extremity; focal sensory symptoms such as a "needles and pins" sensation or numbness; autonomic symptoms such as vomiting, pallor, flushing, sweating, dizziness, erection of body hairs, pupillary dilation, tachycardia, and incontinence; and psychic symptoms such as hallucinations and fear (Ozuna, 2000).

3. **Motor symptoms** of a GTC seizure are easily recognized. The tonic phase is characterized by rigid extension of the arms and legs. The clonic phase follows and is characterized by relaxation of the muscles alternating with contractions (rhythmic jerks). Following the clonic phase, the bladder sphincter relaxes, and urinary incontinence may occur.
4. The **postictal phase** is characterized by sleep with the extent and duration related to the duration of the GTC seizure.

G. Neurodiagnostic Findings

Specific studies to identify the underlying cause of the seizure vary depending on the suspected neuropathology (e.g., an MRI or CT scan for a structural lesion). EEG provides adjunctive data for diagnosing a seizure. Most GTC seizures produce abnormal EEG findings. Specific EEG findings vary with the type of seizure (Table 4-7).

H. Medical Management

Control of seizures with anticonvulsants is the mainstay of therapy. Identify the causes of the seizure, and correct the underlying pathology.

I. Multidisciplinary Management for Status Epilepticus

Potential for injury related to uncontrolled movements of seizure activity

1. **Expected outcome:** The patient will be free of injury after a seizure.
2. **Nursing assessment:** Assess the patient's airway for tongue biting. Describe characteristics of seizure activity. Assess the patient's environment for potential hazards.
3. **Collaborative interventions:** For an unexpected seizure, immediately clear the environment of potentially hazardous materials. In anticipation of seizure activity, maintain seizure precautions (e.g., standby oxygen, padded side rails, suction equipment). The patient should not be restrained during seizures.

TABLE 4-7
Characteristic EEG Features in the Various Seizure Types

Seizure Type	Interictal EEG Abnormalities
PARTIAL SEIZURES	
Simple partial	Variable, spikes over involved area of cortex may be normal
Complex partial	Variable, frontal or temporal lobe spikes
GENERALIZED SEIZURES	
Absence	Generalized spike-wave, often activated by sleep, hyperventilation, or photic stimulation
Generalized tonic-clonic	Variable, frequently normal
Myoclonic	Usually abnormal, generalized spike-wave, multiple spikes
Tonic or atonic	Usually abnormal, generalized abnormalities, spikes, multiple spike-waves

From David RB, ed.: *Pediatric neurology for the clinician.* Norwalk, Conn, 1992, Appleton & Lange.

❖ Ineffective breathing pattern from seizure or anticonvulsants

1. **Expected outcomes:** The patient will maintain a normal range of $Paco_2$ and a Pao_2 greater than 80 mm Hg.
2. **Nursing assessment:** Assess for a patent airway, ventilatory effort, and adequate oxygenation via skin color, arterial blood gases, and pulse oximetry.
3. **Collaborative interventions:** Maintain an open and unobstructed airway using caution to avoid inflicting oral trauma. Provide supplemental oxygen (Fio_2 1.0). Support ventilations as needed, including bag-valve-mask ventilation or tracheal intubation for apnea or prolonged seizure.

❖ Alteration in cerebral tissue perfusion related to a cerebral metabolic rate in excess of substrate and oxygen delivery

1. **Expected outcomes** include control of seizure activity, no significant complications from medication therapy, and resumption of premorbid mental functioning.
2. **Nursing assessment:** Document seizure activity, including information about the prodromal period, aura, duration of the seizure, characteristics of motor behaviors, and characteristics of the postictal phase. Assess mental status following the seizure (Ozuna, 2000).
3. **Collaborative interventions**
   a. Control seizure activity. Secure venous access and administer 25% dextrose (2 to 4 mL/kg) if hypoglycemia is suspected or confirmed by rapid test. Administer anticonvulsants (Table 4-8). Three classifications of anticonvulsants are typically used to control seizures. Benzodiazepines act rapidly and are used as a first-line medication. Lorazepam (Ativan) is frequently used in children because major side effects are infrequent (less respiratory depression). Rectal diazepam (Diastat) is now available and may be given in the field or when IV access is delayed. Phenytoin (Dilantin) is longer acting and is used to maintain seizure

TABLE 4-8
Initial Anticonvulsants to Control Status Epilepticus

Drug	Dose	Rate of Administration	Time to Effect	Side Effects
RAPID-ACTING AGENTS				
Diazepam (undiluted)	Begin 0.25 mg/kg IV and titrate to effect	<1 mg/min	1–2 min	Respiratory depression; thrombophlebitis
Lorazepam 2 mg/ml	0.1 mg/kg max 4 mg single dose	1 mg/min	2–3 min	Drowsiness, confusion, ataxia
Midazolam	0.075 mg/kg IV			Same as above; respiratory depression
LONGER-ACTING AGENTS				
Phenytoin 50 mg/ml; dilute in normal saline 1:10	15 mg/kg, up to 45 mg/kg	20–50 mg/min	~20 min	Heart block; hypotension
Phenobarbital 130 mg/ml	10 mg/kg, up to 30 mg/kg	30 mg/min	10–12 min	Respiratory depression

Modified from Blumer JL: *A practical guide to pediatric intensive care.* St Louis, 1990, Mosby-Year Book.

control. It is cardiotoxic and must be given slowly (0.5 to 1 mg/minute in the child). Fosphenytoin (Cerebyx) is a recently produced water-soluble prodrug of phenytoin that is quickly converted to phenytoin with higher unbound peak levels. Advantages over phenytoin include that it does not precipitate in commonly used IV solutions; it can be administered IM; it can be infused more quickly (in 7 to 10 minutes); and there is reduced risk of extravasation reactions, hypotension, and cardiac dysrhythmias. Both phenytoin and fosphenytoin are not sedating and are useful for patients with an altered mental status. Phenobarbital is often used in combination with other anticonvulsants because it is longer acting (Shafer, 1999; Stewart-Amidei, 2002; The Status Epilepticus Working Party et al., 2000; Winkelman, 1999).

b. If seizures persist despite conventional anticonvulsant therapy, additional interventions may be required, including an increased dosage and frequency of the preceding medications. Barbiturate coma provides chemically induced ECS. When maintained for approximately 48 to 72 hours, it has been successful in arresting seizure activity following discontinuation of the barbiturate (Orlowski and Rothner, 1998). General anesthesia with inhalation gas (e.g., halothane or isoflurane) is also used to achieve ECS and arrest seizure activity. General anesthesia is not used as often as IV anesthesia (i.e., barbiturates) because it requires gas-scavenging equipment and operating room facilities. Guidelines do not exist regarding the depth and duration of inhalation anesthetics. Paraldehyde has been successful in arresting seizure activity; however, the IV form is no longer available and rectal administration is unreliable. The rectal solution can be sterilized and made into a 4% solution for IV use; 0.15 mL/kg is administered over 1 hour. If seizure activity is arrested before the hour is complete, the infusion may be reduced to a level that maintains a seizure-free state (Orlowski and Rothner, 1998).

c. Monitor electrolytes, calcium, glucose, toxic screen, and blood urea nitrogen (BUN). Obtain appropriate neurodiagnostic studies to determine the underlying cause of the seizure.

d. Discuss with the patient and family the potential long-term effects of anticonvulsive therapy. Phenytoin (Dilantin) can cause gingival hyperplasia, lymphadenopathy, hirsutism, acromegaloid facies, ataxia, nystagmus, rickets, and folate deficiency. Phenobarbital can cause hyperkinesis, drowsiness, and rash. Carbamazepine (Tegretol) can cause drowsiness and abdominal distress. Valproic acid (Depakene) can cause drowsiness, alopecia, and abdominal discomfort.

INTRACRANIAL HEMORRHAGE

A. Arteriovenous Malformation

1. **Description:** Arteriovenous malformation (AVM) is an abnormal connection between arteries and veins without an interposed capillary bed. AVMs can occur in any part of the brain and can vary in size from a few millimeters to large formations. Characteristically, they are cone shaped and thin walled and may involve parenchymal or meningeal tissue.
2. **Incidence and etiology:** AVMs are the most common cause of spontaneous intracranial hemorrhage in children (Meyer-Heim and Boltshauser, 2003). The exact incidence is unknown, but approximately 2000 new cases are identified annually. AVMs are occasionally familial (Yokoyama et al., 1991). Most cases are

parenchymal (85% to 90%). AVMs are present at birth, but the patient may not become symptomatic until 10 to 20 years of age; 85% to 90% are supratentorial.

3. **Pathophysiology**
   a. *AVMs* occur early in fetal development from failure of the capillaries to develop. Supply of blood to adjacent brain tissue is diminished or absent (ischemia) because of the diversion of CBF through the AVM without the benefit of capillaries to allow diffusion of oxygen and glucose (i.e., there is a vascular "steal"). Without the inherent resistance to blood flow through a capillary bed, blood flow through the vascular malformation is increased. A pressure gradient develops, and the malformation continues to grow; collateral vessels develop, which add to the mass. Because there are no capillaries, high-pressure arterial blood empties directly into thin-walled veins. Veins are at risk for rupturing with hemorrhage.
   b. *Neurologic dysfunction* can occur from compression of surrounding tissue, ischemia of surrounding tissue and gliosis, hemorrhage, and hydrocephalus from obstruction of CSF.
4. **Defining characteristics** (ApSimon et al., 2002; Hofmeister et al., 2000; Stapf et al., 2003)
   a. The most common presentation in children is from spontaneous hemorrhage, and the incidence of hemorrhage increases with age. Increased ICP occurs from mass effect. Meningeal irritation occurs with subarachnoid hemorrhage. Rapid neurologic deterioration ensues with rupture and bleeding into the ventricles. Focal signs may be present and relate to the location of the hemorrhage.
   b. Seizures are the second most common presenting sign.
   c. Headaches are the third most common presenting sign. They occur from displacement of pain-sensitive arteries and veins. Veins on the scalp or face may be enlarged.
   d. CHF may occur in neonates with a large AVM because of the increased cardiac output necessary to support the AVM blood flow (often seen in vein of Galen aneurysms).
   e. A cranial systolic bruit is heard over the carotid arteries, mastoid bone, or eyes.
5. **Neurodiagnostic studies**
   a. CT scan may be used as a screening procedure and identifies blood collection and ventricular size. A high-resolution scan may reveal an aneurysm.
   b. Cerebral arteriography is usually obtained if surgery is required. It identifies the size, shape, and location of the aneurysm and vessel anatomy.
   c. MRI may be used as a screening procedure and is superior to the CT scan. It identifies hemorrhage, ventricular size, and vasospasm.
6. **Medical management** (Eder et al., 2001; Hongo et al., 2000; Irie et al., 2000; Massager et al., 2000; Nicolato et al., 2002; Zhou et al., 2000)
   a. *Treatment varies* and depends on the size and location of the AVM, the patient's age, cerebral dominance, technical support, condition of the patient, and characteristics of feeder vessels. Often treatment options are used in combination.
   b. *Surgical options* include open total surgical excision as the treatment of choice, but some formations are inoperable.
   c. A *second option* for inoperable or small AVMs (less than 3 cm in diameter) is Gamma knife radiosurgery or proton beam irradiation. Laser therapy uses a light beam to photocoagulate vessels of the AVM. Its advantages include the ability to coagulate small, fragile vessels; provide hemostasis following surgical resection; and clearly define the AVM.

d. The *third treatment option* is embolization of the AVM. It is performed by inserting a catheter into the cerebral circulation (e.g., carotid or vertebral arteries) and depositing a substance (e.g., Silastic sphere, Gelfoam, metallic pellet) to block blood vessels within the lesion. The use of transarterial embolization alone rarely obliterates an AVM in its entirety and is most often used as adjunctive therapy (i.e., staged embolizations can reduce the size of an AVM for surgical resection).

7. **Multidisciplinary management** (See Periventricular and Intraventricular Hemorrhage.)

B. Aneurysm

1. **Description:** An aneurysm represents a weakening in the arterial wall. The size may vary from a few millimeters to 2 to 3 cm. Most aneurysms are located at bifurcations in or near the circle of Willis, in the vertebrobasilar arteries, or within the carotid system.
2. **Incidence** (Guertin, 1998): Presentation during childhood is rare. Aneurysms in childhood account for 1.3% of aneurysms for all ages. Aneurysms are usually diagnosed at the time of rupture. The male-to-female ratio is 2:1 during childhood. Like adults, 10% to 20% of children have multiple aneurysms.
3. **Etiology:** Aneurysms may be congenital (majority), traumatic, arteriosclerotic, or septic in origin. A high percentage of aneurysms are found in the posterior circulation, and 20% occur at the carotid bifurcation. They may be associated with unrepaired coarctation of the aorta and subacute bacterial endocarditis. Aneurysms in children are more distal in origin, are more likely giant or mycotic aneurysms, are less likely to be atherosclerotic, and are located more peripherally (e.g., distal branches of the middle cerebral artery) than in adults (Guertin, 1998).
4. **Pathophysiology**
   a. *Abnormalities* exist in the arterial wall, especially in the elastica and media layers. There are four main types of aneurysms:

❖ A *saccular (berry) aneurysm* is rare in childhood. The sac gradually grows over time, usually rupturing between the third to sixth decade of life.

❖ A *fusiform (giant) aneurysm* results from diffuse atherosclerotic changes. It is commonly found in basilar arteries or terminal ends of internal carotids.

❖ A *mycotic aneurysm* is relatively common in children compared with adults. It results from arteritis caused by bacterial emboli.

❖ A *traumatic aneurysm* is a weakening of the arterial wall that occurs from a bone fracture or penetrating missile. It is rare in childhood.

   b. An *aneurysm* is significant when it ruptures and hemorrhages. Patients usually have acute symptoms with bleeding into the subarachnoid space. A clot forms following rupture of an aneurysm. Seven to 10 days later, the clot dissolves, and the patient is at risk for rebleeding. A rapid injection of blood into the brain may produce an acute increase in ICP. Cerebral hypertension may also result from obstruction of CSF circulation. Hypothalamic disturbances may occur from close proximity of hemorrhage to the hypothalamus. Vasospasm may be seen early following hemorrhage; however, the incidence is far less than in the adult population (Guertin, 1998).

5. **Defining characteristics:** Frequently, children are asymptomatic for many years. Nonspecific findings include nausea, back pain, lethargy, and photophobia. Localized periorbital pain and diplopia or ptosis may indicate third cranial nerve compression. A giant aneurysm may present as a mass effect (increased ICP). Symptoms related to hemorrhage (see the preceding discussion), severe headache, and seizures may occur. Neonates may present with CHF.

6. **Neurodiagnostic studies** are the same as for AVM.
7. **Medical management**
   a. *The goal of treatment* following rupture of an intracranial aneurysm is to prevent rebleeding of the aneurysm and control cerebral vasospasm. Controversy exists as to when an operation is of benefit. Early surgery (i.e., within the first hours or days) carries a high risk because of the critical condition of the patient and cerebral vasospasm, which may occur between 4 and 12 days after the hemorrhage. Postponing surgery until the patient is more stable (e.g., CPP greater than 60 mm Hg, MAP greater than 70 mm Hg, ICP below 20 mm Hg, neurologic status unchanged or improved from baseline) and cerebral vasospasm has been relieved carries a risk of a second bleed (the first 48 hours are associated with the highest incidence of rebleeding). Although vasospasm may occur, the incidence is low in children. Routine nimodipine prophylaxis is not strongly recommended in children.
   b. *Surgical options* include occluding the aneurysm at its neck with clips (most common), occluding the parent vessel on either side of the aneurysm (dependent on collateral circulation), coating the aneurysm with a material after wrapping it in muslin, or embolization of the aneurysm.
8. **Multidisciplinary management** (See Periventricular and Intraventricular Hemorrhage.)

C. Periventricular and Intraventricular Hemorrhage

1. **Description:** Periventricular and intraventricular hemorrhage (PIVH) involves bleeding into the subependymal germinal matrix at the level of the foramen of Monro (periventricular) and bleeding into the lateral ventricles spreading throughout the ventricular system (intraventricular).
2. **Incidence** (Larroque et al., 2003; Mancini et al., 1999): Approximately 20% to 30% of neonates have IVH. The incidence decreases as the weight and age of the neonate increase. Ninety percent of PIVH occurs within the first 72 hours of life.
3. **Etiology**
   a. The presence of subependymal germinal matrix (periventricular region) is characteristic of prematurity. The matrix is a highly vascular, gelatinous area with vessels that lack supporting structure. Glial and neuronal precursor cells are perfused by numerous fragile capillaries. Neonates have an immature vascular autoregulatory system with increased fibrinolytic activity. Before 32 weeks' gestation, there is increased CBF to this area; after 32 weeks' gestation, there is a shift of blood flow to the cerebral cortex and subcortical areas.
   b. Other risk factors include hypoxia, placental abruption, infections that alter the CBF in the periventricular region, respiratory complications such as pneumothorax (or any condition that increases venous pressure and impedes cerebral venous return), and rapid infusion of hyperosmolar infusions.
4. **Pathophysiology**
   a. The pathogenesis of PIVH and IVH relates to three interacting factors. The first is incomplete development of the vascular supply to the cerebral white matter. The second is maturation-dependent impairment of CBF. The subependymal germinal matrix is highly vascular and the vessels are thin walled, fragile, and lack supporting structures. Conditions that alter CBF can cause rupture of vessels and bleeding. Together, these two immature processes place the premature neonate at risk for ischemic injury to the cerebral white matter and bleeding into and around the intracranial ventricles. The third pathogenetic factor is the vulnerability of the oligodendroglia precursor cell that is the

cellular target in PIVH and leukomalacia. These cells are vulnerable to the cellular processes that result from ischemic injury (free radical production) and have deficient antioxidant defenses (Berger et al., 2002; Volpe, 2001).

b. Classification of bleeding is used to assess the location and amount of bleeding present:
   - Grade I: Subependymal hemorrhage only
   - Grade II: Intraventricular hemorrhage without ventricular dilation
   - Grade III: Intraventricular hemorrhage with ventricular dilation
   - Grade IV: Intraventricular and parenchymal hemorrhage

c. Blood clots within the ventricular system may obstruct the flow and absorption of CSF, resulting in progressive hydrocephalus.

5. **Defining characteristics:** Three basic clinical syndromes may be seen.
   a. A *saltatory syndrome* is a subtle deterioration that progresses over hours to days. Clinical features include depressed level of consciousness, hypotonia, irritability, drop in hematocrit, abnormal eye movements and position, and alteration in spontaneous movements.
   b. A *silent syndrome* is clinically undetected and usually diagnosed on routine ultrasound examinations of the head.
   c. A *catastrophic syndrome* is a rapid deterioration progressing in minutes to hours. Clinical features include coma, apnea, generalized seizures, abnormal posturing, unreactive pupils, a drop in hematocrit, and alteration in vital signs (e.g., hypotension, bradycardia) and endocrine function.
6. **Neurodiagnostic** (Maalouf et al., 2001; Ment et al., 2002)
   a. Real-time cranial sonography is the study of choice. It identifies the degree and location of the hemorrhage. Advantages include its portability, low cost, and noninvasive nature.
   b. CT scan and MRI identify structures as listed above. Disadvantages include transporting the patient to another location, maintaining patient stability during the procedure, and the difficulty of doing serial examinations.
7. **Medical management:** No specific surgical treatment is required for non-progressive hydrocephalus. Progressive hydrocephalus may require serial lumbar punctures to remove CSF and external ventricular drainage of CSF.
8. **Multidisciplinary management for intracranial hemorrhages**

❖ Potential for alteration in cerebral tissue perfusion related to hemorrhage, increased ICP, vasospasm, rebleeding, or hydrocephalus
   a. *Expected outcomes* include no hemorrhage, rebleeding, or vasospasm; premorbid baseline neurologic status; and no postoperative complications.
   b. *Nursing assessment:* The frequency of serial neurologic assessments is individualized to the patient; however, a general guideline is every 15 minutes if the patient's condition is deteriorating. Once the patient's condition is stable, assessments can be performed every hour. Monitor ICP, analyze waveforms, and calculate CPP at frequent intervals. Monitor cardiovascular status and assess for CHF (particularly in infants). Postoperative monitoring includes temperature, WBC count, ICP monitoring, and wound condition.
   c. *Collaborative interventions*
      - Prevent or minimize hemorrhage or rebleeding by maintaining a quiet, dark (if appropriate for the child) environment and enforcing strict bed rest. Controlled ventilation with the use of paralytic agents reduces fluctuating CBF velocity in infants and can reduce the incidence of intracranial hemorrhage (Perlman et al., 1985). Neonates who weigh less than or equal to 1250 g and who are clinically stable and lack contraindications for indomethacin should be treated with prophylactic indomethacin to prevent

intraventricular hemorrhage (Ment et al., 1999). Administer analgesics for headache. Administer stool softeners and order soft diet to prevent straining with defecation. Administer sedatives for anxiety and analgesics for pain. Administer anticonvulsants for seizure control.

- Control vasospasm (uncommon). Hyperperfusion consists of volume expansion with crystalloids or colloids to increase CPP and therefore CBF. Induced arterial hypertension consists of increasing the MAP to a level of 20 to 100 mm Hg higher than the pretreatment MAP. Dopamine and dobutamine are usually selected because of the ease of titration. The induced arterial hypertension improves CPP and CBF. Calcium channel blockers are used to inhibit contraction of vascular smooth muscle by blocking the influx of calcium into smooth muscle. The desired effect is reduced vasoconstriction and improved CBF. Nimodipine (Nimotop) is the preferred calcium antagonist because of its affinity for cerebral vessels; however, unlike the adult population, it is not used prophylactically because of the lower incidence of vasospasm in children.
- Provide postoperative craniotomy care (see Space-Occupying Lesions [Tumors] discussion).

❖ Potential for decreased cardiac output and tissue perfusion related to high flow AVM (see Congestive Heart Failure in Chapter 3)

❖ Potential for injury related to seizures (see Seizures discussion)

CENTRAL NERVOUS SYSTEM INFECTIONS

A. Description

1. **Meningitis** is an inflammation of the meninges (the outer coverings of the brain and spinal cord). Bacterial (purulent) meningitis is diagnosed with evidence of a bacterial pathogen in the CSF. *Viral* (aseptic) meningitis is defined as meningitis without evidence of bacterial pathogen in the CSF (by usual laboratory testing).
2. **Encephalitis** is defined as an acute inflammation of brain tissue and occasionally the meninges.

B. Incidence

1. **Bacterial meningitis** is age specific, with the highest incidence in children younger than 1 year of age. Males predominate (Phillips and Simor, 1998). **Viral meningitis** is less common than bacterial meningitis. The highest incidence is in infants younger than 1 year. Most cases occur in younger children.
2. **Encephalitis** occurs most often in children younger than 10 years of age. The incidence decreases after age 10 years and is constant until age 40 years, when it decreases further. It is more common in children who are immunosuppressed.

C. Etiology

1. **Bacterial meningitis:** Since the introduction of hemophilus b conjugate vaccine, the incidence of invasive *Haemophilus influenzae* has decreased significantly. Currently the most common causative agents of bacterial meningitis in North America are *Neisseria meningitidis* and *Streptococcus pneumoniae* (Neuman and Harper, 2003; Phillips and Simor, 1998; Shepard et al., 2003). The most common pathogens for **viral meningitis** are enteroviruses, mumps, herpes simplex (type 1), adenoviruses, and California virus.

2. **Encephalitis** pathogens include arthropod-borne viruses and herpes simplex (type 1). It may also occur from systemic viral infections or following vaccination from a live attenuated virus vaccine.

D. Pathophysiology

1. **Bacterial meningitis** pathogens usually arise from a distant site and colonize. They enter the bloodstream, producing septicemia, and then invade the meninges. Less frequently, pathogens infect the meninges via a direct route (e.g., depressed skull fracture, penetrating missile). Pathogens proliferate and spread into CSF and then invade parenchyma and blood vessel walls, producing vasculitis or cerebral edema. Purulent exudate may obstruct CSF pathways, producing hydrocephalus. Cell necrosis may also occur. **Viral meningitis** pathogenesis remains unclear. It is believed that the port of entry is the nasal pharynx, where the viral pathogen colonizes and spreads to the CNS via the bloodstream. The clinical course is usually self-limiting, with improvement seen in 7 to 14 days.
2. **Encephalitis** viral invasion begins in extraneural tissue (e.g., mastoid) and travels to the CNS via the bloodstream. Once in the CNS, pathogens may enter the CSF circulation through the choroid plexus or through passive transfer through the blood-brain barrier. Less frequently, pathogens may enter the CNS along peripheral nerves or via the olfactory system. Widespread nerve-cell degeneration may occur, as well as cerebral edema, cell necrosis, and increased ICP.

E. Defining Characteristics

1. **Bacterial meningitis** is characterized by nuchal rigidity (stiff neck), Brudzinski's sign (flexion of the hips and knees with passive flexion of the neck), Kernig's sign (back pain and resistance after passive extension of the lower legs), photophobia (abnormal intolerance of light), fever, vomiting, lethargy, headache, and alteration in consciousness. Petechial rash may occur with *N. meningitidis*. Late stages may produce increased ICP and cardiovascular collapse. Symptoms in infants are less specific and include vomiting, lethargy, bulging fontanelle, hypothermia or hyperthermia, diarrhea, and poor feeding. **Viral meningitis** presentation is similar to clinical symptoms seen in bacterial meningitis but usually milder. Most infants younger than 12 months have minimal symptoms.
2. **Encephalitis'** course of illness varies considerably (mild to elevated ICP and death) and depends somewhat on the infectious agent and the specific CNS structures involved. Clinical manifestations include prodromal symptoms of fever, malaise, myalgia, upper respiratory symptoms, nausea, vomiting, and stiff neck. CNS invasion is indicated by lethargy, drowsiness, stupor that may progress to coma, seizures, and localized symptoms. Severe cases may have signs and symptoms of increased ICP. Meningeal signs may be present and depend on the degree of meningeal involvement (compared with cerebral involvement).

F. Neurodiagnostic Studies

1. **CSF analysis** is the gold standard for diagnosing bacterial meningitis. Obstructive hydrocephalus must be ruled out before lumbar puncture can be performed.
   a. *CSF analysis in bacterial meningitis* demonstrates the following:
      - Elevated WBC count; polymorphonuclear cells predominate
      - Elevated protein content (normal 10 to 30 mg/dL)
      - Decreased glucose content (normal 40 to 80 mg/dL)
      - Positive results from Gram stain
      - Positive results from culture for organism

- Color: Turbid or cloudy
- Results are variable in the neonate because the WBC count may be normal, glucose content may be normal (it should be compared to serum), and protein levels are normally higher in neonates (20 to 170 mg/dL).

b. *CSF results in viral meningitis* demonstrate the following:
- Slightly elevated WBC count; lymphocytes predominate
- Normal or slightly increased protein content
- Normal glucose content
- Negative results from Gram stain or culture for bacteria

c. *CSF results in encephalitis* are variable but may be similar to viral meningitis. Viral antibodies may be found. Large amounts of RBCs may be seen with herpes simplex.

2. **CT scan and MRI** may demonstrate abnormal findings in children with meningitis but do not predict outcome or the degree of brain swelling. MRI with diffuse weight imaging magnetic resonance spectroscopy are able to detect early and subtle abnormalities (e.g., vasculitis and soft tissue imaging) (Hunter and Morriss, 2003; Zimmerman et al., 2003).
3. **Adjunctive tests** include Latex particle agglutination test (LPA) and rapid urine antigen assay (Das et al., 2003; Neuman and Harper, 2003). **EEG** is used as an adjunctive study in all CNS infections. Abnormal background EEGs are predictive of outcome in neonates with bacterial meningitis. Chequer et al. (1992) found that infants who had normal or mildly abnormal EEG backgrounds had normal outcomes and infants with markedly abnormal EEG backgrounds had abnormal outcomes (e.g., death or neurologic sequelae). The abnormal EEG backgrounds are generally nonspecific. The EEG is also helpful in identifying focal abnormalities.
4. **Brain biopsy** is the definitive diagnostic study for encephalitis but is rarely performed because the procedure poses risks to the patient and treatment would remain the same (i.e., supportive).

G. Medical Management

Antimicrobial therapy is the mainstay of bacterial meningitis treatment. Chemoprophylaxis is given to close contacts (e.g., family members, day care contacts, and primary caregivers in the hospital) of patients with *H. influenzae* and *N. meningitidis* (Burns and Zimmerman, 2000; Murray and Gilsdorf, 2001). Supportive care is all that is usually available for encephalitis and viral meningitis. ICP monitoring is not routinely used for CNS infections.

H. Multidisciplinary Management

Decreased cerebral tissue perfusion related to increased ICP

1. **Expected outcomes** include a normal ICP, premorbid neurologic status, no complications, and normal CSF analysis.
2. **Nursing assessment:** Provide serial neurologic assessment, including head circumference in infants; assess for increased ICP; and monitor fluid and electrolyte status.
3. **Collaborative interventions**

a. Use the preceding interventions to control increased ICP.

b. Administer antimicrobial therapy for bacterial meningitis. Broad-spectrum antibiotics are used until the pathogen is isolated. Most common antibiotics are third-generation cephalosporins. Ampicillin may be added for neonates to cover *Listeria monocytogenes*. Vancomycin (Vancocin) is added when pencillin-resistant organisms are suspected. Administer antimicrobials immediately following culture collections. Appropriate antimicrobial therapy continues for 10 to 14 days. Administration of dexamethasone (Decadron) is recommended in patients with *H. influenzae* to prevent hearing deficits (American Academy of Pediatrics, 1990; Chaudhuri, 2004; Lutsar et al., 2003; van de Beek et al., 2003). Current dosing guidelines are 0.6 mg/kg daily in four divided doses IV for the first 4 days of antimicrobial therapy. Dexamethasone should be administered at the time of the first antimicrobial dose. It is not used for aseptic meningitis.

c. Respiratory isolation may be used for 24 hours for patients with bacterial meningitis caused by or suspected to be caused by *H. influenzae* or *N. meningitidis.* Maintain enteric precautions for aseptic meningitis for 7 days from the onset of disease.

d. Administer acyclovir (Zovirax) 30 mg/kg daily divided every 8 hours for 10 days or longer for herpes simplex encephalitis.

❖ Potential for ineffective breathing pattern related to increased ICP

1. **Expected outcomes** include normal arterial blood gases, oxygen saturation greater than 95%, normal respiratory effort and rate, and no requirement for supplemental oxygen.
2. **Nursing assessment:** Monitor respiratory rate, work of breathing, arterial blood gases, and SaO_2.
3. **Collaborative interventions:** Administer oxygen as needed; support and maintain ventilations as needed (intubation and mechanical ventilation); perform pulmonary toilet for airway secretions; and perform chest physiotherapy as needed (in the absence of increased ICP).

❖ Potential for injury related to seizures (see Seizures discussion)

❖ Alteration in comfort related to meningeal irritation, headache, photophobia, fever

1. **Expected outcomes** include no complaints of headache, meningeal signs, or fever and normal light tolerance.
2. **Nursing assessment:** Monitor pain using pain scales, assess for meningeal signs (e.g., stiff neck, Brudzinski's sign, Kernig's sign), monitor temperature, and assess effectiveness of comfort measures.
3. **Collaborative interventions**
   a. Maintain body temperature in the normal range by using antipyretics and sponging with tepid water.
   b. Maintain a quiet environment by dimming lights and controlling noise.
   c. Alleviate nausea and vomiting by administering oral care and antiemetics.
   d. Eradicate infection (see preceding).
   e. Control increased ICP (see preceding).
   f. Administer analgesics for complaints of headache, arthralgia, and neck pain.
4. Potential for alteration in fluid and electrolytes is related to SIADH, diabetes insipidus, diuretics, fluid restrictions.
5. **Expected outcomes** include normal serum and urine electrolytes and osmolalities, normal range of urine specific gravity, and central venous pressure and vital signs within normal limits.
6. **Nursing assessment:** Monitor urine output, hemodynamic parameters, and serum and urine electrolytes and osmolality.
7. **Collaborative interventions** (see Chapter 6)

SPACE-OCCUPYING LESIONS (TUMORS)

A. Description

1. Tumors are an abnormal proliferation of CNS cells producing a space-occupying lesion and increased ICP. Because neurons do not have the capability to reproduce (significantly), most CNS tumors arise from support cells (glial cells).

2. Lesions are classified according to histology and location (Brunker and Shah, 2001):
   a. *Infratentorial* (below the tentorium) tumors include *brainstem gliomas* (malignant), *cerebellar astrocytoma* (malignant tumors that enlarge slowly and worsen over several months), *medulloblastomas* (malignant tumors that enlarge quickly, have symptoms detected within 3 months from onset, and are found almost exclusively in children), and *ependymomas* (benign tumors derived from ependymal cells arising from any part of the ventricular system and frequently located in the fourth ventricle in young children and the lateral ventricles in older children and adolescents).
   b. *Supratentorial* (above the tentorium) tumors include *hemispheric tumors* (usually malignant gliomas, low-grade tumors without distinct borders that infiltrate the parenchyma) and *midline tumors*, including *optic chiasm tumors* (malignant), *craniopharyngiomas* (malignant), *pineal-region tumors* (usually malignant), and *germ cell tumors* (malignant).

B. Incidence

Brain tumors are the second most common malignancy and the most common solid tumor in children (Brunker and Shah, 2001; Kline and Sevier, 2003). In the United States, approximately 1700 children were diagnosed with a brain tumor in 1999 (Smith and Gloeckler Ries, 2002). The posterior fossa is the most frequent site of occurrence in children. Infratentorial tumors are the most common location in children up to the age of 5 years (Rickert and Paulus, 2001). The main histologic diagnoses are astrocytomas, medulloblastomas, ependymomas, craniopharyngiomas, and germ cell tumors. Males have a slightly higher incidence than females (Rickert and Paulus, 2001; Surawicz et al., 1999). More than half of all children diagnosed with brain tumors live longer than 5 years (American Cancer Society, 2004).

C. Etiology

The causes are unknown (Baldwin and Preston-Martin, 2004). Risk factors include neurofibromatosis and von Hippel-Lindau disease (for hemangioblastomas). Past cranial irradiation increases the incidence of developing a secondary cancer; the amount of irradiation varies depending on the initial type of cancer and treatment. Another accepted risk factor is immunosuppression.

D. Pathophysiology

Physiologic changes are based on a space-occupying lesion and the effects of increased ICP. Increased ICP develops not only from the tumor mass but also from blockage of CSF flow or tumor-associated edema. If increased ICP is left untreated, ischemia and herniation syndromes may occur.

E. Defining Characteristics (Armstrong and Gilbert, 2000)

1. **Symptoms** vary tremendously in children and depend on location, rate of growth, and age and developmental stage of the child.
2. **General symptoms** include increased ICP caused by obstruction of the CSF pathways (most common). Classic signs and symptoms of increased ICP in verbal children include headache (usually on awakening in the morning; diffuse, dull and steady in quality; and less prominent in supratentorial tumors) and nausea.
3. **Localized symptoms of infratentorial tumors:** *Cerebellar tumors* cause impaired coordination and balance, truncal ataxia (irregular muscular coordination of the upper body), and nystagmus. *Brainstem tumors* cause cranial nerve dysfunction, ataxia, and corticospinal tract dysfunction.

4. **Localized symptoms of supratentorial tumors**
   a. *Tumors located near the cortical surface* cause seizures and focal cerebral dysfunction. Symptoms depend on the area affected but may include motor dysfunction, irritability, and speech dysfunction.
   b. *Deep cerebral hemispheric tumors* cause hemiplegia and visual-field defects.
   c. *Frontal-lobe tumors* provoke behavioral changes, language dysfunction, motor weakness, and seizures with focal motor onset or tonic-clonic movements.
   d. *Occipital-lobe tumors* cause visual field dysfunction (e.g., homonymous hemianopsia, which describes a defect in the right or left halves of the visual fields of the two eyes) and visual hallucinations.
   e. *Temporal-lobe tumors* produce auditory and speech dysfunction such as receptive aphasia, olfactory dysfunction such as involuntary smacking or licking of the lips, and psychomotor seizures.
   f. *Sella turcica–area tumors* produce eating dysfunction, metabolic dysfunction, and autonomic seizures.
   g. *Parietal-lobe tumors* cause reading dysfunction and dysfunction in awareness of contralateral extremities.
5. **Infants and toddlers** usually present with nonspecific symptoms (e.g., vomiting, lethargy, unsteadiness, irritability). Weakness and seizures are less common.

F. Neurodiagnostic Studies

1. **CT scan** is performed with and without contrast in approximately 15 minutes. It is useful for urgent diagnostic studies.
2. **MRI** (Kanan and Gasson, 2003) is the preferred diagnostic study and is performed both with and without contrast. It provides a better definition of tumor than a CT scan and identifies small tumors not seen on CT scan. MRI demonstrates the tumor in all planes and requires about 45 minutes to complete. The child may require sedation. MRI also avoids irradiation.
3. **Human chorionic gonadotropin (hCG) and alpha-fetoprotein (AFP)** may be elevated in a child with a pineal-region tumor. Elevated levels of hCG and AFP usually indicate nongerminomatous germ cell tumor.
4. **CSF polyamines** may be elevated in several types of brain tumors and hydrocephalus.
5. **Brain biopsy** is required to make a tissue diagnosis for specific treatment protocols and is usually done during surgical tumor debulking.

G. Medical Management

1. The **goal** is to eradicate the tumor with minimal morbidity.
2. Therapy usually consists of **three elements.**
   a. *Surgery* is used to obtain tissue for histologic examination, to reduce tumor size (debulk), and to create VP shunts for patients with surgically uncorrectable hydrocephalus. Total resection is rarely possible, and postoperative edema may occur; however, debulking improves the effectiveness of radiation and chemotherapy. Intraoperative MRI has improved the safety and effectiveness of brain tumor resections with minimal damage to surrounding normal tissue (Kanan and Gasson, 2003).
   b. *Irradiation* is the frontline therapy for diffuse tumors. It is delayed as long as possible in infants and toddlers to avoid damage to normal developing brain tissue. Stereotactic techniques have improved the effectiveness of irradiation and have limited damage to normal tissue. Stereotactic procedures include use of a basic frame that attaches to the patient's skull. Side arms (Y axis) and vertical (Z axis) and horizontal (X axis) bars and an arc are attached to the

frame. With the use of a CT scan or MRI and these coordinates, instruments are precisely directed to a specific area of the brain.

c. Traditional *chemotherapy* has been limited in part because the blood-brain barrier limits many systemic drugs from entering the CNS. However, chemotherapy's effectiveness has increased over the last decade. Like most other childhood cancer, combination chemotherapy is more effective than single-agent therapy. Commonly used chemotherapeutic agents include vincristine, cyclophosphamide, cisplatin, carboplatin, etoposide, lomustine, and carmustine. Chemotherapeutic agents are most effective with treating astrocytomas, medulloblastomas, and chiasmal gliomas. Children younger than 2 years of age are treated with radical surgical resection and chemotherapy to delay irradiation for 1 to 2 years to allow brain tissue development.

H. Multidisciplinary Management of Postoperative Craniotomy

Alteration in cerebral tissue perfusion related to increased ICP: Postoperative cerebral swelling, intracranial bleeding.

1. **Expected outcomes** include normal ICP, premorbid or improved preoperative neurologic status, no intracranial bleeding, no complications, and CPP greater than 50 mm Hg or higher, depending on the patient's age and condition.
2. **Nursing assessment:** Perform baseline neurologic assessment followed by serial assessments. Calculate the CPP if an ICP monitor is in place. Assess functioning of the ICP monitoring device. Cerebral swelling usually peaks on the third postoperative day. Monitor side effects of chemotherapeutic agents.
3. **Collaborative interventions** (see Intracranial Hypertension)

- ❖ Alteration in comfort related to incisional pain and headache
- ❖ Potential for injury related to seizures (see Seizures discussion)
- ❖ Potential for infection related to preoperative corticosteroids, immunosuppression, invasive lines, surgical wound (see CNS Infections)
- ❖ Alteration in fluid volume status related to nausea and vomiting, SIADH, and diabetes insipidus (see Chapter 6)
- ❖ Ineffective breathing pattern related to anesthesia, increased ICP, depressed level of consciousness

HYDROCEPHALUS

A. Description

Hydrocephalus refers to a variety of conditions that result in an excess of CSF in the intracranial compartment.

1. **Noncommunicating hydrocephalus** is an obstruction within the ventricular system.
2. **Communicating hydrocephalus** is a blockage to CSF circulation outside the ventricular system in subarachnoid cisterns or poor CSF absorption at the pacchionian granulations.
3. **Normal-pressure hydrocephalus** (low-pressure, adult, or occult hydrocephalus) usually occurs in middle age from arachnoid adhesions or communicating hydrocephalus.
4. **Hydrocephalus ex vacuo** is a ventricular enlargement from loss of brain parenchyma rather than an overproduction of CSF.

B. Incidence

Congenital hydrocephalus occurs in approximately 4 per 1000 live births. The exact incidence of acquired hydrocephalus is unknown but estimated at 1 per 1000 individuals (Andrews and Mooney, 1990).

C. Etiology

Congenital hydrocephalus is present at birth and includes Arnold-Chiari type II deformity, aqueductal stenosis, and congenital arachnoid cysts. *Acquired hydrocephalus* results from obstructive lesions that may include neoplasms, hemorrhage, infection, or trauma.

D. Pathophysiology

The cause of hydrocephalus is most often obstruction of the flow of CSF somewhere along its pathway of circulation (usually congenital aqueductal stenosis). Less often it is due to overproduction or reduced absorption of CSF. Untreated hydrocephalus with increased ICP causes dilation of the ventricles above the site of obstruction, atrophy of the cerebral cortex, and degeneration of the white matter tracts. Untreated cerebral hypertension may decrease CBF, cause cerebral herniation, and compromise brainstem function.

E. Defining Characteristics

1. Clinical presentation depends on how rapidly the ICP increases. Acute hydrocephalus with increased ICP may present with cerebral hypertension and rapid deterioration.
2. Slowly progressing hydrocephalus may have more subtle signs. In the infant, these include poor feeding, increased head circumference, setting-sun sign (sclera of the eyes are visible above the iris), Macewen's sign or "cracked-pot" sound when the skull is percussed, bulging fontanelles, prominent scalp veins, thin and shiny scalp skin, and high-pitched cry with increased ICP. Older children experience nausea and vomiting, headache, unsteady broad-based gait with a history of falling, deterioration in school performance, urinary incontinence, papilledema, diplopia, seizures, and behavioral changes (e.g., irritability, lethargy, personality changes).

F. Neurodiagnostic Studies

1. **Presumptive diagnosis** is based on clinical examination and presenting signs.
2. **CT scan or MRI** demonstrates an enlarged ventricular system and the pathology causing hydrocephalus.
3. **Ultrasound** is used with open fontanelles and demonstrates enlarged ventricles.
4. **Skull radiograph** demonstrates separated sutures or widened sutures, a "beaten silver" appearance on x-ray film from thinning of the skull and widened or split sutures, and the size of the cranial vault.
5. **CSF analysis** may demonstrate the presence of infection or inflammatory process.

G. Medical Management

The cause of obstruction must be corrected (e.g., excision of the tumor compressing the ventricle, antibiotics for inflammation from bacterial meningitis, or third ventriculostomy). Serial lumbar punctures or ventricular taps allow drainage of CSF and are indicated for temporary forms of obstructive hydrocephalus. Surgical insertion of a shunting device may be required. A VP shunt is most commonly used.

H. Multidisciplinary Management

- ❖ Decreased cerebral tissue perfusion related to increased ICP
- ❖ Potential for infection related to invasive surgery
- ❖ Alteration in comfort related to surgical incision pain, headache
- ❖ Alteration in skin integrity related to subcutaneous device with external pressure, large head with minimal muscular control

TRAUMATIC BRAIN INJURY

A. Description

A traumatic brain injury, or TBI, is an insult to the brain caused by an external force and not of a degenerative or congenital nature. It produces a diminished or altered state of consciousness and results in impairment of cognitive abilities or physical functioning, which may be permanent or temporary (National Head Injury Foundation, 1986).

B. Incidence

Beyond the first year of life, multiple trauma is the leading cause of death and disability among children; 60% to 80% of multiple traumas include a head injury. About 100,000 to 250,000 acutely brain-injured children are admitted to hospitals annually. One million children annually are estimated to sustain some type of head injury. Boys are victims almost twice as often as girls. Nationwide 1300 individuals die annually from bicycle-related deaths, half of which involve children and adolescents (Durkin et al., 1998).

C. Etiology

Many causes are age-related (Durkin et al., 1998; Rice, 2003). In all age groups, the most common cause of TBI is from a motor-vehicle accident. Children younger than 2 years who have a TBI are usually occupants of motor vehicles, and they often are not restrained or are improperly restrained. Older children with a TBI are more frequently pedestrians or cyclists. Infants sustain TBIs in falls, walker-related injuries, and nonaccidental injuries. Older children and adolescents are injured in bicycle-related or motorcycle-related accidents, by firearms and assaults, and during recreational activities. Risk factors include young age, substance abuse, and lack of protective devices (e.g., helmets). (See discussion on Multiple Trauma in Chapter 9 for a detailed description of incidence, etiology, risk factors, and prevention.)

D. Pathophysiology

1. **Primary injuries** occur at the time or within seconds of traumatic impact.
   a. *Skull fractures* are usually linear in children and occur along a suture line or perpendicular to a suture line. *Diastasis* (separation of cranial sutures) may occur in infants and small children; the separation may progress to growing fractures (i.e., a gradual erosion and separation of the fracture line) when accompanied by dural tears. Depressed fractures may represent depressed bone fragments or indentation of pliable skull bone without loss of bone integrity ("Ping-Pong" depression in an infant). *Basal fractures* are breaks in the basilar portions of the frontal, ethmoid, sphenoid, temporal, or occipital bones.
   b. A *concussion* is a transient loss of awareness or memory immediately following rapid deceleration of brain tissue. Patients do not always lose consciousness. It usually involves no structural brain damage. Diagnosis is based on history. Diffuse axonal injury and damage to neurons may occur from shearing.
2. **Secondary injuries** develop after the traumatic event and are a consequence of the primary injury.
   a. *Cerebral lacerations* are tears in the brain tissue, often associated with skull fractures. They are less common in children because the smoother inner table of the skull offers less resistance between bone and brain tissue.
   b. *Cerebral contusions* are heterogeneous areas of hemorrhage and edema within the brain tissue. They begin as primary injuries, but swelling, hemorrhage,

and subsequent increased ICP produce secondary injuries. These are less common in young children compared with adolescents and adults.

c. *Extradural hematomas:* Subdural hematoma represents bleeding into the dural space, usually venous in origin, from bilateral bridging of cerebral veins. They are more common than epidural hematomas in children. Epidural hematoma represents a collection of blood (usually arterial in origin) in the extradural space. The most common location is under the temporal bone from the middle meningeal artery. These are less common in children compared with adults.

d. *Diffuse generalized cerebral swelling* is produced by increased blood volume (hyperemia). The basic triggering mechanism is unknown. True cerebral edema (increased water content of brain tissue) may follow with severe injuries, especially surrounding brain contusions and hematomas.

E. Defining Characteristics

1. **Symptoms** depend on the type and severity of the injury. Simple linear fractures are usually asymptomatic.
2. **Basilar fractures** present with specific symptoms.
   a. *Battle's sign* represents postauricular hematoma and swelling from damage to the sigmoid sinus temporal bone.
   b. *The raccoon or panda sign* represents a periorbital blood collection from an anterior skull-base fracture (there is an absence of a subconjunctival hemorrhage).
   c. *Rhinorrhea* represents CSF leakage into the middle-ear cavity with drainage through the eustachian tube into the nose. *Anosmia* is the lack of smell from damage to the olfactory nerve. Both are usually related to middle fossa basilar fracture.
   d. *Hemotympanum* represents a blood collection behind the tympanic membrane from a temporal bone fracture. If the dura mater is torn at the same time, CSF may leak out of the ear canal *(otorrhea).*
   e. *Vertigo* may occur with damage to the inner ear.
   f. *Acute deterioration with associated hemorrhage and increased ICP* is most often seen with occipital transverse fractures because of the close proximity to the vital centers of the brainstem.
3. **Cerebral contusion** presentation depends on the location of the injury. Most injuries occur on the cortical surface of the temporal and frontal lobes from acceleration-deceleration forces, placing the patient at risk for focal seizures. The size of the injury and the shift in brain structures also affect presentation. Large contusions can produce a significant mass effect with shifting of intracranial structures and increased ICP. Clinical signs of increased ICP and herniation may be present. Symptoms also depend on the degree of associated swelling. Swelling occurs around the contusion 3 to 4 days after the injury. Significant swelling can also cause a shifting of brain structures and increased ICP.
4. **Concussion** may result in loss of consciousness, disorientation, retrograde amnesia, headaches, vomiting, fatigue, and posttraumatic seizures. Diaphoresis, pallor, and lethargy may occur in infants.
5. The symptoms of **epidural hematoma** vary. Infants may present with a bulging fontanelle, anemia with significant bleeding, and separation of cranial sutures. Older children demonstrate hemiparesis or hemiplegia and anisocoria. (*Anisocoria* is an inequality of the pupils that is usually greater than a 1-mm difference; some individuals normally have unequal pupils, usually less than a 1-mm difference.) All ages may have symptoms of increased ICP in severe epidural hematoma.

6. The clinical presentation of **subdural hematoma** is usually nonspecific and may include drowsiness, lethargy, and irritability. Retinal hemorrhages and seizures may occur especially in children younger than 3 years of age. Significant bleeding produces tense, bulging, and pulseless fontanelles. Retinal hemorrhages in a child younger than 3 years is highly suggestive of intentional injury.
7. **Generalized cerebral swelling** presents with increased ICP.

F. Neurodiagnostic Studies

1. **CT scan** remains the gold standard for acute evaluation. Mass lesions are identified both with and without shifts in brain structures. Bone windows identify basilar fractures. Epidural hematoma demonstrates a double-convex (lentiform), hyperdense area, and it does not cross suture lines (Figure 4-16 B). Subdural hematoma demonstrates a more diffuse blood collection crossing the suture lines. The acute phase is usually hyperdense and crescent shaped (Figure 4-16, *A*). Cerebral swelling and edema result in changes in density.
2. The disadvantages of **MRI** (see MRI under Neurodiagnostic Monitoring) limit its use as an initial screening study. It is superior to the CT scan in imaging nonhemorrhagic contusions and posterior fossa and small vascular lesions.
3. The **skull radiograph's** routine role in evaluating acute TBI has been supplanted by the CT scan. However, skull radiographs are useful in identifying missile injuries and some depressed skull fractures.
4. **ICP monitoring** is usually recommended for patients with severe injury, including those with a Glasgow Coma Score less than 8, abnormal CT findings with potential for increased ICP, and comatose patients with or without an abnormal CT scan (Brain Trauma Foundation, 2003; O'Sullivan et al., 1994).

G. Medical Management

1. **Surgical management** depends on the type of lesion. In general, children require surgery less often. Extradural hematomas are evacuated. Large intracerebral hemorrhages producing midline shifts are removed. Growing fractures are repaired with cranioplasty.
2. **Medical management** is supportive and directed toward preventing secondary injury, including hypoxia and ischemia, increased ICP, and complications (e.g., seizures, obstructive hydrocephalus, hypotension).

H. Multidisciplinary Management

❖ Alteration in cardiovascular tissue perfusion related to cardiopulmonary arrest

1. **Expected outcomes** include heart rate and rhythm within normal limits; MAP and CPP within normal limits; respiratory rate, pattern, and effort within normal limits; and no complications.
2. **Nursing assessment:** Provide baseline and serial cardiovascular, respiratory, and neurologic assessments.
3. **Collaborative interventions:** Maintain ventilation and oxygenation by controlling ventilation (e.g., intubation, manual ventilation) and administering supplemental oxygen. Support the cardiovascular system (e.g., cardiac compressions, inotropic agents, fluids).

❖ Alteration in cerebral tissue perfusion related to increased ICP

❖ Impaired gas exchange related to increased pulmonary interstitial water content (neurogenic pulmonary edema)

1. **Expected outcomes** include normal arterial blood gases, spontaneous respirations, normal respiratory rate and effort, oxygen saturation greater than 90%, and the absence of adventitious breath sounds.

2. **Nursing assessment:** Monitor heart rate and rhythm, respiratory rate and work of breathing, breath sounds, arterial blood gases and pulse oximetry, and intake and output.
3. **Collaborative interventions:** Administer oxygen to maintain SaO_2 at greater than 95%. Maintain good pulmonary toilet and PEEP when a patient is receiving manual ventilation. Preoxygenate and sedate the patient before suctioning. Limit suction passes to two. Administer fluids as ordered while maintaining adequate perfusion. Administer diuretics as ordered.

❖ Potential for fluid-volume alterations related to SIADH and diabetes insipidus (see Chapter 6)

ENCEPHALOPATHY

A. Description

Encephalopathy is a term used to describe any condition that produces a generalized disturbance in the brain's cellular metabolism, resulting in an alteration of consciousness. In children the list of potential causes is endless; causes may be chronic or acute, static or progressive, and inherited or acquired. The prototypic encephalopathies seen in critically ill children are Reye syndrome and hypoxic-ischemic encephalopathy.

1. **Reye syndrome** is an acute toxic-metabolic encephalopathy associated with hepatic dysfunction. Even though it is rarely seen currently, the principles of its clinical management are used widely.
2. **Hypoxic-ischemic encephalopathy** is a final common pathway for a number of pathologies that produce brain injury from two physiologic abnormalities. Damage to brain tissue from ischemia results from a reduction in blood flow and damage to brain tissue from *hypoxia* (decreased oxygen) or *anoxia* (absence of oxygen).

B. Incidence

The peak incidence of Reye syndrome (DeVivo et al., 1976; Keating, 1987) occurred between 1970 and 1980 at 1 to 8 cases per 100,000 individuals. It rarely recurs in survivors. The exact incidence of hypoxic-ischemic encephalopathy is unknown because the condition is a complication of a number of pathologies.

C. Etiology

The cause of Reye syndrome (Tasker et al., 1996) is unknown. Possible "triggering" factors include antecedent viral infection (most often influenza B) and concurrent aspirin ingestion (Centers for Disease Control, 1984). Hypoxic-ischemic injury can occur from any disorder that compromises cardiopulmonary functioning (e.g., sudden infant death syndrome [SIDS], drowning and near-drowning, cardiopulmonary arrest, prolonged seizures).

D. Pathophysiology

1. **Reye syndrome** produces acute vomiting and alteration in the level of consciousness during recovery from a viral illness. Microscopic liver changes include fatty infiltration (including other viscera) and swelling and disruption of mitochondria (Trauner, 1992). Hepatic dysfunction occurs, resulting in metabolic and enzymatic alterations such as increased liver enzymes; increased ammonia; coagulation disorders; and an alteration in carbohydrate, amino acid, and lipid metabolism. No jaundice is present. Cerebral edema and increased ICP may occur. Multisystem organ failure may develop.

2. **Hypoxic-ischemic encephalopathy** (Rogers and Kirsch, 1989; Traystman et al., 1991) results in damage during the initial hypoxic-ischemic event or during the reperfusion phase. It results from the depletion of vital metabolic substrates and accumulation of toxic by-products. Cellular changes are multifaceted, complex, and interrelated. They include energy depletion and anaerobic metabolism; lactic acidosis contributes to cellular damage, ionic pump failure occurs, and lipid perioxidation develops with free fatty acid accumulation. Another cellular change is loss of ionic homeostasis (resulting in calcium related damage, excitatory amino acid production, and oxygen free radical production). Irreversible cellular damage occurs with cytotoxic edema formation; increased ICP occurs infrequently.

E. Defining Characteristics

1. **Reye syndrome** may progress in one of two ways. A mild, self-limiting course lasts several days, or a severe course demonstrates progressive deterioration with loss of neurologic function. The disease process is staged into four or five categories of symptoms (Chesney, 1992; Owen and Levin, 1991).
   a. Stage I: Lethargic, frightened, and confused but follows commands
   b. Stage II: Stuporous, combative, agitated, and delirious
   c. Stage III: Unresponsive coma, decorticate posturing, and pupils dilated but react to light
   d. Stage IV: Loss of oculocephalic reflex, decerebrate posturing, and dilated pupils
   e. Stage V: Loss of brainstem reflexes (pupillary and oculovestibular), irregular breathing progressing to apnea, and flaccidity
2. The defining characteristics of **hypoxic-ischemic encephalopathy** depend on the cause of the hypoxic-ischemic event. Mild cases may demonstrate no apparent neurologic signs. Severe injury may present with signs such as coma, increased ICP, vegetative state, or death.

F. Neurodiagnostic Studies

1. **Reye syndrome**
   a. *Chemistries* reveal increased transaminases, usually 2 to 3 times normal (normal levels: aspartate aminotransferase [AST] 5 to 55 U/L; alanine aminotransferase [ALT] 5 to 50 U/L), increased prothrombin time (normally 11 to 15 seconds), increased serum ammonia (normally 29 to 70 μg/dL), hypoglycemia (normally 60 to 100 mg/dL), hyperuricemia (normally 1.7 to 6.6 mg/dL, 1 to 11 years), and hypophosphatemia (normally approximately 130 to 500 U/L, 1 to 11 years).
   b. Findings from *CSF analysis* are normal except for possible elevated opening pressure.
   c. *EEG* characteristics depend on the stage of the disease process. The typical pattern is a progressive slowing of electrical activity (Owen and Levin, 1991).
   d. *CT scan* is used to rule out structural causes of coma. It may demonstrate cerebral edema.
   e. *Liver biopsy* is used to differentiate other forms of hepatic disease. It demonstrates mitochondrial swelling, membrane changes, and fatty infiltration of the liver.
   f. *ICP monitoring* is used to manage ICP and CPP.
2. **Hypoxic-ischemic encephalopathy**
   a. *Chemistries* vary and depend on the extent of hypoxic-ischemic damage to other organs.

b. *CSF analysis* reveals normal cell count and routine chemistries. Creatine kinase-BB assay is present (Goe and Massey, 1988).
c. *EEG* findings depend on the extent of cortical damage (Wauquier et al., 1987). Slight to moderate insults demonstrate changes in peak frequency or asymmetric rhythms from homotopic regions in each hemisphere. Severe insults demonstrate progressive slowing of electrical activity.
d. *CT scan* is the same as for Reye syndrome.
e. *ICP monitoring* is not routinely used for encephalopathy from asphyxial arrest. ICP control does not improve outcome (Kochanek et al., 1998).

G. Medical Management

1. **Reye syndrome** has no specific therapy; supportive care is provided (Owen and Levin, 1991). Maintain fluid and electrolyte balance with supplemental glucose ($D_{10}W$ or $D_{15}W$) to maintain glucose at a high normal level, calcium supplements, and reduction of ammonia with neomycin (Mycifradin). Prevent bleeding by treating elevated prothrombin time and partial thromboplastin time with fresh frozen plasma (FFP), 10 mL/kg, before invasive procedures (e.g., liver biopsy, ICP catheter insertion) and vitamin K, 1 mg IV, every 2 to 3 days. Increased ICP is the primary cause of mortality; therefore therapies are directed toward controlling ICP and maintaining CPP (see Intracranial Hypertension discussion).
2. The mainstay of therapy for **hypoxic-ischemic encephalopathy** is to resume oxygenated blood flow as soon as possible to prevent secondary brain injury. Even though increased ICP is rare after global cerebral ischemia, ICP-directed management continues to be used with some exceptions. Barbiturate coma has not been shown to be beneficial (Brain Resuscitation Clinical Trial I Study Group, 1986; Haun et al., 1996). Several cerebral resuscitation therapies have been proposed, but their efficacy remains to be validated in the clinical setting. Improvement of CBF through induced moderate arterial hypertension has been advocated in the past; however, data do not exist to demonstrate its efficacy (Kirsch et al., 1989; Safar, 1986). Decreased coagulation and viscosity of blood (Safar, 1988; Wauquier et al., 1987), administration of calcium antagonists (Steen et al., 1985), and administration of free radical scavengers (Imaizumi et al., 1990; Liu et al., 1989) have been studied as well.

H. Multidisciplinary Management

❖ Alteration in cardiovascular tissue perfusion related to diffuse myocardial ischemia, fatty infiltration (see Chapter 3)

❖ Alteration in cerebral tissue perfusion related to increased ICP, microcirculatory changes (see Intracranial Hypertension discussion)

❖ Alteration in fluid and electrolyte status related to vomiting and hypoglycemia (Reye syndrome), SIADH, and diabetes insipidus

1. **Expected outcomes** include normal electrolytes, serum glucose, serum and urine osmolalities (or expected values if using hypertonic infusions), and urine output.
2. **Nursing assessment** includes monitoring intake and output, serum and urine chemistries and osmolalities, serum glucose, CVP, and urine specific gravity.
3. **Collaborative interventions:** Administer crystalloids to maintain normal hydration. Reduce fluids for SIADH. With central diabetes insipidus, provide fluid resuscitation for hypovolemia and administer desmopressin (DDAVP). Administer supplemental electrolytes to correct imbalances and glucose for hypoglycemia. Administer neomycin for severely elevated serum ammonia.

❖ Potential for infection related to invasive lines

❖ Potential for injury related to seizure activity (see Seizure discussion)

SPINAL CORD INJURY

A. Description

1. **Complete spinal cord injury (SCI)** is the complete loss of motor and sensory function as a result of interruption of nerve pathways below the level of the injury. *Quadriplegia* is the complete loss of leg function and loss or limited use of arms from cervical injury. *Paraplegia* is the loss of leg function alone from high lumbar injury.
2. **Incomplete cord injury** causes some loss of motor and sensory function with some sparing of function below the level of the injury.
   a. *Posterior cord syndrome* is caused by injury to the dorsal columns. There is loss of proprioception but preservation of other sensory and motor function.
   b. *Anterior cord syndrome* from injury to the anterior cord results in loss of motor function below the level of the injury. Sensory function is lost except for proprioception and vibration sense.
   c. *Central cord syndrome* is caused by injury or edema to the central spinal cord in the cervical area. Greater motor deficits occur in the upper extremities compared with the lower extremities. Sensory deficits are variable but are usually greater in the upper extremities. Bowel and bladder dysfunction is common.
   d. *Partial spinal cord syndrome* (Brown-Séquard syndrome) results from injury to one side of the spinal cord, resulting in loss of voluntary motor function on the same side as the injury. Loss of pain, temperature, and touch occurs on the contralateral side.
   e. *Conus medullaris* is an injury to the sacral cord and lumbar nerve roots, resulting in an areflexic bladder, bowel, and lower limb.

B. Incidence

1. Nationwide, 7800 SCI injuries occur annually, most commonly in men (2:1 ratio of males to females) aged 16 to 30 years and less commonly in children. The most frequent sites of injury are the lower cervical region (C4-C7 and T1) and the thoracolumbar region (T12, L1, and L2) (Muir and Town, 2003).
2. Cervical injury is rare in children; the upper cervical spine is more commonly injured in small children than in adolescents and adults (Mann and Dodds, 1993). Children have a higher incidence of SCI without radiographic abnormality (SCIWORA). This condition occurs predominantly in children and is thought to result from severe subluxation and trauma of the vertebral column. Pang and Wilberger (1982) theorized that SCIWORA is more common in young children because immature spines allow for reduction after momentary subluxation. As a result, the spinal cord is stretched or compressed with subsequent ischemia. Compression fractures are the most common SCIs (Mann and Dodds, 1993).

C. Etiology

1. The most common cause of SCI is motor vehicle related. Less common causes include bicycle accidents, sports (especially winter sports and diving) accidents, falls, and violence. Seatbelt-type injuries (flexion-distraction) are almost exclusively seen in children younger than 13 years. Flexion-distraction injuries occur when children are restrained in an automobile with only a lap belt. Intestinal and lumbar spine injuries occur as a result of flexion of the upper body against a fixed lap belt with a high-impact motor-vehicle accident (Muir and Town, 2003).

2. Nontraumatic causes include tumor, disc herniation, infection, spinal stenosis, and congenital abnormalities.

D. Pathophysiology

1. SCI most often occurs from vertebral injury, usually from acceleration-deceleration or deformation forces. Hyperextension causes fracture and dislocation of the posterior elements. Hyperflexion causes fracture or dislocation of the vertebral bodies, discs, or ligaments. Vertical compression causes shattering fractures. Rotational forces cause rupture of the supporting ligaments and fractures (Muir and Town, 2003).
2. **Types of SCIs and consequences**
   a. *Concussion of the cord* is caused by stretching and shearing of the spinal cord without tissue trauma. It causes a temporary disruption of cord-mediated functions.
   b. *Contusion of the cord* is a bruising and swelling of the cord, causing a temporary or permanent loss of cord-mediated function.
   c. *Laceration* is a tearing of neural tissue. The condition is reversible with minimal injury but may result in permanent dysfunction of cord-mediated functions.
   d. *Transection of the cord* is severing of the cord, causing permanent loss of cord-mediated function.
   e. *Hemorrhage of the cord* is blood vessel damage with bleeding into neural tissue. There is no major loss of function, depending on the extent of injury.
   f. *Damage to the blood vessels* that supply the cord results in decreased perfusion of the spinal cord with local ischemia. Alteration in function depends on the severity of ischemia.
3. **Intracellular and extracellular changes from SCI** cause an increase in excitatory amino acids, increase in free oxygen radical formation, alteration in calcium homeostasis, and increase in platelet-activating factor (PAF). Cellular alterations produce edema, damage to cell membranes, ischemia, and cellular death at the level of injury and approximately two segments above and below it. Normal activity is lost at and below the level of the injury.
4. **High cervical injuries** may cause immediate death.
5. **Spinal shock** (complete loss of reflex function) may result from acute SCI. It can occur within 60 minutes of the injury and may last for 7 to 20 days. It results from loss of integrity of the ANS below the level of injury, producing venous pooling, bradycardia, and hypotension.
6. **Autonomic dysreflexia** is a life-threatening complication in SCI. It is rare during the acute phase, but it may occur any time after an SCI. Autonomic dysreflexia results from an uncontrolled, paroxysmal, continuous lower motor neuron reflex arc due to stimulation of the sympathetic nervous system. The response typically occurs from stimulation of sensory receptors (e.g., distended bladder or bowel) below the level of the cord injury. The ANS responds with arteriolar vasospasm resulting in increased blood pressure. Carotid sinus baroreceptors are stimulated and respond with activation of the vasomotor centers in the brainstem via the ninth and tenth cranial nerves. The parasympathetic nervous system (vagus nerve) sends a stimulus to the heart, causing bradycardia and vasodilation. The peripheral vessels and viscera do not respond because the efferent pulse cannot pass through the spinal cord. The vagus nerve is not "turned off," and profound bradycardia may occur (Muir and Town, 2003).
7. **Temperature regulation** is impaired in patients with injuries above T1 because of the loss of connection between temperature centers in the hypothalamus and

sympathetic outflow of the spinal cord. Body temperature is regulated by the ambient temperature.

E. Defining Characteristics

Sensory and motor dysfunction depends on the type and level of the injury.

1. **Complete transection** results in loss of voluntary movement of body parts, loss of sensation to body parts, and loss of autonomic and spinal reflexes below the level of the injury. Reflex activity may return in 1 to 2 weeks.
2. **Incomplete transection** causes variable levels of vasomotor instability and bowel and bladder dysfunction and asymmetric flaccid paralysis, asymmetric loss of reflexes, variable sensory function (e.g., pain, temperature, touch, pressure, proprioception), and variable visceral and somatic responses below the level of injury.
3. **Spinal shock in the acute period** results in loss of vasomotor tone with complete transection causing hypotension, poor venous circulation, and bradycardia; loss of perspiration below the level of the injury; and loss of bladder and rectal control.
4. **Autonomic hyperreflexia** is a complication that usually occurs after the acute phase of an SCI. It results from a continuous, uncontrolled, paroxysmal lower motor neuron reflex arc, a massive sympathetic response that causes vasoconstriction with severe hypertension (systolic pressures of more than 200 mm Hg). The vagus nerve responds with bradycardia and vasodilation above the lesion. It occurs primarily in patients with injuries above T4 through T6 and is absent in patients who have injuries that destroy the preganglionic sympathetic fibers. Stimuli that can trigger this response include bladder dysfunction (e.g., distention, infection, outflow obstruction), surgical procedures, line insertions, tight clothing, pressure sores, and an impacted rectum. Symptoms include paroxysmal hypertension, headache, blurred vision, nausea, bradycardia, nasal congestion, and piloerection.

F. Neurodiagnostic Studies

1. **Radiographic spine films** are examined carefully to determine the integrity of each component of each vertebra and alignment of each segment. Frequently, spinal cord trauma occurs without radiographic findings in children because of their cartilaginous spine.
2. **CT scan** is used when radiographs do not adequately explain the clinical picture. CT scan identifies SCIs and bony lesions.
3. **MRI** is indicated for use the same as a CT scan. It clearly identifies the relationship of the spinal cord and surrounding vertebral elements and readily identifies cord compression. About half of all children with SCI do not demonstrate radiographic abnormalities on plain films, CT scans, or myelograms. However, MRI can usually identify spinal cord pathology with SCIWORA (Pang and Wilberger, 1982). Clinical assessment should be considered when evaluating SCI. MRI is not routinely used in unstable patients but is an excellent study for follow-up care.
4. **Myelography** is used when pathology is unclear and is helpful in identifying spinal cord abnormalities, including cord hematoma, epidural hematoma, swelling, and preexisting disease.

G. Medical Management

Medical management consists of prevention of a secondary injury.

1. **Immobilization of the spine** until it can be surgically stabilized is imperative. During transport, a semirigid cervical collar and spine backboard (ideally with a

head well to keep the head in a neutral position) should be used. Foam blocks or linen rolls and tape help to stabilize the head and shoulders on a backboard.

2. **Spinal canal decompression** is used to prevent secondary injury to the spinal cord. Cervical traction is used to stabilize fractures or when subluxation has occurred. Muscle relaxants are frequently used with traction. Surgical decompression with posterior laminectomy and debridement may be indicated once the patient has stabilized and bleeding and swelling have stopped (usually after 7 to 10 days).
3. **Stabilization of the spine with surgical fixation** is accomplished by the fusion of two or more vertebrae with the insertion of bone grafts, metal rods, or wires. A halo jacket involves the placement of a halo ring around the skull fixated with screws to the skull. The ring is attached to a padded jacket or cast made into a vest via vertical rods and a horizontal articulation device. Traction is adjusted to stabilize cervical fractures.
4. **Pharmacologic prevention of a secondary injury** with methylprednisolone (Solu-Medrol) has neuroprotective effects (Hall, 1992; Hilton and Frei, 1991), including inhibition of lipid perioxidation, inhibition of arachidonic acid release and eicosanoid formation, maintenance of spinal cord blood flow, improvement of ionic pump function, and decreased intracellular accumulation. The clinical effect is a reduction in spinal cord swelling. Accurate administration is critical to the effectiveness of the drug, and guidelines are followed carefully. The loading dose is 30 mg/kg IV over 15 minutes, followed after 45 minutes by the maintenance dose of 5.4 mg/kg per hour IV for 23 hours (continuous). The loading dose is given within 8 hours of the injury, and the maintenance dose is started within 1 hour of the loading dose (Allen et al., 1996). Indications are for evidence of an SCI less than 8 hours old. Relative contraindications include pregnancy, uncontrolled diabetes mellitus, medication allergy, and injury more than 8 hours old.

H. Multidisciplinary Management

❖ Alteration in respiratory function: Breathing pattern related to high cervical injury (lack of innervation of respiratory muscles); ineffective airway clearance related to artificial airway and diminished respiratory muscle innervation

1. **Expected outcomes** include normal arterial blood gases, Sa_{O_2} greater than 95%, adequate ventilation, and no respiratory complications (such as pneumonia, aspiration, edema).
2. **Nursing assessment** is provided to assess for spontaneous or effective ventilations; to monitor oxygenation (e.g., arterial blood gases, Sa_{O_2}); assess effectiveness of cough and ability to mobilize secretions; respiratory rate, pattern, and work of breathing (note acute changes); and breath sounds.
3. **Collaborative interventions:** Maintain the artificial airway, assist with ventilatory support, perform chest physiotherapy and postural drainage, administer effective pulmonary toilet, and maintain aseptic technique with invasive procedures. Decompress the stomach with an indwelling orogastric tube.

❖ Alteration in cardiac output related to ANS dysfunction

1. **Expected outcomes** include a normal blood pressure and heart rate and rhythm, capillary refill in less than 3 seconds, and urine output of 1 to 2 mL/kg per hour.
2. **Nursing assessment:** Monitor heart rate and rhythm, urine output, and systemic arterial pressure. Perform serial measurements of cardiac output and cardiac index (if available), and assess systemic perfusion (e.g., pulses, color, capillary refill).

3. **Collaborative interventions:** Support circulation as needed using fluids, inotropic and vasopressor agents, and elastic stockings. Maintain functioning of invasive lines. Correct bradycardia with atropine, an anticholinergic drug used to increase the rate of cardiac conduction. Eliminate the precipitating cause (e.g., hypothermia, distended bladder).

❖ Potential for impaired gas exchange related to pulmonary emboli from immobility (deep-vein thrombosis [DVT])

1. **Expected outcomes** include normal arterial blood gases, $Sa{O_2} > 95\%$, and no swelling, redness, tenderness, or pain in the lower extremities.
2. **Nursing assessment** includes assessment of the respiratory status for acute deterioration, serial measurements of the legs, and assessment for signs of venous thrombosis (pain, swelling, redness, and tenderness in the lower extremities). With vena cava filter use, assess the venous access site for bleeding, swelling, and hematoma.
3. **Collaborative interventions:** Apply antiembolism stockings or mechanical devices designed to improve venous return from the lower extremities. Consult with physical or occupational therapy to plan appropriate range-of-motion and positioning therapy. Maintain good hydration. Administer subcutaneous heparin or warfarin (Coumadin) as ordered.

❖ Potential for alteration in skin integrity related to immobility, decreased venous blood flow, reduced sensory receptors; children at risk for occipital pressure ulcers

1. **Expected outcome** is the absence of skin breakdown.
2. **Nursing assessment** includes skin assessment (especially heels, elbows, sacral, and occipital areas) for alterations in integrity (including redness, swelling, and breakdown), assessment for the degree of mobility, and assessment of the environment for potential sources of skin trauma (including traction, soiled linens, and patient appliances).
3. **Collaborative interventions:** Change the patient's position frequently, and use a pressure-reduction surface if available; maintain dry and clean bed linens and clothing; provide meticulous skin care; and consult with physical or occupational therapy to plan appropriate range of motion and positioning therapy.

❖ Potential for pulmonary infection related to artificial airway, general debilitated state, and immobility

1. **Expected outcomes** include normal WBC, temperature, and respiratory parameters.
2. **Nursing assessment** includes monitoring oxygenation (e.g., arterial blood gases, $Sa{O_2}$) and assessing effectiveness of cough and ability to mobilize secretions, respiratory rate, pattern, work of breathing (note acute changes), and breath sounds. Monitor for infection (e.g., WBC, temperature, tachycardia) and evaluate tracheal cultures.
3. **Collaborative interventions:** Provide pulmonary toilet, maintain hydration, perform chest physiotherapy and postural drainage, and maintain aseptic technique with invasive procedures.

❖ Alteration in temperature regulation related to poikilothermism (i.e., body temperature is controlled by the environment instead of internal regulatory centers)

1. **Expected outcome** is a temperature within normal range.
2. **Nursing assessment** includes monitoring core temperature frequently.
3. **Collaborative interventions** include adjusting the environmental temperature to maintain normal temperature range, adjusting clothing and bed linens,

correcting hypothermia (e.g., warming blanket, heating lamps, warm linens), and correcting hyperthermia (e.g., remove excessive clothing, sponge with tepid water).

❖ Alteration in elimination patterns related to diminished innervation of viscera

1. **Expected outcomes** are no constipation, impactions, or urinary retention.
2. **Nursing assessment** includes assessment for bladder or abdominal distention; assessment of intake and output; assessment of stools for frequency, consistency, and color; assessment for presence of bowel sounds; and monitoring of urine cultures.
3. **Collaborative interventions** include maintaining urinary drainage with intermittent or indwelling catheterization, obtaining routine urine cultures and renal studies, maintaining good hydration, and administering stool softeners and bulk-forming agents.

SCOLIOSIS AND SPINAL FUSIONS

A. Description

The normal spine has three curves: cervical lordosis, thoracic kyphosis, and lumbar lordosis. *Scoliosis* is defined as a lateral curvature of the spine greater than 10 degrees. The three major types of scoliosis are *congenital* (vertebral abnormalities develop in utero), *neuromuscular* (resulting from muscle weakness or imbalance), and *idiopathic* (unknown by definition).

B. Incidence

The etiology of adolescent idiopathic scoliosis (AIS), the most common form of scoliosis, is unclear. Most likely, the etiology is multifactorial (Ahn et al., 2002). Only 15% of the curves progress. Scoliosis can occur at any age. Early onset is defined as birth to 5 years or described as infantile at birth to 3 years. Juvenile onset is at 4 to 10 years. Adolescent onset is at older than 10 years. Most cases are adolescent onset, and 90% of AIS cases occur in females (Roach, 1999).

C. Etiology

Congenital scoliosis is an embryologic malformation during the third to fifth embryonic week. **Neuromuscular scoliosis** occurs secondary to neuropathic or myopathic diseases, resulting in muscle imbalance. **Idiopathic** infantile scoliosis occurs in the first years of life and is associated with intrauterine position. The cause of idiopathic juvenile scoliosis is unknown. AIS most often is caused by X-linked inheritance (Mason and Wright, 1995). Spine slenderness and ectomorphy in females are thought to be risk factors for AIS (Burwell, 2003).

D. Pathophysiology

Initial pathologic changes begin in the soft tissues, which shorten on the concave side of the curve. Vertebral deformity occurs as a result of unequal forces applied to the epiphyseal center of the ossification (growth plates). Curves progress during growth spurts. A large curve can be physically disabling and may compromise respiratory function.

E. Defining Characteristics

The first sign is often uneven hips and shoulders. Physical changes are most noticeable when the child bends forward and may include one more prominent breast or scapula and posterior humping of ribs or hips.

F. Neurodiagnostic Studies

1. **Serial radiographs** are used to assess the progression of curve and to document whether it is progressive.
2. **Serial pulmonary function tests** may be used to trend lung capacity.

G. Medical Management

Medical management is based on the degree of the curve and the age of the patient (i.e., how much growth remains).

1. **Mild curves** (in a prepubescent patient) require observation. The young child is evaluated every 3 to 12 months and older children and adolescents are evaluated every 3 to 4 months. (Curves usually progress during growth spurts.)
2. **Moderate curves** (20 to 40 degrees) commonly require orthotic braces. Electrical stimulation is used less frequently. An electrical stimulator transmits an electrical pulse to muscles on the convex side of the curvature, causing the muscles to contract at regular and frequent intervals. Muscle contraction counterbalances the opposing forces, preventing further deformity (Maruyama et al., 2003; Wong and Liu, 2003).
3. **Severe curves** (greater than 40 degrees in a growing child) require spinal fusion and instrumentation (Roach, 1999). Numerous spinal implants are available (Helenius et al., 2003). Hardware (series of metal rods, hooks, and screws) is used and attached to the vertebrae to stabilize the spine until the bone grafts have time to form a solid bone mass, which usually takes 10 to 12 months. Posterior fusion with instrumentation is most common and used primarily for thoracic curves. Anterior fusion with and without instrumentation is used for thoracolumbar and lumbar curves, severe curves, or in children who are lacking the posterior portion of the vertebrae (Roach, 1999). High anterior fusions disrupt the thoracic cavity and require thoracostomy tube(s) placement. SSERs are often used intraoperatively to monitor patients for spinal injury.

H. Multidisciplinary Management of Spinal Fusion

❖ Ineffective breathing pattern related to anesthesia, immobilization, pain

1. **Expected outcomes** include normal respiratory rate, pattern, oxygenation parameters (e.g., arterial blood gases, Sao_2), and clear breath sounds bilaterally.
2. **Nursing assessment** includes respiratory ventilation (e.g., rate, depth), work of breathing (e.g., use of accessory muscles, retractions), effectiveness of incentive spirometry, and respiratory physiologic parameters.
3. **Collaborative interventions:** Support ventilation as needed by administering supplemental oxygen to maintain Sao_2 greater than 95%, maintaining pain control, assisting with airway clearance (suctioning, position changes, and cough and deep breathing), and administering bronchodilators as needed. Monitor chest tube drainage (for anterior fusions).

❖ Decreased cardiac output related to hemorrhage (long procedure with long suture lines; depletion of clotting factors) (Edler et al., 2003; Kannan et al., 2002)

1. **Expected outcomes** include balanced intake and output; urine output greater than 2 mL/kg per hour; CVP within normal range; adequate peripheral pulses; normal vital signs for age; normal hemoglobin, hematocrit, and clotting studies; and normal mental status (awake and responsive).
2. **Nursing assessment** includes monitoring of intake and output, vital signs, and hemodynamic pressures; thoracostomy tube drainage for amount and color; hemoglobin and hematocrit; surgical drains for amount and color; and surgical dressing for drainage amount and color.

3. **Collaborative interventions** include administering isotonic fluids or blood products as needed to support circulation and maintaining patency of the thoracostomy tubes. Amicar (epsilon aminocaproic acid), nitroprusside, and nicardipine may be used to reduce perioperative bleeding (Florentino-Pineda et al., 2004; Lustik et al., 2004).

❖ Alteration in comfort related to incisional pain (posterior, anterior, or thoracotomy)

1. **Expected outcomes** include pain relief or control, absent physiologic manifestations of pain (e.g., tachycardia, diaphoresis, elevated blood pressure, facial grimacing, restlessness), and decreased need for narcotic analgesics.
2. **Nursing assessment** should include physiologic indicators of pain, asking patient frequently about pain control, using age-appropriate pain scales, and assessing the effectiveness of interventions.
3. **Collaborative interventions:** Use nonpharmacologic measures individualized to age, culture, and past experiences, including distractors, imagery, and controlled breathing. Encourage parental involvement. Administer analgesics by continuous infusion or patient-controlled analgesia. Position the patient for comfort.

❖ Potential for injury related to SCI

1. **Expected outcome** is the preoperative neurovascular status.
2. **Nursing assessment** includes monitoring neurovascular status in the lower extremities (e.g., sensation to light touch, movement, pulses, color, and capillary refill).
3. **Collaborative interventions** include positioning as ordered and frequent repositioning. Notify the physician for any neurovascular changes.

❖ Potential for infection related to surgical trauma, invasive lines, and skin breakdown

❖ Potential impaired gas exchange related to pulmonary emboli

❖ Alteration in skin integrity related to immobility

❖ Alteration in elimination related to immobility

CONGENITAL NEUROLOGIC ABNORMALITIES

A. Description

1. **Myelodysplasia, spinal dysraphism,** and **spina bifida** are terms that are used interchangeably to describe a collection of disorders characterized by vertebral arch fusion defects and abnormalities of the spinal cord and coverings. These defects, as well as all disorders of the neural tube, are collectively referred to as *neural tube defects* (NTDs).
2. **Spina bifida cystica,** incomplete fusion of one or more vertebral laminae, results in external protrusion of the spinal tissue. Two classifications include *myelomeningocele,* a protruding saclike structure containing meninges, spinal fluid, and neural tissue, and *meningocele,* a protruding sac containing only meninges and CSF.
3. **Spina bifida occulta** is incomplete fusion at one level without a protrusion of neural structures. The defect is not apparent to the naked eye.

B. Incidence

In the United States, 1 to 2 per 1000 live births will have an NTD (Cohen, 1987). In the United Kingdom, 4 to 5 per 1000 live births will have an NTD. Irish and Moslems have the highest occurrence of NTDs. Asians and African Americans have the lowest incidence. Incidence rates may be higher if the defect is related to some stillbirths and spontaneous abortions.

C. Etiology

The cause of congenital neurologic abnormalities is unknown and possibly multifactorial. The abnormality occurs early in embryonic development.

D. Pathophysiology

The most common part of the spine affected is the lower thoracic lumbar and sacral areas (Reigel, 1989). The anterior aspects of the spinal cord are frequently intact with varying degrees of destruction to the dorsal columns. Sometimes it is associated with brain abnormalities, including cellular migration, agenesis of the corpus callosum, arachnoid cysts, and Arnold-Chiari malformations. The degree of functional impairment depends on the extent of the defect and associated neural tissue.

E. Defining Characteristics

1. **Spina bifida occulta** often goes undetected. Possible signs (over the midline of the lumbosacral area) include a palpable mass, dermal sinus, skin discoloration, and a tuft of hair. Spinal cord or nerve involvement may demonstrate asymmetry of the lower extremities, persistent enuresis (late onset), and progressive weakness of one or both legs.
2. **Meningocele** is a visible defect of the cord and covering. It may have minimal to no involvement of the lower extremities.
3. **Myelomeningocele** dysfunction ranges from minimal impairment to total paralysis of the lower extremities. Lumbosacral lesions usually result in some hip, knee, or ankle flexion. Sensory involvement is usually symmetric but patchy. Usually some degree of bowel and bladder dysfunction exists. Arnold-Chiari type II deformity is present in most cases. It consists of elongation and herniation of the cerebellar vermis through the foramen magnum, displacement and distortion of the medulla (including the fourth ventricle), impeded CSF flow and hydrocephalus, and possibly lower bulbar dysfunction producing apnea, vocal cord paralysis, and stridor.

F. Neurodiagnostic Studies

1. **Radiographs** are taken of the entire spine to identify the precise level of deformity and to rule out deformities at other levels.
2. **CT scan or MRI** is done to visualize the ventricular system and brainstem.
3. **Serum AFP** levels are used as a screening tool for open NTDs during the 16th and 18th weeks of gestation. Normal maternal serum AFP at 16 weeks is 38 ng/mL and at 18 weeks is 49 ng/mL. NTD levels vary; therefore any level above the normal range is further evaluated.

G. Medical Management

In recent years, immediate closure of the protruding sac is indicated. The goals of surgery are to preserve all neural tissue, provide a physiologic skin barrier, and control progressive hydrocephalus. Surgical closure involves several steps, including dissection of the exposed sac, closure of the dura over preserved neural tissue, and closure of the skin covering the repair. Skin grafting may be necessary. If hydrocephalus is present, a CSF shunting device is inserted or the foramen magnum is enlarged.

H. Multidisciplinary Management

❖ Potential for infection related to surgical incision, fragility of covering, invasive lines, urinary retention

1. **Expected outcomes** include no signs and symptoms of infection and a healed wound incision.

2. **Nursing assessment** includes monitoring vital signs, WBC count, cultures, and urine studies; assessing the sac's protective barrier (before and after the operation) for drainage, odor, and color; assessing neurologic functioning, including head circumference and fontanelles and signs of increased ICP; and assessing for bladder distention and monitoring urinary output.
3. **Collaborative interventions** include protecting the sac with a sterile saline moist dressing preoperatively and maintaining the child in a prone or side-lying position before and immediately after the operation to promote wound healing. Provide routine postoperative care, maintain sterile dry wound dressings, administer antibiotics as ordered, and prevent contamination of the wound from feces and urine.

❖ Potential for decreased cardiac output related to anaphylactic shock from latex hypersensitivity

1. **Expected outcomes** include no signs and symptoms of anaphylactic shock (e.g., bronchospasm, hypotension, loss of consciousness).
2. **Nursing assessment** includes monitoring for signs and symptoms of contact dermatitis or immediate hypersensitivity (urticaria, faintness, nausea, vomiting, abdominal cramps, bronchospasm, hypotension). Screen patients for latex allergies.
3. **Collaborative interventions** includes prevention and treatment. Provide a latex-free environment for patients at risk for sensitivity (e.g., patients with NTDs) or with a known hypersensitivity to latex: label room "latex safe"; remove all latex products from the patient's immediate environment; check all products for latex content; notify ancillary departments; and disseminate latex allergy protocol.

❖ Alteration in cerebral tissue perfusion related to increased ICP from hydrocephalus

❖ Alteration in elimination related to decreased innervation of bladder, urinary sphincter, lower intestines

REFERENCES

Abhik K et al.: Treatment of acute traumatic brain injury in children with moderate hypothermia improves intracranial hypertension. *Crit Care Med* 30:2742-2751, 2002.

Adelson PD et al.: Guidelines for the acute medical management of severe traumatic brain injury in infants, children, and adolescents. *Crit Care Med* 31(6):5417-5490, 2003.

Ahn UM et al.: The etiology of adolescent idiopathic scoliosis. *Am J Orthop* 31:387-395, 2002.

Allen EM et al.: Head and spinal cord injury. In Rogers MC, editor: *Textbook of pediatric intensive care.* Baltimore, 1996, Williams & Wilkins.

Altman DI et al.: Cerebral blood flow requirement for brain viability in newborn infants is lower than in adults. *Ann Neurol* 24:218-226, 1988.

American Academy of Pediatrics Committee on Infectious Diseases: Dexamethasone therapy for bacterial meningitis in infants and children. *Pediatrics* 86:130-133, 1990.

American Academy of Pediatrics: Provisional Committee on Quality Improvement: Practice parameter: the neurodiagnostic evaluation of the child with a severe febrile seizure. *Pediatrics* 97:769, 1996.

American Cancer Society: What are the key statistics for brain and spinal cord tumors? www.cancer.org. 2004.

Anttila M: Clinical criteria for estimating recovery from childhood bacterial meningitis. *Acta Paediatr* 83:63-67, 1994.

Anttila M, Himberg JJ, Peltola H: Precise quantification of fever in childhood bacterial meningitis. *Clin Pediatr* 31:221-227, 1992.

ApSimon HT et al.: A population-based study of brain arteriovenous malformation: long-term treatment outcomes. *Stroke* 33:2794-2800, 2002.

Arbour R: Aggressive management of intracranial dynamics. *Crit Care Nurse* 18:30-44, 1998.

Armstrong TS, Gilbert MR: Metastatic brain tumors: diagnosis, treatment, and nursing interventions. *Clin J Oncol Nurs* 4:217-225, 2000.

Bader MK: New frontiers in managing pediatric brain injury. Presentation National Teaching Institute. Aliso Viejo, CA, 2003, American Association Critical-Care Nurses.

Baldwin RT, Preston-Martin S: Epidemiology of brain tumors in childhood—a review. *Toxicol Appl Pharmacol* 1:118-131, 2004.

Berger R, Garnier Y, Jensen A: Perinatal brain damage: underlying mechanisms and neuroprotective strategies. *J Soc Gynecol Invest* 9:319-328, 2002.

Betjes MG: Hyponatremia in acute brain disease: the cerebral salt waste syndrome. *Eur J Intern Med* 13:9-14, 2002.

Brain Resuscitation Clinical Trial I Study Group: Randomized clinical study of thiopental loading in comatose survivors or cardiac arrest. *N Engl J Med* 314:397-403, 1986.

Brain Trauma Foundation: Guidelines for the acute management of severe traumatic brain injury in infants, children, and adolescents. *Pediatr Crit Care Med* 4(3): S1-S67, 2003.

Brunker C, Shah S: Systems and diseases. Exploring normal anatomy and physiology. Nervous system 11: brain tumours. *Nurs Times* 97(26):43-46, 2001.

Burn IT, Zimmerman RK: Haemophilus influenzae type B disease, vaccine, and care of exposed individuals. *Fam Pract* 49(9 Suppl):S7-13, 2000.

Burwell RG: Aetiology of idiopathic scoliosis: current concepts. *Pediatr Rehabil* 6:137-170, 2003.

Camfield PR, Camfield CS: Pediatric epilepsy: an overview. In Swaiman KF, Ashwal S, editors: *Pediatric neurology: principles & practice*. St. Louis, 1999, Mosby.

Centers for Disease Control: Reye syndrome—United States. *MMWR Morb Mortal Wkly Rep* 34:13, 1984.

Chaudhuri A: Adjunctive dexamethasone treatment in acute bacterial meningitis. *Lancet Neurol* 3:54-62, 2004.

Chequer RS et al.: Prognostic value of EEG in neonatal meningitis: retrospective study of 29 infants. *Pediatr Neurol* 8:417-422, 1992.

Chesney PJ: Pediatric infectious disease-associated syndromes. In Fuhrman BP, Zimmerman JJ, editors: *Pediatric critical care*. St. Louis, 1998, Mosby.

Cohen F: Neural tube defects: epidemiology, detection, and prevention. *J Obstet Gynecol Neonatal Nurs* 2:105-115, 1987.

Das BK et al.: Bacterial antigen detection test in meningitis. *Ind J Pediatr* 70:799-801, 2003.

DeVivo DC, Keating JP, Haymond MW: Acute encephalopathy with fatty infiltration of the viscera. *Pediatr Clin North Am* 23:527-535, 1976.

Dreifuss FE: Classification of epileptic seizures and the epilepsies. *Pediatr Clin North Am* 36:265, 1989.

Durkin MS et al.: The epidemiology of urban pediatric neurological trauma: evaluation of, and implications for, injury prevention programs. *Neurosurgery* 42(2):300-310, 1998.

Eder HG et al.: The role of gamma knife radiosurgery in children. *Child Nerv Syst* 17:341-347, 2001.

Edler A, Murray DJ, Forbes RB: Blood loss during posterior spinal fusion surgery in patients with neuromuscular disease: is there an increased risk? *Paediatr Anaesth* 13:818-822, 2003.

Fishman RA: Brain edema and disorders of intracranial pressure. In Rowland LP, editor: *Merrit's Textbook of neurology*. Baltimore, Md., 1995, Williams & Wilkins.

Florentino-Pineda I et al.: The effect of amicar on perioperative blood loss in idiopathic scoliosis: the results of a prospective, randomized double-blind study. *Spine* 29, 233-238, 2004.

Freeman JM, Ferry PC: New brain death guidelines in children: further confusion [Editorial]. *Pediatrics* 81:301-303, 1988.

Goe MR, Massey TH: Assessment of neurologic damage: creatine kinase-BB assay after cardiac arrest. *Heart Lung* 17:247-253, 1988.

Gopinath SP et al.: Comparison of jugular venous oxygen saturation and brain tissue PO_2 as monitors of cerebral ischemia after head injury. *Crit Care Med* 27:2569-2570, 1999.

Guertin SR: Neurosurgical intensive care: selected aspects. In Fuhrman BP, Zimmerman JJ, editors: *Pediatric critical care*. St. Louis, 1988, Mosby.

Guidelines for the determination of brain death in children. *Pediatrics* 80:298-300, 1987.

Hall ED: The neuroprotective pharmacology of methylprednisolone. *J Neurosurg* 76: 13-21, 1992.

Haun SE et al.: Theories in brain resuscitation. In Rogers MC, editor: *Textbook of pediatric intensive care.* Baltimore, 1996, Williams & Wilkins.

Helenius I et al.: Harrington and Cotrel-Dubousset instrumentation in adolescent idiopathic scoliosis: long-term functional and radiographic outcomes. *J Bone Joint Surg Am* 85-A:2303-2309, 2003.

Hilton G, Frei J: High-dose methyl-prednisolone in the treatment of spinal cord injuries. *Heart Lung* 20:675-680, 1991.

Hofmeister C et al.: Demographic, morphological, and clinical characteristics of 1289 patients with arteriovenous malformation. *Stroke* 31:1307-1310, 2000.

Hongo K et al.: Surgical resection of cerebral arteriovenous malformation combined with pre-operative embolisation. *J Clin Neurosci* 7(suppl 1):88-91, 2000.

Hunter JV, Morriss MC: Neuroimaging of central nervous system infections. *Semin Pediatr Infect Dis* 14:140-164, 2003.

Imaizumi S et al.: Liposome-entrapped superoxide dismutase reduces cerebral infarction in cerebral ischemia in rats. *Stroke* 21:1312-1317, 1990.

Irie K et al.: Treatment of arteriovenous malformation of the brain-preliminary experience. *J Clin Neurosci* 7(suppl 1): 24-29, 2000.

Jensen D: *The human nervous system.* New York, 1980, Appleton-Century-Crofts.

Johnston MV: Development, structure, and function of the brain and neuromuscular systems. In Fuhrman BP, Zimmerman JJ, editors: *Pediatric critical care.* St. Louis, 1998, Mosby.

Jumah MA et al.: Bulk diffusion apnea test in the diagnosis of brain death. *Crit Care Med* 20:1564-1567, 1992.

Kanan A, Gasson B: Brain tumor resections guided by magnetic resonance imaging. *AORN J* 77:583-589, 2003.

Kannan S et al.: Bleeding and coagulation changes during spinal fusion surgery: comparison of neuromuscular and idiopathic scoliosis patients. *Pediatr Crit Care Med* 3:364-369, 2002.

Keating JP: Reye syndrome. In Feigin RD, Cherry JD, editors: *Textbook of pediatric infectious disease.* Philadelphia, 1987, W. B. Saunders.

Kidd KC, Criddle L: Using jugular venous catheters in patients with traumatic brain injury. *Critical Care Nurse* 21:16-22, 2001.

Kirsch JR et al.: Brain resuscitation: medical management and innovations. *Crit Care Nurs Clin North Am* 1:143-154, 1989.

Kline NE, Sevier N: Solid tumors in children. *J Pediatr Nurs* 18:96-102, 2003.

Kochanek PM et al.: Hypoxic-ischemic encephalopathy: pathobiology and therapy of the postresuscitation syndrome in children. In Fuhrman BP, Zimmerman JJ, editors: *Pediatric critical care.* St. Louis, 1998, Mosby.

Larroque B et al.: White matter damage and intraventricular hemorrhage in very preterm infants: the EPIPAGE study. *J Pediatr* 143:477-483, 2003.

Littlejohns LR, Bader MK, March K: Brain tissue oxygen monitoring in severe brain injury, I. *Crit Care Nurse* 23:17-25, 2003.

Liu TH et al.: Polyethylene glycol-conjugated superoxide dismutase and catalase reduce ischemic brain injury. *Am J Physiol* 256:H589-H593, 1989

Lustik SJ et al.: Nicardipine versus nitroprusside for deliberate hypotension during idiopathic scoliosis repair. *J Clin Anesth* 16:25-33, 2004.

Lutsar I et al.: Factors influencing the anti-inflammatory effect of dexamethasone therapy in experimental pneumococcal meningitis. *J Antimicrob Chemother* 52: 651-655, 2003.

Maalouf EF et al.: Comparison of findings on cranial ultrasound and magnetic resonance imaging in preterm infants. *Pediatrics* 107:719-727, 2001.

Mancini MC et al.: Intraventricular hemorrhage in very low birth weight infants: associated risk factors and outcome in the neonatal period. *Rev Hosp Clin Fac Med Sao Paula* 54:151-154, 1999.

Marion DW et al.: Effect of hyperventilation on extracellular concentrations of glutamate, lactate, pyruvate, and local cerebral blood flow in patients with severe traumatic brain injury. *Crit Care Med* 30:2619-2625, 2002.

Mason KJ, Wright S: Altered musculoskeletal function. In Betz A, Hunsberger M, Wright S, editors: *Family-centered nursing care of children.* Philadelphia, 1995, W. B. Saunders.

Maruyama T et al.: Conservative treatment for adolescent idiopathic scoliosis: can it reduce the incidence of surgical treatment? *Pediatr Rehabil* 6: 215-219, 2003.

Massager N et al.: Gamma knife radiosurgery for brainstem arteriovenous malformation: preliminary results. *J Neurosurg* 93(suppl 3):102-103, 2000.

Ment LR, Keller MS, Duncan CC: Intraventricular hemorrhage of the preterm neonate. In K.F. Swaiman KF, Ashwal S, editors: *Pediatric neurology: principles & practice.* St. Louis, 1999, Mosby.

Ment LR et al.: Practice parameter: neuroimaging of the neonate: report of the Quality Standards Subcommittee of the American Academy of Neurology and the Practice Committee of the Child Neurology Society. *Neurology* 58:1726-1738, 2002.

Meyer-Heim AD, Boltshauser E: Sponetaneous intracranial haemorrhage in children: aetiology, presentation and outcome. *Brain Dev* 25:416-421, 2003.

Muir R, Town DA: Spinal cord injury. In Moloney-Harmon PA, Czersinski SJ, editors: *Nursing care of the pediatric trauma patient.* St. Louis, 2003, W. B. Saunders.

Murray DL, Gilsdorf JR: Chemoprophylaxis for household contacts of index cases of invasive non–type B haemophilus influenzae disease: reply. *Pediatr Infect Dis J* 20:1099-1100, 2001.

National Head Injury Foundation: *Definition of traumatic brain injury.* Southborough, Mass., 1986, National Head Injury Foundation.

Neuman MI, Harper MB: Evaluation of a rapid urine antigen assay for the detection of invasive pneumococcal disease in children. *Pediatrics* 112:1279-1282, 2003.

Nicolato A et al.: Gamma knife radiosurgery in the management of arteriovenous malformations of the basal ganglia region of the brain. *Minim Invasive Neurosurg* 45:211-223, 2002.

Orlowski JP, Rothner AD: Diagnosis and treatment of status epilepticus. In Fuhrman BP, Zimmerman JJ, editors: *Pediatric critical care.* St. Louis, 1998, Mosby.

O'Sullivan MG et al.: Role of intracranial pressure monitoring in severely head-injured patients without signs of intracranial hypertension on initial computerized tomography. *J Neurosurg* 80:46-50, 1994.

Outwater KM, Rockoff MA: Apnea testing to confirm brain death in children. *Crit Care Med* 12:357-358, 1984.

Owen DB, Levin DL: Reye's syndrome. In Levin DL, Morris FC, editors: *The essentials of pediatric intensive care.* St. Louis, Quality Medical Publishers, 1991.

Ozuna J: Seizure disorders and epilepsy. *Primary Care Pract* 420:608-618, 2000.

Palmer J: Management of raised intracranial pressure in children. *Intens Crit Care Nurs* 16:319-327, 2000.

Pang D, Wilberger JE: Spinal cord injury without radiographic abnormalities in children. *J Neurosurg* 57:114-129, 1982.

Pellock JM: Status epilepticus. In Swaiman KF, Ashwal S, editors: *Pediatric neurology: principles & practice.* St. Louis, 1999, Mosby.

Perlman JM et al.: Reduction in intraventricular hemorrhage by elimination of fluctuating cerebral blood flow velocity in preterm infants with respiratory distress syndrome. *N Engl J Med* 312:1353-1357, 1985.

Phillips EJ, Simor AE: Bacterial meningitis in children and adults. *Postgrad Med Online* 103(3), 1998.

Plum R, Posner JB: *The diagnosis of stupor and coma.* Philadelphia, 1982, FA Davis.

Reigel D: Spina bifida. In McLaurin R et al., editors: *Pediatric neurosurgery.* Philadelphia, 1989, W. B. Saunders.

Rice BA: Pediatric injury prevention. In Moloney-Harmon PA, Czersinski SJ, editors: *Nursing care of the pediatric trauma patient.* St. Louis, 2003, W. B. Saunders.

Rickert CH, Paulus W: Epidemiology of central nervous system tumors in childhood and adolescence based on the new WHO classification. *Child Nerv System* 17:503-511, 2001.

Rogers MC, Kirsch JR: Current concepts in brain resuscitation. *JAMA* 261:3143-3147, 1989.

Safar P: Cerebral resuscitation after cardiac arrest: a review. *Circulation* 74(suppl IV):138-153, 1986.

Safar P: Resuscitation from clinical death: pathophysiologic limits and therapeutic potentials. *Crit Care Med* 16:923-941, 1988.

Scott RC, Surtees RAH, Neville BGR: Status epilepticus: pathophysiology, epidemiology, and outcomes. *Arch Dis Child* 79: 73-77, 1998.

Shafer PO: Epilepsy and seizures. Advances in seizure assessment, treatment, and self-management. *Nurs Clin North Am* 34, 743-759, 1999.

Shepard CW et al.: Neonatal meningococcal disease in the United States, 1990-1999. *Pediatr Infect Dis J* 22:418-422, 2003.

Shewmon A: Commentary on guidelines for the determination of brain death in children. *Issues Clin Neurosci* 24:789-791, 1988.

Sieber FE, Traystman RJ: Special issues: glucose and the brain. *Crit Care Med* 20:104-114, 1992.

Slota MC: Neurological assessment of the infant and toddler. *Crit Care Nurse* 3:87-94, 1983.

Slota MC: Pediatric neurological assessment. *Crit Care Nurse* 3:106-112, 1983.

Smith MA, Gloecker Ries LA: Childhood cancer: incidence, survival, and mortality. In Pizzo PA, Poplack DG, editors: *Principles and practice of pediatric oncology.* Philadelphia, 2002, Lippincott-Raven.

Stapf C et al.: Effect of age on clinical and morphological characteristics in patients with brain arteriovenous malformation. *Stroke* 34:2669-2670, 2003.

Steen PA et al.: Nimodipine improves outcome when given after complete cerebral arrest in primates. *Anesthesiology* 62:406-414, 1985.

Stewart-Amidei C: Pharmacology advances in the neuroscience intensive care. *Crit Care Nurs Clin North Am* 14:31-38, 2002.

Surawicz TS et al.: Descriptive epidemiology of primary brain and CNS tumors: results from the central brain tumor registry of the United States, 1990-1994. *Neuro-oncol* 1:14-25, 1999.

Swaiman K: Spinal fluid examination. In Swaiman KF, Ashwal S, editors: *Pediatric neurology: principles & practice.* St. Louis, 1999, Mosby.

Tasker RC, Dean JM, Rogers MC: Reye syndrome and metabolic encephalopathies. In Rogers MC, editor: *Textbook of pediatric intensive care.* Baltimore, 1996, Williams & Wilkins.

The Status Epilepticus Working Party: The treatment of convulsive status epilepticus in children. *Arch Dis Child* 83:415-419, 2000.

Tokutomi T et al.: Optimal temperature for the management of severe traumatic brain injury: effect of hypothermia on intracranial pressure, systemic and intracranial hemodynamics, and metabolism. *Neurosurgery* 52:102-111, 2003.

Trauner DA: Toxic and metabolic encephalopathies. In David RB, editor: *Pediatric neurology for the clinician.* Norwalk, Conn., 1992, Appleton & Lange.

Traystman RJ, Kirsch JR, Koehler RC: Oxygen radical mechanisms of brain injury following ischemia and reperfusion. *J Appl Physiol* 71:1185-1195, 1991.

Unwin DH, Giller CA, Lopitnik TA: Central nervous system monitoring: what helps, what does not. *Surg Clin North Am* 71: 733-747, 1991.

van de Beek D et al.: Corticosteroids in acute bacterial meningitis. *Cochrane Database Syst Rev* 3:CD004305, 2003.

Vernon-Levett P: Intracranial dynamics. In Curley MAQ, Moloney-Harmon PA, editors: *Critical care nursing of infants and children.* Philadelphia, 2001a, W. B. Saunders.

Vernon-Levett P: Neurologic critical care problems. In Curley MAQ, Moloney-Harmon PA, editors: *Critical care nursing of infants and children.* Philadelphia, 2001b, W. B. Saunders.

Volpe JJ: Neurobiology of periventricular leukomalacia in the premature infant. *Pediatr Res* 50:553-562, 2001.

Wauquier A, Edmonds HL, Clincke GHC: Cerebral resuscitation: pathophysiology and therapy. *Neurosci Biobehav Rev* 11: 287-306, 1987.

Welch K: The intracranial pressure in infants. *J Neurosurg* 52:693-699, 1980.

Winkelman C: A review of pharmacodynamics in seizure management. *J Neurosci Nurs* 31:50-53, 1999.

Winkelman C: Effect of backrest position on intracranial and cerebral perfusion pressures in traumatically brain-injured adults. *Am J Critical Care* 9:373-382, 2000.

Wong MS, Liu WC: Critical review on non-operative management of adolescent idiopathic scoliosis. *Prosthet Orthot Int* 27:242-253, 2003.

Yokoyama K, Asano Y, Murakawa T: Familial occurrence of AVM of the brain. *J Neurosurg* 74:585, 1991.

Zimmerman JW et al.: Diffusion-weighted imaging in acute bacterial meningitis in infants. *Neuroradiology* 45:634-639, 2003.

CHAPTER 5

Renal System

LISA MILONOVICH AND ANDREA KLINE

ESSENTIAL DEVELOPMENTAL ANATOMY

A. Anatomic Location

The kidneys are positioned within the retroperitoneal space and are surrounded by adipose tissue and loose connective tissue. The kidneys lie along the lower two thoracic vertebrae and the first four lumbar vertebrae. They are not fixed but move with the diaphragm and are supported by the surrounding vascular system, adipose tissue, and fibrous tissue called the *renal fascia.* The right kidney lies slightly lower than the left.

B. Anatomic Structure

1. **Development:** All nephrons are formed by 28 weeks' gestation. Kidney weight doubles in the first month of life. Filtration and absorption capabilities are not developed until the epithelial cells of the nephrons mature. As the loop of Henle matures and elongates, the ability to concentrate urine improves. Infants are more vulnerable to dehydration and fluid overload because of their inability to concentrate or to excrete urine in response to changes in fluid status. Bladder capacity is age dependent: infants, 15 to 20 mL; adult bladder, 600 to 800 mL. The kidneys of infants and children are relatively large for their body size and age, making them more susceptible to trauma.
2. **Gross structures (Figure 5-1)**
   a. The *capsule* is the thin, fibrous, tough outer covering of the kidney.
   b. The outer portion of the kidney is the *cortex.* It contains all the glomeruli, the proximal and distal convoluted tubules, the first portions of the loop of Henle, and the collecting ducts.
   c. The inner region contains the *medulla* and the *pelvis.* The medulla has a pyramidal shape and contains primarily the collecting ducts and loops of Henle. The pelvis forms the upper end of the ureter. It is formed by the merging of the collecting ducts and tubular structures. It provides the pathway of urine from the kidney to the ureter. The fluid in the pelvis is identical to urine.
3. **Gross renal vasculature:** About 20% to 25% of the total cardiac output is delivered to the kidneys. Two renal arteries branch from the descending aorta, and each renal artery branches repeatedly into arterioles.
4. **Microscopic structure**
   a. The *nephron* is the functional unit of the kidney. Each mature kidney has about 1 million nephrons. The *nephron wall* is composed of a single layer of epithelial cells. The top end (origin) of the nephron is called *Bowman's capsule,* which is found in the cortex of the kidney. The fluid in Bowman's capsule is a filtrate of blood plasma.

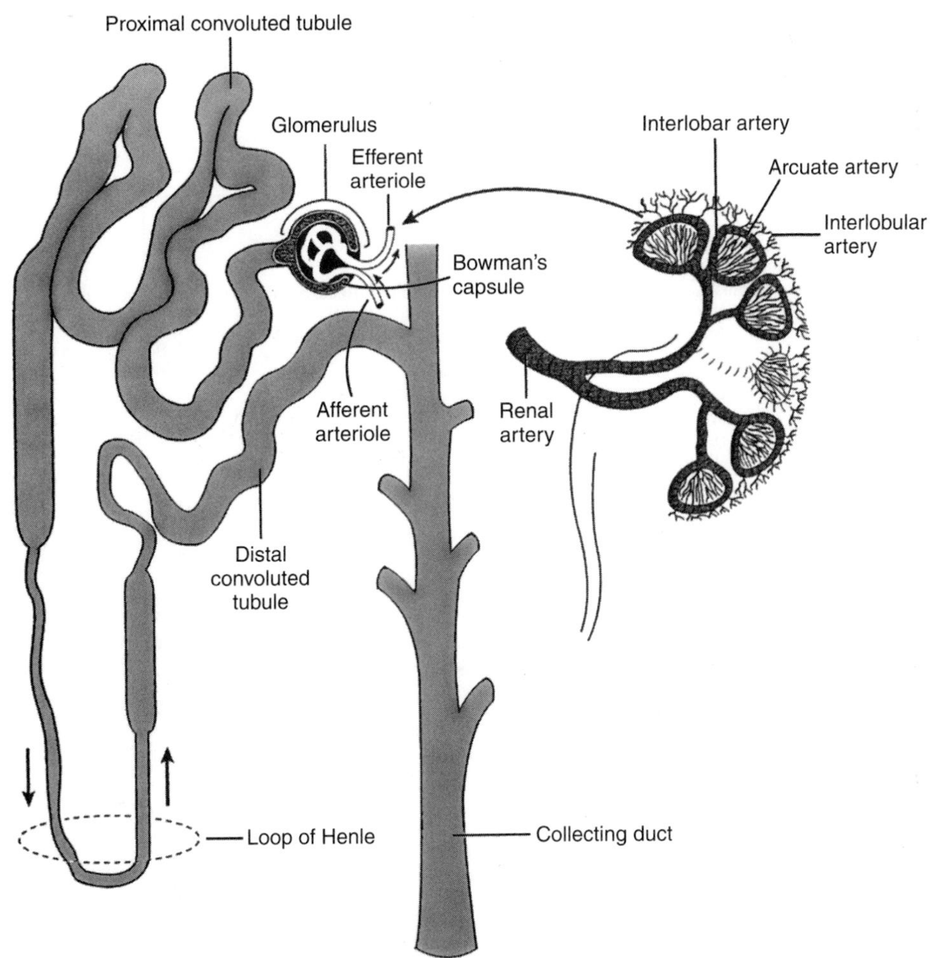

FIGURE 5-1 ■ Gross structure of bisected kidney.
(From Curley MAQ, Moloney-Harmon P: *Critical care nursing of infants and children.* Philadelphia, 2001, W. B. Saunders, p 733.)

b. There are two types of nephrons. *Cortical* nephrons (85% of nephrons) originate in the outer portion of the cortex and have short loops of Henle that reach only the outer region of the medulla. *Juxtaglomerular* nephrons originate closer to the medulla, have very long loops of Henle that reach deep into the medulla, and are important for water conservation in the body.

c. The nephron can be divided into three parts: vascular components, tubular components, and collecting ducts.

- *Vascular components* of the nephron: Within Bowman's capsule, the capillary bed is called the *glomerulus* (Bowman's capsule and the glomerulus may be referred to collectively as the *glomerulus*). Afferent arterioles bring blood to the glomerulus. Efferent arterioles take blood as it exits the glomerulus to the second capillary bed of peritubular capillaries, which supply the proximal and distal tubules in the cortex. Efferent arterioles of juxtaglomerular

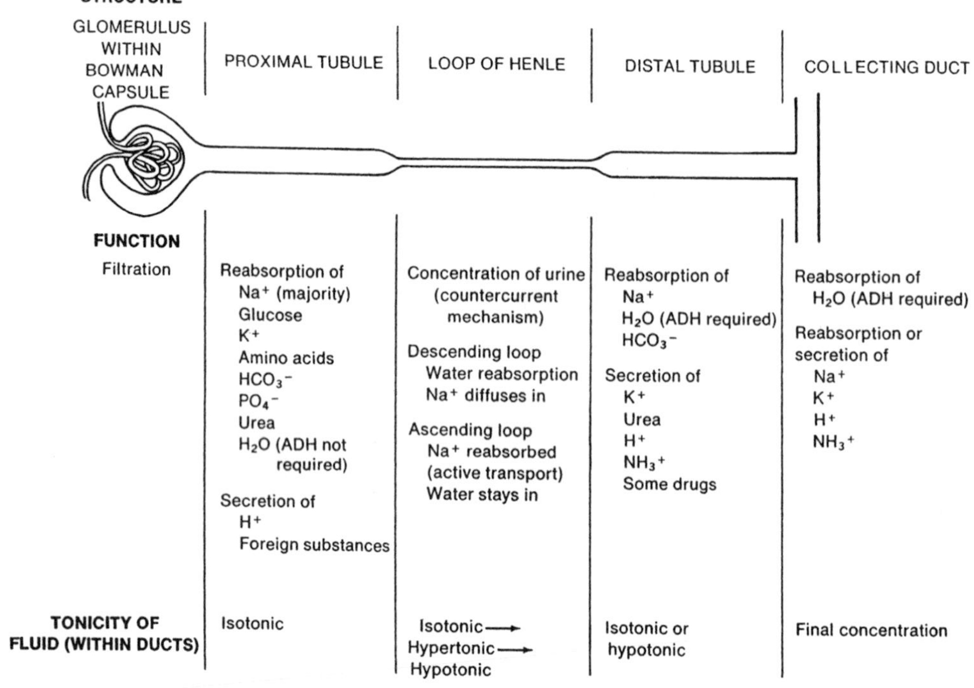

FIGURE 5-2 ■ Tubular components of the nephron.
(From Whaley LF, Wong DL: *Nursing care of infants and children*, ed 6, St. Louis, 1999, Mosby.)

nephrons send off branches to create the *vasa recta*, a loop of straight vessels that stretch deep down to supply the medulla, descending alongside the descending limbs of the loop of Henle and back up toward the cortex.

- *Tubular components* of the nephron (Figure 5-2): The proximal tubule is proximal to Bowman's capsule. The tubule begins as coiled and convoluted (proximal convoluted tubule) and then straightens as it extends into the medulla. The descending limb of the loop of Henle is a long, thin tubule that extends deep into the medulla. At its deepest point in the medulla, it turns sharply upward toward the cortex. The ascending limb of the loop of Henle is considerably thicker than the descending limb. It becomes continuous with the distal tubule. The distal tubule is a coiled, convoluted structure responsible for final adjustments of filtrate.
- Collecting ducts gather fluid from several nephrons and drain into larger ducts, which drain into the minor calices in the renal pelvis.

PHYSICAL ASSESSMENT

A. Medical History

Medical history includes significant prenatal history, pain (frequency, intensity, type, and location), unexplained or frequent itching, edema, unusual thirst or dry mouth, change in urinary patterns (for example, an increase or decrease in number of wet diapers), a change in activity level (lethargy may be secondary to anemia resulting from the lack of erythropoietin production), recent changes in weight, and hypertension.

B. Physical Examination

1. **Cardiorespiratory findings:** Meticulous assessment of cardiovascular volume status includes respiratory rate, blood pressure, and heart rate. Several factors have been implicated in hypertension related to kidney diseases. Factors that can produce hypertension include fluid overload, the renin-angiotensin system, and increased sympathetic nervous system activity. Uncontrolled hypertension can contribute to worsening of kidney function. There is also a reciprocal effect, with hypertension being a major risk factor for kidney disease. If the patient has significant fluid overload, respiratory distress may be present.
2. **Abdominal Findings:** Abdominal inspection and palpation provide a gross assessment of the gastrointestinal and genitourinary systems. Assessment and findings related to the genitourinary system may include abdominal distention or striae (which may indicate fluid retention). Kidneys are rarely palpable except in neonates. Enlarged kidneys may be indicative of tumor, cysts, or hydronephrosis. A distended bladder may be palpable under the symphysis pubis, which may indicate urinary obstruction. Ascites may be observed in patients with severe nephrotic syndrome.
   - *Extremities:* Examine extremities for signs of edema.
   - *Neuropsychiatric features:* Signs of confusion, somnolence, stupor, coma, seizures, or focal neurologic findings may be present if significant uremia or toxic wastes build up.
   - *Skin:* Evaluate turgor as indication of fluid status. A sallow complexion may represent urochrome deposits in the skin. Areas of petechiae or purpura may indicate vascular or infectious etiologies of renal failure.

ESSENTIAL PHYSIOLOGY AND CLINICAL ASSESSMENT OF KIDNEY FUNCTION

A. Basic Transport Mechanisms

1. During **active transport,** substances combine with a carrier and, with the help of adenosine triphosphate (ATP), diffuse against the concentration gradient and through the tubular membrane. Sodium, glucose, amino acids, calcium, potassium, chloride, bicarbonate, and phosphate are reabsorbed from the tubule by active transport.
2. **Passive transport** involves movement of substances in response to changes in the concentration gradient, without the assistance of ATP or a carrier. Diffusion is the spontaneous movement of solutes across a semipermeable membrane from a high concentration to a lesser concentration. As water reabsorbs out of the tubule and the urea concentration in the tubule increases, urea diffuses out of the tubule. Osmosis is the spontaneous movement of water across a semipermeable membrane from an area of lesser solute concentration to an area of greater solute concentration. As sodium is reabsorbed from the tubule and concentration increases outside the tubule, water moves out of the tubule to balance the concentration gradient. Serum colloid osmotic pressure is the opposing pressure preventing free water from moving out of the vascular space.

B. Urine Formation

Urine formation involves the following physiologic processes: filtration, reabsorption, and secretion.

1. **Filtration**
   a. Fluid and various substances, known as the *glomerular filtrate*, are filtered from the plasma through the porous walls of the glomerular capillaries into Bowman's capsule and on to the renal tubules. Glomerular filtrate is primarily composed of water; it is essentially the same substance as blood plasma except for the larger protein molecules.
   b. The pathway for filtration is through capillary fenestrations across the basement membrane and through slit passages. The ability and resistance to passing through filtration pathways depend on size, shape, and electrical charge of the molecules. Albumin (protein) molecules are too large to permeate the glomerular membrane, creating a high osmotic pressure that opposes orthostatic filtration from the vascular space.
   c. The "forcing" pressure, or filtration pressure, is the net pressure acting to force substances out of the glomerulus.
      - The primary force is the hydrostatic pressure of the blood inside the capillaries generated by the pumping action of the heart.
      - The secondary forces are the osmotic pressure of the plasma in the glomerular capillaries and the hydrostatic pressure in Bowman's capsule.
   d. Regulation of glomerular filtration rate (GFR)
      - Renal blood flow (RBF) and glomerular filtration rate (GFR) remain relatively constant over a wide range of perfusion pressures. This is referred to as *autoregulation*. Numerous neural and hormonal factors can alter RBF: renal vasoconstrictors that decrease RBF, including endothelin, angiotensin II, thromboxane, alpha-adrenergic receptor stimulators, vasopressin, and catecholamines. Vasodilators that may relax renal vascular smooth muscle include prostaglandins, atrial peptides, bradykinin, and nitric oxide.
      - Changes in filtration pressure can directly affect GFR. Factors affecting filtration pressure, and thus the GFR, include vasoconstriction or vasodilation of afferent and efferent arterioles, blood flow rate, tubule obstruction, and changes in serum osmotic pressure. RBF is controlled by sympathetic nerve impulses that constrict arterioles. The effect on GFR depends on which arteriole (afferent or efferent) is constricted (Table 5-1).
      - Vasodilation and vasoconstriction are autoregulatory responses to changes in systemic arterial pressure. They occur to maintain constant renal blood flow and a stable GFR. A distal tubular feedback mechanism ensures constant delivery of filtrate to the distal tubule.
      - The effect of shock on GFR and renal function is detailed in Table 5-2.
   e. Measuring filtration: *Clearance* is the volume of a specific substance filtered from the plasma over a designated time, generally:

$$\text{Clearance (mL/min/1.73 m}^2\text{)} = \text{Concentration of Substance in Urine} \times \text{Volume of Urine Collected/Plasma Concentration of that Substance}$$

      - Substances used to assess GFR include creatinine, inulin (nonmetabolizable sugar), and ^{131}I-iothalamate (Glofil; radioactive isotope).
      - GFR is approximately equal to creatinine clearance. *Creatinine* is an endogenous waste product that is produced by the muscles and excreted by the kidneys. Creatinine clearance may slightly overestimate GFR.
      - GFR as measured by creatinine clearance:
        - First week of life: GFR = 15 to 20 mL/min/1.73 m^2

■ **TABLE 5-1**
■ ■ **Factors Affecting Glomerular Filtration Rate (GFR)**

Factors	Physiologic Response	Net Effect on GFR
Afferent arteriole vasoconstriction, efferent arteriole vasodilation, or both	Decreased blood flow Decreased glomerular hydration pressure	Decrease
Afferent arteriole vasodilation or efferent arteriole vasoconstriction	Blood backs up in the glomerulus Increased hydrostatic pressure	Increase
Decrease in plasma protein concentration	Decreased plasma osmotic pressure	Increase
Slow blood flow	Larger proportions of the plasma filter out of the glomerulus Plasma osmotic pressure rises	Decrease
Rapid blood flow	Less change in plasma osmotic pressure	Increase
Tubular obstruction	Fluid backs up in the renal tubules Hydrostatic pressure increases in Bowman's capsule	Decrease

■ **TABLE 5-2**
■ ■ **Renal Response to Shock**

Glomerular hydrostatic pressure falls
↓
Epithelial cells of the tubules do not receive sufficient nutrients to support the high metabolic rate
↓
Cells die; tubular necrosis occurs
↓ ↓
Renal function may be lost   Renal tubular epithelial cells regenerate
↓
Renal function is recovered

- At the second week of life: GFR = 35 to 40 mL/min/1.73 m^2
- At 6 months: GFR = 60 mL/min/1.73 m^2
- At 1 year: GFR = 80 to 120 mL/min/1.73 m^2

- Alteration in GFR occurs with decreased renal perfusion, changes in glomerular perfusion pressures (e.g., shock, glomerular nephritis), and decreases in plasma oncotic pressure (e.g., nephrotic syndrome).
- The filtration fraction is the percent of fluid filtered into Bowman's capsule by the glomerulus in relationship to the total renal plasma flow (normal = 20%).

2. **Tubular reabsorption:** As fluid flows along the nephron, past the cells of the tubular wall, substances are reabsorbed from the renal tubule and returned to the blood via the peritubular capillaries.
   a. Most of tubular reabsorption occurs in the proximal tubule. By the time the filtrate reaches the end of the proximal tubule, two thirds of the water and virtually all the nutrients have been reabsorbed and returned to the blood. The proximal tubules play a role in acid-base balance and regulation of calcium, magnesium, and phosphorus. The proximal tubules have active transport systems for secretion of organic acids and bases from blood to tubule lumen.

b. The tubular cells lining the walls of the proximal tubules are surrounded by two different membranes that aid in water and solute reabsorption. The convoluted portion of the proximal tubule has a brushlike border of microvilli that greatly increases surface area exposed to glomerular filtrate and enhances reabsorption. The basolateral membrane has no microvilli but has an abundance of sodium and potassium pumps and other diffusion transport systems for glucose and amino acids.
c. Segments of the renal tubule use particular modes of transport to reabsorb certain substances. Substances reabsorbed by active transport depend on carriers. If the amount of substance exceeds the number of carriers (renal tubular threshold), the remaining substance will remain in the filtrate and be excreted in urine (e.g., glucosuria).
d. Fluid reabsorption is determined by the net sodium reabsorption. If the GFR decreases, net sodium reabsorption decreases and fluid reabsorption decreases. If the GFR increases, net sodium reabsorption increases and fluid reabsorption increases.
e. Several factors enhance the rate of fluid reabsorption from the renal tubule. The efferent arteriole is narrower than the peritubular capillary; therefore blood flowing from the efferent arteriole to the peritubular capillary is under relatively low pressure. The wall of the renal capillary is more permeable than other capillaries.
f. The prime "mover" for most of the proximal tubular transport is the active transport of sodium. Water is reabsorbed by osmosis in response to the reabsorption of sodium ions by active transport. Amino acids and glucose are cotransported (reabsorbed) with sodium into the interstitial fluid and eventually to capillaries. When sodium is reabsorbed from the tubule, it takes chloride with it, changing the osmotic gradient and favoring the reabsorption of water into the interstitium and eventually to the capillaries. When water is absorbed from the tubule, the concentration of the remaining solutes increases, therefore increasing the diffusion of other solutes into the interstitial space and eventually to the capillaries.
g. Measuring reabsorption: The amount of solute reabsorbed is the difference between the amount of solute filtered into the glomerulus and the amount of solute excreted in the urine (assuming the amount filtered is greater than the amount excreted).

3. **Tubular secretion** is the process by which certain substances are removed from the blood or plasma of the peritubular capillary and added to the fluid of the renal tubule through active or passive transport.
   a. Certain organic compounds (such as penicillin, creatinine, and histamine) are actively secreted into tubular fluid by the epithelium of the proximal convoluted segment.
   b. Hydrogen ions are secreted by the distal segment and the collecting ducts. Hydrogen ion secretion plays an important role in acid-base balance.
   c. Potassium ions are secreted into tubular fluid because of the electrochemical attraction created by sodium reabsorption.
   d. Measuring secretion: The amount of solute secreted is the difference between the amount of solute filtered into the glomerulus and the amount of solute excreted in the urine (assuming the amount filtered is less than the amount excreted).

C. Water and Sodium Balance

1. **Measuring water balance and regulation of urine concentration:** Normal serum osmolarity is 272 to 290 mOsm/L. It is approximately equal to twice the

serum sodium concentration. Normal urine osmolarity is approximately 300 mOsm/L. This usually correlates with a urine specific gravity of 1.010 to 1.015.

2. **Role of countercurrent mechanism in concentrating and diluting**
   a. *Filtrate concentration* changes as it flows from the proximal tubule to the collecting ducts. Filtrate becomes increasingly concentrated as it moves from the proximal tubule through the descending limb to the loop of Henle. Maximum concentration occurs at the tip of the loop of Henle. Filtrate becomes less concentrated as it moves up the ascending limb of the loop and on to the collecting duct.
   b. *Juxtamedullary nephrons* and the medullary portion of the kidney play a major role in this countercurrent mechanism. Sodium and chloride are actively reabsorbed out of the thick portion of the ascending limb into the interstitial space and peritubular capillaries, creating an osmotic gradient between the interstitium and the tubule. This segment of the tubule is impermeable to water, and water cannot be reabsorbed with sodium. In response to this osmotic gradient, water is passively reabsorbed out of the descending limb into the interstitium and peritubular capillaries. A concentration gradient is created, and filtrate is more dilute as it enters the collecting duct. As this dilute urine enters the distal tubule and collecting ducts, antidiuretic hormone (ADH) controls the amount of water reabsorption according to the need for dilute or concentrated urine. Antidiuretic hormone is released from the hypothalamus. If dilute urine is needed, ADH is inhibited. If water conservation or concentrated urine is needed, ADH is secreted.
3. **Hormonal control of water balance**
   a. *Vasopressin, or ADH,* plays a role in water balance. The distal convoluted tubule and collecting duct are impermeable to water; so water may be excreted as dilute urine. If ADH is present, the distal tubule and collecting ducts become permeable, water is reabsorbed, and urine is more concentrated. A rise in the solute concentration of the extracellular fluids and blood plasma stimulates cells in the hypothalamus to increase production of ADH and to cause release of ADH from the posterior pituitary. In the kidney, ADH initiates retention of water and decrease in solute concentration. Decreased solute concentration causes decreased ADH release, which causes dilute urine. Increased solute concentration causes increased ADH release, which causes concentrated urine.
   b. *Aldosterone* is responsible for virtually all sodium and water reabsorption in the collecting duct. This region of the renal tubule fine-tunes sodium excretion. The adrenal cortex releases aldosterone in response to angiotensin II, hyperkalemia, hyponatremia, decreased pulse pressure, or decreased right atrial distention. Aldosterone increases sodium reabsorption by increasing the number of sodium channels in the apical plasma membrane of the principal cell. Aldosterone stimulates the secretion of potassium and hydrogen and decreases potassium reabsorption.
   c. *Other factors* also control renal sodium excretion. Hormones that lead to retention of sodium include growth hormone, cortisol, insulin, and estrogen. These act at the tubular level. Parathyroid hormone (PTH), progesterone, and glycogen inhibit tubular reabsorption of sodium. Atrial natriuretic peptide, a 28-amino peptide produced and secreted in the atria of the heart, is released in response to atrial stretch, for example, in response to expansion of central blood volume. This peptide then enhances sodium excretion in part by inhibiting sodium reabsorption on the collecting duct.

4. Sodium and water reabsorption

a. Sodium concentration is higher in the lumen of the tubule than in the cells lining the tubule, so sodium moves into the tubular cells. Because the proximal tubule's brush border has no sodium pump, the sodium cannot be pumped back into the lumen. Only the basolateral membrane can pump out sodium into the interstitial spaces and then diffuse into the peritubular capillaries. When sodium (positively charged) is reabsorbed, it leaves the tubule and moves into the tubular wall. Negatively charged ions (chloride, phosphate, and bicarbonate) follow.

b. Every sodium or chloride ion that leaves the tubule means the loss of osmotically active particles from the tubule to the interstitium. The movement of particles creates a change in osmotic gradient favoring water reabsorption, and water follows the sodium and chloride into the interstitium. With less sodium in the tubule, the concentration of solutes in the tubule increases, thereby increasing diffusion of other solutes out of the tubule and into the interstitial space. As water is reabsorbed from the filtrate into the peritubular capillaries, substances remaining in the tubule become more concentrated. As a result, water moves into the tubules. As sodium reabsorption increases, water reabsorption increases and vice versa.

c. Alteration in the GFR influences the amount of sodium reabsorbed or secreted. When the GFR decreases (e.g., dehydration, sepsis), sodium and water reabsorption increases. Decreased volume decreases venous, atrial, and arterial pressures. Pressoreceptors decrease the number of impulses to the brainstem, which activates sympathetic impulses to stimulate renin release from the juxtaglomerular cells in the afferent arterioles. Renin is converted to angiotensin I, which is converted to angiotensin II, which causes vasoconstriction and secretion of aldosterone. This creates "thirst" in an effort to increase volume. As water volume increases, ADH is secreted to maintain water and solute balance.

D. Electrolyte Balance

1. Potassium ion (K^+)

a. Potassium has a normal serum value of approximately 3.5 to 5 mEq/L. It is the most abundant solute inside cells (145 mEq/L); a very small amount is present in the serum. The kidney is chiefly responsible for maintaining potassium homeostasis. Potassium is an important factor in the performance of many enzyme systems, playing a role in the maintenance of cell volume, pH, and cell excitability *(membrane potentials).* Decreasing serum potassium depolarizes membranes and raises excitability (e.g., cardiac rhythm deterioration leading to fibrillation). Increasing serum potassium hyperpolarizes membranes and decreases excitability (e.g., skeletal and smooth-muscle weakness and decreased reflexes). Potassium shifts frequently occur secondary to acid-base balance changes, hormone imbalance, and pharmacologic agents.

b. Most potassium is reabsorbed in the proximal tubule and the loop of Henle. The distal tubule and collecting ducts have a high concentration of intracellular potassium owing to the action of the sodium-potassium pumps. Changes in renal regulation of potassium are due to changes in potassium secretion in the distal tubule and collecting duct. Increases in intracellular potassium increase the secretion and excretion of potassium. Increases in plasma potassium stimulate the adrenal cortex to secrete aldosterone, which promotes secretion and excretion of potassium.

c. Any drug that interferes with aldosterone activity (e.g., angiotensin-converting enzyme [ACE] inhibitors, angiotensin II receptor blockers, spironolactone, heparin, and beta-blockers) will inhibit potassium secretion and increase serum potassium levels. Potassium excretion is regulated mainly by the collecting duct.

d. Drugs that block the principal cell sodium channel also inhibit potassium secretion (e.g., trimethoprim, pentamidime, amiloride) and may lead to increased serum potassium levels.

e. In acidosis, potassium excretion decreases. Distal tubular and collecting duct cells lose potassium to the plasma, leakage and secretion of potassium into tubules decrease, and potassium shifts from the cells into the plasma. In alkalosis, potassium excretion increases. Potassium increases in the distal tubule and collecting duct. Leakage and secretion of potassium increase. Potassium shifts into the cells. With a shift from acidosis to alkalosis, serum potassium decreases because of the shift into the cells.

2. Sodium

a. The normal serum value is approximately 135 to 145 mEq/L. Hyponatremia may lead to seizure activity. Excess of sodium leads to edema and hypertension. Dilutional hyponatremia occurs secondary to hypotonic fluid intake and impaired free water excretion. The hyponatremia corrects slowly with free water diuresis.

b. Management may include dialysis or continuous renal replacement therapy for severe or symptomatic hyponatremia (serum Na^+ <125 mEq/L) in the oliguric, hypervolemic patient *or* oliguric, hypernatremia patient (Na^+ >150 mEq/L). Hyponatremia metabolic acidosis may be treated with administration of sodium, partly in the form of sodium bicarbonate. Administer normal saline for fluid loss and dehydration. Administer 3% normal saline if the patient is fluid overloaded and has significant hyponatremia. Hypertonic saline is used until the serum sodium is corrected to a "safe" level, often considered to be greater than 125 mEq/L, and then transitioned to a less hypertonic intravenous (IV) solution.

3. Phosphate (phosphorus, inorganic)

a. Normal serum values in the newborn are 4.2 to 6.5 mg/dL. Normal values in children aged 1 to 5 years are 3.5 to 6.5 mg/dL and in older children range from 2.5 to 4.5 mg/dL. Renal excretion of phosphate is the body's primary mechanism for regulation of phosphate; therefore patients in renal failure are at high risk for hyperphosphatemia.

b. PTH indirectly affects serum phosphate levels by affecting calcium. Phosphate and calcium are reabsorbed from bone. Tubular reabsorption of phosphate is decreased as tubular reabsorption of sodium increases. PTH enhances intestinal absorption of calcium and phosphate. Vitamin D is converted to its active form by the liver and kidneys, thereby regulating phosphate and calcium balance. Active absorption of phosphate (and calcium) by the intestine is stimulated by vitamin D. Reabsorption of phosphate and calcium from bone to extracellular fluid is facilitated by vitamin D. Vitamin D stimulates renal tubular reabsorption of phosphate and calcium.

4. Calcium

a. The normal serum value is 9 to 11 mg/dL (total calcium) and 1.00 to 1.4 mmol/dL (ionized calcium). Calcium exists in two forms: ionized and nonionized. About 45% to 50% is ionized, meaning "free" and not bound to albumin. Ionized calcium is the physiologically active form of calcium. Albumin-bound calcium is not filtered at the glomerulus. Decreased serum albumin levels may affect serum calcium levels.

b. PTH is the most important regulator of calcium. Hypocalcemia stimulates the release of PTH, which decreases renal excretion of calcium and increases urinary excretion of phosphorus. Hypercalcemia inhibits the release of PTH.

5. **Magnesium:** The normal serum values are 1.8 to 2.3 mEq/L. Magnesium is an essential cofactor for many metabolic enzymatic processes in the body. Eighty percent of plasma magnesium is filtered at the glomerulus, and only a small amount of this filtrate is excreted.

E. Regulation of Acid-Base Balance

1. **Definitions:** An *acid* is a source of hydrogen ions. A *base* takes up or absorbs hydrogen ions. A *buffer* combines with an acid or base to maintain a stable pH.
2. In an effort to achieve an **acid-base balance,** the lungs regulate carbon dioxide and the kidneys regulate bicarbonate. With normal digestion, metabolic acids (hydrogen ions) are produced. Metabolic hydrogen ions are picked up by serum bicarbonate and form carbon dioxide. An increased level of carbon dioxide and hydrogen ions stimulates increased respiration, which helps to eliminate carbon dioxide and reverse acidosis. Respiratory regulation of acid-base balance is generally inadequate in severe metabolic acidosis and alkalosis.
3. The kidney regulates acid-base balance through hydrogen secretion and bicarbonate reabsorption. Hydrogen ions are secreted (removed from the blood and plasma of the peritubular capillary and added to the fluid of the renal tubule) at the distal tubule and the collecting duct.
   a. *Renal response in alkalotic conditions:* Potassium excretion increases, chloride is reabsorbed with sodium, and bicarbonate is excreted. If an increase in filtrate bicarbonate is secondary to increased serum concentration, bicarbonate excretion increases. If an increase in filtrate bicarbonate is secondary to hypovolemia (e.g., in persistent vomiting), hydrogen ion secretion and bicarbonate reabsorption from the tubules increase, preventing excretion of excess bicarbonate. Alkalosis is corrected as volume status is restored.
   b. *Renal response in acidotic conditions:* Potassium excretion decreases. Bicarbonate is reabsorbed with sodium, and chloride is excreted. Bicarbonate diffuses into the extracellular compartment and ultimately into the plasma (via the renal vein), resulting in reabsorption of hydrogen ions. Renal excretion of acid (ammonium excretion) increases.

F. Regulation of Arterial Blood Pressure

1. **Maintenance of circulating blood volume:** Circulating blood volume is maintained by sodium and water balance. A countercurrent mechanism plays a role in concentrating and diluting. Hormonal control of water balance is mediated by ADH and aldosterone.
2. **Regulation of peripheral vascular resistance** is via the renin-angiotensin-aldosterone system and the central nervous system (CNS) (Figure 5-3). Juxtaglomerular cells release renin in response to a decrease in glomerular pressure *(kidney perfusion pressure),* an increase in sympathetic nervous system stimulation, decreased sodium in the distal tubule, or vasoconstrictive agents. Renin diffuses into the circulatory system and converts angiotensinogen into angiotensin I. As angiotensin I circulates to the lungs, it converts to angiotensin II (and also produces aldosterone). Angiotensin II is a powerful vasoconstrictor of the peripheral vascular system. Angiotensin II stimulates aldosterone secretion, which causes an increase in water and sodium reabsorption. The sympathetic nervous system also regulates peripheral vascular resistance by causing vasoconstriction.

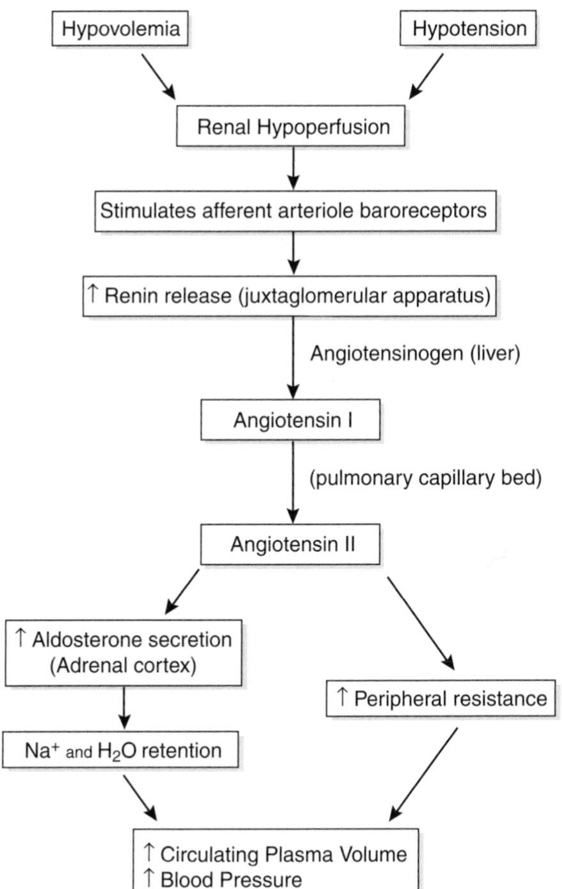

FIGURE 5-3 ■ Renin-angiotensin aldosterone cascade to maintain systemic perfusion pressure.

(From Curley MAQ, Moloney-Harmon PA: *Critical care nursing of infants and children.* Philadelphia, 2001, W. B. Saunders, p 735.)

G. Regulation of Renal Blood Flow

Prostaglandins are vasoactive substances that act by either dilating or constricting renal vessels. Their effect is limited to the renal vasculature. Three prostaglandins are produced by cells in the kidney's cortical and medullary structures. Thromboxane A_2 is a vasoconstrictor. Prostacyclin (PGI_2) and prostaglandin E_2 (PGE_2) are vasodilators. PGI_2 and PGE_2 produce direct vasodilation of afferent arterioles, which helps to maintain renal blood flow and glomerular perfusion. PGE_2 increases urine output by counteracting the actions of ADH. PGE_2 increases sodium excretion by inhibiting its reabsorption from the renal tubules.

H. Elimination of Toxins and Metabolic Wastes

1. **Urea** is produced in the liver as a by-product of amino acid metabolism. Amino acids and proteins are metabolized in the liver and yield ammonia, which is very toxic unless rapidly detoxified into urea. About 50% of urea is passively reabsorbed, and 50% is excreted in the urine. In the presence of ADH, urea is trapped because the upper portions of the collecting duct are impermeable to urea; as water is reabsorbed, the urea becomes concentrated, thus increasing intracellular fluid solute concentration.
2. **Uric acid** is a by-product of metabolism of certain organic bases in nucleic acids. Ninety percent is reabsorbed in the glomerular filtrate, and 10% is secreted into the renal tubule.

3. **Creatinine** is the end product of protein metabolism. Under normal conditions, creatinine is completely filtered by the kidneys and excreted in the urine. Its complete elimination makes it an excellent marker of renal function. The creatinine level is proportional to the blood urea nitrogen (BUN) level. The normal BUN-to-creatinine ratio is 10 to 15:1. An increase in both BUN and creatinine signals renal dysfunction. An increase in BUN without an increase in creatinine may be an indication of dehydration, decreased renal perfusion, or catabolism.

I. Stimulation of Bone Marrow Erythrocyte Production

1. The **anemia** associated with renal failure is due mainly to a deficiency of a hormone called *erythropoietin,* which is produced by the kidneys. In renal failure, production of erythropoietin is insufficient. Erythropoietin stimulates red blood cell production from the bone marrow, and a deficiency of production leads to anemia. However, often the anemia of renal failure can be improved with iron supplementation. Some children with renal failure have iron depletion even when taking iron supplements.
2. IV and subcutaneous recombinant human erythropoietin is available for treatment of anemia secondary to chronic renal failure. Side effects include hypertension, seizures, and vascular access thrombus formation. This is often administered at the time of dialysis if the patient is receiving intermittent dialysis therapy.
3. Uremia shortens the life span of red blood cells and decreases platelet function.
4. Transfusions should be avoided as much as possible, not only because of the infectious risks and risk of fluid overload but also to avoid inhibition of the low, although present, positive feedback on erythropoietin secretion. Other possible deficiencies should be assessed before therapy is initiated, including vitamin B_{12} deficiency, folate deficiency, or aluminum intoxication (the latter leading to microcytic anemia). Throughout the course of therapy, iron stores (serum iron, ferritin, and total iron-binding capacity [TIBC]) should be evaluated frequently because the rapid proliferative response may not be accompanied by an adequate availability of iron. If iron stores prove insufficient during the course of therapy, replacement should be implemented (Table 5-3).

ACUTE RENAL FAILURE

A. Definitions

1. **Acute renal failure** (ARF) is the sudden loss of renal capacity for filtration and tubular reabsorption, resulting in accumulation of wastes, fluid and electrolyte imbalance, and acid-base imbalances. There are many causes of ARF in children, including prerenal disease, intrinsic renal failure, acute tubular necrosis (ATN), and postrenal failure.
2. **Prerenal failure,** the most common cause of ARF, is usually caused by poor perfusion (Table 5-4). A decrease in renal perfusion causes decreased glomerular perfusion and GFR. ARF, by definition, is not associated with any intrinsic parenchymal disease. Impaired renal blood flow may be secondary to impaired cardiac performance, intravascular volume depletion, renal vasoconstriction, or renal artery thrombosis. When reduction of renal blood flow is mild to moderate, kidney blood flow and GFR are maintained by autoregulatory response. This is accomplished by autoregulation of afferent arteriolar dilation and efferent arteriolar vasoconstriction. Prerenal ARF will occur when adaptive mechanisms fail and GFR falls. There is a good prognosis for kidney function if prompt recognition and restoration of adequate renal blood flow is achieved. Two

TABLE 5-3
Pediatric Iron Studies

Total Iron Binding Capacity (TIBC)	Transferrin	Iron	Transferrin Saturation (Tsat)	Ferritin
Direct, quantitative measurement of transferrin	Iron is bound to this globulin protein Carried to the bone marrow for incorporation into hemoglobin Produced in liver	Measurement of the quantity of iron bound to transferrin	Percent saturation of iron bound to transferrin Calculated: tsat (%) = $\frac{\text{Iron}}{\text{TIBC}} \times 100$	Good indicator of available iron stores The major iron storage protein
Normal: 25–420 μg/dL or 43–73 μmol/L	Normal: 200–400 μg/dL	Normal: 60–190 μg/dL or 13–31 μmol/L	Normal: 30%–40%	Normal: Newborn: 25–200 ng/mL 1 mo: 200–600 ng/mL 2–5 mo: 50 – 200 ng/mL 6 mo to 15 y: 7–142 ng/mL
Elevated in iron deficiency Decreased in chronic illness Varies minimally with intake More a reflection of hepatic function (transferrin produced in liver) and nutrition than iron metabolism		Decreased level in iron deficiency Decreased in chronic illness Elevated after massive blood product transfusion	Decreased in iron deficiency Normal in chronic illness	Interfering factors: recent transfusion ingestion of meal high in iron disorders of excessive iron storage hemolytic diseases

common classes of medications, nonsteroidal anti-inflammatory drugs (NSAIDs) and ACE inhibitors, can cause prerenal ARF by impairing renal autoregulation. Hypoxic/ischemic and nephrotoxic acute kidney failure are the most common causes of hospital-acquired kidney failure.

3. **Intrinsic renal failure** is described as acute tubular necrosis related to decreased perfusion to the renal parenchyma as in hemolytic uremic syndrome, acute glomerulonephritis, or acute interstitial nephritis.
4. **Postrenal failure** is usually associated with obstruction of urine flow at any point in the ureters, bladder, or urethral meatus and is caused by such conditions as Wilms' tumor, renal calculi, blood clots, or edema. ARF secondary to postrenal failure is a relatively small percentage of the cases of ARF, but it is an important cause of renal failure in newborn males with posterior urethral valve.

B. Intrinsic Renal Failure (Acute Tubular Necrosis)

1. **Definition:** Acute tubular necrosis (ATN) is the death of tubular cells, which may result when tubular cells are deprived of oxygen *(ischemic ATN)* or when they

TABLE 5-4
Causes of Prerenal Acute Renal Failure

Volume Depletion	Cardiac Dysfunction	Peripheral Vasodilation	Afferent Arteriolar Constriction	Efferent Arteriolar Vasodilation
Inadequate intake	Acute myocardial infarction	Sepsis	Hypercalcemia	ACE inhibitors
Hemorrhage	Cardiomyopathy	Cirrhosis	Sepsis	ARBs
Gastrointestinal losses	Valvular disease	Chronic anemia	Hepatorenal syndrome	
Renal losses	Arrhythmias	Medications: e.g., NSAIDs, amphotericin B, cyclosporine		
Skin losses				
Third spacing				

ACE, angiotensin-converting enzyme; *ARBs*, angiotensin II receptor blockers

have been exposed to a toxic drug or molecule *(nephrotoxic ATN)*. When mean arterial blood pressure drops significantly, renal autoregulatory processes are no longer functional, often leading to development of ATN and uremic syndrome. Multiple factors, including systemic maldistribution of volume and decrease in blood flow secondary to circulating mediators, affect blood and oxygen delivery to the kidneys. Fortunately, new tubular cells usually replace those that have died. The tubular cells of the kidneys undergo a continuous cycle of cell death and renewal, much like the cells of the skin.

2. **Etiology**
   a. *Nephrotoxic* ATN is a toxic insult to the renal tubules secondary to nephrotoxic drugs, radiographic contrast dye, organic solvents, or inappropriate levels of hemoglobin or myoglobin. Tubular epithelium necrosis occurs. The healing process and prognosis are better than that for ischemic ATN because the supporting basement membrane is not affected.
   b. *Ischemic* ATN (hemodynamically mediated renal failure) is a sudden and sustained decline of GFR and necrosis of the tubule cells secondary to nephrotoxic injury. Compensatory and autoregulatory mechanisms are exhausted. Renal oxygen delivery is critically impaired, causing tubular and cellular damage. The body attempts to compensate and maintain adequate renal blood flow and GFR by sodium and water retention, which results in decreased urine output. Oliguric ATN has a much worse prognosis than nonoliguric ATN. Common complications of ARF are noted in Table 5-5.
3. **Pathophysiology**
   a. *Vasoactive factors:* Arteriolar vasoconstriction is induced.
   b. *Tubular factors:* As the hydrostatic pressure increases, there is back leak from the tubular lumen to the vasa recta. Cellular sloughing and casts cause tubular obstruction.

TABLE 5-5
Common Complications of Acute Renal Failure

Metabolic	Cardiovascular	Gastrointestinal	Neurologic	Hematologic	Infectious	Other
Hyperkalemia	Pulmonary edema	Nausea	Neuromuscular irritability	Anemia	Pneumonia	Hiccups
Metabolic acidosis	Arrhythmias	Vomiting	Asterixis	Bleeding	Septicemia	Increased parathyroid hormone
Hyponatremia	Pericarditis	Malnutrition	Seizures		Urinary tract infection	Low total triiodothyronine
Hypocalcemia	Pericardial effusion	Gastrointestinal hemorrhage	Mental status changes			Low thyroxine
Hyperphosphatemia	Pulmonary embolism					Normal free thyroxine
Hypermagnesemia	Hypertension					
Hyperuricemia	Myocardial infarction					

Adapted from Brenner BM: *Brenner & Rector's The Kidney,* 7th ed., Philadelphia, 2004, Saunders.

c. *Vascular factors:* In low blood flow states, nephrotoxins are concentrated in the renal tubular cells. Glomerular capillary permeability increases for proteins and decreases for potassium.

d. *Metabolic factors:* Damage to the cell membrane and impaired cellular function occur as the calcium flux is altered and oxygen free radicals are formed.

4. **The clinical course** of ATN can be divided into four phases:

a. The *onset,* or *initiating phase,* is the time from the precipitating event until cell injury occurs. The duration is hours to days. It may correspond with prerenal failure. Renal failure is reversible at this point. The time course may be *hours* for postischemic ATN compared with *days* for nephrotoxic ATN.

b. The *oliguric phase* is the time from cell injury to the development of uremia. Duration is 1 to 2 weeks. Oliguria (urine output of less than 1 mL/kg per hour) is more common in postischemic ATN. *Anuria* (no urine output) is uncommon in ATN, more common in postrenal obstruction. The following events characterize development of severe nephron dysfunction and uremia or uremic syndrome during this phase:
- GFR is significantly decreased.
- Hypervolemia occurs.
- BUN and plasma creatinine increase.
- Electrolyte imbalances occur.
- Metabolic acidosis is present.
- Side effects of the accumulation of uremic toxins are evident (sluggishness, insomnia, itching, slurring of speech, anorexia, nausea, vomiting, confusion, asterixis, seizures, coma).

c. The *diuretic phase* is the beginning of recovery characterized by improved urine output, increased urea excretion, and solute excretion. Duration is 7 to 14 days. Signs of gradual improvement of overall renal function are seen. In the early part of the phase, urine output dramatically increases each day. In the beginning of the diuretic phase, "dumb" urine is excreted; "dumb" urine is similar to filtrate and shows little function of reabsorption or secretion. Throughout the diuretic phase, urea excretion and solute reabsorption and secretion improve. By the end of this phase, the BUN has fallen and stabilized, electrolyte balance and acidosis are improved, and GFR begins to return to normal. Renal replacement therapy may be indicated during this phase until kidney function has returned enough to control fluid and electrolyte balance. Administration of fluid to replace urine output may be necessary if the patient's volume status and assessment indicate.

d. During the *recovery phase,* renal function slowly reoccurs. It may take years for renal function to return to normal. There may be residual damage and a certain percentage of unrecoverable renal function. Children may have some degree of chronic renal failure for months or years after the insult but generally have steadily improving renal function as months and years pass. Intermittent monitoring of renal function will be required.

C. Invasive and Noninvasive Diagnostic Tools

1. **Prerenal failure vs. ATN:** Diagnostic laboratory values (urine and serum) are detailed in Table 5-6.

2. **Radiologic consultation** may be helpful if serum and urine laboratory values are inconclusive.

a. The risk *of intravenous pyelography (IVP)* outweighs its benefit in acute phase.

b. *Ultrasonography* should be performed if urinary tract obstruction is suspected. It is readily available, accurate, reliable, and noninvasive. Increased echogenicity of the renal parenchyma is a common nonspecific indicator of intrinsic renal

TABLE 5-6
Diagnostic Laboratory Values (Urine and Serum)

Diagnostic Labs	Prerenal	ATN
Urine output	Decreased	Decreased or normal
Urine sediment	Normal	Red blood cell casts, cellular debris
Specific gravity	High (>1.020)	Low (≤1.010)
Osmolality (urine-to-plasma ratio)	>1.5 (>1.2 in neonates)	<1.2
Urine sodium	Low (<10 mEq/L)	High (>30 mEq/L) (>25 mEq/L in neonates)
Creatinine (urine-to-plasma ratio)	>15:1	<10:1
FEN_a (%)*	<1 (<2.5 in neonates)	>2 (>3 in neonates)
Creatinine	Normal or slowly increasing	High and increasing
BUN	High	High and increasing

*Excreted fraction of filtered sodium. Diuretic administration may affect results or measurement of urine sodium.

disease. In some cases of ATN, renal parenchymal echogenicity may be normal. RBF is generally reduced in ARF, and Doppler flow ultrasound can detect low blood flow. Low RBF or abnormal blood flow associated with renal artery stenosis can also be detected. Complete absence of flow suggests complete thrombosis of the renal circulation (Toto, 2004).

c. *A MAG3 renal scan* can distinguish ATN from prerenal or other intrinsic renal disease.

d. *Computed tomography (CT) and magnetic resonance imaging (MRI)* may be helpful in detecting parenchymal renal disease and obstructive uropathy. In most cases they do not provide more information than ultrasonography.

e. *Kidney angiogram* is helpful in patients with ARF caused by vascular disorders, including renal artery stenosis and renal artery emboli.

3. **Kidney biopsy** should be performed only when clinical, biochemical, and noninvasive imaging studies are insufficient for diagnosis and there is reasonable belief that the test results will alter therapy. This is the "gold standard" for diagnostic accuracy in ARF, but in clinical practice it is not routinely performed. Patients with clinical syndrome of rapidly progressing glomerulonephritis may require renal biopsy unless there is an overt contraindication because kidney-preserving therapy may be available for these patients (Toto, 2004).

D. Laboratory Findings in ARF

1. **Urinalysis:** Common findings in ARF
   - a. *Urinary sediment*
     - Intrinsic kidney failure
   - b. *Color*
     - "Dirty" brown: Intrinsic kidney failure
     - Reddish brown: Acute glomerulonephritis
     - Bilious tinge: Mixed hepatic and renal failure
   - c. *Proteinuria*
     - Glomerulonephritis
     - Interstitial nephritis
     - Toxic and infectious causes
   - d. *Casts*
     - Red blood cell (RBC) casts: Glomerulonephritis or vasculitis
     - White blood cell (WBC) casts: Interstitial nephritis

- Granular casts: Glomerulonephritis
- Uric acid crystals: Tumor lysis syndrome
- Calcium oxylate crystals: Ethylene glycol ingestion
- Acetaminophen crystals: Acetaminophen toxicity (acute)

2. **Urine chemistries**
   a. *Urine electrolyte measurement* in ARF is performed to test functional integrity of the renal tubules.
   b. *The most informative urine test* is the fractional excretion of sodium (FENa) (results are inaccurate if the patient is on diuretics).

$$\text{FENa} = \frac{\text{Urine Na} \times \text{Plasma Cr}}{\text{Urine Cr} \times \text{Plasma Na}} \times 100$$

   - Results: less than 1%—prerenal renal failure; greater than 1%—intrinsic or chronic renal failure; less than or greater than 1%—obstructive renal failure.

3. **Hyperkalemia**
   a. *Hyperkalemia* occurs secondary to decreased renal excretion. Oliguric patients do not excrete sufficient potassium to maintain a normal balance. Hyperkalemia may be exacerbated by metabolic acidosis, which causes a shift of potassium from the intracellular space. Continued acid production occurs from catabolic cellular metabolism, despite loss of renal excretory function. Multiple blood transfusions and RBC hemolysis release potassium. The longer the blood is stored, the higher the potassium content of the blood as a result of cell lysis and potassium release. Blood banks generally release the oldest unit of blood first. In an infant or child with hyperkalemia requiring blood transfusion, a specific request should be made for a fresh unit of blood.
   b. *Electrocardiographic (ECG)* changes secondary to hyperkalemia can range from peaked T waves, prolonged PR interval, and complete heart block to ventricular fibrillation as the potassium level increases.
   c. *Other clinical manifestations* may include muscle cramps, muscle weakness, muscle twitching, abdominal cramps, diarrhea, and ileus.
   d. *Management of hyperkalemia* depends on the severity of electrolyte imbalance. Patients with a serum potassium level greater than 7 mEq/L and evidence of myocardial toxicity are at an extremely high risk for lethal arrhythmias. Prompt, aggressive intervention is critical for survival.
   - Treatment measures include the administration of insulin (0.1 units/kg regular insulin) and hypertonic glucose (0.5 to 1 mL/kg 50% dextrose) to promote cellular uptake of potassium. These medications essentially "move" the potassium around in the body and are *not* causing true potassium excretion. The effects of cellular shifts on serum potassium are short lived and require frequent monitoring of serum sodium and potassium. These medications may need to be redosed until potassium excretion occurs.
   - Albuterol is another pharmacologic strategy to shift serum potassium into the cellular space, although it is not as potent as IV strategies. Its peak action is 90 to 120 minutes. Patients with hyperkalemia may be placed on continuous inhaled albuterol.
   - Movement of the potassium into the cells can be facilitated by hyperventilation and administration of sodium bicarbonate (1 to 3 mEq/kg). (*Caution:* Do not mix calcium and bicarbonate in IV solutions because precipitation will occur.)

- Stabilize the myocardium with IV calcium (10-20 mg/kg per dose calcium chloride [infants and children] or 50-100 mg/kg per dose calcium gluconate [infants and children]).
- Eliminate exogenous sources of potassium (potassium-free hydration).
- Remove potassium from the patient using resin exchange via the gastrointestinal tract with a sodium polystyrene sulfonate (Kayexalate) enema (1 g/kg per dose). (*Note:* Repeat the enema two or three times per 24-hour period if necessary.) Sodium polystyrene sulfonate (Kayexalate) exchanges sodium for potassium in the gastrointestinal tract. It must be retained in the gastrointestinal tract to cause the renin exchange and ultimate removal of potassium. If it is not retained, the dose should be repeated. It may be instilled high in the rectum using red rubber tube. Full effect is usually seen in 4 hours.
- If kidney function is absent or severely impaired, or if hyperkalemia is severe, consider hemodialysis. Hemodialysis against a potassium-free dialysate can decrease serum potassium as rapidly as 1.5 mEq/hour. Continuous renal replacement therapy without potassium in the replacement fluid or dialysate is also an option if the patient is too hemodynamically unstable to tolerate hemodialysis.

e. *Desired patient outcomes*
- Maintain normative K^+ values.
- Maintain adequate urine output.
- Absence of acidosis.
- Absence of dysrhythmia.

4. Hyperphosphatemia

a. *Hyperphosphatemia* occurs as a result of the kidney's inability to excrete phosphate in mild to moderate renal insufficiency. Phosphorus homeostasis is maintained by an increase in phosphorus excretion per nephron through the action of PTH. As renal failure progresses and GFR is less than 30 mL per minute, elevated phosphorus level will ensue. Hyperphosphatemia may also be secondary to tumor lysis syndrome, rhabdomyolysis, bowel infarction, ileus, or the use of sodium phosphate enemas in the presence of gastrointestinal tract abnormalities.

b. *Hyperphosphatemia may not produce signs and symptoms* until levels are very high (above 10 mEq/L); however, a secondary hypocalcemia may develop as an attempt to compensate. See clinical manifestations in the discussion of hypocalcemia.

c. *Management of hyperphosphatemia* may include IV fluid therapy to increase phosphorus excretion or administration of IV calcium. Use of enteral calcium-based phosphate binders should be considered. Administration of phosphorus-containing agents and dietary phosphorus intake should be minimized. Acute situations can be managed initially with the administration of insulin and glucose by shifting phosphorus from the extracellular space to the intracellular space. Management of severe hyperphosphatemia (greater than 10 to 12 mEq/L) may include hemodialysis or renal replacement therapy to decrease phosphate levels.

d. *Long-term sequelae* include increased risk of mortality, cardiovascular disease, bone disease, and extraskeletal calcification of soft tissues, including blood vessels, lungs, kidneys, and joints.

5. Hypocalcemia

a. *Pathophysiology:* Serum calcium declines reciprocally as phosphorus rises. Alterations in calcium most often occur secondary to hyperphosphatemia. Other reasons for hypocalcemia include induced resistance to the action of

PTH, crush injury (occurs early), severe muscle damage, large transfusions of citrate-containing blood products, sepsis, and hypomagnesemia.

   b. *Clinical manifestations of calcium or phosphate imbalance* include CNS changes (anxiety, tetany, and seizures), muscle cramps, hypotension, and Trousseau's and Chvostek's signs.

   c. *Management of hypocalcemia* includes decreasing the serum phosphate levels and replacing magnesium, if indicated, to increase PTH release. If the patient is symptomatic, administer IV 10% calcium gluconate (50 to 100 mg/kg per dose; maximum dose, 2 g). If a more rapid response is required, use calcium chloride (10 to 20 mg/kg per dose [infants and children] and 37 to 74 mg/kg per dose [neonates]; maximum dose, 1 g). Infuse slowly (do not exceed 1 mL per minute), and monitor for bradycardia and asystole with IV calcium infusion. Because of high osmolar content, extravasation with IV administration can cause severe tissue damage.

   d. *In ARF,* PTH's ability to serve as a regulator of phosphorus and calcium balance is compromised because of the alteration in the renal absorption of calcium and excretion of phosphate. Decreased synthesis of the active form of vitamin D results in hypocalcemia.

6. **Hypermagnesemia**

   a. *Mild hypermagnesemia* may occur in ARF secondary to decreased renal excretion of magnesium. It may be secondary to the use of magnesium-containing antacids (Maalox) or total parenteral nutrition (TPN).

   b. *Clinical manifestations:* Acute elevations may depress the CNS, peripheral neuromuscular junction, and deep-tendon reflexes. There is an increased potential for hypotension, hypoventilation, and cardiac arrhythmias.

   c. *Management of hypermagnesemia* usually does not require intervention other than discontinuing magnesium-containing substances (e.g., Maalox). Calcium acts as a direct antagonist to magnesium. In life-threatening situations, IV calcium may be administered. Dialysis may be used for removal of magnesium because loop diuretics in particular enhance magnesium excretion. PTH stimulates reabsorption of magnesium from the tubules.

7. **Glucose intolerance** may develop secondary to decreased peripheral sensitivity to insulin when renal excretion is decreased. Renal replacement therapy can remove glucose.

8. **Uremia** is related to the accumulation of toxins and waste products normally excreted in the urine and is measured as BUN.

   a. *Azotemia* refers to a high serum concentration of nitrogenous wastes. Build-up of creatinine is not harmful to the body; however, uremia can have deleterious effects. Uremic pericarditis occurs only in the presence of prolonged severe renal failure and results from chemical irritation of the pericardium secondary to the metabolic abnormalities. It may culminate in cardiac tamponade or cause recurrent hypotension during hemodialysis. If adequate relief of uremic pericarditis does not occur with hemodialysis, pericardiectomy is recommended.

   b. *Clinical manifestations* are due to toxic effects of substances such as urea and ammonia. Neurologic symptoms include lethargy, confusion, seizures, and coma. Gastrointestinal tract symptoms include anorexia, nausea, vomiting, diarrhea, and gastrointestinal tract bleeding. Cardiovascular symptoms include hypervolemia and hypotension secondary to shifts of fluid into the extracellular space. Hematologic compromise involves anemia, thrombocytopenia, platelet dysfunction, and increased bleeding time. Skin symptoms include pruritus and discoloration. Immunosuppression may result.

c. *Management* for symptomatic patients may include renal replacement therapy. BUN level is often a marker for indication for therapy as well as response to treatment.

9. **Acid-base imbalance**
   a. *Metabolic acidosis* occurs in ARF because of alterations in renal function, including a decrease in GFR, decreased hydrogen ion secretion, decreased bicarbonate reabsorption, decreased ammonia (NH_3) synthesis, and ammonium (NH_4) excretion. Acidosis in ARF results in an increase in the anion gap.

$$\text{Anion Gap} = \text{Sodium} - (\text{Chloride} + \text{Bicarbonate})$$

   b. *Clinical manifestations of acidosis* secondary to ARF include increased minute ventilation, a change in mental status as ammonium excretion decreases, and hyperkalemia as potassium excretion decreases, causing an increased potential for lethal dysrhythmias.
   c. *Management* involves the correction of metabolic acidosis. Minor adjustments may be made by hyperventilation. IV administration of bicarbonate is necessary for significant correction (Table 5-7).

10. **Hematologic changes** include anemia and abnormal platelet function. Anemia is related to decreased erythrocyte production, changes secondary to volume status (i.e., hemoconcentration or hemodilution), frequent blood sampling, and bleeding. Patients with chronic renal failure require erythropoietin supplementation because of decreased erythrocyte production. Although platelet number is generally

TABLE 5-7
Renal Response to Changes in Acid-Base Balance

Change in Acid-Base Balance	Renal Response
RESPIRATORY ACIDOSIS	
Retaining of carbon dioxide and bicarbonate	Increase bicarbonate in plasma to take up hydrogen ions
Plasma hydrogen ions rise	Excretion of acid in urine
RESPIRATORY ALKALOSIS	
Increased elimination or blowing off of carbon dioxide Decreased plasma hydrogen ion concentration	Increase excretion of bicarbonate to conserve hydrogen ions
METABOLIC ACIDOSIS	
Decreased plasma bicarbonate and increased plasma hydrogen ion concentration	Replenish bicarbonate
METABOLIC ALKALOSIS	
Increased plasma bicarbonate	Less intracellular hydrogen ion available for secretion
Decreased plasma and intracellular hydrogen ion concentration	Some bicarbonate escapes into the urine (alkaline urine)
CHRONIC ACIDOSIS	Increase production of ammonia (NH_3) to bind with hydrogen ions and excrete ammonium (NH_4^+) in urine

normal in uremia, the bleeding time is prolonged because of defective platelet activation and adhesiveness. Coagulation tests are normal in ARF. Skin bleeding time is the best predictor of clinical bleeding. Uremic bleeding is usually mild mucocutaneous bleeding. If a uremic patient bleeds, consider a structural or other hemostatic abnormality. If the hemostatic defect is thought to be related solely to the renal failure, peritoneal or hemodialysis can usually reverse the hemostatic disorder. Uremic patients who undergo surgery are always at risk for bleeding. Consider administration of desmopressin (DDAVP) before surgery.

10. **Infection** is a risk for ARF patients, who have an altered immune response secondary to the suppression of macrophages by uremic toxins. Invasive lines increase the risk. Prophylactic antibiotic therapy is generally not indicated.

E. Potential Patient Problem List

- Hypervolemia secondary to fluid retention during the oliguric or anuric phase of ATN
- Hypovolemia secondary to fluid loss during the diuretic phase of ATN
- Decreased cardiac output related to dysrhythmias and alteration in volume status
- Electrolyte imbalance related to change in filtration or change in tubular secretion and excretion
- Multisystem complications related to electrolyte imbalance
- Alteration in skin integrity secondary to uremic toxins (pruritus, dryness, fragile capillaries, easy bruising)
- Alteration in mucous membranes secondary to uremic toxins on mucous membranes
- Alteration in cardiac function (dysrhythmias, increased potential for hypotension or hypertension)
- Alteration in musculoskeletal system (muscle twitching, muscle weakness, depressed deep-tendon reflexes)
- Alteration in acid-base balance
- Increased risk for infection related to invasive catheters and altered immune response
- Alteration in comfort related to pain, multiple procedures, changes in skin integrity, and nausea or vomiting
- Alteration in nutrition related to decreased intake, intake restriction, and altered metabolism of nutrients.
- Potential multisystem complications (Table 5-8)

F. Renal Diseases or Conditions That May Lead to ARF

1. **Hemolytic uremic syndrome (HUS)** is the simultaneous occurrence of hemolytic anemia, thrombocytopenia, and renal failure.
   a. *Pathophysiology* is characterized by microangiopathy with platelet aggregation and fibrin deposition in small vessels in the kidney, gut, and CNS. Hemolytic anemia is believed to be a result of the shearing of red cells as they pass through narrowed vessels.
   b. *"Typical" HUS* peaks from June through September with gastrointestinal prodromes (vomiting, diarrhea, abdominal pain) during the days to weeks preceding onset. HUS is characteristically a disease of young children. *Escherichia coli* 0157:H7 causes a large number of cases of typical HUS.
   c. *Atypical HUS* is an extremely rare group of disorders of the kidneys and is distinctly different from the HUS syndrome caused by *E. coli* 0157:H7. It occurs year round and there is generally no gastrointestinal prodrome. It is

TABLE 5-8
Clinical Manifestations of Potential Multisystem Complications Secondary to Acute Renal Failure (ARF)

System	Clinical Manifestations
Cardiovascular	ECG changes secondary to hyperkalemia
Respiratory	Pneumonia, pulmonary edema
Gastrointestinal	Hemorrhage, abdominal cramping, nausea and vomiting, diarrhea, malnutrition
Neurologic	Altered mental status
Metabolic	Acidosis, hypercalcemia, hyperkalemia, uremia, hypermagnesemia, hyperphosphatemia, hyperuricemia
Hematologic	Anemia, coagulopathy
Infection	Sepsis, pneumonia

ECG, electrocardiogram.

rare in children younger than 2 years. Relapses can occur, and these cases may evolve to terminal renal failure. Children with atypical HUS are much more likely to develop chronic complications such as kidney failure and severe high blood pressure. Familial occurrence is possible. There is substantial evidence that atypical HUS is a genetic disorder.

d. *Clinical symptoms of HUS* include bloody diarrhea (more common in typical HUS), mild to moderate hypertension, fever, lethargy, decreased urine output, and paleness.
e. *Laboratory findings* reveal increased schistocyte number on peripheral smear, anemia (age specific), and an elevated reticulocyte count. Other indicators of intravascular hemolysis include elevated lactate dehydrogenase (LDH), increased indirect bilirubin level, and low haptoglobin level. The Coomb's test is negative. Mild leukocytosis may accompany hemolytic anemia. Thrombocytopenia is uniformly present, and the platelet count is generally less than 60,000/mm^3. Prothrombin time, partial thromboplastin time, fibrinogen level, and coagulation factors are normal.
f. *Significant renal failure* is seen in more than 90% of patients with HUS. Dialysis is required for many of these patients.
g. *Management* is primarily focused on general supportive care and treatment of complications such as ARF, anemia, CNS symptoms, and abdominal symptoms.

2. **Acute glomerulonephritis** refers to a specific set of renal diseases (such as lupus nephritis and poststreptococcal nephritis) that result from immunologic mechanisms triggering inflammation and proliferation of glomerular tissue.
   a. *Acute glomerulonephritis* is currently described as a clinical syndrome that frequently manifests as a sudden onset of hematuria, proteinuria, and red cell casts. With the exception of poststreptococcal glomerulonephritis, the exact triggers for the formation of the immune complexes are unclear. In streptococcal infection, involvement of derivatives of streptococcal proteins has been reported. A streptococcal neuraminidase may alter host immunoglobulin G (IgG). IgG combines with host antibodies. IgG/anti-IgG immune complexes are formed and then collect in the glomeruli. In addition, antibody titers to other antigens, such as antistreptolysin O or antihyaluronidase, DNAase-B, and streptokinase, provide evidence of a recent streptococcal infection and may be elevated. Antigen-antibody complexes mediate glomerular injury.

Hypofiltration occurs as a result of decreased glomerular blood flow. Glomerular blood flow decreases as a result of arteriolar vasoconstriction, capillary obstruction by thrombi, and endothelial cell edema from proliferation of endothelial cells and WBC infiltration.

b. *Clinical signs and symptoms* include salt and water retention secondary to decreased GFR, RBC or granular casts in the urine, declining renal function, hypertension, hematuria, oliguria, and other nonspecific symptoms such as fever, malaise, abdominal discomfort, nausea, or vomiting.

c. *Management* includes sodium and water restriction and treatment of underlying disease as well as management of declining renal function.

d. *Outcome.* Sporadic cases of acute nephritis progress to a chronic form. This progression occurs in as many as 30% of adult and 10% of pediatric patients. The mortality rate of acute glomerulonephritis has been reported at 0% to 7%. The male-to-female ratio is 2:1. Most cases of acute glomerulonephritis occur in patients aged 5 to 15 years.

3. **Nephrotic syndrome** is a pediatric disorder that is characterized by proteinuria greater than 40 mg/m^2 per hour, hypoalbuminemia, edema, and hyperlipidemia that occurs secondary to glomerular damage. It can be a primary or secondary disease.

   a. *Nephrotic syndrome* in children is primarily "idiopathic" (90%), and its presentation and relapses are often associated with a recent upper respiratory infection. It usually presents between 2 and 6 years of age and affects males more often than females. Idiopathic nephrotic syndrome can be divided into three morphologic patterns: (1) minimal-change disease (85%), (2) mesangial proliferation (5%), or (3) focal sclerosis (10%). Presenting signs and symptoms include periorbital edema, dependent edema, ascites, foamy appearance of the urine, weight gain, irritability, pleural effusions, and decreased appetite.

   b. *Secondary nephrotic syndrome* can be induced by membranous nephropathy, glomerulonephritis, lupus nephritis, malaria, hepatitis B, and human immunodeficiency virus (HIV). It has also been associated with malignancy and can occur as a result of exposure to numerous renal toxic drugs and chemicals.

   c. *Diagnosis:* Urinalysis that reveals +3 or +4 protein with occasional microscopic hematuria, decreased creatinine clearance, low serum albumin, elevated cholesterol, and triglycerides.

   d. *Treatment* includes diuretics, antihypertensive, and dietary salt restriction to manage symptoms. Patients with minimal-change disease may be responsive to corticosteroid therapy; however, if the proteinuria persists for longer than a month, a renal biopsy may be indicated to determine the precise cause of the disease. Many patients require low-dose steroid therapy for 3 to 6 months and if a relapse occurs. Patients who are resistant to steroids or have frequent relapse may be treated with cyclophosphamide.

4. **Hepatorenal syndrome** is renal failure that develops in the presence of end-stage liver disease in absence of intrinsic kidney disease. Hepatorenal failure may accompany liver failure related to fulminant hepatic failure, hepatic malignancy, liver resection, hepatitis, or biliary tract obstruction.

   a. *Kidney dysfunction* is characterized by intense constriction of the renal cortical vasculature leading to oliguria and avid sodium retention. Portal hypertension and resultant splanchnic sequestration may occur.

   b. *Signs and symptoms* include increased renal vascular resistance, decreased glomerular filtration, increased sodium and water retention (secondary to hyperaldosteronism), decreased urine output, and electrolyte and coagulation abnormalities.

c. *Management* includes treatment of the hepatic failure and support of renal function as well as avoidance of intravascular volume depletion and nephrotoxic agents.
d. *Prognosis* is poor for patients without subsequent liver transplant. The only established therapy that improves renal failure in this syndrome is liver transplantation.

5. **Tumor lysis syndrome** (TLS) typically occurs after effective chemotherapy or radiation, but it may occur after treatment with glucocorticoids, antiestrogen tamoxifen, and interferon. It is most likely to occur in patients with poorly differentiated leukemias and lymphomas, a high WBC, or bulky lymphoma. During tumor lysis, rapid release of intracellular metabolites exceeds the excretory capacity of the kidneys.
   a. *Potential effects* of tumor lysis include hyperuricemia, hypocalcemia, hyperphosphatemia, hyperkalemia, and hyperxanthinemia. These electrolyte imbalances lead to crystallization, tubular obstruction, decreased urine output, and renal failure. The severity of the condition is proportional to the tumor burden. A previous history of renal impairment increases the likelihood for developing tumor lysis syndrome. Prevention of complications from cell breakdown is the optimal goal.
   b. *Management* of TLS ideally is prevention. At risk patients should receive vigorous hydration and allopurinol before cancer treatment is begun. Urate oxidases and urinary alkalinization should be considered. Electrolyte imbalances should be treated promptly. Hypocalcemia should not be treated unless the patient is symptomatic because administration of calcium may precipitate metastatic calcifications in a patient with hyperphosphatemia. Peritoneal dialysis is not as effective as hemodialysis because the clearance rates for phosphate and uric acid are significantly lower. Severe electrolyte disturbances may require hemodialysis or continuous renal replacement therapy.
6. **Cardiac failure:** Changes in renal function may be attributed to hypovolemia or hypervolemia, hypotension, and electrolyte imbalance. Decreased cardiac output may lead to decreased renal flow and decreased GFR, decreased flow to the parenchyma, and ATN.
7. **Rhabdomyolysis:** Rhabdomyolysis can be caused directly by muscle injury or indirectly by several medical conditions (Table 5-9).
   a. *Diagnosis:* Myoglobinuria is present in most patients. Myoglobin is a small, bright red protein that is common in muscle cells. It gives the muscle much of its red coloration. Myoglobin stores oxygen for use when muscles are exercised. The cellular release of myoglobin is often accompanied by an increase of creatine kinase (CK). When excreted into the urine, it is called myoglobinuria, which is a monomer containing a heme molecule similar to hemoglobin. Myoglobin can precipitate, causing tubular obstruction and acute renal insufficiency. Clinical features of myoglobinuria include weakness, discomfort, pain, tenderness, swelling, tea-colored urine, kidney dysfunction, fever, and leukocytosis. It can be recognized clinically by urinalysis with a dipstick strongly positive for heme and urine sediment with few or no red cells. A more sensitive and diagnostic finding is an elevated creatine phosphokinase (CPK). ARF seldom occurs until CPK levels exceed 15,000 to 20,000.
   b. *Renal failure* may ensue from myoglobinuria resulting from ferrihemate toxicity, tubular obstruction, altered GFR, hypotension, and crystal formations. Aspartate aminotransferase and alanine aminotransferase may also be elevated as they are released from necrotic muscle.

TABLE 5-9
Causes of Rhabdomyolsis and Myoglobinuria

Traumatic	Infections	Fluid and Electrolyte Disorders	Drug Abuse	Medications	Thermoregulatory
Crush syndrome	Bacterial	Hypophosphatemia	Cocaine	Statins	Hyperthermia
Compression injury	Viral, most commonly influenza	Hypokalemia	Heroin	Clofibrate	Heat stroke
Compartment syndrome	Fungal (e.g., Candida, aspergillus)	Hypo/hypernatremia	Alcohol		Malignant hyperthermia (anesthesia induced)
Vascular occlusion	Malaria	Ketoacidosis	Amphetamines		
		Hyperosmolar coma	Ecstasy		

c. *Prevention of renal failure* hinges on prompt and aggressive treatment that includes volume depletion and maintenance of high urine output. Mannitol and alkalinization of the urine may also be considered.

G. Desired Patient Outcomes for the Child in ARF

1. Urine output remains adequate.
2. Laboratory values indicate resolving ARF (e.g., stabilized or decreasing BUN and creatinine).
3. Cardiac output remains adequate.
4. Intake and output balance is maintained.
5. Fluid and electrolyte balance is maintained.
6. Nutritional status is optimized.
7. No signs of infection exist.
8. The child remains comfortable and anxiety is minimized.

H. Management of ARF

1. **Response to treatment** is related to the extent of nephron damage and ATN.
   a. *In prerenal failure,* there is no actual nephron damage and the kidneys respond well to treatment for symptoms of decreased urine output, electrolyte abnormalities, or both.
   b. *In true intrinsic ATN,* actual nephron damage has occurred and response to therapy to treat the underlying problem of renal dysfunction is often futile.
2. **The plan of care** to support renal function includes eliminating the cause of AKF, if known, and discontinuing or altering the dose of potentially nephrotoxic medications. All drugs excreted by the kidneys require an alteration of the dosage based on the level of renal function. Serum concentrations of potentially

toxic drugs should be closely monitored. Creatinine clearance and serum creatinine should be monitored when using potentially nephrotoxic agents. Drug dosage alteration is indicated with increased levels of serum creatinine. If a patient is receiving renal replacement therapy, drug supplementation may be necessary to restore the drug that is removed or filtrated.

3. **Maintain adequate intravascular volume** and maintain adequate blood pressure.
4. **Pharmacologic support** includes diuretics and other agents. Common indications for diuretic therapy include pulmonary edema, hypertension, hypercalcemia, hyperkalemia (furosemide), generalized edema, hypervolemia, and increased intracranial pressure. Diuretics promote renal excretion of water, either directly or indirectly by acting on different segments of the tubules.
   a. *Loop diuretics* inhibit reabsorption of sodium and chloride in the ascending loop of Henle and distal renal tubule, interfering with the chloride-binding cotransport system. This leads to increased excretion of water, potassium, sodium, chloride, magnesium, and calcium. Furosemide (Lasix) and bumetanide (Bumex) are two of the most potent loop diuretics. Potential complications include hypovolemia, hypokalemia, hyponatremia, metabolic alkalosis, hypercalciuria, hypomagnesemia, hyperglycemia, ototoxicity, renal calculi, and thrombocytopenia.
   b. *Thiazide diuretics* inhibit sodium reabsorption in the distal tubules, leading to excretion of sodium, chloride, potassium, bicarbonate, magnesium, phosphate, calcium, and water. Chlorothiazide (Diuril) or hydrochlorothiazide (HydroDIURIL) is frequently used as a secondary or adjunct agent in diuretic therapy. Potential complications are similar to loop diuretics. Potassium supplemental therapy may be indicated.
   c. *Nonthiazide, sulfonamide diuretics* inhibit sodium reabsorption in the cortical diluting site and proximal tubules, leading to increased excretion of sodium and water as well as potassium and hydrogen ions. Metolazone (Zaroxolyn) is frequently used as a secondary agent in conjunction with loop diuretics.
   d. *Potassium-sparing diuretics* compete with aldosterone for binding sites in the distal tubule, increasing sodium chloride and water excretion while conserving potassium and hydrogen ions. Spironolactone (aldosterone antagonist) is the most commonly used agent. Potassium-sparing diuretics are used in conjunction with a potassium-depleting diuretic agent to decrease the occurrence of hypokalemia. They also have minimal side effects but may block the effect of aldosterone on arteriolar smooth muscle.
   e. *Osmotic diuretics* increase the osmotic pressure in the glomerular filtrate, which inhibits tubular reabsorption of water and electrolytes, thus increasing urinary output. Mannitol is a sugar that is relatively inert and freely filtered by the glomerulus; however, it is not greatly reabsorbed by the renal tubule. The transient pulling of fluid into the intravascular space can increase the intravascular volume significantly; therefore, mannitol should not be used with patients in congestive heart failure and hypervolemia or in those with renal failure.
   f. *Acetazolamide (Diamox)* acts by competitively inhibiting carbonic anhydrase, resulting in increased excretion of sodium, potassium, bicarbonate, and water. It also results in a decrease in the formation of aqueous humor. Metabolic acidosis can result secondary to the limitation of secretion of hydrogen ions from the tubule and subsequent decreased reabsorption of bicarbonate and sodium.
   g. *Low-dose dopamine* (0.5 to 3 mcg/kg per minute) stimulates dopaminergic receptors located on the afferent arterioles. Afferent arterioles dilate, increasing

blood flow to the glomerulus, which increases the GFR, resulting in increased urine output. In addition, it binds to the DA-1 receptor in the proximal tubule, loop of Henle, and cortical collecting duct, inhibiting the Na-K-ATPase pump and thus promoting naturesis. Inhibition of the Na-K-ATPase pump also decreases oxygen demand and may be protective against ischemic damage. Dopamine promotes the excretion of free water by inhibiting the release of ADH. The role of low-dose dopamine in the prevention of ARF remains controversial. Data on the use of low-dose dopamine do not support improved outcomes, improvement in renal function, or decreased need for dialysis; thus its use is being discouraged in clinical practice. In addition, the deleterious effects of dopamine add to the controversy. These include hormonal effects, an increase in oxygen demand to the renal medulla secondary to increase naturesis/diuresis, and potential cardiorespiratory effects.

I. Replacement Therapy

Consider renal replacement therapy if function cannot be adequately supported using the preceding measures.

J. Complications

Complications of end-stage renal disease (ESRD) include hypertensive disease, hyperlipidemia, and hyperparathyroidism because of poor control of calcium and phosphate levels.

RENAL REPLACEMENT THERAPIES

Renal replacement therapies for infants and children include peritoneal dialysis (PD), hemodialysis, and continuous renal replacement therapy.

A. Methods of Solute Clearance and Water Removal: Convection, Diffusion, Ultrafiltration

1. **Convective transport** occurs when water and small particles are carried through membrane pores into ultrafiltrate by a moving stream of fluid containing large protein molecules. The important determinants of convective transport are the direction and rate of the solvent flux across the membrane. Unlike diffusion, it is not influenced by any solute concentration gradient.
2. **Diffusion** is the removal of a solute from a higher concentration to a lower concentration to establish equilibrium. If adequate clearance is not obtained by convection alone, it may be necessary to influence clearance by diffusion as well.
3. **Ultrafiltration** is the removal of extracellular fluid. The rate of removal is determined by the surface area of the filter membrane, the permeability coefficient of the membrane to water, and the transmembrane pressure gradient.

B. Peritoneal Dialysis

1. **Indications** for PD include an inability to tolerate anticoagulation, ATN, renal cortical necrosis, renal agenesis, bilateral renal dysplasia, and other renal dysfunction requiring long-term, nonemergent therapy. PD is often used for infants and children in either ARF or chronic renal failure.
2. **Types** of PD include continuous ambulatory PD (CAPD), manual PD, or continuous-cycling PD using a computerized cycler device. Access is via a soft

catheter placed in the peritoneal space. Catheter placement can be performed in the operating room or at the bedside.

a. *Process:* An ordered amount of dialysate is instilled via a catheter into the peritoneal cavity. The removal of water and solutes *(ultrafiltrate)* is adjusted by raising the osmolarity of the dialysate (increasing the glucose concentration) or increasing the dwell time. Dwell times impact waste and fluid removal. Long dwell times may achieve good waste and solute clearance but poor fluid removal. Short dwell times have poor waste and solute clearance but remove a significant amount of fluid. The amount of dialysate placed into the peritoneal space *(inflow volume)*, is determined by gradually increasing volumes from 15 to 50 mL/kg of body weight as tolerated. Standard dialysate solution contains dextrose, sodium, calcium, magnesium, chloride, and lactate (which is metabolized to produce bicarbonate). Potassium, heparin, or antimicrobial medications can be added to the peritoneal fluid as needed. CAPD or manual PD may be needed in infants and small children when inflow volumes are less than 50 mL. Excessive inflow volume can be assessed by monitoring for signs of pain, discomfort, or respiratory compromise on inflow. The dialysate solution must be warmed to or near body temperature to prevent hypothermia.

b. *Manual PD* is more time consuming than the cycler method. It involves manual timing of dwells, exact measurement of inflow and outflow volumes, calculation of net ultrafiltration after each dwell time, and cumulative ultrafiltrate tabulation. Inflow is initiated, the catheter is clamped, and a timer is set to mark dwell time completion. Clots, kinks, and catheter position can affect the ability to inflow adequately. Dwell cycles generally range from 30 to 120 minutes and include fill, dwell, and drain times. On completion of the dwell time, the catheter is unclamped and the outflow drains to a urine collection bag to be measured. Drain times are dependent on catheter patency. The net ultrafiltrate is calculated (outflow volume minus inflow volume). The cycle is repeated at ordered intervals.

c. *CAPD* via a cycler utilizes the same principles as manual PD, but it requires less hands-on nursing time, has a decreased incidence of infection because of having a closed system, provides a programmable automated ultrafiltrate calculation, and has a built-in mechanism for dialysate warming.

3. **Potential complications** of PD include peritonitis, which can be indicated by cloudy dialysate, abdominal pain, tenderness, or sepsis. Mechanical and iatrogenic catheter problems may also occur and include leakage at the insertion site, bowel perforation, retroperitoneal hemorrhage, increased intra-abdominal pressure resulting from obstruction of the catheter, and hernia. Other complications include impaired pulmonary function related to abdominal distention or fluid overload, decreased cardiac output and stroke volume related to fluid status, hypoproteinemia resulting from protein losses in the dialysate, and hyperglycemia related to absorption of dextrose from the dialysate. Hyperglycemia may require treatment with insulin.

C. Hemodialysis

1. **Indications** for hemodialysis may include symptomatic electrolyte imbalance, hypervolemia, pulmonary edema, severe acidosis, anuria not responsive to other therapy, severely elevated BUN and creatinine, cardiac failure, TLS, hepatic failure, hyperammonemia, drug intoxication, and other conditions that require rapid, efficient correction of the abnormality.
2. **Process:** An extracorporeal circuit carries blood from the patient via a large-bore venous catheter through a filter or artificial kidney and back to the patient. The

filter is a semipermeable membrane through which water, solutes, and other substances are filtered (ultrafiltrate). Removal of solutes occurs through the filter by diffusion, which is created by infusion of the dialysate into the filter (the opposite side of the semipermeable membrane) countercurrent to the flow of blood. Negative pressure is added to the dialysate side of the circuit to increase the fluid and solute removal from the blood. Positive pressure is generated via a roller pump on the venous side of the blood circuit, increasing removal of excess fluid. Blood access is obtained via a double-lumen central venous catheter via two single-lumen central venous catheters or via an arterial-venous fistula. It is important to consider the extracorporeal circuit volume in relation to the child's circulating blood volume to prevent hypovolemia. If the extracorporeal circuit volume is greater than 10% of the child's circulating blood volume or if the child weighs less than 10 kg, the circuit may be primed with a colloid substance. Small-volume artificial kidneys and circuit sizes have enabled hemodialysis to be an option for small infants.

3. **Potential complications** include hypovolemia, hypervolemia, systemic bleeding, filter rupture or circuit disconnection, infection, and transfusion reaction.
4. **Nursing implications:** Vital signs, oxygenation, hemodynamic parameters, fluid status, electrolyte balance, and physiologic response to treatment must be closely monitored. Inadequately treated intravascular hypovolemia, rapid electrolyte and pH changes, and hypoxemia will significantly affect cardiac function and lead to severe compromise. Volume expanders such as albumin or isotonic crystalloid products should be readily available during treatment. Rapid decrease in the patient's nitrogenous waste load may also result in osmotic changes that lead to an altered level of consciousness known as *disequilibrium syndrome*. Hemodialysis removes drugs along with the solutes, water, and toxins; therefore drug dosing must be adjusted for the patient receiving hemodialysis. A hemodynamically unstable child may not tolerate the rapid fluid removal associated with hemodialysis and may require a more gentle therapy such as PD or continuous renal replacement therapy (CRRT).

D. Continuous Renal Replacement Therapy

1. **Indications** for CRRT include ARF with hemodynamic instability, azotemia, severe electrolyte imbalance, hypervolemia, and symptomatic metabolic abnormalities. CRRT may also be initiated in patients who would otherwise not be able to receive adequate nutrition owing to fluid restriction. CRRT is appropriate for hemodynamically unstable patients who are unable to tolerate hemodialysis and patients who are not candidates for PD.
2. **Process**
   a. *CRRT* uses a double-lumen venous catheter or two single-lumen venous catheters. It offers a highly efficient circuit that is driven by a roller-head pump and is the preferred method of renal replacement therapy for the hemodynamically unstable patient in many neonatal and pediatric intensive care units. A number of different pumps are commercially available for hemofiltration, but they all work in a similar fashion. A roller-head pump drives the blood through the hemofilter, and one or more other roller-head pumps control the ultrafiltration rate, replacement fluid, and dialysis rate. Several methods of CRRT can be used to accomplish the goal of fluid or solute removal. The method used is dictated by the patient's condition as well as the institutional policies and preferences.
   b. *Continuous venovenous hemofiltration (CVVH)* uses the principles of ultrafiltration and convection to allow for fluid and solute removal. Blood is drawn

from one port of a venous catheter, propelled through a hemofilter using a roller-head pump, and returned to the other port of the venous catheter. Ultrafiltration and convection are accomplished as the blood moves through the semipermeable membrane of the hemofilter. The ultrafiltration rate is controlled by programming the hemofiltration pump's fluid controller for an ordered amount each hour. To obtain adequate clearance, large volumes of ultrafiltrate are removed and replacement fluid is infused to maintain the desired fluid balance. The replacement rate is also controlled via the hemofiltration pump's fluid-control module.

c. *Continuous venovenous hemofiltration with dialysis (CVVH-D)* is similar to CVVH but uses a diffusion gradient instead of convection to provide clearance. The process of blood removal is the same as with CVVH, but a dialysate solution is infused into the outside compartment of the hemofilter, countercurrent to the blood, to provide diffusive transport of solutes and water. As with CVVH, the ultrafiltration rate and the dialysate rate are both controlled by the hemofiltration pump's fluid controller or additional infusion pumps. Little or no replacement fluid is used.

d. *Continuous venovenous hemodiafiltration (CVVH-DF)* uses the principles of ultrafiltration, convection, and diffusion to remove fluid and solutes. The process is similar to CVVH-D, but it also utilizes high ultrafiltration rates with replacement fluid, as in CVVH. This method of continuous renal replacement therapy may be used for patients in whom one of the other methods is not providing adequate clearance.

e. *Slow continuous ultrafiltration (SCUF)* may be used to remove a set amount of fluid from a patient each hour. This method of CRRT utilizes the principles of ultrafiltration and convection. It is effective for fluid removal, but it does not utilize a high ultrafiltration rate or replacement fluid and therefore will not provide adequate clearance of solutes.

3. Methods for measuring filtration capability or performance of the filter and circuit

a. *Clearance* is removal of solutes from the plasma and is dependent on the filter's capability for removing individual molecules, the size of the solute, the solute's protein-binding capacity, and the rate of blood flow through the hemofilter. Clearance for a particular molecule can be expressed by the ultrafiltrate-to-plasma ratio, known as the *sieving coefficient.*

$$\text{Sieving Coefficient} = \frac{\text{Concentration of } x \text{ in Ultrafiltrate}[(x)\text{Uf}]}{\text{Concentration of } x \text{ in Plasma } [(x) \text{ Plasma}]}$$
$$(1 = 100\% \text{ Clearance})$$

b. Another indicator of the efficiency of the system is the *filtration fraction (FF).* The FF is reflective of the fraction of plasma water being removed by ultrafiltration. Optimum FF is a percentage that is high enough to provide adequate solute and fluid removal needs but not so high that blood viscosity and increased oncotic pressure impact filter performance.

$$\text{Filtration Fraction } (\%) = \frac{(\text{Qf})\text{Ultrafiltration Rate (mL/min)}}{(\text{QP}) \text{ Plasma Flow Rate at the Inlet (mL/min)}}$$

4. Nursing implications for the hemodynamically unstable infant or child during CRRT

a. *Limited vascular access sites and catheter diameter* often limit blood pump speed and therefore impact circuit efficiency and solute clearance. The challenges of vascular access are greatest in infants and small children because of the small size of the vessels in relation to the catheter. Access may also be difficult in patients with an underlying coagulopathy because of concerns of bleeding during placement of these large-bore catheters. It may be necessary to attempt to correct the coagulopathy before access placement. Optimal placement in an infant or small child would be an internal jugular or subclavian catheter with the tip at the junction of the right atrium, thus preventing "pulling of the vessel wall" and subsequent obstruction to flow. A femoral catheter may be used, however, and the pump speed is adjusted accordingly. As with all indwelling lines, infection is also a risk factor.

b. *Thermoregulation* is a significant issue with infants and small children. Depending on the extracorporeal volume of the circuit compared with the child's size, a significant amount of heat may be lost via the circuit. Fluid- and blood-warmer systems or external heat sources should be used to maintain normothermia. Many of the hemofiltration pumps now available have a blood- or fluid-warming device incorporated. Small-volume extracorporeal tubing sets are ideal if they are available for the pump that is being used.

c. *Anticoagulation* is often necessary to maintain patency of the circuit. Heparinization or citrate regional anticoagulation are the two most commonly used methods of anticoagulation.

- Heparinization involves infusing a heparin solution into the prefilter side of the circuit with the goal of maintaining activated clotting times (ACTs) at 1 to 1.5 times normal. In the absence of a coagulopathy, a heparin bolus is given to the patient before initiation of therapy. In the presence of coagulopathy, heparin administration may be contraindicated, and the life span of the circuit may be decreased. Heparinization is an effective method of anticoagulating the circuit, but precautions must be taken as the patient is also systemically anticoagulated.
- Citrate regional anticoagulation is gaining popularity as the circuit may be anticoagulated without systemic effects. Sodium citrate is infused via the "arterial limb" of the circuit to chelate calcium and prevent clotting. The goal of the therapy is to keep the ionized calcium level of the circuit below 0.5 mmol/L. A calcium infusion is given to the patient via a separate line or via the distal "venous return limb" to maintain the patient's ionized calcium in the normal range (1.1-1.3 mmol/L). Citrate anticoagulation has certain inherent concerns in the pediatric population, the most common of which are the development of a metabolic alkalosis, hypocalcemia, hyperglycemia, and "citrate lock." These problems are seen because the blood flow rate per weight of the pediatric patient is greater than in adults; thus the citrate load is often significantly higher. *Citrate lock* is a phenomenon in which the patient's total calcium level rises as the ionized calcium level decreases. This is the result of infusing the citrate solution at a rate that exceeds the hepatic metabolism and CRRT clearance of citrate. Stopping the citrate infusion for a number of hours and restarting at a lower rate should remedy the situation. Metabolic alkalosis results from the breakdown of citrate to bicarbonate at a rate greater than it can be cleared. Hypocalcemia results from inadequate repletion of calcium to the patient and should be treated by increasing the calcium infusion. Hyperglycemia may result from the large infusion of citrate, which is in a glucose-based solution, or from the high flow of glucose containing dialysate solutions. Prompt recognition of these potential complications can prevent untoward effects to the patient. Citrate regional anticoagulation has generally been performed with diffusive clearance using a calcium-free dialysate solution

to allow for the removal of the large citrate load; however, recent information in the literature suggests that ultrafiltration and convection alone might be adequate to clear citrate by-products.

- The benefit of routine flushes of normal saline, lactated Ringer's, or filter replacement solution to maintain circuit patency and decrease clotting is debatable.

d. *Hemodynamic stability:* The CRRT circuit volume should be considered in relationship to the child's circulating blood volume. In small infants and children, it may be necessary to prime the circuit with whole blood or another colloid substance. If the circuit is primed with a blood product preserved with citrate, assess the serum calcium level before CRRT initiation and treat if necessary to decrease the risk of hypotension secondary to hypocalcemia. Because of drug clearance by the hemofilter, it may be necessary to titrate the infusion of vasoactive agents just before or in the first few minutes after initiation of CRRT. If the preceding precautions are taken, the incidence of hemodynamic instability during initiation of CRRT is rare.

e. *Fluid balance:* It may be necessary to begin at an ordered zero fluid balance and slowly adjust the fluid removal as tolerated. Strict fluid intake and output are recorded hourly. In a child receiving multiple blood products or fluid boluses, it is important to determine what is to be included in the formula as fluid to be removed. The formula for determining the hourly fluid balance is:

(Total intake) – (Total output) +/- (Desired hourly change) = Fluid to be removed

All pumps now available have slightly different calculations for fluid removal and manufacturer recommendations should be followed. Example:

(Total intake) – (Total output) – (Desired hourly change) = Fluid to be removed
(100) – (10) – (–20) = 110 mL to be removed

f. *The extracorporeal circuit:* Plasma-free hemoglobin levels may be measured before initiation of CRRT and daily to monitor RBC destruction. Elevated plasma-free hemoglobin levels indicate the necessity to change the circuit.

RENAL TRANSPLANTATION

A. Criteria for Transplantation

1. **All candidates must have ESRD or rapidly approaching ESRD.** Preemptive transplants, that is, those performed before dialysis is needed, have better long-term outcomes.
2. **Common causes of ESRD** requiring transplantation include congenital renal disorder, glomerulonephritis, and ESRD secondary to other disease states or treatment.
3. **Pretransplantation evaluation criteria:** Transplant is considered at the time of ESRD diagnosis. Urologic issues should be addressed before transplantation, and the patient should be free of any major multisystem complications (malignancy, advanced cardiopulmonary disease) and active infection. Nutritional status should be optimized, and psychiatric and socioeconomic parameters should be viewed as appropriate.
4. **Postoperative management**
   a. *Minimize the risk for infection* by observing strict handwashing and other institutional infection-control guidelines and by using strict aseptic techniques with all dressing changes.

b. *Maintain pulmonary toilet.*
c. *Closely monitor urinary output* and observe for signs and symptoms of infection.
d. *Monitor and maintain metabolic and electrolyte balance* (BUN, creatinine, ionized calcium, phosphorus [low], magnesium, glucose, serum albumin [low if recurrence of disease], urinary protein-creatinine ratio).
e. *Maintain comfort for the patient,* and administer medications as needed to decrease pain or anxiety.
f. *Administer the daily immunosuppressive medication* regimen as ordered, and monitor serum drug levels as necessary.
g. *Potential complications* include ATN, rejection, infection, obstruction to urinary flow, hypovolemia, renal artery stenosis, renal vein thrombosis, and ureteral leaks.
h. *Intermediate term follow-up* consists of monitoring for hyperparathyroid hormone and hypercalcemia. Parathyroid may still be "revved up" from pretransplant and parathyroid resection may be required.
i. *Long-term complications:* Posttransplant lymphoproliferative disease and infections (particularly Epstein-Barr virus [EBV], cytomegalovirus [CMV], herpes simplex virus [HSV], BK virus, varicella, and Pneumocystis carinii pneumonia [PCP]).
j. *Outcomes:* Living donated kidney's long-term outcomes are better than cadaveric. Kidney transplants in general have 90% to 95% success rate at 5 years.

RENAL TRAUMA

A. Etiology and Risk Factors

1. Renal trauma is the most common traumatic genitourinary injury in the pediatric population. Contusion or laceration constitutes the majority of renal injuries and are often seen in association with other more life-threatening injuries.
2. The most common source of renal trauma is blunt trauma, primarily from motor-vehicle accidents. The two types of blunt trauma causing most renal injuries are direct compression from external force or deceleration injury. With deceleration injury, there is a concern for laceration of the renal artery. In addition, acute renal trauma may occur as a result of decreased perfusion. Lumbar scoliosis and fracture of the body or transverse processes of the spine transmit significant injury to the retroperitoneal region. Penetrating trauma is a rare but increasing cause of renal injury in children.
3. Children are at greater risk than adults for blunt force renal trauma because of the larger size of a child's kidney in relation to abdomen size, underdevelopment of a child's abdominal wall muscles, and lack of protection from the lower ribs. Children with underlying renal abnormalities are at greater risk of injury from mild blunt force trauma than those with normal kidneys.

B. Clinical Manifestations

1. **Signs and symptoms** of genitourinary trauma include blood at the urethral meatus; high-riding prostate; gross hematuria; and labial, scrotal, or perianal ecchymosis or hematoma. Hematuria occurs in 90% of cases. If the patient is hypovolemic, hematuria may not manifest until after fluid replacement. There is no correlation between the magnitude of injury and the degree of hematuria. These signs and symptoms are contraindications to bladder catheterization.
2. In **penetrating trauma,** proximity of the wound to the genitourinary area increases suspicion of renal trauma.

3. In **blunt trauma** the child may be asymptomatic or complain of abdominal or flank pain.

C. Interpretations from Diagnostic Studies

1. **Computed tomography (CT)** is the gold standard imaging study for renal trauma in children. Advantages include more accurate demonstration of renal injury, visualization of nonvascularized regions, and simultaneous visualization of the other intra-abdominal organs. **Abdominal or kidney, ureter, and bladder (KUB) film** demonstrating obliteration of the renal shadow is suggestive of renal trauma. Up to 85% of plain abdominal films demonstrate normal findings despite proven renal trauma.
2. **IVP** may be done if an isolated urogenital injury is suspected. This examination allows evaluation of all genitourinary structures.
3. **Ultrasonography** has limited application in evaluation of renal trauma but may have utility in a rapid initial screen. Doppler-enhanced ultrasound gives information related to renal perfusion and the integrity of vascular pedicles of the kidney.
4. **Arteriography** may assist in planning surgical intervention if vascular disruption has occurred.
5. **Radionucleotide renal scan** demonstrates renal function, perfusion, and urinary extravasation. It is useful if there is a contraindication to contrast dye.
6. Use of **MRI** is limited because of the technique and the amount of information gained.

D. Classification

Renal injuries are classified as grade I through V (Table 5-10).

E. Desired Patient Outcomes

1. Absence of hematuria
2. Adequate urine output
3. Absence of hypertension
4. Negative results from radiographic studies

TABLE 5-10
Renal Injury Scale

	Grade	Injury Description
RENAL INJURY SCALE		
I	Contusion	Microscopic or gross hematuria; urologic studies normal
	Hematoma	Subcapsular, nonexpanding without parenchymal laceration
II	Hematoma	Nonexpanding perirenal hematoma confined to the renal retroperitoneum
	Laceration	<1 cm parenchymal depth of renal cortex without urinary extravasation
III	Laceration	>1 cm parenchymal depth of renal cortex without collecting-system rupture or urinary extravasation
IV	Laceration	Parenchymal laceration extending through the renal cortex, medulla, and collecting system
	Vascular	Main renal artery or vein injury with contained hemorrhage
V	Laceration	Completely shattered kidney
	Vascular	Avulsion of renal hilum, which devascularizes kidney

Adapted from Moore E, Shackford S, Packter H, et al.: Organ injury scaling: spleen, liver and kidney, *J Trauma* 29: 1664-1666, 1989.

F. Plan of Care

1. Most **penetrating renal injuries** require surgical exploration and potential intervention.
2. **Management of blunt trauma** is dependent on the stability of the child and the extent of injury. Eighty-five percent of blunt trauma cases are minor injuries (grades I-III), requiring only observation and bed rest until gross hematuria resolves. If results from initial radiographic studies are abnormal, continued follow-up for a year or longer might be necessary.
3. **Management of major renal trauma can be divided into two groups**: operative or nonoperative. Patients who are hemodynamically unstable despite transfusion must be managed surgically. However, controversy remains about whether to treat patients with major injury involving urinary extravasation or renal fracture conservatively (nonoperatively) or aggressively (operatively). Data exist to support both approaches.
4. **Long-term follow-up** (i.e., 6 months to 1 year) is important because hypertension is subtle yet frequently associated with vascular trauma.

REFERENCES

Andreoli SP: Acute renal failure. *Curr Opin Pediatr.* 14(2):183-188, 2002.

Awazu M et al.: "Maintenance" therapy and treatment of dehydration and overhydration. In Ichikawa I, editor: *Pediatric textbook of fluid and electrolytes.* Baltimore, Md., 1989, Williams & Wilkins, pp 417-428.

Berstein D: Diseases of the pericardium. In Behrmanm RE, Kliegman RM, Jenson HB, editors: *Nelson textbook of pediatrics,* ed 7. Philadelphia, 2004, Elsevier, p 1580.

Brady HR, Clarkson MR, Lieberthal W: Acute renal failure. In Brenner BM, editor: *Brenner & Rector's: the kidney,* ed 7. Philadelphia, 2004, Elsevier, pp 1215-1258.

Brem AS: An overview of renal structure and function. In Fuhrman BP, Zimmerman JJ, editors: *Pediatric critical care.* St. Louis, 1998, Mosby, pp 692-702.

Brigli AE, Anani FA: Hepatorenal syndrome: definition, pathophysiology, and intervention. *Crit Care Clin* 18(2):345-373, 2002.

Bunchman TE et al.: Pediatric hemofiltration: normocarb dialysate solution with citrate anticoagulation. *Pediatr Nephrol* 17: 150-154, 2002.

Chadha V, Garg U, Warady BA, Alon US: Citrate clearance in children receiving continuous venovenous renal replacement therapy. *Pediatr Nephrol* 17:819-824, 2002.

Davis ID, Avner ED: Introduction to glomerular diseases. In Behrmanm RE, Kliegman RM, Jenson HB, editors: *Nelson textbook of pediatrics,* ed 17. Philadelphia, 2004, Elsevier, pp 1731-1735.

Eknoyan G, Levin A, Levin NW: Bone metabolism and disease in chronic kidney disease. *Am J Kidney Dis* 42(4):1-201, 2003.

Fishman JA: BK virus nephropathy—polyoma virus adding insult to injury. *N Eng J Med* 347:527-530, 2002.

Friedman AL: Acute renal disease. In Fuhrman BP, Zimmerman JJ, editors: *Pediatric critical care.* St Louis, 1998, Mosby-Year Book, pp. 723-737.

Grehn LS, Kline A, Weishaar J: Renal critical care problems. In Curley MAQ, Maloney-Harmon PA, editors: *Critical care nursing of infants and children.* Philadelphia, 2001, W. B. Saunders, pp 731-764.

Hazinski MF: *Manual of pediatric critical care.* St. Louis, 1999, Mosby.

Hole JW: *Human anatomy and physiology.* Dubuque, Iowa, 1984, William C. Brown, pp 747-778.

Kennedy J: Renal disorders. In Hazinski MF, editor: *Nursing care of the critically ill child.* St. Louis, 1992, Mosby, pp. 629-713.

Lancaster LE: Acute renal failure. In Huddleston VB, editor: *Multisystem organ failure: pathophysiology and clinical implications.* St. Louis, 1992, Mosby, pp 222-235.

Kapoor M, Chan GZ: Fluid and electrolyte abnormalities. *Crit Care Clin* 17(3):503-529, 2001.

Margenthaler JA, Weber TR, Keller MS: Blunt renal trauma in children: experience with conservative management at a pediatric trauma center. *J Trauma* 52(2): 928-932, 2000.

Marik PE, Iglesias J, The NORASEPT II Study Investigators: Low-dose dopamine does not prevent acute renal failure in patients with septic shock and oliguria. *Am J Med* 107(4):387-390, 1999.

Marieb EN, Mallatt J, Wilhelm PB: *Human anatomy,* ed 4. San Francisco, 2005, Benjamin Cummings.

McCormick A, Sterk MB: Acute renal failure of the neonate. *Dimens Crit Care Nurs* 5:155-161, 1986.

Moore E, Shackford S, Packter H et al.: Scaling: spleen, liver and kidney. *J Trauma* 29:1664-1666, 1989.

Moritz ML, Ayus JC: Disorders of water metabolism in children: hyponatremia and hypernatremia. *Pediatr Rev* 23(11): 371-280, 2002.

Mylonakis E et al.: BK virus in solid organ transplant recipients: an emerging syndrome. Transplantation 72:1587-1592, 2001.

Peixoto AJ: Critical issues in nephrology. *Clin Chest Med* 24(4):561-581, 2003.

Peterson NE: Genitourinary trauma. In Mattox KL, Feliciano DV, Moore EE, editors: *Trauma.* New York, 2000, McGraw-Hill, pp 839-878.

Quigley RP, Alexander SR: Acute renal failure. In Levin DL, Morriss FC, editors: *Essentials of pediatric intensive care.* New York, 1997, Churchill-Livingstone, pp 509-531.

Russel RS et al.: Management of grade IV renal injury in children. *J Urol* 166(3):1049-1050, 2001.

Schneider RE: Genitourinary tract. In Marx JA, editor: *Rosen's emergency medicine: concepts and clinical practice.* St. Louis, 2002, Mosby, pp 448-452.

Schwarz A: New aspects of the treatment of nephrotic syndrome. *J Am Soc Nephrol* 12(17):544-547, 2001.

Shuman M: Hemorrhagic disorders: abnormalities of platelet and vascular function: structure and function of the kidneys. In Goldman L, Bennett JC, editors: *Cecil textbook of medicine,* ed 21. Philadelphia, 2000, W.B .Saunders, pp 1001-1003.

Simone S: Abdominal/genitourinary trauma. In Maloney-Harmon PA, Czerwinski SJ, editors: *Nursing care of the pediatric trauma patient.* St. Louis, 2003, W. B. Saunders, pp 227-247.

Slatopolsk E: New developments in hyperphosphatemia management. *J Am Soc Nephrol* 14(9 suppl 4) S297-S299, 2003.

Taketomo CK, Hodding JH, Kraus DM: *Pediatric dosage handbook.* Hudson, Ohio, 2001, Lexi-Comp.

Tisher CC: Structure and function of the kidneys. In Goldman L, Bennett JC, editors: *Cecil textbook of Medicine,* ed 21. Philadelphia, 2000, W.B. Saunders.

Toto RD: Approach to patient with kidney disease. In Brenner BM, editor: *Brenner & Rector's: the kidney,* ed 7. Philadelphia, 2004, Elsevier, pp 1079-1086.

Vogt BA, Avner ED: Conditions particularly associated with proteinuria. In Behrmanm RE, Kliegman RM, Jenson HB, editors: *Nelson textbook of pediatrics,* ed 17. Philadelphia, 2004, Elsevier, pp 1753-1757.

Wood EG, Lynch RE: Fluid and electrolyte balance. In Fuhrman BP, Zimmerman JJ, editors: *Pediatric critical care.* St Louis, 1998, Mosby, pp 703-722.

CHAPTER

6 Endocrine System

DEB TEMPLIN

Two types of endocrine problems are seen in the pediatric intensive care unit (PICU): (1) specific endocrine abnormalities that occur in normal children (diabetes mellitus, hypothyroidism) and (2) endocrine dysfunction secondary to critical illness (diabetes insipidus, syndrome of inappropriate antidiuretic hormone [SIADH], adrenal insufficiency).

ENDOCRINOLOGY CONCEPTS

A. Role of the Endocrine System

1. Maintain the internal environment, including fluid and electrolyte balance; blood pressure; and maintenance of fat, muscle, and bone.
2. Functions of the endocrine system involve control and regulation of metabolism and energy stores, growth and development, reproduction and sex differentiation, and coordination of the body's response to stress (e.g., trauma, critical illness, major surgery) (Guyton and Hall, 2001). The hormonal response to prolonged stress or critical illness is poorly understood and may be maladaptive in some cases.
3. Integrated functions include central nervous system (CNS) input to the endocrine system via the hypothalamic-pituitary complex. The immune system contributes to endocrine regulation via the biologic response modifiers (cytokines, interleukin-1, tumor necrosis factor) (Chrousos, 2002).
4. Endocrine diseases occur as a result of hypersecretion/hyperfunction or hyposecretion/hypofunction, although the specific cause is a problem in the target cell (Thibodeau and Patton, 2003).
5. Many of the most powerful therapies used in the PICU are mediators of the neuroendocrine system: epinephrine, norepinephrine, vasopressin, insulin, steroids, and octreotide.

B. Endocrine Glands

These glands or organs consist of specialized cells that synthesize and secrete biochemical messengers (hormones) in response to specific signals (e.g. hyperglycemia, hyperosmolality, hypocalcemia).

1. **Endocrine glands** secrete hormones directly into the bloodstream (e.g., adrenal glands, endocrine pancreas, thyroid gland).
2. **Exocrine glands** secrete biochemical substances that are released into ducts to be delivered to target organs (e.g., salivary glands, sebaceous glands, exocrine pancreas, sweat glands).
3. **Major glands:**
   a. *Hypothalamus-pituitary complex* (anterior and posterior pituitary gland)

b. *Thyroid gland*
c. *Parathyroid glands*
d. *Adrenal glands*
e. *Islets of Langerhans in the pancreas*
f. *Gonads*
g. *Other sources:* Cells that are normally considered outside the endocrine system can manufacture and secrete hormones in certain circumstances (e.g., pulmocytes may secrete adrenocorticotropic hormone [ACTH]). Cardiac myocytes secrete atrial natriuretic peptide (ANP) and brain or B-type natriuretic peptide (BNP) in response to myocardial stretch and overload. ANP and BNP cause natriuresis (salt loss) and diuresis. ANP is released by the atrial myocyctes, and BNP is released from atrial and ventricular myocytes. BNP levels are elevated in left ventricle dysfunction and heart failure (Adams et al., 2003; Zap et al., 2004).

C. Hormones

1. **Hormones** (Table 6-1) are chemical messengers that are released directly into the bloodstream from endocrine glands in response to specific stimuli or signals that cause:
   a. *Tremendous effects* in extremely small quantities
   b. *Binding* with the specific **receptor, target cell, or organ**, which initiates specific cell response. Cells that do not possess this specific receptor do not respond (Guyton and Hall, 2001; Piano and Huether, 2002) (Figure 6-1, p. 451). Receptors are located on the cell membrane, in cell cytoplasm, or in the nucleus of the target cell.
   c. *Facilitation* of communication between cells, both locally and distally.

TABLE 6-1
Summary of the Endocrine System

Gland/Hormone	Effect	Hypofunction	Hyperfunction
ADENOHYPOPHYSIS (ANTERIOR PITUITARY)*			
Somatotropic hormone (STH) or growth hormone (GH) (somatotropin) Target tissue: bones	Promotes growth of bone and soft tissues Has main effect on linear growth Maintains a normal rate of protein synthesis Conserves carbohydrate utilization and promotes fat mobilization Is essential for proliferation of cartilage cells at epiphyseal plate Is ineffective for linear growth after epiphyseal closure Has hyperglycemic effect (antiinsulin action)	Epiphyseal fusion with cessation of growth Prepubertal dwarfism Pituitary cachexia (Simonds disease) Generalized growth retardation Hypoglycemia	Prepubertal gigantism Acromegaly (after full growth is attained) Diabetes mellitus Postpubertal hypoproteinemia
Thyrotopin (thyroid-stimulating hormone [TSH]) Target tissue: thyroid gland	Promotes and maintains growth and development of thyroid gland Stimulates thyroid hormone secretion	Hypothyroidism Marked delay of puberty Juvenile myxedema	Hyperthroidism Thyrotoxicosis Graves disease

*For each anterior pituitary hormone there is a corresponding hypothalamic-releasing factor. A deficiency in these factors caused by inhibiting anterior pituitary hormone synthesis produces the same effects.

Continued

TABLE 6-1
Summary of the Endocrine System (*cont'd*)

Gland/Hormone	Effect	Hypofunction	Hyperfunction
Adrenocorticotropic hormone (ACTH) Target tissue: adrenal cortex	Promotes and maintains growth and development of adrenal cortex Stimulates adrenal cortex to secrete glucocorticoids and androgens	Acute adrenocortical insufficiency (Addison disease) Hypoglycemia Increased skin pigmentation	Cushing syndrome
Gonadotropins Target tissue: gonads	Stimulate gonads to mature and produce sex hormones and germ cells	Absent or incomplete spontaneous puberty	Precocious puberty Early epiphyseal closure
Follicle-stimulating hormone (FSH) Target tissue: ovaries, testes	Male: Stimulates development of seminiferous tubules Initiates spermatogenesis Female: Stimulates graafian follicles to mature and secrete estrogen	Hypogonadism Sterility Absence or loss of secondary sex characteristics Amenorrhea	Precocious puberty Primary gonadal failure Hirsutism Polycystic ovary Early epiphyseal closure
Luteinizing hormone (LH)[†] Target tissue: ovaries, testes	Male: Stimulates differentiation of Leydig cells, which secrete androgens, principally testosterone Female: Produces rupture of follicle with discharge of mature ovum Stimulates secretion of progesterone by corpus luteum	Hypogonadism Sterility Impotence Absence or loss of secondary sex characteristics Ovarian failure Eunuchism	Precocius puberty Primary gonadal failure Hirsutism Polycystic ovary Early epiphyseal closure
Prolactin (luteotropic hormone) Target tissue: ovaries, breasts	Stimulates milk secretion Maintains corpus luteum and progesterone secretion during pregnancy	Inability to lactate Amenorrhea	Galactorrhea Functional hypogonadism
Melanocyte-stimulating hormone (MSH) Target tissue: skin	Promotes pigmentation of skin	Diminished or absent skin pigmentation	Increased skin pigmentation
NEUROHYPOPHYSIS (POSTERIOR PITUITARY)			
Antidiuretic hormone (ADH) (vasopressin) Target tissue: renal tubules	Acts on distal and collecting tubules, making them more permeable to water, thus increasing reabsorption and decreasing excretion of urine	Diabetes insipidus	Syndrome of inappropriate secretion of ADH Fluid retention Hyponatremia
Oxytocin Target tissue: uterus, breasts	Stimulates powerful contractions of uterus Causes ejection of milk from alveoli into breast ducts (letdown reflex)		
THYROID			
Thyroxine (T_4) and triiodothyronine (T_3)	Regulates metabolic rate; controls rate of growth of body cells	Hypothyroidism Myxedema	Exophthalmic goiter (Graves disease)

[†]In the male. LH is sometimes known as interstitial cell–stimulating hormone (ICSH).

TABLE 6-1
Summary of the Endocrine System (*cont'd*)

Gland/Hormone	Effect	Hypofunction	Hyperfunction
	Especially important for growth of bones, teeth, and brain Promotes mobilization of fats and gluconeogenesis	Hashimoto thyroiditis General growth is greatly reduced; extent depends on age at which deficiency occurs Mental retardation in infant	Accelerated linear growth Early epiphyseal closure
Thyrocalcitonin	Regulates calcium and phosphorus metabolism Influences ossification and development of bone		
PARATHYROID GLANDS			
Parathyroid hormone (PTH)	Promotes calcium reabsorption from blood, bone, and intestines Promotes excretion of phosphorus in kidney tubules	Hypocalcemia (tetany)	Hypercalcemia (bone demineralization) Hypophosphatemia
ADRENAL CORTEX			
Mineralocorticoids Aldosterone	Stimulate renal tubules to reabsorb sodium, thus promoting water retention but potassium loss	Adrenocortical insufficiency	Electrolyte imbalance Hyperaldosteronism
Sex hormones (androgens, estrogens, progesterone)	Influence development of bone, reproductive organs, and secondary sexual characteristics	Male: feminization	Adrenogenital syndrome
Glucocorticoids Cortisol (hydrocortisone and compound F) Corticosterone (compound B)	Promote normal fat, protein, and carbohydrate metabolism In excess, tend to accelerate gluconeogenesis and protein and fat catabolism Mobilize body defenses during period of stress Suppress inflammatory reaction	Addison disease Acute adrenocortical insufficiency Impaired growth and sexual function	Cushing syndrome Severe impairment of growth with slowing in skeletal maturation
ADRENAL MEDULLA			
Epinephrine (adrenaline), norepinephrine (noradrenaline)	Produces vasoconstriction of heart and smooth muscles (raises blood pressure) Increases blood sugar via glycolysis Inhibits gastrointestinal activity Activates sweat glands		Hyperfunction caused by: pheochromocytoma neuroblastoma ganglioneuroma

Continued

TABLE 6-1
Summary of the Endocrine System (*cont'd*)

Gland/Hormone	Effect	Hypofunction	Hyperfunction
ISLETS OF LANGERHANS OF PANCREAS			
Insulin (beta cells)	Promotes glucose transport into the cells Increases glucose utilization, glycogenesis, and glycolysis Promotes fatty acid transport into cells and lipogenesis Promotes amino acid transport into cells and protein synthesis	Diabetes mellitus	Hyperinsulinism
Glucagon (alpha cells)	Acts as antagonist to insulin, thereby increasing blood glucose concentration by accelerating glycogenolysis Able to inhibit secretion of both insulin and glycogen		Hyperglycemia May be instrumental in genesis of diabetic ketoacidosis (DKA) in diabetes mellitus
Somatostatin (delta cells)	Able to inhibit secretion of both insulin and glycogen		
OVARIES			
Estrogen	Accelerates growth of epithelial cells, especially in uterus following menses Promotes protein anabolism Promotes epiphyseal closure of bones Promotes breast development during puberty and pregnancy Plays role in sexual function Stimulates water and sodium reabsorption in renal tubules Stimulates ripening of ova	Lack of or repression of sexual development	Precocious puberty: early epiphyseal closure
Progesterone	Prepares uterus for nidation of fertilized ovum and aids in maintenance of pregnancy Aids in development of alveolar system of breasts during pregnancy Inhibits myometrial contractions Has effect on protein catabolism Promotes salt and water retention, especially in endometrium		
TESTES			
Testosterone	Accelerates protein anabolism for growth Promotes epiphyseal closure Promotes development of secondary sex characteristics Plays role in sexual function Stimulates testes to produce spermatozoa	Delayed sexual development or eunuchoidism	Precocious puberty: early epiphyseal closure

From Hockenberry MJ: *Wong's nursing care of infants and children*, 7th ed. St. Louis, 2003, Mosby.

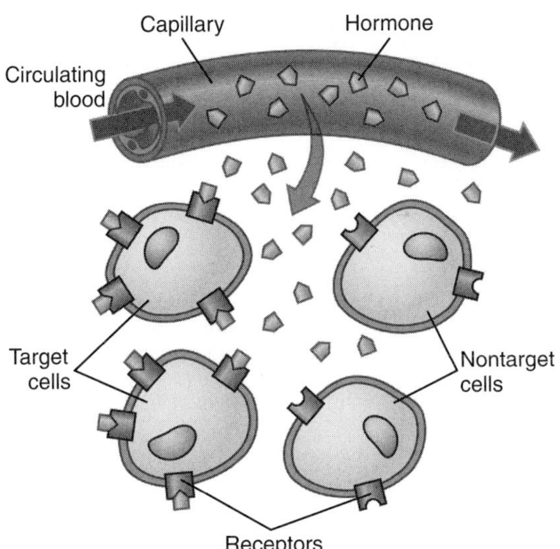

FIGURE 6-1 ■ The target cell concept. A hormone acts only on cells that have receptors specific to that hormone because the shape of the receptor determines which hormone can react with it. This is an example of the lock-and-key model of biochemical reactions.
(From Thibodeau GA, Patton KT: *Anatomy and physiology*, ed 5. St. Louis, 2003, Mosby.)

2. **Chemical structures** of hormones (Guyton and Hall, 2001; Piano and Huether, 2002)
   a. *Proteins and polypeptides* (water-soluble) are synthesized from amino acids. They bind to cell surface membranes. Examples are anterior and posterior pituitary hormones, ACTH, insulin, and parathyroid hormone.
   b. *Steroids* (lipid soluble) are synthesized from cholesterol. They diffuse through plasma membrane and enter the cytoplasm. Examples are cortisol, aldosterone, estrogen, progesterone, and testosterone.
   c. *Amino acid derivatives* are derived from a single amino acid molecule (tyrosine). Thyroxine (T_4) and tri-iodothyronine (T_3) from the thyroid gland are synthesized by adding iodine to tyrosine. Epinephrine, norepinephrine, and melatonin are modified from tyrosine (Thibodeau and Patteon, 2003).
3. A considerable amount of information is not known about hormones, their interactions with each other, and their interactions with the nervous system and immune system.
4. **Hormones** can be exogenously administered to critically ill patients.

D. Feedback Mechanism

1. **Negative feedback** is the primary mechanism controlling hormonal regulation, thereby preventing oversecretion of the hormone (Guyton and Hall, 2001; Piano and Huether, 2002). Negative feedback occurs when the specific cell response has been achieved or exceeded and the information is relayed to the secreting gland to inhibit secretion (Figure 6-2).
2. This mechanism is responsible for maintaining constant homeostasis.

DEVELOPMENTAL ANATOMY AND PHYSIOLOGY

A. Hypothalamic-Pituitary Complex (Neuroendocrine System)

1. **Embryology**
   a. The *hypothalamus* arises from the diencephalon after a proliferation of neuroblasts. The fibers of the supraoptic tract are present by 12 weeks' gestation with maturation of the neurons by 30 weeks (Settle, 2000).

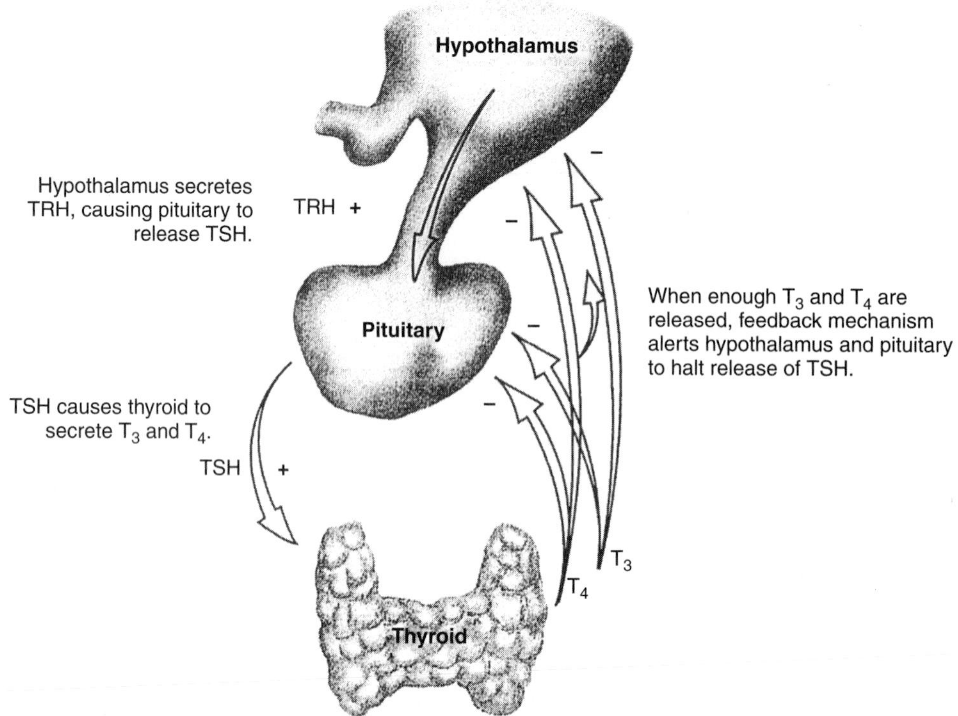

FIGURE 6-2 ■ Feedback control in hormone production.
(From James SR, Ashwill JW, Droske SC: *Nursing care of children: principle & practice,* ed 2. Philadelphia, 2002, W. B. Saunders, 2002.)

- Antidiuretic hormone (ADH) and oxytocin production begins at about 12 weeks' gestation.

b. The *pituitary gland* has a double embryonic origin, which contributes to the differentiation of the anterior and posterior lobes. Pituitary development begins between week 4 and 5 of gestation (Dorton, 2000). Pituitary hormones are present at 8 weeks' gestation, and secretion can be detected as early as 12 weeks' gestation (Rosenblum and Connor, 2003).

c. *Anterior pituitary* is recognizable at 4 to 5 weeks' gestation and rapidly matures at 20 weeks. It originates from *Rathke's pouch,* which is ectodermal tissue from the oropharynx that migrates to join the posterior pituitary. By week 5 of gestation, a connection between Rathke's pouch and the infundibulum is present (Aron et al., 2004; Dorton, 2000).
- Production of ACTH occurs by 8 weeks' gestation, TSH by 15 weeks' gestation, somatotropin by 10 or 11 weeks' gestation, prolactin by 12 weeks' gestation, and follicle-stimulating hormone (FSH) and luteinizing hormone (LH) by 11 weeks' gestation. (Rosenbloom and Connor, 2003).

d. *Posterior pituitary* originates from the neuroectoderm of the diencephalon (hypothalamus). It develops during week 5 or 6 of gestation (Dorton, 2000).
- The fetal posterior pituitary is capable of maintaining fetal osmolality and blood volume. In the fetus and newborn, increased levels of ADH are found secondary to hypoxia and stress. Serum levels of ADH in the newborn correlate with the length of labor. Data indicate that ADH

secretion is fully mature in the newborn; however, renal responsiveness may be decreased.

2. **Role of the hypothalamus:** The hypothalamus functions as a center to integrate incoming stimuli from the CNS and the peripheral nervous system. It translates neurotransmitter hormonal signals into appropriate endocrine responses (Aron et al., 2004; Guyton and Hall, 2001). Secretion of pituitary hormones is under the control of the hypothalamus, through either hormonal or electrical signals. The anterior pituitary is under the control of hormones secreted by the hypothalamus. The stimulating and inhibiting hormones from the hypothalamus are carried to the anterior lobe of the pituitary gland via the hypothalamic-hypophyseal portal vessels (Figure 6-3, *A*). The posterior pituitary is controlled by the hypothalamus via nerve fibers that terminate in the posterior pituitary (Figure 6-3, *B*). The hypothalamus synthesizes ADH and transports it to the posterior pituitary.
3. **Anatomic location** (Figure 6-4): The *hypothalamus* is anterior and below the thalamus. It forms the floor and the walls of the third ventricle. The *pituitary gland* (also called the *hypophysis*) is located in the sella turcica below the optic chiasm, on the superior surface of the sphenoid bone, and covered by dura. The pituitary gland is connected to the hypothalamus by the pituitary stalk and is called *infundibulum.* The pituitary gland can be accessed surgically through the back of the nose. The pituitary gland has two distinct lobes that produce different hormones.

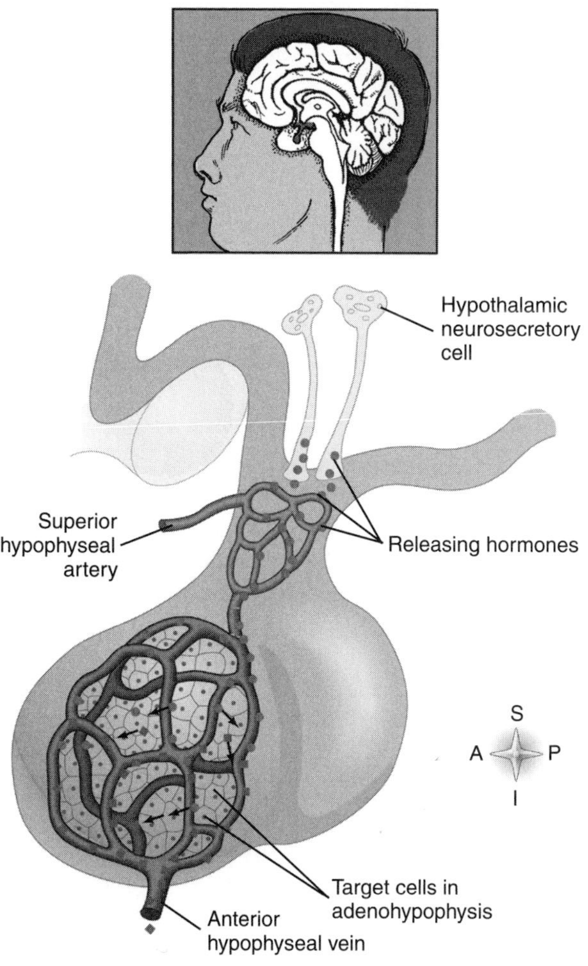

FIGURE 6-3, A ■ Hypophyseal portal system. Neurons in the hypothalamus secrete releasing hormones into veins that carry the releasing hormones directly to the vessels of the adenohypophysis, thus bypassing the normal circulatory route. (From Thibodeau GA, Patton KT: *Anatomy and physiology*, ed 5. St. Louis, 2003, Mosby.)

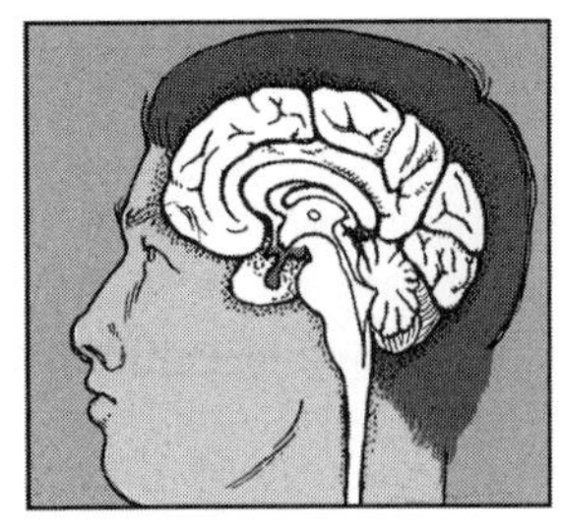

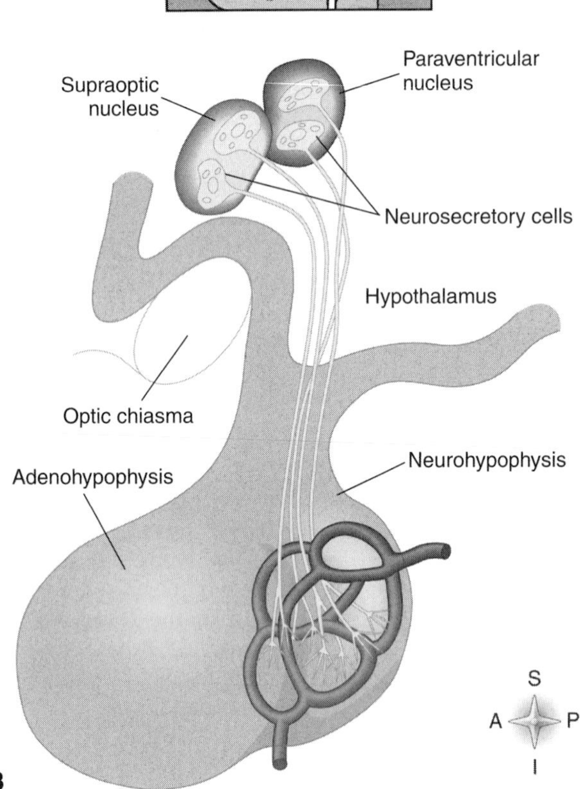

FIGURE 6-3, B ■ Relationship of the hypothalamus and neurohypophysis. Neurosecretory cells have their cell bodies in the hypothalamus and their axon terminals in the neurohypophysis. Thus hormones synthesized in the hypothalamus are actually released from the neurohypophysis.

(From Thibodeau GA, Patton KT: *Anatomy and physiology*, ed 5. St. Louis, 2003, Mosby.)

- **a.** *Anterior pituitary (adenohypophysis)* constitutes two thirds of the pituitary gland (Aron et al., 2004). Hypothalamic-releasing hormones control hormone secretion. The anterior pituitary secretes growth hormone (GH), ACTH, thyroid-stimulating hormone (TSH), prolactin, FSH, and LH.
- **b.** *Posterior pituitary (neurohypophysis)* hormones are controlled by nerve fibers in the hypothalamus called the *hypothalamohypophysia tract* (which contains approximately 100,000 nerve fibers) (Aron et al., 2004). The posterior pituitary secretes ADH and oxytocin. These hormones are synthesized in the hypothalamus, transported via nerve tracts in the pituitary stalk, and stored in the posterior pituitary.

4. Cell types of the hypothalamus, neurohypophysis, and adenohypophysis

- **a.** The *supraoptic and paraventricular nuclei* originate in the hypothalamus. *Thirst receptors* and *osmoreceptors* are located in the hypothalamus close to the supraoptic nucleus. ADH is formed primarily in the supraoptic nucleus, but small amounts of ADH are produced in the paraventricular nucleus. Oxytocin is formed primarily in the paraventricular nucleus (Guyton and Hall, 2001).

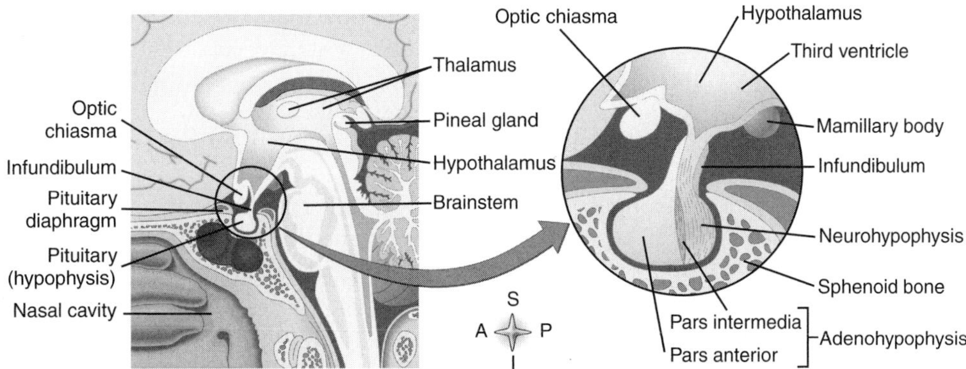

FIGURE 6-4 ■ Location and structure of the pituitary gland (hypophysis).
The pituitary gland is located within the sella turcica of the skull's sphenoid bone and is connected to the hypothalamus by a stalklike infundibulum. The infundibulum passes through a gap in the portion of the dura mater that covers the pituitary (the pituitary diaphragm). The inset shows that the pituitary is divided into an anterior portion, the adenohypophysis, and a posterior portion, the neurohypophysis. The adenohypophysis is further subdivided into the pars anterior and pars intermedia. The pars intermedia is almost absent in the adult pituitary.
(From Thibodeau GA, Patton KT: *Anatomy and physiology,* ed 5. St. Louis, 2003, Mosby.)

b. The *posterior pituitary* is composed of pituicytes, described as "glial-like cells." They are support structures for the nerve fibers that come from the hypothalamus. The pituicytes do not secrete hormones (Guyton and Hall, 2001).
c. The *anterior pituitary* consists of five different types of secretory cells (Aron et al., 2000; Dorton, 2000).
   - Somatotrophs secrete GH and constitute 50% of anterior pituitary cells.
   - Lactotrophs secrete prolactin and constitute 10% to 25% of anterior pituitary cells. These cells proliferate during pregnancy secondary to elevated estrogen levels.
   - Corticotrophs secrete ACTH and constitute 15% to 20% of anterior pituitary cells.
   - Gonadotrophs secrete LH and FSH and constitute 10% to 15% of anterior pituitary cells.
   - Thyrotrophs secrete TSH and constitute less than 10% of anterior pituitary cells.

5. **Hypothalamic hormones**
   a. *Growth hormone-releasing hormone* (GHRH) stimulates release of growth hormone.
   b. *Thyrotropin-releasing hormone* (TRH) stimulates release of thyroid-stimulating hormone.
   c. *Corticotropin-releasing hormone* (CRH) stimulates release of ACTH.
   d. *Gonadotropin-releasing hormone* (GnRH) stimulates release of LH and FSH.
   e. *GH inhibitory hormone,* also called *somatostatin,* inhibits release of GH and decreases secretion of TSH, renin, parathyroid hormone, glucagons, and insulin.
   f. *Prolactin inhibitory hormone* (PIH), which is the same as the catecholamine dopamine, inhibits secretion of prolactin.
   g. These hormones are transported to the *anterior pituitary* by the hypophysial portal vessels. The releasing/inhibitory hormones regulate the stimulation

and secretion of the anterior pituitary hormones (Aron et al., 2004; Guyton and Hall, 2001; Piano and Huether, 2002).

6. **Anterior pituitary hormones** (Figure 6-5)
   a. *Growth hormone*
      - *Biosynthesis:* GH is a polypeptide hormone secreted by the somatotroph cells.
      - *Regulation:* The strongest stimulus for release is growth hormone-releasing hormone (GHRH) secreted by the ventromedial nucleus in the hypothalamus. GHRH is transported to the anterior pituitary via the hypothalamic-hypophysial portal vessels. Starvation, hypoglycemia, stress, exercise, and low blood levels of fatty acids can stimulate GH release. Hypoglycemia stimulates the ventromedial nucleus, the same center that causes the sensation of hunger.
      - The *inhibition of GH release* occurs secondary to growth hormone-inhibitory hormone (GHIH), also known as *somatostatin; hyperglycemia; exogenous GH; and corticosteriods.* GHIH is secreted by cells in the periventricular region (located above the optic chiasm) in the hypothalamus and the delta cells of the pancreas (Aron et al., 2004; Guyton and Hall, 2001).
      - *Secretion:* Fifty percent of circulating GH is bound to growth hormone-binding proteins and has a plasma half-life of 20 to 50 minutes (Aron et al., 2004). GH is released in a pulsatile fashion with increased levels occurring during early hours of deep sleep.
      - *Effects:* GH is an anabolic hormone that facilitates linear growth in all tissues of the body through increased mitosis and increased cell size. GH, via insulin-like growth factor 1, increases protein synthesis through increased RNA replication (Aron et al., 2004). GH increases the mobilization of fatty acids from adipose tissue and enhances their conversion to acetyl coenzyme A to be utilized for energy. GH decreases carbohydrate utilization and increases blood glucose levels through the diminished use of glucose by the cell inducing "insulin resistance" (Guyton and Hall, 2001). GH stimulates bone, cartilage, and tissue growth. GH may have immune stimulating effects.
      - *Abnormalities of GH secretion:* In growth hormone deficiency (GHD), the anterior pituitary fails to produce enough GH; consequently, stature is less than genetic determination would indicate. Most GHD is idiopathic. An excessive level of GH produces gigantism, usually caused by pituitary adenoma. Gigantism is due to excessive GH secretion after the epiphyses of the long bones have closed.
      - *Role in critical illness:* Acute illness is thought to induce a state of GH resistance resulting in a catabolic state that is compounded by the stress response (Van den Berghe, 2003). Circulating GH levels are increased. The normal pulsatile release of GH is altered. In chronic critical illness, GH secretion is suppressed and there may be a "relative GH deficiency" (Van den Berghe, 2003).

   b. *Adrenocorticotropic hormone* (ACTH)
      - *Biosynthesis:* ACTH is a polypeptide hormone secreted by corticotroph cells.
      - *Regulation:* The stimulation for the release of ACTH is CRH, which is secreted by the hypothalamus. Pain, stress, trauma, hypoxia, low cortisol levels, and vasopressin administration also stimulate release of ACTH (Aron et al., 2004).
      - Inhibition to release of ACTH is primarily through negative feedback secondary to increased cortisol levels, which in turn will decrease the

formation of CRF. Exogenous steroids decrease ACTH secretion, leading to adrenal insufficiency.
- *Secretion:* ACTH has a diurnal pattern and plasma levels vary. Highest levels occur in the early morning and decrease over the day. Diurnal pattern is lost during times for stress. ACTH has melanocyte-stimulating abilities, which determine the concentration of melanin in the skin (Guyton and Hall, 2001).
- *Effects:* ACTH stimulates the secretion of the adrenocortical hormones (glucocorticoids, mineralocorticoids, and adrogenic steroids) to produce and secrete cortisol and aldosterone (refer to cortisol and aldosterone under Adrenal Glands).
- *Abnormalities of ACTH secretion:* Long-term ACTH oversecretion stimulates hypertrophy, proliferation, and hyperfunction of the adrenal cortex (Guyton and Hall, 2001). Undersecretion of ACTH leads to adrenal insufficiency.
- *Role in critical illness:* Relative adrenal insufficiency is seen in critical illness, especially in sepsis. Hydrocortisone therapy to treat relative adrenal insufficiency is reserved for children with catecholamine resistance and suspected or proven adrenal insufficiency (Carcillo and Fields, 2002). Children on chronic steroids require stress doses of steroids when under going surgery or any "stressful" event.

c. *Thyroid-stimulating hormone*
- *Biosynthesis:* TSH, also known as *thyrotropin,* is a glycoprotein hormone secreted by the thyrotroph cells.
- *Regulation:* Stimulations for the release of TSH include thyrotropin-releasing hormone (TRH), which is secreted by the hypothalamus; exposure to severe cold; and decreased level of thyroid hormone. Somatostatin and negative feedback from increased blood levels of thyroid hormones inhibit TSH. Dopamine inhibits TSH secretion.
- *Effects:* TSH stimulates the thyroid gland to release tri-iodothyronine (T_3) and thyroxine (T_4), increase glucose uptake and oxidation, stimulate iodide metabolism, and increase thyroid cell size and vascularity (Greenspan, 2004).
- *Abnormalities of TSH secretion:* Hypersecretion of TSH induces hyper-thyroidism. Hyposecretion of TSH induces hypothyroidism and delay of puberty.
- *Role in critical illness:* Nonthyroidal illness syndrome or sick euthyroid syndrome refers to abnormalities in thyroid function that occur in patients with illness, surgery, or fasting not caused by thyroid or pituitary dysfunction (Langton and Brent, 2002). T_3 or T_4 levels or both are generally decreased during times of illness, and TSH may be normal or reduced secondary to a decreased response to TRH. It is unclear whether these changes reflect a protective response or a maladaptive process because the abnormalities generally disappear when the illness resolves (Fliers et al., 2001; Langton and Brent, 2002). There is debate over whether to supplement with thyroid hormone or not; most authorities agree that these patients should not have supplementation because the normal TSH reflects a euthyroid state. Thyroid testing should be repeated once the illness has resolved.

d. *Follicle-stimulating hormone*
- *Biosynthesis:* FSH is a glycoprotein hormone that is secreted by the gonadotroph cells.
- *Regulation:* The stimulus for FSH release is gonadotropin-releasing hormone (Gn-RH) secreted by the hypothalamus. FSH secretion is inhibited through negative feedback secondary to increased levels of estrogen secreted by the ovaries and increased levels of inhibin secreted by the testes.

- *Effects:* In males, FSH stimulates testicular growth; following puberty, FSH promotes spermatogenesis. In females, FSH stimulates the growth of the ovarian follicles and the secretion of estrogen.
- *Role in critical illness:* Unknown.

e. *Luteinizing hormone* (LH)

- *Biosynthesis:* LH is a glycoprotein hormone that is secreted by the gonadotroph cells.
- *Regulation:* The stimulus for release of LH is GnRH secreted by the hypothalamus. Inhibition for the release of LH is negative feedback secondary to increased levels of estrogen, progesterone, and testosterone.
- *Effects:* In males, LH stimulates the production of testosterone from the Leydig cells and maturation of spermatozoa. In females, LH stimulates estrogen and progesterone production. LH is responsible for ovulation and maintenance of the corpus luteum.
- *Role in critical illness:* Unknown.

f. *Prolactin*

- *Biosynthesis:* Prolactin is a polypeptide hormone that is secreted by the lactotroph cells.
- *Regulation:* The stimulus for the release of prolactin is oxytocin, which is secreted by the posterior pituitary, TRH, and prolactin-releasing hormone (PRH) from the hypothalamus (Piano and Huether, 2002). Immune-derived cytokines and stress also stimulate prolactin release. Inhibition of the release of prolactin is with dopamine, which is secreted by the hypothalamus.
- *Effects:* Prolactin stimulates lactation and during pregnancy increases the growth of the ductal system in the breast and the production of breast milk. It maintains the corpus luteum and progesterone production during pregnancy. Prolactin stimulates immune function by supporting the growth and survival of lymphocytes.
- *Role in critical illness:* Exogenous dopamine blocks prolactin production and may be associated with clinically significant effects on the immune system.

7. Posterior pituitary hormones (Figure 6-5)

a. *Antidiuretic hormone* (*ADH,* also referred to as *arginine vasopressin*)

- *Biosynthesis:* ADH is a polypeptide. The prohormone is carried in vesicles through the axons to the posterior pituitary. Final synthesis of the prohormone to ADH occurs in the vesicles during axonal transport.
- *Regulation:* Osmoreceptors in the hypothalamus are in close proximity to the supraoptic nucleus. When serum osmolality increases, the cells in this area begin to shrink, stimulating the release of ADH (Figure 6-6).
- The most potent *stimulus for ADH release* is a serum osmolality exceeding 275 to 280 mOsm/kg (Moritz and Ayus, 2002). Osmotic changes as small as 1% stimulate the release of ADH (Cheetham and Baylis, 2004; Muglia and Majzoub, 2002; Wong and Verbalis, 2002). These small changes in osmolality also stimulate the thirst mechanism, a protective mechanism to maintain water balance and prevent dehydration. A decrease in circulating blood volume perceived by the baroreceptors in the carotid sinus of the aortic arch also stimulates ADH release (Terpstra and Terpstra, 2000). Infants, small children, patients who are comatose or disoriented, or individuals who have abnormal thirst response are not able to meet these physiologic demands; therefore, they are dependent on others to ensure an adequate intake of water. Hemorrhage (10% to 20% circulating blood volume), hypotension, nausea, hypercapnia, morphine, nicotine, and hypoxemia can activate the release of ADH (Guyton and Hall, 2001; Wong and Verbalis, 2002).

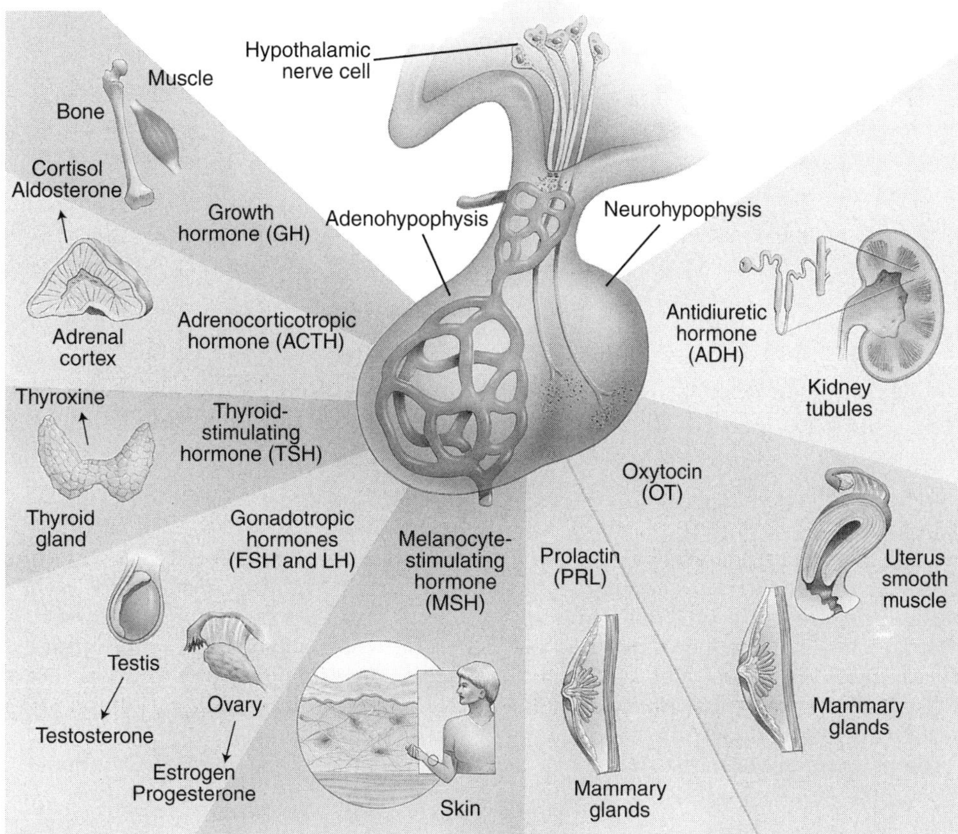

FIGURE 6-5 ■ Pituitary hormones and their target organs. Adrenocorticotropic hormone *(ACTH)*, thyroid-stimulating hormone *(TSH)*, follicle-stimulating *(FSH)*, luteinizing hormone *(LH)*, male analog of LH, interstitial cell-stimulating hormone *(ICSH)*, melanocyte-stimulating hormone *(MSH)*, growth hormone *(GH)*.
(Modified from Thibodeau GA, Patton K: *Anatomy and physiology*, ed 4, St Louis, 1999, Mosby.)

Catecholamines and angiotensin II can modulate the release of ADH, which is a powerful stimulus to ACTH and to prolactin release.

- *ADH release* is inhibited by a serum osmolality below 275 mOsm/kg (Moritz and Ayus, 2002). The baroreceptors in the carotid sinus and the volume receptors in the left atrium send signals to the brainstem via the vagus and glossopharyngeal nerves. The stimulus is then carried to the hypothalamus. This pathway is primarily inhibitory; however, a fall in pressure or volume decreases the amount of inhibition, facilitating the release of ADH. Vincristine, cyclosphosphamide, alcohol, and glucocorticoids inhibit ADH release (Guyton and Hall, 2001; Moritz and Ayus, 2002). Atrial natriuretic factor (ANF) inhibits ADH release and its effect on the kidney.
- *Effects:* Three receptors are responsive to ADH: V_1, V_2, and V_3. V_1 receptors are located in blood vessels and hepatocytes. When stimulated, they produce smooth-muscle contraction, which leads to powerful vasoconstriction. V_2 receptors are located in the kidney, primarily in the collecting tubule and the ascending loop of Henle. V_3 receptors are located in the pituitary and

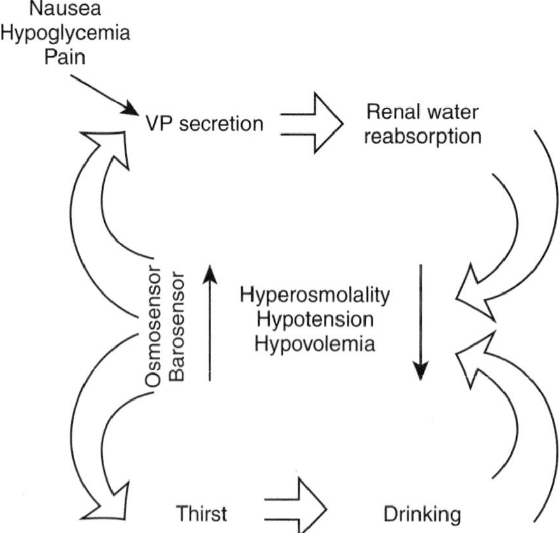

FIGURE 6-6 ■ Regulation of vasopressin secretion and serum osmolality. Hyperosmolality, hypovolumia, and hypotension are sensed by osmosensors, volume sensors, and barosensors, respectively. These stimulate both vasopressin *(VP)* secretion and thirst. Vasopressin, acting on the kidney, causes increased reabsorption of water (antidiuresis). Thirst causes increased water ingestion. The result of these dual negative-feedback loops is a reduction in hyperosmolality or hypotension/hypovolemia. Additional stimuli for vasopressin secretion include nausea, hypoglycemia, and pain.
(From Sperling MA: *Pediatric endocrinology,* ed 2. Philadelphia, 2002, W. B. Saunders.)

potentiate the action of CRH, thereby adding to the release of ACTH (Aron et al., 2004; Breault and Majzoub, 2004; Muglia 2002). ADH increases the permeability of the distal renal tubules and the collecting ducts to water, which is therefore reabsorbed back into the circulation, increasing circulating blood volume. Antidiuresis is the primary action of V_2 stimulation. ADH enhances sodium chloride transport out of the ascending limb of the loop of Henle. This serves to maximize the interstitial osmotic gradient in the renal medulla, facilitating water reabsorption and urine concentration.

- *Abnormalities of ADH:* Deficiency results in diabetes insipidus (DI). Excess ADH results in syndrome of inappropriate antidiuretic hormone (SIADH).
- *Role in critical illness:* Vasopressin is administered to patients who have refractory hypotension with vasodilatory shock or after cardiac bypass to increase systemic vascular resistance (Liedel et al., 2002; Rosenzweig et al., 1999). SIADH and diabetes insipidus are discussed later in this chapter.

b. *Oxytocin*

- *Biosynthesis:* Oxytocin is a polypeptide that is almost identical to ADH except for the placement of two of the amino acids in the peptide chain. Like ADH, the prohormone for oxytocin is carried in vesicles through axons from the hypothalamus to the posterior pituitary, where the final synthesis of oxytocin occurs during neuronal transport.
- *Regulation:* The stimulus for oxytocin release is an increase in estrogen, the onset of labor with stretching and stimulation of the cervix and vagina (labor can occur in women with oxytocin deficiency, although the duration is prolonged), suckling stimuli on the nipple, hemorrhage, or psychologic

stress. Oxytocin is inhibited by pain, heat, or loud noises (Guyton and Hall, 2001).

- *Effects* include contraction of the uterus in pregnancy (levels are highest during the last stage of labor) and contraction of the myoepithelial cells in the alveoli of the mammary gland, stimulating the release of breast milk.
- *Role in critical illness:* Unknown.

B. Thyroid Gland

1. **Embryology:** The thyroid gland is the first fetal endocrine gland to develop. Twenty-four days after fertilization, development of the thyroid gland begins from the endodermal floor of the primitive pharynx. As the embryo grows, the thyroid gland descends into the neck, passing the laryngeal cartilages. This process is complete by 7 weeks' gestation. Fetal brain development is dependent on thyroid hormones. The fetal thyroid gland is able to concentrate iodine by 10 to 12 weeks' gestation. T_3 and T_4 are present by the end of the first trimester; however, low levels of thyroid hormones and TSH suggest a relative pituitary hypothyroidism during fetal development. Thyroid hormone levels peak at 24 hours of life and slowly decrease over the next few weeks. Serum calcitonin is high at birth and slowly decreases over the first week of life, possibly contributing to neonatal hypocalcemia (Fisher, 2002; Kemper and Foster, 2003; Kirsten, 2000; Moore and Persaud, 2003; Palma Sisto, 2004).
2. **Location:** The thyroid gland consists of two lobes located on each side of the trachea below the larynx. A band of tissue called the *isthmus,* which lies over the second to fourth tracheal cartilages, connects the lobes.
3. **Cell types:** The thyroid gland consists of a large number of follicles filled with colloid. The main constituent of colloid is thyroglobulin, a glycoprotein containing the thyroid hormones. Follicular cells and a basal membrane constitute the outer boundary of the follicle. Cuboidal epithelioid cells secrete colloid. Between the follicular cells are parafollicular cells that secrete calcitonin. The thyroid gland is highly vascular; follicles are in close contact with blood and lymphatic vessels (Guyton and Hall, 2001; Kirsten, 2000; Steffensrud, 2000).
4. **Regulation of thyroid hormone:** The thyroid gland secretes T_3, T_4, and calcitonin. The negative feedback mechanism involving the hypothalamus (TRH), anterior pituitary gland, and the thyroid hormones regulate the thyroid gland.
5. **Synthesis of thyroid hormone:** Synthesis of the thyroid hormones is complex and dependent on iodine and tyrosine. Tyrosine is an amino acid present in the body but iodine must be ingested and absorbed by the GI tract into the blood. The thyroid iodide pump actively transports iodide across the follicular cell membrane to be oxidized into iodine then bind with tyrosine in the thyroglobulin molecule. TSH stimulates the iodide pump. Thyroid hormones are synthesized within the thyroglobulin molecule. The thyroid gland is unique in its ability to store hormones in the follicular colloid for several months until released into the blood stream; therefore when synthesis stops the physiological effects of hyposecretion are not seen for several months. Thyroglobulin is not released into circulating blood; the thyroid hormones must split from the thyroglobulin molecule before being released (Kirsten, 2000; Guyton and Hall, 2001; Piano and Huether, 2002).
6. **Thyroxine (T_4)**
   a. *Biosynthesis:* Ninety percent of the thyroid hormone production is T_4, which is a precursor to T_3), and 99% is bound to plasma proteins (Kirsten, 2000).

b. *Regulation:* TSH, low iodide levels, and extreme cold stimulate the release of T_4. Release of T_4 is inhibited by excess iodide and negative feedback resulting from increased levels of thyroid hormones that decrease the anterior pituitary secretion of TSH. Stimulation of the sympathetic nervous system causes a decrease in the secretion of TSH with a subsequent decrease in thyroid hormone secretion.

c. *Effects:* T_4 is a prohormone necessary for the production of T_3. The effects of T_4 are similar to the effects of T_3, although these effects are less potent and have a longer duration of action (Kirsten, 2000).

d. *Factors that impair peripheral conversion of T_4 to T_3:* propranolol, amiodarone, glucocorticoids (at anti-inflammatory doses), liver failure, renal insufficiency, malnutrition, and major illness (Kirsten, 2000).

e. *Role in critical illness:* Dopamine administration decreases the response of TSH to TRH and suppresses TSH secretion. In a retrospective cohort study, T_4 infusions in brain-dead children decreased vasopressor requirements (Zuppa, 2004). Sick euthyroid syndrome is discussed under TSH role in critical illness.

7. **Triiodothyronine (T_3)**

a. *Biosynthesis:* T_3 constitutes 10% of the hormones released by the thyroid gland, and the remaining is produced by extrathyroidal deiodination of T_4 (Langton and Brent, 2002). T_3 is four times more potent than T_4; 99% is bound to plasma proteins (Kirsten, 2000).

b. *Regulation* of T_3 is the same as for T_4.

c. *Effects:* On release into the bloodstream, the thyroid hormones bind with plasma proteins. Because of their high affinity for the plasma-binding proteins, the thyroid hormones are released into the peripheral cells very slowly. Once they enter the cell, these hormones bind with intracellular proteins and are stored. Intracellular activity may last days or weeks. T_3 maintains basal metabolic rate and promotes tissue growth through the stimulation of almost all aspects of carbohydrate and fat metabolism. T_3 promotes protein synthesis, regulates body temperature, and stimulates oxygen consumption through an increase in metabolic rate. In addition, T_3 maintains cardiac output, heart rate, and strength of myocardial contraction through increased metabolism and direct effect on the heart. T_3 increases the rate and depth of respiration secondary to increased metabolism and increased carbon dioxide production. An increase in gastrointestinal (GI) tract motility and secretion of digestive enzymes occurs with T_3 (Guyton and Hall, 2001; Greenspan, 2004).

d. *Role in critical illness:* Cardiopulmonary bypass (CPB) for cardiac surgery reduces circulating thyroid hormones. T_3 supplementation has been given as an adjunct to improve cardiac function in neonates after cardiac surgery (Bettendorf, 2000). Currently there is a multicenter double-blind, randomized, placebo-controlled trial to evaluate the safety and efficacy of T_3 supplementation in children younger than 2 years of age undergoing cardiac surgery when CPB is utilized (Portman et al., 2004). Sick euthyroid syndrome is discussed under the section of the role of TSH in critical illness.

8. **Abnormalities of T_3 and T_4 secretion**

a. *Hypothyroidism* is caused by low levels of thyroid hormones (T_3 or T_4) and elevated TSH levels; resulting in lowered metabolic rate, subnormal temperature, low heart rate, hypotension, weight gain, fatigue, and constipation. Infants with untreated congenital hypothyroidism become mentally handicapped (Holcomb, 2003).

b. *Hyperthyroidism* is caused by high levels of thyroid hormones and results in a hypermetabolic state with weight loss, tachycardia, hypertension, irritability, increased GI tract motility, and restlessness (Holcomb, 2003). Hyperthyroidism is rarely seen in the pediatric population.

9. **Calcitonin**
   a. *Biosynthesis:* Calcitonin is a polypeptide. It is manufactured by the parafollicular cells of the thyroid gland.
   b. *Regulation:* The stimulus for release of calcitonin is an increase in serum calcium and gastrin. A low serum calcium level inhibits release of calcitonin.
   c. *Effects:* Calcitonin plays a minor role in calcium and phosphorus regulation (Figure 6-7). It opposes the action of PTH, stimulates osteoblasts to deposit calcium and make new bone, enhances renal excretion of calcium, decreases active vitamin D formation to lower serum calcium, and enhances renal excretion of calcium (Steffersrud, 2000).

C. Parathyroid Glands

1. **Embryology:** The third and fourth pharyngeal pouches differentiate into the thymus and parathyroid glands during the fourth to sixth week of gestation. During gestation the mother is the sole source of minerals for the fetus. Following birth, the newborn must rapidly adapt to this loss of support. Ionized calcium and PTH levels remain low for 48 hours after birth. Infants develop an

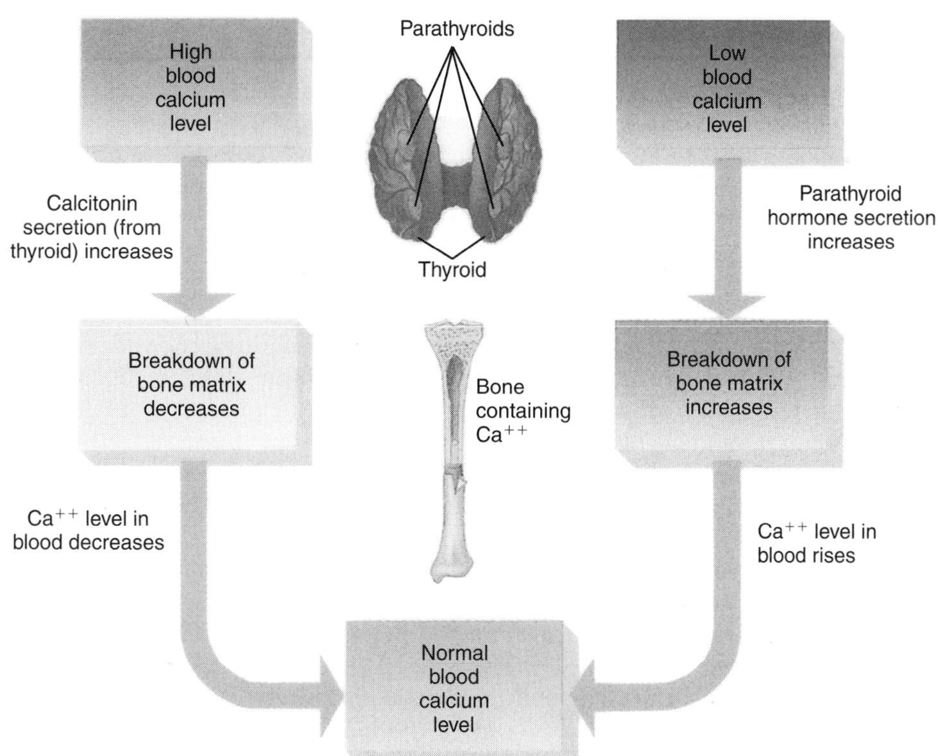

FIGURE 6-7 ■ Regulation of blood calcium levels. Calcitonin and parathyroid hormones have antagonistic (opposite) effects on calcium concentration in the blood. (From Thibodeau GA, Patton KT: *Anatomy and physiology*, ed 5, St Louis, 2003, Mosby.)

appropriate PTH response to hypocalcemia during the first weeks of life, although the response is slow (Moore and Persaud, 2003; Steffensrud, 2000).

2. **Location:** There are usually four parathyroid glands, although 12% to 15% of the population will have a fifth parathyroid gland (Shoback, 2004). Two pairs are located behind the thyroid gland on each side of the trachea.
3. **Cell types:** The parathyroid gland contains mostly chief cells, which secrete most of the PTH. A small to moderate amount of oxyphil cells are present in the parathyroid gland; their function is not understood. It is speculated that they might be chief cells that are modified but no longer secrete PTH. The oxyphil cells are absent in infants and children (Guyton and Hall, 2001).
4. **Parathyroid hormone**
   a. *Biosynthesis:* PTH is an amino acid. A prohormone is synthesized on the ribosomes and cleaved to form PTH. It is stored in the secretory granules in the cytoplasm of the chief cells (Steffensrud, 2000).
   b. *Regulation:* The stimulus for release of PTH is hypocalcemia (Figure 6-7) and mild hypomagnesemia. Release of PTH is inhibited by increased ionized calcium, hypermagnesemia, and severe or chronic hypomagnesemia (Shobach, 2004).
   c. *Effects:* PTH is the major hormone in the regulation of serum calcium. In the kidney, PTH increases calcium reabsorption and phosphorus excretion (there is an inverse relationship between calcium and phosphorus). PTH stimulates the conversion of vitamin D, increases GI tract calcium and phosphate absorption, and promotes bone resorption of calcium (movement out of the bone into the extracellular fluid).

5 **Abnormalities of parathyroid function**
   a. *Hyperparathyroidism* is a rare disorder in which elevated levels of PTH cause hypercalcemia.
   b. *Hypoparathyroidism* is the absence of PTH, resulting in hypocalcemia and hyperphosphatemia.
   c. *Role in critical illness:* Impaired calcium metabolism resulting from abnormalities of parathyroid function may be seen in infants and lead to profound hypocalcemia with seizures and shock.

D. Pancreas

1. **Embryology**
   a. *Dorsal and ventral pancreatic buds* arise from the primitive endoderm at week 5 of gestation and fuse at 17 weeks' gestation (Werlin, 2003). Acini (secretory cells) develop from cells around the primitive ducts in the pancreatic buds. The islets of Langerhans develop from cell groups that separate from the primitive buds and form next to the acini. The islets of Langerhans appear at 12 to 16 weeks' gestation. (Moore and Persaud, 2003; Werlin, 2003).
   b. *Insulin secretion* begins at approximately 10 weeks' gestation and glucagon at 15 weeks' gestation. The main determinant of fetal glucose uptake is maternal blood glucose level. Glucose passes through the placenta to the fetus, although the placenta is relatively impermeable to insulin; therefore, the fetal pancreas must secrete insulin (Moore and Persaud, 2003; Sperling and Menon, 2004).
   c. *Maturation of the beta and alpha cells* increases progressively after birth, and fasting levels of insulin rise progressively during the first 3 months of life. Glucagon levels rise sharply after birth, remain stable during the first 48 hours of life, and then rise progressively throughout the next days of life.

d. The high content of body fat in the term newborn is a buffer against hypoglycemia during periods of fast. Premature or small-for-gestational-age infants have less body fat, and therefore, during the first month of life, these infants have lower blood glucose levels than term infants. The neonate and young child also exhibit hypoglycemia when fasting for shorter periods than the older child or adult. Counterregulatory hormonal responses to hypoglycemia are immature and the enzymes of the gluconeogenic pathway are not completely functional in the newborn.

e. *External sources* of glucose are more important in the young child because of limited glycogen stores, which is related to the small muscle mass and large glucose consumption rate. Liver glycogen stores are depleted 4 to 8 hours after a meal in the young child (Stanley et al., 2002).

f. *Lipase and amylase secretion* is low in infants. Digestion of starch is dependent on salivary amylase, which travels to the duodenum; therefore, when an infant is fed formula high in starch, diarrhea occurs (Werlin, 2003).

2. Location

The pancreas is shaped like a tadpole, with a head, body, and tail, and it lies across the posterior abdominal wall between the spleen and duodenum.

3. Cell types

a. The *exocrine* function involves the acini cells, which secrete enzymes that are important in the digestive process. These enzymes eventually drain into the duodenum.

b. The *endocrine function* is a ductless system that directly secretes insulin, glucagon, and somatostatin into the portal circulation. It constitutes less than 2% of the total pancreatic volume. The islets of Langerhans have four cell types:
- Alpha cells, which secrete glucagons, constitute 25% of islet cells.
- Beta cells, which secrete both insulin and amylin, constitute 60% of islet cells.
- Delta cells, which secrete somatostatin, constitute 10% of islet cells.
- Polypeptide cells, which secrete pancreatic polypeptide and gastrin, constitute 5% of islet cells (Guyton and Hall, 2001).

4. Insulin

a. *Biosynthesis:* Insulin is an anabolic hormone, a hormone of fuel storage. Synthesized on the ribosomes of the beta cells, proinsulin is stored in secretory granules and converted to insulin when the signal comes for its secretion. Insulin's circulatory half-life is approximately 6 minutes (Guyton and Hall, 2001).

b. *Secretion:* The two types of secretions are (1) a meal-related secretion that controls the after-meal increase in glucose levels and (2) a basal secretion that manages the glucose production that occurs overnight and between meals (Rosenstock, 2001).

c. *Regulation*: Release of insulin is predominantly stimulated by an increase in the blood glucose level and amino acid levels and occurs in two stages (Table 6-2). Other factors that potentiate the release of insulin are GI tract hormones (gastrin, secretin), cortisol, growth hormone, and glucagon (Guyton and Hall, 2001). Inhibition of insulin release is hypoglycemia and the α-adrenergic effects of catecholamines, somatostatin, and some pharmacologic agents (prostaglandins) (Piano and Huether, 2002). Once blood glucose levels fall to fasting levels, insulin secretion halts (Figure 6-8).

d. *Effects*
- *Carbohydrate metabolism:* Insulin increases glucose uptake by the liver, muscle, and adipose tissue and stimulates glycogen synthesis and storage

■ TABLE 6-2
■ ■ Stages of Insulin Release

STAGE 1

Within 5 min of an acute elevation of serum glucose, there is an immediate release of preformed insulin into the blood; insulin levels increase tenfold. This high level of release is not maintained, and secretion drops by approximately one half.

STAGE 2

Fifteen minutes after an elevation in serum glucose, insulin secretion increases a second time and reaches a plateau during the next 2–3 h. This is secondary to the synthesis of new insulin, as well as the continued release of preformed insulin by the beta cells.

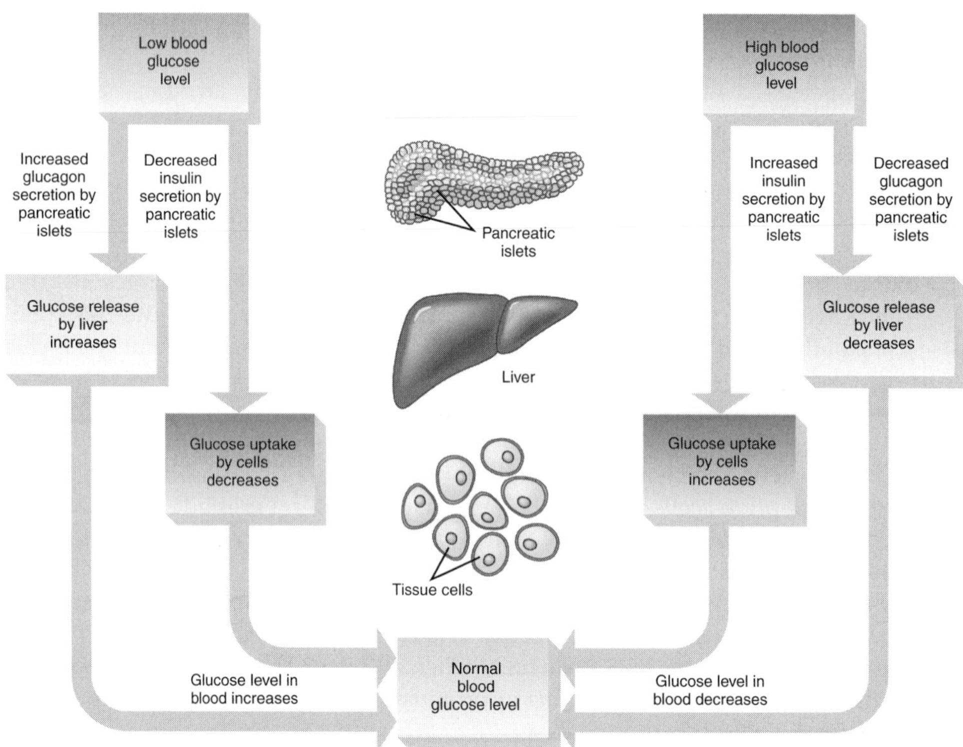

FIGURE 6-8 ■ Regulation of blood glucose levels. Insulin and glucagon, two of the major pancreatic hormones, have antagonistic (opposite) effects on glucose concentration in the blood.

(From Thibodeau GA, Patton KT: *Anatomy and physiology,* ed 5, St. Louis, 2003, Mosby.)

in the liver and muscle *(glycogenesis).* Insulin inhibits gluconeogenesis (formation of glucose from noncarbohydrate sources) and glycogenolysis (breakdown of glycogen to glucose). Insulin is not necessary for glucose uptake by the brain (Guyton and Hall, 2001).

- *Fat metabolism:* Insulin stimulates triglyceride synthesis, transport of fatty acids across the cell membrane, and storage in adipose tissue. Insulin inhibits lipolysis (fat breakdown) and ketogenesis (making of ketones from fat) (Guyton and Hall, 2001; Piano and Huether, 2002).

- *Protein metabolism:* Insulin facilitates transport of amino acids into the cells, works synergistically with GH to promote growth, and stimulates protein synthesis. Insulin inhibits proteolysis (protein breakdown) (Guyton and Hall, 2001).
- *Secondary effects of insulin on other cellular functions* (relatively minor role) involve transport of potassium, magnesium, and phosphate into the cell.

e. *Effects of lack of insulin:* Lack of insulin markedly reduces the rate of transport of glucose across the cell membrane. Reduced insulin secretion also increases the amount of stored triglycerides in the liver; increases serum triglycerides, fatty acids, and cholesterol; and increases serum levels of acetoacetic acid, acetone, and ketone bodies because of increased oxidation of fat *(lipolysis).* Liver and muscle glycogen is converted to glucose and released into the blood *(glycogenolysis).* Gluconeogenesis includes the breakdown of proteins *(proteolysis)* to form glucose (Guyton and Hall, 2001; Piano and Huether, 2002).

f. *Role in critical illness*: Recently tight control of serum glucose (80-110) utilizing insulin infusions has shown improved outcomes in adult trauma patients (Van den Berghe et al., 2001). These data have not been validated in children, in whom the risk of iatrogenic hypoglycemia may be more important. Insulin also has a role in the treatment of hyperkalemia.

5. Glucagon

a. *Biosynthesis:* Glucagon is a large peptide that is synthesized and secreted by the alpha cells of the islet cells and by cells in the GI tract.

b. *Regulation:* Hypoglycemia, amino acids, proteins, sympathetic stimulation, and vigorous exercise are stimulants for the release of glucagon. Hyperglycemia, high levels of circulating fatty acids, and somatostatin suppress release of glucagon (Masharani et al., 2004; Piano and Huether, 2002).

c. *Effects:* Glucagon is a catabolic hormone, a hormone of fuel mobilization. It is an insulin antagonistic hormone that directs the breakdown of liver glycogen (glycogenolysis), increases gluconeogenesis in the liver, and increases the availability of fatty acid to make energy available to the tissues (Guyton and Hall, 2001; Piano and Huether, 2002).

d. *Role in critical illness:* Glucagon has been used as treatment in the overdose of calcium channel blockers. Glucagon increases cyclic adenosine monophosphate (cAMP) production and acts as an inotrope (Abbruzzi, 2002).

6. Somatostatin

a. *Biosynthesis:* Somatostatin is a polypeptide synthesized and secreted by the delta cells of the islet cells. It is present in the hypothalamus, pancreas, and GI tract.

b. *Regulation:* Glucose, amino acids, fatty acids, and GI tract hormones stimulate the release of somatostatin.

c. *Effects:* Somatostatin inhibits the secretion of insulin, glucagon, GH, and TSH; it decreases the production of gastric acid and gastrin; decreases GI tract motility and absorption; and decreases splanchnic blood flow (Guyton and Hall, 2001; Masharani et al., 2004).

d. *Role in critical illness:* Octreotide, which is a somatostatin analog, is used to decrease GI bleeding and to control bleeding associated with portal hypertension. Octreotide is being used in the management of chylothorax (Pratap et al., 2001).

E. Adrenal Glands

1. Embryology:

a. The adrenal glands develop from two different origins: the *cortex,* arising from the mesoderm, and the *medulla,* arising from the neural crest cells.

Differentiation of the adrenal medulla occurs late in gestation. The zona reticularis is not developed until the end of the third year of life and is not fully developed until puberty. The mesoderm is involved in the development of the gonads (Levin and White, 2003).

b. *Fetal cortisol* is necessary for the enzymatic maturation of the fetal liver. Newborn blood cortisol levels are increased as a result of increased cortisol secretion and less conversion to cortisone (Levin and White, 2003). Cortisol progressively decreases over the next 2 months of life.

c. Early in the fetus' development there is no *epinephrine*. Norepinephrine is dominant at birth (Levin and White, 2003).

d. The *sympathetic nervous system* is immature in the newborn and infant. α-Adrenergic and β-adrenergic receptors are decreased in number, density, and responsiveness in the infant (Moore and Persaud, 2003).

2. **Location**

The adrenal glands are small glands that lie atop the kidneys. Each gland has two distinct parts, the cortex, constituting 80% of the gland, and the medulla, constituting 20% of the gland (Guyton and Hall, 2001).

3. **Anatomic Structure**

The adrenal gland is surrounded by a fibrous capsule. The adrenal cortex has three zones: *zona* glomerulosa, the outermost layer (beneath the capsule), constituting 15% of the cortex; *zona fasciculate,* the middle layer (next to the medulla), constituting 78% of the cortex; and the *zona* reticularis, the inner layer, constituting 7% of the cortex. The adrenal medulla has sympathetic and parasympathetic innervation but the adrenal cortex does not. The right adrenal veins drain into the inferior vena cava while the left adrenal vein drains into the renal vein (Piano and Huether, 2002).

4. **Cell types**

a. The *adrenal cortex* is responsible for the secretion of corticosteroids. These hormones are synthesized from cholesterol.
   - The zona glomerulosa is responsible for the secretion of aldosterone.
   - The zona fasciculata is responsible for secreting glucocorticoids, mainly cortisol and a small amount of androgen secretion.
   - The zona reticularis is responsible for secreting androgen and small amounts of glucocorticoid secretion.

b. The *adrenal medulla* is responsible for the secretion of the catecholamines epinephrine and norepinephrine.

5. **Aldosterone**

a. *Biosynthesis:* Aldosterone is a steroid compound synthesized from cholesterol absorbed from the blood. Synthesis is catalyzed by a number of specific enzymes. Because of the similar structure of all the steroids, an alteration in one enzyme can produce significant changes in the steroids being formed.

b. *Regulation:* The renin-angiotensin system, volume depletion, decreased renal perfusion, ACTH, increased levels of angiotensin II, and hyperkalemia increase aldosterone release (Figure 6-9). A small increase in serum potassium will triple aldosterone release (Guyton and Hall, 2001). Inhibition to aldosterone release is secondary to volume expansion, hypokalemia, and low angiotensin levels (Guyton and Hall, 2001).

c. *Effects:* Aldosterone is responsible for 90% of mineralocorticoid activity (Guyton and Hall, 2001). It acts on the distal tubule, collecting tubule, and collecting duct of the kidney to promote sodium reabsorption and potassium excretion. Along with renal reabsorption of sodium, there is a concurrent movement of water into the vascular bed. The net effect is an increase in

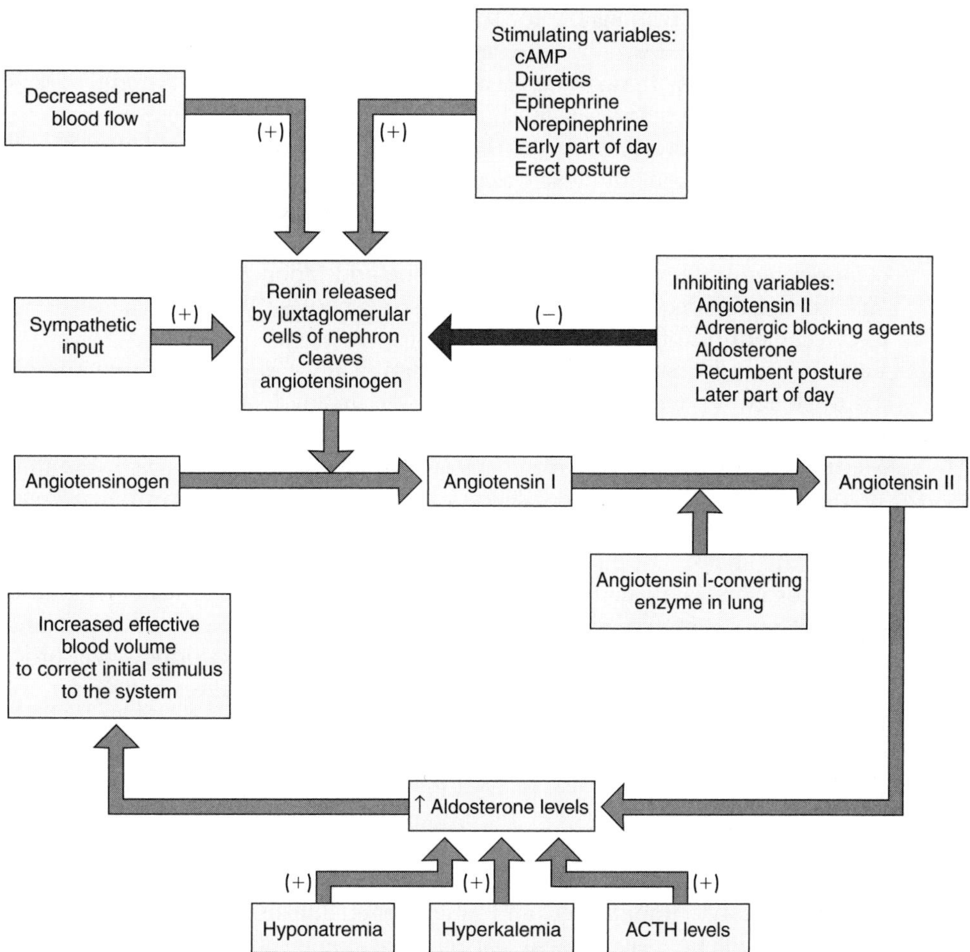

FIGURE 6-9 ■ The feedback mechanisms regulating aldosterone secretion. *cAMP,* Cyclic adenosine monophosphate; *ACTH,* adrenocorticotropic hormone.
(From McCance K, Huether SE: *Pathophysiology: the biologic basis for disease in adults and children,* ed 4. St. Louis, 2002, Mosby.)

extracellular sodium, an increase in extracellular volume, and a decrease in extracellular potassium. Aldosterone promotes reabsorption of sodium and excretion of potassium by the sweat and salivary glands and promotes hydrogen ion excretion by the kidney (Guyton and Hall, 2001). Spironolactone competes with aldosterone for distal renal tubules receptor sites.

d. *Role in critical illness:* Aldosterone increases most likely secondary to the renin-angiotensin system (Van den Berghe, 2003).

6. **Cortisol**
   a. *Biosynthesis:* Cortisol is a steroid compound. Synthesis of cortisol is similar to that of aldosterone.
   b. *Regulation:* The primary stimulus for secretion of cortisol is ACTH. Stress is another strong stimulus. Release of cortisol is inhibited by negative feedback to the anterior pituitary secondary to increased cortisol levels, producing a decrease in ACTH release.
   c. *Secretion:* Cortisol has a diurnal rhythm that mimics ACTH release.

d. *Effects:* Cortisol is responsible for 95% of glucocorticoid activity (Guyton and Hall, 2001). Cortisol increases gluconeogenesis and decreases the peripheral use of glucose. The net effect of the preceding two actions leads to hyperglycemia. Protein synthesis decreases, and catabolism of protein increases. Cortisol promotes mobilization of fatty acids from the tissues. Anti-inflammatory effects include stabilization of lysosomal membranes, a decrease in capillary permeability, block of allergic reactions, and reduction of the intensity of the inflammatory reaction. Cortisol sensitizes the vascular bed to the alpha effects of norepinephrine to support vascular tone and blood pressure and protects against stress. Adequate circulating cortisol is necessary for normal response to catecholamine infusions.

e. *Role in critical illness:* Absolute adrenal insufficiency is rare. Relative adrenal insufficiency, in which cortisol production is inadequate to the level of stressful stimuli, can be seen in sepsis. The American College of Critical Care Medicine (ACCM) defines adrenal insufficiency as a total cortisol less than 18 mg/dL (Carcillo and Fields, 2002). Clinically, patients with relative adrenal insufficiency demonstrate impaired response to catecholamines with persistent shock despite dose escalation of vasopressive medication. Hydrocortisone is recommended by the ACCM guidelines for catecholamine-resistant shock in patients with specific risk factors (purpura fulminans, chronic steroid use) (Carcillo and Fields, 2002). Many practitioners will order a cortisol level but empirically give hydrocortisone while waiting for the results.

7. **Abnormalities of adrenal cortical function**

a. *Adrenal insufficiency:* Primary adrenal insufficiency (Addison disease; rare in children) is due to an absent or damaged adrenal gland. Symptoms are secondary to absent or insufficient glucocorticoids and mineralocorticoids. Chronic deficiency produces weakness, weight loss, anorexia, hyperpigmentation, electrolyte imbalances, and altered metabolism. Adrenal crisis due to an acute depletion of adrenal cortical hormones (secondary to stress or infection) precipitates vomiting, diarrhea, convulsions, coma, hypotension, hyperpyrexia, tachycardia, and cyanosis. Adrenal insufficiency can also result from exogenous suppression with oral or IV steroids. High levels of circulating steroids suppress ACTH release, and abrupt withdrawal of steroids results in symptoms previously described. Adrenal insufficiency can cause profound shock.

- *Risk factors for adrenal insufficiency:* Use of etomidate, severe sepsis, fungal sepsis, prematurity, and age less than 6 months

b. *Hyperfunction of the adrenal cortex* (Cushing syndrome) results in growth retardation; weight gain; moon facies; striae on the hips, abdomen, and thighs; bruises; bone demineralization; emotional lability; and increased blood volume.

8. **Epinephrine**

a. *Biosynthesis:* Epinephrine is a catecholamine derived from the amino acid tyrosine. Tyrosine is converted to dopamine in the sympathetic nerve endings. Dopamine is converted to norepinephrine, which is converted to epinephrine in the adrenal medulla. Eighty percent of the catecholamine secreted by the adrenal medulla is epinephrine (Guyton and Hall, 2001).

b. *Regulation:* Preganglionic sympathetic nerves pass from the spinal cord to the adrenal medulla. These nerve tracts end on secretory cells that secrete epinephrine and norepinephrine directly into the blood. The secretory cells are embryologically derived from nerve cells. Any stress or stimulus that produces a sympathetic ("fight-or-flight") response stimulates secretion of epinephrine from the adrenal medulla. ACTH and cortisol also stimulate release of epinephrine. Inhibition of epinephrine is through negative feedback. High levels of circulating catecholamines produce a down-regulation of sympathetic receptors.

c. *Effects:* Epinephrine mediates the "fight or flight" response. Epinephrine stimulates the β-adrenergic receptors in the end-organs. The greatest effect is due to stimulation of the sympathetic β_1-adrenergic receptors in the heart, resulting in increased cardiac contractility, conduction velocity, and heart rate. The net result is an increase in cardiac output and blood pressure. In isolation, stimulation of the β_2-adrenergic receptors of the vascular bed promotes relaxation; however, during stress the vasoconstricting effects of norepinephrine counteract significant vasodilation. Other effects of stimulation of the β-adrenergic receptors are intestinal, bladder and uterine relaxation and bronchial dilation. Epinephrine increases metabolic activity to a much greater degree than norepinephrine. It increases glycogenolysis and glucose release, resulting in elevations of blood glucose to supply fuel substrates. Circulating epinephrine accounts for 10% of the sympathetic activity during the stress response (Guyton and Hall, 2001).

d. *Role in critical illness:* Epinephrine is used in low-blood-pressure cold shock (Carcillo and Fields, 2002).

9. **Norepinephrine**
   a. *Biosynthesis:* Norepinephrine is synthesized in the nerve endings of the sympathetic nervous system. The precursor is dopamine, which is converted in nerve ending vesicles to norepinephrine.
   b. *Regulation* is the same as for epinephrine.
   c. *Effects* are secondary to stimulation of the α-adrenergic receptors in the end-organs. The most significant effect during stress is peripheral vasoconstriction supporting blood pressure. Stimulation of the α-adrenergic receptors also produces dilation of the iris, contraction of the bladder and intestinal sphincters, and pilomotor contraction.
   d. *Role in critical illness:* Norepinephrine is used in low-blood-pressure warm shock (Carcillo and Fields, 2002).
10. The most significant abnormality of adrenal medulla function is **hyperfunction**. *Pheochromocytoma* is a catecholamine-secreting tumor arising from the adrenal medulla that produces hypertension, tachycardia, diaphoresis, tremors, and headaches (Vaughan, 2004).

CLINICAL ASSESSMENT OF ENDOCRINE FUNCTION

Many endocrine disorders develop over time, so they may not become apparent immediately. Often in hindsight it becomes apparent that a child has had an endocrine disorder for years. Assessment and documentation of past medical conditions, growth patterns, developmental milestones, physical examinations, and family history are critical to the accurate diagnosis of endocrine disorders.

A. History

1. **Prenatal history** includes complications of pregnancy; prenatal exposure to infections, drugs, radiation, and alcohol; and gestational diabetes.
2. **Neonatal history** includes gestational age, complications of labor and delivery, method of delivery, Apgar scores, hospitalization as a newborn, congenital anomalies, feeding difficulties, and postnatal complications.

3. **Growth and development** factors to evaluate include height and weight, recent changes in weight, and developmental milestones and growth patterns.
   a. *Diet* is assessed, including food preferences and aversions, content and time of typical meals, snacking behaviors, changes in appetite, and anorexia. Problems with digestion such as nausea, bloating, food intolerances, abnormal stool patterns, diarrhea, or constipation are noted.
   b. *School performance and problems* or recent changes in performance are discussed. Assessment of personality and behavioral traits includes recent changes in behavior, irritability, sluggishness, disinterest, lethargy, emotional lability, attention deficits, increased aggressiveness, altered self-esteem, perceptions of body image, family roles, and socialization issues.
   c. *Sleep and rest patterns,* including normal bedtimes, incidence of insomnia, ease of falling asleep, restlessness, snoring, bed-wetting, and nightmares are evaluated. Also, note activity and exercise patterns, including the types of exercise normally engaged in, stamina, strength, outside interests, and hobbies.
   d. *Sexual maturation*, including the age of development, any abnormalities, timing and character of menarche, and sexual activity is recorded.
4. **Past medical history** includes known endocrine disorders, neurosurgery, trauma or stress, and previous hospitalizations.
   a. *Medication history* can be significant.
      - High-dose steroids can induce hyperglycemia, inhibit normal physiologic release of steroids from the adrenal cortex (this adrenal insufficiency can cause profound shock), suppress ACTH release, and alter serum electrolytes.
      - Nonsteroidal anti-inflammatory agents (NSAIDs) enhance renal responsiveness to ADH.
      - Sedatives, narcotics, and anesthetics can stimulate the thirst mechanism and alter ADH release.
      - Phenytoin inhibits insulin release.
      - Chemotherapy alters ADH release.
      - Stimulants stimulate the thirst mechanism, alter glucose metabolism, and can modulate release of catecholamines.
      - Ethanol stimulates the thirst mechanism, alters serum osmolality and ADH release, and alters glucose metabolism by inhibiting insulin.
      - Tricyclic antidepressants stimulate the thirst mechanism and alter ADH release.
      - Hypoglycemic agents alter glucose metabolism and serum glucose levels.
      - Hormone replacements alter normal feedback mechanisms for hormone release.
      - Diuretics stimulate the thirst mechanism, alter serum electrolytes and osmolality, and alter renal response to ADH.
      - Propranolol, amiodarone, and glucocorticoids (at anti-inflammatory doses) impair peripheral conversion of T_4 to T_3.
   b. *Other diseases* can have a relationship with endocrine disorders. Cystic fibrosis can be an underlying cause of diabetes mellitus (DM). Pancreatitis constitutes part of the differential diagnosis for pancreatic disorders. Renal disease can be an underlying cause of diabetes insipidus (DI) and part of the differential diagnosis for ADH abnormalities. Lung disease can be an underlying cause of SIADH. Pheochromocytoma is a catecholamine-secreting tumor.
5. **Family history** includes the parents' ages; height, weight, and body proportions of family members; the parents' age at puberty; familial and genetic diseases; health of parents and siblings; presence of known endocrine disorders in other family members; the child and family's perception of any known endocrine

disorders in the family; and the impact of known endocrine disorders on the family's lifestyle.

B. Physical Assessment (Haas, 2000; Pandian and Nakamoto, 2004)

1. **Height and weight** are measured.
2. **Body size and proportion,** fat distribution, upper and lower body ratios, chest circumference, and arm span are compared with previous measurements, if those are available.
3. **Temperature, blood pressure, and heart rate** are recorded.
4. **Head** circumference and percentiles on age- and sex-related growth charts are plotted.
5. **Intake and output** are monitored.
6. The **head, eyes, ears, nose and throat (HEENT)** survey includes observation for sunken or protruding eyes, periorbital edema, gaze, pupil symmetry, and visual acuity. The thyroid gland and neck are palpated for masses or thrills, and the neck is auscultated for bruits. The mucous membranes are assessed for moisture and color, and the oral cavity is inspected for abnormalities of the lips and palate, the presence of caries, and abnormalities in dentition. Observe for obvious dysmorphic features.
7. **Skin assessment** includes turgor and moisture; color, including hyperpigmentation, depigmentation, nevi, and café au lait spots; texture of the skin, including the presence of excess oil, rough or dry skin, acne, and temperature; hair texture and distribution; and brittle nails.
8. **Neurologic assessment** includes the level of consciousness (irritability, lethargy, hyperactivity), cranial nerves, size and shape of the head, palpation of the fontanelle and of suture lines, pupil responses, fine and gross motor movement, abnormal gait or stance, the presence of tremors, reflexes, abnormal deep tendon reflexes, and the presence of seizure activity.
9. **Cardiovascular evaluation** includes rate, rhythm, and character of heart tones; peripheral pulses; perfusion, capillary fill time, warmth, and mottling of skin; palpation for thrills, heaves, and point of maximal impulse (PMI); edema; and blood pressure (hypertension or hypotension, orthostasis).
10. **Respiratory assessment** includes the rate and depth of respiration, odor of breath (acetone), chest excursion, chest symmetry and deformities, and characteristics of breath sounds (coarse or fine crackles, areas of diminished breath sounds).
11. **Abdominal assessment** notes the presence of bowel sounds (hypoactive or hyperactive), tenderness and pain, size, and shape (central obesity with thin arms and legs, distribution and character of fat) and includes palpation of the liver, spleen, and masses.
12. **Genitourinary survey** includes the development of external sexual organs and testicular size, palpation of the kidneys, and the Tanner stage of pubic hair and breast development.
13. **Musculoskeletal survey** includes disproportionate growth (body habitus, length of extremities), the presence of genu valgum or genu varum, short or unusually long metacarpals, and palpation of muscles.

C. Diagnostic Studies

1. **Laboratory** (Table 6-3)
   a. *Blood chemistries* are performed for screening and include electrolytes (magnesium, phosphorus, calcium), glucose, pH, osmolality, blood urea nitrogen (BUN), creatinine, and cortisol levels to assess the pituitary-adrenal

TABLE 6-3
Laboratory Abnormalities in Endocrine Disease

Disorder	Laboratory findings
Diabetes insipidus	Low urine specific gravity (<1.005) Low urine osmolarity (50-200) Low vasopressin (<0.5 pg/mL)
Syndrome of inappropriate antidiuretic hormone (SIADH)	Low serum Na^+ and chloride with normal HCO_3^- Hypouricemia Inappropriately concentrated urine
Hypoparathyroidism	Low serum calcium High serum phosphorus Normal or low alkaline phosphatase Low 1,25-hydroxy-vitamin D_3 Low PTH (may be normal or elevated in pseudohypoparathyroidism)
Hyperparathyroidism	High serum calcium Low serum phosphorus Normal or high alkaline phosphatase High parathyroid hormone (PTH)
Congenital adrenal hyperplasia (classic 21-hydroxylase deficiency)	Low serum Na^+ and chloride High serum potassium High renin Low cortisol Elevated androgens and cortisol precursors Hypoglycemia

From Gunn VL, Nechyba C: *The Harriet Lane handbook*, ed 16. Philadelphia, 2002, Mosby.

axis (plasma levels vary with age and time of day). Screening is done for inborn errors of metabolism (part of the differential diagnosis of endocrine dysfunction); inborn errors of metabolism alter fat and glucose metabolism and normal growth. Screening is done for enzyme deficiencies; various enzyme deficiencies may be the underlying cause of alterations in metabolism and growth. Hormone levels are sent to the laboratory to evaluate the endocrine gland and the target cell or organ. Glycosylated hemoglobin is measured to assess blood glucose control. Vasopressin levels determine the type of DI.

b. *Urine* is tested for electrolytes, fractional excretion of sodium, specific gravity, osmolality, glucose, ketones, and pH.

c. *Dynamic tests of function:*

- The water-deprivation test is described later within the discussion of DI.
- With a glucose tolerance test (rarely obtained), an oral or intravenous (IV) glucose load is administered following an overnight fast, and serial blood glucose determinations are made, which can help in the diagnosis of DM type 1.
- An insulin tolerance test is used to assess the hypothalamic-pituitary-adrenal axis. Following overnighting fast, regular insulin is administered IV to produce hypoglycemia, and serial blood sampling is performed to determine cortisol, blood glucose, and GH levels (Pandian and Nakamoto, 2004). This test requires continuous patient monitoring and is hazardous to those with panhypopituitarism.

- TRH stimulation is used to assess the hypothalamic-pituitary-thyroid axis. TRH is administered IV, and serial blood determinations of T_3, T_4, and TSH are obtained to diagnose thyroid dysfunction.
- An ACTH stimulation test is used to assess the hypothalamic-pituitary-adrenal axis. Following an IV dose of ACTH, serial cortisol levels are obtained to diagnose adrenal insufficiency.
- GH stimulation is used to diagnose growth hormone deficiency (GHD). Insulin, clonidine, arginine, or glucagon may be administered to stimulate the release of GH (Pandian and Nakamoto, 2004).

2. **Pitfalls in the interpretation of endocrine function tests:** Many hormones are secreted according to a specific diurnal rhythm. Plasma hormone levels are dependent on the time and circumstances of measurement. A single measurement of blood levels may not accurately reflect mean levels. Additionally, the hormone levels that are labeled "normal" may be appropriate for the healthy person but not to the person in a state of critical illness. Factors that interfere with endocrine tests include drug therapy, nutritional status, stress, and pathology.
3. **Radiologic tests**
   a. *Chest radiographs* are used to evaluate for pleural effusions or congestive heart failure (CHF).
   b. *Computed tomography (CT)* scan of the head and neck determines the presence of cerebral edema, tumors, or midline defects. CT scan of the abdomen is used to determine the presence of pancreatic or renal tumors.
   c. *Magnetic resonance imaging (MRI)* of the head is used to determine the presence of tumors.
   d. *Ultrasound* of the neck and abdomen is used to determine renal and pancreatic function, to evaluate for pancreatic tumors, and to determine thyroid function.
   e. *Bone age* evaluates normal growth patterns.
4. An **electrocardiogram (ECG)** is used to evaluate myocardial function and the presence of dysrhythmias.

DIABETES MELLITUS

A. Definitions

1. **Type 1: Insulin-dependent diabetes mellitus (IDDM):** IDDM (10% of the DM population [Jones and Huether, 2002] and more than 90% of cases of childhood diabetes [Wraight et al., 2003]) is an autoimmune disease that results in the T-cell-mediated destruction of the beta pancreatic cells (Wraight et al., 2003; Kaufman, 2003). The process may be slow because some children maintain a limited ability to secrete insulin for up to 5 years (Sperling, 2002). IDDM (DM type 1) occurs in genetically susceptible children, usually in response to an environmental agent that triggers the autoimmune process (Wraight et al., 2003). Clinical symptoms manifest when the beta cells secretion is 20% or less (Sperling, 2002). IDDM is the most common form of diabetes in infants and children and requires insulin replacement therapy. IDDM is associated with ketoacidosis.
2. **Type 2: Non-insulin-dependent diabetes mellitus (NIDDM):** NIDDM (90% of the DM population) was previously referred to as *adult-onset diabetes*. NIDDM is associated with obesity, a strong family history, and older age. It is not an autoimmune process but instead is due to insulin resistance (Sperling, 2002; Wraight et al., 2003). Enough insulin is produced to prevent ketoacidosis, so onset is slow. It can often be treated with oral hypoglycemic agents, diet, or exercise. Increasing NIDDM diagnosis among adolescents is due to being

overweight secondary to high-calorie diets and sedentary lifestyles (Fagot-Campagna, 2000; Fajans et al., 2001).

B. Diabetic Ketoacidosis

1. Pathophysiology

a. *Diabetic ketoacidosis (DKA)* is a relative or absolute insulin deficiency (Figure 6-10). In the absence of insulin, stored fuel substrates are mobilized, cellular uptake of glucose is inhibited, and glucose production by the liver is increased, resulting in hyperglycemia. Glycogenolysis, proteolysis, and lipolysis occur (Guyton and Hall, 2001; Sperling, 2002).

b. An increase in *counterregulatory hormones* (glucagon, cortisol, catecholamines, and growth hormone) contributes to hyperglycemia. Hyperglycemia results from increased glucose production and decreased glucose utilization. Glycosuria occurs when the renal threshold for glucose is exceeded, and polyuria results from an osmotic diuresis resulting from glycosuria. Passive electrolyte losses occur secondary to diuresis. Hyperosmolality is secondary to

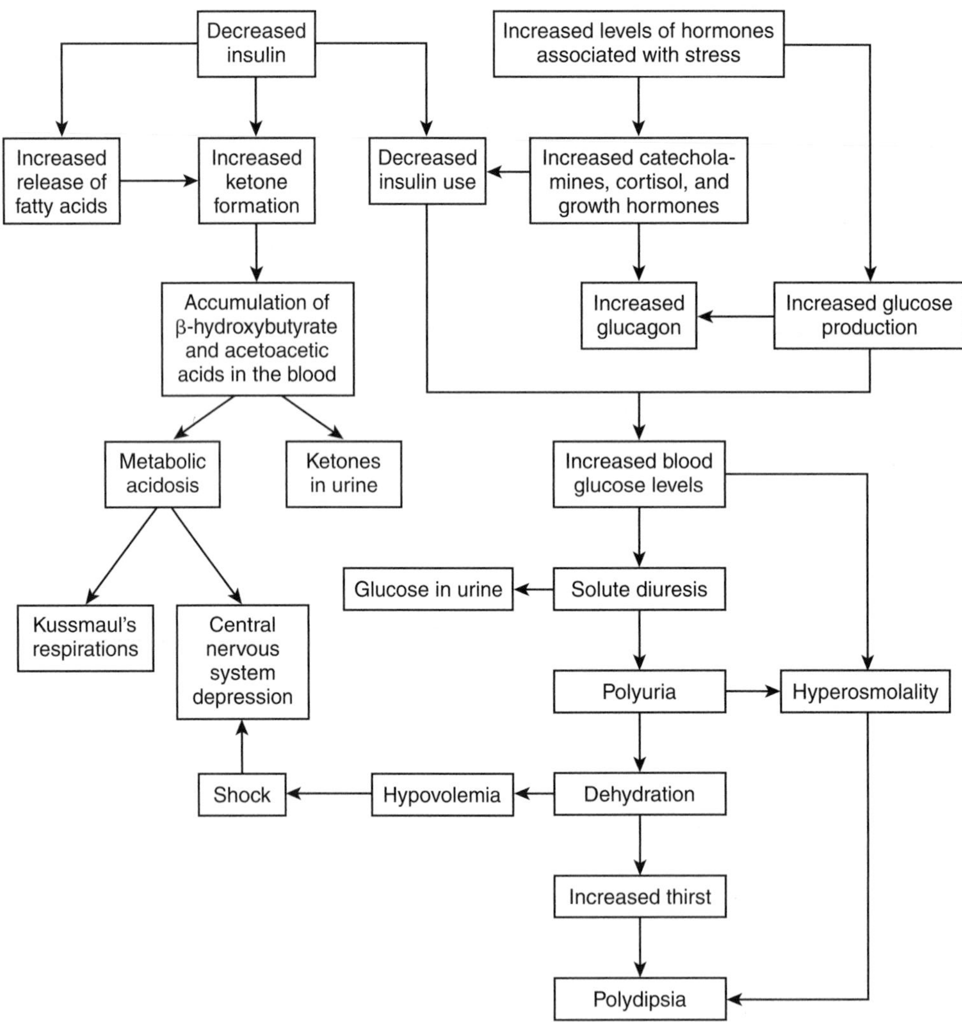

FIGURE 6-10 ■ Diabetic ketoacidosis.
(From Lewis SM, Heitkemper MM, Dirksen SR: *Medical surgical nursing: assessment and management of clinical problems*, ed 5. St. Louis, 2000, Mosby.)

hyperglycemia and free water loss with diuresis. There is a fluid shift from the intracellular space to the extracellular space (Dunger et al., 2004). Nausea and vomiting occur secondary to ketoacidosis, electrolyte imbalances, and possible viral illness. Dehydration occurs secondary to osmotic diuresis and vomiting (Dunger et al., 2004; Guyton and Hall, 2001; Sperling, 2002). Serum osmolarity can be very high, putting patients at risk for cerebral edema and stroke.

c. *Lack of insulin* results in mobilization and incomplete oxidization of fatty acids. There is a resulting increase in ketone bodies (acetoacetic acid, β-hydroxybutyric acid, and acetone), which contributes to the development of metabolic acidosis (Dunger et al., 2004; Guyton and Hall, 2001; Sperling, 2002). Metabolic acidosis contributes to the extracellular movement of potassium with a resultant depletion of total body potassium, although serum levels may be normal or even high.

2. **Etiology** is related to inadequate endogenous insulin secretion (DM initially presents as DKA in 25% to 50% of children newly diagnosed with diabetes [Menon and Sperling, 2003]); deliberate or inadvertent omission of insulin; or acute stress, infection, or steroid use in patients with IDDM. DKA at initial diagnosis of IDDM is more common in children younger than 4 years (Dunger et al., 2004).
3. **Risk factors** include a previous history of IDDM with poor metabolic control. Initial presentation of IDDM precipitated by stress, emotional problems, acute infection, or trauma (Menon and Sperling, 2003); adolescents with diabetes who do not comply with their treatment plan; stress (personal or family) or acute illness in patients with diabetes; cystic fibrosis; and high-dose steroids (Dunger et al., 2004; Menon and Sperling, 2003).
4. **Signs and symptoms** (Table 6-4) include polyuria, polydipsia, polyphagia, and hyperglycemia, generally with a serum glucose level greater than 200 mg/dL. However, DKA can occur with normoglycemia or hypoglycemia if severe vomiting is present, pH is less than 7.30, and serum bicarbonate is less than

TABLE 6-4
Signs and Symptoms of Diabetic Ketoacidosis

Symptoms	Underlying mechanisms
Hyperglycemia	Relative or absolute insulin deficiency
Metabolic acidosis (gap acidosis)	Build up of B-hydroxybutyrate, acetoacetic acids, and acetone in the serum from incomplete oxidization of fatty acids
Dehydration, shock	Osmotic diuresis secondary to hyperglycemia, vomiting
Kussmaul breathing	Deep, rapid breathing; a compensatory mechanism to blow off carbon dioxide and normalize pH
Cardiac arrhythmia	Hypokalemia, hyperkalemia
Sodium imbalance	Total body sodium depleted secondary to sodium loss from osmotic diuresis
	Dilutional hyponatremia secondary to hyperglycemia, fluid drawn into extracellular space, decreasing sodium content
Potassium imbalance	In acidosis, potassium shifts from intracellular space into extracellular space.
	Insulin and acidosis correction shifts potassium intracellular
	Total body potassium depletion secondary to losses from osmotic diuresis
Mental status changes	Cerebral edema, level of acidosis, degree of dehydration
Hyperosmolality	Hyperglycemia, osmotic diuresis
Ketonuria	Ketones rise above the renal threshold and spill into the urine
Glucosuria	Glucose spills into the urine when blood glucose exceeds renal threshold

15 mmol/L (Dunger et al., 2004; Monon, 2003; Sperling, 2002). Hyperosmolality is present. Serum sodium levels may be high, low, or normal with total body sodium depletion secondary to urinary losses or dilutional hyponatremia (fluid shifts from intracellular space to extracellular space) secondary to hyperglycemia. Serum potassium may be high, low, or normal with total body potassium depletion. In acidosis, potassium shifts from intracellular space to extracellular space (increasing potassium levels). Insulin and acidosis correction shifts potassium back into the intracellular space. Elevated serum triglycerides are present. The white blood cell (WBC) count is elevated with a shift to the left (Sperling, 2002). Other symptoms include weight loss, weakness and lethargy, nausea and vomiting, abdominal pain, dehydration, tachycardia, hypovolemia, poor perfusion, shock, glycosuria, ketonuria, rapid deep respiration (Kussmaul's breathing) and lethargy, stupor, or coma.

5. **Categories** of DKA (Dunger, 2004)
   a. *Mild:* pH <7.30 and bicarbonate <15 mmol/L
   b. *Moderate:* pH <7.20 and bicarbonate <10 mmol/L
   c. *Severe:* pH <7.10 and bicarbonate <5 mmol/L
6. **Interpretation of diagnostic studies**
   a. *Hyperglycemia* is due to insulin deficiency, decreased glucose uptake, gluconeogenesis, and an increase in the counterregulatory hormones.
   b. *Glycosuria* occurs secondary to hyperglycemia.
   c. *pH* level less than 7.30 and bicarbonate less than 15 mmol/L are due to acetoacetic acid and β-hydroxybutyrate dehydrogenase (ketones) production.
   d. *Ketonuria* is due to the high levels of acetone in the urine. *Ketonemia* is due to high serum acetone levels.
   e. *Serum osmolality* is greater than 300 mOsm/kg because of hyperglycemia and osmotic diuresis *(dehydration).*
   f. *Electrolyte disturbances* are related to electrolyte loss with osmotic diuresis and metabolic acidosis. Sodium levels can be falsely low as a result of hyperglycemia, which increases serum osmolality, drawing fluid into the extracellular fluid (ECF), and artificially decreasing serum sodium concentration. To correct for pseudohyponatremia, add 1.6 mEq/LNa for each 100 mg/dL of serum glucose greater than 100 mg/dL.
   g. *Islet cell antibodies and insulin autoantibodies* may offer a screening tool for detecting patients with pre-type I IDDM in the future, but they are not diagnostic for DKA.
   h. A *glucose tolerance test* can be used to diagnose glucose intolerance in a child with glucosuria and normal or mildly elevated serum glucose. This test may be useful in diagnosing type 2 diabetes, but it has no role in the diagnosis of DKA.
   i. *Glycosylated hemoglobin (HbA_1)* reflects blood glucose control over the last 120 days. Elevated levels are correlated with high serum glucose concentrations, usually less than 8% (Sperling, 2002).
   j. *CT scan* is used to diagnose cerebral edema, an uncommon but ominous manifestation of DKA.
7. **Diagnoses**
   a. *Differential diagnoses* include adrenocortical dysfunction, use of high-dose steroids, pheochromocytoma, pancreatitis, cystic fibrosis, exogenous catecholamines, stress response, DI, alcoholic ketoacidosis, starvation, hyperglycemia, hyperosmolar nonketotic syndrome, and inborn errors of metabolism.
   b. *Collaborative diagnoses*
      - ❖ Fluid-volume deficit related to osmotic diuresis secondary to hyperglycemia
      - ❖ Low cardiac output related to fluid volume deficit

- ❖ Potential for cerebral edema related to treatment
- ❖ Arrythmias related to electrolyte imbalances
- ❖ Acid-base imbalance related to ketoacidosis
- ❖ Electrolyte imbalances related to osmotic diuresis or treatment or both
- ❖ Potential for hypoglycemia related to treatment
- ❖ Potential for self-care deficits related to lifelong treatment and monitoring, with possible noncompliance
- ❖ Alteration in body image related to chronic illness and future complications
- ❖ Alteration in nutrition related to poor metabolic control
- ❖ Potential for infection related to secondary complications
- ❖ Potential for knowledge deficit regarding home management

8. Treatment goals

- **a.** *Correct fluid and electrolyte imbalances slowly.*
- **b.** *Correct metabolic acidosis.*
- **c.** *Provide insulin to treat and prevent ketosis and to lower serum glucose.*
- **d.** *Prevent neurologic complications.*
- **e.** *Maintain good metabolic control (long term).*
- **f.** *Treat underlying disorders.*
- **g.** *Educate about and prevent recurrence.*

9. Management

- **a.** *Fluid:* Reestablishing intravascular volume is a priority. Administer normal saline (NS) 20 mL/kg during the first 1 to 2 hours as volume expansion. Reassess and administer another fluid bolus, if needed, to treat poor perfusion (Dunger, 2004). Calculate the fluid deficit based on weight before the illness (Table 6-5). If the information is not available, calculate fluid deficit by clinical observation (Table 6-6), or generally one can assume that children in DKA are minimally 10% dehydrated (Menon and Sperling, 2003; Sperling, 2002). Replace fluid deficit, daily fluid requirement, and ongoing losses (urine, vomiting) over the next 48 hours. Although normal saline is an isotonic fluid, the child in DKA is hyperosmolar, and therefore normal saline is hypotonic compared with the child's osmolality.
- **b.** *Electrolytes:* Potassium and phosphate replacement is required. If hyperkalemia is present, wait until urine output is achieved. If a normal potassium level is present, initiate replacement in a combination of KCl, KPO_4, or K acetate because insulin will drive potassium and phosphate back into the cell, thus decreasing serum of potassium and phosphorous levels (Sperling, 2002). Phosphate replacement is necessary, usually given as KPO_4 in the replacement fluids. Bicarbonate replacement in children is a controversial step and should be instituted only if pH is less than 7.10 or if shock, cardiac insufficiency, or renal failure is present. If sodium bicarbonate is given, it should be given *slowly* (i.e., over 2 hours); then clinical status should be reassessed. Sodium bicarbonate

TABLE 6-5
Deficit Therapy

The most precise method of assessing fluid deficit is based on preillness weight, calculated as follows:

$$\text{Fluid deficit (L)} = \text{Preillness weight (kg)} - \text{Illness weight (kg)}$$

$$\%\ \text{Dehydration} = \frac{\text{Preillness weight} - \text{Illness weight}}{\text{Preillness weight}} \times 100\%$$

From Gunn VL, Nechyba C: *The Harriet Lane handbook*, 16th ed. Philadelphia, 2002, Mosby.

TABLE 6-6
Clinical Observations in Dehydration*

	Older Child: 3% (30 mL/kg)	6% (60 mL/kg)	9% (90 mL/kg)
Examination	**Infant: 5% (50 mL/kg)**	**10% (100 mL/kg)**	**15% (150 mL/kg)**
Dehydration	Mild	Moderate	Severe
Skin turgor	Normal	Tenting	None
Skin (touch)	Normal	Dry	Clammy
Buccal mucosa/lips	Moist	Dry	Parched/cracked
Eyes	Normal	Deep set	Sunken
Tears	Present	Reduced	None
Fontanelle	Flat	Soft	Sunken
CNS	Consolable	Irritable	Lethargic/obtunded
Pulse rate	Normal	Slightly increased	Increased
Pulse quality	Normal	Weak	Feeble/impalpable
Capillary refill	Normal	≈2 sec	>3 sec
Urine output	Normal	Decreased	Anuric

From Gunn VL, Nechyba C: *The Harriet Lane handbook*, ed 16. Philadelphia, 2002, Mosby.
CNS, central nervous system.
*For the same degree of dehydration, clinical symptoms are generally worse for hyponatremic dehydration than for hypernatremic dehydration.

should not be given as a bolus (Menon and Sperling, 2003; Sperling, 2002). Sodium bicarbonate administration is not without potential problems: CNS acidosis, hypokalemia, too rapid correction of acidosis, increased sodium load, increasing serum osmolality, and impaired tissue oxygenation (Dunger, 2004; Menon and Sperling, 2002; Sperling, 2002).

c. *Insulin:* (Table 6-7) Rehydration will cause serum glucose to decrease and improve insulin sensitivity to the tissues (Menon and Sperling, 2003). Insulin is needed to normalize serum glucose levels, to suppress ketogenesis and lipolysis, and to resolve ketoacidosis. Insulin infusion is initiated at 0.1 unit per kilogram of body weight per hour, and steady state is achieved in 60 minutes (Dunger, 2004). Blood glucose should drop to 80 to 100 mg/dL per hour, not to exceed 100 mg/dL per hour (Moff and Peterson, 2002; Sperling, 2002). When the blood glucose falls to 250 to 300 mg/dL with continued acidosis, add 5% or 10% dextrose to fluids administered IV (Dunger, 2004; Menon and Sperling, 2003; Sperling, 2002). Do not stop insulin if the blood glucose falls or if persistent acidosis or ketosis occurs. Decrease the insulin dose if the blood glucose continues to fall despite the addition of dextrose to the IV fluids. IV insulin should continue until the pH is greater than 7.25, bicarbonate is greater than 15 mmol/L, and the child is tolerating oral intake. Transition to subcutaneous insulin when acidosis has been corrected and the child can tolerate food. Give subcutaneous insulin 30 to 60 minutes before discontinuing the continuous infusion.

The goal of insulin therapy is to mimic the pancreas. Humalog (Lispro) and Novolog (Aspart) are fast acting-insulins that replace meal-related insulin. Ultralente insulin has been used as a basal insulin replacement, although peaks were variable, thus causing hypoglycemia. Lantus (Glangine) effect is

TABLE 6-7
Insulin Preparations

Insulin	Onset (hr)	Peak (hr)	Duration (hr)
RAPID ACTING			
NovoLog	0.17-0.33	1-3	3-5
Humalog	0.25-0.5	0.5-1.5	6-8
SHORT ACTING			
Regular	0.5-1	1-5	3-10
INTERMEDIATE ACTING			
NPH	1-4	4-14	10-24
Lente	1-4	4-14	12-24+
LONG-ACTING			
Ultralente	4–10	8-30	18-36
BASAL			
Lantus	5	No pronounced peak	20-24+

Data from Taketomo CK, Hodding JH, Kraus DM: *Pediatric dose handbook*, ed 11. Cleveland, Ohio, 2004, Lexi-Comp.
NPH, Isophane insulin suspension.

for 24 hours without a peak action (Rosenstock, 2001) to replace the basal secretion from the pancreas. There is a "honeymoon period" in which there is residual beta-cell function (in type 1 diabetes), although secretion is inadequate and exogenous insulin is required to prevent ketoacidosis. This period varies from weeks to months and rarely lasts up to 1 or 2 years (Sperling, 2002).

d. *Monitoring:* Vital signs, blood pressure, intake and output, cardiovascular assessment, and neurologic checks are done hourly. Hourly glucometer determination of blood glucose is done at the bedside if glucose is not outside the range of the glucometer. Initial laboratory tests should include complete blood count (CBC), electrolytes, BUN, creatinine, glucose, and pH. Electrolytes and pH are monitored every 2 hours until stable. A gradual rise in serum sodium as the glucose levels fall can help to prevent rapid changes in serum osmolality, thus maintaining normal serum osmolality. BUN and creatinine are assessed every 12 hours. Intake and output, daily weights, and urine ketones (every void) are monitored (Dunger, 2004).

10. Complications

a. *Acute*

- Hypoglycemia is due to infrequent blood glucose monitoring and delayed glucose replacement.
- Persistent acidosis can be related to inadequate insulin dose or an ineffective method of delivery (Sperling, 2002).
- Hypokalemia can occur because of inadequate potassium replacement.
- Cerebral edema can be present on presentation, or it sometimes develops 4 to 12 hours after treatment has been initiated (Dunger, 2004). Symptoms include headache, decreased or deteriorating neurologic status, increased blood pressure, bradycardia, and vomiting (Dunger, 2004; Menon and Sperling, 2003). Risk factors include the duration and severity of symptoms before therapy, high serum BUN at presentation (reflective of the degree of dehydration), a lack of rise in sodium level with therapy, hypocapnia,

bicarbonate treatment (Dunger, 2004; Glaser et al., 2001; Marcin et al., 2002; Menon and Sperling, 2003; Quintana, 2004; Sperling, 2002), and rapid correction of hyperglycemia with resultant decreased serum osmolality. Mortality from DKA is related to cerebral edema and herniation.

- Fluid overload and CHF can occur as a result of treatment.
- Aspiration is possible if the level of consciousness is depressed.

b. *Chronic*

- Chronic complications can include poor metabolic control with episodes of hypoglycemia and hyperglycemia, poor growth, insulin resistance, hypertrophy and lipoatrophy (lipoatrophy is rare with purified insulins) of injection sites, limited joint mobility, vaginitis and candidiasis, retinopathy, nephropathy, neuropathy (rare in childhood), and macrovascular disease.

HYPERGLYCEMIC, HYPEROSMOLAR, NONKETOTIC SYNDROME

A. Pathophysiology

The occurrence of hyperglycemic, hyperosmolar, nonketotic syndrome (HHNS) is rare in children, although with the increase in type 2 diabetes in children and adolescents, the incidence of HHNS probably will increase (Goldberg and Inzucchi, 2003). Insulin secretion is present but inadequate, or insulin actions are diminished, producing hyperglycemia without ketogenesis and ketoacidosis. The absence of ketosis in the presence of profound hyperglycemia is the most puzzling component of HHNS. Postulated mechanisms for this phenomenon include the following: (1) insulin secretion is adequate to prevent ketosis but not hyperglycemia; (2) counterregulatory hormone levels are lower, and therefore lipolysis and ketogenesis are suppressed; and (3) dehydration with hyperosmolality may suppress ketogenesis (Delaney et al., 2000; Goldberg and Inzucchi, 2003; Masharani et al., 2004). Marked hyperosmolality with significant dehydration is present. Polyuria is secondary to osmotic diuresis that results from hyperglycemia. Electrolyte losses occur secondary to osmotic diuresis. The degree of hyperglycemia, hyperosmolality, and dehydration is much greater in HHNS than in DKA. Because of the absence of ketoacidosis and the associated physical symptoms (e.g., Kussmaul's breathing, anorexia, nausea and vomiting), treatment may be delayed; therefore these patients often present with profound cardiovascular collapse and neurologic sequelae (e.g., coma) (Goldberg and Inzucchi, 2003). Shock and neurologic deficits are secondary to progressive and profound dehydration.

B. Precipitating Factors

Preexisting cardiovascular and renal disease has been associated with HHNS. Infections (commonly urinary and respiratory), trauma, burns, pancreatitis, thyrotoxicosis, pneumonia, type 2 diabetes, heat stroke, dialysis (peritoneal dialysis and hemodialysis), IV hyperalimentation, and poor glucose control may precipitate HHNS. Phenytoin has been associated with HHNS because of its inhibition of insulin release. Corticosteroids, β-blockers, and thiazide diuretics have been associated with HHNS (Goldberg and Inzucchi, 2003; Masharani et al., 2004).

C. Signs and Symptoms

Signs and symptoms (Table 6-8) include polyuria, polydipsia, serum glucose greater than 600 mg/dL, serum osmolality greater than 330 mOsm/kg, normal pH or mild

TABLE 6-8
Differentiation Between Diabetic Ketoacidosis (DKA) and Hyperglycemic, Hyperosmolar, Nonketotic Syndrome (HHNS)

	DKA	HHNS
Nausea and vomiting	Present	Absent
Neurologic changes	Present	Present
Polyuria	Present	Present
Respiratory rate	Kussmaul's breathing	Normal
Blood glucose	Usually >200 mg/dL	>600 mg/dL
Blood ketones	Elevated	Normal
Urine ketones	Present	Absent
Blood HCO_3^-	<18 mmol/L	>18 mmol/L
Blood pH	<7.30	>7.30
Serum osmolality	>300 mOsm/kg	>330 mOsm/kg
Sodium deficits	4–11 mEq/kg	2–8 mEq/kg
Potassium deficits	1–10 mEq/kg	0.5–3 mEq/kg
Water deficits	50–100 mL/kg	60–170 mL/kg

metabolic acidosis, and serum bicarbonate of 18 to 24 mmol/L. Serum sodium levels may be high, low, or normal with total body sodium depletion secondary to urinary losses or dilutional hyponatremia secondary to hyperglycemia. Serum potassium levels may be high, low, or normal with total body depletion. Tachycardia, hypotension, low central venous pressure, shock, and glycosuria without ketonuria may occur. Lethargy, stupor, or coma also may occur. Neurologic impairment is significantly higher in children with HHNS than in those with DKA because of the severity of hyperosmolality. Mortality rate increases with higher levels of hyperosmolality (Delaney et al., 2000).

D. Interpretation of Diagnostic Studies

1. **Hyperglycemia** is due to decreased release or action of insulin. Insulin levels are adequate to prevent ketosis.
2. **Glycosuria** is secondary to hyperglycemia.
3. Hyperosmolality is secondary to hyperglycemia and loss of free water with osmotic diuresis.
4. **Mild metabolic acidosis** is secondary to dehydration, low cardiac output, renal insufficiency, and lactic acidosis.
5. **Electrolyte disturbances** are due to urinary losses.

E. Diagnoses

1. **Differential diagnoses** include DM, pancreatitis, renal insufficiency, and adrenocortical dysfunction.
2. **Collaborative diagnoses**

- ❖ Fluid volume deficit related to osmotic diuresis
- ❖ Low cardiac output related to fluid-volume deficit
- ❖ Potential for arrhythmias related to electrolyte disturbances
- ❖ Acid-base imbalance related to low cardiac output and lactic acidosis
- ❖ Electrolyte imbalances related to osmotic diuresis and treatment
- ❖ Potential for cerebral edema related to treatment
- ❖ Potential for hypoglycemia related to treatment

F. Treatment Goals

1. **Treat** underlying disorder.
2. **Correct** hyperglycemia and hyperosmolality.
3. **Correct** fluid and electrolyte deficits.
4. **Prevent** neurologic complications.
5. **Educate** about and prevent recurrence.

G. Management

1. **Fluid and electrolyte therapy** involves volume resuscitation of poorly perfused, hypovolemic, or hypotensive (blood pressure is the last to fall) patients with isotonic fluid. Once blood pressure is normalized, IV fluids can be changed. Calculate the fluid volume deficit (see Tables 6-5 and 6-6); replace half during the first 12 hours and the remainder during the next 24 hours in addition to daily maintenance fluid. Because of the frequency of renal insufficiency with HHNS, potassium is not added until renal function is known, urine output is adequate, and serum potassium levels are less than 4.5 mmol/L. Potassium levels decrease rapidly when insulin therapy is initiated secondary to potassium and glucose entering the cell. Potassium replacement can be added to the IV fluids as a combination of KCl and KPO_4 or as KCl alone, depending on laboratory values (Delaney et al., 2000). Once serum glucose reaches 300 mg/dL, dextrose should be added to the IV fluids.
2. **Insulin therapy:** Often hyperglycemia is corrected with fluid therapy alone. Insulin therapy should be used with caution in HHNS. Low-dose insulin therapy can be used to achieve a gradual decline in hyperglycemia and osmolality, often after the institution of fluid therapy. Continuous infusion of 0.5 unit/kg per hour is usually adequate to decrease blood glucose levels and should be discontinued to prevent hypoglycemia once blood levels fall below 300 mg/dL.
3. **Monitoring:** Physical assessment of cardiovascular system, vital signs, blood pressure, and neurologic checks are done every 30 to 60 minutes. Hourly determination of blood glucose is performed at the bedside. Initial laboratory studies include CBC, electrolytes, BUN, creatinine, glucose, and pH. Electrolytes and pH are monitored every 2 hours until they become stable, and BUN and creatinine measurements are done every 12 hours until they are stable. Intake and output and daily weights are also monitored.

H. Complications

Complications include hypoglycemia (from treatment), neurologic deficits (resulting from hyperosmolality), and cerebral edema and death from rapid correction of the hyperosmolar state. Mortality averages 14% to 17% (Jones and Huether, 2002).

ACUTE HYPOGLYCEMIA

A. Pathophysiology

Hypoglycemia is defined as serum glucose less than 50 mg/dL (Sperling and Menon, 2004; Thornton et al., 2002; Wolfsdorf and Weinstein, 2003). Energy failure may contribute to rapid cell death, particularly in the brain. Nonketotic hypoglycemia is associated with hyperinsulinism; 60% present within the first week of life (Thornton et al., 2002). Ketotic hypoglycemia is secondary to metabolic derangements associated with lack of glucose for metabolism, with resulting fat metabolism. The body utilizes many systems to prevent hypoglycemia (Figure 6-11).

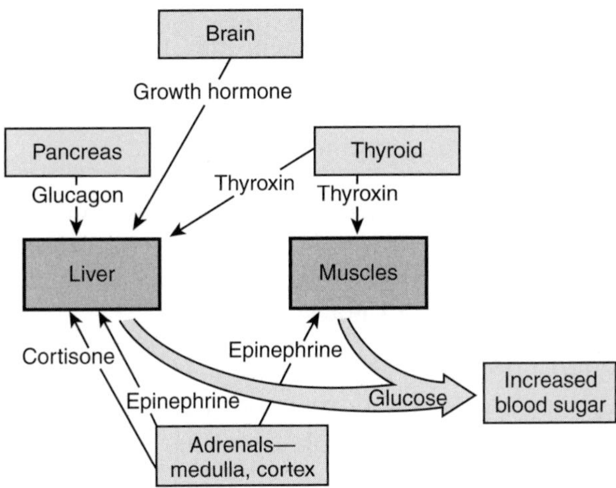

FIGURE 6-11 ■ Body systems respond to hypoglycemia in various ways to increase blood glucose levels.

(From Hockenberry MJ: *Wong's nursing care of infants and children,* ed 7. St. Louis, 2003, Mosby.)

B. Etiology

1. **Neonatal hypoglycemia** can be transient (days to weeks), caused by immature fasting adaptation, depletion of glycogen stores, hyperinsulinemia (e.g., in infants of diabetic mothers), or lack of exogenous supply. Hypopituitarism, inborn errors of metabolism (defective gluconeogenesis), congenital hyperinsulinism, or adrenocortical deficiency would demonstrate persistent hypoglycemia (Sperling and Menon, 2004; Stoll and Kliegman, 2003; Wolfsdord, 2003). Ten percent of normal newborns will have hypoglycemia with a 6-hour delay in first feeding, which demonstrates the immaturity of the fasting mechanism. Poorly feeding breastfed newborns are at risk for hypoglycemia (Palma Sisto, 2004).
2. **Childhood hypoglycemia** can be caused by inborn errors of metabolism, growth hormone deficiency, cortisol deficiency, stress, hepatic dysfunction, excessive insulin in IDDM, severe malnutrition, infections, or drugs.

C. Risk Factors

1. Infants of diabetic mothers
2. Small-for-gestational-age infants
3. Stress or acute illness
4. Insulin infusion
5. Infants or children with compromised IV access and nothing-by-mouth (NPO) status
6. Increased metabolism
7. Poor nutrition
8. Medications: β-blocker (blocks the response or release of epinephrine), angiotensin-converting enzyme (ACE) inhibitors
9. Liver disease

D. Sign and Symptoms

1. **Associated with autonomic nervous system stimulation** and epinephrine release (to prevent hypoglycemia), these symptoms are associated with rapid fall of glucose levels: Shakiness or trembling, tachycardia, sweating, anxiety, weakness, hunger, nausea, and vomiting (Sperling and Menon, 2004; Thornton et al. 2002).
2. **Associated with diminished glucose to the brain,** these symptoms are related to severe hypoglycemia: Lethargy, irritability, confusion, seizure, coma, twitching, personality or behavioral changes, visual changes and inability to concentrate (Sperling and Menon, 2004; Thornton et al., 2002).

E. Interpretation of Diagnostic Studies

1. **Blood glucose** is less than 50 mg/dL. If glucose is measured by a glucometer, confirm the results with a serum sample sent to the laboratory. Glucose tolerance test is of little value.
2. **Low plasma carnitine levels** can indicate medium-chain acyl-CoA deficiency (although this is a very rare occurrence).
3. **Low plasma levels of GH** indicate GH deficiency.
4. **Low cortisol levels** are due to cortisol deficiency.
5. **Elevated blood insulin** levels indicate hyperinsulinemia.
6. **Urine-reducing substances** indicate fructose intolerance or galactosemia.
7. **Urinary ketones** can differentiate between ketotic and nonketotic hypoglycemia.
8. **Abdominal CT** scan is used to determine the presence of a pancreatic tumor.
9. **Abdominal ultrasound** can identify insulinoma.

F. Diagnoses

1. **Differential diagnoses** include hepatic failure, pancreatic tumors, cardiovascular disease, neurologic disease, endocrine deficiencies, inborn errors of metabolism, tumors, and sepsis.
2. **Collaborative diagnoses**

- ❖ Potential for alterations in nutrition resulting from low blood glucose, decreased substrate for metabolism, or altered metabolic pathways.
- ❖ Potential for neurologic alterations resulting from decreased amounts of the primary metabolic substrate of the brain (glucose).

G. Treatment Goals

1. **Correct** and maintain normal blood glucose.
2. **Support** cellular metabolic requirements.

H. Management

1. **Newborns** may need early feedings; consider initiation of nutritional support (hyperalimentation or parental feedings).
2. **IV boluses** of 10% or 25% glucose (0.5 to 1 g/kg over 1 to 3 minutes).

$$0.5 \text{ to } 1 \text{ g/kg} = 5 \text{ to } 10 \text{ mL/kg of } D_{10} \text{ or } 2 \text{ to } 4 \text{ mL/kg of } D_{25}$$

3. **Continuous infusion** of dextrose (usually 10% dextrose).
4. **Identification** and treatment of underlying cause.
5. **Maintain** normothermia and decrease environmental stress.
6. **Monitor** glucose levels.
7. In **patients with DKA**, add dextrose or decrease insulin infusion.
8. **Treat** underlying metabolic disorders (Sperling and Menon, 2004; Stoll and Kliegman, 2003; Thornton et al., 2002).

H. Complications

Complications include neuronal death, coma, seizures, neurologic deficits, and death.

SYNDROME OF INAPPROPRIATE ANTIDIURETIC HORMONE (SIADH)

A. Pathophysiology

SIADH is characterized by inappropriate, excessive secretion of ADH in the absence of a hypovolemic stimulus. SIADH occurs in the face of low serum sodium and low serum osmolality that would normally serve to inhibit ADH secretion through negative feedback (Mortitz, 2002), which results in water retention and expansion of extracellular volume. Hyponatremia is secondary to hemodilution, although total body sodium stores are normal (Figure 6-12). Renal function is normal. Clinical signs and symptoms are secondary to increased blood volume and hyponatremia.

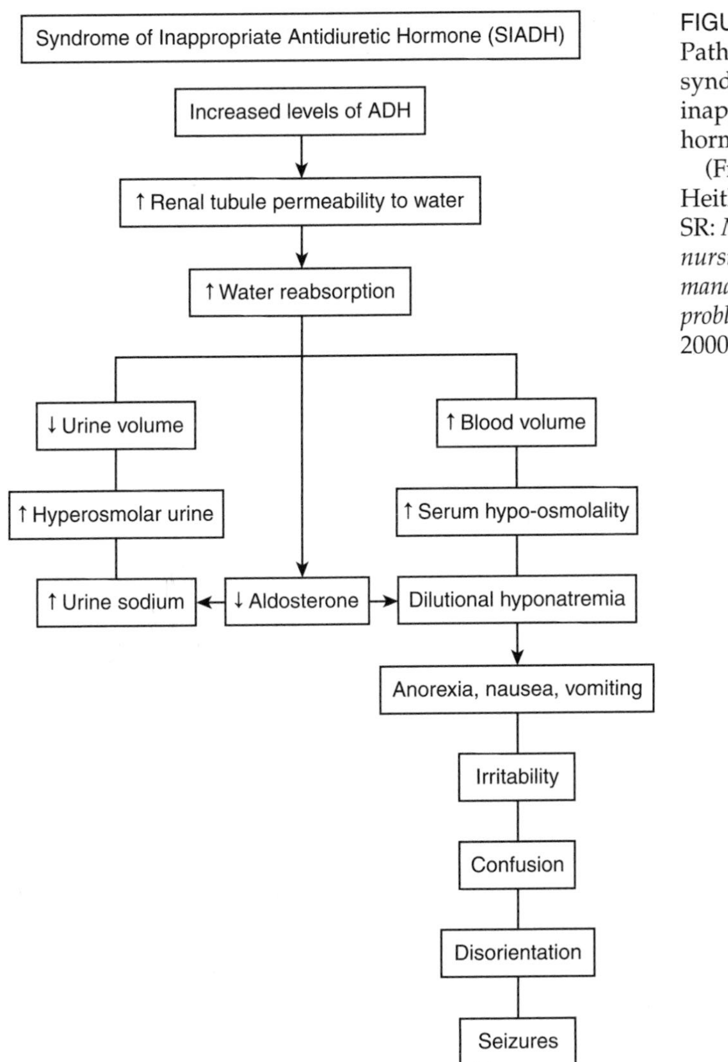

FIGURE 6-12 ■ Pathophysiology of syndrome of inappropriate antidiuretic hormone (*SIADH*). (From Lewis SM, Heitkemper MM, Dirksen SR: *Medical-surgical nursing: assessment and management of clinical problems*, ed 5. St. Louis, 2000, Mosby.)

B. Etiology and Risk Factors

1. **Conditions associated with SIADH**
   a. *Meningitis* (Moritz, 2002)
   b. *Head trauma*
   c. *Cerebral tumors:* Germ cell tumors, craniopharyngiomas, pituitary tumors, hypothalamic gliomas, and third-ventricle tumors. Often children who have tumors fluctuate between SIADH and DI.
   d. *Cerebral hemorrhage*
   e. *Pulmonary disease:* Tuberculosis, pneumonia, abscesses.
   f. *Chronically ill or malnourished* children may develop chronic increased ADH secretion because of a downward resetting of the osmotic receptors. Hyponatremia is chronic, and ADH secretion occurs at a lower serum osmolality.
   g. *Spinal surgery*
2. **Medications associated with SIADH** include analgesics, vincristine, cyclophosphamide, carbamazepine, serotonin reuptake inhibitor antidepressants, ACE inhibitors, and barbiturates (Miller, 2001; Moritz, 2002).
3. **Other precipitating conditions** include severe pain, temperature changes, and mechanical ventilation or positive pressure ventilation, which causes a decrease in atrial natriuretic peptide (ANP) production, thereby stimulating ADH release (Langfeldt and Cooley, 2003).

C. Signs and Symptoms (Table 6-9)

1. The **severity** of the clinical presentation depends on the degree and rapidity with which hyponatremia occurs (Miller, 2001; Moritz and Ayus, 2002).
   a. The first symptom is *low urine output and the absence of hypovolemia.*
   b. *Headache, confusion, lethargy, altered level of consciousness, coma, or seizures* may occur.
   c. *Nausea and vomiting* are often seen.
   d. *Weight gain* may occur, but skin turgor is normal and there is no peripheral edema.
   e. *Filling pressures* are either normal or increase.
   f. *Hypertension and tachycardia* are late signs.

D. Laboratory Data

1. **Serum osmolality** is less than 275 mOsm/kg. Urine osmolality is elevated inappropriately relative to serum osmolality (Moritz and Ayus, 2002).

TABLE 6-9
Differentiation Between Diabetes Insipidus (DI) and Syndrome of Inappropriate Antidiuretic Hormone (SIADH)

	DI	SIADH
Serum sodium	>145 mEq/L	<135 mEq/L
Urine sodium	Low	High
Serum osmolality	>300 mOsm/kg	<275 mOsm/Kg
Urine osmolality	<300 mOsm/L	>800 mOsm/L
Urine specific gravity	<1.005	>1.020
Urine output	High	Low

Data gathered from Holcomb SS: Diabetes insipidus. *Dimens Crit Care Nurs* 21(3):94-98, 2002; Langfeldt LA, Cooley ME: 2003). Syndrome of inappropriate antidiuretic hormone secretion in malignancy: review and implications for nursing management. *Clin J Oncol Nurs* 7 (4):425-430, 2003; Terpstra TL: Syndrome of inappropriate antidiuretic hormone secretion: recognition and management. *Med Surg Nurs* 9(2):61-70, 2000.

2. **Serum sodium** is less than 135 mEq/L. Continued renal excretion of sodium occurs with urine sodium greater than 30 mEq/L.
3. **Urine specific gravity** is greater than 1.020 in the absence of hypovolemia.

E. Interpretation of Diagnostic Studies

1. **Hyponatremia and hypo-osmolality** occur secondary to water retention and hemodilution.
2. **Excessive concentration of urine** occurs with high specific gravity and increased osmolality because of ADH's effect on the renal tubules, resulting in increased water reabsorption by the kidney. Increased fractional excretion of sodium is noted.
3. **Clinically euvolemic**
4. **Renal, thyroid, and adrenal function** tests are normal.

F. Diagnoses

1. **Differential diagnoses** include congestive heart failure, water intoxication, glucocorticoid deficiency, hypothyroidism, renal failure, nephrotic syndrome, third space losses, heat exhaustion (increased sweating), GI tract losses, laboratory error, and cerebral salt wasting (a syndrome of hyponatremia, natriuresis, and hypovolemia without elevated ADH levels that requires fluid replacement [Ferry et al., 2001]).
2. **Collaborative diagnoses**

❖ Fluid and volume excess related to excessive ADH secretion and water retention
❖ Alteration in mental state related to underlying conditions (e.g., meningitis, brain tumors), rapid development of hyponatremia, or acute increases in serum osmolality
❖ Potential for seizures related to serum sodium less than 120 mmol/L
❖ Potential for cerebral hemorrhage that results from rapid correction of hypo-osmolar state

G. Treatment Goals

1. **Normalize** serum sodium.
2. **Normalize** serum osmolality.
3. **Decrease** extravascular fluid volume.
4. **Treat** underlying disorder or discontinue offending medication.
5. **Prevent** neurologic sequelae.

H. Management

1. **Serum sodium** should be normalized over 24 to 48 hours to prevent neurologic sequelae. Acute increases in serum sodium and osmolality can cause the brain cells to shrink, precipitating cerebral hemorrhage, central pontine myelinolysis, and brain injury (Aron et al., 2004; Miller, 2001). Treatment is based on the degree of hyponatremia and hypo-osmolality. Usually fluid restriction to insensible losses (or 800 to 1000 L/m^2 per day) is sufficient to decrease blood volume and increase serum sodium (Moritz and Ayus, 2002). If serum sodium is less than 120 mEq/L and the child is symptomatic (seizures or other mental status abnormality), 3% sodium chloride (NaCl) can be administered by IV push to correct serum sodium to 125 mEq/L. To calculate sodium correction: sodium in mEq = [desired sodium (mEq/L) − patient's actual sodium (mEq/L)] × 0.6 × weight (in kilograms) (Taketomo et al., 2003). Once serum sodium level is greater than 135 mmol/L, fluid restriction may be liberalized to a maintenance fluid rate.
2. **Monitoring** includes intake and output, specific gravity with every void, serum electrolytes and osmolality (every 4 to 6 hours until normal), and daily weights.

Urine electrolytes and osmolality may be obtained to help make the initial diagnosis; however, frequent monitoring may not be necessary. Central venous pressure is obtained if possible; heart rate, blood pressure, and neurologic status are monitored (Langfeldt and Cooley, 2003).

I. Complications

Complications include seizures (if serum sodium is less than 120 mEq/L), cerebral edema (if serum sodium falls too rapidly), cerebral dehydration and hemorrhage (if corrected too quickly), muscle cramps or weakness (secondary to hyponatremia), cerebral dymelination (occurs several days following correction of hyponatremia due to magnitude of correction and underlying illness), and pulmonary edema or hypertension (secondary to fluid overload).

DIABETES INSIPIDUS

A. Pathophysiology

1. **Diabetes insipidus (DI)** is a clinical condition that is characterized by a decrease in both urine concentrating ability and water conservation, resulting in excessive diuresis and low urine osmolality (Figure 6-13). The two types of DI are central (or neurogenic) and nephrogenic. DI can be transient; it occurs in many neurosurgical patients, or it can be a permanent condition (Wong and Verbalis, 2002).
2. **Central** DI is the most common form of DI in children and in the critical care environment. Deficiency of ADH is due to failure of the hypothalamus to synthesize, or failure of the posterior pituitary to secrete, or both.
3. **Nephrogenic** DI is characterized by normal secretion of ADH by the posterior pituitary. The distal tubule and the collecting duct in the kidney, however, are resistant to the effects of ADH. Nephrogenic DI is the most difficult form of DI to treat.

B. Etiologies and Risk Factors

1. **Central DI** results from pituitary and suprasellar surgery, midline defects (septooptic dysplasia and agenesis of the corpus callosum), head trauma (usually an ominous sign that indicates absent pituitary function), CNS infections, cerebral edema, cerebral hemorrhage or infarct; or it may be congenital, familial, or idiopathic (Holcomb, 2002; Wong and Verbalis, 2002).
2. **Nephrogenic DI** is related to chronic renal disease, polycystic kidney disease, familial tendency, pregnancy, chronic hypokalemia, chronic hypercalcemia, starvation, and medications such as lithium, amphotericin B, phenytoin, ethanol, diuretics, and gentamicin. Sickle cell nephropathy can also cause DI (Holcomb, 2002; Wong and Verbalis, 2002).

C. Signs and Symptoms (see Table 6-9)

1. **A large quantity of dilute urine** is the first sign of DI.
2. **Hypernatremia** (serum sodium is greater than 145 mmol/L)
3. **Serum hyperosmolality** (greater than 300 mOsm/kg)
4. **Polyuria,** dilute urine with specific gravity is less than 1.005
5. **Urine osmolality** less than 200 mOsm/kg
6. **Polydipsia**
7. **Signs of dehydration** include low central venous pressure, tachycardia, hypotension, poor skin turgor, dry mucous membranes, and weight loss.

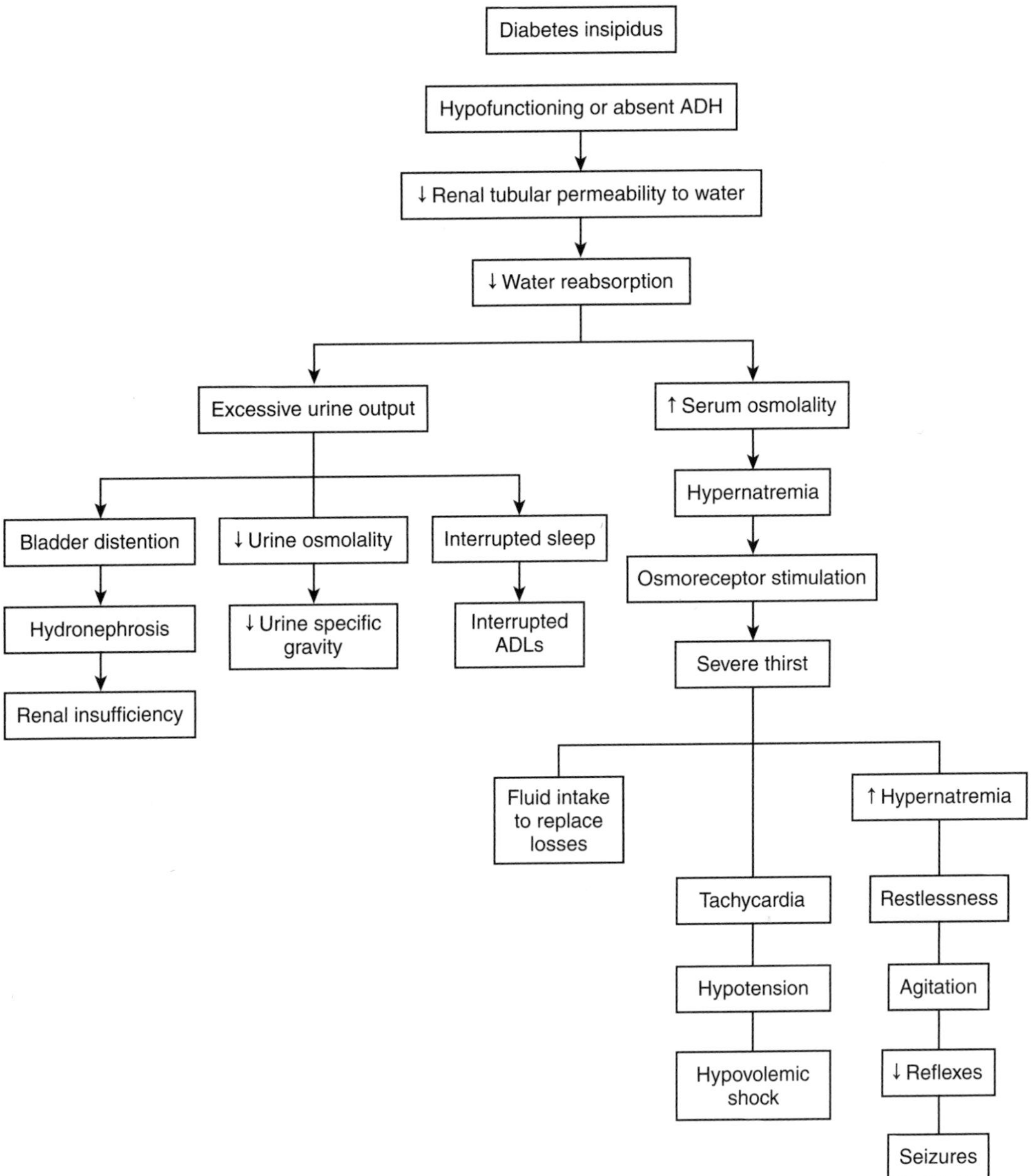

FIGURE 6-13 ■ Pathophysiology of diabetes insipidus (DI). *ADH,* antidiuretic hormone; ADLs, activities of daily living.

(From Lewis SM, Heitkemper MM, Dirksen SR: *Medical surgical nursing: assessment and management of clinical problems,* ed 5. St. Louis, 2000, Mosby.)

8. **Altered mental status:** Lethargy, confusion, and coma (see lab values in Table 6-9)

D. Interpretation of Diagnostic Studies

1. **Hypernatremia and hyperosmolality** are due to water loss and hemoconcentration.
2. **Low specific gravity and urine osmolality** are due to the kidney's inability to reabsorb water and concentrate urine.

3. **Vasopressin levels** are low or unmeasurable in central DI. Vasopressin levels are normal or high in nephrogenic DI.
4. **MRI or CT** scan is used for the diagnosis of cerebral edema or underlying conditions such as cerebral tumors, calcifications, hypopituitarism, or midline defects.
5. **Pituitary function** tests determine GH or ACTH defects.
6. A **water deprivation test** can be used to diagnosis DI, but it is not typically done in critically ill children (Holcomb, 2002). This test requires careful supervision and monitoring. All medications that can interfere with the secretion or action of ADH should be discontinued before the test (including alcohol and tobacco). Unrestricted access to fluids should be allowed until the test starts. At the beginning of the study, a baseline weight, serum sodium and osmolality, urine osmolality, and volume are recorded. Over the next 6 to 8 hours, all fluids and foods are withheld. The child is weighed every hour, and urine volume and osmolality are measured with every void. At the end of the study, serum laboratory specimens are redrawn. The test is terminated if body weight falls 3% to 5%. If serum osmolality remains high and hypotonic polyuria continues in spite of water deprivation, the diagnosis of DI is made (Holcomb, 2002).
7. An **ADH test** can to useful to differentiate between central and nephrogenic DI. The patient is given a dose of vasopressin or desmopressin (DDAVP). If urine volume falls and becomes more concentrated, the patient has central DI; if there is no response to vasopressin, the patient has nephrogenic DI (Holcomb, 2002).

E. Diagnoses

1. **Differential diagnoses** include DM, sodium excess (improperly mixed formula or iatrogenic sodium administration), overuse of diuretics, adipsia, increased insensible water loss, and primary polydipsia.
2. **Collaborative diagnoses**

❖ Potential for low cardiac output secondary to hypovolemia related to diuresis and intravascular volume loss

❖ Potential for neurologic insult related to underlying causes (e.g., midline defects, head trauma) or a rapid rise in serum osmolality

❖ Potential for the development of cerebral edema related to rapid correction of hyperosmolar state

❖ Fluid and electrolyte imbalance related to excessive diuresis

F. Treatment Goals

1. **Correct** dehydration and fluid deficits.
2. **Correct** hypernatremia slowly.
3. **Control** free water loss by the kidney.
4. **Prevent** neurologic sequelae.

G. Management

1. In **central DI,** the decision to use fluid, or ADH replacement therapy, or both is often based on the severity of the illness, the patient's condition, and the underlying cause. Hypernatremia is corrected slowly; rapid correction will alter osmolarity and can result in cerebral edema. Sodium levels should fall no faster than 1 mg/dL per hour. If dehydration is severe and shock is present, treat the shock with fluid resuscitation. Patients who are dehydrated will need fluid volume deficits replaced with hypotonic fluids (normal saline will be

TABLE 6-10
Antidiuretic Hormone (ADH) Replacement Therapies

Name	Dose	Onset	Duration (hr)
Aqueous vasopressin, IM, sub-Q	2.5-10 units 2-4 times a day (range: 5-30 mcg/day)	1 hr	2-8 hr
Aqueous vasopressin, IV	0.5 milliunits/kg/hr (0.0005 units/kg/hr) Double dose every 30 min as needed to maximum 0.01 units/kg/hr	30 min	No information available
Desmopressin (DDAVP), Intranasal	5 mcg/day in 1-2 divided doses	Within 1 hr	5-21 hr
Oral	0.05 mg twice daily (range, 0.1-0.8 mg daily)	1 hr	6-8 hr

Data from Taketomo CK, Hodding JH, Kraus DM: *Pediatric dose handbook,* ed 11. Cleveland, Ohio, 2004, Lexi-Comp.

hypotonic in a patient with hypernatremia) over 48 hours. In acute, sudden-onset DI, urine replacement milliliter per milliliter with hypotonic fluids in addition to maintenance fluids normalizes serum electrolytes and blood volume, *or* ADH replacement therapy is titrated to keep specific gravity at a level greater than 1.010 and urine output at 2 mL/kg per hour with normal serum sodium. ADH replacement may be administered intranasally, IV, intramuscularly (IM), subcutaneously, orally, or by continuous infusion (Table 6-10). Children with an intact thirst mechanism are allowed unlimited access to oral fluids, and IV fluids are discontinued. Infants, comatose patients, or children with an abnormal thirst response require careful monitoring of their fluid intake (enteral or parental or both).

2. **Nephrogenic DI** is difficult to treat. A sodium-restricted diet may help to decrease the solute load to the kidneys. Hydrochlorothiazide (diuretic) paradoxically reduces polyuria by causing excessive sodium reabsorption in the proximal tubule, with resultant reduction of volume delivered to the distal tubule and less urine formed, thus reducing the glomerular filtration rate (Cheetham and Baylis, 2004). This mechanism is not well understood. NSAIDs inhibit renal production of prostaglandin, thereby enhancing renal responsiveness to ADH. ADH replacement therapy is of no value.
3. **Monitoring** includes intake and output, daily weights, frequent hemodynamic and neurologic assessments, urine specific gravity, urine osmolality, and serum sodium and osmolality. In severe cases, serum sodium may need to be monitored frequently (i.e., every 1 to 2 hours) until normal.

H. Complications

Complications include cardiac collapse and shock from rapid diuresis; neurologic sequelae from a rapid rise in serum osmolality; cerebral edema, herniation, and possible death due to rapid correction of hyperosmolar state; electrolyte imbalances secondary to inadequate monitoring of serum electrolytes during therapy; and water intoxication and fluid overload related to overtreatment with ADH replacement therapy.

REFERENCES

Abbruzzi G, Stork CM: Pediatric toxicologic concerns. *Emerg Med Clin North Am* 20(1):223-247, 2000.

Adams KF, Mathur VS, Gheorghiade M: B-type natriuretic peptide: from bench to bedside. *Am Heart J* 145(2):34-46, 2003.

Aron DC, Findling JW, Tyrrell JB: Hypothalamus and pituitary gland. In Greenspan FS, Gardner DG, editors: *Basic & clinical endocrinology,* ed 7. New York, 2004, Lange Medical Books/McGraw-Hill.

Bettendorf M et al.: Tri-iodothyronine treatment in children after cardiac surgery: a double-blind, randomized, placebo-controlled trial. *Lancet* 356(9229):529-534, 2000.

Breault DT, Majzoub JA: Diabetes insipidus. In Behrman RE, Kliegman RM, Jenson HB, editors: *Nelson textbook of pediatrics,* ed 17. Philadelphia, 2004, W. B. Saunders.

Carcillo J, Fields A: Clinical practice parameters for hemodynamic support of pediatric & neonatal patients in septic shock. *Crit Care Med* 30(6):1365-1378, 2002.

Cheetham T, Baylis PH: Diabetes insipidus in children: pathophysiology, diagnosis and management. *Paediatr Drugs* 4(12): 785-796, 2004.

Chrousos GP: Organization and integration of the endocrine system. In Sperling MA, editor: *Pediataric endocrinology,* ed 2. Philadephia, 2002, W. B. Saunders.

Delaney MF, Zisman A, Kettyle WM: Diabetic ketoacidosis and hyperglycemia hyperosmolar nonketotic syndrome. *Endocrinol Metab Clin* 29(4):683-705, 2000.

Dorton AM: The pituitary gland: embryology, physiology and pathophysiology. *Neonatal Network* 19(2):9-17, 2000.

Dunger DB et al.: European Society for Paediatric Endocrinology/Lawson Wilkins Pediatric Endocrine Society Consensus Statement on Diabetes Ketoacidosis in Children and Adolescents. *Pediatrics* 113(2):e133, 2004. http://www.pediatrics.org/cgi/content/full/113/2/e133.

Fagot-Campagna A et al.: Type 2 diabetes among North American children and adolescents: an epidemic review and a public health perspective. *J Pediatr* 136(5): 664, 2000.

Fajans SS, Bell GI, Polonsky KS: Molecular mechanisms and clinical pathophysiology of maturity-onset diabetes of the young. *N Engl J Med* 345(13):971-980, 2001.

Ferry RJ et al.: Hyponatremia and polyuria in children with central diabetes insipidus: challenges in diagnosis and management. *J Pediatr* 138(5):744-747, 2001.

Fisher DA: Disorders of the thyroid in the newborn and infant. In Sperling MA, editor: *Pediataric endocrinology,* ed 2. Philadelphia, 2002, W. B. Saunders.

Fliers E, Alkemake A, Wiersinga WM: The hypothalamic-pituitary-thyroid axis in critical illness. *Best Pract Res Clin Endocrinol Metab* 15(4):453-464, 2001.

Glaser N et al.: Risk factors for cerebral edema in children with diabetic ketoacidosis. *N Engl J Med* 344 (4):264-269, 2001.

Greenspan FS: The thyroid gland. In Greenspan FS, Gardner DG, editors: *Basic and clinical endocrinology,* ed. 7. New York, 2004, Lange Medical Books/McGraw-Hill.

Goldberg PA, Inzucchi SE: Critical issues in endocrinology. *Clin Chest Med* 24(4): 583-606, 2003.

Guyton AC, Hall JE: *Textbook of medical physiology,* ed 10. Philadelphia, 2001, W. B. Saunders.

Hass LB: Nursing assessment endocrine system. In Lewis SM, Heitkemper MM, Dirksen SR, editors: *Medical surgical nursing assessment and management of clinical problems,* ed 5. St. Louis, 2000, Mosby.

Holcomb SS: Diabetes insipidus. *Dimens Crit Care Nurs* 21(3):94-98, 2002.

Holcomb SS: Detecting thyroid disease, part 1. *Nursing* 33(8):32cc1-32cc4, 2003.

Jones RE, Huether SE: Alterations of hormonal regulation. In McCance K, Huether SE, editors: *Pathophysiology: the biologic basis for disease in adults & children,* ed 4. St. Louis, 2002, Mosby.

Kaufman FR: Diabetes mellitus. *Pediatr Rev* 24(9):291-299, 2003.

Kemper AR, Foster CM: Congenital hypothyroidism: a guide for the general pediatrician. *Contemp Pediatr* 20(6):32-42, 2003.

Kirsten D: The thyroid gland: physiology and pathophysiology. *Neonatal Network* 19(8):11-26, 2000.

Langfeldt LA, Cooley ME: Syndrome of inappropriate antidiuretic hormone secretion in malignancy: review and implications for nursing management. *Clin J Oncol Nurs* 7(4):425-430, 2003.

Langton JE, Brent GA: Nonthyroidal illness syndrome: evaluation of thyroid function in sick patients. *Endocrinol Metab Clin* 31(1):159-172, 2002.

Levin LS, White PC: Disorders of the adrenal glands. In Behrman RE, Kliegman RM, Jenson HB, editors: *Nelson textbook of pediatrics,* ed 17. Philadelphia, 2004, W. B. Saunders.

Liedel JL et al.: Use of vasopressin in refractory hypotension in children with vasodilatory shock: five cases and a review of the literature. *Pediatr Crit Care Med* (3)1:15, 2002.

Marcin JP et al.: Factors associated with adverse outcomes in children with diabetic ketoacidosis-related cerebral edema. *J Pediatr* 141(6):793-797, 2002.

Masharani U, Karam J, German M: Pancreatic hormones & diabetes mellitus. In Greenspan FS, Gardner DG, editor: *Basic and clinical endocrinology,* ed 7. New York, 2004, Lange Medical Books/McGraw-Hill.

Menon RK, Sperling MA: Diabetic ketoacidosis. In Menon RK, Sperling MA, editors: *Pediatric diabetes.* Boston, 2003, Kluwer Academic Publishers.

Miller M: Endocrine and metabolic dysfunction syndromes in the critically ill: syndromes of excess antidiuretic hormone release. *Crit Care Clin* 17(1):11-23, 2001.

Moff I, Peterson R: Endocrinology. In Gunn VL, Nechyba C, editor: *The Harriet Lane handbook,* ed 16. Philadelphia, 2002, Mosby.

Moore KL, Persaud TVN: *The developing human,* ed 7. Philadelphia, 2003, W. B. Saunders.

Moritz ML, Ayus JC: Disorders of water metabolism in children: hyponatremia and hypernatremia. *Pediatr Rev* 23(11): 371-379, 2002.

Muglia LJ, Majzoub JA: Disorders of the posterior pituitary. In Sperling MA, editor: *Pediataric endocrinology,* ed 2. Philadelphia, 2002, W. B. Saunders.

Palma Sisto PA: Endocrine disorders in the neonate. *Pediatr Clin North Am* 51(4):1141, 2004.

Pandian R, Nakamoto JM: Rational use of the laboratory for children and adult growth hormone deficiency. *Clin Lab Med* 24(1):141-174, 2004.

Piano M, Huether SE: Mechanisms of hormonal regulation. In McCance K, Huether SE, editors: *Pathophysiology: the biologic basis for disease in adults & children,* ed 4. St. Louis, 2002, Mosby.

Portman MA, Fearneyhough C, Karl TR et al.: The triiodothyronine for infants and children undergoing cardiopulmonary bypass (TRICC) study: design and rationale. *Am Heart J* 148(3):393-398, 2004.

Pratap U, Slavik Z, Ofoe VD et al.: Octreotide to treat postoperative chylothorax after cardiac operations in children. *Ann Thorac Surg* 72:1740-1742, 2001.

Quintana EC: Factors associated with adverse outcomes in children with diabetic ketoacidosis-related cerebral edema. *Ann Emerg Med* 43(6):2539-2543, 2004.

Rosenbloom AL, Connor EL: Hypopituitarism and other disorders of the growth hormone and insulin-like growth factor axis. In Lifshitz F, editor: *Pediatric endocrinology,* ed 4. New York, 2003, Marcel Dekkel.

Rosenstock J: Insulin therapy: optimizing control of type 1 and type 2 diabetes. *Clin Cornerstone* 4(2):50-64, 2001.

Rosenzweig EB, Starc TJ, Chen JM et al.: Intravenous arginine-vasopressin in children with vasodilatory shock after cardiac surgery. *Circulation* 100:11.182–11.186, 1999.

Settle M: The hypothalamus. *Neonatal Network* 19(6):9-14, 2000.

Shobach D, Marcus R, Bikle D: Metabolic bone disease. In Greenspan FS, Gardner DG, editors: *Basic & clinical endocrinology,* ed 7. New York, 2004, Lange Medical Books/McGraw-Hill.

Sperling MA: Diabetes mellitus. In Sperling MA, editor: *Pediataric endocrinology,* ed 2. Philadephia, 2002, W. B. Saunders.

Sperling MA, Menon RK: Differential diagnosis and management of neonatal hypoglycemia. *Pediatr Clin North Am* 51(3):703-723, 2004.

Stanley CA et al.: Hypoglycemia in neonates and infants. In Sperling MA, editor: *Pediataric endocrinology,* ed 2. Philadelphia, 2002, W. B. Saunders.

Steffensrud S: Parathyroids: the forgotten glands. *Neonatal Network* 19(1):9-16, 2000.

Stoll BJ, Kliegman RM: The endocrine system. In Behrman RE, Kliegman RM, Jenson HB, editors: *Nelson textbook of pediatrics,* ed 17. Philadelphia, 2004, W. B. Saunders.

Taketomo CK, Hodding JH, Kraus DM: *Pediatric dose handbook,* ed 11. Cleveland, Ohio, 2004, Lexi-Comp.

Terpstra TL: Syndrome of inappropriate antidiuretic hormone secretion: recognition and management. *Med Surg Nurs* 9(2): 61-70, 2000.

Thibodeau GA, Patton KT: *Anatomy and physiology*, ed 5. St. Louis, 2003, Mosby.

Thornton PS et al.: Hypoglycemia in the infant and child. In Sperling MA, editor: *Pediataric endocrinology*, ed 2. Philadelphia, 2002, W. B. Saunders.

Van den Berghe G: Endocrine evaluation of patients with critical illness. *Endocrinol Metab Clin* 32(2):385-410, 2003.

Van den Berghe G, Wouters P, Weekers F et al. Intensive insulin therapy in critically patients. *N Engl J Med* 345(19):1359-1367, 2001.

Vaughan ED: Diseases of the adrenal gland. *Med Clin North Am* 88(2):443-466, 2004.

Werlin SL: Exocrine pancreas. In Behrman RE, Kliegman RM, Jenson HB, editors: *Nelson textbook of pediatrics*, ed 17. Philadelphia, 2004, W. B. Saunders.

Wolfsdorf JI, Weinstein DA: Hypoglycemia in children. In Lifshitz F, editor: *Pediatric endocrinology*, ed 4. New York, 2003, Marcel Dekker.

Wong LL, Verbalis JG: Systemic diseases associated with disorders of water homeostatis. *Endocrinol Metab Clin* 31(1): 121-140, 2002.

Wraight PR et al: Genetics of diabetes in childhood. In Menon RK, Sperling MA, editors: *Pediatric diabetes*. Boston, 2003, Kluwer Academic Publishers.

Zap LB, Mukerjee D, Timms PM et al.: Natriuretic peptides, respiratory disease, and the right heart. *Chest* 126(4):1330-1336, 2004.

Zuppa AF et al. The effect of a thyroid hormone infusion on vasopressor support in critical ill children with cessation of neurological function. *Crit Care Med* 32(11): 2318-2322, 2004.

CHAPTER

7 Gastrointestinal System

SARAH A. MARTIN AND SHARI SIMONE

DEVELOPMENTAL ANATOMY AND PHYSIOLOGY

A. Embryologic Development of the Digestive Tract (Figure 7-1)

1. The **digestive tract** develops from the primitive gut, which differentiates into the foregut, midgut, and hindgut by the third week of gestation (Kenner and Lott, 2003).
   a. *Foregut:* Buccal cavity, salivary glands, pharynx, esophagus, stomach, proximal duodenum, liver, pancreas, and bile duct system
   b. *Midgut:* Distal duodenum, jejunum, ileum, cecum, appendix, ascending colon, and proximal part of transverse colon
   c. *Hindgut:* Remainder of the colon and rectum
2. The **esophagus and trachea** are a single tube until the fourth week of gestation, at which time the tracheoesophageal septum begins to separate the structures.
3. **Development of the gut** is nearly complete by week 20 of gestation.

B. Gastric Activity

1. **Gastric motility** in infants is decreased and somewhat irregular compared with the adult. Gastric emptying is increased.
2. **Gastroesophageal reflux** is common during the first 6 months because of a complex set of factors, including pressure-volume changes and anatomic relationships causing inappropriate relaxation of the lower esophageal sphincter.

C. Immature Neonatal Liver

The liver matures in function during the first year of life. Toxic substances are inefficiently detoxified. Synthesis of liver enzymes and degradation are impaired. Adjust therapeutic drug dosing for hepatotoxicity as necessary.

D. Metabolic Rate in Children

1. **Caloric requirements** per kilogram of weight are greater in children than in adults. The basal metabolic rate (BMR) is highest during the first 2 years of life and increases during growth spurts.
2. **Children** require baseline calories, regardless of their activity level, to promote growth and development and require additional calories during acute illness (i.e., disease, surgery, fever, and pain) (Table 7-1). The BMR increases 12% with each centigrade degree of temperature increase above 37° C. Paralyzed children have decreased caloric needs. Caloric needs can be supplied by enteral or parenteral feedings.

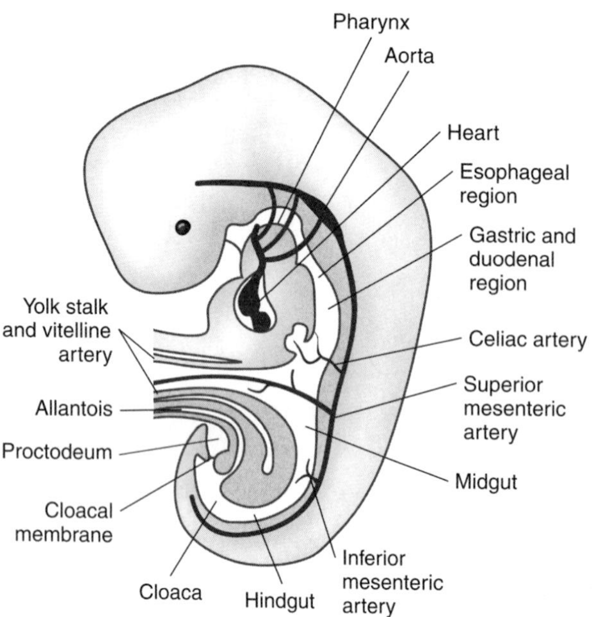

FIGURE 7-1 ■ Primitive gut. (From Kenner C, Lott JW: *Comprehensive neonatal nursing*, ed 3. Philadelphia, 2003, W. B. Saunders.)

TABLE 7-1
Caloric Requirements in Critically Ill Children

Age	kcal/kg/d
High-risk neonate	120–150
0–6 mo	120
6–12 mo	100
1–2 y	90–100
2–6 y	80–90
7–9 y	70–80
10–12 y	50–60
>12 y	40

E. General Anatomic Considerations

1. The **abdominal wall** is less muscular in the infant and toddler, making the abdominal organs easier to palpate. In the infant, the liver can be palpated 1 to 2 cm below the right costal margin (RCM) at the midclavicular line.
2. In **younger children,** the contour of the abdomen is protuberant because of immature abdominal musculature. After 4 years of age, the abdomen is no longer protuberant when the child is in a supine position; but, because of lumbar lordosis, the abdomen remains protuberant when the child stands.

ANATOMY AND PHYSIOLOGY

A. Structure and Function (Figure 7-2)

1. **Oral cavity:** The oral cavity serves as a reservoir for chewing and mixing food with saliva. *Salivary glands* include the submandibular, sublingual, and parotid glands. Saliva is composed of water, small amounts of mucus, sodium bicarbonate, chloride, potassium, and amylase. Amylase begins carbohydrate digestion.

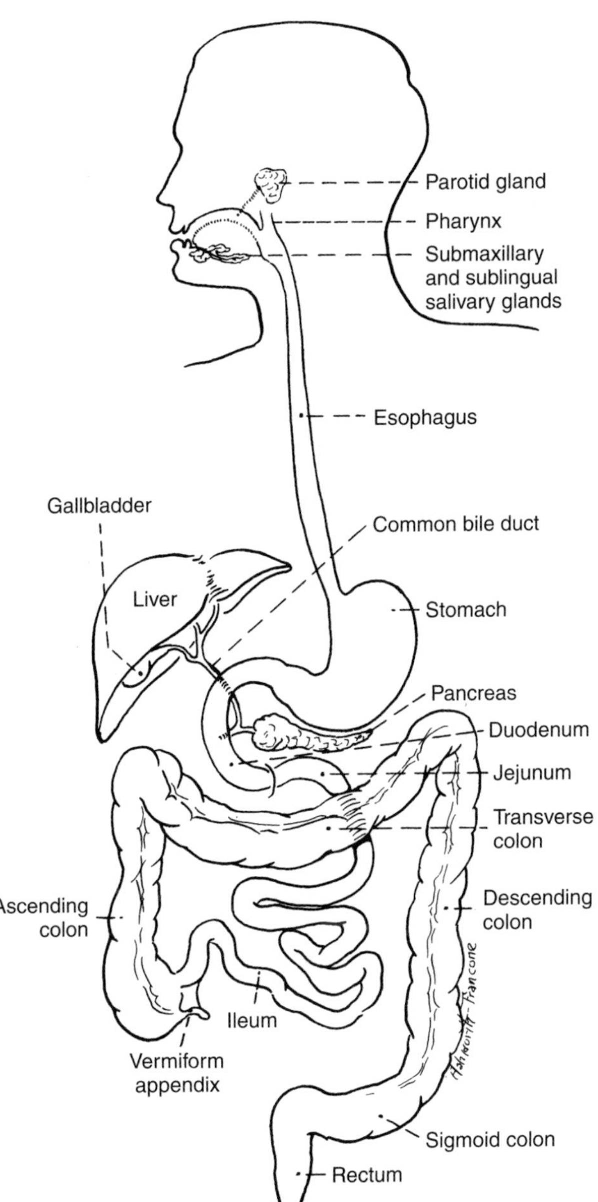

FIGURE 7-2 ■ Gastrointestinal tract and associated structures.
(Reprinted with permission from Jacob SW, Francone CA: *Elements of anatomy and physiology*, ed 2. Philadelphia, 1989, W. B. Saunders.)

2. The **esophagus** propels swallowed food to the stomach. The upper esophageal sphincter prevents air from entering the esophagus during respiration. The lower esophageal sphincter closes after swallowing to prevent reflux of gastric contents into the esophagus.
3. **Stomach**
   a. The *stomach* is a hollow, muscular organ that acts as a reservoir for ingested food. It secretes digestive juices that mix with digested food (chyme). *Parietal cells* secrete hydrochloric acid and intrinsic factor. Intrinsic factor is a glycoprotein that is required for vitamin B_{12} absorption. The secretion is regulated by stimuli (i.e., H_2 histamine receptors). *Chief cells* secrete pepsinogen, which combines with hydrochloric acid to break down protein.

b. *Gastric emptying* is affected by the volume of food, osmotic pressure, and chemical composition of the contents. Emptying is controlled by the pyloric sphincter. Delayed emptying is caused by foods with high fat content, solid foods, sedatives, sleep, and specific hormones (i.e., secretin and cholecystokinin). Accelerated emptying is caused by foods with high carbohydrate content, liquids, and increased volume.

4. The **small intestine** is the primary site for digestion and absorption of fats, amino acids, sugars, proteins, carbohydrates, and vitamins. The small intestine is anatomically adapted to increase surface digestion and absorption due to folds of mucosa lined with villi and the brush-border membrane. The brush border contains digestive enzymes and contributes to the transfer of nutrients and electrolytes. The epithelial absorptive cells are called *enterocytes*. Glutamine (amino acid) stimulates the proliferation of enterocytes. The gastrointestinal tract (GI) continuously renews the cells lining its surface.
   a. The *duodenum* is the primary site for the absorption of iron, trace metals, and water-soluble vitamins.
   b. The *jejunum* is the principal absorption site for proteins and sugar carbohydrates. Ninety percent of nutrients and 50% of water and electrolytes are absorbed here.
   c. The *ileum* is responsible for absorption of bile salts and vitamin B_{12}. The ileoceccal valve controls the entry of digested material from the ileum into the large intestine and prevents reflux into the small intestine. Digestion in the ileum continues by the action of pancreatic enzymes, intestinal enzymes, and bile salts. Carbohydrates are broken down into monosaccharides and disaccharides and are absorbed by villous capillaries. Proteins are degraded to peptides and amino acids and are absorbed by villous capillaries. Fats are emulsified and reduced to fatty acids and monoglycerides.
5. **Colon:** The anatomic segments of the colon or large intestine include the cecum, ascending colon, transverse colon, descending colon, sigmoid colon, and rectum. Water and electrolytes are reabsorbed in the descending colon. Feces are stored in the rectum. The greatest growth of anaerobic and gram-negative aerobic bacteria is in the ascending colon. *Bacteroides fragilis* (anaerobic) and *Escherichia coli* (aerobic) play a role in metabolizing bile salts and synthesizing vitamins.
6. **Pancreas:** The pancreas's exocrine function is to secrete bicarbonate and enzymes (e.g., amylase, lipase) for digestion and absorption of fats, carbohydrates, and proteins. The pancreas's endocrine function involves islet cells, which function in glucose homeostasis by synthesizing and secreting insulin.
7. **Liver**
   a. *Liver functions* include the following:
      - Formation of clotting (coagulation) factors I, II, V, VII, IX, X, and XI
      - Synthesis of plasma proteins (albumin, fibrinogen, and 60% to 80% of globulins)
      - Synthesis and transportation of bile (bile salts, pigment, and cholesterol)
      - Storage of glycogen, fat, and fat-soluble vitamins
      - Metabolism of fats, carbohydrates, and proteins
      - Metabolism and deactivation of bilirubin and many toxins by oxidation or conjugation reactions
   b. Three fourths of the blood supply to the liver is supplied by the *portal venous system* (blood rich in nutrients) and one fourth by the hepatic artery (blood rich in oxygen).

c. *Nutrients* are absorbed from the GI tract and transported by either the portal or lymphatic circulation. The lymphatic system plays a pivotal role in transporting lipid-soluble substances.

8. **Biliary tree and gallbladder:** The biliary tree serves as the conduit for bile flow from the liver to the duodenum. The gallbladder provides a storage and concentration site for bile.
9. **Splanchnic circulation:** The splanchnic circulation supplies blood to the stomach, small intestine, and colon. It receives one fourth of the body's cardiac output. The major arterial branches are the celiac, superior mesenteric, and inferior mesenteric. Venous drainage from the stomach, pancreas, small intestine, and colon flows to the portal vein to the liver and then to the heart through the hepatic vein and inferior vena cava.

B. Regulation of Fluid and Electrolyte Movement

Large volumes of water, electrolytes, proteins, and bile salts are secreted and reabsorbed throughout the GI tract, resulting in massive fluid and electrolyte shifts. Fluid and electrolyte movement occurs concurrently with digestion and absorption of nutrients.

CLINICAL ASSESSMENT

A. General Principles of Abdominal Assessment

Examination of the abdomen is difficult in a child. A frightened child will not cooperate with the examination. A child suffering from multisystem trauma will be unable to localize pain. The preferred order of assessment is inspection, auscultation, palpation, and percussion.

B. Abdominal Examination Assessment Techniques

1. **Inspection:** Evaluate for size, contour, symmetry, integrity, visible peristalsis, umbilicus, masses, and wounds. Underdeveloped abdominal musculature in children allows easier visualization of masses and fluid waves. Abdominal distention (the abdomen is normally rounded in infants and toddlers) is the hallmark sign of obstruction.
2. **Auscultation**
   a. Determine the *absence, presence, and character of peristalsis or bowel sounds.* Bowel sounds are absent in paralytic ileus and peritonitis. A venous hum heard over the upper area of the abdomen suggests portal obstruction. A bruit (caused by turbulent blood flow through a partially occluded artery) suggests an arteriovenous malformation (AVM). High-pitched or hyperactive bowel sounds suggest an obstruction.
   b. *Bowel sounds* should be heard every 5 to 30 seconds. Listen to all four quadrants for a few minutes to confirm absent bowel sounds.
3. **Palpation:** Begin with light palpation and assess for guarding and tenderness. With deep palpation, assess for abdominal tone, masses, pulsations, fluid, and organ enlargement. The liver is normally palpated at the RCM or is nonpalpable. The spleen is not normally palpable.
4. **Percussion:** Percussion is used to estimate the size of organs and aids in the diagnosis of ascites, obstruction, and peritonitis. Assess for abdominal distention, fluid, masses, or organ enlargement. Percussion of solid organs (liver and spleen) and ascites elicits dullness. Absence of dullness over the liver may be found with free air in the abdomen secondary to perforation. The stomach is

tympanic when empty. Depending on contents, the intestines' tone is hyperresonant to tympanic.

INVASIVE AND NONINVASIVE DIAGNOSTIC STUDIES

Serial laboratory and diagnostic studies are obtained for all patients with a GI disorder. Table 7-2 summarizes common laboratory tests indicating GI dysfunction. Diagnostic studies commonly used to determine GI pathology are summarized in Table 7-3.

PHARMACOLOGY

A. Antibleeding Agents

1. **Vasopressin (Pitressin) (Taketomo et al., 2003)**
   a. *Action:* Nonselective, short-acting vasoconstrictor. It decreases splanchnic blood flow and portal hypertension.
   b. *Uses:* GI hemorrhage.
   c. *Dosage:* Continuous intravenous (IV) infusion—Initial 0.002 to 0.005 units/kg per minute; double as needed every 30 minutes to a maximum of 0.01 units/kg per minute. Maximum recommended dose is 0.01 units/kg per minute.
   d. *Side effects* include hypertension, bradycardia, arrhythmias, wheezing, bronchospasm, abdominal cramping, vomiting, decreased urine output, and hyponatremia.
2. **Octreotide acetate (Sandostatin) (Taketomo et al., 2003)**
   a. *Action:* Decreases splanchnic blood flow; inhibits gastrin synthesis and gastric acid output.
   b. *Uses:* For GI hemorrhage and intractable diarrhea. This agent has been used for the treatment of chylothorax. Somatostatin is used when conservative treatment fails.
   c. *Dosage:* 1 mcg/kg IV bolus; infusion rate 1 mcg/kg per hour (IV) for GI hemorrhage, titrating the rate to response. Dosage of 1 to 10 mcg/kg every 12 hours (IV, subcutaneous [SC]) is used for intractable diarrhea. Dose reductions are recommended for patients with renal failure.
   d. *Side effects* include bradycardia, chest pain, hypertension, abdominal cramps, nausea, diarrhea, headache, fat malabsorption, hypoglycemia or hyperglycemia, and hypothyroidism.
3. **Vitamin K_1, phytonadione (AquaMEPHYTON, Mephyton) (Taketomo et al., 2003)**
   a. *Action:* Provides vitamin K activity and can be used as a cofactor in the liver synthesis of clotting factors II, VII, IX, and X.
   b. *Uses:* Prevents and treats hypoprothrombinemia caused by drug- or anticoagulant-induced vitamin K deficiency.
   c. *Dosage:* 1 to 2 mg per single dose SC, IV, or intramuscular (IM). IM should be used only when SC administration is not feasible. Dosages up to 10 mg daily have been used. Dilute in 5 to 10 mL of IV fluid for IV infusion over 15 to 30 minutes. The maximum rate of IV administration should not exceed 1 mg per minute in adults or 0.5 mg per minute in children at a maximum concentration of 10 mg/mL.
   d. *Side effects* include a transient flushing reaction, rare hypotension, rare dizziness, rash, and urticaria. Vitamin K_1 may cause anaphylaxis or hypersensitivity (rare).

TABLE 7-2
Liver Function Tests (LFTs)

LFT	Function	Pediatric Reference Value	Changes with Hepatic Failure
Alanine aminotransferase (ALT)	ALT catalyzes the reversible transfer of an amino group between the amino acid alanine and α-glutamic acid.	<37 IU/L	ALT initially increases with cell destruction. Following cell necrosis, enzyme level peaks and then decreases. It may be an ominous sign if the enzyme level peaks and falls rapidly. ALT is more hepatic specific as compared to AST. Isolated increases are characteristic of hepatitis.
Aspartate aminotransferase (AST)	AST catalyzes the reversible transfer of the amino group between the amino acid aspartate and α-ketoglutamic acid.	<34 IU/L	AST initially increases with cell destruction. Following cell necrosis, enzyme level peaks and then decreases. It is an ominous sign if the enzyme level peaks and falls rapidly. Isolated increases are characteristic of hepatitis.
Alkaline phosphatase (ALP)	ALP cleaves phosphates from compounds with a single phosphate group. The hepatic isoenzymes are believed to be largely derived from the epithelium of the intrahepatic bile ducts, rather than from hepatocytes.	Newborn: <310 IU/L 1 mo–1 yr: <360 IU/L 1–10 y: <290 IU/L 10–15 y: <400 IU/L >15 y: <110 IU/L	ALP levels increase with inflammation or obstruction of the hepatobiliary tract.
γ-Glutamyl transpeptidase (GGTP)	GGTP is an isoenzyme of ALP. GGTP catalyzes the transfer of glutamyl groups among peptidase and amino acids.	<120 IU/L	Hepatobiliary causes should be considered with increased levels. Significantly increased levels reflect hepatobiliary obstruction, whereas moderately elevated levels may suggest hepatocellular destruction.
Bilirubin	Bilirubin is a by-product of the heme portion of the breakdown of the hemoglobin molecule. Fat-soluble bilirubin binds to albumin as indirect bilirubin for transport to the liver. In the liver, fat-soluble bilirubin is detached from the albumin and conjugated with glucuronic acid, rendering it water	Total bilirubin Newborn: 1–12 mg/dL Child: 0.2–1.3 mg/dL Direct: 0.1–1.3 mg/dL Indirect: 0.1–0.3 mg/dL	Increased indirect bilirubin levels occur as the liver is unable to conjugate the bilirubin with impaired synthetic function or in the presence of an excessive load of bilirubin in cases of hemolysis. Impaired excretion of direct bilirubin into the bile ducts or biliary tract results in increased levels of direct bilirubin with increased amounts absorbed into the blood. Impaired

Continued

■ **TABLE 7-2**
■ ■ **Liver Function Tests (LFTs) (*cont'd*)**

LFT	Function	Pediatric Reference Value	Changes with Hepatic Failure
Bilirubin—cont'd	soluble. Direct bilirubin is excreted into the hepatic ducts and eventually into the intestinal tract.		synthetic function and obstruction increase total bilirubin levels.
Prothrombin time (PT)	PT is the laboratory measure of the time for a fibrin clot to form after tissue thromboplastin (factor III) and calcium are added to the sample. PT allows for clinical evaluation of the extrinsic clotting cascade.	10.5–13.5 s	A prolonged PT reflects poor utilization of vitamin K due to parenchymal disease or low levels of vitamin K due to obstructive jaundice. With clinical hepatic failure, the failure of the PT to respond after the administration of IV vitamin K reflects significant parenchymal injury.
Albumin	Albumin is the major circulating plasma protein responsible for maintaining plasma oncotic pressure. Albumin levels reflect a component of liver synthetic function.	3.8–5.4 g/d	The half-life of albumin is 21 d; therefore, hypoalbuminemia is present with chronic hepatic failure. Interpret with caution, as protein intake and albumin administration may alter the albumin level.
Ammonia	Ammonia is formed from the deamination of amino acids during protein metabolism and is a by-product of the breakdown of colonic bacteria proteins.	Newborn: 50–84 mcg/dL Child: 12–38 mcg/dL	Increased ammonia levels reflect decreased synthetic function. Elevated ammonia levels can occur in the presence of acute or chronic hepatic failure. Elevated ammonia levels may alter neurologic status.

Adapted from Martin SA: The ABCs of pediatric LFTs. *J Pediatr Nurs* 18(5):445–449, 1992.

B. Antiulcer Agents

1. **Cimetidine (Tagamet) (Crill and Hak, 1999; Rudolph et al., 2001; Taketomo et al., 2003)**
   a. *Action:* Histamine-2 receptor antagonist; decreases the secretion of acid.
   b. *Uses:* Short-term treatment of active duodenal ulcers and gastric ulcers, gastroesophageal reflux disease (GERD), or for long-term prophylaxis and prevention of upper GI tract bleeding.
   c. *Dosage:* Neonate—5 to 10 mg/kg daily IV, IM, or PO in divided doses every 8 to 12 hours. Infant: 10 to 20 mg/kg daily IV, IM, or PO in divided doses every 6 to 12 hours. Child—20 to 40 mg/kg daily IV, IM, or PO in divided doses every 6 hours; maximum dose 800 to 1200 mg per dose two or three times daily. Continuous IV infusion is used with GI tract bleeding. The IV dose should be titrated to maintain pH greater than 5.0. Dose reductions are recommended for patients with renal impairment.

TABLE 7-3
Common Diagnostic Studies for GI Disorders

Procedure	Purpose	Disorder
ABDOMINAL X-RAY: Flat plate; Cross table lateral; Lateral decubitus	Evaluate organ size, position, gas patterns, air-fluid levels	TEF, bowel obstruction, perforation, ileus, NEC
FLUOROSCOPY:		
Barium swallow	Examine the integrity of the esophagus, diagnoses structural abnormalities	Malrotation, esophageal or small bowel strictures
Upper GI series	Examine the esophagus, stomach, and duodenum, diagnose structural abnormalities; delayed gastric emptying	GE reflux, malrotation, volvulus, ulcerative disease
Upper GI with small bowel follow-through	Same as upper GI with follow-up films of esophagus to small intestine	Small bowel disorders
ENDOSCOPY:		
Flexible upper endoscopy	Directly visualize upper GI mucosa, diagnose lesions, source of bleeding	Esophageal varices, severe gastritis
Endoscopic retrograde cholangiopancreatography (ERCP)	Directly visualize the biliary pancreatic ducts	Pseudocyst, stones, chronic pancreatitis
Flexible colonoscopy	Directly visualize mucosa of large intestine, diagnose mucosal injury, bleeding source	Polyp, inflammatory bowel disease
BIOPSY		
Percutaneous liver biopsy	Obtain liver specimens	Biliary atresia, hepatitis
NUCLEAR SCANS		
Hepatobiliary excretion scan (HIDA)	Determine liver excretory function	Biliary atresia
Meckel scan	Evaluate location of bleeding (radioactive isotope is taken up by parietal cells)	Meckel's diverticulum
ABDOMINAL ULTRASOUND	Visualize organ structure, diagnose tissue abnormalities rapidly	Liver disease, hepatic AVM, trauma in unstable child, pancreatitis
ABDOMINAL CT SCAN WITH CONTRAST	Evaluate for vascular disorders, definitive imaging of solid organs, evaluate for infection, abcess	Organ trauma, liver disease, pancreatitis, pseudocyst
MAGNETIC RESONANCE IMAGING (MRI)	Definitively image abdominal organs in stable child	Hepatic hemangioma, hepatic AVM

Modified from Simone S: Gastrointestinal critical care problems. In Curley MAQ, Moloney-Harmon PA, editors: *Critical care nursing*, ed 2. Philadelphia, 2001, WB Saunders.

d. *Side effects* include bradycardia, tachycardia, hypotension, diarrhea, nausea, vomiting, dizziness, headache, agitation, gynecomastia, elevated serum creatinine, elevated aspartate aminotransferase (AST) and alanine aminotransferase (ALT), neutropenia, and thrombocytopenia.

2. **Ranitidine (Zantac) (Crill and Hak, 1999; Rudolph et al., 2001; Taketomo et al., 2003)**
   a. *Action:* Histamine-2 receptor antagonist; decreases the secretion of acid.
   b. *Uses:* Short-term treatment of active peptic ulcer disease, GERD, or long-term prophylaxis and prevention of hypersecretory states and bleeding.
   c. *Dosage:* Premature and term infant younger than 2 weeks—1.5 to 2 mg/kg daily IV divided every 12 hours. Child—2 to 4 mg/kg daily IV divided every 6 to 8 hours, for a maximum of 200 mg daily; 0.08–0.17 mg/kg per hour continuous IV infusion; 4 to 10 mg/kg daily divided twice daily; maximum GERD dosing is 300 mg daily. Dose reduction is recommended for patients with renal impairment.
   d. *Side effects* include bradycardia, tachycardia, headache, dizziness, nausea, vomiting, elevated serum creatinine, hepatitis, arthralgia, leukopenia, and thrombocytopenia.
3. **Famotidine (Pepcid) (Rudolph et al., 2001; Taketomo et al., 2003)**
   a. *Action:* Histamine-2 receptor antagonist; decreases the secretion of acid.
   b. *Uses:* Therapy and treatment of peptic ulcer disease, GERD, and hypersecretory states.
   c. *Dosage:* 0.5 to 1 mg/kg daily orally (PO), IV in divided doses every 12 hours and at bedtime to a maximum of 40 mg/day. Dose reductions are recommended for patients with renal impairment.
   d. *Side effects* include bradycardia, tachycardia, headache, dizziness, constipation, diarrhea, thrombocytopenia, and pancytopenia.
4. **Omeprazole (Prilosec) (Rudolph et al., 2001; Taketomo et al., 2003)**
   a. *Action:* Proton-pump inhibitor (PPI); direct inhibitor of hydrochloric acid secretions at the cellular level.
   b. *Uses:* Treatment of severe erosive esophagitis and short-term treatment of severe GERD and peptic ulcer disease.
   c. *Dosage:* 1 mg/kg/day PO every 12 hours or every day. The capsule form of the medication is a sustained-release capsule. The capsule can be opened, and the beads should be mixed with an acidic medium such as apple juice for delivery through a gastric tube or with sodium bicarbonate through a jejunal tube. The beads of medication should *not* be crushed.
   d. *Side effects* include bradycardia, tachycardia, nausea, diarrhea, abdominal cramps, headache, dizziness, skin rash, elevated liver enzymes, hematuria, proteinuria, and thrombocytopenia.
5. **Pantoprazole (Protonix) (Rudolph et al., 2001; Taketomo et al., 2003)**
   a. *Action:* PPI; a direct inhibitor of hydrochloric acid secretions at the cellular level. This PPI has a more direct inhibition of acid secretion that differs compared with other PPIs. It demonstrates antimicrobial activity against *Helicobacter pylori.*
   b. *Uses*: GERD, pathological hypersecretory conditions, and as an adjunct to duodenal ulcer treatment. Currently no pediatric studies have been performed evaluating the use for acid-related disease, including GERD (Patel et al., 2003).
   c. *Dosage:* Children—20 mg PO every 24 hours; 0.5 to 1 mg/kg daily was used in 15 children aged 6 to 13 years.
   d. *Side effects* include hypotension, hypertension, headache, urticaria, pruritus, hyperglycemia, nausea, vomiting, diarrhea, constipation, urinary frequency, elevated liver enzymes, cough, and dyspnea. With IV administration, anaphylaxis has been reported.
6. **Lansoprazole (Rudolph et al., 2001; Taketomo et al., 2003)**
   a. *Action:* PPI; a direct inhibitor of hydrochloric acid secretion at the cellular level.

b. *Uses*: Short-term treatment (up to 4 weeks) for duodenal ulcers, erosive esophagitis, and hypersecretory conditions.
c. *Dosage*: Child—For GERD in patients weighing less than 10 kg, 7.5 mg PO once daily; for children who weigh less than 10 to 30 kg, 15 mg PO once or twice daily; for those who weigh more than 30 kg, 30 mg PO once or twice daily.
d. *Side effects* include hypertension, hypotension, nausea, dyspepsia, diarrhea, constipation, elevated liver enzymes, and tinnitus.

7. **Sucralfate (Carafate) (Rudolph et al., 2001; Taketomo et al., 2003)**
   a. *Action:* Gastric protectant; paste formation and ulcer adhesion occur within 1 to 2 hours and last up to 6 hours.
   b. *Uses:* Short-term management of duodenal ulcers and gastritis.
   c. *Dosage:* 40 to 80 mg/kg daily PO in divided doses every 6 hours. Administer before meals or on an empty stomach.
   d. *Side effects* include facial edema, constipation, diarrhea, nausea, dry mouth, rash, pruritus, and respiratory difficulty. Decreased absorption of concurrently administered drugs may occur. Safety and efficacy in children have not been established.
8. **Magnesium hydroxide and aluminum hydroxide (Maalox), aluminum hydroxide (Amphojel), and calcium carbonate (Titralac) (Taketomo et al., 2003)**
   a. *Action:* Antacid that neutralizes gastric acid.
   b. *Uses:* Prophylaxis against GI tract bleeding or in the treatment of peptic ulcer disease.
   c. *Dose:* Infant—0.5 mL/kg per dose PO every 1 to 4 hours; titrate to gastric pH between 3.5 and 4.0. Child—2.5 to 5 mL PO per dose up to four times per day or 5 to 15 mL/day PO every 1 to 4 hours; titrate to gastric pH greater than 4.0. In peptic ulcer disease, 5 to 15 mL per dose PO every 3 to 6 hours; 5 to 15 mL per dose PO 1 to 3 hours after meals and at bedtime.
   d. *Side effects* are usually related to the salt constituent of the antacid. Magnesium can cause diarrhea, aluminum can cause constipation and seizures, and sodium can cause fluid retention.

C. Prokinetics

1. **Metoclopramide (Reglan) (Sandritter, 2003; Taketomo et al., 2003)**
   a. *Action:* Potent dopamine receptor antagonist; blocking dopamine receptors in the chemoreceptor trigger zone, preventing emesis; accelerating gastric emptying and intestinal transit time.
   b. *Uses:* GERD, prevention of postoperative and chemotherapy-related nausea and vomiting.
   c. *Dosage:* 0.1 to 0.4 mg/kg IV every 6 to 8 hours; 0.4 to 0.8 mg/kg daily PO divided four times daily. Maximum dose is 10 to 15 mg IV or PO. Dose reductions are recommended in patients with renal impairment.
   d. *Side effects* include extrapyramidal reactions, seizures, hypertension, hypotension, arrhythmias, constipation, diarrhea, neutropenia, and leukopenia.
2. **Erythromycin (EES) (Sandritter, 2003; Taketomo et al., 2003)**
   a. *Action:* Works as a motilin receptor agonist and increases lower esophageal sphincter tone.
   b. *Uses:* Macrolide antibiotic and prokinetic agent.
   c. *Dosage:* Child—Erythromycin lactobionate or gluceptate: Initial 3 mg/kg IV, followed by 20 mg/kg daily orally in three or four divided doses before meals and at bedtime.

d. *Side effects* include ventricular arrhythmias, bradycardia, skin rash, abdominal pain, nausea, vomiting, diarrhea, eosinophilia, and cholestatic jaundice.

D. Other Agents

1. **Lactulose (Cephulac) (Taketomo et al., 2003)**
   a. *Action:* Hyperosmotic laxative; ammonia detoxicant.
   b. *Uses:* Used to prevent and treat portal-systemic encephalopathy. This treatment is controversial because the benefit of this therapy can be diminished relative to potential fluid and electrolyte disturbances.
   c. *Dosage:* Infant—2.5 to 10 mL/day PO divided three or four times per day. Child—40 to 90 mL/day PO divided three to four times per day. Adjust dosage to produce two to three stools per day.
   d. *Side effects* include abdominal discomfort, diarrhea, nausea, and vomiting.
2. **Magnesium hydroxide (Milk of Magnesia) (Taketomo et al., 2003)**
   a. *Action:* Cathartic and laxative.
   b. *Uses:* Bowel evacuation and treatment of hyperacidity; contraindicated in patients with appendicitis, intestinal obstruction, ileostomy, or colostomy.
   c. *Dosage:* As a laxative in children younger than 2 years—0.5 mL/kg PO per dose. Ages 2 to 5 years—5 to 15 mL/day PO or in divided doses. Ages 6 to 12 years—15 to 30 mL/day PO or in divided doses. As an antacid, 2.5 to 5 mL PO as needed.
   d. *Side effects* include hypotension, diarrhea, respiratory depression, and hypermagnesemia.
3. **Polyethylene glycol-electrolye solution (GoLYTELY, MiraLax) (Taketomo et al., 2003)**
   a. *Action:* Induces catharsis with strong electrolyte and osmotic effects.
   b. *Uses:* As a bowel preparation for procedures and for treatment of constipation.
   c. *Doses:* For bowel preparation 25 to 40 mL/kg per hour PO until rectal effluent is clear. For constipation, 4.25 g ($^1/_4$ capful) to 17 g (1 capful) PO may be used once or twice daily.
   d. *Side effects* include metabolic acidosis, potential for electrolyte disturbances, nausea, cramps, and abdominal distension.

E. Immunosuppressive Therapy

1. **Basic principles:** Combination therapy is used to maximize therapeutic benefit of agents while minimizing associated toxicities. Institution of specific protocols and organ-specific therapies exist. Generally, when the patient exhibits toxicities of the therapy, the patient is receiving excessive amounts of the drugs. Drug doses are decreased in the posttransplant period as tolerated.
2. **Tacrolimus (Prograf) (Taketomo et al., 2003)**
   a. *Action:* Blocks the production of interleukin-2 and other lymphokines that promote T-cell proliferation.
   b. *Dose:* 0.03 to 0.15 mg/kg daily via a continuous IV infusion; 0.15 to 0.3 mg/kg daily PO in divided doses twice a day. Dosing is variable depending on the organ transplanted and may be based on drug levels.
   c. *Side effects:* With IV use, greater toxicity is observed, including hypertension, renal impairment, central nervous system (CNS) effects (insomnia, headache, tremor, seizure, paresthesia), hyperkalemia, hypomagnesemia, hyperglycemia, GI tract symptoms, and lymphoproliferative disease.
3. **Cyclosporine (Sandimmune) (Taketomo et al., 2003)**
   a. *Action:* Inhibits T-cell proliferation through inhibition of interleukin-2 synthesis.

b. *Dose:* 2 to 10 mg/kg daily IV in divided doses every 8 to 24 hours for maintenance; 5 to 15 mg/kg daily PO divided every 12 to 24 hours. Dosing is variable depending on the organ transplanted and may be based on drug levels.
c. *Side effects* include hypertension, renal impairment, CNS toxicity (headache, tremor, seizure, paresthesia), hypomagnesemia, GI tract symptoms, gum hyperplasia, hirsutism, and lymphoproliferative disease.

4. **Corticosteroids: Methylprednisolone (Solu-Medrol) and prednisone**
   a. *Action:* Depress the immune system by decreasing lymphocytes, macrophage motility, and leukocyte chemotaxis.
   b. *Dosage*
      - Methylprednisolone: 0.5 to 1.7 mg/kg daily in divided doses every 6 to 12 hours administered PO, IM, or IV.
      - Prednisone: 0.05 to 2 mg/kg daily PO in divided doses one to four times daily.
   c. *Side effects* include glucose intolerance, hyperglycemia, ulcers, weight gain, hypertension, sodium and water retention, infection, and acne.
5. **Mycophenolate mofetil (Cellcept) (Taketomo et al., 2003)**
   a. *Action:* Inhibits T- and B-cell proliferation by inhibiting the inosine monophosphate dehydrogenase pathway.
   b. *Dosage:* IV dosing is not available for children; 600 mg/m^2/dose twice daily PO.
   c. *Side effects* include hypertension, headache, rash, nausea, vomiting, dyspepsia, cough, leukopenia, neutropenia, thrombocytopenia, and anemia.
6. **Azathioprine (Imuran) (Taketomo et al., 2003)**
   a. *Action:* Inhibits DNA synthesis.
   b. *Dosage:* Initial dose is 2 to 5 mg/kg daily administered either PO or IV. Maintenance is 1 to 3 mg/kg per day taken once daily.
   c. *Side effects* include bone marrow suppression (anemia, leukopenia), pancreatitis, nausea and vomiting, and mucosal ulceration.
7. **Muromonab-CD3 (Orthoclone OKT3) (Taketomo et al., 2003)**
   a. *Action:* Monoclonal antibody that complexes with CD3 receptor of the T cell and blocks cell function involved in organ rejection.
   b. *Uses:* Generally used in the treatment of intractable rejection.
   c. *Dosage:* Children less than 12 years—0.1 mg/kg daily IV for 10 to 14 days; or for children who weigh less than 30 kg—2.5 mg IV once daily for 10 to 14 days; for children who weigh ≥ 30 kg—5 mg IV once daily for 10 to 14 days.
   d. *Side effects:* The first dose should be administered in an intensive care unit (ICU) because of the potential adverse reactions. Administration of methylprednisolone sodium succinate before the first dose and hydrocortisone sodium succinate 30 minutes after the first dose is recommended to decrease the incidence of reactions. A first-dose effect (flulike symptoms, anaphylactic-type reaction) may occur in 30 minutes to 6 hours or up to 24 hours after the first dose. Administration may result in infection, pulmonary edema with fluid overload, hypotension, anaphylaxis, and the need for cardiopulmonary resuscitation.
8. **Daclizumab (Zenapax) (Taketomo et al., 2003)**
   a. *Action:* Humanized immunoglobulin G-1 (IgG-1) monoclonal antibody that binds specifically to the alpha subunit and interleukin-2 (IL-2) receptors, thus inhibiting IL-2 activation of lymphocytes involved in organ rejection.
   b. *Uses:* Used in immunosuppressive combinations (with Cyclosporin, Prograf, or Imuran) to prevent rejection.
   c. *Dose:* Dosing may be center specific based on protocol. Initial dose is 1 mg/kg IV administered no more than 24 hours before transplant, followed by 1 mg/kg dose IV every 14 days for a total of five doses. Maximum dose is not to exceed 100 mg.

d. *Side effects* include edema, hypertension, hypotension, headache, impaired wound healing, tremors, tubular necrosis, hematuria, congestion, and diaphoresis.

ACUTE ABDOMINAL TRAUMA

A. Pathophysiology, Etiology, and Risk Factors

1. **General principles:** Acute abdominal trauma is the most common potentially lethal injury and is often associated with other traumatic injuries (Gaines and Ford, 2002). Anatomic differences in children compared with adults include a body size that allows greater distribution of injury, a larger body surface area that allows for greater heat loss, abdominal organs that are more anterior with less subcutaneous fat protection, and a smaller blood volume resulting in hypovolemia with relatively smaller volume losses.
2. **Mechanism of injury**
   a. *Blunt* injuries are caused by compression of solid or hollow viscous organs against the spine; rapid acceleration and deceleration with subsequent tearing of structures; or increased abdominal pressure resulting in contusion, laceration, or bursting of organs with subsequent hemorrhage. Solid organs are injured more commonly than hollow organs, and the most commonly injured organ is the spleen. Blunt trauma can result in lethal injury without visible signs of trauma.
   b. *Penetrating* injuries are most often caused by gunshot or stab wounds. The most common injury is to the hollow viscera. Major vascular injuries are common. The onset of peritonitis may be immediate. Wounds that penetrate the abdomen require surgical exploration (Stafford et al., 2002).

B. Signs and Symptoms of Acute Abdominal Trauma

1. **Significant injuries** to the head and extremities may overshadow abdominal injuries.
2. **Signs of injury** are often subtle and include rebound tenderness, pain, rigidity, pallor, grunting respirations, hypotension, failure to respond to fluid resuscitation, and increasing abdominal girth. Acute abdominal distention occurs even with minor trauma, especially in infants and often in children as a result of crying and swallowing air. Distention may lead to vomiting and aspiration.
3. **Signs of retroperitoneal bleeding** include Cullen's sign (ecchymosis around the umbilicus) and Turner's sign (ecchymosis over the flank).

C. Diagnostic Studies

1. **Abdominal x-rays, supine and cross-table,** are useful for determining intraperitoneal free air, ground-glass appearance (suggests intraperitoneal blood or urine), associated lower-rib fractures (indicates severe force), and signs of an ileus.
2. **Ultrasound,** or FAST (focused abdominal sonography for trauma), is a rapid diagnostic tool to identify intraperitoneal fluid in the hemodynamically unstable child with blunt trauma. However, FAST is poor at identifying organ-specific injury and therefore does not replace the abdominal CT as a tool for definitive diagnosis of abdominal injury (Coley et al., 2000).
3. **Abdominal CT scan** is the standard of care for evaluation of the peritoneal cavity and retroperitoneum in the hemodynamically stable child. The use of IV contrast is recommended to evaluate organ perfusion, bowel integrity, and the

presence of intraperitoneal fluid (Nastanski et al., 2001). The use of oral contrast in addition to IV contrast remains controversial (Rothrock et al., 2000; Stafford et al., 2002). Some experts suggest that oral contrast poses no benefit over IV contrast and may increase the risk of aspiration (Sanchez and Paidas, 1999).

4. **Diagnostic peritoneal lavage (DPL)** is a technique that involves the insertion of a catheter into the peritoneal cavity. Aspiration of blood is a positive tap. If no blood is obtained, then 10 mL/kg of normal saline (NS) or lactated Ringer's solution (LR) is infused through the catheter and the effluent is drained by gravity. Cell count and chemistries are obtained. White cell counts greater than 500 cells/mL, red cells counts greater than 100,000 cells/mL, amylase greater than 175 mg/dL, and aspirating stool or blood is a positive tap. A tap positive for blood indicates hemoperitoneum but provides no information on the bleeding source. The FAST provides the same limited information as the DPL and is not invasive (Gaines and Ford, 2002).
5. **Complete blood count (CBC) and coagulation studies** are used to evaluate bleeding.
6. The utility of other laboratory tests in the diagnosis of intra-abdominal injury is controversial. Elevated **AST and ALT** suggest liver injury (see Table 7-2). Elevated **amylase and lipase** suggest pancreatic injury.
7. **Urinalysis** should be obtained to evaluate for the presence of blood, which indicates kidney or bladder injury.
8. **Nuclear scan** is the gold standard for follow-up evaluation of hepatic and splenic injuries.

D. Nursing and Collaborative Diagnoses

- ❖ Potential fluid-volume deficit related to bleeding resulting from blunt or penetrating trauma
- ❖ Potential for infection related to impaired viscera integrity
- ❖ Potential alteration in nutrition, less than body requirements related to inadequate nutritional intake
- ❖ Pain related to abdominal injury

E. Desired Patient Outcomes

1. Child will maintain adequate intravascular volume. Treat hypovolemic shock with adequate volume resuscitation, and prevent or control bleeding.
2. Child will demonstrate no signs of infection. Observe for signs of peritonitis, which include abdominal distention or rigidity, diffuse pain, rebound tenderness, guarding, absent bowel sounds, erythema, fever, leukocytosis (elevated white blood cell count [WBC]), tachycardia, and tachypnea. Monitor vital signs, and perform a physical examination and laboratory studies, including CBC with differential and chemistries. Administer antibiotic therapy as ordered.
3. Child will maintain adequate nutrition and positive nitrogen balance. Calculate daily caloric requirements and notify the physician if the child's caloric intake is inadequate (see Table 7-1). Monitor serum glucose as appropriate while the child is on nothing by mouth (NPO). Administer peripheral or central parenteral nutrition while the child is NPO. Maintain a warm environment to prevent cold stress in infants.
4. The child's pain will be controlled. Assess for signs and symptoms of pain. Give analgesics as needed. Position the child to maximize comfort. Use techniques appropriate for the child's developmental age.

F. General Patient Care Management

1. Early management of airway, breathing, and circulation (ABCs) has the most direct impact on survival. The critically ill child may require intubation and mechanical ventilation for stabilization of the airway and breathing. Circulatory stabilization requires the placement of large-bore IV lines and fluid resuscitation. Inadequate airway and fluid resuscitation are the leading causes of preventable death. Central venous pressure and arterial blood pressure lines are placed to allow close monitoring of the child's intravascular volume and blood pressure.
2. Serial monitoring of vital signs and abdominal girth is the key to appreciating the progression of findings associated with abdominal injury. Avoid deep palpation because it may cause further injury.
3. Insertion of a nasogastric (NG) or orogastric (OG) tube allows for gastric decompression, minimizes aspiration risk, and maximizes respiratory effort.
4. Serial laboratory studies are necessary for evaluation of injury, especially following the hematocrit, which is imperative to assess for ongoing bleeding.
5. Most solid-organ abdominal injuries are managed nonoperatively. The blood volume of a child is approximately 80 mL/kg. Fluid resuscitation guidelines include administering up to 40 mL/kg of saline or LR solution. If the child remains hemodynamically unstable, a blood transfusion should then be given (Rothrock et al., 2000). Indications for surgical exploration include massive fluid resuscitation (>40 mL/kg of blood transfusions or more than 50% of blood volume), penetrating trauma, signs of peritonitis, radiographic evidence of pneumoperitoneum, and certain blunt injuries (e.g., diaphragmatic injury or bladder rupture).

G. Specific Injuries

1. The **spleen** is the most commonly injured abdominal organ.
   a. *Signs and symptoms* include left upper quadrant (LUQ) tenderness, bruising, or abrasion, positive Kehr's sign (LUQ pain radiating to the left shoulder), signs of decreased perfusion (pallor, tachycardia, delayed capillary refill, and hypotension), and nausea and vomiting. Other signs may include Cullen's or Turner's sign.
   b. *Diagnostic studies:* Abdominal x-ray examinations are rarely helpful but may demonstrate an elevated left hemidiaphragm or a medially displaced lateral stomach border suggesting splenic laceration. The hematocrit may be decreased related to bleeding, or leukocytosis may be noted. Definitive diagnosis is made by abdominal computed tomography (CT) scan with contrast. FAST ultrasound may be useful to evaluate injury to other organs.
   c. *Classification* is based on location and extent of injury (Table 7-4).
   d. *Management:* The standard of care is nonoperative treatment in hemodynamically stable patients. Care involves strict bed rest for 4 to 7 days, frequent monitoring of vital signs and physical examinations, and serial hematocrits until transfusions have not been required for more than 48 hours. Patients are NPO until stable. Surgery may include a *splenectomy* or *splenorrhaphy*. In most instances, suturing the injury or *splenorrhaphy* results in salvage of the spleen. The ultimate goal is preservation of the immune function of the spleen. Massive splenic injury requires a *splenectomy*. Postoperative care includes monitoring for potential complications such as atelectasis, bleeding, ileus, pain, and infection.
   e. *Complications* include rebleeding or splenic laceration 3 to 5 days after the initial injury. Splenectomized children are at risk for overwhelming postsplenectomy infection (OSI). The mortality associated with OSI is

TABLE 7-4
Splenic Injury Scale

Grade	Injury Description
I	
Hematoma	Subcapsular, nonexpanding, <10% of surface area
Laceration	Capsular tear, nonbleeding, <1 cm of parenchymal depth
II	
Hematoma	Subcapsular, nonexpanding, 10%-50% of surface area Intraparenchymal, nonexpanding, <5 cm in diameter
Laceration	Capsular tear, 1-3 cm of parenchymal depth that does not involve a trabecular vessel
III	
Hematoma	Subcapsular, >50% of surface area or expanding, ruptured subcapsular or parenchymal hematoma, intraparenchymal hematoma, >5 cm or expanding
Laceration	>3 cm of parenchymal depth or involving trabecular vessels
IV	
Hematoma	Ruptured intraparenchymal hematoma with active bleeding
Laceration	Laceration involving segmental or hilar vessel producing major devascularization (>25% of spleen)
V	
Laceration	Completely shattered spleen
Vascular	Hilar vascular injury that devascularizes spleen

Adapted from Lynch JM, Meza MP, Newman B et al.: Computed tomography grade of splenic injury is predictive of the time required for radiographic healing, *J Pediatr Surg* 32:1093-1096, 1997.

approximately 50% (Davidson and Wall, 2001). *Streptococcus pneumoniae* is the most common causative agent. Vaccination against encapsulated bacteria, including *S. pneumoniae, Haemophilus influenzae* type b, and *Neisseria meningitides,* is recommended after splenectomy. Daily penicillin prophylaxis is recommended in children younger than 5 years (Potoka et al., 2002; Stylianos, 2000). Parents should be taught signs and symptoms of infection and when to seek medical attention. Children who sustain an isolated splenic injury are restricted from contact sports and strenuous physical activity for a period consisting of the grade of injury plus 2 weeks.

2. The **liver** is second only to the spleen as a major source of hemorrhage and is the most common source of lethal hemorrhage (Morgan, 2000). Bleeding stops spontaneously with most injuries.
   a. *Signs and symptoms* include right upper quadrant (RUQ) tenderness, ecchymosis, abrasion, enlarging abdominal girth, signs of shock, and associated injuries such as lower rib fractures, pelvic fracture, or head injury.
   b. *Diagnostic studies:* Definitive diagnosis is made with abdominal CT scan with contrast. Elevated transaminases are highly suggestive of liver injury, especially AST greater than 200 IU/L and ALT greater than 100 IU/L (Puranik et al., 2002). A rapidly falling hematocrit suggests severe liver injury. Serial CT scans are performed to assess healing or continued bleeding.

c. *Classification:* Injuries are graded according to increasing severity (Table 7-5). Outcome after liver injury correlates more strongly with the injury severity score and associated injuries than with the grade of liver injury (Hackam et al., 2002).

d. *Management* is similar to the treatment of splenic injury and involves supportive care with a nonoperative approach (Gaines and Ford, 2002). Nonoperative management requires close monitoring of vital signs and physical examinations. Fever, leukocytosis, and abdominal tenderness remote from the liver injury may indicate an occult injury. Serial hematocrits, coagulation studies, chemistries, and transaminase levels should be monitored for significant liver dysfunction and monitored until stable. Close monitoring for ongoing bleeding is necessary, and patients should remain on strict bed rest until they are stable. Surgery is indicated for the hemodynamically unstable child, signs of peritonitis, or transfusion requirements exceeding 50% of the estimated blood volume during the first 24 hours (Garcia and Brown, 2003; Pryor et al., 2001; Rothrock et al., 2001). Children with isolated hepatic injury are restricted from contact sports and strenuous physical activity for a period consisting of the grade of injury plus 2 weeks.

e. *Complications* of operative management include delayed bleeding, abscess formation, abdominal compartment syndrome, biliary obstruction, and biloma.

TABLE 7-5
Liver Injury Scale

Grade	Injury Description
I	
Hematoma	Subcapsular, <10% of surface area
Laceration	Capsular tear, <1 cm parenchymal depth
II	
Hematoma	Subcapsular, 10%-50% of surface area, intraparenchymal, <10 cm in diameter
Laceration	1-3 cm parenchymal depth, <10 cm in length
III	
Hematoma	Subcapsular, >50% of surface area or expanding, ruptured subcapsular or parenchymal hematoma Intraparenchymal hematoma >10 cm or expanding
IV	
Laceration	Parenchymal destruction involving 25% to 75% of hepatic lobe
V	
Laceration	Parenchymal destruction >75% of hepatic lobe
Vascular	Juxtahepatic venous injuries (retrohepatic cava/major hepatic veins)
VI	
Vascular	Hepatic avulsion

Adapted from Moore EE, Cogbill TH, Jurkovich GJ et al.: Organ injury scaling: spleen and liver (1994 revision), *J Trauma* 38(3):323-324, 1995.

3. The **pancreas** is located deep in the upper abdomen and is infrequently injured unless a significant sustained force compresses it against the spine. The classic injury is compression by bicycle handlebars in which the child flips over the bike and is impaled in the epigastrium by the handlebars. Other mechanisms include motor-vehicle collisions and child abuse.
   a. *Signs and symptoms* include diffuse abdominal tenderness, deep epigastric pain radiating to the back, and bilious vomiting.
   b. *Diagnostic studies*
      - Amylase is elevated (reference range 0 to 88 IU/L). The extent of amylase increase alone does not correlate with the severity of injury and may be a nonspecific finding occurring with blunt injury in the absence of pancreatic injury.
      - Lipase (reference range, 20 to 180 IU/L). Elevation of amylase to greater than 200 IU/L and lipase greater than 1800 IU/L correlates with significant pancreatic injury (Nadler et al., 1999).
      - Diagnosis is usually made by abdominal CT scan with IV or oral contrast. Overall accuracy of diagnosis is between 60% and 70% (Canty and Weinman, 2001).
      - Ultrasound is useful for diagnosis of pseudocyst and ascites.
      - Endoscopic retrograde cholangiopancreatography (ERCP) may be necessary to visualize ductal disruption or posttraumatic stricture.
   c. *Classification:* Injury is graded based on the extent of parenchymal injury and the degree of disruption of the duct (Table 7-6).
   d. *Management* is nonoperative if there is no ductal disruption. Supportive care interventions include NPO, NG tube for gastric decompression, IV fluids, and pain management. Parenteral nutrition should be considered if NPO longer than 3 days. Children are monitored for signs of infection. If a pancreatic pseudocyst (a loculated collection of pancreatic juices) develops, patients require 6 to 8 weeks of bowel rest with parenteral nutrition. Surgery is indicated for the treatment of distal transection of the pancreas. Surgery involves drainage, partial resection, or repair of lacerated ducts.
   e. *Complications* include the development of pancreatic fistula or pseudocyst formation. Large cysts that have not resolved after 4 to 6 weeks require drainage. The standard of practice is surgical drainage, but percutaneous and endoscopic drainage has been successful (Patty et al., 2001; Shilyansky et al., 1998). Because the pancreas is stimulated with oral intake, feeding tolerance must be evaluated before pulling surgical drains. Somatostatin or octreotide have been used to decrease pancreatic secretions following pseudocyst formation (Fanta et al., 2003).

TABLE 7-6
Pancreatic Injury Severity Scale

Class	Injury Description
I	Contusion or laceration without duct injury
II	Ductal transection or parenchymal injury with probable duct injury
III	Proximal transection or parenchymal injury with probable duct injury
IV	Combined pancreatic and duodenal injury

Adapted from Jobst MA, Canty TG, Lynch FP: Management of pancreatic injury in pediatric blunt abdominal trauma, *J Pediatr Surg* 34(5):818-823, 1999.

4. **Stomach**
   a. *Signs and symptoms* of injury include abrasion or contusion in the upper abdomen and bloody gastric drainage. A boardlike abdomen with severe pain suggests perforation. Perforation leads to signs and symptoms of peritonitis within hours of injury.
   b. *Diagnostic studies:* Abdominal x-ray detects free air or abnormal NG tube position.
   c. *Management* includes surgical repair.
5. **Small and large intestine:** Small bowel injuries are the third most common site of abdominal organ injury in blunt trauma (Wise et al., 2002). Common mechanisms include the lap-belt syndrome and abuse. The **colon and rectum** are rarely injured in children, and injuries to these organs usually occur in the presence of abuse.
   a. *Signs and symptoms* include bloody gastric drainage, absent bowel sounds, tympanic sounds on percussion, midabdominal ecchymosis, seat belt mark, and pain that increases as peritonitis develops. Signs and symptoms of peritonitis include severe abdominal pain, tenderness, guarding, distension or rigidity, redness, absent bowel sounds, fever, leukocytosis, and respiratory distress. Evaluation of a rectal injury requires rectal examination by the physician and is often done with the patient under general anesthesia.
   b. *Diagnostic studies:* Abdominal x-rays with supine and lateral decubitus views may reveal air fluid levels, dilated loops of bowel, bowel wall thickening, or a Chance fracture (lumbar spine fracture). Helical CT scan has improved the accuracy in detecting bowel and mesenteric injuries over the standard CT scan with contrast (Garcia and Brown, 2003; Killeen et al., 2001).
   c. *Management* requires surgical repair and generally involves segmental resection with primary anastomosis. Supportive care includes frequent monitoring, NG decompression, replacement of excessive gastric output, stress ulcer prophylaxis, antibiotic therapy, fluid and electrolyte management, parenteral nutrition, and pain management.
   d. *Complications:* Delayed perforation, stricture formation, adhesions, and short bowel syndrome.

ACUTE GI TRACT HEMORRHAGE

A. Pathophysiology

The child presenting with sudden massive blood loss is at risk for hemodynamic instability. The first priority is to determine the extent of the blood loss and establish whether perfusion is compromised. Greater than 15% circulating blood volume (CBV) loss results in stimulation of autonomic cardiovascular responses to maintain blood pressure and perfusion. Greater than 20% CBV loss results in decreased systolic blood pressure and metabolic acidosis. Rapid fluid resuscitation is required, or cardiovascular collapse and death may occur.

B. Etiology

Etiology is based on age. Tables 7-7 and 7-8 outline the presentations of upper and lower GI bleeding (Fox, 2000).

C. Signs and Symptoms (Table 7-9)

1. The **location of bleeding** can be identified by the color and source of the bleeding. Upper GI bleeding is defined as bleeding that originates proximal to

TABLE 7-7
Causes of Upper GI Bleeding in Infants and Children

Neonates	Infants-Adolescents
Esophagitis	Esophagitis
Gastritis	Gastritis
Gastroduodenal ulcer	Gastroduodenal ulcer
Coagulaopathy associated with infection	Esophageal varices
Vascular anomaly	Gastrointestinal duplication
Hemorrhagic disease (Vitamin K deficiency)	Mallory-Weiss tear
	Vascular anomaly
	Coagulopathy
	Caustic ingestion

TABLE 7-8
Causes of Lower GI Bleeding in Infants and Children

Age	Causes
Neonates (<1 mo)	Milk protein allergy Necrotizing enterocolitis Hirschprung's enterocolitis Midgut volvulus Coagulopathy
Infant (1 mo-2 yr)	Milk protein allergy Anal fissure Intussusception Infectious enterocolitis Meckel's diverticulum Vascular anomaly
Child (2-10 yr)	Anal fissure Juvenile polyps Infectious enterocolitis Henoch-Schonlein purpura Hemolytic-uremic syndrome Vascular anomaly
Adolescent (11-18 yr)	Anal fissure Infectious enterocolitis Inflammatory bowel disease Vasculitis Hemorrhoids Intestinal duplication

the ligament of Treitz. Lower GI bleed occurs distally to ligament of Treitz. **Hematemesis** is the result of acute blood loss from the upper GI tract and presents as coffee grounds emesis or frank blood. **Hematochezia** is bright or dark red blood per rectum. **Melena** is caused by the digestion of blood in the GI tract and presents as black, tarry stools and indicates an upper GI source of bleeding. **Occult bleeding** is the result of chronic blood loss.

2. Signs and symptoms of **hypovolemic shock** occur with acute bleeding and include tachycardia, weak peripheral pulses, pallor and mottled color, and cool

TABLE 7-9
Presentations of GI Tract Bleeding

Presentation	Definitions
ACUTE BLEEDING	
Hematemesis	Bloody vomitus; either fresh, bright red blood or dark, grainy digested blood with "coffee ground" appearance
Melena	Black, sticky, tarry, foul-smelling stools caused by digestion of blood in the GI tract (seen in both upper GI and lower GI tract bleeding)
Hematochezia	Fresh, bright red blood passed from the rectum
CHRONIC BLEEDING	
Occult	Trace amounts of blood in normal-appearing stools or gastric secretions; detectable only with a guaiac test

Modified from Huether SE, McCance KL, Tarmina MS: Alterations of digestive function. In McCance KL, Huether SE, editors: *Pathophysiology: the biological basis for diseases in adults and children*, ed 2. St Louis, 1994, Mosby–Year Book Inc.

skin. Blood pressure may be normal despite significant blood loss; hypotension is a late sign of shock.

3. **Other signs and symptoms** include jaundice, hepatosplenomegaly, ascites, abdominal tenderness, guarding, absent or high-pitched bowel sounds, and perianal fissure.

D. Nursing and Collaborative Diagnoses

- Fluid volume deficit related to bleeding
- Potential ineffective breathing patterns related to elevation of the diaphragm from intra-abdominal bleeding
- Potential alteration in nutrition, less than body requirements related to NPO status
- Alteration in comfort related to multiple invasive procedures

E. Desired Patient Outcomes

1. Child will maintain adequate intravascular volume as evidenced by effective peripheral perfusion. Treat hypovolemic shock with volume resuscitation. Prevent or stop bleeding.
2. Child will maintain effective breathing pattern and rate. Maintain airway patency, monitor respiratory status and effort, and maintain the position of comfort to maximize diaphragm excursion. Optimize oxygenation by providing oxygen, and prepare for intubation as needed.
3. Child will maintain adequate nutrition and positive nitrogen balance. Monitor serum glucose as appropriate while the child is NPO. Administer peripheral or central parenteral nutrition while the child is NPO. Calculate daily caloric requirements, and notify the physician if the child's caloric intake is inadequate.
4. Child will achieve a maximal level of comfort. Allow the child's parents to be present as much as possible. Use pain-control measures appropriate for the child's developmental age.

F. Diagnostic Studies

1. **Laboratory studies:** Arterial blood gas (ABG) is measured to monitor for metabolic acidosis; CBC to evaluate for anemia and thrombocytopenia; prothrombin time (PT) and partial thromboplastin time (PTT) to evaluate for

coagulopathies; serum fibrinogen and fibrin split products to evaluate for disseminated intravascular coagulation (DIC); type and crossmatch for potential blood transfusion; guaiac test to evaluate for blood in stool or gastric fluid; chemistries, ammonia, and liver function tests (LFTs) to screen for renal and liver dysfunction; and pancreatic enzymes to assess for pancreatic injuries. If bloody diarrhea is present, send stool culture and fecal leukocytes. CBC, peripheral smear, platelet count, urinalysis, blood urea nitrogen (BUN), and creatinine should be obtained in patients with suspected hemolytic-uremic syndrome.

2. **Abdominal x-ray examination** involves a supine and lateral decubitus view to evaluate for distorted bowel gas pattern suggesting bowel obstruction, air-fluid levels, or pneumoperitoneum. Bowel-wall thickening suggests colitis.
3. **Endoscopy** provides direct visualization of the GI tract to determine injury, structural defects, or source of bleeding. An upper endoscopy is the preferred diagnostic procedure to evaluate bleeding of the upper GI tract and for therapeutic treatment (sclerotherapy, band ligation, heater therapy) of esophageal varices (Fox, 2000; Rayhorn et al., 2000a). Colonoscopy is performed for lower GI bleeding.
4. **Radionuclide studies** are indicated for midintestinal bleeding (Rayhorn et al., 2000b) and are effective tests for locating subacute or intermittent bleeding. Two types are used: technetium-labeled sulfur colloid (more sensitive) and technetium-pertechnetate-labeled red blood cells. Demonstration of IV Tc-99m pertechnetate uptake by ectopic gastric mucosa in a Meckel's scan is helpful in diagnosing Meckel's diverticulum (a congenital remnant located 2 feet from the ileocecal valve).
5. **Angiography** is used selectively in children when a vascular anomaly is suspected, such as arteriovenous malformations, hemangiomas, and telangiectasias.

G. General Patient Care Management

1. Assess for signs of respiratory distress.
2. Secure two large-bore IVs for fluid resuscitation. Administer fluid (20 mL/kg of NS or LR) or blood transfusion (15 mL/kg) until peripheral circulation is adequate. After central line and arterial line placement continuously monitor central venous pressure (CVP) and blood pressure for response to fluid resuscitation and the need for continued therapy. The initial hematocrit may be misleading with acute bleeding.
3. Monitor PT, PTT, and fibrinogen for coagulopathies. Administer vitamin K (AquaMephyton), platelets, or fresh frozen plasma (FFP) as necessary.
4. Monitor electrolytes, BUN, and creatinine for potential renal dysfunction. Monitor urine output via a Foley catheter.
5. Monitor serum ionized calcium following transfusion for potential hypocalcemia.
6. Monitor for signs of further bleeding including poor perfusion, abdominal pain, increased abdominal girth, decreased bowel sounds, hematemesis, and hematochezia.
7. Assess for signs and symptoms of abdominal perforation including fever, severe or persistent abdominal pain, and abdominal rigidity.
8. Place NG tube and administer room temperature saline lavage until bleeding stops.
9. Monitor gastric pH. Administer antacid if pH is less than 4. Antacids, H_2-histamine receptor antagonists, proton-pump inhibitors, and sucralfate may have some preventive effect on rebleeding (Fox, 2000).

H. Esophageal Varices

1. **Acute treatment** involves the administration of vasopressin (Pitressin), or octreotide (Sandostatin) (see Pharmacology section). Insertion of a Sengstaken-Blakemore tube may be performed if endoscopy is not available. The tube has three separate lumens for gastric suction, inflation of gastric balloon, and inflation of esophageal balloon. Balloons must be deflated every 12 to 24 hours. Ensure patency of the gastric suction lumen by irrigating frequently. Frequent serious complications, including perforation or erosion of the esophagus or stomach (from hyperinflation or prolonged inflation of the balloons), limit its usefulness.
2. **Endoscopic variceal sclerosis** is the current treatment of choice. The sclerosing agent is injected directly into or alongside varices through a flexible fiberoptic endoscope. Complications include ulceration with rebleeding, perforation, and stricture formation.
3. **Ligation** (banding) of esophageal varices is as effective as sclerotherapy and has fewer side effects.
4. **Transjugular intrahepatic portosystemic shunt (TIPS) (Figure 7-3).** This is a nonsurgical approach to palliate portal hypertension. It is effective but associated with a high rate of shunt thrombosis, and its use is contraindicated in the presence of heart disease. Repeated injection sclerotherapy may also be used as alternative therapy.
5. **Surgery** is considered if other therapies are ineffective. Shunting procedures divert blood flow from the liver and allow decompression of the portal system with portal hypertension. Specific entities requiring surgery include Meckel's diverticulum, duplication cyst, Hirschsprung enterocolitis, midgut volvulus, necrotizing enterocolitis, and intussusception (if barium reduction not effective), and a refractory bleeding ulcer.
6. **Complications** include rebleeding, shock, sepsis, and hepatic encephalopathy.

GI TRACT ABNORMALITIES

Anatomical GI abnormalities occur when the GI tract fails to develop normally in utero. Disorders of the intestine, including malrotation and intussusception, can occur in infants and children at any time. See Table 7-10.

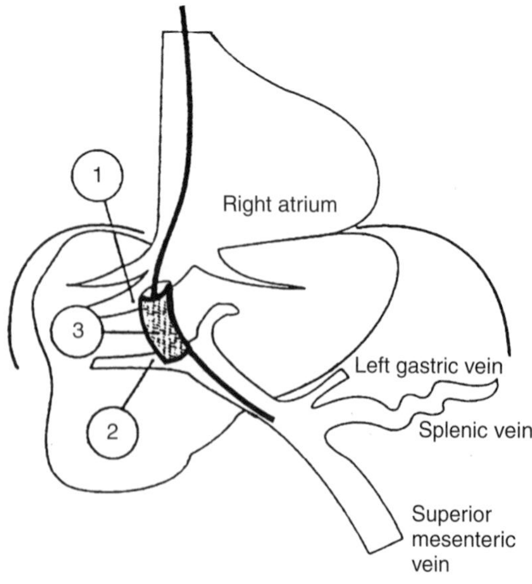

FIGURE 7-3 ■ Technique of transjugular intrahepatic portal-systemic shunt (TIPS).

Following transjugular catheterization of a hepatic vein (*1*) and puncture of a main branch of the portal vein (*2*), the shunt is established by implanting a stent spanning the hepatic parenchyma between sites *1* and *2*.

(Reprinted with permission of *The New England Journal of Medicine* from Rossle M, Haag K, Ochs A et al.: The transjugular intrahepatic portosystemic stent-shunt procedure for variceal bleeding. *N Engl J Med* 330:165, 1994.)

Text continued on p. 528.

TABLE 7-10
Gastrointestinal Abnormalities

Diagnosis	Etiology and Risk Factors	Pathophysiology	Signs and Symptoms	Nursing Diagnoses	Patient Care Management	Complications
Omphalocele	Cause unknown; may be caused during the second stage of rotation of the midgut with incomplete return of the bowel into the abdomen at 8-10 wk gestation	Herniation of abdominal viscera into the umbilical cord usually covered by a peritoneal sac with the umbilical arteries and veins inserting into the apex of the defect Associated anomalies include cardiac defects, neurologic abnormalities, genitourinary abnormalities, skeletal abnormalities, chromosomal abnormalities, malrotation of the intestine, Beckwith-Wiedman syndrome	Size of the defect is variable Dehydration, hypothermia, hypoglycemia, and respiratory distress (dependent on lesion size)	Potential for alteration in breathing patterns: ineffective r/t abdominal hernia Potential for fluid volume deficit: actual r/t increased insensible water loss and third spacing Potential for alteration in nutrition: actual r/t NPO status Impairment of skin integrity: actual r/t abdominal hernia Alteration in comfort r/t postoperative pain	1. Cover exposed abdominal hernia with warm, moist dressing; cover dressing with plastic Defect may be covered with bowel bag 2. Maintain NPO status 3. Place OG/NG tube 4. Maintain neutral thermal environment 5. Monitor I & Os 6. Monitor electrolyte status 7. Provide IV hydration (may require 1.5-2 times maintenance fluids) 8. Administer IV antibiotics 9. Preoperative evaluation for associated anomalies: cardiac echo, renal ultrasound, chromosomal analysis 10. Repair of defect: primary surgical closure, staged silo closing, or secondary epithelization of defect	Intestinal obstruction Respiratory distress Sepsis Wound infection Feeding intolerance Gastroesophageal reflux disease (GERD) Sac rupture Vascular compromise of abdominal contents and lower extremities once the defect is reduced

Continued

TABLE 7-10
Gastrointestinal Abnormalities (*cont'd*)

Diagnosis	Etiology and Risk Factors	Pathophysiology	Signs and Symptoms	Nursing Diagnoses	Patient Care Management	Complications
Omphalocele—cont'd					11. Postoperative care a. TPN with enteral feeds when ileus resolved b. Management of fluid and electrolyte status c. Monitor for infection d. Encourage pulmonary toilet e. Pain management	
Gastroschisis	Increased worldwide incidence—cause unknown; proposed etiologies include an intrauterine vascular accident involving the omphalomesenteric artery with subsequent disruption of the abdominal ring, deficiency of embryonic mesenchyme	Evisceration of abdominal contents usually lateral and to the right of the umbilicus, may the small and large intestine; no protective membranes Associated anomalies include intestinal stricture and atresia	Size of defect usually smaller than an omphalocele Intestine may be edematous and inflamed due to exposure to amniotic fluid Bowel exposure precursors to prolonged ileus	Potential for alteration in breathing patterns: ineffective r/t abdominal hernia Potential for fluid volume deficit: actual r/t increased insensible water losses and third spacing Alteration in nutritional status: actual r/t NPO status and post-op ileus Impairment of skin integrity: actual r/t abdominal hernia	1. Cover exposed abdominal hernia with warm, moist dressing; cover dressing with plastic Defect may be covered by a bowel bag 2. Maintain NPO status 3. Place OG/NG tube 4. Maintain neutral thermal environment 5. Monitor I & Os 6. Monitor electrolyte status 7. Provide IV hydration 8. Administer IV antibiotics	Intestinal obstruction Respiratory distress Sepsis Wound infection Feeding intolerance (GERD) Partial/complete bowel infarction with resultant short gut syndrome (SGS)

				Alteration in comfort: r/t surgical procedure	9. Repair of defect: primary closure or silo staged reduction with surgical repair of the abdominal wall after the herniated bowel has been returned to the abdominal cavity 10. Postoperative care a. TPN b. Management of fluid and electrolyte status c. Monitor for infection d. Encourage pulmonary toilet e. Pain management	
Volvulus	Abnormal rotation and fixation of the intestine; most commonly occurs in infancy; however, may occur at any age	Complication of malrotation The intestine returns from the umbilical cord about week 10 gestation, undergoes a counterclockwise rotation about the axis of the superior mesenteric artery,	Bilious vomiting Melena or currant-jelly stools Abdominal distension X-ray can reveal variable findings: normal gas pattern, duodenal obstruction, multiple dilated bowel loops	Alteration in nutrition: actual r/t NPO status Alteration in comfort: actual r/t pain associated with vascular compromise and associated postoperative pain	1. Maintain NPO status 2. Provide IV hydration 3. Administer IV antibiotics 4. Prepare child for emergency surgery 5. Postsurgical care a. TPN b. Management of fluid and electrolyte status	Sepsis Bowel infraction with resultant SGS

Continued

TABLE 7-10
Gastrointestinal Abnormalities (*cont'd*)

Diagnosis	Etiology and Risk Factors	Pathophysiology	Signs and Symptoms	Nursing Diagnoses	Patient Care Management	Complications
Volvulus—cont'd		followed by fixation to the posterior abdominal wall; abnormal twisting causes vascular obstruction, with development of midgut necrosis, unless immediate diagnosis and surgery occur	An upper GI with small bowel follow-through evaluates the position of the ligament of Treitz, duodenal obstruction, and proximal jejunum in the right abdomen		c. Monitor for infection d. Encourage pulmonary toilet e. Pain management	
Intestinal atresia	Etiology thought to be related to in utero vascular accident (e.g., volvulus, intussusception) due to constriction of the superior mesenteric artery Obliteration of the intestinal lumen due to occlusion or total absence	Four types: Type 1: Intact mucosal membrane obstructs the intestinal lumen Type 2: Gaps in bowel continuity, short fibrotic bands connect proximal and distal segments Type 3: No connective tissue between gaps on the intestine Type 4: Atretic segments that are numerous and continuous	Signs of bowel obstruction: bilious vomiting, abdominal distension	Alteration in nutritional status: actual r/t NPO status Alteration in comfort r/t associated postoperative pain	1. Maintain NPO status 2. Provide IV hydration 3. Administer IV antibiotics 4. Prepare for palliative/ corrective surgery 5. Postoperative care a. TPN b. Management of fluid and electrolyte status c. Monitor for signs and symptoms of infection d. Encourage pulmonary toilet e. Pain management	Intestinal perforation Ileus

Intussusception	Frequently preceded by gastroenteritis, lead point intussusception is caused by a specific anatomic instigator (e.g., polyp, enlarged lymph node, tumor); most commonly occurs in children of age 6 to 18 mo	One segment of the intestine invaginates into another (usually the ileum into the cecum); the entrapped bowel initially develops venous obstruction with eventual arterial obstruction and gangrene	Recurrent and severe abdominal pain Bloody stool Signs of bowel obstruction: bilious vomiting, abdominal distension, RUQ may have sausage-shaped mass	Alteration in nutrition: actual r/t NPO status Alteration in comfort: pain associated with lesion	1. Provide IV fluids 2. Maintain NPO status 3. Nonsurgical repair with barium enema 4. Surgical repair, if radiologic intervention unsuccessful 5. Postsurgical care a. Provide IV hydration b. Administer IV antibiotics c. Monitor for infection d. Encourage pulmonary toilet e. Pain management	Intestinal perforation Intestinal infarction Shock
Tracheoesophageal fistula (TEF)	History of maternal polyhydramnios Abnormal separation of the esophagus in relation to the trachea	Five types of the anomaly can occur: Type A: Isolated esophageal atresia (EA) Type B: EA with proximal TEF Type C: EA with distal TEF (most common type) Type D: EA with proximal and distal TEF	Dependent on type of anomaly Dysphagia Inability to pass OG/NG tube Choking/cyanosis with feeding Recurrent pneumonia	Potential for ineffective airway clearance r/t dysphagia Potential for fluid volume deficit r/t continuous suctioning of oral/gastric secretions Alteration in nutritional status: actual r/t feeding difficulties, NPO status	1. Maintain NPO status 2. Provide IV hydration 3. Maintain the HOB elevated 4. Constant suctioning of upper airway to clear oral secretions 5. Surgical repair/palliation of defect 6. Postoperative care a. Management of fluid and electrolyte status	Respiratory distress Aspiration Esophageal stricture Anastamotic leak

Continued

TABLE 7-10
Gastrointestinal Abnormalities (*cont'd*)

Diagnosis	Etiology and Risk Factors	Pathophysiology	Signs and Symptoms	Nursing Diagnoses	Patient Care Management	Complications
Tracheoesophageal fistula (TEF)—cont'd		Type E: Isolated TEF (referred to as an H-type)			b. Monitor for infection c. Wound care d. Encourage pulmonary toilet e. Pain management	
Diaphragmatic hernia (see Chapter 2 for pulmonary complications)	Failure of diaphragm closure or return of the intestine prior to diaphragmatic closure	Herniation of the abdominal organs into the thoracic cavity Herniation of the intestine into the thorax with resultant lung hypoplasia (usually left; right may be affected if there is displacement of the mediastinum)	Respiratory distress Heart tones shifted to the right Scaphoid abdomen	Alteration in breathing patterns: ineffective r/t pulmonary hypoplasia Alteration in nutritional status: actual r/t NPO status	1. Maintain NPO status 2. Place NG tube for gastric decompression 3. Place right-side down to augment pulmonary perfusion 4. Pulmonary management: mechanical ventilation; ECMO may be indicated 5. Prepare for emergent surgical repair	Respiratory failure Pneumothorax Sepsis
Hirschsprung's disease	Failure of innervation of GI tract around 5-12 wk gestation	Peristalsis in lower GI tract ceases	Newborn: fails to pass meconium Signs of intestinal obstruction: bilious vomiting, abdominal distension	Potential for fluid volume deficit r/t NPO status, vomiting Alteration in nutritional status: actual r/t feeding difficulties, NPO status	Neonate 1. Maintain NPO status 2. Provide IV hydration 3. Pass NG tube 4. Prepare for surgical correction	1. Obstruction 2. Malnutrition

	Child: constipation, ribbonlike stool, abdominal distension, visible peristalsis	Impairment of skin integrity: actual r/t colostomy Alteration in comfort r/t postoperative pain	5. Postoperative care a. Management of fluid and electrolyte status b. Monitor for infection c. Wound care, colostomy usually present d. Encourage pulmonary toilet e. Pain management Child 1. May benefit from low-residue, high-calorie, and high-protein diet 2. See management for neonate for additional interventions

BOWEL INFARCTION, OBSTRUCTION, AND PERFORATION

A. Etiology and Risk Factors

1. **Acute abdomen** refers to the sudden onset of abdominal pain and tenderness that warrant evaluation for surgical intervention.
2. **Etiology:** Causes in neonates include necrotizing enterocolitis (NEC), intussusception, midgut volvulus, birth trauma, and Hirschsprung disease (see Table 7-10). Causes in children and adolescents include appendicitis (common cause of peritonitis), Meckel's diverticulum, inflammatory bowel disease, and trauma. Indwelling catheters such as ventriculoperitoneal shunt or peritoneal dialysis catheter are also risk factors.

B. Pathophysiology

1. **Peritoneal inflammation (peritonitis)** occurs as a result of injury or contamination. Primary peritonitis occurs with no obvious cause of contamination, but infection is indirectly introduced into the peritoneal cavity from the bloodstream or lymphatics. Secondary peritonitis occurs as a result of direct GI tract injury, such as with trauma. The inflammatory response causes exudation of fluid into the peritoneal cavity. Hypovolemia occurs as fluid shifts into the peritoneal cavity.
2. **Upper GI tract perforations** result in leakage of hydrochloric acid, digestive enzymes, or bile causing chemical peritonitis.
3. **Lower GI tract perforation** results in the leakage of fecal material, which releases aerobic and anaerobic bacteria into the peritoneum. Endotoxins may be released and cause bacterial peritonitis and sepsis.
4. **Injury** to the peritoneum causes decreased bowel motility and usually results in an ileus.

C. Signs and Symptoms

1. **Obstruction** results in abdominal distention, tenderness, bilious vomiting, fever, and absent or hyperactive bowel sounds.
2. **Perforation** causes signs of respiratory distress, including tachypnea, retractions, flaring, grunting, cyanosis, hypoxemia, and acidosis.
3. Signs of **third spacing** include increased abdominal girth and hypovolemia (tachycardia, decreased peripheral perfusion, decreased urine output, and hypotension [late sign]).
4. Symptoms of **peritonitis** include fever, nausea, marked abdominal distention or rigidity, erythema over the abdomen, absent or hypoactive bowel sounds, diffuse abdominal pain, guarding of the abdomen, and rebound tenderness.

D. Diagnostic Studies

1. **Abdominal x-ray examination** may reveal a paucity of gas, dilated loops of bowel, or air-fluid levels with a bowel obstruction. A lateral or cross-table view reveals the presence of free air with bowel perforation. Bowel wall thickening or intraluminal air (pneumatosis) is seen with NEC.
2. **Contrast enema** is a diagnostic and therapeutic treatment for intussusception. Typically, air enema results in successful reduction of the obstructed bowel (McCollough and Sharieff, 2003).
3. **Upper GI Series** (usually with small bowel follow-through) is the gold standard for making the diagnosis of small bowel obstruction (McCollough and Sharieff, 2003).

4. **Abdominal CT scan** with IV contrast is used to evaluate suspected abscess or mass.

E. Nursing and Collaborative Diagnoses

- ❖ Potential for infection related to impaired bowel integrity
- ❖ Alteration in nutrition; less than body requirements related to inadequate nutritional intake
- ❖ Alteration in fluid-volume deficit related to third spacing
- ❖ Potential alteration in electrolyte status related to fluid losses from the GI tract and third spacing
- ❖ Alteration in comfort related to multiple invasive procedures or injury

F. Desired Patient Outcomes

1. Child will demonstrate **no signs of infection.** Monitor vital signs for fever, tachycardia, and tachypnea. Monitor CBC for leukocytosis and thrombocytopenia. Observe for signs of peritonitis including abdominal distention, diffuse pain and tenderness, fever, and tachycardia. Observe for signs of an abscess, including localized pain, fever, and leukocytosis. Administer broad-spectrum antibiotics.
2. Child will maintain **adequate nutrition** and **positive nitrogen balance.** Monitor serum glucose as appropriate while the child is NPO. Administer total parenteral nutrition (TPN) while the child is NPO. Calculate daily caloric requirements and notify the physician if the child's caloric intake is inadequate.
3. Child will maintain **adequate intravascular volume.** Monitor intake and output closely for signs of dehydration. Provide volume resuscitation for hypovolemic shock.
4. Child will maintain **normal electrolyte balance.** Monitor serum electrolytes frequently. Provide electrolyte replacement as needed.
5. Child will achieve a maximal level of **comfort.** Allow the parents to remain with the child. Provide pharmacologic intervention as appropriate. Use age-appropriate techniques for coping with pain.

G. Patient Care Management

1. Provide frequent **vital sign monitoring** with assessment for respiratory distress. Elevate the head of the bed 30 to 45 degrees to enhance respiratory effort. Prepare for intubation and ventilation if respiratory failure is evident.
2. Place an **NG tube** for gastric decompression and drainage.
3. **Surgical intervention** may be indicated for persistent abdominal pain, evidence of localized peritonitis (erythema over a portion of the abdomen), and the presence of free air on abdominal x-ray examination.

H. Complications

Complications include decompensated shock, perforation, infarction, or death.

NECROTIZING ENTEROCOLITIS

A. Etiology and Risk Factors

1. NEC is a disease of the **newborn** and is characterized by abdominal distention, bloody stools, and the presence of gas in the wall of the intestine. NEC is seen

primarily in premature infants following a hypoxic or hypoperfusion insult. Infrequently it occurs in full-term infants, usually within the first 10 days of life (Ostlie et al., 2003).

2. **Risk factors** include history of an anoxic episode at birth and other neonatal stressors, such as hypotension, shock, sepsis, and cold stress. Other risk factors include umbilical artery catheters, early feedings, hyperosmolar feedings, and congenital heart disease.

B. Pathophysiology

1. Three essential precipitating factors act either individually or together to produce NEC: ischemic damage to the intestine, bacterial colonization of the intestine, and enteral feeding (Neu and Weiss, 1999).
2. Bowel ischemia leads to injury and disruption of the intestinal mucosal epithelium. Bowel wall injury allows entry of bacteria and leads to tissue damage, including necrosis and ulceration.
3. The introduction of feeding produces hydrogen gas. Hydrogen gas penetrates the perforated intestinal wall. The entry of hydrogen gas into the submucosal tissue is called *pneumatosis intestinalis;* it can be seen on plain abdominal film and is diagnostic of NEC.

C. Signs and Symptoms

1. Initially, symptoms of NEC are nonspecific and include unexplained apnea, bradycardia, hypoglycemia, electrolyte imbalance, lethargy, temperature instability, and poor feeding. The **classic triad** is abdominal distention, bilious vomiting, and blood in the stools.
2. Signs of progressive NEC include discoloration of the abdominal wall, respiratory distress, hypotension, leukopenia, thrombocytopenia, and a WBC count reflecting a shift to the left.
3. Staging criteria are detailed in Table 7-11.

TABLE 7-11
Staging Criteria for Necrotizing Enterocolitis (NEC)

STAGE I (SUSPECT)

a. History of perinatal stress
b. Systemic manifestations: temperature instability, lethargy, apnea, bradycardia
c. GI tract manifestations: poor feeding, increasing gastric residuals, emesis (may be bilious or have positive results for occult blood), mild abdominal distention, occult blood in stool

STAGE 2 (DEFINITE)

a. Above history and signs and symptoms plus persistent occult or gross GI tract bleeding
b. Marked abdominal distention
c. Abdominal radiographs show significant intestinal distention with ileus, small bowel separation, pneumatosis cystoides intestinalis

STAGE 3 (ADVANCED)

a. Same signs and symptoms as in stage 2 plus deterioration in vital signs
b. Evidence of septic shock or marked GI tract hemorrhage
c. Abdominal radiographs show pneumoperitoneum

Modified from Bell MJ, Ternberg JL, Reign RD et al.: Neonatal necrotizing enterocolitis: therapeutic decisions based upon clinical staging. *Ann Surg* 1:187, 1978.

D. Diagnostic Studies

Abdominal x-ray examination with supine and lateral views may reveal pneumatosis intestinalis, dilated loops of small bowel, and pneumoperitoneum if perforation has occurred.

E. Patient Care Management

1. Infants are kept **NPO** with an NG tube to low intermittent suction for gastric decompression. Fluids and electrolytes are monitored, and parenteral nutrition is provided. Umbilical catheters are discontinued. Broad-spectrum antibiotic therapy is prescribed.
2. **Respiratory and cardiac status** are closely monitored with frequent monitoring of vital signs and abdominal girth.
3. **Guaiac stool testing** is used to detect occult bleeding. Serial platelet counts and serial abdominal x-ray examinations are used to monitor progression.
4. **Surgery** is indicated if signs of perforation, peritonitis, or clinical deterioration are evident.

F. Complications

Complications include short-gut syndrome, neurologic impairment, shock, and death.

HYPERBILIRUBINEMIA

A. Etiology and Risk Factors

1. **Bilirubin** is the by-product of the heme portion of the breakdown of the hemoglobin molecule.
2. **Hyperbilirubinemia** is an elevated level of serum bilirubin. Indirect prehepatic-unconjugated bilirubin elevations may be physiologic rather than pathologic. Direct posthepatic-conjugated bilirubin elevations are always pathologic. The terms *direct* and *indirect* are used interchangeably with conjugated and unconjugated hyperbilirubinemia. Direct hyperbilirubinemia includes conjugated and delta bilirubin measurements.
3. Premature neonates; infants with traumatic births and increased hemolysis; breast-fed infants; infants of East Asian, Native American, and Greek descent; ABO incompatibilities; Rh isoimmunization; and infants of diabetic mothers are at higher risk for developing neonatal or physiologic jaundice or hyperbilirubinemia (Dennery et al., 2001).

B. Pathophysiology

1. **Fat-soluble bilirubin** binds to albumin as indirect (prehepatic-unconjugated) bilirubin for transport to the liver. In the liver, fat-soluble bilirubin is detached from albumin and conjugated with glucuronic acid, rendering the bilirubin water soluble. Increases in indirect bilirubin result when the liver is not able to conjugate the bilirubin with impaired synthetic function.
2. **Direct (posthepatic-conjugated) bilirubin** is excreted into the hepatic ducts and eventually into the intestine. Impaired excretion of direct bilirubin into the bile ducts leads to increased levels of conjugated bilirubin as increased amounts are reabsorbed into the blood.
3. **Impaired synthetic function** and obstruction increase total bilirubin.
4. Three types of jaundice (prehepatic, hepatocellular, cholestatic) can occur. **Prehepatic** is usually caused by hemolysis. The total bilirubin is increased with

the majority of the bilirubin in the indirect form. **Hepatocellular** jaundice results from liver dysfunction characterized by hepatic inflammation (infection, hepatitis, drug induced). The total bilirubin is increased. **Cholestatic** jaundice results from failure of biliary excretion. An increase in direct bilirubin is present.

5. **Physiologic jaundice** is a transient hyperbilirubinemia that is frequently observed in otherwise completely healthy newborns. Bilirubin values peak at day 3 of life and usually normalize by 2 weeks of age.

C. Signs and Symptoms

Indirect, direct, and total bilirubin levels are elevated. **Jaundice** is an accumulation of yellow pigment in the skin and other tissues and is evident when total bilirubin is greater than 3 mg/dL. **Kernicterus** is the presence of yellow pigment in the basal ganglia of the brain and is a complication of severe unconjugated hyperbilirubinemia. Bilirubin can enter the brain if it is not bound to albumin (unconjugated) or if there has been damage to the blood-brain barrier. Signs of kernicterus include a sluggish Moro's reflex, opisthotonus, hypotonia, vomiting, high pitched cry, seizures, and paresis of gaze (sun-setting sign). Dark-colored urine and pale-colored stool may occur in conjugated hyperbilirubinemia.

D. Nursing and Collaborative Diagnosis

❖ Potential for altered neurologic status related to kernicterus

E. Desired Patient Outcome

Child's hyperbilirubinemia will resolve without long-term sequelae.

F. Patient Care Management

1. Management of **indirect hyperbilirubinemia** includes phototherapy by bilirubin lights or bilirubin blankets. As much skin surface as possible should be exposed. Cover eyes to protect from light and provide eye care every 4 hours. Fluid requirements are increased up to 20% because of increased insensible water losses. With excessive hyperbilirubinemia, exchange transfusion and pharmacologic interventions (i.e., phenobarbital administration) are required.
2. Management of **direct hyperbilirubinemia** depends on the etiology.

G. Complications

Indirect hyperbilirubinemia can result in brain damage.

HEPATIC FAILURE

A. Etiology and Risk Factors of Acute Hepatic Failure

1. **Hepatitis (inflammation of the liver)** is the most frequent cause of hepatic failure. Hepatotropic viral infectious causes include the following:
   a. *Hepatitis A virus (HAV)*
      - On average the incubation period is 28 days.
      - Serologic markers for HAV include hepatitis A antibodies of the IgM class (anti-HAV IgM), whose presence reflects active or recent HAV infection, and hepatitis A antibodies of the IgG class (anti-HAV IgG), whose presence reflects immunity.
      - The Advisory Committee on Immunizations Practices recommends routine vaccination for children at age 2 years living in communities with high

rates of hepatitis A (Alaska, Arizona, Oregon, New Mexico, Utah, Washington, Oklahoma, South Dakota, Idaho, Nevada, and California), for those who have planned travel to endemic areas, and day care workers.

- Disease transmission is via the oral-fecal route. Food, water, and shellfish contaminated by the virus are the usual sources.
- In countries with poor sanitation, nearly 100% of preschool children are seropositive. In the Unites States, about 10% of preschool children are seropositive, with most infections occurring from ages to 5 to 14 years (Marsano, 2003).

b. *Hepatitis B virus (HBV)*

- The incubation period is on average 80 days.
- Synthetic hepatitis B vaccine is available and is part of the American Academy of Pediatrics recommended immunization schedule.
- Serologic markers of HBV include hepatitis B surface antigen (HbsAg), whose presence reflects acute or chronic infection; hepatitis B e antigen (HbeAg), whose presence reflects active HBV infection with active viral replication and high infectivity; and antibody to hepatitis B surface antigen (anti-HBs), whose presence reflects clinical recovery and immunity.
- Disease transmission occurs through the exchange of blood or body fluids. Neonates can acquire the virus via maternal transmission.
- Disease presentation varies and may consist of a prodrome, followed by insidious onset, with symptoms usually resolving within 1 to 3 months (Marsano, 2003). Of patients with chronic disease, 30% to 50% have a history of acute disease (Marsano, 2003); 90% of affected infants develop chronic hepatitis and a chronic carrier state. A small percentage of infected individuals develop fulminant hepatic failure (FHF).

c. *Hepatitis D virus (HDV)*

- Incubation period is 21 to 90 days.
- HDV is caused by an incomplete virus and requires the helper function of the HBV for replication; therefore only individuals infected with HBV can be HDV positive. HDV is directly cytopathic to the liver cells and tends to cause more severe hepatitis compared with HBV.
- Serologic markers for HDV include antibody to HDV (anti-HDV), whose presence reflects exposure to the delta virus, and RNA of HDV (HDV RNA), whose presence reflects active replication of HDV. Coinfection can be identified by simultaneous detection of antibody of the IgM class to the hepatitis B core antigen (anti-HBc IgM) plus HbsAg, which establishes acute HBV infection.

d. *Hepatitis C virus (HCV)*

- Incubation time is 2 to 26 weeks (Marsano, 2003).
- Serologic markers for HCV include anti-HCV antibody, indicating exposure to HCV and polymerase chain reaction (PCR), whose presence reflects HCV infection. Approximately 240,000 children are exposed or infected in the United States (Jonas, 2001).
- Children who have been multiply transfused (e.g., childhood malignancies, hemodialysis, open-heart surgery) have infection rates reported to be 50% to 90% (Jonas, 2001). Transfusion-related infection has been virtually eliminated with screening of the blood supply for HCV antibody since 1992.
- Perinatal transmission is now the most common mode of acquiring HCV in children.

e. *Clinical presentation of hepatitis* involves three stages (Barnard and Hazinski, 1992).

- *Preicteric stage* has a duration of approximately 1 week. Signs and symptoms include fever, chills, anorexia, malaise, abdominal pain, nausea, vomiting, joint pain, hepatomegaly, and lymphadenopathy. HAV is characterized by nonspecific features of viral illness, including fever, headache, anorexia, and nausea. HBV is characterized by arthralgia, arthritis, transient skin rash, and later malaise, nausea, vomiting, and low-grade fever. Jaundice usually occurs 10 to 12 days after the onset of symptoms.
- *Icteric stage* has a duration of 2 to 6 weeks. Signs and symptoms include weakness, fatigue, pallor, jaundice, dark urine, pale-colored stool, and pruritus.
- During the *posticteric stage,* there is resolution of the jaundice, darkening of the stools, and normalization of LFT values. Complete recovery occurs in most cases.

f. *Other viral causes* include hepatitis E, herpes simplex virus, Epstein-Barr virus, adenovirus, varicella, and cytomegalovirus (which may be congenitally acquired). Infants are at risk if the mother is infected with a primary infection and active infection is present at birth.

2. **Neonatal "giant cell" hepatitis** is a histologically descriptive term. The disease is characterized by large cells with many nuclei. The cause is unknown, and giant cells are a feature of many liver diseases.
3. **Drug-induced acute hepatic failure**
   a. The *liver* is the most common site for drug metabolism. Children receiving drugs known to be hepatotoxic should have serial LFT monitoring while receiving therapy. The risk of developing FHF increases with continued use of the drug in the presence of developing hepatitis.
   b. The *most common toxic drugs* are acetaminophen (Tylenol), nonsteroidal anti-inflammatory drugs, ecstasy (methyldioxymethamphetamine), anticonvulsants (phenytoin [Dilantin] and valproate [Depakene]), methotrexate, halothane, and isoniazid (Sass and Shakil, 2003).
4. **Wilson's disease** is an autosomal recessive disorder that results in excessive accumulation of copper in the organs. The biochemical disorder of copper metabolism is a defect in the copper adenosine triphosphatase transporter, with decreased copper excretion, defective incorporation of copper into ceruplasmin, and copper accumulation (Carlson et al., 2004). Liver dysfunction manifestations are variable and the child may present with FHF. Medical therapy includes administration of *d*-penicillamine and dietary restrictions of copper. Liver transplantation is indicated in the presence of FHF or cirrhosis with decompensation.
5. **Reye syndrome** is a multisystem disease characterized by severe encephalopathy with fatty changes to the viscera (particularly the liver). The disorder is associated with viral illnesses treated with aspirin.

B. Etiology of Chronic Hepatic Failure

1. The **difference between acute and chronic disease** presentation relates to the rate of parenchymal (organ-specific tissue) injury. Fibrosis leads to cirrhosis with development of portal hypertension evident by the presence of hepatosplenomegaly, varices, and ascites.
2. **Most children** have a chronic presentation of hepatic failure vs. an acute presentation. (See the chronic disease etiologies in the Hepatic Failure discussion.)

C. Pathophysiology of Acute Hepatic Failure

1. **Pathophysiology** of acute hepatic failure is presumed to be multifactorial. Portal-systemic shunting (caused by progressive liver destruction) allows blood

flow from the intestine to be shunted around the liver, bypassing any remaining viable hepatocytes. The liver is unable to remove toxic metabolites normally formed by intestinal bacterial degradation of proteins, amino acids, and blood (e.g., ammonia). Altered blood-brain permeability is hypothesized to be related to toxin(s) of intestinal origin bypassing the portal filtration, resulting in a disruption of the blood-brain barrier.

2. **Fulminant hepatic failure** is diagnosed in children who develop signs of encephalopathy within 8 weeks of the onset of liver disease and in whom there is no evidence of previous liver dysfunction. Multiple-organ or system failure occurs.
3. **Neurologic pathophysiology:** Etiology remains unclear, although vasogenic and cytotoxic mechanism are thought to be involved with the development of cerebral edema (Sass and Shakil, 2003).
4. **Renal pathophysiology**
   a. More than one type of *renal failure* may be present. Careful differentiation of the type of renal failure must be made before appropriate therapy can be initiated.
   b. *Prerenal azotemia* occurs when prerenal blood flow and renal perfusion are compromised. Treatment includes addressing the cause of decreased renal perfusion (i.e., fluid resuscitation).
   c. *Acute tubular necrosis* is related to parenchymal damage to the kidney associated with a chronic prerenal or postrenal condition (e.g., toxic chemical exposure or glomerulonephritis). It may occur with concomitant sepsis, hemorrhage, and ischemia.
   d. *Hepatorenal syndrome* (functional renal failure of liver disease) is likely to be related to an unidentified substance causing oliguric renal failure in the presence of hepatic failure. Renal failure resolves with improvement of the hepatic dysfunction; however, the associated mortality is high.
5. **Hematologic pathophysiology**
   a. *Coagulopathy* is related to an abnormal production of prothrombin and other clotting factors produced by the liver, signifying impaired hepatic synthetic function and ineffective removal of activated clotting factors.
   b. *Hypersplenism* results from increased portal venous pressures delaying the blood flow through the splanchnic bed with resultant congestion and enlargement of the spleen. Splenic overactivity increases destruction of red blood cells (RBCs), platelets, and WBCs. The sequela of splenomegaly includes anemia, platelet dysfunction (quantitative and qualitative), leukopenia, and DIC.

D. Signs and Symptoms of Acute Hepatic Failure

1. **Staging** of hepatic encephalopathy
   a. *Stage I:* Normal level of consciousness, periods of lethargy and euphoria
   b. *Stage II:* Disorientation, increased drowsiness, and agitation with mood swings
   c. *Stage III:* Marked confusion, sleeping most of the time
   d. *Stage IV:* Coma
2. **Jaundice:** Yellow discoloration of the skin, mucous membranes, and sclera is caused by excessive bilirubin levels.
3. **Renal failure symptoms** depend on the type of renal failure the child is experiencing. Azotemia should be evaluated carefully in the presence of hepatic failure, as nitrogenous wastes cannot be metabolized appropriately. Increased serum creatinine levels and oliguria are present.

4. **Coagulopathy** is recognized by an elevated PT. A PT that is uncorrectable despite IV vitamin K (AquaMephyton) administration reflects significant parenchymal disease. In addition, there will be platelet dysfunction. Other signs include bruising and bleeding from mucosal surfaces and the presence of petechiae.

E. Signs and Symptoms of Chronic Hepatic Failure

1. **Hepatosplenomegaly:** The liver becomes firm and enlarged with regeneration, and the liver and spleen become enlarged due to vascular engorgement.
2. **Varices:** With intrahepatic fibrosis there is obstruction of blood flow with formation of collaterals in the esophagus and rectum. These veins are thin walled and prone to the development of varicosities (i.e., rectal, esophageal) and GI tract bleeding.
3. **Ascites** is related to the accumulation of fluid in the abdomen related to altered plasma oncotic pressure (decreased albumin production) and increased portal venous pressure. Increased abdominal girth, everted umbilicus, bulging flanks, positive fluid wave, and respiratory distress are noted.
4. **Malnutrition** is evident because of inadequate bile salts and the child's inability to absorb fat-soluble vitamins (A, D, E, and K). Poor weight gain and deficiencies of vitamin A (causing atrophy of the epithelial tissue and night blindness when severe), vitamin D (causing rickets), vitamin E (causing muscle degeneration, megaloblastic anemia, hemolytic anemia, creatinuria, target cell anemia, spur cell anemia, and peripheral neuropathy), and vitamin K (causing hypoprothrombinemia resulting in coagulopathy) are noted. Adequate glucose is necessary to maintain normal blood glucose levels.
5. **Pruritus** is related to bile salt deposition on the epidermis. Constant itching can be accompanied with skin breakdown.
6. **Asterixis:** "Liver flap" is a flapping tremor of the hand noted when both arms are raised with forearms fixed and the hands dorsiflexed.
7. **Fetor hepaticus** is a fecal breath that is intestinal in origin.
8. **Rickets** are caused by an abnormal bone formation related to a deficiency of vitamin D, calcium, and phosphorus. Pathologic fractures and bone malformations result.
9. **Telangiectasis** (vascular spiders, spider angiomas, spider nevi) are skin lesions consisting of a central arteriole from which smaller vessels radiate. Spontaneous bleeding from lesions can occur.
10. **Xanthomas** are fatty nodules that develop in the subcutaneous skin layer due to the accumulation of cholesterol.

F. Invasive and Noninvasive Diagnostic Studies

Comprehensive blood chemistries, hematology and coagulation studies, ultrasound, CT scan, liver biopsy, endoscopy, and LFTs (see Table 7-2) may be useful in the determination of pathology as described above.

G. Nursing and Collaborative Diagnoses

- Potential for altered thought processes and cerebral perfusion related to hepatic encephalopathy with resultant increased intracranial pressure (ICP)
- Potential for alteration in fluid and electrolyte status related to acute tubular necrosis, prerenal azotemia, and hepatorenal syndrome
- Potential for bleeding and GI tract bleeding related to coagulopathy, portal hypertension, and the presence of varices
- Potential for altered nutritional status and less than body requirements related to altered fat, protein, and carbohydrate metabolism

❖ Potential for sepsis related to impaired immune function and potential for intestinal bacterial translocation.

H. Patient Care Management

1. Management of **encephalopathy**
   a. *Monitor* for signs of increased ICP or neurologic dysfunction. Placement of an ICP monitoring device may be contraindicated in the presence of coagulopathy. Provide intubation when appropriate for airway control and hyperventilation.
   b. *Intervene* to decrease serum ammonia with administration of neomycin to decrease GI tract ammonia formation and lactulose (Cephulac) to acidify colonic flora and promote ammonia elimination. Restrict dietary protein.
2. Management of **hepatorenal syndrome:** Monitor fluid and electrolyte status and correct electrolyte imbalances. Dialysis may be indicated (hemodialysis or continuous venovenous hemofiltration).
3. Management of **coagulopathy:** Administration of blood products (FFP by bolus or continuous infusion, platelets, packed RBCs, and factor VII), and IV vitamin K (AquaMephyton) therapy may be required.
4. Management of **portal hypertension**
   a. *Variceal bleeding* is treated with pharmacologic agents (i.e., vasopressin [Pitressin], octreotide (Sandostatin) and propranolol [Inderal]), endoscopic injection of a sclerosing agent into or endoscopic band ligation of varices, the Sengstaken-Blakemore tube (see Acute Treatment of Esophageal Varices in Acute GI Tract Hemorrhage section), or surgical intervention with a portosystemic shunt, or any combination of these. Currently endoscopic variceal sclerotherapy is the most common initial treatment for children with hemorrhagic complications of variceal bleeding, although variceal ligation is being done with increased frequency (Kato et al., 2000). However, these procedures do not treat the cause of portal hypertension, and for many children portosystemic shunting is appropriate.
   b. The *goal of portosystemic shunts* is to redirect portal blood flow into the systemic venous circulation, decreasing the portal venous pressure (Ryckman and Alonso, 2001). Central shunts (portacaval shunt) are created by anastomosis of the portal vein to the inferior vena cava. Distal splenorenal shunts are created by anastomosis of the splenic vein to the left renal vein. Nonshunt surgical procedures, including the Sugiura procedure (devascularization of the upper and lower two thirds of greater and lesser curvature of the stomach and ligation of select gastric vessels), are not as successful as shunt procedures (Ryckman and Alonso, 2001). Complications of shunting procedures include thrombosis of the anastomotic vessel, elevated ammonia levels, peptic ulcers, aggravated hepatic failure, and ascites.
5. Management of **splenomegaly:** A spleen guard is a custom-fitted plastic device to cover and protect the spleen. Children must avoid contact sports.
6. Management of **ascites:** Sodium restriction and diuretic therapy (IV furosemide [Lasix], bumetanide [Bumex]) or acetazolamide can help to control fluids. Paracentesis may be used when respiratory compromise occurs. It may precipitate fluid shifts. Complications include infection and hemorrhage.

I. Complications

Complications of acute hepatic failure include encephalopathy; cerebral edema, which is a major cause of mortality for children with FHF; hepatorenal syndrome; and coagulopathies resulting in GI tract, cerebral, and pulmonary hemorrhage. Associated mortality for children is as high as 70% to 90%.

LIVER TRANSPLANTATION

A. Etiologies and Risk Factors

1. **Biliary atresia** is the most common indication for pediatric liver transplantation. The incidence is 1 per 8,000 to 13,000 white infant births (Askin anad Diehl-Jones, 2003). Biliary atresia is a congenital defect of unknown cause that involves the absence or obstruction of the intrahepatic and extrahepatic ducts of the biliary system. With the development of fibrosis, bile flow is obstructed. Progressive disease with resultant fibrosis and eventual cirrhosis occurs.
2. **Metabolic diseases**
   - a. *Alpha-1 antitrypsin (α_1AT) deficiency* is transmitted via an autosomal-recessive trait. Only 5% to 20% of α_1AT-deficient children develop liver disease. The disorder involves a deficiency of α_1AT, which is a polymorphic glycoprotein synthesized by the liver. Liver dysfunction is usually evident as cholestasis during the neonatal period, and cirrhosis develops in later childhood. Children with α_1AT deficiency are at increased risk for developing hepatocellular carcinoma.
   - b. *Tyrosinemia* is an autosomal-recessive trait that results in deficiency of fumarylacetoacetate hydrolase (FAH) activity. Children with tyrosinemia have an increased risk for developing hepatocellular carcinoma.
3. **Intrahepatic cholestasis**
   - a. *Progressive familial intrahepatic cholestasis (PFIC)* is of probable autosomal-recessive inheritance and constitutes a group of disorders with varied clinical characteristics and familial patterns of occurrence. It is characterized by a paucity of bile duct development. Symptoms usually develop before 6 months of age with severe pruritus and moderate jaundice (Whitington et al., 1994). Effective treatment includes surgical biliary diversion and liver transplantation.
   - b. *Alagille syndrome (arteriohepatic dysplasia)* is an autosomal-dominant trait (Alagille et al., 1987). The syndrome's characteristics include a broad forehead, indented chin, vertebral defects, pulmonary artery stenosis, and congenital heart disease. Cholestasis may resolve in infancy with recurrence in childhood.
4. **Metastatic disease**
   - a. *Hepatoblastoma* usually occurs as a single-mass lesion composed of epithelial cells or a mixture of epithelial and mesenchymal components. Seventy-five percent of these cases occur before age 3 years. The abdomen enlarges with the presence of an abdominal mass.
   - b. *Hepatocellular carcinoma* is a highly malignant tumor characterized by anaplastic hepatocytes. It has a peak incidence in infancy, with another peak between the ages of 10 and 15 years. Signs and symptoms include abdominal swelling with associated pain and discomfort, fever, nausea, vomiting, weight loss, lethargy, and jaundice.

B. Contraindications to Transplantation

There are no absolute contraindications to liver transplantation. The presence of metastatic disease or sepsis is a relative contraindication.

C. Pretransplant Considerations

1. **Pretransplant considerations** involve a medical workup that includes a thorough history and examination, laboratory tests, assessment for evidence of

portal hypertension, and assessment of portal vein patency. Family preparation and education are extensive.

2. The **pediatric end-stage liver disease (PELD) model** was recently developed to score the severity of a child's liver disease as a means of assessing his or her chances of dying before transplantation (Ascher, 2003). The child's PELD score is based on age, growth failure, bilirubin level, international normalized ratio (INR), and albumin and is currently used to determine a child's status with the United Network for Organ Sharing. Children with FHF, primary graft dysfunction, metabolic disease causing brain damage, and malignancies continue to receive priority when an organ becomes available for transplantation.

D. Nursing and Collaborative Diagnoses

- ❖ Airway clearance: Ineffective related to the lengthy abdominal procedure, large transverse abdominal incision, and postoperative pain
- ❖ Impaired gas exchange: Potential related to postsurgical atelectasis
- ❖ Altered breathing patterns: Related to ascites, large donor organ, bleeding, and phrenic nerve paresis
- ❖ Potential for hemodynamic instability related to hypertension associated with the use of immunosuppressive agents or hypotension associated with graft dysfunction or surgical bleeding
- ❖ Potential for vessel thrombosis related to small vessel size

E. Desired Patient Outcomes

1. Child will be extubated after recovering from anesthesia.
2. The child will not experience hemodynamic instability (hypertension or hypotension).
3. All existing coagulopathies will resolve in the immediate postoperative period.
4. All vascular anastomoses (portal vein, hepatic artery, and caval anastomoses) will remain patent.

F. Patient Care Management

1. Promote **pulmonary toilet.** After resolution of the existing coagulopathies, initiate chest physiotherapy. Evaluate diaphragm function with an ultrasound if the child fails extubation twice.
2. Treat **hypertension** with antihypertensives. The first-line drug in the immediate postoperative period is institution specific; sodium nitroprusside, sublingual nifedipine (Procardia), or hydralazine are drugs that may be used when necessary.
3. Monitor **Jackson-Pratt drainage.** Bloody drainage greater than 30 mL/kg per hour may indicate surgical bleeding. The presence of bile in a surgical drain could indicate a bile leak.
4. Avoid rapid correction of **coagulopathies.** Hematocrit is maintained at approximately 30%. Subclinical anticoagulation is used for vessel thrombosis prophylaxis and is initiated when the PT is less than 17 seconds. Aspirin decreases platelet aggregation. Dipyridamole (Persantine) is a platelet adhesion inhibitor. Dextran decreases blood viscosity and platelet adhesiveness. Heparin is used as a prophylactic anticoagulant.
5. Other **commonly used medications** include immunosuppressive therapy (see Pharmacology section) and drugs for infection prophylaxis. Broad-spectrum IV antibiotics are given for the first 48 hours. If the patient is afebrile, the antibiotics are discontinued. Co-trimoxazole (Bactrim) is prescribed indefinitely for

Pneumocystis carinii prophylaxis. Nystatin (Mycostatin) is an antifungal agent used for thrush prophylaxis while steroids are prescribed. Ganciclovir (Cytovene) is administered intravenously for 14 days for cytomegalovirus and Epstein-Barr virus prophylaxis.

G. Complications

1. **Rejection**
   a. *Signs and symptoms* include fever, RUQ tenderness, lethargy, light-colored stools, dark-colored urine, and elevated liver enzymes.
   b. *Liver biopsy* is used for definitive diagnosis. Before the biopsy, check platelet count and PT. Ultrasound marking is used when necessary (e.g., may be done in the presence of abnormal anatomic findings, as in the presence of a reduced-size graft following liver transplantation). Monitoring for complications of the biopsy includes frequent assessment of vital signs for the assessment of hemorrhage, chest x-ray examination to rule out pneumothorax, and serial hematocrit measurements.
   c. Treatment is augmentation of the child's immunosuppression.
2. **Infection** is the leading cause of morbidity and mortality following transplantation.
   a. *Bacterial infections* occur most often within the first 30 days. Common causes include preexisting disease conditions, central lines, surgical intervention, and posttransplantation factors, including transfusion requirements and dosing of immunosuppressive agents. Treatment is antibiotic therapy.
   b. *Viral infections* usually occur from 31 to 180 days following transplantation. Primary infections occur when the patient becomes infected with a virus with no previous exposure. Secondary infection involves the reactivation of a latent virus. Recovery from a secondary infection is usually easier than recovery from a primary infection. Common organisms include cytomegalovirus and Epstein-Barr virus (EBV). Early diagnosis of CMV infection can be made with pp65 antigenemia and for EBV with the EBV-PCR in the blood (Reyes, 2001). Treatment is antiviral therapy. Acyclovir (Zovirax) inhibits viral DNA synthesis of the herpesviruses. Ganciclovir (Cytovene) inhibits DNA polymerase. Side effects include impaired renal function, neutropenia, thrombocytopenia, confusion, and nausea.
3. **Lymphoproliferative disease (LPD) and EBV infection:** LPD is characterized by the development of continually proliferating B lymphocytes, presumably stimulated under the influence of EBV. LPD is diagnosed by clinical, laboratory, and pathologic examination. Tissue biopsy with histologic evidence is necessary to confirm the diagnosis. Treatment involves reducing or discontinuing the child's immunosuppression and initiating antiviral therapy.

INTESTINE TRANSPLANTATION

A. Etiologies and Risk Factors

1. **Short gut syndrome** is the most common indication for intestine transplantation. A child is rendered short gut if the loss of absorptive function of the intestine necessitates parenteral nutrition support because of malabsorption and malnutrition. Short gut occurs because of congenital and acquired disease processes.
   a. *Congenital conditions* include gastroschisis, volvulus, intestinal atresias, and extensive Hirschsprung disease (see Table 7-10).

b. *Acquired conditions* include NEC (see NEC section) and traumatic injuries.
c. *Parenteral nutrition–induced cholestasis* is a possible complication of intestinal failure in patients with resultant concomitant liver and intestinal failure.

2. **Other indications,** according to Reyes (2001), include intestinal motility (intestinal pseudo-obstruction and aganglionosis) and enterocyte absorptive impairment (microvillous inclusion disease and autoimmune enteropathy), and malignancies in the abdominal cavity.

B. Contraindications to Transplantation

1. There are no absolute contraindication to intestinal transplantation. The presence of metastatic disease or sepsis is a relative contraindication.
2. No evidence of efforts at intestinal rehabilitation.

C. Pretransplant Considerations

1. Pretransplant considerations involve a medical workup that includes a thorough medical, surgical, and psychosocial history. In addition, because intestine candidates usually have a history of multiple central line sites, an ultrasound is done to assess great vessel patency. An upper GI and small bowel follow-through are done to assess GI anatomy and function and to ascertain the length of remaining intestine.
2. Kato et al. (2003) found that older patients (i.e., older than 2 years), patients with a higher body weight, those not hospitalized at the time of transplant, and those without concomitant liver failure had better survival.
3. Depending on the child's diagnosis and clinical course, an isolated intestine graft, liver-intestine graft, or multivisceral graft (a graft that also includes the stomach) will be the operation of choice and is determined after the child is evaluated.

D. Nursing and Collaborative Diagnoses

- ❖ See Liver transplant section.
- ❖ Potential for impairment in skin integrity related to the ostomy and abdominal wounds
- ❖ Potential for alteration in nutrition: Less than body requirements related to need for intestinal adaptation and postoperative recovery
- ❖ Potential for graft-versus-host disease related to the large lymphoid load in the intestine

E. Desired Patient Outcomes

1. Child will be extubated after recovering from anesthesia.
2. The child will not experience hemodynamic instability (hypertension or hypotension).
3. The child's transplanted intestine will adapt, and enteral feeds will be tolerated.
4. Immunosuppression will be titrated to prevent rejection and to minimize infectious complications, including sepsis related to bacterial translocation and graft-versus-host disease.

F. Patient Care Management

1. See liver transplant section in addition to the following patient care considerations.
2. Assessment of bowel integrity is done initially by stomal appearance and outputs.

G. Complications

1. **Rejection**
   a. The *intestinal allograft* of all the organs transplanted has the highest rate of rejection between 70% and 95% (Reyes, 2001).

b. *Signs and symptoms* include fever related to translocation, pale or dusky stoma, an increase or decrease in enteric output, abdominal pain, and guaiac positive enteric output.
c. *Serial intestinal biopsies* are done through the ileostomy. Histologic criteria for rejection include presence of crypt cell destruction (apoptosis) in the presence of lymphocyte infiltration (Reyes, 2001).
d. *Treatment* is augmentation of the child's immunosuppression.

2. **Infection** is the leading cause of morbidity and mortality following transplantation. Causes include bacterial, viral, and fungal infections (Green and Michaels, 2005).
   a. *Cytomegalovirus* can be particularly problematic for the intestine recipient.
   b. *Bacterial overgrowth*
3. **Lymphoproliferative disease** and EBV infection: See Complications in Liver transplant section.
4. **Graft-versus-host disease** is diagnosed by the presence of a rash confirmed by skin biopsy. Diarrhea and an elevated bilirubin level may also be observed. Treatment involves augmentation of immunosuppression.

REFERENCES

Abu-Elmagd K, Reyes J, Bond G et al.: Clinical intestinal transplantation: a decade of experience at a single center. *Ann Surg* 234(3):404-417, 2001.

Askin DF, Diehl-Jones WL: The neonatal liver part III: pathophysiology of liver dysfunction. *Neonat Network* 22(3):5-15, 2003.

Alagille D, Estrada A, Hadchouel M, et al.: Syndromic paucity of the interlobular bile ducts (Alagille syndrome or arteriohepatic dysplasia): review of 80 cases. *J Pediatr* 110:195-200, 1987.

Ascher NL: What's new in general surgery: transplantation. *J Am Coll Surg* 196(5): 778-783, 2003.

Barnard JA, Hazinski MF: Pediatric gastrointestinal disorders. In Hazinski MF, editor: *Nursing care of the critically ill child.* St. Louis, 1992, Mosby, pp 715-801.

Bell MJ, Ternberg JL, Feign RD et al.: Neonatal necrotizing enterocolitis: therapeutic decisions based upon clinical staging. *Ann Surg* 1:187, 1978.

Canty TG Sr, Weinman D: Management of major pancreatic duct injuries in children. *J Trauma* 50(6):1001-1007, 2001.

Carlson MD, Al-Mateen M, Brewer GJ: Atypical childhood Wilson's disease. *Pediatr Neurol* 30(1):57-60, 2004.

Coley BD, Mutabagani KH, Martin LC et al.: Focused abdominal sonography for trauma (FAST) in children with blunt abdominal trauma. *J Trauma* 48(5):902-906, 2000.

Crill CM, Hak EB: Upper gastrointestinal tract bleeding in critically ill pediatric patients. *Pharmacotherapy* 19(2):162-180, 1999.

Davidson RN, Wall RA: Prevention and management of infections in patients without a spleen. *Clin Microbiol Infect* 7: 657-660, 2001.

Dennery PA, Seidman DS, Stevenson DK: Neonatal hyperbilirubinemia. *N Engl J Med* 344(8):581-590, 2001.

Fanta K, Cook BS, Schweer L: Traumatic injury to the pancreas: the challenges of care in the pediatric patient. *J Trauma Nurs* 10(3):72-78, 2003.

Fox VL: Gastrointestinal bleeding in infancy and childhood. *Gastroenterol Clin North Am* 29(1):37-66, 2000.

Gaines BA, Ford HR: Abdominal and pelvic trauma in children. *Crit Care Med.* 30(11):S416-S423, 2002.

Garcia VF, Brown RL. Pediatric trauma beyond the brain. *Crit Care Clin* 19: 551-561, 2003.

Green M, Michaels MG: New kids on the block: an old problem for a growing pediatric population. *Pediatr Transplant* 116:160-7, 2005.

Gross RE: *The surgery of infancy and childhood.* Philadelphia, 1953, W. B. Saunders.

Hackam DJ, Potoka D, Meza M et al.: Utility of radiographic hepatic injury grade in predicting outcome for children after blunt abdominal trauma. *J Pediatr Surg* 37: 386-389, 2002.

Huether SE, McCance KL, Termina MS: Alterations of digestive function. In

McCance KL, Huether SE, editors: *Pathophysiology: the biological basis for disease in adults and children*, ed 2. St Louis, 1994, Mosby-Year Book Inc.

Jobst MA, Canty TG, Lynch FP: Management of pancreatic injury in pediatric blunt abdominal trauma. *J Pediatr Surg* 34(5): 818-823, 1999.

Jonas MM: Challenges in the treatment of hepatitis C in children. *Clin Liver Dis* 5(4):1063-1071, 2001.

Kato T, Mittal N, Nishida S et al.: The role of intestinal transplantation in the management of babies with extensive gut resections. *J Pediatr Surg* 38(2):145-149, 2003.

Kato T, Romero R, Koutouby R et al.: Portosystemic shunting in children during the era of endoscopic therapy: improved postoperative growth parameters. *J Pediatr Gastroenterol Nutr* 30(4):419-424, 2000.

Kenner C, Lott JW: Assessment and management of gastrointestinal system. *Comprehensive neonatal nursing*, ed 3. Philadelphia, 2003, W. B. Saunders, pp 448-485.

Killeen KL, Shanmuganathan K, Boyd-Kranis R et al.: CT findings after embolization for blunt splenic trauma. *J Vasc Interv Radiol* 12:209-14, 2001.

Lynch JM, Meza MP, Newman et al.: Computed tomography grade of splenic injury is predictive of the time required for radiographic healing. *J Pediatr Surg* 32: 1093-1096, 1997.

Marsano LS: Hepatitis. *Primary Care Clin Office Pract* 30(1):81-107, 2003.

McCollough M, Sharieff GQ: Abdominal surgical emergencies in infants and young children. *Emerg Med Clin North Am* 2003;21:909-935, 2003.

Morgan R: Abdominal trauma in infants and children: prompt identification and early management of serious and life-threatening injuries. Part 1: injury patterns and initial assessment. *Pediatr Emerg Care* 16(2):106-115, 2000.

Nadler EP, Gardner M, Schall LC et al.: Management of blunt pancreatic injury in children. *J Trauma* 47:1098-1103, 1999.

Nastanski F, Cohen A, Lush SP et al.: The role of oral contrast administration immediately prior to the computed tomographic evaluation of the blunt trauma victim. *Injury* 32:545-549, 2001.

Neu J, Weiss MD: Necrotizing enterocolitis: pathophysiology and prevention. *JPEN J Parenter Enter Nutr* 23:S13-S17, 1999.

Ostlie DJ, Spilde TL, St. Peter SD, et al.: Necrotizing enterocolitis in full-term infants. *J Pediatr Surg*. 2003;38(7):1039-1042, 2003.

Patel AS, Pohl JF, Easley DJ: Proton pump inhibitors and pediatrics. *Pediatr Rev* 24(1):12-15, 2003.

Patty I, Kalaoui M Al-Shamali M et al.: Endoscopic drainage for pancreatic pseudocyst in children. *J Pediatr Surg* 36:503-505, 2001.

Potoka DA, Schall LC, Ford HR: Risk factors for splenectomy in children with blunt splenic trauma. *J Pediatr Surg* 37(3):294-299, 2002.

Pryor JP, Stafford PW, Nance ML: Severe blunt hepatic trauma in children. *J Pediatr Surg* 36(7):974-979, 2001.

Puranik SR, Hayes JS, Long J et al.: Liver enzymes as predictors of liver damage due to blunt abdominal trauma in children. *South Med J* 95:203-206, 2002.

Rayhorn N, Thrall C, Silber G: A review of the causes of upper gastrointestinal tract bleeding in children. *Gastroenterol Nurs* 24(1):23-27, 2000a.

Rayhorn N, Thrall C, Silber G: A review of the causes of lower gastrointestinal tract bleeding in children. *Gastroenterol Nurs* 24(2):77-82, 2000b.

Reyes J: Intestinal transplantation for children with short bowel syndrome. *Semin Pediatr Surg* 10(2):99-104, 2001.

Rothrock SG, Green SM, Morgan R: Abdominal trauma in infants and children: prompt identification and early management of serious and life-threatening injuries. Part II: specific injuries and ED management. *Pediatr Emerg Care* 2000;16(3):189-195, 2000.

Rudolph CZ, Mazur LJ, Liptak GS, et al.: Guidelines for the evaluation and treatment of gastroesophageal reflux in infants and children. *J Pediatr Gastroenterol Nutr* 32 (suppl 2):S1-S31, 2001.

Ryckman FC, Alonso MH: Causes and management of portal hypertension in the pediatric population. *Clin Liver Dis* 5(3):789-818, 2001.

Sanchez JL, Paidas CN: Childhood trauma: now and in the new millennium. *Surg Clin North Am* 79:1503-1535, 1999.

Sandritter T: Gastroesophageal disease in infants and children. *J Pediatr Health Care* 17(4):198-203, 2003.

Sass DA, Shakil AO: Fulminant hepatic failure. *Gastroenterol Clin* 32(4):1195-1211, 2003.

Shilyansky J, Sena LM, Kreller M et al.: Nonoperative management of pancreatic injuries in children. *J Pediatr Surg* 33: 343-349, 1998.

Stafford PW, Blinman TA, Nance ML: Practical points in evaluation and resuscitation of the injured child. *Surg Clin North Am* 82:273-301, 2002.

Stylianos S: Evidence-based guidelines for resource utilization in children with isolated spleen or liver injury: the APSA Trauma Committee. *J Pediatr Surg* 35: 164-167, 2000.

Taketomo CK, Hodding JH, Kraus DM: *Pediatric dosage handbook,* ed 10. Hudson, Ohio, 2003, Lexi-Comp.

Whitington PF, Freese DK, Alonso EM et al.: Clinical and biochemical findings in progressive intrahepatic cholestasis. *J Pediatr Gastroenterol Nutr* 18(2):131-141, 1994.

Wise BV, Mudd SS, Wilson ME: Management of blunt abdominal trauma in children. *J Trauma Nurs* 9(1):6-14, 2002.

CHAPTER

8 Hematology and Immunology

KATHRYN ROBERTS, DEBBIE BRINKER, AND BARBARA MURANTE

DEVELOPMENTAL ANATOMY AND PHYSIOLOGY

A. Hematopoiesis

1. **Hematopoiesis** is the process by which blood cells are formed.
2. **Anatomic sites** of hematopoiesis vary with age.
   a. *During embryonic and fetal life,* the yolk sac, liver, spleen, thymus, lymph nodes, and bone marrow are all involved (Nathan et al., 1998; Tortora and Grabowski, 2002).
   b. *At birth,* hematopoiesis takes place in the bone marrow, called red marrow, of all bones.
   c. *After birth,* there is the gradual replacement of red (blood-forming) marrow by yellow (fatty) marrow. By adulthood, red marrow exists only in the pelvis, vertebrae, cranium, and sternum.
3. **Mature blood cells** arise by a developmental process called **differentiation.**
   a. *Pluripotent hematopoietic stem cells* give rise to many differentiated blood cells and also replenish themselves.
   b. Pluripotent hematopoietic stem cells differentiate into *committed stem cells.* These cells are committed to, develop, and differentiate into a certain cell type (i.e., red cells, platelets, white cells).
   c. *The process of development and differentiation* is guided and stimulated by a variety of important growth factors and cytokines: erythropoietin (stimulates red cells), thrombopoetin (platelets), and granulocyte colony-stimulating factor (G-CSF) stimulates white cells.
4. **Five types of cells** arise from the stem cell. Each of these cells end with *-blast,* which refers to a nucleated precursor cell (Tortora and Grabowski, 2002). *Proerythroblasts* form the mature erythrocyte (red blood cells [RBCs]). *Myeloblasts* form the mature neutrophils, eosinophils, and basophils (a type of white blood cell [WBC]). *Monoblasts* form the mature monocytes (a type of WBC). *Lymphoblasts* form the mature lymphocytes (a type of WBC). *Megakaryoblasts* form the mature thrombocytes (platelets) (Figure 8-1).
5. **Development of the pluripotential stem cell** into a mature hematopoietic cell (RBC, WBC, or platelet) occurs in approximately 1 to 2 weeks.
6. Alterations in the development of blood cell lines include **aplasia,** in which the bone marrow completely fails to develop stem cells, and **hypo-plasia,** where the bone marrow develops an abnormally low number of stem cells.

B. The Immune System

1. Functionally and anatomically, there is overlap with the **hematopoietic system and hematopoiesis.**

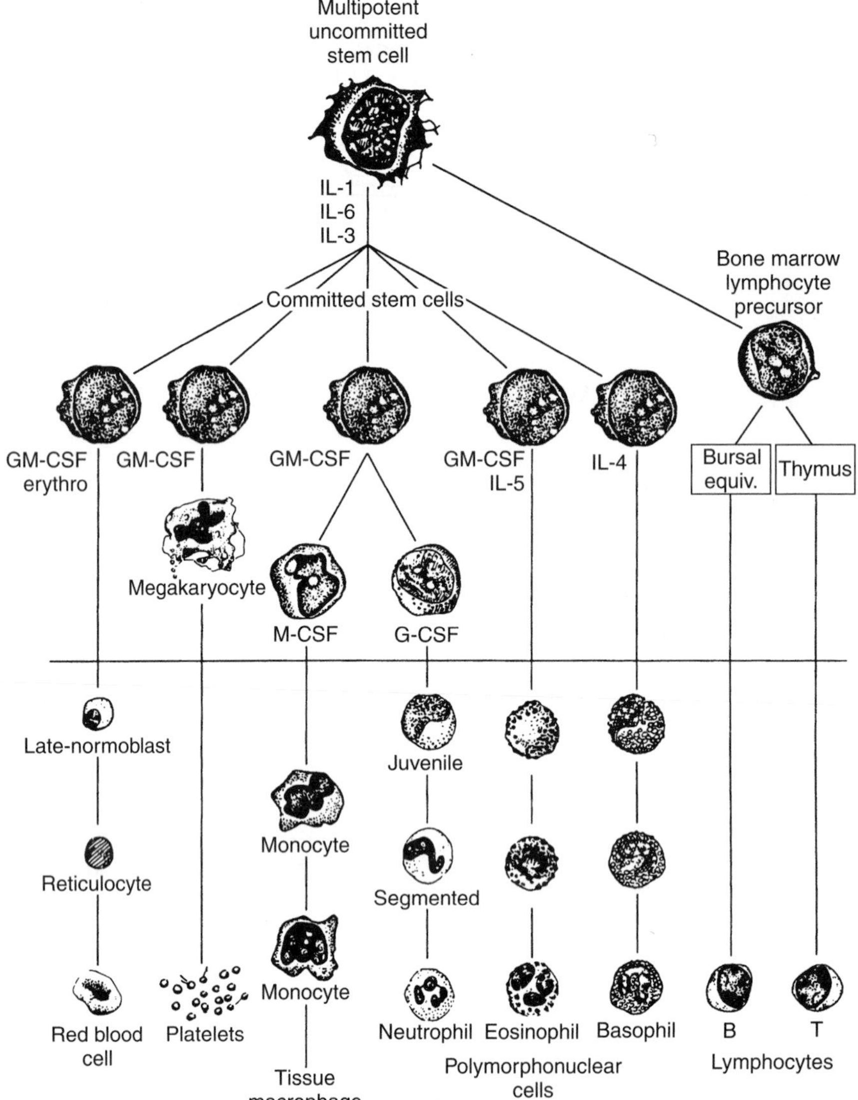

FIGURE 8-1 ■ Cell differentiation from stem cells. The process of hematopoiesis in which the most primitive cells differentiate and ultimately give rise to erythrocytes, granulocytes, thrombocytes, and macrophages. Colony-stimulating factors (CSFs) act on blood precursors to stimulate the production of specific cell lineages; the principal sites of action of these CSFs are indicated. Cells below the horizontal line are found in normal peripheral blood. *G,* granulocyte; *M,* macrophage; *IL,* interleukin.

(From Ganong WF. Circulating body fluids. In Ganong WF, editor: *Review of medical physiology,* ed 16. Norwalk, Conn, 1993, Appleton & Lange, p 471.)

2. **Lymphocyte**
   a. A *type of WBC* whose role is to provide protection to the organ via development of various types of immunity.
   b. There are two main types of lymphocytes: *B cells* (involved with humoral immunity; the production of antibodies); and *T cells* (involved with cellular immunity).

c. Key sites of development of lymphocytes include the bone marrow (for B lymphocytes) and the thymus, situated behind the sternum, (for T lymphocytes). These sites of development are called *primary lymphocyte tissue organs.*

d. *Secondary lymphoid tissue or organs* are sites for storage, division, and activation of lymphocytes.

- The spleen is important for humoral immunity and for cellular immunity as well. It is also rich in macrophages (phagocytic cells) and serves as a normal site for destruction of old or damaged red cells.
- Lymphatic channels transport fluid from the interstitium around the cells in the body, through lymph nodes, and eventually empty into a large lymphatic vessel called the *thoracic duct.*
- Lymph nodes are bean-shaped structures located along the length of the lymphatic vessels (Figure 8-2). Distribution is throughout the body and clustered in groups, both superficial and deep. Lymph nodes function as filters and are important sites of lymphocyte activation and differentiation.
- Mucosa-associated lymph tissues (MALT) are dispersed throughout the body and line mucosal surfaces (i.e., the gastrointestinal [GI] tract, lungs,

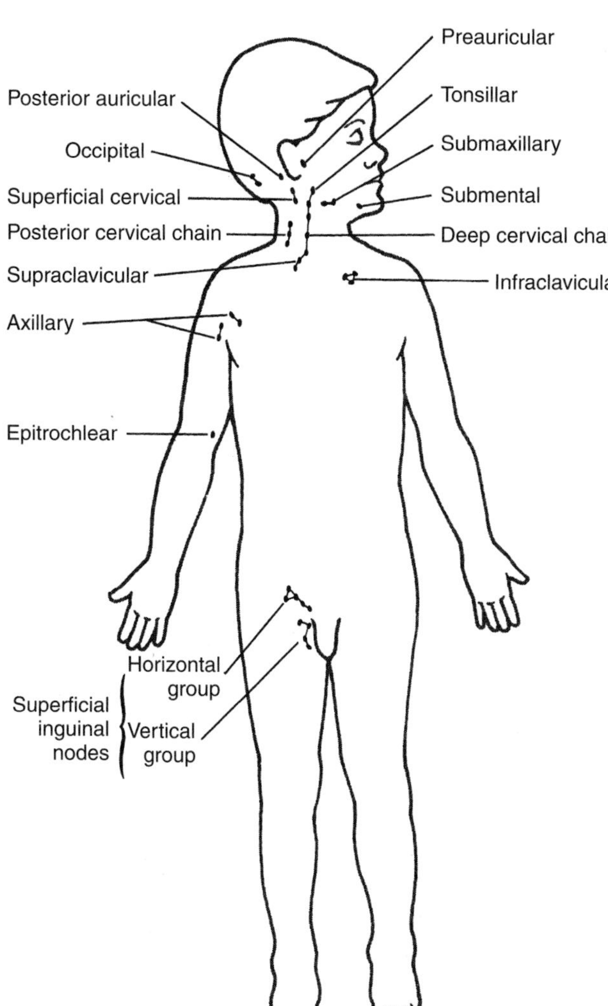

FIGURE 8-2 ■ Lymph nodes of the body. (From Betz CL, Hunsberger, MM, Wright S, editors: *Family-centered nursing care of children,* ed 2. Philadelphia, 1994, W. B. Saunders, p 474.)

skin). They are located within or close to sites of potential invasion by bacteria or foreign substances.
- The liver is rich in a particular type of macrophage called *Kupffer's cells.* These have filtering functions similar to, although less effective than, the spleen.

C. Committed Hematologic Lines

1. **Red blood cells** (RBCs, or erythrocytes)
   a. *RBCs* develop from erythroid precursor cells under the influence of erythropoietin.
   b. *Reticulocytes* represent the stage of maturation just before the mature erythrocyte. Reticulocytes are normally present in small numbers in the peripheral blood and are increased during states of erythroid stimulation. They quickly (in 24 to 48 hours) mature into RBCs.
   c. *Mature RBCs* have a life span of 120 days. Their main function is to pick up oxygen as they transit the pulmonary capillaries and deliver that oxygen to the tissues.
   d. *Hemoglobin* is a large, complex, iron-containing protein that fills RBCs and is responsible for the RBCs' oxygen-carrying abilities.
      - Normal adult hemoglobin is called Hgb A.
      - Hemoglobin F (fetal Hgb) is present in large concentrations in the fetus, but it rapidly declines after birth and is present in only minimal amounts in children and adults.
      - Normal RBC production requires adequate amounts of iron, folic acid, and vitamin B_{12}.
      - Anemia represents a decreased number of red cells or hemoglobin, with a resultant decrease in oxygen-carrying capacity. Anemia can result from decreased production of red cells, increased destruction, or blood loss. Anemia is measured as a decrease in hematocrit and hemoglobin; it is usually defined as a hemoglobin level below 11 g/dL during childhood. Gradual losses can be compensated with few clinical signs and symptoms until the hemoglobin falls to 8 g/dL. Aplastic anemia is associated with decreased RBCs, platelets, and WBCs.
      - The RBCs carry a variety of important surface antigens that are important in transfusion medicine. The most important antigens are A and B. The presence or absence of these determine one's blood group. Other antigen groups are also important; the Rh system is of considerable significance in pediatrics, where maternal sensitization to the D antigen can lead to hemolytic disease of the newborn.
2. **Leukocytes** (white blood cells [WBCs])
   a. The *WBCs* are a heterogeneous group of cells that serve in a variety of ways to protect the organism. Phagocytosis, humoral and cellular immunity, and mediators of the inflammatory response are all important components of host defense. Granulocytes (neutrophils), lymphocytes (discussed separately), monocytes, eosinophils, and basophils are the different types of WBCs.
   b. *Neutrophils* account for the largest component of total circulating WBCs, usually 60% to 70% (age related). Neutrophils are the most active in phagocytosis.
      - Neutrophils originate and mature in the bone marrow and can be found in blood vessel walls, intravascular spaces, tissues, and bone marrow. The adult bone marrow reserve is approximately 10 times the quantity of the neutrophils in the circulation and tissue and body cavities (Guyton and Hall, 2000). The infant and young child have smaller bone marrow reserves of neutrophils and are less able to replenish these cells rapidly (Grant, 2001).

- The mature form of the neutrophil is polymorphonucleated (PMNs or "poly"). PMNs normally constitute the majority of the circulating neutrophils and are phagocytic and active in inflammation and tissue damage. PMNs are the first WBCs to respond to infection and the most numerous WBCs at the site of infection.
- The immature form of the neutrophil has an unsegmented-appearing nucleus and is referred to as a *band*. The immature form lacks complete phagocytic ability and normally constitutes less than 10% of the circulating neutrophils.
- *Neutrophilia* is an increased number of circulating neutrophils, often accompanied by an increase in the number of immature *neutrophils* (bands). Neutrophilia is associated with infections; situations that increase cardiac output (stress response associated with surgery, hemorrhage, or emotional distress such as intense crying); or increased release of epinephrine, adrenocorticotropic hormone (ACTH), or adrenal corticosteroids. Neutrophilia is also sometimes seen following administration of G-CSF.
- Neutropenia is a decreased number of circulating neutrophils ($<1500/mm^3$); it is often associated with malignant conditions and marrow hypoplasia or aplasia.
- WBCs mature in the bone marrow for approximately 10 days. WBCs then are released into the circulation, circulate in the blood for 4 to 8 hours, and then circulate another 4 to 5 days in the tissues. The life span of WBCs is shortened in the presence of an infection.

c. *Eosinophils* normally account for 2% to 5% of the circulating WBC and have weak phagocytic activity. Eosinophils may have a role in "turning off" the immune response because the eosinophil is the last to arrive at the site of infection. Cytoplasmic granules contain chemical substances that destroy parasitic worms and act on immune complexes involved in allergic responses.

- Eosinophilia is an increased number of eosinophils that is greater than normally present. The eosinophil count may increase to as high as 50% of the circulating WBCs with parasitic infection and less often with allergic conditions. *Eosinopenia* is a decreased number of eosinophils; this decrease is not clinically significant.
- From the bone marrow, eosinophils are released into the circulation and migrate to tissues. Unlike other granulocytes, eosinophils may recirculate back and forth between the circulation and the tissues.

d. *Basophils* represent the smallest proportion of granulocytes, accounting for fewer than 1% of circulating WBCs. Cytoplasmic granules contain chemical substances (e.g., histamine, heparin, and probably serotonin) that are released and participate in inflammation and allergic responses.

- Production and life span of the basophil is not thoroughly understood. *Basophilia* is an increased number of circulating basophils. *Basopenia* is a decreased number of circulating basophils; it is not clinically significant.

3. Mononuclear phagocytes (monocytes and macrophages)

a. *Monocytes* normally constitute 3% to 8% of circulating WBCs. Produced in the bone marrow and spending only a brief time in the circulation, most monocytes migrate into the tissues and differentiate into macrophages.

- *Monocytosis,* an increase in the number of circulating monocytes, is observed in patients with viral, parasitic, or rickettsial infections.
- *Monocytopenia,* a decrease in the number of circulating monocytes, is not clinically significant. It is sometimes seen with human immunodeficiency virus (HIV) infection or in patients receiving prednisone therapy.

b. *Macrophages* are not quantified in the serum and have a long life span; some live for years. Macrophages commonly reside in a specific tissue, although a small percentage may wander. Examples of fixed macrophages include alveolar macrophage, Kupffer's cells in the liver, microglial cells of the brain, and spleen sinus macrophages. Macrophages play a primary role in *nonspecific* defenses through the ability to phagocytose. They are capable of phagocytosing larger and greater numbers of particles than the neutrophil or the monocyte. Macrophages also play a primary role in *specific* defense through processing and presentation of the antigen to the helper T cell.

4. **Lymphocytes** (lymphoid lineage) are the primary immune cells associated with humoral and cell-mediated immunity (CMI), although a small portion of lymphocytes (natural killer [NK] cells) are nonspecific in nature.
   a. *Lymphocytes* account for 10% to 40% of the circulating WBCs. They are produced in the bone marrow and then migrate to other parts of the body to differentiate and mature into several distinct subsets. Cells that migrate to the thymus differentiate into T lymphocytes (T cells) and mediate CMI. Cells that migrate to the bursa equivalent in the human (thought to be the bone marrow) differentiate into B lymphocytes (B cells) and mediate humoral immunity (involving antibody production). NK cells constitute a subset of lymphocytes that is nonspecific in nature.
      - *Lymphocytosis,* an increase in the number of circulating lymphocytes, is often noted in patients with viral infections (such as infectious mononucleosis or infectious hepatitis) or lymphocytic leukemia or lymphoma.
      - *Lymphopenia,* a decrease in the number of circulating lymphocytes, is often noted in patients with congenital immunodeficiency, acquired immunodeficiency syndrome (AIDS), uremia, or following administration of corticosteroids or ACTH.
   b. *T lymphocytes, or T cells,* normally constitute 65% to 85% of all lymphocytes. T cells mediate CMI, which confers a component of specific, acquired immunity and protects from infections with intracellular organisms, such as viruses, fungi, protozoa, and helminthic parasites. T cells are involved in the elimination of mutated or tumor cells and the immune response triggered during tissue graft or organ transplantation.
      - Subsets of T lymphocytes have been identified through the identification of specialized molecules of the cell membrane surfaces, referred to as *clusters of differentiation (CD).*
      - **Helper T cells** (CD4) send chemical signals (via lymphokines) to the cytotoxic T cells, macrophages, and NK cells. They have an important role in the activation of B cells.
      - **Suppressor T cells** (CD8) send a signal to inhibit actions of B cells, helper T cells, and killer T cells.
      - **Cytotoxic or killer T cells** (CD8) eliminate targets *directly* by chemical destruction and play a role in the rejection of tissue transplantation.
   c. *B lymphocytes, or B cells,* normally constitute up to 35% of circulating lymphocytes. B cells mediate humoral immunity (HI) through transformation into a plasma cell, which then secretes immunoglobulin. HI confers a component of specific, acquired immunity and protects the host from bacterial infection and viral invasion.
   d. *NK cells* normally constitute 5% to 10% of the total lymphocyte count. NK cells have neither B- nor T-cell markers and are referred to by many other names (e.g., non-B, non-T cells, null cells). The target for the NK cell is the tumor cell or virally infected cell. The NK cells' cytotoxic abilities are

nonspecific in nature because they can destroy the target without prior sensitization.

e. *Memory cells* have cluster differentiation (CD) according to the various distinct cell types (helper, suppressor, or cytotoxic T cell or B cell). They are programmed to recognize the original invading microorganism on subsequent invasions. Memory cells initiate a secondary response and may result in elimination before any signs or symptoms of infection are seen.

D. Platelets (Thrombocytes)

1. *Megakaryoblasts* mature into **megakaryocytes.**
   a. Megakaryocytes break into pieces (budding) forming platelets, which are released into the blood stream. Granulocyte-macrophage colony-stimulating factor (GM-CSF), stem cell factor, and interleukin-3 (IL-3) have been shown to stimulate the growth of megakaryocytes but are ineffective clinically. Thrombopoietin may be effective, but it is unavailable for clinical use in humans at this time.
   b. Two thirds of *mature platelets* circulate in the bloodstream, and one third are stored in the spleen but released if needed to maintain hemostasis. The life span of platelets produced in vivo is 7 to 10 days; transfused platelets have a shorter life span, usually 3 to 4 days. Thrombocytes usually are removed by the spleen or incorporated into a clot.
2. **Characteristics:** Thrombocytes are minute, round, or oval discs. Platelet performance depends on the quantity of platelets (platelet count: 150,000 to 400,000/mm^3) and the quality of function. *Adhesiveness* is stickiness, the ability to attach to blood vessel walls and surfaces. *Aggregation* is the process in which first platelets release substances that further recruit platelets so that a platelet plug is formed. Aggregation is increased with secretion of epinephrine and serotonin, substances found on the surface of platelets. Functions are decreased in the presence of antiprostaglandins such as aspirin (see Relevant Pharmacology section). Newly produced platelets are more effective than those that have been in the circulation for a few days.

E. Plasma Factors

More than 40 substances or protein molecules in blood and tissues are involved in the clotting cascade.

1. **Procoagulants,** also known as plasma clotting factors (Table 8-1), promote coagulation. Clotting factors lead to the formation of a fibrin clot. They are referred to by Roman numerals and the name of the substance. Anticoagulants are produced in the liver except for factor VIII (formation site unknown). Vitamin K is required for production of factors II, VII, IX, and X. Factors are circulated in inactive form until stimulated to initiate clotting (see Plasma Factors discussion). All factors act in concert in vivo to respond to tissue or blood-cell injury. Consumption of the substances results in their destruction.
2. **Anticoagulants** inhibit coagulation.
   a. *Circulating anticoagulants* are antithrombin III, protein C, and protein S. Antithrombin III inactivates thrombin and inhibits factor X. Protein C inactivates factors V and VIII, stimulates fibrinolysis, and elevates levels of tissue plasminogen activator (tPA). Protein activates protein C.
   b. The fibrinolytic system's major component is *plasminogen*. Plasminogen is produced in the liver and circulated in the plasma. Concentrations increase in response to inflammatory states. Plasminogen is converted to plasmin, which has the ability to digest fibrinogen and fibrin. A by-product is D-dimer, an

■ **TABLE 8-1**
■ ■ **Nomenclature for Coagulation Factors**

Factor	Synonym
I	Fibrinogen
II	Prothrombin
III	Tissue thromboplastin
IV	Calcium
V	Proaccelerin
VI	Not assigned
VII	Proconvertin
VIII	Antihemophilic factor (AHF)
IX	Plasma thromboplastin component (Christmas factor)
X	Stuart factor (Stuart-Prower factor)
XI	Plasma thromboplastin antecedent (PTA)
XII	Hageman factor
XIII	Fibrin-stabilizing factor (FSF)

Modified from Gordon JB, Bernstein ML, Rogers MC: Hematologic disorders in the pediatric intensive care unit. In Rogers M, editor: *Textbook of pediatric intensive care*, ed 2. Baltimore, 1992, Williams & Wilkins.

indicator of the breakdown of cross-linked fibrin. tPA further stimulates the conversion of plasminogen to plasmin. It is synthesized by endothelial cells of the vessels and is stimulated by tissue anoxia or damage to the endothelial lining of vessels. tPA will not activate plasminogen in the absence of fibrin.

c. The *antithrombin system* involves a plasma protein that inactivates thrombin, and active clotting factors not used in the clotting process.

3. **Coagulation** depends on a balance between the procoagulants and the anticoagulants. A balance is needed to maintain blood as a fluid when the vasculature is intact and uninjured. Anticoagulants usually predominate until a blood vessel or tissue is injured.

FUNCTION AND PHYSIOLOGIC MECHANISMS

A. Red Blood Cells

1. **RBC** function is to transport oxygen from the lungs to the tissues. Oxygen-carrying capacity is determined by the amount of hemoglobin available to combine with the oxygen.
2. **White blood cells (WBCs)**
   a. *Functions* (Mandell et al., 2004)
      - Defense: WBCs protect the body's internal environment from "nonself" antigens or microorganism invasion by inactivating, destroying, or eliminating "nonself" antigens.
      - A DNA code at the molecular level assists the immune system in discriminating "self" from "nonself" or "altered self." Nonself is composed of foreign or alien molecular structures and is referred to as *antigenic* or as an *antigen*. Antigens are identified by characteristic shapes on their cell surfaces, referred to as *epitopes*. Antigens carry numerous epitopes, sometimes hundreds, on their cell surface (Mudge-Grout, 1992).
      - Major histocompatibility complex (MHC) molecules serve as the genetic blueprint. The MHC molecules specific to the human species are human leukocyte antigens (HLA) and are located on chromosome 6. HLA antigens

are located on the surfaces of most nucleated cells in the body as well as on platelets. HLA antigens are inherited according to mendelian laws, with an individual's genotype determined by one paternal and one maternal haplotype. Close relatives share some of these antigens, whereas identical twins share all these antigens.

- HLA antigens of the MHC are divided into three classes (I, II, and III) based on function, types of cell antigens expressed on the cell membrane surfaces, and structure.
- *Class I* includes HLA-A, -B, and -C antigens and is found on all nucleated cell surfaces and platelets. Class I antigens serve as identification markers of self, assist in the elimination of cells infected with intracellular microorganisms and of mutated or malignant cells, and are involved in the rejection of tissue grafts. Class I antigens are the target antigens recognized by the cytotoxic T cells.
- *Class II* includes HLA-D and HLA-DR antigens and is located nearly exclusively on the surfaces of certain immune cells (macrophages and B lymphocytes). Class II antigens serve as identification markers of exogenous antigens and assist in the elimination of extracellular microorganisms.
- *Class III* antigens are located between class I and class II antigens on chromosome 6 and are involved in the alternative and classical pathways of complement (Mandell et al., 2004; Mudge-Grout, 1992).

b. *Homeostasis:* WBCs remove old or damaged debris from the circulation.

c. *Surveillance:* WBCs recognize and guard against the development, growth, and dissemination of abnormal cells.

3. **Physiologic mechanisms** of WBCs are usually categorized by three lines of defense, each representing increasingly more complex and sophisticated means of protection and methods of elimination.

a. The *first line of defense* involves the child's natural, innate barriers with unique physical, chemical, and mechanical capabilities. This provides a nonspecific or generic defense with immediate onset.

- Physical and mechanical barriers prevent or minimize entry and attachment of antigen. These include the phenomenon of colonization and bacterial interference, mucous traps in the respiratory and GI tract, hair and cilia traps, saliva, tears, and urine (dilution and washing away of antigens), defecation and vomiting (expulsion of invading organisms), and an intact GI lining. Many factors associated with critical illnesses are thought to threaten the barrier role of the gut mucosa and increase the risk of translocation of gram-negative bacteria or endotoxin.
- Chemical barriers deter attachment, survival, and replication of antigen. These include the acid pH of the skin; lysozymes present in saliva, tears, and nasal secretions; gastric secretions; and unsaturated fatty acids in sweat and sebaceous glands.
- The first line of defense has distinct developmental implications.
  - Skin: The newborn's skin is about 1 mm thick at birth and increases to approximately twice that thickness at maturity. The newborn has scant amounts of stratum corneum, the barrier component of the skin, resulting in increased skin permeability (Malloy and Perez-Woods, 1991). The stratum corneum develops quickly and is considered an adequate barrier at 2 weeks of age (Harpin and Eutter, 1983). After the neonatal period, the sebaceous glands involute and produce only small amounts of sebum until puberty. The differences noted in sweating may be related to the immaturity of autonomic (sympathetic) control of sweating rather than to the structural immaturity of the glands. Complete neural control

of sweat glands is noted between 2 and 3 years of age. Diminished sweat production may result in lower quantities of bactericidal and fungicidal substances and, in some, alteration in the physical barrier of the infant or young child's skin.

- Respiratory: The small airways of the infant and young child make a significantly greater contribution to airway resistance compared to the adult (Bellanti and Kadlec, 1990). This increased resistance to flow places the child at greater risk for airway occlusion secondary to edema or inflammatory exudate. Normal defense mechanisms of the respiratory tract may be disrupted by such narrowing or obstruction.
- GI tract: Newborn saliva contains no secretory IgA. At birth the gastric pH is approximately 6, but it normally reaches a pH of 2 to 3 within the first 24 hours of life (Mandell et al., 1990). Acidity of the stomach gradually increases through childhood and then plateaus to adult levels at 10 years of age. The newborn's intestinal epithelium allows certain molecules to pass into the systemic circulation. The maturation of the intestinal epithelium is thought to occur in response to hormones and a variety of growth factors, but the specifics are unknown (Bousvaros and Walker, 1990).
- Ophthalmologic: Tearing is present by approximately 6 weeks of age, and lysozyme levels in the infant and the normal adult are comparable.

b. The *second line of defense* involves the inflammatory response, phagocytosis, and complement activation. It is nonspecific or generic in nature with immediate onset once triggered if the first line of defense is ineffective.

- The local inflammatory response is a sequential reaction to injury hallmarked by the release of numerous chemical mediators such as histamine, bradykinin (and other kinins), serotonin, and prostaglandins. The goals of inflammation include localization, dilution, and destruction of the offending antigen, maintenance of vascular integrity, minimization of tissue damage, and transportation of cells and substances to the area.
- Vascular response is characterized by immediate vasoconstriction, which facilitates fibrin plug formation and WBC, RBC, and platelet margination. Vasodilation facilitates cell and cell products to move close to the area of injury. Capillary permeability assists in cell and cell-product movement from the vascular space into the tissues. Local increases in hydrostatic pressure and increased oncotic pressure of proteins in the interstitium leads to edema (Guyton and Hall, 2000).
- Cellular response involves **margination** or pavementing the lining of cells along the capillary endothelium to prepare for movement from the intravascular space to the tissue. Margination is facilitated by the vascular response because fluid leakage into the interstitium results in an increased blood viscosity and a decreased blood flow. **Diapedesis** is an ameboid type movement of WBCs through the junctions between the endothelial lining from the intravascular space to the site of injury (Guyton and Hall, 2000). The sequence of cell movement is neutrophils first, followed by monocytes and, much later, lymphocytes. **Chemotaxis** involves chemical signals to attract cells to the site of injury. Substances that serve as chemotactic chemicals include microbial products, components of damaged WBCs and tissue, activated complement proteins, and others. Once WBCs are in the area of injury, phagocytosis may begin.
- Other components of the inflammatory response, biochemical mediators, and plasma enzyme cascades facilitate the inflammatory response through diverse but complementary actions. Numerous biochemical mediators

have been identified, such as prostaglandins, leukotrienes, endorphins, and histamine. The primary nonspecific plasma enzyme cascades include complement, coagulation (involved in the vascular response via hemostasis; see Coagulation Cascade), fibrinolysis (primary activity is the degradation of fibrin clot; see Fibrinolytic System), and kallikrein or kinin (bradykinin; enhances inflammatory response by promoting vasodilation, increased capillary permeability, neutrophil chemotaxis, and other actions).

- Phagocytosis: Phagocytes include granulocytes (especially neutrophils) and monocytes or macrophages. The purpose of phagocytosis is to capture, engulf, and destroy the antigen. Additionally, phagocytosis may eventually present the antigen to the helper T lymphocyte. The process of phagocytosis is complex and involves several mechanisms:
  - Recognition of the antigen as nonself.
  - Adherence or attachment of the phagocyte to the antigen or invader.
  - Ingestion or engulfment is performed through the use of pseudopods. Eventually the antigen is taken into the phagocyte's cytoplasm, where it is enveloped in a sac (phagosome).
  - Killing and degradation: The antigen-containing sac is subjected to lysozyme and the process known as the *respiratory (oxidative) burst,* containing hydrogen peroxide, superoxide anion, and hydrochlorite anion. Some microorganisms are ingested but not necessarily killed. For instance, the toxins from staphylococci may in turn kill the phagocyte. Others, such as tubercule bacilli, may multiply within the phagosome and eventually destroy the phagocyte.
- The *complement system* is a complex group of more than 20 enzymes and proteins that, like the coagulation system, react sequentially in a cascading manner. There are 11 principal proteins labeled C1 through C9 (Nathan et al., 1998). Complement system activation can occur through two separate, but interrelated, pathways. However, both pathways lead to the generation of C3 and C3b and a final common pathway. The classic pathway activation is stimulated by antigen-antibody interaction. The alternate pathway activation is stimulated without antigen-antibody interaction, but with more generic activators; it is a slower process than classic pathway activation (Nathan et al., 1998). The final common pathway of complement activation is various events that limit the damage posed by the antigen, including enhancement of inflammation, chemotaxis, opsonization (the process of coating an organism with antibodies or proteins to increase its palatability to phagocytes), and target cell membrane lysis.
- Developmental distinctions in the second line of defense
  - Local inflammatory response: Infants and young children are less able to localize infection, perhaps because of the following: The newborn's neutrophil chemotaxis is altered (Anderson et al., 1983; Masuda et al., 1989); this chemotactic activity remains unchanged for the first 24 months of life and may not reach adult activity until approximately 16 years of age (Klein et al., 1977). The infant's neutrophils have less ability to aggregate and are less deformable than the adult's (Miller, 1983). It appears that the neutrophil surface is more rigid, which may impair the cell's movements though capillary walls and bone marrow sinusoids. This may partially explain impaired chemotaxis and thus the inability to localize infection.
  - Systemic response to infection: The infant has considerably smaller numbers of stored neutrophils per kilogram of body weight than the

adult (Abramson et al., 2004). Because of the smaller neutrophil storage pool, there is less ability to replace repeatedly the number of circulating neutrophils. Infants and young children may display neutropenia rather than neutrophilia in the presence of infection, and increased release of immature neutrophils in the presence of infection may be exaggerated in the infant and young child (Christensen and Rothstein, 1980).

- Phagocytosis: Some evidence indicates that phagocytosis in the newborn is deficient (Goldman et al., 1985), whereas others report that phagocytic activity is normal (Abramson et al., 2004; Miller, 1980).
- Complement proteins gradually increase to 60% to 80% of normal adult levels at birth for the classical pathway and lower percentages for the alternative pathway (Berger and Frank, 1989; Goldman et al., 1985), but it is not until about 3 to 6 months of age that serum complement levels are within normal adult range (Goldman et al., 1985). Low levels may lead to relative and subtle deficiencies in complement system function and at birth may contribute to the newborn's afebrile and absent leukocytic response to infection (Berger and Frank, 1989).

c. The *third line of defense* involves specific, acquired immunity and is triggered if the first and second lines of defense are ineffective in eliminating or containing the antigen. The immune response is a highly complex sequence of events that are triggered by an antigen and integrally associated with other physiologic events including, but not limited to, complement activation and the clotting and fibrocytic systems (Mudge-Grout, 1992). Hallmarks of the third line of defense include specificity, the ability of a lymphocyte to respond to a single antigen for which it was designed, and memory (i.e., the ability of a lymphocyte to recall prior exposure to an antigen and respond in an accelerated, potentiated manner). Specific, acquired immunity may be obtained either passively or actively and naturally or artificially (Table 8-2).

- *Specific acquired immunity* occurs in phases. Recognition and processing of the antigen are the primary responsibilities of the macrophage, although the B lymphocyte may participate. Once identified as nonself or foreign, the macrophage ingests the antigen and through an enzyme-mediated reaction begins "antigen processing." When "antigen processing" is complete, the macrophage re-expresses the processed antigen on its membrane surface in conjunction with HLA antigen. Antigen presentation to the B or T lymphocyte occurs (Mudge-Grout, 1992). Processing and presentation of the antigen trigger the immune response to facilitate elimination.
- *Acquired immunity* comprises two different, but closely interrelated, antigen-specific immune responses (Figure 8-3): (1) Humoral immunity (HI), which is mediated by B lymphocytes, results in the synthesis and secretion of immunoglobulins and *indirectly* eliminates or impedes the antigen. HI provides protection primarily from encapsulated pyogenic bacterial infections. (2) Cell-mediated immunity (CMI), which is mediated by T lymphocytes, *directly* eliminates the antigen. CMI protects from viral, fungal, protozoal, and mycobacterial infections; plays a role in the response to malignancies; and participates in the rejection of transplanted tissues and in hypersensitivity reactions (Mudge-Grout, 1992).
- HI: B lymphocytes can be activated without the help of the T lymphocyte, as in T-cell-independent antigen response, but most commonly are activated with the assistance of the T lymphocyte, as in the T-cell-dependent antigen response. B cells transform into plasma cells, which synthesize and secrete immunoglobulins and subsequently interact with the antigen for which it

TABLE 8-2
Acquired, Specific Immunity: Definition, Acquisition, and Characteristics

Types of Acquired, Specific Immunity	Definition and Acquisition	Characteristics
PASSIVE IMMUNITY		
Natural	Acquired through natural contact with *antibody* transplacentally or through colostrum and breast milk (e.g., IgG and IgA from mother to fetus or neonate)	No participation of the host; a transfer of preformed substances or sensitized cells from an immunized host to a nonimmunized host
Artificial	Acquired through the administration of *antibody* or antitoxin (e.g., γ-globulin, tetanus)	Onset is immediate, but duration is temporary
ACTIVE IMMUNITY		
Natural	Acquired through natural infection; the body is exposed to an *antigen* and mounts an immune response to that antigen (e.g., chickenpox)	Active participation of the host following exposure to an antigen either naturally (subclinical or clinical disease) or artificially through immunization
Artificial	Acquired through inoculation with a variant *antigen*, but usually not the entire antigen (e.g., immunization, attenuated virus)	Provides slow antigen-specific development of antibody, but provides permanent or long-lived immunity to that antigen

Adapted from Mudge-Grout CL: *Immunologic disorders.* St Louis, 1992, Mosby-Year Book Inc.

was made. Immunoglobulins (antibodies) are glycoproteins produced by plasma cells in response to an antigen. The nature of the antibody response varies with the chemical and physical nature of the antigen, the antigen's route of entry, and the immunization history of the child (Mudge-Grout, 1992). There are five major classes of immunoglobulins (Table 8-3).

- Outcomes of *antigen-antibody interaction* include *neutralization* (antibody binds the antigen, causing the antigen to be ineffective or promoting removal by phagocytes), *agglutination* (antibody combines with the antigen to form clumps), *precipitation* (antibody combines with the antigen to make an insoluble lattice formation that precipitates), *opsonization* (antibody coats the antigen, enhancing phagocytosis), *complement* (antibodies activate complement, thus causing target cell lysis), and *antibody-dependent cytotoxicity* (antibody facilitates lysis of the antigen by another immune cell).
- *Primary response:* Antibody production occurs 2 to 10 days after the first exposure, and the response peaks in 1 to 3 weeks. Immunoblobulin M (IgM) is followed by an IgG response.
- *Secondary response* is the response that occurs with exposure to a previously encountered antigen. Memory cells are responsible for the rapid (in 1 to 2 days), prolific, sustained response to the familiar antigen. Antibody response is primarily IgG at much higher titers for a shorter period compared with the primary response (Mudge-Grout, 1992).
- CMI involves T-lymphocyte recognition and activation. T lymphocyte binds to the antigen *and* to a class I or class II protein on the surface of an antigen presenting cell (usually the macrophage). Class I HLA antigens are

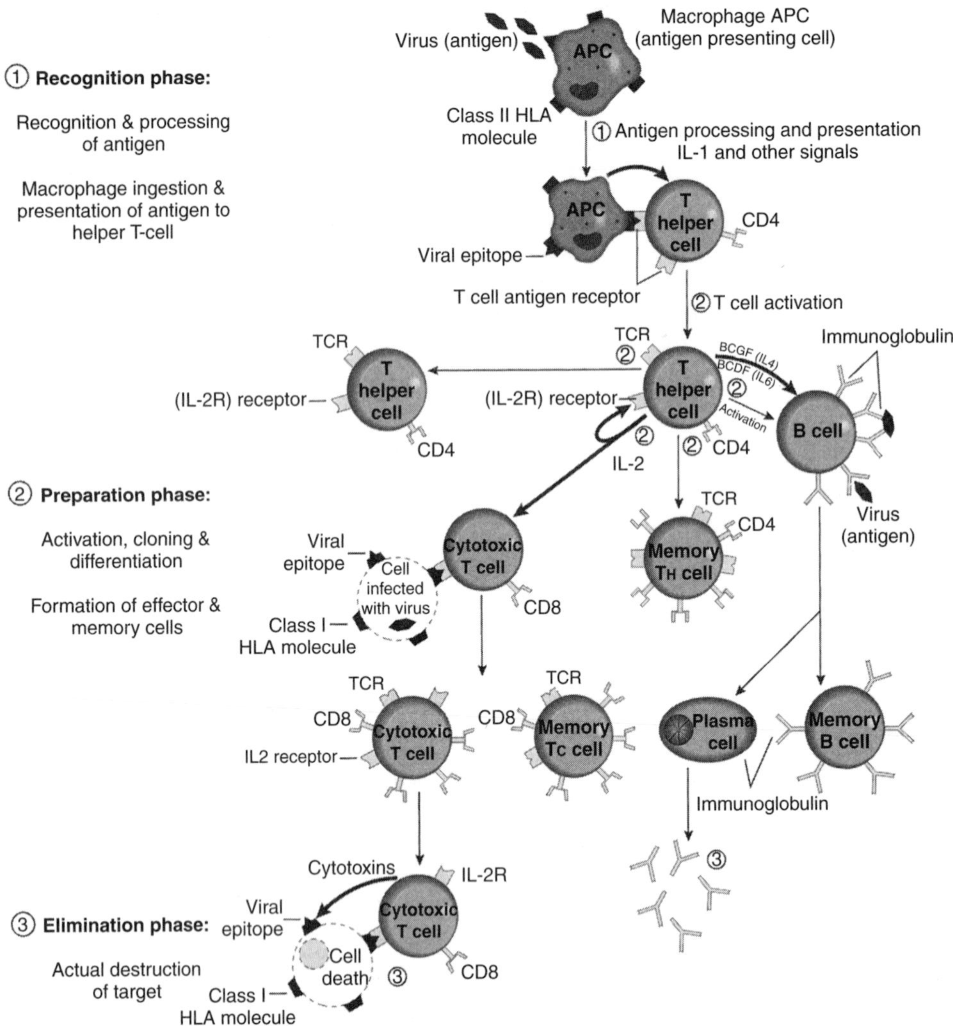

FIGURE 8-3 ■ Overview of specific acquired immunity. The grand scheme of specific acquired immunity is composed of humoral (immunoglobulin) immunity (HI) orchestrated by the B cell and cell-mediated immunity (CMI), orchestrated by the T cell. Note the interdependence between the B and T cells. The three phases of the specific immune response are indicated by numbers in the figure: *1,* recognition phase; *2,* preparation phase, and *3,* elimination phase.

(Adapted from Goodman JW: The immune response. In Stites DP, Terr AI, Parslow TG, editors: *Basic and clinical immunology,* ed 9. Norwalk, Conn, 1997, Appleton & Lange.)

required for cytotoxic T-lymphocyte activation. Class II HLA antigens are required for helper T-lymphocyte activation.

- Communication among all the cells participating in the immune response is facilitated through the secretion of cytokines. Cytokines are hormone-like substances that function to up-regulate and down-regulate immunologic, inflammatory, and reparative host responses. Cytokines secreted by lymphocytes are referred to as *lymphokines.* Cytokines secreted by monocytes or macrophages are referred to as *monokines.* Cytokines are distinct from endocrine hormones in that they are produced by a number of cells rather than by a specialized gland, they do not usually present in the serum, and

TABLE 8-3
Human Immunoglobulins

Ig	Percentage in Serum	Location	Activity and Function
IgG	75%	Most abundant intravascularly Also in extravascular spaces (e.g., lymph, colony-stimulating factor)	Only immunoglobulin to cross placenta Primary antibody class Activates complement Takes 10–14 d after antigen stimulation to develop sufficient IgG titer in primary response; only 4 d in secondary response Appears 1 wk after IgM and peaks in 1–3 wk or longer after IgM peaks Promotes phagocytosis via opsonization
IgA	15%	Found in mucous membrane secretions Intravascular	Two types: serum and secretory Primary defense against local invasion of body surfaces and orifices
IgM	10%	Intravascular only	Promotes phagocytosis Can activate complement Participates in blood transfusion reactions; makes antibodies for "nonself" ABO blood groups Made in utero and may indicate the presence of an intrauterine infection or ABO incompatibility First made in response to an antigen Predominant in a primary infection Peaks 1–2 wk after infection Increases in chronic infections
IgE	0.1%	Found in serum bound to mast cells and basophils	Triggers release of histamine and other mediators from mast cells and basophils Involved in type I immediate hypersensitivity or anaphylactic reactions Defense against parasite infections
IgD	<1%	Found in serum located on surface of B cells	Function not yet defined May participate in B-cell differentiation Increases in chronic infection

Data from Grady C: Host defense mechanisms: an overview, *Sem Oncol Nurs* 4(2):92, 1988; Mudge-Grout C: *Immunologic disorders.* St Louis, 1992, Mosby–Year Book Inc; and Selekman J: Pediatric problems related to the immunologic system. In Feeg VD, Harbin RE, editors: *Pediatric nursing: core curriculum and resource manual.* Pitman, NJ, 1991, Anthony Jannetti, Inc.

they act in a paracrine (locally near the producing cell) or autocrine (directly on the producing cell) fashion rather than on distant target cells. Selected cytokines are described in Table 8-4.

- Developmental distinctions in the third line of defense: The infant's B cells are deficient in producing comparable adult levels and subclasses of immunoglobulins. Serum immunoglobulin levels, the degree of synthesis at birth, and the age at which the levels are comparable to the adult are reflected in Table 8-5. The IgG level seems comparable between the newborn and the adult, but this level reflects the transplacental acquisition of maternal antibody during primarily the third trimester of gestation. The infant is lowest in immunoglobulin concentrations at about 4 to 5 months of

TABLE 8-4
Selected Cytokines: Source and Functions

Type	Source	Functions
INTERLEUKINS (ILs)		
IL-1 (endogenous pyrogen)	T cell, B cell, macrophage, endothelium, tissue cell	Enhances T-cell growth and function; stimulates macrophages; immuno-augmentation
IL-2 (T-cell growth factor)	T cells	Promotes T-cell and B-cell growth; activates T cell; enhances NK activity
IL-3 (multi-CSF)	T cells, mast cells	Stimulates growth of immature hematopoietic precursor cells (e.g., granulocytes, macrophages, RBCs, platelets, and mast cells)
BCGF (IL-4)	T cells	Enhances B-cell growth and function
BCDF (IL-6)	T cells	Enhances B-cell growth and function
INTERFERONS		
Interferon alfa	Lymphocytes, NK cells, macrophages, fibroblasts, epithelial cells	Enhances NK activity; provides antiviral protection; induces HLA-I expression; induces fever; generates cytotoxic T lymphocytes; induces macrophage killing of tumor cells
Interferon beta	Fibroblasts, macrophages, epithelial cells	Provides antiviral protection
Interferon gamma	T cells, NK cells	Activates macrophages; induces macrophage killing of microorganism and tumor cells; regulates action of certain cytokines; increases NK cell activity; increases expression of Fc receptor and HLA-I antigens
TUMOR NECROSIS FACTOR	Macrophages, T cells, and others	Enhances destruction of tumor cells
COLONY-STIMULATING FACTORS (CSFs)		
G-CSF	Monocytes, macrophages, endothelial cells, and fibroblasts	Stimulates growth and activation of neutrophils
M-CSF	Monocytes, macrophages, endothelial cells, and fibroblasts	Stimulates growth and activation of monocytes
GM-CSF	T cells, endothelial cells, and fibroblasts	Stimulates growth and activation of neutrophils, eosinophils, and macrophages

Data from Mudge-Grout CL: *Immunologic disorders.* St Louis, 1992, Mosby–Year Book Inc; and Plaeger SF: Principal human cytokines. In Stiehm ER, editor: *Immunologic disorders in infants and children*, ed 4. Philadelphia, 1996, WB Saunders Co.

HLA, human leukocyte antigen; *NK*, natural killer; *RBCs*, red blood cells.

age, when maternal IgG begins to decrease through natural catabolism and when infant synthesis of immunoglobulin is low. This period is referred to as physiologic hypogammaglobulinemia. During this time, the infant is most susceptible to infections caused by viruses, candida, and acute inflammatory bacteria (*Staphylococcus aureus, Streptococcus pyogenes,*

TABLE 8-5
Serum Immunoglobulins: Developmental Perspectives

Ig	Synthesis by Fetus (Gestation wk)	Percentage of Adult Levels at Birth	Age at Which Adult Levels Are Achieved
IgM	10.5	10%	1–2 y
IgD	14	Small amount	1 y
IgG*	12	110%†	4–10 y
IgA	30	Small amount or none	6–15 y
IgE	10.5	Small amount	6–15 y

From Rosenthal CH: Immunosuppression in the pediatric critical care patient, *Crit Care Nurs Clin North Am* 1(4):779, 1989.
*Crosses placenta.
†Greater than or equal to maternal level.

Streptococcus pneumoniae, Haemophilus influenzae type B, and *Neisseria meningitidis*). This state can be prolonged to such an extent that the young child suffers from recurrent and severe infections.

B. Platelets

1. The **function of platelets** is to maintain normal hemostasis and vascular integrity when a blood vessel wall is injured.
2. **Hemostasis** is a complex interaction among three responding systems:
   a. *Blood vessel walls* have a "nonstick" lining that normally repels platelets and keeps blood cells flowing smoothly.
   b. *Injury to a vessel wall* leads to constriction of the injured vessel within seconds. The sympathetic nervous system responds with a catecholamine surge. The vessel immediately constricts, cutting off the blood supply.
   c. *Hemostatic response of platelets:* Circulating platelets rush to the injured area to form a protective plug. Platelets change to become "sticky" with hairlike projections and adhere to the injured area. As platelets aggregate, they release substances (prostaglandin, serotonin, thromboxane A_2) that attract additional platelets to the area (Figure 8-4). Formation of a platelet plug or clot occurs within 1 to 3 minutes. Further activation of platelets is influenced by plasma clotting proteins, particularly thrombin. This process is referred to as *primary hemostasis* and is completed in minutes to about an hour. Secondary hemostasis involves the plasma clotting factors (see section on Plasma Factors).
3. **Physiologic conditions** influencing platelet response can be quantitative (increase or decrease in number) or qualitative (abnormal function).
   a. An increase in the number of *circulating platelets (platelet count)* usually occurs after acute blood loss to enhance hemostasis.
   b. *Thrombocytopenia,* defined as a platelet count lower than $150{,}000/mm^3$, can result from decreased production, increased destruction, or increased trapping in the spleen (splenic sequestration). Causes of thrombocytopenia include medications (see Relevant Pharmacology discussion), renal or liver disease, cardiopulmonary bypass or hemodialysis, aplastic anemia, autoimmune or idiopathic thrombocytopenic purpura (ITP), viral diseases, disseminated intravascular coagulation (DIC), radiation to the bones, and malignancies involving the bone marrow (displacement of normal stem cells with malignant cells). Thrombocytopenia may also result from congenital

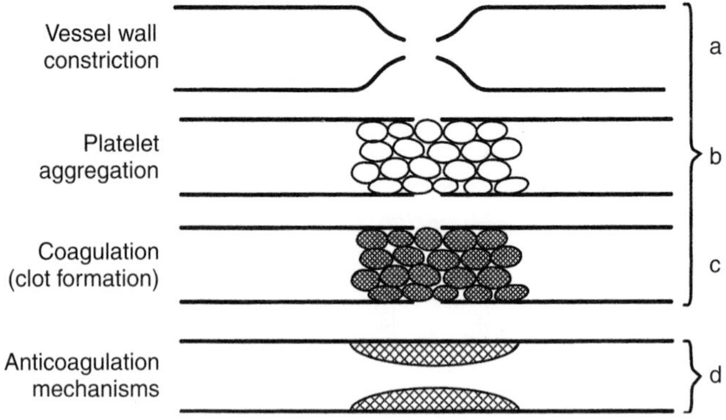

FIGURE 8-4 ■ Hemostatic response of platelets. Major mechanisms involved in primary hemostasis (*a* through *c*). Injury results in vessel wall constriction, platelet aggregation, and clot formation. Anticoagulation mechanisms *(d)* reestablish blood flow by lysing the clot.
(From Harvey M: *Study guide to core curriculum for critical care nursing*. Philadelphia, 1986, W. B. Saunders, p 162.)

disorders, such as thrombocytopenic absent radii (TAR), Wiskott-Aldrich syndrome, and May-Hegglin anomaly.

c. *Platelet function* can be impaired by medications (e.g., aspirin, nonsteroidal anti-inflammatory drugs [NSAIDs)]; see Relevant Pharmacology discussion) and renal disease. Uremia causes reversible impairment of qualitative platelet function. Impaired platelet function results in bleeding in areas abundant in capillaries, such as the mucous membranes in the GI tract, the vagina, the bladder, and the nasopharynx, producing petechiae or ecchymosis or both.

d. Most *platelet problems* in critical care are due to thrombocytopenia rather than to decreased function of the platelets. Hemostasis begins to be affected when the platelet count is below 80,000 to 100,000/mm^3, but bleeding is unlikely until the platelet count is less than 25,000/mm^3. If the platelet count is less than 50,000/mm^3, easy bruising may occur. If the platelet count is less than 10,000 to 20,000/mm^3, spontaneous bleeding may occur, especially if the child is anemic or febrile. If the platelet count is 10,000/mm^3, severe spontaneous or intracranial bleeding may occur.

C. Plasma Factors

1. **Procoagulants** contribute to the process of secondary hemostasis, which is represented by the formation of a fibrin clot and trapping of RBCs at the site of the initiating primary hemostatic plug.
2. Different substances **(enzymes and proteins)** amplify initial activation of a soft clot to an appropriately sized, fully developed clot (Figure 8-5).
3. **Factors** play a role in initiating primary nonspecific plasma enzyme cascades.
4. **Coagulation cascade** starts within the bloodstream itself *(intrinsic)* or outside the bloodstream *(extrinsic)*. The process results in blood changing from a liquid to a gel state by the ultimate conversion of fibrinogen to insoluble fibrin polymers. Contraction of the fibrin network follows, causing the plug to retract, the walls of the damaged vessel to come together, and the injured vessel wall to seal shut.
   a. The *intrinsic pathway* is activated when platelets contact collagen or damaged endothelium. Its function is screened by partial thromboplastin time (PTT).

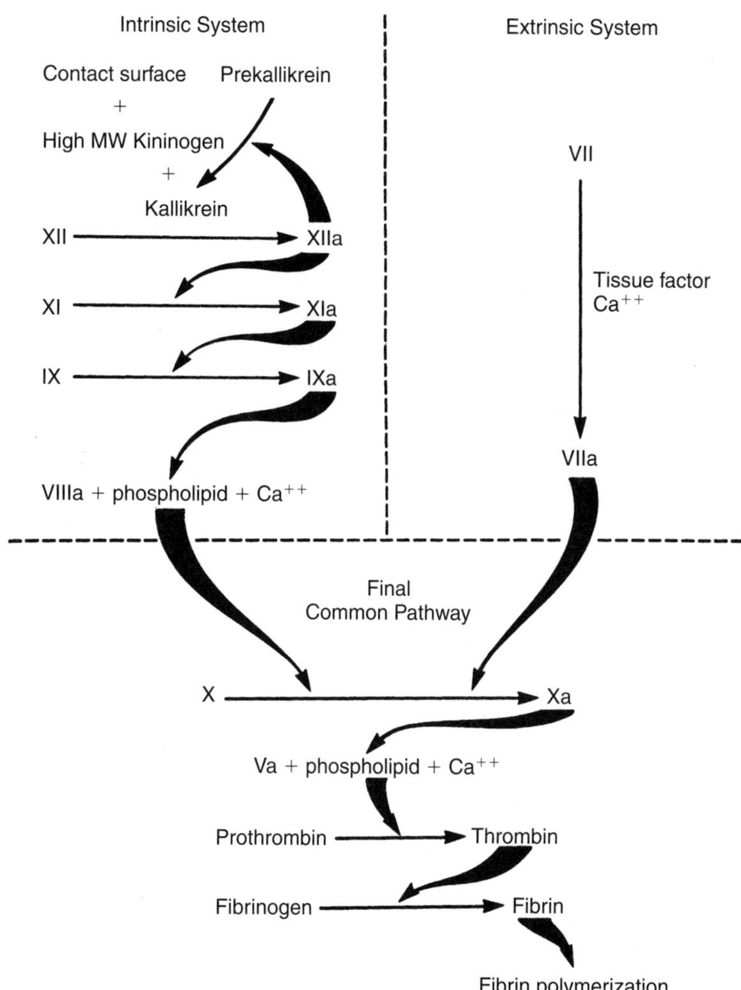

FIGURE 8-5 ■ Platelet clotting factors. Secondary hemostasis. The coagulation cascade starts within (intrinsic) or outside (extrinsic) the bloodstream, both leading to a common pathway. Inactive components and factors become active indicated by the *a*.
(From Farmer JC, Parker RI: Coagulation disorders. In Civetta JM, Taylor RW, Kirby RR, editors: *Critical care*, ed 2. Philadelphia, 1992, JB Lippincott, p 1701.)

b. The *extrinsic pathway* is activated when tissue factor is released from injured tissues, such as when tissues have been cut in surgery. Its function is screened by prothrombin time (PT).
c. The *common pathway* is the part of the coagulation cascade that is activated by the intrinsic or extrinsic pathway. The final step is a fibrin mesh within the platelet plug. Thrombin stimulates the platelets to further aggregate. Fibrin is an essential portion of a clot, soluble until polymerized by factor XIII, which converts it to a stable (insoluble) clot. The function of the common pathway is screened by both the PT and PTT.

5. **Anticoagulant mechanisms** function to maintain blood as a fluid to maintain vascular patency. The system must turn off the various coagulation pathways to reestablish blood flow through an injured vessel, maintain vascular patency, and modulate the balance between the clotting and lysing systems.

a. The *fibrinolytic system* involves the process of lysing a clot. Plasminogen is the precursor to the active part, which is plasmin. It is produced in the liver and circulated in the plasma. The conversion to plasmin is increased in states such as inflammation and coagulation or in the presence of tPA. Plasmin lyses fibrin clots by digesting fibrin or fibrinogen. Plasmin splits fibrin into smaller elements called fibrin split products (FSPs) or fibrin degradation products (FDPs). FSPs impair platelet aggregation, reduce prothrombin, and interfere with polymerization of fibrin.

b. The *antithrombin system* defends against excessive clotting and maintains blood as a fluid. The blood vessel wall has sites that allow thrombin to be inactivated by antithrombin III. Disorders of antithrombin mechanism include congenital thrombotic disorders (thrombophilia) and hepatic failure.

CLINICAL ASSESSMENT

A. History

1. **Chief complaint** is noted in the patient's or the primary caretaker's own words.
2. **History of present illness**
   a. Activity intolerance, fatigue, and weakness; shortness of breath and dyspnea; and "racing heart"
   b. Fever or chills, chronic or recurrent infection, lymphadenopathy, skin rash, and joint pain
   c. Petechiae, bruising, or abnormal bleeding (either prolonged after a minor injury or spontaneous)
3. **Patient health history**
   a. Record *immunizations* and previous immunologic testing.
   b. The patient's *diet and nutrition history* is described, including recent weight gain or loss, dietary restrictions, food dislikes and intolerance, and routine dietary intake, including cultural adherence. All blood cell lines are dependent to some extent on adequate nutritional intake. In particular, iron, vitamin B_{12}, and folic acid are needed for RBC development.
   c. *Allergies and hypersensitivities* are noted, including allergies to inhalants (e.g., animal dander, pollens), contactants (e.g., fibers, chemicals, latex), injectables (e.g., drugs, blood transfusions), or ingestants (e.g., foods, food additives, drugs) and the symptoms accompanying the allergic or hypersensitivity reaction.
   d. *Previous surgeries* that may impair hematologic or immunologic status are noted, including organ or tissue transplantation, thymectomy, or splenectomy.
   e. Inquire about *medical conditions* that might impair hematologic or immunologic status. Abnormalities of RBCs are seen with anemia or malabsorption syndromes. Liver or spleen disorders (functional splenectomy), chronic or recurrent infections, mononucleosis, or problems with wound healing may impact WBC function or numbers. Platelets may be abnormal with prolonged or excessive bleeding or menorrhagia. Plasma factors may be implicated in hemarthrosis. Cancer, bone marrow abnormalities, congenital blood disorders, and immunodeficiency all can affect hematologic and immune status.
   f. *General symptoms* include fatigue, change in level of activity, weakness, headache, chills, fever, weight loss, failure to thrive, night sweats, poor wound healing, malaise, pain, prolonged or excessive bleeding, excessive bleeding related to dental extractions, and menorrhagia.
   g. *Specific symptoms:* See Table 8-6 for specific symptoms of concern.

TABLE 8-6
Symptoms of Concern

System	Symptoms of Concern
Neurologic	• Confusion, restlessness, syncope, irritability, impaired consciousness or somnolence • Deficits in sensory and/or motor function; altered cranial nerve function (cough, gag, swallow, blink)
Skin	• Prolonged bleeding, bruising easily, petechiae, jaundice, pallor, lesions, ulcers, decreased skin turgor, rhinitis, dermatitis, urticaria, eczema
Eyes	• Visual disturbances, retinal hemorrhages, pallor, erythema of conjunctivae
Nose and mouth	• Epistaxis, gingival bleeding, sore or ulcerated tongue, mucositis, candidiasis, vesicular crusting lesions
Lymph nodes	• Adenopathy (enlargement) or tenderness
Respiratory	• Tachypnea, respiratory tract infection, respiratory distress, dyspnea, orthopnea, cough, hemoptysis, sputum, chest pain • Bleeding from nose or endotracheal tube
Cardiovascular	• Hemodynamic instability • Oozing from venipuncture, intraarterial, or intravenous sites • Pale skin and mucous membranes, vasculitis
GI	• Frank or occult bleeding in GI contents • Anorexia, altered bowel sounds, diarrhea, constipation, melena, vomiting, hematemesis, protruberant abdomen (not age-related), abdominal pain, masses, hepatosplenomegaly
GU	• Hematuria, menorrhagia, urinary tract infection
Mobility	• Ataxia, paresthesias • Altered level of activity • Muscle weakness • Pain in joints, back, shoulders, bones • Hemarthrosis

   h. *Psychosocial history* should include recent stresses or life-changing events, response to stress, and coping methods.

4. **Family history** of RBC, WBC, platelet, and coagulation factor abnormalities is noted.
   a. *RBC abnormalities* include jaundice, anemia, and RBC dyscrasia, such as sickle cell anemia.
   b. *WBC abnormalities* include malignancies; frequent, recurrent, or chronic infections; congenital immunodeficiencies; acquired immunodeficiencies; and autoimmune disorders.
   c. *Platelet abnormalities* include any bleeding disorders or predisposition to bleeding or clotting.
   d. *Congenital bleeding disorders* include hemophilia, von Willebrand disease, and clotting disorders (thrombophilia).
   e. Any *symptoms of blood disorders* similar to the patient's symptoms are noted.
5. **Medication history**
   a. *Prescription agents* used to treat existing hematologic or immunologic conditions may include multivitamins, iron preparations (oral or parenteral), vitamin B_{12}, folic acid, or erythropoietin (EPO) for RBC deficiencies. A wide variety of agents used to treat infection, autoimmune disorders, and

malignancies affect WBC number and function and the ability of the body to mount an inflammatory response. Examples of such agents include antineoplastic agents, antibiotics, antivirals or antiretrovirals, antifungals, NSAIDs, and colony stimulating factors. Anti-platelet agents such as aspirin may compromise clotting functions. Anticoagulants affect plasma factors. Evaluate agents used to treat nonhematologic or immunologic conditions that adversely affect hemopoietic function (see Relevant Pharmacology discussion).

b. *Nonprescription* drugs include common agents such as aspirin, but also recreational use of substances.

6. Social-cultural history

a. *Environmental exposures* may include radiation, either inadvertent exposure or radiation therapies (total or localized), or inadvertent exposure to chemicals such as benzene, lead, and insecticides.

b. Discuss *recent travel*, especially outside the United States.

c. Determine whether the *patient is sexually active* (including nonconsensual sex). Evaluate sexual preference, safer sex practices, and multiple partners.

d. Determine *tobacco and alcohol use*. Alcohol consumption reduces the intake of essential nutrients and vitamins and may affect RBC production, platelet function, and clotting mechanisms.

e. Evaluate the *use of complementary therapies* and other interventions used by the patient and family.

B. Physical Examination of the Patient

1. Inspection (see Table 8-6)

2. Auscultation

a. Heart sounds, including gallop, rhythm, and pericardial rubs (may indicate an inflammatory process)

b. Lung sounds, including rales, rhonchi, and pleural rubs

3. Palpation

a. Palpate *superficial lymph nodes* for location, size, tenderness, fixation, and texture (see Figure 8-2). In pediatric patients, "shotty" lymph nodes are often palpable along the cervical chain. This may not always be of clinical significance.

b. Examine for *sternal or rib tenderness*, joint mobility and tenderness, and bone or abdominal tenderness.

c. Palpate *liver and spleen* for size and tenderness. Tenderness may be indicative of an inflammatory process or an enlarged organ with stretching of the capsule secondary to bleeding or malignancy. Assess for complications of portal hypertension (hepatomegaly or splenomegaly). Hepatosplenomegaly may also be noted in patients with numerous hematologic and oncologic disorders (e.g., hemolytic anemia, immunodeficiency disorders, and cancer).

NONINVASIVE AND INVASIVE DIAGNOSTIC TESTS

A. Complete Blood Cell Count (CBC)

1. Red blood cell (RBC) count

a. *Normal* is approximately 4.5 to 6×10^6 million/mm^3 (varies with age) (Table 8-7).

b. RBCs are *reduced* in anemia from any cause and relatively with fluid overload.

c. RBCs are *increased* in chronic hypoxemia, high altitude, and polycythemia.

TABLE 8-7
Hematologic Values During Infancy and Childhood

Age	Hemoglobin (g/dL)		Hematocrit (%)		Reticulocytes (%)	MCV (fl)	Leukocytes (WBC/mm^3)		Neutrophils (%)		Lymphocytes (%)	Eosinophils (%)	Monocytes (%)
	Mean	Range	Mean	Range	Mean	Lowest	Mean	Range	Mean	Range	Mean*	Mean	Mean
Cord blood	16.8	13.7–20.1	55	45–65	5	110	18,000	(9,000–30,000)	61	(40–80)	31	2	6
2 wk	16.5	13–20	50	42–66	1		12,000	(5,000–21,000)	40		63	3	9
3 mo	12.0	9.5–14.5	36	31–41	1		12,000	(6,000–18,000)	30		48	2	5
6 mo–6 y	12.0	10.5–14	37	33–42	1	70–74	10,000	(6,000–15,000)	45		48	2	5
7–12 y	13.0	11–16	38	34–40	1	76–80	8,000	(4,500–13,500)	55		38	2	5
Adult													
Female	14	12–16	42	37–47	1.6	80	7,500	(5,000–10,000)	55	(35–70)	35	3	7
Male	16	14–18	47	42–52		80							

From Christensen RD, Ohs RK: Development of the hematopoietic system. In Behrman RE, Kliegman RM, Arvin AM, editors: *Nelson textbook of pediatrics*, ed 15. Philadelphia, 1996, WB Saunders Co.

*Relatively wide range.

fl, femtoliters; *MCV*, mean corpuscular volume; *WBC*, white blood cells.

2. **Hemoglobin** (Hgb) measures the oxygen-carrying capacity of the RBC and gives it the red color.
   a. *Normal:* (See Table 8-7).
   b. *Hgb* × *3* is an approximation of the patient's hematocrit.
   c. *Hgb is reduced* in anemia from any cause and relatively with fluid overload.
   d. *Hgb is increased* in polycythemia and relatively with severe dehydration.
3. **Hematocrit** (Hct) compares the volume of RBCs with the volume of plasma; it is measured as percent of total RBC volume.
   a. *Normal:* (See Table 8-7).
   b. *Hct is reduced* in anemia from any cause and relatively with fluid overload.
   c. *Hct is increased* in polycythemia and relatively with severe dehydration.
4. **Peripheral smear** enables a more exact evaluation of blood cell size, shape, and composition and is especially useful in evaluating anemia and confirmation of thrombocytopenia.
5. **Reticulocyte count** is the number of young RBCs. It indicates the proportion of immature RBCs in the circulation and is helpful in determining the cause of anemia in some children. The reticulocyte count measures the responsiveness and potential of the bone marrow to respond to bleeding or hemolysis.
   a. *Normal:* 0.5% to 2% (may vary from one laboratory to another)
   b. The *reticulocyte count is reduced* after a blood transfusion, in aplastic conditions, or in nutritional anemias.
   c. The *reticulocyte count is increased* in hemolytic anemia, after blood loss, and with bone marrow recovery as a compensatory mechanism.
6. **Total white blood cell (WBC) count**
   a. *Normal* is approximately 5000 to 10,000/mm^3 (age specific) (see Table 8-7).
   b. Variations in the total WBC count include *leukocytosis,* an elevation in WBC count above normal range, and *leukopenia,* a reduction in WBC count below normal range.
   c. *Total WBC count reflects only* those WBCs in the intravascular space (excluding the marginal pool). WBCs are also located in the following:
      - Marginal pool: Cells are temporarily sequestered in small vessels or adhere to the walls of large blood vessels.
      - Tissues: Nearly twice as many neutrophils are found in the tissues as intravascularly.
      - Bone marrow: The bone marrow is the primary storage area for mature neutrophils. However, infants and young children have smaller bone marrow reserves of neutrophils and are less able to replenish these cells repeatedly (Scott, 2000).
7. **Differential WBC count** measures the five subcategories of circulating WBCs and is reported as a percentage of the total WBC count. It evaluates the bone marrow's ability to produce those particular cells (see Table 8-7). Neutrophil shifts are the number of "segs," "polys," or "bands" as reported in the differential WBC count, which may be interpreted in two ways:
   a. As an indication of the *cell's maturity,* a "shift to the left" indicates predominantly immature neutrophils (bands), as seen in overwhelming infection or use of colony stimulating factors. A "shift to the right" indicates an increased number of mature neutrophils (polys or segs), which can be observed in patients experiencing pernicious anemia (vitamin B_{12} deficiency), folate deficiency, and morphine addiction.
   b. The *differential count* also is an indication of the type of cell that is excessively prominent.

8. **Absolute cell counts** specifically quantifies a particular cell line and may be derived for any cell line.
   a. Following is an example calculation of an *absolute neutrophil count (ANC):*
      - Obtain patient's total WBC count (i.e., WBC = 5 k/mm^3).
      - Translate the total WBC count into an absolute number (*k* means 1000 cells; therefore 5 × 1000 = 5000 or an absolute WBC count of 5000/mm^3).
      - Obtain WBC differential and add the percentages of "polys" plus "bands" (polys = 60% plus bands = 10%; therefore 60% + 10% = 70%).
      - Translate the percentage of "polys" plus "bands" into an absolute number by dividing by 100 (70% ÷ 100 = 0.7).
      - Multiply the absolute WBC count by the absolute "polys" plus "band" count (5000 × 0.7 = 3500; therefore, absolute neutrophil count = 3500/mm^3).
9. **Absolute neutrophil count (ANC)**
   - *Normal:* 1500 to 7200/mm^3 (may vary in infants and with race).
   - *Interpretation:*

ANC <1000: Moderate risk for infection
ANC <500: High risk for infection

10. **Absolute lymphocyte counts** were once thought to be comparable across ages. Although total lymphocyte count and subsets of lymphocytes are equivalent percentages of the WBC count in all ages, the young child's higher WBC count yields greater absolute numbers of lymphocytes and subsets of lymphocytes.
    a. A *lymphocyte count of less than 15% to 20%* of the differential WBC count is considered abnormal.
    b. *Lymphocyte subset determinations* are capable through monoclonal antibody technology. Quantifying lymphocyte subsets is useful in monitoring a patient's response to immunosuppressive therapy during the organ transplant process, an infectious process or an immune disorder, and the effect of medications on the patient's immune system.
       - CD4 count (helper T lymphocyte): Cytomegalovirus (CMV) and Epstein-Barr virus (EBV) may result in a transient decrease in CD4 helper cells (LexiComp, 2004).
       - CD8 count (suppressor or cytotoxic T lymphocyte): Viral illnesses may result in a marked increase in CD8 suppressor or cytotoxic cells (LexiComp, 2004).
       - CD4:CD8 (helper-to-suppressor or cytotoxic) lymphocyte ratio: Normally there are more helper than suppressor or cytotoxic T lymphocytes. The normal ratio is greater than 1.0 (LexiComp, 2004). Patients initially diagnosed with AIDS commonly demonstrate an elevation of CD8 suppressor or cytotoxic cells below 400 and a decrease of CD4 helper cells, resulting in a low CD4:CD8 ratio (LexiComp, 2004).

B. Other Immune-Related Diagnostic Testing

1. **Erythrocyte sedimentation rate (ESR)** is a nonspecific indicator of acute inflammatory response. In many cases, the ESR is so nonspecific that it has little clinical utility as a single value, but following trends is helpful to assess the effectiveness of therapies. In the immunocompromised child, it may be one of the few objective measurements of response to therapy or relapse.
   a. ESR measures the amount of RBCs that settle in 1 hour: Normal values for the modified Westergren technique range from 0 to 10 mm/hour for a child, 0 to 15 mm/hour for adult males, and 0 to 20 mm/hour for adult females (LexiComp, 2004).

b. *Elevated rates* occur in many conditions, including acute and chronic inflammatory conditions, such as Kawasaki syndrome, juvenile arthritis, and rheumatic fever; hypersensitivity conditions, such as Stevens-Johnson syndrome; and malignancy (LexiComp, 2004).
c. *Decreased rates* occur in hypofibrinogenemia, sickle cell anemia, and congestive heart failure.

2. **C-reactive protein** is a nonspecific indicator of active inflammation.
   a. *C-reactive protein,* produced by the liver during periods of inflammation, enhances phagocytic activity of phagocytes, particularly of the neutrophil.
   b. *Normal value is less than 6 mg/mL.* Levels increase exponentially within 6 to 8 hours of the onset of infection or injury. Following the implementation of appropriate antimicrobial therapy, levels will fall rapidly (Grant, 2001).
3. **Histocompatibility testing** identifies the HLA antigens, the child's genetic blueprint. Although HLA antigens are present on all nucleated cells, lymphocytes are commonly used (Grant, 2001).
   a. *Histocompatibility testing* is used for tissue typing for transplantation, paternity testing, and the diagnosis of various autoimmune diseases (Grant, 2001).
   b. Two methods are used for histocompatibility testing: *tissue typing* and *crossmatching.*
      - *Tissue typing* is the determination of an individual's HLA class I and II specificities. This is routinely performed for organ and tissue transplantation using complement-dependent cytotoxic assay.
      - *Crossmatching* is performed before solid-organ transplantation to prevent (*or* minimize) risk of rejection after surgery.
      - Crossmatching detects the presence of antibodies in the recipient's serum that are directed against the HLA antigens of the potential donor. Various methods are used to complete HLA testing, with most patients awaiting transplantation undergoing four initial crossmatching tests, including lymphocytes, T or B lymphocyte-enriched preparations, preformed antibodies, and auto-crossmatch.
   c. *Molecular typing* (only available in some centers) can be performed to define further DNA sequencing and assist in the selection of a more complete or precise match between the donor and recipient bone marrow cells.
4. **Complement assays** evaluate the primary complement components of the classic pathway and some of the components of the alternate pathway (Mudge-Grout, 1992). Total complement hemolytic 50 (CH50) is used to test the integrity of the entire complement system because the entire cascade must be intact to reflect a normal level. The individual complement components (both from a total and functional perspective) also are measured.
5. **Total immunoglobulin level** and levels for the various classes and subclasses are measured. Normal Immunoglobulin levels vary with age; therefore it is imperative that age-adjusted values be used for all comparisons. Immunoglobulin levels can be diagnostic of congenital or primary immunodeficiencies (quantitative testing). If immunoglobulin levels are normal, in spite of suspected immunodeficiency, evaluation of the function and effectiveness of the immunoglobulin responding to an antigen may be indicated (qualitative testing).
6. **Coombs' test or antiglobulin test** will determine the presence of antibody-coated RBCs by using a solution of antiimmunoglobulins (Scott, 2002). Agglutination or clumping occurs if the RBCs are coated with antibodies or complement. The greater the quantity of antibodies against the RBCs, the more clumping will occur. Any clumping is read as a positive result using a scale of

trace to +4. Coombs' test differentiates types of hemolytic anemia and detects immune antibodies (Scott, 2002).

a. *Direct Coombs' test* is an antiglobulin test that determines that serum antibodies (IgG) have attached to RBCs. It is used to detect newborn hemolytic disease, autoimmune processes in newborns and children, or hemolytic transfusion reactions. After transfusion, a positive result may indicate an antibody-mediated hemolytic reaction, but a negative result does not rule out such a condition because the transfused RBCs may have been completely destroyed in the recipient's bloodstream by the time the sample was drawn. A normal response is negative.

b. *Indirect Coombs' test* is a type of antibody screening that detects specific serum antibodies (IgG) to RBC antigens that are in the serum but not attached to the RBCs. It is used to detect IgG-positive antibodies in maternal blood and the newborn and is performed before RBC transfusions to detect any incompatibilities other than major ABO groups. A normal response is negative.

7. **Detection of antibody and antigens** is accomplished through a variety of in vitro techniques such as immunodiffusion, agglutination, enzyme-linked immunosorbent assay (ELISA), monoclonal antibodies, radioimmunoassay (RIA), and others.

a. *ELISA:* See use of ELISA in the diagnosis of HIV infection.

b. *Monoclonal antibodies* are laboratory-produced antibodies for a single "destiny" antigen that are used for prevention, diagnosis, and treatment of graft rejection and graft-versus-host disease (GvHD).

- Anti-T-lymphocyte monoclonal antibodies, such as muromoab-CD3 (Orthoclone OKT3), are often given in rejection episodes unresponsive to steroid therapy. Muromonab-CD3 blocks T-lymphocyte function and clears T-lymphocyte infiltrates from graft sites of rejection (Miller, 2001). Muromonab-CD3 may be administered to prevent the child's mature T lymphocytes from rejecting the grafted or transplanted organ. To prevent GvHD in bone marrow transplant patients, the donor marrow may be incubated with anti-T-lymphocyte monoclonal antibodies before the marrow is infused into the recipient to purge the donor marrow of immunocompetent T cells.
- Monoclonal antibodies can also be used to monitor subsets of T lymphocytes at the site of organ graft to assist in the diagnosis or monitoring of graft rejection.
- Monoclonal antibodies are used on serum, urine, sputum, and stool samples (among others) to diagnose infections with microorganisms such as herpes simplex virus, streptococci, *Chlamydia*, and *Pneumocystis carinii.*
- Monoclonal antibodies assist in the identification of cells and tissues (e.g., B- and T-lymphocyte differentiation, or HLA or blood typing) and are used in the diagnosis of various diseases (e.g., cancer, autoimmune disease). Monoclonal antibodies to various tumor antigens or tumor products can be used in vitro to confirm the diagnosis of certain types of cancers. A radioactive tracer can be attached to monoclonal antibodies so that after the monoclonal antibodies are administered, a body scan may reveal where the cancer is located.

C. Coagulation

1. **Platelet count**

a. *Normal:* 150,000 to 400,000/mm^3

b. *50,000/mm^3* is usually adequate for hemostasis.

2. **Bleeding time** is the time needed for a standard skin wound to stop bleeding spontaneously. It is an indicator of platelet function if platelet number is adequate.

It measures primary hemostasis. Bleeding time is sensitive to qualitative defects in platelet function but is nonspecific as to type of defect. A standardized incision is made on a relatively vascular area of the forearm and the time required for bleeding to stop is measured.

a. *Normal:* Less than 10 minutes
b. *Bleeding time* is prolonged in thrombocytopenia or abnormal platelet function. It is difficult to interpret in the presence of a low platelet count.

3. **Closure time** assesses platelet-related hemostasis with better accuracy and reliability than bleeding time. Closure times are performed on an instrument that simulates a vascular injury in vitro to evaluate platelet function using anticoagulated whole blood.
   a. *Normal:* COL/EPI test, 84-175 seconds; COL/ADP test, 65-117 seconds
   b. *Higher values* indicate abnormal platelet function.
   c. A *normal COL/EPI test* excludes significant platelet function defects; no further testing is performed. If repeat analysis with the COL/ADP test reveals a normal time, the prolonged COL/EPI may be related to a medication-induced platelet dysfunction. If the COL/ADP is also abnormal, there may be a true platelet defect requiring a complete platelet function analysis.
4. **Prothrombin time** (PT): Assesses the extrinsic coagulation system by measuring factor VII and the common pathway or factors X, V, II (prothrombin), and I (fibrinogen).
   a. *Normal:* Control is usually 12 to 15 seconds (normal controls are established by the individual laboratory).
   b. *PT is prolonged* with oral anticoagulants, DIC, liver disease, long-term use of antibiotics, vitamin K deficiency, and phenytoin use.
5. **International normalization ratio** (INR): Minimizes variation in PT results. It is calculated as the patient PT/control PT to the power of the international sensitivity index. Normal INR is typically 1.0 units/mL with some variation with age (Andrew and Montgomery, 1998).
6. **Activated partial thromboplastin time** (aPTT) assesses the intrinsic coagulation system by measuring the kinins; factors VIII, IX, XI, and XII; and the common pathway (II, V, X). aPTT measures the time needed for a fibrin clot to form after an activating agent (calcium) and phospholipid have been added to a blood sample. It is used frequently to monitor heparin therapy.
   a. *Normal:* Usually 25 to 40 seconds (normal controls are established by the individual laboratory).
   b. *aPTT is prolonged* with heparin therapy, DIC, severe vitamin K deficiency, liver disease, hemophilia, and some von Willebrand disease.
   c. *Any sample with heparin contamination* falsely elevates the PTT, thrombin time (TT), and FSPs. Research has questioned the accuracy of using heparinized indwelling catheters for obtaining samples for PTT measurement (Hoste et al., 2002). Venipuncture is a more reliable method for obtaining accurate values, although accurate samples may be obtained from arterial catheters as follows (not studied for pediatric, systemically heparinized, pulmonary artery, central venous, or Hickman catheters):
      - Withdraw a quantity of blood that is a minimum of six times the dead space of the catheter or tubing the blood is passing through (Laxon and Titler, 1994). Then draw the sample for coagulation tests.
      - Any results in contradiction to the patient's clinical status should result in repeated coagulation tests from a nonheparinized site.
7. **Thrombin time (TT)** reflects the time for thrombin to convert fibrinogen to fibrin.

a. *Normal:* 10 to 15 seconds
b. *Results are normal* in factor VIII deficiency.
c. *Results are prolonged* when coagulation is inadequate due to decreased thrombin activity, DIC, antithrombin activity such as heparin therapy, insufficient or abnormal fibrinogen, or uremia.

8. **Fibrinogen**
   a. *Normal:* 200 to 400 mg/dL; only 70 to 100 mg/dL is needed for hemostasis to occur.
   b. *Decreased values* reflect a risk of bleeding and are also seen in hepatic dysfunction.
   c. *Increased values* may reflect a hypercoagulable state or inflammatory conditions secondary to activation of plasma enzyme cascades.
9. **D-dimer:** Measurement of the degradation of cross-linked fibrin; a specific test for DIC.
   a. *Normal:* (0.5 μg/mL)
   b. *Increased values* seen in DIC and inflammatory states.
10. **Specific factor assays** measure amounts of each of the various plasma proteins such as II, V, VII, VIII, and IX.
11. **Activated clotting time (ACT)** is the time it takes a patient's whole blood to clot using a bedside ACT instrument. ACT provides a rapid measurement useful in titrating heparin infusions safely because the ACT responds linearly to changes in heparin levels.
    a. *Normal:* 90 to 150 seconds
    b. The *goal* of heparinization is to have ACT twice the preheparinization measurement. ACTs correlate directly with a patient's aPTT. Blood sample must be fresh, thus requiring the test to be done at the bedside with fresh whole blood.

D. Blood Typing

1. **More than 300 different antigens** have been identified against human blood cells, each of which can cause antigen-antibody reactions.
2. **ABO** is one system for typing the antigens for individuals.
   a. There are four blood groups (phenotypes). An individual inherits a specific type of blood; each type of blood has a specific antigen makeup with the antibodies described.
      - Group A: Natural anti-B antibodies are present in the plasma.
      - Group B: Natural anti-A antibodies are present in the plasma.
      - Group AB: No natural anti-A or anti-B antibodies are present in the plasma.
      - Group O: Both natural anti-A and anti-B antibodies are present in the plasma.
   b. ABO compatibility is essential for blood transfusion.
3. **Rh system** is a second important blood antigen grouping system involving several other antigens found on RBCs.
   a. The most potent and easy to detect is the Rh D antigen. Absence of the D antigen is termed *Rh negative.* If the Rh D antigen is detected, the blood is termed *Rh positive.*
   b. A person first must be *exposed to Rh antigen* before a significant reaction will occur. IgG antibodies can develop to the Rh antigens after sensitization by prior transfusion or pregnancy. A transfusion of Rh-positive blood to a sensitized Rh-negative person can provoke acute hemolysis.
   c. *Coombs' test* is used to determine the presence of IgG antibodies (Rh factor antibodies in an Rh negative person).
4. **Cold agglutinins:** IgM antibodies present in the plasma of some persons can cause RBCs to clump when blood plasma temperature is below normal body

temperature. Antibodies react to RBCs regardless of the blood type of donor blood and may lead to circulatory impairment and RBC hemolysis. Screening is done by indirect agglutination tests and actual measurement by the antiglobulin test. The reaction is often not significant clinically because optimal activation of these antibodies is at 4°C. Reduce potential for reactions by administering blood through a warming system.

E. Radiologic Examination

1. The **chest x-ray examination** is commonly valuable in detecting and tracking various inflammatory or malignant processes. However, just as other signs and symptoms of infection are masked during neutropenia, the chest x-ray examination also *might* be unreliable in revealing pneumonia in some immunocompromised children. The immune response in the neutropenic child may be so diminished that even in the presence of a fulminant pneumonia the chest radiographic examination may inadequately reflect this process (Maschmeyer, 2001). Thoracic computed tomography produces a much higher yield and is recommended in those neutropenic patients at risk for a complicated pulmonary infection. It has been observed in some neutropenic patients that once the neutrophil count begins to increase to a near-normal level, the chest x-ray results may worsen, revealing the existing pneumonia.
2. **Diagnostic imaging studies** of other areas of the body are indicated by the child's history and physical examination.

F. Biopsies

1. **Bone marrow:** Aspiration of the fluid bone marrow and needle core biopsy of the bone.
   a. *Purpose:* Histologic and hematologic examination of cellular components of the blood
   b. *Technique:* The patient is usually sedated, and the patient's respiratory status is closely monitored. Preferred sites are the anterior and posterior iliac crests (Leonard, 2002). If the patient is less than 1 month of age, the preferred site is the tibia.
   c. A *contraindication* is respiratory compromise such that positioning the patient for the procedure would exacerbate the compromise.
   d. *Complications* include bleeding and infection at the site.
   e. *Transfusions* given just before a biopsy is done will not affect bone marrow results.
2. **Lymph node biopsy or excision**
   a. *Purpose:* To evaluate the architectural structure and histologic characteristics.
   b. *Techniques:* The patient is usually under general anesthesia. Areas other than the inguinal area are preferred as less risk for infection. Use the inguinal site only if other sites do not demonstrate enlargement.
   c. *Contraindication:* Bleeding
   d. *Complications* include bleeding and infection at the site.

RELEVANT PHARMACOLOGY

Numerous medications affect the hematologic and immunologic systems of the body. Mechanisms by which pharmacologic agents directly affect the hematologic and immunologic systems include those that increase production of cell lines (e.g., colony-stimulating factors or growth factors) or that decrease production or increase destruction of cell lines or entire bone marrow production (e.g., chemotherapeutic agents). Side effects of pharmacologic agents on the hematologic and immunologic systems vary in intensity and range of cells affected (one cell line versus the entire bone marrow function).

A. Therapeutic Modalities That Enhance the Functions of the Hematologic and Immunologic Systems

1. **Erythropoetin** (EPO)
   a. *Indications* include anemia of prematurity, zidovudine (AZT)-induced anemia, anemia associated with chronic renal failure, or anemia from bone marrow suppression following chemotherapy or medication administration and bone marrow transplant. EPO is useful in other conditions for which transfusions are to be avoided, such as those not consenting to transfusions for religious reasons.
   b. *Mechanisms of action:* EPO promotes RBC production by stimulating the division and differentiation of erythroid progenitor cells (Lexi-Comp, 2004). EPO increases hematocrit but requires adequate iron stores.
   c. *Side effects* are generally well tolerated.
      - Irritation at the injection site may occur.
      - Self-limiting side effects include nausea, vomiting, and flu-like syndrome.
      - In adult patients who have had long-term hemodialysis therapy, hypertension, thrombosis, and seizures have been reported to be associated with EPO.
2. **Myeloid growth factors:** Filgrastim (G-CSF), sargramostim (GM-CSF) (see Table 8-4 and Figure 8-1)
   a. *Indications:* To reduce the duration of neutropenia (and associated infection risk) associated with bone marrow transplantation or administration of chemotherapy or immunosupppressants. These growth factors are also being used in patients with severe chronic neutropenia due to congenital neutropenia, cyclic neutropenia, or idiopathic neutropenia, and in the treatment of neonatal neutropenia, and in AIDS patients receiving AZT (Lexi-Comp, 2004).
   b. *Mechanism of action:* Growth factors stimulate maturation of myeloid precursors.
      - G-CSF effects are more selective than those of GM-CSF because G-CSF produces an increase in the neutrophil count without affecting monocytes or eosinophils. Other activities of G-CSF include the increase of neutrophil phagocytosis.
      - GM-CSF is multipotent or has the potential to stimulate and differentiate several cell lineages including neutrophils, monocytes, eosinophils, and macrophages. Other biologic activities include the induction of mature neutrophils and monocytes to increase phagocytosis, antibody-dependent cytotoxicity, and enhanced monocyte tumor necrosis factor.
   c. The most common *side effect* is a flu-like syndrome including low-grade fever, bone pain, chills and rigor, myalgias, and headache. The severity of symptoms is variable and is influenced by the dose, route of administration, and schedule. Symptoms are reversible once the agent is discontinued, and recovery time is variable, ranging from days to several weeks. "First-dose effect" can occur with symptoms that include hypotension, tachycardia, flushing, and syncope. This is rare and limited to the first dose.

B. Therapeutic Modalities That Depress the Functions of the Hematologic and Immunologic Systems

1. **Marrow suppressive agents** given for another purpose that suppress RBC and WBC production and activity:

a. *Chemotherapeutic agents*

- Indications include cancer and immunologically mediated diseases such as rheumatoid arthritis.
- Mechanisms of action: Chemotherapeutic agents interfere with the normal cycle of the cell replication, especially affecting cells with short life spans or in a constant state of reproduction such as blood cells, hair cells, and cells lining the GI tract.
- Hematologic side effects involve failure of the bone marrow to develop the cell line. Such aplasia is dose dependent and usually reversible.

b. *Antibiotics, antivirals, and antiretrovirals*

- Chloramphenicol (Chloromycetin): Classic example
  - Indications include infection from a wide variety of bacteria, including gram-positive, gram-negative, aerobic, and anaerobic organisms; and from spirochetes, rickettsiae, *Chlamydia,* and mycoplasmas. Chloramphenicol crosses the blood-brain barrier and is particularly effective in central nervous system (CNS) infections caused by susceptible organisms. Newer cephalosporins, however, have largely replaced chloramphenicol for *H. influenzae* meningitis.
  - Mechanism of action is through inhibition of bacterial protein synthesis. It is usually bacteriostatic but can be bacteriocidal against common meningeal pathogens *(H. influenzae, N. meningitidis, S. pneumoniae).*
  - Hematologic side effects are both dose related and idiosyncratic (e.g., aplastic anemia). Reversible bone marrow suppression, which is primarily characterized by anemia (with or without thrombocytopenia and leukopenia), is believed to be *dose related.* It is more likely to occur in patients receiving large doses, prolonged therapy, or serum concentrations ≥25 mcg/mL. It is more common than aplastic anemia and is reversible within 1 to 3 weeks after the drug is discontinued. Hemolysis has occurred in patients with G6PD deficiency who receive chloramphenicol. *Bone marrow aplasia* is rare, *idiosyncratic,* and frequently fatal. It is not dose related and occurs weeks to months after the drug is discontinued. The mechanism of action is unknown.
- Trimethoprim-sulfamethoxazole (co-trimoxazole, TMP-SMZ, Bactrim, Septra)
  - Indications include *P. carinii* pneumonia (PCP) prophylaxis and treatment.
  - Mechanisms of action: TMP-SMZ interrupts thymidine synthesis by inhibiting sequential enzymatic processes. These two folate antagonists are combined for synergism. Most bacteria are more susceptible to the combination of agents than to either agent used alone. Individual agents at therapeutic levels are bacteriostatic, but the combination is usually bacteriocidal.
  - Side effects: Most common are rash (secondary to a hypersensitivity to the sulfonamide component), fever, nausea and vomiting, and neutropenia. Less common are thrombocytopenia, hepatitis, azotemia, bone marrow aplasia, and hemolytic anemia (secondary to hypersensitivity and G6PD deficiency). Discontinuation of medication is associated with complete resolution of neutropenia.
- Zidovudine (previously known as azidothymidine, AZT) (see HIV/AIDS section) was the first licensed antiretroviral drug for HIV infection.
- Mechanisms of action: AZT, a nucleoside reverse transcriptase inhibitor, belongs to a family of compounds called *dideoxynucleosides* and acts by terminating the growth of the DNA chain produced by the viral RNA

template. Other dideoxynucleosides are commonly used in children (e.g., didanosine (or ddI), stavudine, lamivudine) and have less hematologic toxicity than zidovudine.

- Hematologic side effects involve anemia, neutropenia, and thrombocytopenia.
- Ganciclovir
  - Indications include prophylaxis and treatment of CMV in the immunosuppressed patient.
  - Mechanisms of action: Ganciclovir is a derivative of acyclovir that belongs to a class of agents called purine nucleosides. This purine analog acts by incorporation into nucleic acids of DNA. This leads to abnormal transcription and translation and the loss of viral infectivity.
  - Hematologic side effects: Neutropenia is common and appears to be related to the dose and duration of therapy. Thrombocytopenia is less common.

2. **Marrow suppressive agents** given to suppress one or more types of WBCs (therapeutic immunosuppression) that have dose-related effects leading to an increased risk of infection.
   a. *Corticosteroids*
      - Indications include malignancies, treatment of acute or chronic GvHD, and prevention and treatment of rejection of transplanted tissue. The use of steroids in combination with co-trimoxazole is now the standard of care for the management of HIV-infected children with PCP or in children with lymphocytic interstitial pneumonitis (LIP). Debate exists over the use of dexamethasone in the management of pediatric bacterial meningitis (El Bahir et al., 2003). Corticosteroids do not reduce hemolysis in transfusion reactions, but they ameliorate drug-induced hemolysis. In ITP corticosteroids are thought to act by inhibiting the phagocytosis of antibody-associated coated platelets, thus increasing platelet life span.
      - Mechanisms of action: Corticosteroids alleviate temporary lymphocytopenia and reduce the migration of neutrophils and monocytes to sites of inflammation. Other actions include decreasing the number of cells available to participate in the inflammatory response; stabilizing the vascular beds by decreasing capillary permeability, thus inhibiting the movement of cells from the vascular space to the tissues; and reducing the functional capabilities of immunologically active cells. Corticosteroids increase the neutrophil count secondary to mature neutrophil release from the bone marrow and a decrease of movement of the neutrophils from the blood to the tissues.
      - Side effects are significant, especially with long-term use, and include hyperglycemia, hypertension, sodium and water retention, depression and sleep disturbances, increased risk of infection (especially viral and opportunistic infection), acne, and delayed wound healing.

   b. *Cyclosporine A (CSA)*
      - Indications include the prevention and treatment of GvHD and the prevention of rejection of transplanted tissue, stem cells or bone marrow.
      - Mechanisms of action: CSA depresses the body's natural response to "non-self," antigenic tissue. CSA binds to cyclophilin intracellularly, forming an active, protein-drug complex. CSA inhibits the production and activation of the cytotoxic T lymphocytes secondary to calcineurin inhibition. Once T cells are activated, however, CSA cannot suppress T-cell proliferation. Thus, CSA works well at preventing but not treating rejection of transplanted tissues. CSA inhibits macrophage release but has little effect on function of B lymphocytes or T suppressor cells and antibody production.

- Administration: CSA is given intravenously or orally. Absorption of oral preparations was unpredictable and incomplete. However, utilization of cyclosporine microemulsion (Neoral) has greatly reduced the absorptive variability associated with Sandimmune (Nevins, 2000). Continuous IV infusion is less toxic than bolus infusions and is often given in combination with steroids.
- Side effects include nephrotoxicity, hypertension, hepatotoxicity, neurologic disturbances (seizures), hyperglycemia, gynecomastia, hirsutism, and gingival hypertrophy.

c. *Tacrolimus*
- Indications: Tacrolimus (Prograf) is a potent immunosuppressant (100X CSA on a weight basis) that is increasingly being used in pediatric patients who have undergone solid-organ transplants.
- Mechanism of action: Tacrolimus is a calcineurin inhibitor that suppresses the first phase of T-cell activation by blocking the production of calcineurin and IL-2 production.
- Side effects: Side effects occur commonly with tacrolimus, including nephrotoxicity, neurotoxicity, GI disturbances, and infectious complications. The most common toxicity involves the CNS, including headache, insomnia, tremor, and rarely, seizures. Nephrotoxicity includes increased BUN, serum creatinine, hyperkalemia, and hypomagnesemia. GI disturbances include nausea and diarrhea. Ileus has occurred in postoperative patients on IV tacrolimus. Glucose intolerance requiring long-term insulin therapy can occur in up to 10% of patients (Nevins, 2000). Posttransplant lymphoproliferative disorder (PTLD) is the most severe complication associated with tacrolimus. It is believed that PTLD occurs as the result of active Epstein-Barr virus replication.

d. *Sirolimus* (Rapamune)
- Indications: Initial use of sirolimus in pediatric patients was that of a rescue therapy in patients intolerant to tacrolimus or with resistant rejection. Sirolimus appears to be less nephrotoxic than either tacrolimus or cyclosporine, and its use as a component of routine immunosuppressant therapy in patients who have received solid-organ transplants is currently under investigation (Sindhi, 2003; Vilalta et al., 2003).
- Mechanism of action: The mechanism of action for sirolimus differs from that of tacrolimus and cyclosporine. Sirolimus suppresses the second phase of T-cell activation.
- Side effects: Generally, side effects are dissimilar to the calcineurin inhibitors and include bone marrow suppression and hyperlipidemia. Significant hyperlipidemia has been reported in adults and has been reported anecdotally in pediatric patients with improvement noted following dose reduction (Nevins, 2000).

e. *Mycophenolate mofetil* (MMF, Cellcept)
- Indications include prevention of rejection of transplanted tissues; MMF is almost always used in conjunction with other immunosuppressive therapies.
- Mechanism of action: MMF is hydrolyzed to form mycophenolic acid (MPA). MPA causes a depletion of certain amino acids within the purine biosynthesis pathway, resulting in the inhibition of T- and B-cell proliferation, cytotoxic T-cell generation, and antibody secretion.
- Side effects occur as the result of GI dysfunction (diarrhea, hemorrhage, anorexia, ulcers, pancreatitis) and bone marrow suppression (leukopenia, neutropenia, anemia, thrombocytopenia).
- About 60% of patients do not tolerate MMF in therapeutic doses.

f. *Azathioprine* (AZA, Imuran)

- Indications include prevention of acute rejection of transplanted tissues and treatment of rejection (less effective than as a preventive agent).
- Mechanisms of action: AZA is a purine synthesis inhibitor. It blocks RNA and DNA synthesis, thus preventing cytotoxic T-cell proliferation and antibody production. It inhibits promyelocyte proliferation within the bone marrow.
- Side effects include bone marrow suppression, GI tract disturbances (nausea, vomiting, anorexia, diarrhea), fever, chills, hepatotoxicity, increased risk of other cancers, and thrombocytopenia.
- Special considerations: Serious drug interactions can occur with allopurinol (Zyloprim), which inhibits the metabolism of AZA, causing increased serum levels of AZA's active metabolite (mercaptopurinol), leading to increased toxicity. Therefore a reduced dose of AZA is required if a patient is receiving both of these medications.

g. *Lymphocyte immune globulin* preparations

- Production: Purified polyclonal immune globulins are derived from animal sources, which are injected with human thymus or lymphoid cells. Antibodies are formed against these cells and accumulate in the animal's serum. Extraction of the antibodies from the animal's serum is done followed by purification to yield the immune globulin.
- Indications include prevention or treatment of acute rejection of transplanted tissue, prevention and treatment of GvHD following bone marrow transplantation, and aplastic anemia.
- Mechanisms of action: A purified, concentrated, and sterile γ-globulin (IgG) reduces the number of circulating lymphocytes, making them susceptible to phagocytosis by macrophages.
- Preparations:
  - Antithymocyte globulin (ATGAM), also known as *lymphocyte immune globulin,* is produced from the serum of horses immunized with human thymus lymphocytes. It reduces the number of circulating, thymus-dependent lymphocytes.
  - Antithymocyte globulin (Thymoglobulin) is derived from the serum of rabbits.
- Side effects of ATGAM and Thymoglobulin are similar and include fever, chills, anemia, thrombocytopenia, skin reactions (rash, pruritus, urticaria, wheal), and serum sickness–like symptoms (dyspnea; arthralgia; chest, back, and flank pain; diarrhea; nausea and vomiting). Anaphylaxis is uncommon but may occur anytime during therapy. Observe the child continuously for possible allergic reactions throughout the infusion. Preinfusion treatment with an antipyretic, antihistamine, or steroid is highly recommended. An intradermal skin test before administration to rule out serious allergic reactions is recommended before the administration of ATGAM. The patient may require ATGAM desensitization if the patient has positive results from a skin test. A test dose is not administered before the initiation of thymoglobulin; however, premedication with an antipyretic, antihistamine, and steroid is necessary. Other effects may include reactivation of CMV, herpes simplex virus, or EBV or antigen- or antibody-induced glomerulonephritis.

h. *Monoclonal antibodies:* Muromonab-CD3 (Orthoclone, OKT3)

- Production: Mouse spleen cells are harvested and injected with human peripheral T-cells. Immunologically active B-cells are isolated and then cloned. Monoclonal antibodies are derived from a single antibody-producing clone as opposed to ATGAM, which is polyclonal in origin. This results in less variability between different lots of the drug. The monoclonal antibodies are also more selective in action than immune globulins.

- Indications include rejection of transplanted tissues unresponsive to steroids.
- Mechanisms of action: Muromonab binds to the CD3 structure on T-lymphocytes, leading to significant T-cell depletion. It has no direct effect on B lymphocytes or antibody production.
- Side effects include a cytokine-release syndrome with influenza-like symptoms (fever, chills, tremors, headache, nausea, vomiting, diarrhea), dyspnea, pulmonary edema, or anaphylaxis. Preinfusion treatment with a steroid is required. Diphenhydramine and acetaminophen are also used as premedication therapy. Muromonab may reactivate CMV, herpes simplex infections, or EBV 2 to 3 weeks after therapy.

3. **Platelet suppressive agents** given for another purpose that result in the suppression of platelet activity.
   a. *Aspirin (ASA)*
      - Indications include the need for antipyretic, anti-inflammatory, analgesic, or antiplatelet effects.
      - Mechanisms of action: ASA inhibits platelet aggregation by inhibiting thromboxane A_2 for the life of an exposed platelet (7 to 10 days). Effects do not disappear with drug clearance. ASA also inhibits prostacyclin.
      - Hematologic side effects include the prolongation of bleeding time to one to three times normal. If aspirin is given to those with liver disease or to those receiving anticoagulant therapy, the effects are amplified.

   b. *NSAIDs* (e.g., Ibuprofen, Naproxen)
      - Indications include the need for anti-inflammatory, analgesic, and antipyretic actions.
      - Mechanism of action involves a decrease in function of platelets, which is reversible on the affected platelet when the NSAID is eliminated from the blood.
      - Hematologic side effects include prolonged bleeding time.

4. **Agents affecting plasma clotting factors**
   a. *Heparin* is an anticoagulant made from porcine intestinal mucosa or bovine lung.
      - Indications include deep-vein thrombosis, pulmonary embolism, mural thrombosis, and minimization of clotting during cardiopulmonary bypass surgery, hemodialysis or hemofiltration, cardiac catheterization, or hemodynamic monitoring. Heparin may also be used for selected causes of DIC, such as acute promyelocytic leukemia, and to maintain patency of vascular access devices.
      - Mechanisms of action: Heparin inhibits clot formation but has no effect on formed clots. It dramatically accelerates the body's own anticoagulant mechanism, particularly that provided by antithrombin III (enhances the inactivation of thrombin II, inhibits X). Heparin promotes the destruction of factor X and has a direct inhibitory effect on factors IX and X and thrombin. It also interferes with in vitro platelet aggregation, increases plasminogen activation levels (thereby promoting fibrinolysis), and inhibits thrombin.

- For acute thrombosis, continuous IV infusion is preferred. Titrate to maintain the PTT or APTT 1.5 to 2 times normal. After acute anticoagulation is achieved, initiate concomitant oral therapy with warfarin (Coumadin); however, continue heparin for the first 3 to 5 days of warfarin therapy.
- Side effects are reversed with protamine sulfate, which binds heparin to a complex that lacks anticoagulant activity. Bleeding occurs, especially with children who have deficiencies of coagulation factors such as hemophilia or those with liver disease, platelet dysfunction syndromes (such as with aspirin therapy), peptic ulcer disease, and severe hypertension. Heparin-induced thrombocytopenia is a potential side effect. See Heparin-Induced Thrombocytopenia for more information.

b. *Warfarin* (Coumadin) is an anticoagulant.
- Indications include chronic anticoagulant therapy, such as long-term oral treatment of deep venous thrombosis and prevention of intracardiac clot formations associated with decreased wall motion, such as chronic atrial fibrillation.
- Mechanisms of action: Warfarin inhibits the liver's activation of factor VII, followed by depression of factors II, IX, and X. It also increases plasma antithrombin III levels. Effectiveness is dependent on absorption from the GI tract, vitamin K status of the patient, and rate of hepatic metabolism of warfarin.
- Administration: The oral route is used and dose is titrated to achieve an INR in the 2 to 3 range. Warfarin must be given for 5 to 7 days, overlapping with heparin before adequate anticoagulation is assumed.
- Side effects: Minor to life-threatening GI tract bleeding may occur. Side effects are reversed with vitamin K. Many drug interactions are possible, resulting in excessive anticoagulation; therefore, the nurse should consult with the pharmacist about any possible drug interactions before administration of warfarin.

c. *Fibrinolytic agents:* Drugs that dissolve clots (thrombus).
- Indications include great vein, atrial, arterial, and renal vein thromboses; occlusion of grafts; superior vena cava syndrome; and obstruction of vascular access devices such as central lines.
- Mechanisms of action: Fibrinolytic agents promote conversion of plasminogen into plasmin and induce systemic fibrinolysis. Plasmin is a proteolytic enzyme that reacts with proteins other than fibrin being lysed.
- Specific agents
  - Streptokinase, a biologic product of certain strains of streptococci, is antigenic in nature. Repeat exposures to this drug increase the risk of anaphylaxis and are not recommended.
  - Urokinase, initially isolated from urine and fetal kidney cells, is produced using recombinant DNA technology and is not antigenic. This enzyme directly activates plasminogen. It has a lower incidence of allergic reactions than streptokinase, but availability varies.
  - Alteplase (tPA) activates plasminogen in the presence of fibrin. It binds to fibrin in the clot and converts entrapped plasminogen to plasmin. Concurrent heparin or antiplatelet therapy is sometimes given. It has the advantage of relatively selectively activating only the plasminogen bound to fibrin.

- Monitor fibrinogen levels, fibrinogen degradation products, hematuria, and gingival bleeding.
- Side effects: There is an increased risk of bleeding in children who have had major surgery within the preceding 10 days, a biopsy, or a history of active bleeding, especially from the GI tract. As with heparin, risks of bleeding must be weighed against the risks of the thrombosis. Effects can be reversed with the administration of fresh frozen plasma (FFP).

BLOOD COMPONENT THERAPY

A. Blood products

Blood products commonly used for pediatric critically ill patients, indications, dosages, and nursing implications are outlined in Table 8-8.

B. Special Donor Designation and Cross-Matching Issues

1. **Knowledge** regarding special donor requirements or individual patients is vital. Document the number of products available for immediate transfusion and when to send blood for type and cross.
2. **Donor-directed (designated) blood** is the donation of blood by family or friends for a specific patient.
    a. This is *not possible* for emergent needs.
    b. This has *not offered a safety advantage* over volunteer donors. There is a potential for clerical errors resulting from the additional steps in the donation process as well as from inaccurate history disclosure.
    c. *Directed donation from parents* to neonates isn't recommended due to maternal alloantibodies and maternal antibodies in the infant's circulation.
    d. *Directed donation from family members* is not recommended for any patient who is a candidate for bone marrow transplantation.
3. **Human leukocyte antigen (HLA)–matched platelets** are needed when a patient has developed antibodies to antigens on platelets (e.g., multiple transfusions). This minimizes the chance of reaction to donor platelets so that the patient achieves an adequate rise in platelet count.
4. **Patients who require life-long transfusions** (e.g., sickle-cell disease patients) may develop multiple alloantibodies to donor blood antigens, which make cross-matching difficult.
5. **O-negative unmatched blood** may be given to patients with an urgent, life-threatening need for red blood cells.

C. Modification of Blood Products

1. **The goal of modification** before transfusion is to minimize the risks of transfusions for patients with special needs.
2. **Leukodepletion**
    a. *Indications* include patients who have previously experienced a febrile transfusion reaction, prevention of alloimmunization in recipients of frequent platelet transfusions, and prevention of CMV when CMV-negative products are not available.
    b. The *goal* of leukodepletion is to decrease nonhemolytic febrile reactions. This is achieved by *prestorage or bedside filtration*, which removes 70% to 90% of WBCs. It is also *accomplished less often* by washing RBCs, freezing, and deglycerolizing RBCs (AABB, 2002; Manno, 1996).

Text continued on p. 587.

TABLE 8-8
Blood Products Commonly Used in the PICU

Blood product	Indication	Dosage	1) Must be ABO Compatible 2) Compatibility Tested	Expected Response/ Estimated Change	Rate of Administration	Available Modifications	Special Considerations
Whole blood 500 mL/U	Symptomatic deficit of oxygen-carrying capacity plus hypovolemic shock Massive blood loss Exchange transfusions	20 mL/kg initially, followed by volume necessary to stabilize child's condition	1) Yes (must be ABO identical; Rh positive may receive Rh negative) 2) Yes	6mL/kg →↑ Hgb by 1g/dL	As fast as tolerated	Warmed Irradiated Leukocyte-depleted CMV neg, frozen, deglycerolyzed	Rarely used, usually for massive acute blood loss Platelets, WBCs, and clotting factors within stored whole blood are not functional
Packed red blood cells (PRBC) 200-350 mL/U	Anemia/symptomatic deficit of oxygen-carrying capacity ± hypovolemia	10-20 mL/kg	1) Yes 2) Yes	3 mL/kg →↑ Hgb by 1 g/dL 10 mL/kg →↑ Hct by 10%	2-4 h (not greater than 6 h 5mL/kg/h (2mL/kg/h if child has cardiac dysfunction)	Washed Warmed Irradiated Leukocyte-depleted CMV neg, frozen, deglycerolyzed	Multiple transfusions may result in dilution of coagulation factors Wait 4-6 h after transfusion to check hematocrit
Platelets 50-75 mL/U (random donor); 200-300 mL for pheresed units*	Thrombocytopenia (usually platelet count <10,000-20,000 or <50,000 with active bleeding) Abnormal platelet function	1-2 units/ 10 kg	1) Yes (preferred) 2) No	1 U/10 kg should ↑ plt 50,000 mm^3	As fast as tolerated, but usually not faster than 1 mL/kg/min	Irradiated Leukocyte-depleted CMV neg Volume-reduced Single donor HLA matched	Premedicate with acetaminophen or diphenhydramine for prevention of reaction Do not use microaggregate filters High risk of alloimmunizations with repeated transfusion Transfusion not indicated in platelet-destruction conditions, except in emergency

*May give low volume.

Continued

TABLE 8-8
Blood Products Commonly Used in the PICU (*cont'd*)

Blood product	Indication	Dosage	1) Must be ABO Compatible 2) Compatibility Tested	Expected Response/ Estimated Change	Rate of Administration	Available Modifications	Special Considerations
Fresh frozen plasma 200-250 mL/U	Deficit of plasma coagulation factors (prolonged PT, PTT) Provides plasma for volume expansion plus all coagulation factors Provides low levels of factor V and VIII	Clotting deficiency: 10-15 mL/kg Acute hemorrhage: 15-30 mL/kg	1) Yes 2) No		Depends on patient tolerance; not faster than 1 mL/kg/min, not slower than 4 hours	Irradiated	Should not be used for hypovolemia/ hypoproteinemia unless coagulation values are prolonged Must be used within 6 hours of thawing
WBC granulocyte transfusion 200-500 mL/U	Adjunct to infection measures in high-risk patients and neonates Questionable benefit, but newer techniques include priming donor with G-CSF	10-15 mL/kg Given every day for 4 d	1) Yes 2) Yes	No increase to a minimal increase of WBCs	Infuse over 2-4 h Slower rates may ↓ reaction	No leukocyte depletion Irradiated to prevent GVHD	Febrile reaction is common Prime donor with G-CSF Premedicate 1 hour prior to transfusion (acetaminophen, diphenhydramine, or steroids) Administer WBCs greater than 4 to 12 h between amphotericin B doses Caution when receiving amphotericin B due to pulmonary reaction

Cryoprecipitate 10-40 mL/bag	Hemophilia A, only in special situations with directed donors Hypofibrinogenemia Factor XIII deficiency Von Willebrand disease	1 unit per 5 kg DIC 1-2 bags/ 10 kg Additional doses at 8-12 h intervals based on Factor VIII levels and clinical status of patient	1) No 2) No		As fast as tolerated; usually not faster than 1 mL/kg/min	Irradiated	Must be used within 4 h of thawing for pooled units; 6 h for single unit Transmission of infections such as HIV and hepatitis B and C can occur Large doses in patient with normal fibrinogen may lead to hyperfibrinogenemia leading to acute thrombosis and DIC
Factor VIII Concentrate[†]	Hemophilia A	Dosage 10-50 u/kg Administer 20 u/kg for mild hemorrhage; 40 u/kg for severe hemorrhage	1) No 2) No	1 U/kg factor will ↑ level about 1%-2%	Rate of administration per manufacturer	Stable with refrigeration weeks to months Most patients receive recombinant factor to decrease risk of virus transmission	Patient may develop antibodies to Factor VIII resulting in less effectiveness of product
Albumin 5% and 25%	Hypovolemia Hypoproteinemia 25% severe burns and cerebral edema	5%: 10-20 mL/kg 25%: 2-4 mL/kg	1) No 2) No		5%: as fast as tolerated 25%: 20-60 min	NA	No infectious risk Risk of circulatory overload secondary to increased osmotic pressure, especially with 25% albumin Use within 6 h of entering container

[†]Dose dependent on manufacturer and patient weight.

Continued

TABLE 8-8
Blood Products Commonly Used in the PICU (*cont'd*)

Blood product	Indication	Dosage	1) Must be ABO Compatible 2) Compatibility Tested	Expected Response/ Estimated Change	Rate of Administration	Available Modifications	Special Considerations
Plasma protein factors (Plasmanate) 250 mL bottle	Volume expansion Hypoproteinemia	10-15 mL/kg per dose	1) No 2) No		5-10 mL/min		
IVIG Pools of plasma (>1000) donors 90%-95% is IgG	Antibody deficiency disorders: congenital and acquired, including high-risk, LBW infants; patients post-transplant	(Dose varies per manufacturer)	1) No 2) No		Per individual manufacturing preparation; infuse slowly over 15-30 min and then gradually increase to max rate as tolerated		Reactions occur in 10%-15% of IVIG infusions, usually mild, not anaphylactic

3. **Irradiation**
   a. This process *destroys the leukocytes' ability to engraft* in the immunosupressed patient at risk for transfusion-associated graft-versus-host disease (TA-GVHD).
   b. It is *indicated for patients who are susceptible to TA-GVHD* including posttransplantation, severely immunocompromised, lymphoma, or leukemia patients.
   c. *Irradiated blood products* pose no danger to health care personnel (AABB, 2002).
4. **Filtration at the bedside**
   a. *170- to 200-unit filters* are standard in blood administration and platelet recipient sets.
   b. *Each filtered set* can be used for up to 4 units and should hang no longer than 4 hours.
   c. *WBC filters* may be used if indicated and if leukofiltration is not accomplished before storage at the blood bank.

D. Administration of Blood Products

1. **Blood warmer** is indicated for transfusions of more than 1 unit of blood every 10 minutes, exchange transfusions in neonates, hypothermic patients, and those who have cold agglutinin disease.
   a. *Warming* prevents severe hypothermia, dysrhythmias, and cardiac arrest.
   b. *Devices* should be temperature controlled and heated through an inline system only.
   c. RBCs heated above 37°C may hemolyze.
2. **Mechanical pumps** (e.g., volumetric or syringe pumps) may be used to administer RBCs at a specific rate with minimal hemolysis. Pumps should be tested and validated for use with blood components (AABB, 2002).
3. **Reduced-volume blood** products (i.e., platelets) may be available from the blood bank and used for infants and children who need small-volume infusions.
   a. RBC volumes may be ordered in small aliquots. Several aliquots may be prepared from a single donor unit, thus limiting donor exposure and risks.
   b. Pedi-paks (~80 mL) and syringe aliquots with specific amounts may be provided by the blood bank.

E. Complications

Primary prevention includes meticulous verification of the patient's identification and specific unit cross-matching. Table 8-9 summarizes reactions, signs and symptoms, and treatments for transfusion reactions. Early detection of reactions includes staying with the patient and starting the transfusion at a slow rate during the first 15 minutes before increasing to the ordered or desired rate.

1. **Acute hemolytic reactions**
   a. *Most serious reaction* occurs when the patient has antibodies to an antigen on the transfused RBCs (e.g., ABO incompatibility from mismatched blood).
   b. *Reactions may be immediate* (fever, hematuria), or delayed (3 to 5 days up to weeks) after transfusion with anemia and hematuria resulting from lower antigen titers.
2. **Nonhemolytic reactions**
   a. *Febrile reactions* result from an immune response to infused WBCs or plasma proteins.
      - Rarely serious, but can be the initial manifestation of life-threatening hemolytic reaction.

TABLE 8-9
Transfusion Reactions to Blood or Blood Products

Reaction	Cause	Signs and Symptoms	Treatment
Anaphylaxis (occurs with infusion of only a few mL of product)	• Most often caused by antigen-antibody complexes involving antibodies to IgA • IgA deficiency	• Bronchospasm • Cough • Respiratory distress • Hypotension* • Urticaria • Vomiting	• Discontinue transfusion • Keep vein open with NS (completely new tubing set) • Notify physician • Administer epinephrine, steroids • Respiratory support • Deglycerolized (washed) red cells in future transfusions
Acute hemolytic transfusion reaction	• Transfusion of ABO-incompatible blood resulting in hemolysis of red cells	• Fever, chills* • Hypotension* • Hemoglobinemia • Hemoglobinuria • Lumbar pain (classic sign) • Shock • Dyspnea • Diaphoresis • Anxiety (impending sense of doom) • Chest pain • Restlessness • DIC	• Stop transfusion • Keep vein open with NS (completely new tubing set) • Notify physician • Treat shock and/or respiratory distress • Osmotic diuresis to prevent acute tubular necrosis • Treat DIC
Nonhemolytic	• Recipients reacting to poorly defined transfused antigens or recipient's antibodies reacting to transfused leukocytes and/or plasma proteins	• Fever (mild to severe)* • Chills • Headaches • Palpitations • Hives • Local erythema • Itching	• Stop transfusion • Keep vein open with NS (completely new tubing set) • Notify physician • Relieve symptoms (antipyretics, antihistamines) • If reaction mild such as urticaria and/or slight fever and chills, may consider continuing transfusion after antihistamine; may also consider premedication and/or leukocyte-depleted products for future transfusions

*Consider bacterial contamination of product.

- Discontinue transfusion if patient's temperature rises 1°C or more above baseline.
- Prevented with leukocyte-depleted blood products.

b. *Allergic reaction*

- If the reaction is mild (local erythema, pruritis), transfusion is temporarily stopped, antihistamine is given, and infusion may be restarted if symptoms are resolving. Patient is pretreated with antihistamine before subsequent transfusions.

- Anaphylactic reactions with more severe symptoms of bronchospasm and hypotension are rare. Reaction typically occurs after a few millilters of blood product is transfused, almost exclusively in IgA-deficient recipients. Interventions include discontinuing product, administration of epinephrine, fluids, and corticosteroids (AABB, 2002; Manno, 1996).

3. **Alloimmunization**
   - a. *Risk* is in patients who receive multiple transfusions with the patients developing antibodies against antigens on surface of donor cells. These antibodies destroy future transfused cells that possess targeted antigens.
   - b. Alloimmunized patients who receive platelet transfusions receive no therapeutic effect. Single-donor or HLA-matched platelets may offset this problem.
   - c. Patients who are alloimmunized against red cell antigens may hemolyze donor cells.
   - d. Leukocyte-depleted blood components reduce risk of alloimmunization.
4. **Circulatory overload** occurs when transfusion volume exceeds circulatory system capacity.
   - a. *Blood bank* can divide red cells (aliquots) and provide "volume-reduced" platelets for volume-sensitive patients.
   - b. *Volumes and rates of transfusion* should be based on patient's size and clinical status.
   - c. *Increased respiratory support* and diuretics may be necessary to treat circulatory overload.
5. **Citrate toxicity**
   - a. *CPDA (citrate-phosphate-dextrose-adenine)* is still used in some blood centers to preserve blood. Citrate in this preservative binds with serum calcium, potentially causing hypocalcemia.
   - c. Patients who receive *very rapid transfusions or multiple transfusions* over a short period and patients with existing hepatic or renal dysfunction are at risk.
   - d. For *at-risk patients,* check serum calcium before and during transfusions and treat with IV calcium chloride or calcium gluconate if toxicity in presence of hypocalcemia is anticipated.
6. **Transmission of infectious diseases** is greatest with paid donors, multiple transfusions, and pooled plasma fractions. Mandatory screening of donor blood for hepatitis (B and C), HIV, and CMV before it is transfused decreases the risk.
   - a. *Risk of hepatitis (B and C) infection:*
     - Hepatitis B: 1:200,000/unit of transfused products
     - Hepatitis C: 1 in 1.9 million units of transfused products
     - Cases of hepatitis vary in severity and may be fatal or result in chronic liver disease.
   - b. *Risk of HIV infection: 1:2.1 million units of transfused products*
     - All blood banks screen products for HIV antibody and antigen; however, the virus (antigen) may be present in the donor's blood for 25 days before antibodies are detectable. Risk of infection is also decreased by screening donors for lifestyles associated with HIV infection.
   - c. *Risk of CMV infection* is decreased if patients are given products not containing WBCs.
     - Approximately 50% of donors are CMV positive, indicating a prior or current CMV infection. The virus may persist in the WBCs, leading to a

carrier state despite the presence of antibody; for this reason, blood from antibody-negative donors is less likely to transmit CMV.

- Clinical symptoms range from mild febrile illness to extensive disseminated disease resulting in death, particularly in immunocompromised patients and neonates.
- If possible, transfuse very high-risk CMV-negative patients (e.g., post-bone marrow transplant) with CMV antibody-negative blood. If the patient is CMV antibody-positive, no additional benefit will occur from transfusing CMV antibody-negative blood. Irradiation does not prevent CMV transmission from the donor to the recipient.

7. The risk of **bacterial contamination** is 1 in 50,000 for platelets and 1 in 500,000 for RBC transfusions. It is more likely for products that require thawing in a water bath or those stored at room temperature, such as platelets.
   a. *Contamination* is confirmed by prompt Gram staining of the residual blood in the blood bag. Also, culturing the blood bag and filter may provide further evidence of the specific organism.
   b. *Clinical symptoms* are noted in Table 8-9. Management includes broad-spectrum antibiotics plus supportive treatment with fluids and vasopressors.
8. **Coagulopathy** can occur during massive transfusion (replacement of more than 1 blood volume).
   a. The *patient's body* cannot replace more than a small fraction of coagulation factors and platelets, and stored blood has lost activity for platelet and coagulation factors.
   b. *It is recommended* that for every 3 units of RBCs administered, the child also receives 1 unit of FFP and 1 unit of platelets. Coagulation studies may be done to determine specific component requirements.
9. **TA-GVHD** occurs when T lymphocytes present in donated blood react against recipient's tissues. It occurs most often in immunocompromised patients or after bone marrow transplantation. It can be prevented by irradiation of donor blood.
10. **Metabolic complications** are associated with massive transfusion or when a patient has severe liver or kidney disease. Hypothermia and hypocalcemia can occur and are addressed in previous sections.
11. **Iron overload** occurs with chronic infusions over an extended period (years) in patients with severe chronic anemia (e.g., sickle cell anemia). It is due to the quantity of iron administered by transfusion being greater than that which is excreted. Overload results in deposits of iron in the cells of the myocardial, endocrine, and liver cells, leading to organ damage. It is managed by giving an iron-chelating agent (deferoxamine mesylate).

IMPLICATIONS OF SYSTEM DYSFUNCTION

A. Anemia

1. **Anemia** is defined as a reduction in red cell mass or blood hemoglobin concentration or a combination of the two. Pediatric anemia most frequently occurs as the result of a decrease in RBC production, an increase in RBC destruction, a combination of the two, or blood loss.
2. The **most significant problems** seen in PICU patients with anemia include altered gas exchange, altered tissue perfusion, and altered fluid volume. Nursing assessment and management are targeted at these three key problems.

3. **Assessment:** Signs and symptoms of anemia vary with the rapidity of its onset and with the underlying cause. If anemia develops rapidly, signs and symptoms may be more pronounced. If anemia develops more slowly, compensatory mechanisms such as expanding plasma volume decrease the cardiovascular symptoms. The patient may have only slight dyspnea on exertion despite significant anemia. Young children will self-regulate dyspnea by decreasing their activity level.
   a. *Clinical signs and symptoms* include tachycardia, tachypnea, diminished level of consciousness, lightheadedness, postural hypotension, and pallor of skin and mucous membranes.
   b. *Laboratory data:* Hemoglobin less than 2 standard deviations below the mean for the normal population is considered consistent with anemia (Oski et al., 1998).
4. **Interventions**
   a. *Administer blood products* as ordered.
   b. *Improve oxygenation.* Reduce fear and anxiety to minimize oxygen demand. Assist in activities to reduce physiologic oxygen demand. Administer supplemental oxygen as ordered (only effective if adequate hemoglobin is present to carry the oxygen). Use semi-Fowler's position for maximum ventilation-perfusion match.
   c. *Administer EPO* in selected situations to promote endogenous RBC production.
5. Prevent **iatrogenic anemia** caused by large quantities of blood required for diagnostic procedures. Use smaller blood collection tubes; modern blood chemistry analyzers can perform a number of tests on a few drops of serum. Monitor and document cumulative total volume of blood drawn. Use fingerstick techniques to obtain capillary blood for testing whenever practical.

❖ Decreased gas exchange related to decreased red cell mass or decreased hemoglobin production.

B. White Blood Cells: Hypoactivity

1. **Assessment**
   a. *Local signs and symptoms of inflammation* include erythema, edema, warmth, pain, and decreased function of an affected area. Also note the presence and characteristics of exudate (serous versus suppurative).
   b. *Systemic clinical signs and symptoms of infection* include body temperature below 36°C or above 38°C, tachycardia, tachypnea, altered mental status (e.g., confusion, irritability), diaphoresis, rigors or chills, and generalized symptoms such as change in activity level, fatigue, or malaise.
   c. *Laboratory data*
      - Alterations in WBC count: leukocytosis, leukopenia, increased number of bands
      - Positive blood or body fluid cultures
      - Significant findings in site-specific diagnostic tests (e.g., pneumonia demonstrated on a chest radiograph)
2. **Interventions**
   a. Critically ill children have a higher risk of developing *skin compromise* related to compromised nutritional status, diminished sensation, immobility, diminished oxygenation and perfusion, immunosuppression, use of medical devices or procedures (Quigley and Whitney, 2001). The goal of nursing care is to promote skin integrity.
   b. *Assess and monitor* skin integrity, body orifices, IV sites, and pressure areas for evidence of inflammation, infection, or skin breakdown.
   c. See Box 8-1 for detailed *skin care practice guidelines.*

d. *Assess for and differentiate between inflammation and infection,* which are not synonymous terms. Although all infections occur in the presence of inflammation, not all inflammation indicates infection. *Infection* is the pathologic process caused by the invasion of normally sterile tissue, fluid, or body cavity by pathogenic or potentially pathogenic microorganisms (Levy et al., 2003). Special attention must be paid to patients in whom the cardinal signs of the local inflammatory response may be diminished or absent (e.g., immunocompromised patients, patients receiving medications suppressing the inflammatory response, newborns with a delayed or limited ability to localize infection). In these patients, the most reliable signs of the local inflammatory response are often pain and fever.

e. *Assess and monitor specific sites* for infectious processes.
- Pulmonary or lower respiratory tract infection: Note tachypnea, any change in level of consciousness, feeding, behavior or activity level, presence of cough, signs of respiratory distress, and abnormal breath sounds (see Chapter 2).
- Bacteremia, both primary and catheter related: Note systemic signs and symptoms of infection.

f. *Assess for and differentiate between systemic infection and a systemic inflammatory response syndrome (SIRS).* SIRS is the acute development of two or more of the following (American College of Chest Physicians [ACCP] and Society of Critical Care Medicine [SCCM], 1992):
- Fever (>38°C) or hypothermia (<36°C)
- Tachycardia (outside age-appropriate range)
- Tachypnea (outside age-appropriate range)
- Alteration in WBC count, either leukocytosis (WBC >12,000/mm^3; use age-appropriate range [see Table 8-6]), leukopenia (WBC <4000/mm^3), or greater than 10% bands.

g. *Administer prescribed antimicrobial agents* and monitor response. Dilute medication per formulary guidelines to diminish venous irritation and ensure complete administration by following antibiotic with an adequate flush.

BOX 8-1
SKIN CARE PRACTICE GUIDELINES

Assess and individualize skin care practices.
- Bathe daily with pH-balanced cleanser.
- Keep skin surfaces dry.
- Use moisture barrier products on incontinent infants and children.
- Hydrate skin.
- Avoid products that contain perfumes, alcohol, or latex.
- Minimize the use of adhesives.
- Minimize the impact of medical devices.
- Keep mucous membranes clean and moist.
- Keep eyes moist and protected.
- Maximize nutritional status.
- Support tissue perfusion and oxygenation.
- Promote immunocompetence.
- Minimize the hazards of immobility.

From Quigley SM, Whitney DE: Skin integrity. In Curley MAQ, Moloney-Harmon PA, editors: *Critical care nursing of infants and children,* ed 2. Philadelphia, 2001, W. B. Saunders, p 515.

Establish a schedule to maximize pharmacologic effects and minimize late administration. Assess for superinfections that may occur with long-term antibiotic use. Accurately obtain drug levels (serum drug concentrations, or SDC) as ordered.

h. *Administer granulocytes or biologic response modifiers* as ordered.

i. *Institute measures to decrease the patient's risk of infection* with endogenous organisms. Assist in personal hygiene measures (oral care, etc.) as indicated. In collaboration with the physician, explore the possibility of using the patient's GI tract for feeding to minimize the risk of bacterial translocation.

3. **Prevention:** Institute good handwashing and universal precautions for all individuals who may have contact with the patient. Use proper technique for initiating and maintaining all intravascular lines and during all invasive procedures. Promote optimal fluid and nutritional intake. Ensure a clean environment and restrict the patient's contact with individuals who may have infectious processes. Use a health screening tool for siblings wishing to visit the patient. Prevent the spread of infectious processes through the use of appropriate isolation procedures.

❖ Actual or potential for infection resulting from unintentional stressors (e.g., immunodeficiency, malnutrition, iatrogenic interventions such as placement of multiple invasive devices, immobility, or environmental pathogens) or intentional stressors (e.g., bone marrow suppression in preparation for transplantation or therapeutic regimens, including chemotherapy or radiation).

1. **Assessment**

a. *Differentiate between hyperthermia and fever:*

- *Hyperthermia* occurs when body temperature exceeds the set point. This typically occurs as the result of the body or some external condition creating more heat than the body can eliminate (as in heat stroke, aspirin toxicity, hyperthyroidism) (Algren and Arnow, 2003).
- *Hyperpyrexia* or fever is an elevation in set point such that the body temperature is regulated at a higher level and typically occurs as the result of an infectious process.

b. *Clinical signs and symptoms of fever* include elevated temperature of 38° to 41°C. Young infants and immunocompromised patients may respond with hypothermia in the presence of infection. Other symptoms include tachycardia; tachypnea; cloudy or altered mentation, confusion, or irritability; warm, dry skin with flushed cheeks; and diaphoresis.

c. *Positive implications of increased* temperature include enhanced activity of cells of the immune system and a nonconducive environment for the growth and activity of invading microorganisms (antigens). Negative implications of increased temperature include increased metabolic demand, increased insensible water loss and potential dehydration, and fatigue.

2. **Interventions**

a. *Monitor and document fever pattern.* In collaboration with the physician, determine the cause of fever. **Fever may be the *only* sign of infection in the immunocompromised patient, and the patient is presumed to have an infection until proven otherwise.**

b. *Monitor for dehydration.* Estimate insensible water losses. In collaboration with the physician, evaluate the need for adjustment of fluid requirements.

c. *Identification of the source of infection* is a primary concern in a febrile patient. Indwelling catheters should be sampled for culture. If possible, two peripheral blood samples should be obtained from separate venipuncture sites. Other cultures that may be obtained include sputum, tracheal, routine urinalysis and culture, and a stool examination and culture (especially if diarrhea is present).

d. In collaboration with the physician, consider the *administration of antipyretics* (only after the fever is evaluated) and broad-spectrum antibiotic therapy (until the specific cause of the infection is determined).

e. *Institute measures to decrease the temperature* when the patient is febrile. Remove excess clothing or bed linens. Apply cool moist compresses, especially to the forehead and axilla. Use a cooling blanket but discontinue use if shivering ensues. Prevent chills or shivering because the associated peripheral vasoconstriction may actually further increase body temperature. Shivering raises basal metabolic rate and increases heat production and body temperature (Algren and Arnow, 2003).

f. *Institute measures to increase comfort* when the patient is febrile. Change wet bed linens in the presence of diaphoresis or with the use of a cooling blanket. Cool the patient's room if possible. Provide rest periods.

g. If possible, *discontinue medications that may cause fever* as an adverse reaction.

❖ Elevated temperature due to infectious processes

1. **Assessment**

a. *Definitions* (Kline, 2002)

- *Mucositis:* Generalized inflammation of the oral mucosa
- *Esophagitis:* Inflammation of the mucous membranes of the esophagus

b. This is a common, dose-limiting *toxicity* caused by chemotherapy, radiation and neutropenia.

c. *Clinical signs and symptoms* are variable and range from reddened areas to deep ulcerations. Other manifestations include pain; dysphagia; thick oral secretions; the presence of white patches; cracked, dry lips; and drooling. The risk of infection increases greatly with impaired tissue integrity within the oral cavity. The fungal infection candidiasis (moniliasis or thrush) is identified by the presence of white plaques with indurated borders (Panzarella et al., 2002). The tongue may also be swollen and cracked. A specimen should be cultured and the prophylactic regimen supplemented with an antifungal agent.

d. *Implications of altered oral mucous membranes* include impaired integrity and increased risk of infection, inadequate nutritional intake or absorption, pain, and difficulty swallowing or speaking (if not intubated).

2. **Interventions:** Assess and monitor the condition of the oral mucosa. Institute measures to prevent inflammation (mucositis) or to prevent further injury to existing inflammation. Avoid exposure to chemical or physical irritants, and provide adequate fluid intake. Provide oral hygiene measures at least 3 times a day. Provide treatment based on assessment findings, and institute measures to increase comfort (Table 8-10).

❖ Altered integrity of mucous membranes resulting from oral infection or the side effects of chemotherapy or radiation

C. White Blood Cells: Hyperactivity

1. **Hypersensitivity reactions** are classified according to the source of the antigen that stimulates the immune response (Table 8-11). Type I immediate hypersensitivity reaction or anaphylaxis results in hyperactivity of the surveillance function of the immune system

a. *Assessment:* Clinical signs and symptoms typically occur within seconds or minutes of exposure to the antigen and are the result of the action of

TABLE 8-10
Example of Oral Care Guidelines

Assessment	Treatment
NORMAL MUCOSA AND GINGIVAE: GRADE 0 (NO MUCOSITIS)	
Oral mucosa is pink, moist; no lesions, crusts, or debris; gingivae are pink, firm, and stippled	1. Aid and encourage brushing, flossing, and rinsing after meals, particularly in evenings. 2. Use soft bristle brush, fluoride toothpaste, and 1/2-strength Cepacol.
MUCOSITIS AND GINGIVITIS: GRADE I (EARLY, MILD FORM)	
Oral mucosa or gingivae are red, shiny, with possible white patches; gingivae may appear swollen; patient may complain of a burning sensation or general discomfort in the mouth; tongue may appear coated, red, dry, or swollen	1. Rinse with alkaline-saline solution q2-4h while awake. 2. Debride teeth and gingivae b.i.d. using an Ultra-Suave toothbrush dipped in 1/2-strength Peroxyl. Rinse with water. 3. Swish and hold 5–10 mL of 1/2-strength S.T. 37 for 30 sec; then spit. Use 4 times per day. 4. If white patches are present, candidiasis should be considered and cultures done. Add Nilstat to the regimen.
MUCOSITIS WITH ULCERATION: GRADE II (MODERATE FORM)	
Mucositis and gingivitis as previously described, but with the addition of focal ulceration; patient hesitates to eat because of pain from chewing or swallowing	On a 3 times per day schedule: 1. Debride teeth and gingivae using an Ultra-Suave toothbrush dipped in 1/2-strength Peroxyl. Rinse copiously with alkaline-saline solution. For pain relief: 1. For isolated, small ulcers, apply Kank-A solution with provided applicator directly to the ulcer. 2. For more extensive and numerous ulcers, swish and hold 5–10 mL of Ulcer-Ease solution in the mouth for 30 sec; then spit out.
MUCOSITIS WITH SEVERE ULCERATION: GRADE III (SEVERE FORM)	
Severe erythema and ulceration or white patches present; patient complains of severe pain and cannot eat, drink, or swallow; saliva may appear thick and viscid with much drooling	1. Rinse for 30 sec with Ulcer-Ease to anesthetize mucosa. 2. Debride teeth and gingivae using an Ultra-Suave toothbrush dipped in alkaline-saline solution. Rinse copiously with alkaline-saline solution. *Do not use Peroxyl in grade III mucositis.* 3. For pain relief: Use Ulcer-Ease solution or 1/2-strength Dyclone (1%). Use systemic analgesia if not effective.
MOUTH DRYNESS (XEROSTOMIA)	
Thick "ropy" saliva (early sign) or an obviously dry mouth	1. Mucositis mouth care (see "Mucositis" above). 2. Rinse mouth with saline, ad lib. 3. Swab mouth with Moi-Stir oral swabsticks several times daily. 4. Administer artificial saliva (Xero-Lube) p.r.n. 5. Lip care (see "Lip care") p.r.n.

Continued

TABLE 8-10
Example of Oral Care Guidelines (*cont'd*)

Assessment	Treatment
LIP CARE	
Lips dry, chapped, rough, but free of crusts and debris	Treatment varies based on assessment: Moisten lips with lanolin q2-4h
Lips cracked, ulcerated, or crusted	Clean q2-4h with gauze saturated with saline. Pat dry and apply Lanoline or K-Y jelly.
Fissuring or cracking at the corners of the mouth (usually indicates candidiasis)	Apply Mycolog ointment q.i.d.
DEBRIS ON TEETH	
Platelet count >20,000 and no or minimal pain on brushing	Gentle brushing of teeth and gingivae with a *soft* bristle brush. Hold brush under hot water to further soften brush bristles.
Platelet count <20,000; patient unable to tolerate brushing or spontaneous bleeding noted from gingivae	1. Rinse mouth with alkaline-saline solution. 2. An Ultra-Suave toothbrush dipped in very dilute Peroxyl or alkaline-saline solution can be used. Rinse copiously with either water or more alkaline-saline solution. 3. A moistened gauze wrapped over a finger may also be used to debride teeth and gums. Toothettes are *not* effective.

Modified from Hopkins K: *Oral care guidelines for patients receiving chemotherapy and radiation therapy.* Memphis, 1993, St Jude Children's Research Hospital.

inflammatory mediators on surrounding tissues and blood vessels (Sevier and Kline, 2003). Increased capillary permeability can lead to profound hypotension, circulatory collapse, and facial edema. Constriction of smooth muscle can result in wheezing, crackles, and progressive difficulty in breathing and stridor. An influx of eosinophils can produce erythema and pruritus.

b. *Interventions:* Diagnosis and management of anaphylaxis are based on clinical manifestations.
- Maintain oxygenation and ventilation. Administer supplemental oxygen as needed. Intubation and mechanical ventilation may be necessary. In the presence of tracheal or laryngeal edema, intubation may be difficult and there is a possibility that the patient may require an emergency tracheotomy. Epinephrine 1:1000 is administered for treatment of bronchoconstriction.
- Support circulation with fluid administration and epinephrine administration to counteract vasodilation. Other vasoactive medications (e.g., dopamine, norepinephrine) may be required.
- Administer prescribed medications. Antihistamines serve as antagonists to most of the effects of histamine. Bronchodilators relax bronchial smooth muscle. Corticosteroids are anti-inflammatory agents that serve to enhance the effects of bronchodilators.
- Identify the antigen and avoid future exposures.

2. Autoimmune disease represents the hyperactivity of the homeostasis function of the immune system.

a. The *homeostasis* function of the immune system removes old and damaged "self" components from the body.

TABLE 8-11
Hypersensitivity Reactions

Type	Description	Example
Type I (anaphylactic reaction)	Triggered in response to an exposure to an environmental antigen. Mediated by IgE antibodies that bind to specific receptors on the surface of mast cells and basophils. Results in the release of a host of mediators to produce a classic anaphylactic response.	Anaphylaxis Asthma Allergic rhinitis, hay fever
Type II (tissue specific hypersensitivity)	Triggered by the presence of an antigen found only on a cell or tissue. Mediated by antibody (usually IgM, but also IgG) through two different mechanisms (complement and Fc receptors on phagocytes). Results in the destruction of the antibody-coated cell with consequences dependent on the cell that is destroyed (e.g., RBC, WBC, or platelet).	ABO incompatibility Rh incompatibility Drug-induced thrombocytopenia
Type III (immune complex reaction)	Triggered by the formation of antigen-antibody complexes that activate the complement cascade. Immune complexes are formed in the circulation and are later deposited in blood vessels or healthy tissue. Multiple forms of the response exist depending on the type and location of the antigen. Results in local edema and neutrophil attraction and thus degradative lysosomal enzymes resulting in tissue injury.	Serum sickness Glomerulonephritis
Type IV (delayed hypersensitivity)	Triggered by the recognition of an antigen. Mediated by activated T lymphocytes and release of lymphokines, which then stimulate the macrophage to phagocytize foreign invaders and some normal tissue. Results in a delayed onset. Does not have an antibody component; this response is strictly a cellular reaction.	Contact sensitivities such as poison ivy and dermatitis Tuberculin reactions Graft rejection

RBC, red blood cell; *WBC*, white blood cell.

b. The *immune system* mistakenly identifies itself as "nonself" and begins to form antibodies *(autoantibodies)* against its own healthy cells *(autoantigens)*. This results in the development of immune complexes that are deposited in tissues (e.g., skin, joints, kidneys) and in tissue damage.

c. Examples of *autoimmune disease* in children are juvenile-onset diabetes mellitus and systemic lupus erythematosus.

3. **Malignancy**

The *surveillance function* of the immune system identifies and destroys cells that are "nonself" or "self" cells that have undergone mutation.

❖ Increased inflammatory response related to increased immune system activity

D. Platelets and Plasma Factors

1. **Assessment** should include vital signs (tachycardia and hypotension), fluid and electrolyte status (decreased urine output, emesis, diarrhea), characteristics of fluid losses (assess for gross or occult blood), perfusion status, capillary refill, mental status, and urine output. Use urine and stool tests to detect the presence of blood.
2. **Interventions**
   a. *Volume replacement:* Administer crystalloids or colloids or both, blood products, and vasoactive infusions as ordered.
   b. *Control of bleeding:* Apply direct pressure or cold compresses, and elevate the extremity. Apply topical hemostatic agents such as an absorbable gelatin sponge (Gelfoam).
3. **Prevention**
   a. *Identify which patients are at increased risk for bleeding.*
   b. *Avoid intramuscular and subcutaneous injections;* if necessary, apply pressure for 10 minutes. If intravascular access is needed, peripheral IV access rather than central access poses less risk for trauma and bleeding to the patient.
   c. *Provide a safe environment,* such as padding the side rails and other firm surfaces, especially if the child is combative or at risk for seizure activity.
   d. *Do not administer aspirin or NSAIDs* because of their effects on platelets. Parents should be taught to read nonprescription medication labels to avoid giving the child aspirin.
   e. *Prevent intracranial bleeding* related to increased intracranial pressure. Teach the patient to avoid the Valsalva maneuver and to cough, sneeze, and blow nose gently. Administer stool softeners.
   f. *Provide mouth care* with foam swabs and a mild saline or bicarbonate and peroxide solution.
   g. *Administer vitamin K* (normally obtained from diet and enteric bacterial synthesis). Vitamin K deficiency is the most common cause of prolonged PT in the intensive care unit (ICU) (Chakraverty et al., 1996). Vitamin K is needed for factors II, VII, IX, and X to be effective. Deficiencies are seen with malnutrition, obstructive biliary disease, liver disease, and with use of certain cephalosporins, such as cefamandol. At the first sign of PT prolongation, administer vitamin K IV or subcutaneously or add to TPN. PT should correct within 24 hours. Anaphylactoid reactions are rare but are seen more often with the IV route.

❖ Hypovolemia related to bleeding

RED BLOOD CELL DISORDERS: SICKLE CELL DISEASE

A. Pathophysiology

1. **Sickle cell disease (SCD)** is the general term used to describe a group of genetic disorders that are characterized by mutations in the hemoglobin gene. These mutations lead to sickling of the RBCs in response to deoxygenation.
2. *When the oxygen saturations fall,* RBCs with HbSS (an abnormal form of hemoglobin associated with SCD) become crescent or sickle shaped. These sickled

RBCs become trapped in small vessels, leading to erythrostasis and occlusion of the microvasculature. Hypoxemia, acidosis, hypothermia or hyperthermia, and dehydration lead to further sickling and increased viscosity of the blood.

3. *Masses of sickled RBCs* occlude blood vessels, leading to thrombosis, ischemia, and infarction. Specific organs involved will present with signs of hypoperfusion, vascular occlusion, and tissue ischemia. The body recognizes and hemolyzes the abnormal RBC structure. Sickled RBCs may return to normal shape when the blood is more oxygenated (such as in the pulmonary vein). However, after repeated occasions, a portion of RBCs released into free circulation will be more sensitive to mechanical trauma, even normal trauma experienced during circulation, or they will not return to their nonsickled shape even when the blood is well oxygenated.

B. Etiology and Risk Factors

1. **SCD** is a serious, chronic, autosomal-recessive, hemolytic disease. The most common forms are hemoglobin SS disease (HbSS), hemoglobin SC disease (HbSC), hemoglobin S-beta thalassemia (HbSβthal), and other rare variants. Clinical manifestations will vary in type and severity between each of these phenotypes. See Table 8–12 for more detail.
2. **SCD** occurs almost exclusively in individuals of African descent and typically manifests after 6 months of age when most of the fetal hemoglobin (HbF) has been replaced with HbSS or HbSC.

C. Clinical Manifestations

Clinical manifestations occur secondary to the anemia and organ dysfunction caused by vascular occlusion. Specific symptoms include aching bones, especially hands and feet in infants, sudden severe abdominal pain, chest pain, and splenomegaly in young children. The spleen is nonfunctional in children with HbSS disease even if the spleen is enlarged. SCD is not associated with bleeding. Impaired growth and development, failure to thrive, and increased tendency to develop serious infections are results of decreased splenic function (Table 8-13).

D. Interpretation of Diagnostic Studies

1. **Peripheral blood smear** will show sickle cells. If only the sickle cell trait is present, smear will be normal. Hemoglobin electrophoresis indicates the precise type of hemoglobinopathy.
2. **CBC** reflects hemolytic anemia with reduced hemoglobin, hematocrit, and RBC count because the spleen has destroyed sickled cells. Platelets and reticulocyte count may be elevated as a compensatory response to anemia.
3. **Bilirubin** may be elevated because of the hemolysis of the sickled cells.
4. **Radiologic findings**
   a. *Bone x-rays* may show no abnormality in the face of severe bone pain.
   b. *Chest x-rays* may show cardiomegaly and pulmonary infiltrate with acute chest syndrome.
   c. *Computed tomography (CT)* scan and magnetic resonance imaging (MRI)/magnetic resonance angiography (MRA) should be performed after stabilization if a cerebral vascular accident (CVA) is suspected.

E. Nursing and Collaborative Diagnosis

- ❖ Potential for impaired gas exchange
- ❖ Activity intolerance
- ❖ Pain

TABLE 8-12
Comparison of Sickle Cell Syndromes

Genotype	Clinical Condition	Percent Hemoglobin					Other Findings
		Hb A	Hb S	Hb A_2	Hb F	Hb C	
SA	Sickle cell trait	55–60	40–45	2–3	—	—	Usually asymptomatic
SS	Sickle cell anemia	0	85–95	2–3	5–15	—	Clinically severe anemia; Hb F heterogeneous in distribution
S-B° thalassemia	Sickle cell-beta° thalassemia	0	70–80	3–5	10–20	—	Moderately severe anemia; splenomegaly in 50%; smear: hypochromic, microcytic anemia
S-B$^+$ thalassemia	Sickle cell-beta$^+$ thalassemia	10–20	60–75	3–5	10–20		Hb F distributed heterogeneously; mild microcytic anemia
SC	Hb SC disease	0	45–50	—	—	45–50	Moderately severe anemia; splenomegaly; target cells
S-HPFH	Sickle-hereditary persistence of Hb F	0	70–80	1–2	20–30	—	Asymptomatic; Hb F is uniformly distributed

From Scott JP: Hematology. In Behrman RE and Kliegman RM, editors: *Nelson's essentials of pediatrics*. Philadelphia, 2000, W. B. Saunders.

TABLE 8-13
Clinical Manifestation of Sickle Cell Anemia*

Manifestation	Comments
Anemia	Chronic, onset 3–4 mo of age; may require folate therapy for chronic-1 hematocrit usually 18%–26%
Aplastic crisis	Parvovirus infection, reticulocytopenia; acute and reversible; may need transfusion
Sequestration crisis	Massive splenomegaly (may involve liver), shock; treat with transfusion
Hemolytic crisis	May be associated with G6PD deficiency
Dactylitis	Hand-foot swelling in early infancy
Painful crisis	Microvascular painful vaso-occlusive infarcts of muscle, bone, bone marrow, lung, intestines
Cerebrovascular accidents	Large- and small-vessel occlusion → thrombosis/bleeding (stroke); requires chronic transfusion
Acute chest syndrome	Infection, atelectasis, infarction, fat emboli, severe hypoxemia, infiltrate, dyspnea, absent breath sounds
Chronic lung disease	Pulmonary fibrosis, restrictive lung disease, cor pulmonale
Priapism	Causes eventual impotence; treated with transfusion, oxygen, or corpora cavernosa-to-spongiosa shunt
Ocular	Retinopathy
Gallbladder disease	Bilirubin stones; cholecystitis
Renal	Hematuria, papillary necrosis, renal-concentrating defect; nephropathy
Cardiomyopathy	Heart failure (fibrosis)
Skeletal	Osteonecrosis (avascular) of femoral or humeral head
Leg ulceration	Seen in older patients
Infections	Functional asplenia, defects in properdin system; pneumococcal bacteremia, meningitis, and arthritis; deafness from meningitis in 35%; *Salmonella* and *Staphylococcus aureus* osteomyelitis; severe *Mycoplasma* pneumonia
Growth failure, delayed puberty	May respond to nutritional supplements
Psychologic problems	Narcotic addiction (rare), dependence unusual; chronic illness, chronic pain

From Scott JP: Hematology. In Behrman RE and Kliegman RM, editors:. *Nelson's essentials of pediatrics.* Philadelphia, 2000, WB Saunders.

CMV, Cytomegalovirus; *EBV*, Epstein-Barr virus; *G6PD*, glucose-6-phosphate dehydrogenase; *HIV*, human immunodeficiency

*Clinical manifestations with sickle cell trait are unusual but include renal papillary necrosis (hematuria), sudden death on intraocular phyphema extension, and sickling in unpressurized airplanes.

F. Goals and Desired Patient Outcomes: Prevention of Complications

1. Promote early diagnosis through **newborn screening.**
2. Encourage **follow-up** in a comprehensive sickle cell clinic.
   a. Educate the family regarding the importance of *mandatory prophylactic penicillin* starting at 2 months of age. Discontinuation of pencillin prophylaxis is controversial.
   b. Teach parents that *fever* (temperature >38.5°C) must be promptly evaluated to determine the source of the fever and the need for treatment.
   c. Teach parents to *palpate the spleen* for possible enlargement.
3. Prevent **crises** through prevention of dehydration, hypoxemia, and acidosis.
4. Prevent **infection** with vaccines such as for pneumococcal organisms and *H. influenzae.* Infants should receive the heptavalent conjugated pneumococcal vaccine at regular intervals. Children older than 2 years must receive the 23-

valent pneumococcal vaccine with a booster at 5 years (Wethers, 2000). Children with SCD can begin to receive yearly influenza vaccines after 6 months of age.

G. Patient Care Management

1. **Pain management:** Supportive interventions
   a. *Prevent pain* by rapid recognition and management of dehydration, hypoxemia, and acidosis to prevent sickling.
   b. *Obtain a history* of past and present pain management.
   c. *Conduct frequent, ongoing pain assessments* using the appropriate pain scale for age, developmental level, and clinical condition.
   d. *Use analgesics and anti-inflammatory agents* as indicated and ordered. Monitor effectiveness in decreasing pain.
      - Patient-controlled analgesia (PCA)
   e. *Use nonpharmacologic pain management techniques* as indicated (e.g., heat, massage, distraction, guided imagery).
   f. In selected clinical situations (e.g., severe acute chest syndrome) *RBC transfusion or exchange transfusion* is given to "dilute out" HbSS-containing RBCs. Goal is usually a hematocrit of 25% to 30% with <30% HbS. Avoid raising the hematocrit more than 35% because this will increase the viscosity of the blood and promote increased sickling.
2. **Bed rest** minimizes oxygen demand and consumption.
3. **Hydroxyurea:** Although considered routine therapy for adult patients with SCD who have severe recurrent pain, Hydroxyurea, a cytotoxic agent, is not used routinely in pediatric patients due to concerns about its possible mutagenic and carcinogenic effects (Jenkins, 2002). Hydroxyurea enhances the production of HbF, thereby decreasing the ability of the RBCs with HbSS to sickle. The response is quite variable from patient to patient. Use is limited to only those children most severely affected by SCD.
4. **Steroid Therapy:** The effectiveness of steroid therapy in the management of pain associated with vaso-occlusive crises is not considered standard care, although a number of studies have noted a decreased duration of hospitalization, decreased opiod requirements, and a reduced number of blood transfusions in children with acute chest syndrome who received steroid therapy (Bernini, 1998; Griffin et al., 1994).
5. **Bone marrow** or stem cell transplant is the only current therapy that may provide a cure for SCD.
6. **Gene therapy** may offer a future cure for SCD. Gene transfer to correct the molecular defect in the hemoglobin is under investigation as a future treatment.

H. Complications of Sickle Cell Disease

1. **Infections** are a major cause of morbidity and mortality for children with SCD.
   a. *Compromised function* of the spleen leads to an increased susceptibility to encapsulated bacteria. There is an increased risk of *S. pneumoniae* (pneumococcus) and *H. influenzae* type b infections. *S. pneumoniae* is a leading cause of death in the first 3 years of life; it can progress from onset of fever to death in less than 12 hours. *H. influenzae* infections have an insidious onset. Any clinical pneumonia decreases the effectiveness of oxygenation, thereby increasing sickling of RBCs.
   b. *Assess* for infections requiring immediate attention and admission to the hospital. Note significant pain, fever, and chills. Patients with SCD typically have a slightly elevated WBC count; but with infection, the WBC count further increases to greater than 30,000/mm^3. Chest radiographic examination demon-

strates significant pulmonary infiltrates if infection involves the pulmonary system.

c. *Management:* Obtain blood cultures and immediately begin antibiotics, including coverage for pneumococcus and *H. influenzae* if the child is younger than 5 years of age. Transfuse with RBCs only to give sufficient volume to alleviate signs or symptoms of inadequate tissue oxygenation.

2. **Splenic sequestration crisis** is a life threatening complication. It is the second most common cause of morbidity and mortality in SCD during the first decade of life. The exact cause is unknown, but often it is associated with viral illnesses and prior sequestration crises. Acute pooling of blood in the splenic sinuses results in a rapid decrease in Hgb. This results in acute splenic enlargement, significant anemia, and, if severe, can progress rapidly to hypovolemic shock and death. Splenic sequestration is typically seen in children between the ages of 6 months and 3 years; however, it has been seen in children as young as 2 months (Jakubik and Thompson, 2000; Jenkins, 2002). Children with HbSC and Hbβthal may have issues with splenic sequestration into their later childhood years.
   a. *Assessment:* Clinically, pallor of the mucosal surfaces, tachycardia, abdominal fullness, splenomegaly, left upper quadrant pain, and weakness are noted. Laboratory results demonstrate a rapid fall in hemoglobin and hematocrit.
   b. *Management*
      - A mild crisis (moderate increase in spleen size, a decrease in hemoglobin of less than 2 g/dL) may resolve spontaneously without treatment. Provide adequate hydration, monitor splenic size, and assess for recurrent symptoms or further deterioration of status.
      - For a severe crisis (massive splenomegaly, a decrease in hemoglobin of more than 2 g/dL, signs of hypovolemia), administer oxygen and rapidly transfuse RBCs to correct hypovolemia. Serial CBCs are monitored to prevent transfusion of an excessive volume of blood. Usually when hypovolemia is corrected, sequestered RBCs are released from the spleen.
      - Splenic sequestration has a recurrence rate of 50%. Long-term management involves initiation of a chronic transfusion program to maintain HbSS at less than 30%. In children with recurrent crises, a partial or full splenectomy may be performed. Full splenectomy will prevent further sequestration and partial may reduce the recurrence of splenic sequestration crises (Owusu-Ofori and Riddington, 2004). Following a splenectomy or if the spleen fibroses, the child will need preventive strategies for infection. Adults are not susceptible to these crises, as their spleens are atrophied (called *autosplenectomy*) because of repeated infarctions.

3. **Aplastic crisis** is a transient episode of failure of RBC production that can be life threatening. It is usually associated with human parvovirus B19, leading to transient suppression of erythropoiesis.
   a. *Assessment:* Clinical manifestations of severe anemia, including fever, anorexia, lethargy, tachypnea, tachycardia, nausea, vomiting, abdominal pain, and headache are noted (**not** splenomegaly). Laboratory results show a rapid decrease in hemoglobin, low reticulocyte count (<1%) in peripheral blood, and low RBC precursors in the bone marrow aspirate. A concurrent episode of acute chest syndrome may be seen.
   b. *Management:* Transfuse with RBCs slowly to alleviate signs or symptoms of inadequate tissue oxygenation. Protective isolation may be used. All caretakers must adhere to isolation guidelines. Repeat transfusions to maintain the hemoglobin baseline levels (usually 8 to 10 g/dL) until bone marrow function resumes, usually within a few days to 2 weeks.

4. **Acute chest syndrome**
   a. *Acute chest syndrome (ACS)* is defined as respiratory symptoms associated with a pulmonary infiltrate. In children, ACS is often associated with infection. In adults, ACS is usually seen after a severe, bony, painful crisis. Contributing causes include infection, sickling of RBCs in pulmonary vasculature, and bone marrow/fat embolism. The major concern is that a vicious cycle of pulmonary vaso-occlusion, poor oxygenation of blood, increased RBC sickling, and more vaso-occlusion will ensue. Vascular occlusion of branches of the pulmonary artery leads to infarction of the lung. The syndrome may be self-limited, particularly when it involves a small area of pulmonary parenchyma, but it can rapidly progress and become massive and fatal. A chronic pattern of this syndrome will lead to chronic scarring of the lung seen on x-ray examination. Repeated episodes lead to restrictions of vital capacity, pulmonary hypertension, and cor pulmonale.
   b. *Assessment:* Clinical course is variable, ranging from mild symptoms to a rapidly progressing and fatal respiratory failure.
      - Clinical appearance: Fever accompanied by chest pain, cough, dyspnea, tachycardia, and tachypnea.
      - X-ray: Pulmonary infiltrate may not be prominent, especially if the patient is dehydrated; it may progress to a complete "white-out."
      - Laboratory results: Blood and sputum cultures may be positive for organisms.
      - Arterial blood gases: Variable degrees of hypoxia may be seen.
   c. *Management:* Because of the potential for rapid deterioration, the child should be hospitalized and carefully monitored.
      - Presence of pneumonia must be ruled out. However, it is usually very difficult to distinguish between pulmonary infarction and pneumonia, and the processes are likely to coexist. In younger patients, pneumonia is more likely to be the cause of symptoms. In older patients, pulmonary infarction is the more common cause.
      - Initiate broad-spectrum antibiotics for *S. pneumoniae, H. influenzae,* and *Mycoplasma pneumoniae* immediately if new pulmonary infiltrates are seen on radiographic examination.
      - Administer supplemental oxygen to maintain an oxygen saturation of greater than 95%. Administer RBCs to ensure a Hb of 10 to 11 g/dL. Consider a partial exchange transfusion if signs of respiratory failure (PaO_2 <75 mm Hg) are present, if multiple lobes are affected, or if the patient's condition continues to deteriorate.
5. **Vaso-occlusive crisis (pain crisis)** is one of the most debilitating problems for SCD patients. It can occur in any organ system and is characterized by obstruction of small arterioles by sickled RBCs, resulting in ischemia of tissues, organ dysfunction, and pain. Onset is unpredictable with varied frequency, intensity, duration, and severity. Precipitating factors include infection, fever, dehydration, trauma, or exposure to cold. It is self-limited and may last as briefly as a few minutes or may be prolonged, lasting as long as 2 to 3 weeks (usually 4 to 5 days).
   a. *Assessment:* Diagnosis is by history, not by laboratory test or radiographic examination. Clinical appearance demonstrates severe deep pain at any site, commonly musculoskeletal, extremities, back, chest, or abdomen. Chest radiographic examination is used if chest pain is present to rule out acute chest syndrome. During infancy the syndrome is characterized by a "hand-foot" syndrome with soft tissue swelling, heat, and pain of the dorsum of the hands, feet, fingers, and toes.

b. *Management*

- Management of vaso-occlusive disease requires disruption of the cycle of hypoxemia and sickling by providing adequate hydration, oxygenation, antibiotic therapy if infection is suspected, and pain control (Jenkins, 2002).
- Initially rule out other causes of pain, such as osteomyelitis, bone infarction, and other causes for chest or abdominal pain.
- Hydration: Administer $D_5$1/2NS at one to two times normal maintenance rate.
- Administer supplemental oxygen if $Pa{O_2}$ is less than 80 mm Hg. This will not be effective in reducing pain.
- If fever is higher than 38.5°C, blood cultures should be obtained and IV antibiotics begun.
- Pain control measures: It is important not to withhold analgesics because of excessive concern about possible addiction. Acetaminophen with codeine may be used to treat mild pain. Morphine sulfate is typically the drug of choice for the treatment of moderate to severe pain associated with vaso-occlusive disease. Patient-controlled analgesia (PCA) allows for pain control while decreasing anxiety and minimizing the adverse effects of narcotic administration (Jenkins, 2002). If PCA is not an option, use around-the-clock dosing versus a PRN schedule, as PRN scheduling may promote cycles of recurring pain. Reevaluate the pain control plan at least every 12 hours; taper and switch to oral analgesics after pain control has been achieved.

6. **Cerebrovascular accident (CVA)** is usually caused by in situ vaso-occlusion. Stroke affects about 10% of children with SCD (Riddington and Wang, 2003). The exact cause is age related, with cerebral ischemia/thrombosis as the usual cause in children and intracranial bleeding in adults. Monitoring of intracranial arterial blood flow by transcranial Doppler has been shown to predict patients at high risk for stroke. TCD monitoring should start in early childhood (at age 2-4 years).

   a. *Assessment:* Clinical appearance demonstrates hemiparesis, severe unilateral headache, dizziness, lethargy, aphasia, seizures, or change in school performance as signs of increased intracranial pressure.
      - Radiologic studies: CT is initial study followed by MRI/MRA. MRI results may be normal initially because several days of evolution are necessary to detect an edematous infarcted area. Arteriogram is not commonly used, but when it is performed, administration of hyperosmolar contrast requires preparation with hydration and transfusion to lower HbSS to less than 30% before the scan is done. Contrast material may increase sickling. Low-ionic strength contrast medium is preferable.

   b. *Management:* The goal is to prevent progression of the CVA. Emergent management includes monitoring for increased intracranial pressure and exchange transfusion to decrease HbSS level to less than 30%. Use strategies to maintain normal intracranial pressure. Administer anticonvulsants if seizures occur. Patients are at risk for recurrence of CVA. Therefore a chronic RBC transfusion program may be initiated to maintain HbSS levels at less than 30%. Patients may require iron chelation therapy to treat iron overload.

7. **Bone marrow necrosis and fat embolism** are caused by microinfarctions of bone or marrow. Secondary embolization of fat or marrow particles leads to pulmonary infarction or fat globules in the coronary, cerebral, and renal microvasculature, resulting in renal, neurologic, or respiratory failure, which is frequently fatal.

a. *Assessment:* Clinically, severe bone pain, fever, neurologic abnormalities, or respiratory distress are noted. Lipid or fat may be present in sputum specimens.
b. *Management* includes administration of supplemental oxygen, exchange transfusion, and ventilatory support as needed.

8. **Multiorgan system failure (MOSF)** is an unusual clinical condition for patients with SCD resulting from several of the above complications. Episodes of pain complicated by the acute failure of at least two of three organs (lung, liver, or kidney) may result in a severe, life-threatening complication of pain episodes in patients with otherwise mild SCD. It is associated with an unusually severe vaso-occlusive crisis for the child and a high baseline hemoglobin level, which may or may not be associated with an infection. The cause is undefined but is assumed to be from the diffuse microvascular occlusion and tissue ischemia simultaneously in multiple organs and the sequestration and destruction of RBCs, leading to further tissue ischemia from the decreased oxygen-carrying capacity.
   a. *Assessment:* Clinically the child has fever, a rapid fall in hemoglobin and platelet count, nonfocal encephalopathy (confusion, lethargy), and rhabdomyolysis. Laboratory results show hypoxia and elevation of liver enzymes, bilirubin, PT, and creatinine. Radiographic findings include pulmonary infiltrates.
   b. *Management:* Transfusion, if aggressive and prompt, may reverse the syndrome. Exchange transfusion may be necessary for young children. Provide hydration and IV analgesia.
9. **Priapism,** a painful, involuntary erection of the penis, occurs as sickled cells are trapped in the penis. Although it may resolve spontaneously and require only analgesics, management may involve hydration, exchange transfusion (if condition does not resolve in 4 to 6 hours), and surgery to evacuate the stagnant blood.

WHITE BLOOD CELL DISORDERS

Despite the type of stressor (e.g., congenital, acquired, intentional, unintentional), the final common pathway or outcome of immunodeficiency or immunosuppression is impaired immune function or immunocompromise.

A. Definition of Terms

1. **Immunodeficiency:** A permanent state of impaired immune function that is usually genetic or congenital in nature.
2. **Immunosuppression:** A state of impaired immune function that can be intentional or unintentional and is usually temporary.

B. Congenital Immunodeficiency Diseases

1. Disorders are characterized by an **inadequate number or inadequate function** of one or more of the components of the immune system resulting from a genetic or congenital condition. Disorders are divided by involvement of B lymphocytes, T lymphocytes, phagocytes, complement, or a combination of these components.
2. **B-lymphocyte disorders** are characterized by a diminished ability to form immunoglobulins, thus resulting in an inability to generate effective antibody-antigen interactions (Makhoul et al., 2003).
   a. These are a diverse group of *immunodeficiencies* that may manifest as a deficiency in all classes of immunoglobulins (panhypogammaglobulinemia), as a deficiency in only one class of immunoglobulin (hypogammaglobulinemia),

or as a combination of deficiencies in some classes with overproduction of immunoglobulin in another class.

b. *IgA deficiency* is the most common B-lymphocyte disorder and results in increased incidence of early, recurrent infections, allergies, and autoimmune conditions. Another example of a B-lymphocyte disorder includes X-linked agammaglobulinemia.

c. *B-lymphocyte deficiencies* are frequently interrelated with T-lymphocyte dysfunction. (See Combined B- and T-lymphocyte Disorders.)

d. *Etiology and pattern of infections:* Upper respiratory infections, lower respiratory infections, meningitis, bacteremias, and abscesses are commonly seen in patients with B-lymphocyte disorders (Makhoul, et al., 2003). Because of the inability of antibodies to form from mature plasma cells, reinfection from the same organism is common, even following normal childhood immunization.

3. **T-lymphocyte disorders** are characterized by an inadequate number or function of T lymphocytes. These patients have a limited ability to produce mature T lymphocytes, resulting in the inability to assist in the activation of the immune response.

   a. *T-lymphocyte disorders* are associated with the survival and replication of intracellular organisms inside host immune cells. There is an increased incidence of lymphoproliferative disease and malignancies because patients with certain T-lymphocyte disorders may have uncontrolled T-lymphocyte regulation of B-lymphocyte growth (O'Neill Shigeoka, 2002). These disorders are usually associated concomitantly with antibody deficiencies.

   b. Examples of T-lymphocyte disorders include *DiGeorge syndrome* and *chronic mucocutaneous candidiasis.*

   c. *Etiology and pattern of infections* most often are viruses, fungi, protozoa, and intracellular bacteria. Opportunistic infection with organisms such as *Candida albicans* and *P. carinii* pose a risk to these patients.

4. **Phagocyte dysfunction disorders** (e.g., chronic granulomatous disease [CGD]) are disorders resulting from diverse extrinsic or intrinsic factors.

   a. *Extrinsic factors*
      - Deficiency in opsonization related to decrease in either antibody or complement
      - Suppression of neutrophils or altered chemotaxis of neutrophils related to deficiency or alteration in complement
      - Decreased circulating lymphokines
      - Medications with immunosuppressive effect on phagocyte function or number

   b. *Intrinsic factors:* Defects in the metabolic pathway of phagocytes.

   c. *Etiology and pattern of infection* demonstrate an increased incidence of staphylococcal infections. Patients with phagocytic disorders are considered at risk for infection with gram-negative bacterial and fungal infections despite a "normal" WBC count.

   d. Patients with inadequate numbers of phagocytes are referred to as *neutropenic* (total WBC number is decreased) or *granulocytopenic* (number of PMNs and bands decreased). These are clinical states rather than immunodeficiency disorders.

5. **Complement disorders** are characterized by the absence of an inhibitor or a deficiency in one or more of the specific complement components.

   a. *Deficiencies* for each of the key components of complement have been described; however, an increase in the susceptibility to infection is commonly noted for deficiencies in C2, C3, C5, C6, C7, and C8 (Grant, 2001).

b. *Pattern of infection* varies with the complement component that is deficient and can range from recurrent infection to autoimmune.

6. **Combined B- and T-lymphocyte disorders** (e.g., SCID, Wiskott-Aldrich syndrome)
   a. *Incidence* of combined B- and T-lymphocyte disorders is 1 in 50,000 to 70,000 live births (Fischer and Notarangelo, 2004).
   b. This is the most severe of all the *immunodeficiencies* because the patient is unable to form antibody (B lymphocyte), orchestrate the immune response (T lymphocyte), and destroy virally infected cells and cells infected with intracellular microorganisms (T lymphocyte).
   c. *Etiology and pattern of infection* include infection from all types of microorganisms (bacterial, fungal, viral, and protozoal). Infections are often severe and recurrent.

C. Severe Combined Immunodeficiency (SCID)

1. **Etiology and risk factors:** SCID is the most severe form of combined B- and T-lymphocyte disorders and has an estimated incidence of approximately 1 in 50,000 to 1 in 70,000 live births (Gennery and Cant, 2001; O'Neil Shigeoka, 2003). SCID is considered an immunologic emergency, and survival depends on expeditious stem cell transplantation (O'Neil Shigeoka, 2003).
   - Most cases (70%) are inherited in an autosomal or X-linked recessive pattern (Fischer and Notarangelo, 2004). Many variants of the disorder exist and range from partial to almost complete loss of T-lymphocyte function. About 50% of the autosomal recessive inherited cases involve a deficiency of the enzyme adenosine deaminase (Fischer and Notarangelo, 2004).
2. **Pathophysiology**
   a. SCID occurs as the result of a number of autosomal-recessive mutations or as the result of de novo mutations in the y-chain of the IL-2 receptor (O'Neill Shigeoka, 2003).
   b. SCID can occur as a consequence of ADA deficiency. B and T lymphocytes produce chemicals that can accumulate to toxic levels within these cells. Normally these cells produce an enzyme (ADA) that destroys the excess amount of the toxins. When this key "detoxifying enzyme" is missing, these toxins accumulate, poisoning the B and T lymphocytes.
3. **Signs and symptoms**
   a. SCID is initially characterized by an unusual frequency of common infections. If SCID is not recognized, recurrent and life-threatening opportunistic infections of bacterial, fungal, protozoal, or viral origin are seen, with onset within the first year of life (O'Neil Shigeoka, 2003). Infants are particularly susceptible to *Candida, P. carinii,* and CMV (Gennery and Cant, 2001).
   b. Infection is not present at birth because the infant is protected from bacterial infections by transplacental delivery of maternal IgG antibody; but signs and symptoms of infection and failure to thrive develop soon after birth.
   c. Infections are characteristic in terms of severity, recurrence (persistent in nature), type of organism, and location (common sites include the respiratory tract, mucous membranes, liver, GI tract, and blood). Oral candidiasis is resistant to therapy. Chronic diarrhea responds poorly to alterations in diet and may become life threatening.
4. **Interpretation of findings** from invasive and noninvasive diagnostic studies
   a. *WBC count and differential* (Gennery and Cant, 2001)
      - *Total lymphocyte count:* Decreased but variable
      - *Absolute lymphocyte count:* Decreased, usually less than 1500/mm^3; in newborns, less than 2800 is abnormal.
   b. *Cell-mediated immunity*

- *Lymphocyte subsets:* Helper T lymphocytes (CD4): Low to absent; Suppressor or cytotoxic T lymphocytes (CD8): Low to absent
- *Lymphocyte function:* There is diminished or absent lymphocyte response to antigens.

c. *Erythrocyte and leukocyte enzymes,* such as ADA and nucleoside phosphorylase, are assessed to determine the cause of SCID. ADA is not detectable in ADA-deficiency SCID and will be normal in X-linked SCID.

d. *Chest x-ray* examination demonstrates a small or absent thymus.

5. **Nursing and collaborative diagnoses**

❖ Altered protection related to primary immunodeficiency

❖ Potential for infection related to primary immunodeficiency, effects of prescribed medications, and malnutrition

❖ Potential for hyperthermia due to infectious processes

❖ *Potential for impaired gas exchange* related to pulmonary infections (e.g., PCP, other opportunistic infections)

❖ *Potential for fluid-volume deficit* due to infectious processes, chronic and unresponsive diarrhea, and fever

❖ *Potential for altered nutrition,* less than body requirements, related to frequent or chronic infectious processes, and chronic and unresponsive diarrhea

❖ *Potential altered growth and development* related to prolonged or repeated illness or hospitalization

6. **Goals and desired patient outcomes**

a. Augment or improve the child's immune system.

b. Protect from acquisition of infection (avoid live virus immunizations).

c. Detect, identify, and eradicate infections or neoplastic disease.

7. **Patient care management**

a. *Stem cell transplantation* is considered to be first-line therapy for the treatment of SCID. See Stem Cell Transplantation section for further information.

b. *Pretransplant management* includes isolation to prevent infection and meticulous skin and mucosal hygienic care. Patients must be monitored closely for indications of infection (fever may be the only sign). Antibiotics, antivirals, and antifungal agents are administered as appropriate. All RBC transfusions must be irradiated to prevent transfusion-related GvHD.

c. *Immune reconstitution* involves palliative enhancement of immune function. Intravenous immune serum globulin (IVIG) administration (see IVIG section) is used in severely ill children: 100 to 400 mg/kg IV every 1 to 4 weeks.

d. Enzyme-replacement therapy remains controversial. Replacement therapy with polyethylene glycol-modified bovine ADA (PEG-ADA) administered subcutaneously once weekly has resulted in clinical and immunologic improvement for children with SCID associated with ADA deficiency (O'Neil Shigeoka, 2003).

e. Gene therapy is a revolutionary means of replacing defective genes within the body. Successful use of gene therapy in the treatment of x-linked SCID has been reported (Hacein-Bey-Abina et al., 2002), although one patient developed leukemia (Hacein-Bey-Abina et al., 2003). This therapy is currently not available in the United States.

8. **Complications**

a. Infection can progress to sepsis, septic shock, and death (see Septic Shock discussion in Chapter 9).

b. Failure to thrive and malnutrition may require the use of parenteral nutrition.

c. The following increase the risk of these patients developing GvHD:

- Immunocompetent lymphocytes are transfused from the mother to the fetus or infant during gestation or delivery.
- Nonirradiated blood is administered.

d. Progressive poliomyelitis and death may occur if diagnosis is not made early and the child receives the live attenuated poliovirus immunization (O'Neill Shigeoka, 2003). No live attenuated vaccines should be given.

D. Acquired Immunodeficiency Syndrome (AIDS)

1. Definition of terms (American Academy of Pediatrics, 2003)

a. *HIV infection* is the presence of the human immunodeficiency virus, which causes a wide spectrum of disease and a varied clinical course.

b. *AIDS* is the portion of the HIV disease that represents the most severe end of the clinical spectrum.

c. The *incubation or latency stage* is the period from HIV infection to clinical manifestations of the disease; shorter incubation periods in children with perinatally acquired HIV have been noted than for children or adults with other modes of transmission.

2. Pathophysiology

a. *HIV,* an RNA retrovirus, causes AIDS. When a retrovirus infects a cell, the viral RNA is transcribed backward ("retro-") into the host DNA. The virus then uses the host cell's enzymes to direct the synthesis of new viral RNA and proteins to assemble new virus particles. The HIV interrupts normal cellular activity and function and ultimately causes the host cell to die, thereby releasing new virus into the circulation and infection of more host cells.

b. The principal, but not exclusive, target of the HIV is the *helper T lymphocyte,* which orchestrates both cell-mediated immunity (CMI) and humoral immunity (HI). HIV causes the number and function of the helper T lymphocytes to decline, creating a decline in immune function and response and an imbalance in the ratio of helper T lymphocytes to suppressor or cytotoxic T lymphocytes (CD4 to CD8). As the number of CD4 (helper T lymphocytes) declines, the patient becomes increasingly immunocompromised and at risk for opportunistic infection or malignancy.

3. Etiology and risk factors

a. *AIDS* in children was first described in 1982, but retrospective evaluation of previously existing medical records revealed undiagnosed cases as early as 1979 (Lott and Kenner, 1994).

b. *Incidence:* The total number of children with AIDS in the United States decreased 81% in 2000 compared with the numbers reported in 1992. This represents about 1% of the total cases of AIDS in the United States. This is due primarily to the standard use of antiretroviral therapy in HIV infected pregnant women (American Academy of Pediatrics, 2003).

- Estimated AIDS diagnoses through 2002 (CDC, 2002)
  - Children younger than 13 years of age: 9300 cases
  - Children 13 to 14 years: 839 cases
  - Children between 15 and 24 years: 35,460 cases
- More than 90% of the cases reported in children younger than 13 years of age resulted from perinatal transmission (Weinberg, 2000).

c. *Mode of transmission:* Children are most commonly infected by HIV through one of the following means:

- Intrapartum transmission is thought to be the most prevalent mode because of exposure to maternal blood and secretions. Transmission can also occur in utero or postpartum through breast-feeding (Hanson and Shearer, 1998).

Perinatal HIV transmission has been shown to occur between 13% and 39% in infants born to HIV infected women not taking antiretroviral therapy (Weinberg, 2000). Standard of care for an HIV-infected pregnant woman is to take at least AZT during her pregnancy, receive IV AZT during labor, and for the infant to receive 6 weeks of oral AZT. Perinatal transmission is believed to be less than 2% in women who take a combination of antiretroviral medications during their pregnancy (Weinberg, 2000).

- Exposure to infected blood or blood products or sexual contact with an infected individual accounts for less than 5% of cases. The latter is applicable primarily to sexually active adolescents, although younger children may be at risk if they are victims of child abuse (Weinberg, 2000).

4. **Classification system** for HIV in children (Table 8-14): Children are classified into mutually exclusive categories. Once classified, the child may not be reclassified in a less severe category despite improvement in the child's immunologic or clinical condition.
5. **Signs and symptoms**
   a. *Clinical course and manifestations* are very different from those manifested in adult patients. The course of the disease is more accelerated, with most children symptomatic before 2 years compared with 8 to 10 years for adults. The pattern of disease also varies with the age of the patient, with children experiencing a higher incidence of bacterial infections compared with adult patients, neurodevelopmental alterations (including developmental delay), failure to thrive, and different types of cancers rather than Kaposi sarcoma (e.g., lymphoma) (Weinberg, 2000).
   b. *Clinical signs and symptoms* are nonspecific (Grossman, 1988; Lott and Kenner, 1994). The child who is HIV infected may remain asymptomatic for several years. However, on average a perinatally infected infant will show symptoms by approximately 1 year of age (Weinberg, 2000). Symptoms include oral candidiasis, recurrent bacterial infections, chronic diarrhea, lymphadenopathy, hepatosplenomegaly, failure to thrive, eczematous rash, neurologic abnormalities (e.g., microcephaly, encephalopathy, dementia, developmental delay, loss of attained milestones), fever, and salivary gland (parotid) enlargement.

TABLE 8-14

Centers for Disease Control and Prevention (CDC) 1994 Revised Classification System for Human Immunodeficiency Virus in Children*

	Clinical Categories			
Immunologic Categories	**N: No Signs and Symptoms**	**A: Mild Signs and Symptoms**	**B†: Moderate Signs and Symptoms**	**C†: Severe Signs and Symptoms**
1: No evidence of suppression	N1	A1	B1	C1
2: Evidence of moderate suppression	N2	A2	B2	C2
3: Severe suppression	N3	A3	B3	C3

From Centers for Disease Control and Prevention: 1994 revised classification system for human immunodeficiency virus in children less than 13 years of age, *MMWR* 43(RR-12):1–10, 1994.

*Children whose HIV infection status is not confirmed are classified by using the above grid with a letter E (for perinatally exposed) placed before the appropriate classification code (e.g., EN2).

†Both category C and lymphoid interstitial pneumonitis in category B are reportable to state and local health departments as acquired immunodeficiency syndrome.

6. **Interpretation of findings** from invasive and noninvasive diagnostic studies
   a. *Diagnostic considerations*
      - Serum antibodies that are produced in response to the HIV serve as the basis for routine HIV testing (Lott and Kenner, 1994). The following tests are used to detect HIV antibody, (American Academy of Pediatrics, 2003):
        - ELISA is highly sensitive and specific to the HIV antibody. A positive ELISA is always repeated because other antibodies may produce a false-positive result.
        - Western blot is highly sensitive and specific to the HIV antibody. It is usually performed to confirm the result of a positive ELISA.
        - There are challenges with the diagnosis of HIV in infancy because maternal antibody is present in infants born to HIV-infected mothers due to passive transfer of maternal antibody. It is not possible to differentiate between maternal and infant HIV antibody; therefore, more specific viral testing is needed for diagnosis in children younger than 18 months, as described below (Weinberg, 2000). Polymerase chain reaction (PCR) is commonly used to look for the presence of HIV DNA. It is highly sensitive and specific. If a test is positive, the child is considered HIV infected, but it must be repeated for confirmation (Hanson and Shearer, 1998).
        - P24 antigen is the base antigen of HIV. The test is specific but less sensitive than PCR and culture. Therefore some HIV-infected individuals may have a negative p24 antigen result. If p24 is positive, the child is considered HIV infected, but it must be repeated for confirmation (Weinberg, 2000).
        - HIV culture indicates reverse transcriptase activity of the HIV in T cells. It is specific and sensitive, but it requires a long incubation time (60 days) (American Academy of Pediatrics, 2003).
   b. *Immune response to HIV:* HIV, especially vertically transmitted HIV, not only destroys mature and immature immune cells, but it also interferes with the normal development and maturation of the immune system (Weinberg, 2000). Children may or may not have a profound lymphopenia (lymphopenia is uncommon in early infancy [Hanson and Shearer, 1998]).
      - HI is decreased. Especially with vertical (prenatal) transmission, B-cell dysfunction may be evident. During fetal life, the B-cell system matures after the T-cell system and is thought to be more vulnerable to damage by the HIV infection (Hanson and Shearer, 1998). Congenital HIV infection presents with profound defects in HI and *initially* spares CMI (Landor and Rubinstein, 1993). Markedly elevated serum immunoglobulin is the most frequent pattern in pediatric HIV infection; it may denote a relatively mild disease course (Landor and Rubinstein, 1993). Hypogammaglobulinemia, when present, is associated with progressive disease (Landor and Rubinstein, 1993). Antibody synthesis is impaired after immunization. Secondary antibody response is more profoundly compromised than the primary response is (Landor and Rubinstein, 1993), thereby leading to repeated infections with the same organism. Dysregulation of HI is manifested by the formation of autoantibodies directed against platelets, neutrophils, lymphocytes, and RBCs (Landor and Rubinstein, 1993).
      - CMI is affected. Suppressor or cytotoxic T lymphocytes (CD8) are increased. Helper T lymphocytes (CD4) are decreased. The helper-to-suppressor or cytotoxic T lymphocyte ratio (T4/T8 ratio) is decreased, first reflecting an increase in suppressor T lymphocytes and then later a helper T lymphocyte depletion (Landor and Rubinstein, 1993). Lymphocyte function is

decreased. In skin testing, there is a defective or complete failure of delayed hypersensitivity (DH) reactions because of a decreased lymphocyte response to antigens. IL-2 receptor expression is abnormal, and IL-2 secretion is diminished (Landor and Rubinstein, 1993), as is nonspecific cytotoxicity (decreased NK cell function) (Hanson and Shearer, 1998, Landor and Rubinstein, 1993).

c. *CBC may reveal* anemia and thrombocytopenia.

d. *Lymph node biopsies* often reveal marked follicular hyperplasia with an abundance of B cells.

7. **Nursing and collaborative diagnoses**

❖ Potential for infection related to the HIV/AIDS disease process, immunodeficiency, effects of prescribed medications, and malnutrition

❖ Potential for impaired gas exchange related to pulmonary infections (e.g., PCP, other opportunistic infections)

❖ Potential for fluid volume deficit as a result of chronic diarrhea and fever

❖ Potential for altered nutrition, less than body requirements, related to the HIV/AIDS disease process, nausea, vomiting, diarrhea, and effects of prescribed medications

❖ Potential neurologic status changes related to HIV/AIDS disease process

❖ Potential altered parenting related to chronicity of diagnosis and critical illness

❖ Potential for ineffective coping (parent, child, sibling) related to the chronicity of the disease, repeated hospitalizations, critical illness, death of a family member, or anxiety and fear of infection or stigma

❖ Potential for transmission of the disease related to high-risk-taking behavior and lack of knowledge regarding mode of transmission

8. **Goals and desired patient outcomes**

a. *Suppress* retroviral replication.

b. *Augment* or improve the child's immune system.

c. *Detect, identify, and eradicate* infections or neoplastic disease.

9. **Patient care management**

a. *Suppress or inhibit* viral replication and prevent the development or progression of immunodeficiency.

- Several classes of antiretroviral medications work on suppressing viral replication at different points in the life cycle of HIV (Table 8-15).

b. *Management* of children with HIV/AIDS in the intensive care unit (ICU) varies with the reason for their admission.

- Respiratory failure secondary to PCP (*Pneumocystis carinii* pneumonia)
  - PCP with respiratory failure is one of the most common serious opportunistic infections in children with AIDS and is associated with a high mortality rate (American Academy of Pediatrics, 2003). *Pneumocystis carinii* is classified as a fungus; however, it has biologic similarities to protozoa (American Academy of Pediatrics, 2003). It is ubiquitous and benign to the healthy individual. In the immunocompromised host, the organism is an aggressive pathogen with a corresponding high risk of respiratory failure and death (American Academy of Pediatrics, 2003). Infection with *P. carinii* is thought to spread by the respiratory route from person to person. The organism targets the pulmonary tissue and once in the alveolus adheres to the epithelial cell surface. The immunocompetent individual is thought to undergo an asymptomatic infection, and the organism may persist indefinitely (American Academy of Pediatrics, 2003). If the patient is immunocompromised, pneumonitis is characterized by diffuse, bilateral, interstitial, and alveolar infiltrates (Hughes and

TABLE 8-15
Antiretroviral Medications

	Drug Name [Trade Name]	Available Preparations	Major Toxicities
NUCLEOSIDE ANALOG REVERSE TRANSCRIPTASE INHIBITORS	**Abacavir** (ABC, 1592U89) [Ziagen]	300 mg tablets 20 mg/mL syrup	Nausea, vomiting, diarrhea, fever, chills, achiness, extreme tiredness, and skin rash. Patients must be cautioned about the risk of serious hypersensitivity reaction. Hypotension and death have occurred upon rechallenge of the drug. Lactic acidosis has also been reported.
	Didanosine (ddI, dideoxyinosine) [Videx; sustained release *Videx EC*]	25, 50, 100, 150 mg chewable tabs 10 mg/mL pediatric solution *Videx EC*: 125, 200, 250, 400 mg capsules	Diarrhea, abdominal pain, and nausea. Less common: peripheral neuropathy and lactic acidosis. It is also rarely associated with pancreatitis.
	Emtricicitabine (FTC) [Emtriva]	200 mg capsules	Headache, diarrhea, nausea, rash, and hyperpigmentation of palms or soles. Less common: lactic acidosis.
	Lamivudine (3TC) [Epivir]	150 mg tablets 10 mg/mL syrup	Headache, fatigue, abdominal pain, and nausea. Less common: pancreatitis, lactic acidosis, and neutropenia.
	Stavudine (d4T) [Zerit; sustained release *Zerit XR*]	15, 20, 30, 40 mg capsules 1 mg/mL syrup *Zerit XR*: 37.5, 50, 75, 100 mg capsules	Headache, GI disturbances, and skin rash. Less common: pancreatitis, peripheral neuropathy, and lactic acidosis.
	Tenofovir [Viread]	300 mg tablets	Nausea, diarrhea, vomiting, and flatulence. Less common: lactic acidosis and severe hepatosplenomegaly.
	Zalcitabine (ddC, dideoxycytidine) [Hivid]	0.375, 0.75 mg tablets	Headache, malaise, and GI disturbances. Less common: peripheral neuropathy, oral ulcers, hematologic toxicities, pancreatitis, hepatic toxicity, and lactic acidosis.
	Zidovudine (ZDV, AZT, azidothymidine) [Retrovir]	100 mg capsules, 300 mg tablets 10 mg/mL syrup	Granulocytopenia, anemia, and headache. Less common: lactic acidosis and liver toxicity.
	Combination NRTI tablets	**Combivir** = ZDV/3TC (300/150) **Trizivir** = ZDV/3TC/ABC (300/150/300) **Epzicom** = ABC/3TC (300/150) **Truvada** = FTC/viread (200/300)	

TABLE 8-15
Antiretroviral Medications (*cont'd*)

	Drug Name [Trade Name]	Available Preparations	Major Toxicities
NONNUCLEOSIDE ANALOG REVERSE TRANSCRIPTASE INHIBITORS	**Delavirdine** (DLV) [Rescriptor]	100, 200 mg tablets	Headache, fatigue, GI complaints, and rash. There is a potential for multiple drug interactions because it is metabolized by cytochrome P450.
	Efavirenz (DMP266) [Sustiva]	50, 100, 200 mg capsules 600 mg tablets	Rash and CNS effects, such as insomnia, abnormal dreams, hallucinations, and amnesia. Best given in evening. Many drug interactions; check for specifics prior to administration.
	Nevirapine (NVP) [Viramune]	200 mg tablets 10 mg/mL syrup	Rash, nausea, headache, and less often hepatitis and granulocytopenia. Must be dose escalated to decrease hypersensitivity reaction.
PROTEASE INHIBITORS	**Amprenavir** (APV) [Agenerase]	50, 150 mg soft gel capsules 15 mg/mL syrup	Nausea, vomiting, perioral paresthesias, and rash. Less common side effect of Stevens-Johnson syndrome. Potential for multiple drug interactions.
	Atazanavir (ATV) [Reyataz]	100, 150, and 200 mg capsules	Asymptomatic elevations in indirect bilirubin, headache, insomnia, and dizziness. Less common: prolongation of PR interval of electrocardiogram. Potential for multiple drug interactions.
	Fosamprenavir (f-APV) [Lexiva]	700 mg tablets 50 mg/mL syrup	Nausea, vomiting, headache, diarrhea, and perioral parethesia. Rarely, life threatening rash, hyperglycemia, and hemolytic anemia. Potential for multiple drug interactions.
	Indinavir (IDV) [Crixivan]	200, 400 mg capsules	Nausea, headache, dizziness, and hyperbilirubinemia. Less common: nephrolithiasis, hyperglycemia, and hemolytic anemia. Potential for multiple drug interactions.
	Lopinavir/Ritonavir (LPV/RTV) [Kaletra]	133.3/33.3 mg soft gel capsules 80/20 mg/mL elixir	Nausea, vomiting, diarrhea, headache, and asthenia. Less common: lipid abnormalities and hyperglycemia.
	Nelfinavir (NFV) [Viracept]	50 mg/level scoop powder 250, 625 mg tablets	Diarrhea. Less common: asthenia, abdominal pain, rash, and lipid abnormalities.
	Ritonavir (RTV) [Norvir]	100 mg soft gel capsules	Nausea, vomiting, diarrhea, and abdominal pain. Less common:

Continued

■ **TABLE 8-15**
■ ■ **Antiretroviral Medications (*cont'd*)**

	Drug Name [Trade Name]	Available Preparations	Major Toxicities
		80 mg/mL elixir	increased liver enzymes, lipid abnormalities, and circumoral paresthesia.
	Saquinavir (SQV) [Invirase HG, Fortovase SG]	Invirase: 200 mg hard gel capsules Fortovase: 200 mg soft gel capsules	Diarrhea, abdominal pain, headache, rash, and paresthesias. Less common: fat redistribution, hyperglycemia, and ketoacidosis.
FUSION INHIBITOR	**Enfuvirtide** (T20) [Fuzeon]	Lyophilized single-use vial; resuspension supplies 90 mg/mL for subcutaneous injection	Most patients have local reaction at injection site, which includes redness, itching, pain, induration, and the development of nodules. There are no specific drug interactions.

Data excerpted from *Guidelines for the Use of Antiretroviral Agents in Pediactric HIV Infection*, January 2004. This is a living document that is continually updated, and the website (http://aidsinfo.nih.gov/guidelines/pediatric/PED_113004.pdf) should be consulted for details and revisions.

Anderson, 1998). The incidence of PCP in adults with AIDS is closely correlated with the number of absolute helper T lymphocytes (CD4), but this relationship is less so in infants and young children (Hughes and Anderson, 1998).

- Signs and symptoms: PCP is characterized by a tetrad of symptoms in all ages of patients and in all immunocompromised patients (with or without AIDS), but they vary in intensity: cough (unproductive), tachypnea, dyspnea (or a change in the young child's level of activity), and fever (with or without chills). Breath sounds are often clear. The child may demonstrate an acute onset with respiratory distress (without wheezing) and progressive respiratory failure. Blood gases are helpful in evaluating the severity of the pneumonitis (Hughes and Anderson, 1998). Blood gases often reveal hypoxemia, respiratory alkalosis, and decreased diffusing capacity.
- Diagnostic findings: Definitive diagnosis is made when clinical symptoms are accompanied by evidence of the organism. Chest radiographic findings initially may be normal or reveal only mild interstitial infiltrates. Early findings typically begin in the perihilar region, progress peripherally, and finally to the apical portions of the lung (Hughes and Anderson, 1998). Bilateral diffuse alveolar disease appears as pulmonary involvement worsens (Hughes and Anderson, 1998). A late finding is diffuse and extensive bilateral pulmonary consolidation ("white-out"). Diagnosis is made by obtaining evidence of the organism (Hughes and Anderson, 1998). Lower respiratory tract secretions are obtained by bronchoscopy with bronchoalveolar lavage (BAL) or by sputum induction, which is less sensitive but also less invasive than BAL, but may obviate the need for bronchoscopy. If an adequate specimen can be obtained and properly evaluated, diagnosis may be confirmed by sputum induction in older

children (Hanson and Shearer, 1998). Pulmonary parenchyma is obtained via transbronchial lung biopsy or open lung biopsy. Results are most sensitive and specific (Hughes and Anderson, 1998), and although this remains the gold standard, lung biopsy is rarely needed to confirm the diagnosis (Hanson and Shearer, 1998).

- Treatment: Definitive treatment is aimed at eradicating the organism. Two major drugs are available to treat *P. carinii*. Both are equally effective but differ in their adverse effects (Hughes and Anderson, 1998). Trimethoprim-sulfamethoxazole (TMP-SMZ, Bactrim, Septra) is preferred over pentamidine because it has fewer adverse effects. It is recommended for initial treatment of PCP. TMP-SMZ initially is administered intravenously in all but the mildest of cases but may progress to oral doses once the infection is resolving (Hughes and Anderson, 1998). The IV dose is trimethoprim 15 to 20 mg and sulfamethoxazole 75 to 100 mg/kg daily divided in three to four equal doses and infused over 1 hour. PO dose (tablets or suspension) is trimethoprim 20 mg and sulfamethoxazole 100 mg/kg daily divided in three to four equal doses (American Academy of Pediatrics, 2003). The course of treatment is 2 to 3 weeks. At completion of treatment, doses are reduced to prophylactic range but are continued indefinitely (Hughes and Anderson, 1998). Adverse effects occur with both the IV and the PO route of administration. The most common adverse effect is a transient erythematous maculopapular rash that resolves following withdrawal of the drug. Less common adverse effects include nausea and vomiting, neutropenia, diarrhea, anemia, and methemoglobinemia. Indications for discontinuing TMP-SMZ and considering another medication are side effects in the absence of clinical improvement after 3 to 5 days, no clinical improvement after 5 to 7 days, and urticarial rash or Stevens-Johnson syndrome (American Academy of Pediatrics, 2003).
- Pentamidine isethionate is the next drug of choice (Hughes and Anderson, 1998). It is given IM or IV; IV is the preferred route because it is associated with fewer adverse effects. IM use is uncommon and very painful. The IV dose is 4 mg/kg daily. The course of treatment is 2 to 3 weeks. Adverse effects are frequent and include hypotension, hypoglycemia or hyperglycemia, hepatic and renal toxicity, rash, thrombocytopenia, and anemia (Hughes and Anderson, 1998).
- Use of steroids may prevent or suppress the inflammatory response and reduce pulmonary edema secondary to PCP (Mudge-Grout, 1992; American Academy of Pediatrics, 2003).
- Supportive treatment is provided. Most patients require oxygen administration. Mechanical ventilation is indicated with respiratory failure if $Pa{O_2}$ cannot be maintained at 60 mm Hg or greater with inspired O_2 fraction of 50% or greater.
- Prognosis: During early days of treatment, the best indicator of clinical response was blood gas results (American Academy of Pediatrics, 2003). Patients with an alveolar-arterial oxygen gradient less than 30 mm Hg at the time of therapy have a better prognosis than those with ≥30 mm Hg gradient (Hughes, 1994). Chest x-ray examination is less helpful in revealing clinical improvement or deterioration. Subsequent episodes of *P. carinii* infection greatly diminishes the child's chances of survival; therefore lifelong prophylaxis is instituted regardless of clinical status or CD4 counts (American Academy of Pediatrics, 2003). Studies are in progress to determine safety of discontinuing secondary PCP prophylaxis in children

who have had immune reconstitution on highly active antiretroviral therapy. Prophylaxis regimens include *one* of the following (Hughes and Anderson, 1998): TMP-SMZ (Bactrim, Septra) twice daily taken 3 days per week, *or* aerosolized pentamidine once a month, *or* dapsone daily.

- Prophylaxis is initiated in infants born to HIV-infected women. Prophylaxis should begin at approximately 6 weeks of age, regardless of CD4 counts. All HIV-infected infants and infants whose infection status has not yet been determined should remain on prophylaxis until 12 months of age (Hughes and Anderson, 1998). HIV-infected children older than 12 months of age should have regular CD4 monitoring to determine the need for *P. carinii* prophylaxis (Hughes and Anderson, 1998): HIV-infected 1- to 5-year-old children require prophylaxis if the CD4 count is less than 500 cells/mcL or CD4 percentage is less than 15%. HIV-infected 6- to 12-year-old children require prophylaxis if the CD4 count is less than 200 cells/mcL or CD4 percentage is less than 15%.

- Respiratory failure secondary to lymphocytic interstitial pneumonitis (LIP) or pulmonary lymphoid hyperplasia (PLH)
  - LIP/PLH is defined as diffuse infiltration of alveolar walls by mature lymphocytes, plasma cells, and reticuloendothelial cells. Although associated with other immunodeficiencies and autoimmune diseases, it affects up to 51% of children with HIV infection (Weinberg, 2000). In the child with AIDS, LIP is characterized by atypical, rather than mature, lymphocytes invading the bronchioles and creating the pulmonary infiltrate (Weinberg, 2000). The cause of LIP is unknown. It is unclear whether LIP and PLH are two extremes of the same disease or two unrelated entities (Landor and Rubinstein, 1993). EBV DNA has been isolated in the lung tissue of children with LIP/PLH, suggesting persistent EBV infection as a cause (Landor and Rubinstein, 1993; Weinberg 2000).
  - Signs and symptoms present as chronic and progressive. Respiratory symptoms are nonproductive cough, tachypnea, dyspnea, and normal to decreased breath sounds; basilar rales are possible. Other symptoms are generalized lymphadenopathy, digital clubbing and parotid gland enlargement (Weinberg, 2000).
  - Diagnostic findings: Chest radiographic examination discloses diffuse miliary pattern similar to that seen in tuberculosis (Weinberg, 2000) and diffuse reticulonodular infiltrates, at times with hilar and mediastinal adenopathy. Nodular densities are distributed throughout the lung (Hanson and Shearer, 1998). Pulmonary physiology resembles that of PCP and includes hypoxemia, respiratory alkalosis, decreased diffusing capacity, and restrictive lung volumes. The lack of fever, acute respiratory distress, and significant auscultatory findings assist in the distinction between LIP/PLH and PCP (Hanson and Shearer, 1998). Diagnosis is most often made using clinical findings with the exclusion of infectious pathogens but may be confirmed with an open lung biopsy (Hanson and Shearer, 1998).
  - Treatment: LIP/PLH has been known to resolve spontaneously in some HIV-infected children. Because outcomes are variable, treatment is not clearly defined. Antiretroviral therapy has been shown to be beneficial in addition to corticosteroids (Hanson and Shearer, 1998).
  - Prognosis: The child with AIDS experiencing LIP has a better prognosis than a child with a documented opportunistic infection (Hanson and Shearer, 1998).

10. **Transmission precautions**
    a. Although HIV is detected in many body fluids, the single most infectious medium for HIV is blood (American Academy of Pediatrics, 2003). Universal blood and body fluid precautions should be used for *all* patients, including those children who are HIV infected. Use gloves when handling any body secretions including blood, stool, vomitus, or nasogastric (NG) drainage or performing invasive procedures. Use barrier precautions or protective wear (gown and protective eyewear) to prevent skin and mucous membrane contamination. Hands should be washed following glove removal.
    b. Parenteral exposure to infected blood by accidental needlestick injury is the overwhelming cause of HIV in health care workers (American Academy of Pediatrics, 2003). There is a decreased risk with the use of needleless systems, placement of needles and other "sharps" in puncture-resistant containers for disposal, and avoidance of recapping, bending, or removing needles from disposable syringes (American Academy of Pediatrics, 2003). It is important to report all exposures to an employee's occupational health department to be counseled on the risk of aquiring HIV and other blood-borne illnesses. In addition, postexposure prophylaxis (PEP) for HIV may be offered to the health care worker. PEP should begin as soon as possible, preferably within 2 hours of exposure (New York State Department of Health, 2003).
11. **Impact of HIV on other organ systems**
    a. *Respiratory system:* In addition to PCP, there is a high frequency of LIP/LPH in HIV infected children, which causes significant morbidity (Weinberg, 2000).
    b. *Cardiovascular system:* Left ventricular dysfunction and cardiomyopathy are seen frequently by electrocardiography, but are generally not clinically significant. These may be related to the occurrence of congestive heart failure and arrhythmias (Weinberg, 2000). HIV encephalopathy may be related to cardiomyopathy (Weinberg, 2000). Ongoing clinical trials are attempting to understand the incidence of cardiac problems in HIV-infected children, (Hanson and Shearer, 1998).
    c. *CNS*: CNS complications in pediatric HIV are common. It is estimated that progressive encephalopathy occurs in about 20% to 40% of children with HIV infection (Weinberg, 2000). Cerebral atrophy and bilateral calcification of the basal ganglia and frontal white matter are commonly seen by neuroimaging (Weinberg, 2000). Cerebral toxoplasmosis and cryptococcal meningitis are seen rarely in children.
    d. *Hematologic system* (Wilkinson and Greenwald, 1988): The most common disorders are autoimmune thrombocytopenia and drug-induced (therapy) granulocytopenia.
    e. *Recurrent bacterial infections*: Children with HIV are at risk for recurrent, invasive bacterial infections with organisms that include *S. pneumoniae, H. influenzae,* and *Salmonella* spp. (Weinberg, 2000).

E. Secondary Immunodeficiency

1. A large percentage of children admitted to the ICU are *immunocompromised* as a result of an acquired defect in immune function.
2. *Secondary immunodeficiency* is caused by a variety of stressors including, but not limited to, anesthesia, tissue injury (e.g., surgery, trauma, thermal injuries), medications (see Relevant Pharmacology section), malignancy, and malnutrition (acute and chronic).

3. Although the *pathophysiology of the defects in immune function* differs slightly with each of the aforementioned stressors, the implications of these are the same as found in the section on White Blood Cells: Hypoactivity.

COAGULOPATHIES AND PLATELET DISORDERS

A. Disseminated Intravascular Coagulation (DIC)

DIC is a serious bleeding disorder resulting from accelerated normal clotting with a subsequent decrease in clotting factors and platelets, leading to uncontrolled bleeding.

1. **Pathophysiology:** Coagulation mechanisms are abnormally stimulated.
   a. *Clotting component:* Widespread and rapid formation of fibrin thrombi in the microcirculation results in the consumption of certain clotting factors and platelets. The presence of fibrin thrombi in the microcirculation (microclots) leads to ischemic tissue injury. If significant microinfarction occurs, organ function is impaired, leading to brain, kidney, liver, or lung injury.
   b. *Hemorrhagic component:* As the clots are lysed and clotting factors, fibrinogen, and platelets are consumed, blood loses its ability to clot (consumptive coagulopathy). A stable clot, therefore, cannot be formed at injury sites, thus predisposing to hemorrhage. Clotting factors and platelets cannot be made by the body as fast as they are used.
2. **Etiology and risk factors:** DIC is not a primary disease or primary bleeding disorder. DIC is always a result of another disease or condition. It is often associated with shock, infections, hemolytic processes (such as transfusion of mismatched blood), and severe tissue damage (such as extensive burns or trauma, rejection of transplants, and postoperative damage, especially after extracorporeal circulation). Possible additional causes are neoplastic disorders (especially acute promyelocytic leukemia), fat and pulmonary embolisms, snake bites, acute anoxia, hepatic insufficiency or splenectomy, obstetric emergencies and complications, fresh-water near drowning, and heat stroke.
3. **Signs and symptoms:** Two categories of symptoms occur; however, many patients may have laboratory evidence of DIC without clinical signs.
   a. *Clotting* is related to the microvascular thromboses. Symptoms include spontaneous, easy, or disproportionately severe bruising; intramuscular hematoma (spontaneous or trauma related); cool, mottled skin; pallor; and circulatory failure. Thrombosis of peripheral or central veins leads to absent popliteal, posterior tibial, or pedal pulses; cyanosis of fingers, toes, earlobes, or tip of the nose; and tissue necrosis and gangrene.
   b. *Bleeding* in a patient with no previous bleeding history or out of proportion to the degree of thrombocytopenia is noted as a range from prolonged oozing from venipuncture sites and bleeding around intranasal, endotracheal, and urethral catheters to profuse hemorrhage from all orifices. Subtle to occult bleeding occurs. Systemic signs include the following:
      - Skin: Petechiae, ecchymosis, purpura, and hematoma
      - Head: Gingival bleeding and epistaxis
      - Genitourinary: Hematuria
      - GI tract: Hematemesis and melena
      - Neurologic: Headache and altered level of consciousness
      - Cardiovascular: Symptoms of shock
4. **Interpretation of findings** from invasive and noninvasive diagnostic studies: No single laboratory test confirms the diagnosis of DIC.

a. *Platelet count* is decreased.
b. *Coagulation tests*
   - PT is prolonged.
   - PTT is prolonged.
   - Fibrinogen level is decreased.
   - FSP is elevated (>40 mcg/mL) as is D-dimer.

5. **Nursing and collaborative diagnoses**

❖ Potential for bleeding and hemorrhage
   a. *Maintain* mucous membrane and skin integrity.
   b. *Monitor* internal bleeding and control overt bleeding.

❖ Impaired cardiac output due to blood loss

❖ Potential for impaired gas exchange related to blood loss
   a. *Maintain* hemoglobin above 10 g/dL.
   b. *Treat* hypoxemia.

6. **Goals and desired patient outcomes**
   a. *Correct* the primary problem.
   b. *Perfuse* vital organs until primary problem and DIC are controlled.
7. **Patient care management:** Early detection and prompt management can prevent complications and death. Primary disorders associated with DIC must be treated.
   a. *Supportive treatment:* If the symptoms of thrombosis or bleeding are mild, no specific therapy is needed. Begin specific treatments only when significant bleeding or organ dysfunction related to DIC occurs.
      - Administer blood products, replacing coagulation factors. Provide platelet transfusion if platelet count is less than 20,000/mm^3. FFP provides clotting factors; give with packed RBCs if the platelet count is greater than 50,000/mm^3 and the patient is still bleeding. Cryoprecipitate provides needed fibrinogen and factor VIII. Use in addition to FFP or whole blood as needed. Administer if fibrinogen is below 75 g/dL. Fresh whole blood is used if bleeding is profuse to supply all clotting factors and platelets. This will also serve as a volume expander and will increase the oxygen-carrying capacity by increasing the hemoglobin. If, after 6 to 8 hours of aggressive treatment and the patient is still in shock and bleeding, consider double-volume exchange transfusion with heparinized fresh blood, reconstituted FFP, and packed RBCs.
      - Supportive strategies aimed at the inhibition of coagulation activation (i.e., administration of recombinant human activated protein C, recombinant activated factor VII, have been reported to be of benefit (Levi et al., 2004; Tancabelic and Haun, 2004).
      - Heparin by continuous infusion is a controversial treatment unless there is endogenous damage (e.g., purpura fulminans). The goal is to tip the balance within the microcirculation toward physiologic fibrinolysis and allow reperfusion of the vital organs. Although it may stop the clotting, it may initially worsen the bleeding. Administer 10 to 20 U/kg per hour as a continuous infusion after an initial loading dose of 50 U/kg while continuing supportive treatment with blood products. Titrate the infusion to decrease bleeding and increase the fibrinogen with a decrease in the D-dimer. Oral anticoagulants are of no benefit or substitute for heparin.
      - Provide normal perfusion by fluid replacement.
   b. *Improvement* is reflected by increased fibrinogen concentrations and platelet count. Any increase in fibrinogen or platelet count is an encouraging indication that the consumption process has been interrupted and bleeding will be under control.

8. **Complications** are related to end-organ hypoxic or ischemic changes. Multifocal neurologic defects are due to multiple small brain infarcts. Thrombosis of blood vessels supplying the kidney cortex may result in renal failure. Pulmonary embolism and adult respiratory distress syndrome (ARDS) may occur. Acute ulceration and GI bleeding, intra-abdominal bleeding, intrahepatic hemorrhage, and mesenteric thrombosis may occur.

B. Immune Thrombocytopenic Purpura (ITP)

1. **Pathophysiology:** The decreased platelet count is immune-mediated, and purpura means bruises caused by bleeding into the skin. ITP is also called *idiopathic* thrombocytopenic purpura because the exact cause of the disease is not known.
   a. The body develops *antibodies* against its own platelets. These antibodies coat the surface of the platelets and cause the immune system to see the platelet as "foreign" or "nonself" and destroy it. Antibodies directed against specific platelet antigens lead to platelet destruction. Bleeding may occur when platelets are less than $50{,}000/mm^3$. The spleen is the site of antibody production and of destruction of sensitized platelets. Bone marrow produces platelets as rapidly as possible, but the platelets are quickly destroyed (in a few hours). Increased sequestration of platelets in the spleen further limits the availability of platelets to the circulation.
   b. *Exact cause* is often not known; other possible causes of the thrombocytopenia must be ruled out, such as a toxin or drug exposure. Viral illnesses precede the onset of symptoms in most cases in children.
2. **Etiology and risk factors:** Children usually have had a viral-induced upper respiratory tract infection, measles, mumps, or chickenpox a few weeks before the onset of ITP. Clinical course is generally a severe but self-limited thrombocytopenia in children younger than age 12 years. Most cases resolve within 6 weeks to 6 months; 10% go on to develop chronic ITP.
3. **Signs and symptoms:** Patients present with bleeding and thrombocytopenia, particularly in their skin and mucous membranes. The bleeding may be seen in all body parts and may be severe enough to result in shock. Splenomegaly is rare.
4. **Diagnosis**
   a. *Exclude* other causes of accelerated platelet destruction or decreased production of platelets by the bone marrow. Rule out leukemia, meningococcal meningitis, sepsis, systemic lupus erythematosus, and DIC.
   b. The *history* of the child indicates previous good health; some report a recent viral illness.
   c. *Examination* reveals bruises and petechiae appearing almost overnight, with no apparent cause.
5. **Interpretation of findings** from invasive and noninvasive diagnostic studies
   a. *CBC*: Platelet count is decreased.
   b. *PT and PTT* are usually normal.
   c. *FSP levels* are normal.
   d. *Bone marrow aspirate* is usually not performed in typical childhood ITP. When obtained, it is to see whether the bone marrow is producing enough platelets. In ITP it will reveal increased megakaryocytes.
6. **Nursing and collaborative diagnoses**
   ❖ Potential for impaired skin and mucous membrane integrity
   ❖ Potential for hemorrhage
7. **Goals and desired patient outcomes:** Individualization of the treatment plan.

a. *Protection* from sources of trauma. Parents should be taught to make the environment as safe as possible (bumper pads on the crib, avoid toys with sharp or hard surfaces). Older children should not play contact sports; restrict bicycles.
b. *Avoid* other platelet-damaging drugs such as aspirin.
c. *Control* bleeding.
d. *Maintain* adequate platelet count.

8. **Patient care management:** Acute ITP is usually self-limited with most pediatric patients recovering without treatment. Life-threatening bleeding occurs only rarely.
   a. *Steroids* produce an increase in platelets in most cases. They have been shown to decrease the removal of the sensitized platelets from the circulation and to increase production and mobilize platelets from the platelet pool. Steroids prevent bleeding by decreasing the rate of platelet destruction in the spleen and will result in a platelet increase within 5 to 21 days.
   b. The *IVIG mechanism of action* is the same as that of steroids in that it increases the platelet count by blocking the antibodies that destroy the sensitized platelets in the spleen. High doses (1 g/kg) have been shown to elevate the platelet count to higher than 30,000/mm^3 within 3 days. Few patients may not require further doses of IVIG with a permanent increase of their platelet counts. Other patients may require repeated doses of IVIG because of transient increases in their platelet counts.
   c. *Splenectomy* may be used if ITP does not respond to medical treatment and bleeding continues. It is generally avoided in the young child because of the association with a risk of sepsis after splenectomy.
   d. *Platelets* are transfused only if life-threatening bleeding such as CNS or GI tract bleeding occurs. Platelets will be destroyed by antiplatelet antibodies. When platelets are transfused, they are complexed with antibody and rapidly removed from the circulation by the spleen. This can range from minutes to days of the transfusion.
   e. *Immunosuppressive agents* such as vincristine and azathioprine may be given to patients with chronic ITP to suppress the immune system, reducing the platelet antibody with variable success.
   f. *Rh_o(D)* is used for treatment of ITP in nonsplenectomized Rh_o(D) antigen-positive patients. Injection of anti-D coats the patient's D-positive RBCs with antibody, saturating the capacity of the spleen to clear antibody-coated cells, thereby transiently increasing the platelet count in most patients (Lexi-Comp, 2004).
9. **Complications**
   a. *Intracranial bleeding* is the most serious complication, occuring in fewer than 1% of patients with ITP.
   b. *Bleeding from nose or gums* is not as severe but occurs more frequently.
   c. *GI tract and kidney bleeding*
10. **Differentiation from hemolytic-uremic syndrome (HUS)**
    a. *HUS is a triad of hemolytic anemia, thrombocytopenia, and renal failure,* all of which involve diffuse endothelial cell damage, activation of platelets, and widespread involvement of multiple organ systems.
    b. *HUS is similar to ITP* in that HUS is usually associated with infection or viral illness and that many children have bruising and petechiae from severe thrombocytopenia.
    c. *HUS is different from ITP* in that HUS is associated with oliguria or anuria with elevated BUN and with neurologic symptoms such as seizures or coma.
    d. The *average course of illness* for HUS is 4 to 6 weeks.

C. Heparin-Induced Thrombocytopenia (HIT)

Heparin-induced thrombocytopenia is typically characterized by a 50% or greater decrease in platelet count after 5 or more days of unfractionated (standard) heparin therapy. A rapid-onset-pattern can occur if a patient has been exposed to heparin in the recent past (i.e., less than 100 days), with symptoms occurring within the first 24 hours of reexposure. The platelet count nadir is usually around 50,000 mcL.

1. **Pathophysiology**: HIT is caused by an antibody-antigen reaction on the surface of platelets with unfractionated heparin.
   a. *Production* of platelet-derived microparticles that are released in the circulation and activate the coagulation system produce thromboemboli. HIT is an intensely prothrombotic condition.
2. **Etiology and risk factors:** Risk factors are noted previously. Incidence is about 5% in adults but unknown in pediatric patients. Twenty percent of patients with HIT can have paradoxical thrombotic complications, which may include loss of limb or death. An unexplained drop in the platelet count in a patient receiving heparin should raise the suspicion of HIT.
3. **Signs and symptoms:** Signs of clotting (increased bruising, thrombus formation) or bleeding if the platelet count is extremely low. An unexplained drop in platelet count should raise the suspicion of HIT.
4. **Diagnosis:** Blood samples are tested for the presence of specific antibodies. This is correlated with clinical signs and symptoms of thrombosis.
5. **Nursing and collaborative diagnoses**

❖ Potential for thrombosis of major vessels leading to venous, arterial, and intracardiac thromboembolism. Pulmonary embolism and major bleeding are rarely described.
   a. *Monitor* for thrombosis and control overt bleeding.
   b. *Maintain* mucous membrane and skin integrity.

6. **Goals and desired patient outcomes**
   a. *Prevent* thrombus formation.
   b. *Control* bleeding if present.
   c. *Restore* the platelet count/function after stopping heparin.
   d. *Treat* the child with thrombosis with alternative anticoagulation to heparin.
7. **Patient care management:** Any source of heparin, including low-molecular-weight heparin, is discontinued. This includes arterial and central-line flush solutions. If there is no evidence of thrombosis and no indication for continuation of anticoagulants, discontinuation of heparin will result in the platelet count returning to normal.
   a. *If a thrombus is present,* alternative anticoagulation with danaparoid, lepirudin, and argatroban appears to improve outcome because they have minimal cross-reactivity with heparin-induced antibody.
   b. *Patients with severe circulatory compromise* may require limb amputation. An unfavorable outcome (death/limb amputation) was reported in 42.1% of patients without therapy and in 18% of patients treated with alternative anticoagulation (Risch et al., 2004).

PLASMA CLOTTING–FACTOR DISORDER: HEMOPHILIA

A. Pathophysiology

Hemophilia is a disorder of hemostasis of one or more clotting factors.

1. **Types**
   a. *Hemophilia A:* Deficient in factor VIII; also called *Classic Hemophilia.*
   b. *Hemophilia B:* Deficient in factor IX; also called *Christmas Disease.*

2. **Formation of a normal clot** at sites of bleeding is prevented. The degree of bleeding is related to the degree of factor deficiency. Hemophiliacs are susceptible to persistent bleeding or severe hematoma formation following relatively minor trauma. Severe hemophilia is more likely to be associated with spontaneous bleeding.

B. Etiology and Risk Factors

1. **Sex-linked recessive traits** occur almost exclusively in males; female carriers transmit the disease. In hemophilia A, inheritance of an abnormal gene results in decreased or absent factor VIII production. Hemophilia B is caused by a defective factor IX gene and deficient factor IX production.
2. About 15% to 20% of affected individuals do not have a **family history.**
3. **Carriers** on average will have factor activity of 50%; those who have less than 30% activity level may be symptomatic. Therefore carriers should have their factor levels checked.
4. **Diagnosis** can be done during pregnancy for some females identified as at risk for transmitting the disease.
5. The **diagnosis** can be made on a sample of blood obtained at birth (including cord blood).

C. Signs and Symptoms

1. **Bleeding** can occur anywhere in the body following trauma or normal activity or spontaneously.
2. **Specific signs and symptoms** include the following:
   a. *Slow, persistent, prolonged bleeding* from minor injuries and small cuts
   b. *Uncontrollable hemorrhage* subsequent to dental extraction or irritation of the gums
   c. *Epistaxis,* especially after a facial injury
   d. *Hematuria*
   e. *Ecchymosis and subcutaneous hematomas* (petechiae are rare)
   f. *Neurologic manifestations* from bleeding near peripheral nerve leading to compression of the nerves
   g. *Bleeding into joints* (hemarthrosis), which may lead to severe joint deformity, especially knees, ankles, and elbows; it causes permanent crippling.

D. Interpretation of Findings from Invasive and Noninvasive Diagnostic Studies

1. **Hemophilia A**
   a. *Factor VIII assay:* Decreased levels and increased PTT
      - Less than 1% of normal level represents severe hemophilia: Child is at risk for spontaneous and trauma-induced hemorrhage from infancy.
      - 2% to 5% of normal level: Child will have a moderate clinical course except with trauma or surgery, when supportive treatment will be necessary.
      - Greater than 5% of normal level: A mild clinical course; supportive treatment is not often needed.

   b. *Factor VIII* activity levels should be assessed.
   c. *CBC:* Normal results, including platelet count.
2. **Hemophilia B**
   a. *Factor IX assay:* Decreased levels
      - Less than 1% of normal level represents a severe bleeding tendency.
      - 1% to 3% of normal level represents a moderate degree of bleeding tendency.

- 5% to 25% of normal level represents a mild degree of bleeding tendency.
- Greater than 25% of normal level represents significant bleeding only if trauma or surgery.

b. *PT* is normal, and PTT is prolonged (usually at least 60 seconds in children with severe deficiencies).

c. *CBC* results are normal, including platelet count.

3. **Radiographic findings:** Major joint destruction following repeated hemorrhages.

E. Nursing and Collaborative Diagnosis

❖ Potential for hemorrhage related to deficiency of factor VIII or IX

1. **Provide immediate and often repeated administration of factor VIII or IX,** depending on the diagnosis. Only recombinant factor products should be used. Occasionally patients will develop inhibitors or antibodies to their factors. Other activated factor products may be indicated.
2. **Local control of hemarthrosis** includes elastic wraps and ice packs to the affected limb to reduce swelling, bleeding, and pain. Elevation of the extremity, restriction of normal activity for 48 hours to prevent rebleeding, and pain control are important.

❖ Potential for impaired skin and mucous membrane integrity

1. **Prevent** injury. Venipunctures should be only antecubital, external jugular, or other superficial veins. Hold pressure for a minimum of 15 minutes and avoid intramuscular injections. Counseling should include the appropriate level of activity for the child, including contact sports.
2. **Avoid** NSAIDs and aspirin.
3. **Teach** the needs of parents.
4. **Provide** genetic counseling.
5. **Teach** how to recognize a bleeding episode, which measures should be done first, and how to differentiate between episodes that can be controlled at home and those that require hospital care.

F. Goals and Desired Patient Outcomes

1. **Restore** normal clotting activity. *Hemophilia A and B:* For mild hemorrhages, 40% to 50% of normal level is needed to control bleeding. For major bleeding, correction to 100% activity is recommended.
2. **Minimize** tissue and joint damage
3. **Preparation** for the child in need of surgery is 80% to 100% of normal factor level. Keep the level above 30% to 50% during the postoperative course.

G. Patient Care Management

1. **Blood products** for children with hemophilia A:

   a. For *severe bleeding,* give recombinant factor VIII (AHF) concentrate. Half-life is 10 to 12 hours; subsequent transfusions are needed every 8 to 24 hours, depending on the response and severity of bleeding. One to several days of maintenance therapy will be needed for advanced lesions to resolve. The initial dose should not be delayed, and all subsequent doses should be administered on time to ensure that hemostasis is achieved quickly and maintained.

   b. *FFP* requires more quantity than factor VIII concentrates to control bleeding and is not recommended.

   c. For *less severe bleeding* in mild hemophilia (factor VIII greater than 5% to 10%), the use of desmopressin (DDAVP) should be considered. DDAVP causes release of factor VIII from endothelial cells.

2. **Blood products** for children with hemophilia B: *Recombinant factor IX* concentrate should be used. Half-life is 18 to 24 hours; subsequent transfusions are needed every 12 to 48 hours, depending on response and severity of bleeding. One to several days of maintenance therapy are needed for advanced lesions to resolve. The initial dose should not be delayed, and all subsequent doses should be administered on time to ensure that hemostasis is achieved quickly and is maintained. DDAVP is not effective in hemophilia B.

H. Complications

1. **Hematoma formation,** which can be large, results in compression of vital structures. Hematomas may produce fever, leukocytosis, severe pain, and hyperbilirubinemia as a result of RBC degradation.
2. **Progressive arthropathy:** Inflammatory and hypertrophic changes occur in the synovial tissue. Over time this results in erosion of cartilage and bone.
3. **Intracranial bleeding** associated with trauma may be associated with subdural, epidural, intracerebral, subarachnoid, or rarely intraspinal sites.
4. **Inhibitor to factor VIII** may develop.

STEM CELL (BLOOD OR BONE MARROW) TRANSPLANTATION

A. Definition

1. **Stem cell transplantation** (SCT) involves the transplantation of pluripotential hematopoietic stem cells capable of self-renewal and terminal differentiation, giving rise to an entirely new hematopoietic system for the patient.
2. **SCT** is a primary therapy in the treatment of cancer, diseases that affect the immune and hematopoietic systems, and certain inherited diseases such as severe combined immunodeficiency disease (SCIDs) (Gonzales-Ryan et al., 2002).
   a. *Leukemia:* Acute lymphoblastic in relapse, acute myelogenous, chronic myelogenous
   b. *Solid tumors:* Lymphoma, neuroblastoma, other tumors
   c. *Hematopoietic stem cell defect:* Aplastic anemia, congenital severe immunodeficiencies (e.g., SCID), osteopetrosis, thalassemia, sickle cell anemia.
   d. *Other:* Metabolic disorders
3. **Success** of this treatment is related to elimination of the underlying problem, prevention of rejection, prevention of GvHD, and appropriate control over the potential multiorgan complications that occur in the weeks after transplant while waiting for the return of the transplanted bone marrow function.
4. **Purposes of conditioning regimens:** Chemotherapy with or without radiation is used to eliminate the tumor from the recipient, to ablate the recipient's marrow in preparation for the donated marrow, and to suppress the recipient's immunity to prevent rejection of the graft (donated marrow).

B. Types

1. **Autologous transplant** uses stem cells from the patient's own marrow or peripheral blood. Stem cells are harvested during a period in which the malignancy does not involve the blood or bone marrow. The stem cells are then treated and frozen to preserve viability of the cells. After very high doses of chemotherapy and radiation to remove cancer cells from the patient's body, the

stem cells are thawed and reinfused into the patient as a hematopoietic "rescue" from the marrow ablation secondary to high doses of chemotherapy. Autologous transplants are used in the treatment of metabolic disorders and recurrent pediatric solid tumors.

2. **Allogeneic transplant** is the transplantation of cells from an external donor. This type of transplant is performed to correct congenital or acquired defects in marrow production, immune function, or a combination of the two.
   a. *Several types of donors* undergo a bone marrow harvest.
      - *Genotypic match* (sibling): A family member who has demonstrated histocompatibility (similar HLA antigens).
      - *Related mismatched* (parent): A family member who has demonstrated partial HLA matching.
      - *Unrelated phenotypic match:* Marrow from a nonrelative that is HLA matched at the major loci. Donor is found through bone marrow donor registries. At some centers, removal of the T lymphocytes from the marrow before reinfusing the marrow into the donor may minimize the incidence of GvHD.
      - *Unrelated mismatched:* Partially HLA matched and from a different gene pool. A donor is found through bone marrow donor registries. Donor marrow preparation involves removal of the T lymphocytes per unrelated phenotypic matches.

   b. The *donated stem cells* are infused into the patient who has undergone intense chemotherapy or irradiation as part of the treatment of the disease and ablation of the marrow in preparation for transplanted stem cells (also known as the conditioning regimen).
   c. *Engraftment* typically occurs in 2 to 4 weeks in an HLA-matched allogeneic SCT. RBC and platelet function return when normal laboratory values return. Normal WBC count may return in a few weeks; however, effective function of the WBCs may take up to 1 year. If the transplanted stem cells are of a different RBC type, close collaboration with the blood bank is needed to administer the appropriate product as outlined in Table 8-16.
3. An **allogeneic transplant** using stem cells taken from an identical twin and reinfused into the ill twin is termed a **syngeneic transplant.** Usually there are few complications because of identical gene makeup. A less aggressive conditioning regimen is required because only removal of the tumor is needed, not ablation of the marrow to prevent graft rejection.

C. Post-Transplant Management

1. **Reconstitution** of a near-normal immunologic status takes place progressively over a period that may last several months to more than 1 year following the SCT.
   a. To *prevent GvHD,* patients are given immunosuppressive drugs (see section on Relevant Pharmacology).
   b. *Supportive care* is needed to manage electrolyte imbalances and nutritional deficits, deficient blood components, and infections. Total parenteral nutrition and fluid replacements may be needed. RBC transfusions are administered to maintain a hematocrit greater than 25%. Platelet transfusions are administered to maintain a platelet count greater than $20{,}000/mm^3$ unless the patient is actively bleeding or an invasive procedure is planned; then the platelet count should be in the 50,000 to $100{,}000/mm^3$ range. Clotting factors should be replaced with appropriate blood products,

TABLE 8-16
Blood Product Transfusion Guidelines for Bone Marrow Transplantation (BMT)

Donor	Recipient	Packed RBCs	WBCs	Platelets and Plasma
ABO COMPATIBLE				
O	O	O	O	O
A	A	A	A	A, AB
B	B	B	B	B, AB
AB	AB	AB	AB	AB
MAJOR ABO INCOMPATIBILITY				
A	B	O	O	AB
A	O	O	O	A, AB
B	A	O	O	AB
B	O	O	O	B, AB
AB	A	A	A	AB
AB	B	B	B	AB
AB	O	O	O	AB
MINOR ABO INCOMPATIBILITY				
O	A	O	O	A, AB
O	B	O	O	B, AB
O	AB	O	O	AB
A	AB	A	A	AB
B	AB	B	B	AB

Modified from Quinones RR: Bone marrow transplantation. In Fuhrman BP, Zimmerman JJ: *Pediatric critical care.* St Louis, 1992, Mosby.

such as FFP when the PT or PTT is greater than 1.5 times the control value, if the fibrinogen level is less than 100 mg/dL, or if there is active bleeding. Antibiotics may be required.

c. *Pain* related to severe mucositis and liver enlargement usually is effectively managed through the use of continuous narcotic infusions, often in the form of PCA.

D. Acute Complications

1. **Infection** is the leading cause of morbidity and mortality in the post-transplantation patient.
   a. For weeks after the transplant, these *neutropenic and immunosuppressed patients* are highly susceptible to bacterial, viral, and fungal infections despite aggressive antibiotic and antifungal therapy and protective environments. A routine strategy for prevention of infection is high-efficiency particle air (HEPA) filtered air and positive pressure rooms to decrease risk of fungal infections. Some centers use reverse isolation particularly for transplants for children with congenital immunodeficiency diseases. Other requirements include strict handwashing techniques, meticulous central venous catheter care, prophylactic antibiotics, antivirals and antifungals, and daily mouth care. CMV-negative blood products are used if both the donor and recipient of the marrow are CMV-negative.
   b. Identification of the *signs and symptoms* of infection must be immediately followed by prompt and aggressive treatment to avoid septic shock and

death. Signs and symptoms may be obscured in neutropenic patients. Therefore all fevers are regarded as infectious in nature until proven otherwise (Gonzales-Ryan et al., 2002).

c. *Management* includes antibiotics and antiviral agents.

2. **Hepatic dysfunction:** Veno-occlusive disease (VOD) is seen in the first few days up to 2 to 3 weeks after a SCT.
   a. *VOD* is caused by obliteration of small hepatic venules resulting from hepatotoxicity of intensive chemotherapy and radiation. Deposits of fibrous material plug the small venules in the liver. Pressure and fluids back up into the sinusoids of the liver, leading to liver engorgement as venous outflow becomes more and more occluded. Anoxia leads to further injury and necrosis of hepatic tissue with the result that hepatic blood flow and function are even more impaired.
   b. *Diagnosis:* VOD must be differentiated from GvHD, drug-induced liver injury, and hepatitis. Portal Doppler flow studies may reveal reversal of normal flow in VOD. Liver biopsy assists in definitive diagnosis; however, this is a high-risk procedure in the critically ill post-SCT patient because of a high risk of bleeding. Signs and symptoms range from moderate liver dysfunction to hepatic coma. Clinical symptoms include jaundice or hyperbilirubinemia, right upper quadrant pain, hepatomegaly, and ascites or early unexplained weight gain.
   c. *Management:* Presently there are no treatments to prevent or reverse VOD. Clinical efforts are directed toward supportive and symptomatic care until VOD runs its course and the regenerative capabilities of the liver have a chance to repair the damage. Supportive management includes maintenance of intravascular volume to optimize hepatic and renal perfusion, correction of electrolyte imbalances, minimizing the adverse effects of ascites, monitoring for and treating coagulopathies, and frequent adjustment of medications to reflect changes in hepatic clearance.
3. **GI tract dysfunction**
   a. *GI tract dysfunction* is caused by direct toxicity of chemotherapy and radiation, which provides a portal of entry for infection from the denuding of the epithelial lining of the entire GI tract mucosa. Many SCT patients suffer from a breakdown in the integrity of the mucosal defense system.
   b. *Diagnosis*
      - Signs and symptoms include mucositis (inflammation of all mucous membranes, which is quite painful); nausea, vomiting, and diarrhea (hypovolemia and significant electrolyte imbalances); and hemorrhage from a site in the GI tract.
      - Endoscopic procedures
   c. *Management*
      - *Mucositis:* Often peaks 10 to 14 days post-transplant. The severity of swelling and pain is variable. Use appropriate antibiotics, meticulous oral hygiene, and pain control.
      - *Nausea and vomiting:* Aggressive use of antiemetics, especially in combinations individualized to patient response, is indicated.
      - *Diarrhea:* Maintain fluid and electrolyte balance; provide symptomatic relief; and protect the skin in the rectal area from severe excoriation and breakdown.
      - *Hemorrhage:* Maintain hemodynamic stability and find and treat the source; angiography and surgery may or may not be performed, depending on the determination of the risks compared with the benefits.

4. **Renal dysfunction**
   a. *Renal dysfunction* is a frequently seen complication and is caused by toxicities of chemotherapy, antibiotics, antifungals, and CSA and is aggravated by any prerenal problems such as decreased renal perfusion from hypovolemia.
   b. *Diagnosis,* signs and symptoms, and laboratory results are detailed in Chapter 5.
   c. *Specific differences* regarding renal dysfunction in the SCT patient include the following:
      - Hyperkalemia may or may not occur.
      - Hypokalemia frequently occurs, often requiring IV potassium replacement. In patients receiving CSA or amphotericin B, potassium continues to be wasted in the urine unless the patient becomes anuric.
      - Increased BUN is difficult to interpret, as it is influenced by processes other than decreased glomerular filtration rate. Steroids and the presence of blood in the GI tract can significantly increase BUN without any alteration in renal function.
   d. *Hemofiltration* or dialysis is occasionally required to correct life-threatening electrolyte imbalances, eliminate waste products, and restore fluid balance.
5. **Pulmonary complications** are the most common cause of death in patients following a SCT, with interstitial pneumonitis being a major cause. Patients who require mechanical ventilation have a poorer prognosis than those who do not (Jacobe et al., 2003).
   a. *Interstitial pneumonitis* is a general term referring to an inflammatory process involving the interalveolar lining of the lung. Risk factors include immunocompromise of the host from pretransplant and post-transplant immunosuppressive therapy, lung damage from conditioning regimens such as radiation or chemotherapy or interaction of both radiation and chemotherapy, and the presence of an infection, many of which are opportunistic microorganisms (often CMV). It can be confirmed by lung biopsy, but this is a high-risk procedure for the post-SCT patient and is not done often. Interstitial pneumonitis is often described as idiopathic, a pulmonary process that does not yield a positive culture, similar to ARDS.
   b. *Diagnosis:* Although distinguishing radiation-induced pneumonitis from other causes of the symptoms would be useful, this process is difficult by diagnostic imaging or other studies. Signs and symptoms include dry cough, rales, dyspnea, nasal flaring, fever, and restricted ventilatory capacity resulting from decreased pulmonary compliance.
      - Laboratory results: Arterial blood gases indicate hypoxia.
      - Radiographic findings: Diffuse interstitial infiltrates are noted on the chest x-ray film.
   c. *Management:* Prompt recognition of the condition is followed by treatment. If interstitial pneumonitis is radiation induced, steroids are used. If it is infection induced (with or without a positive culture), broad-spectrum antibiotics are used; therapy can be more specific if a pathogen is identified by bronchoalveolar lavage or transbronchial biopsy during bronchoscopy, thoracentesis, or open-lung biopsy (rarely done because of the high risk for the SCT patient). If the child's condition deteriorates, intubation and mechanical ventilation may be required. Recovery is slow, and aggressive supportive care is required. Toxicity to the lungs is exacerbated by high oxygen and airway pressure settings.
6. **Cardiac complications**
   a. *Cardiac complications* are caused by cancer therapy, especially anthracyclines or cyclophosphamide or radiation to the chest, as part of the conditioning

regimen or given before SCT. Heart failure often leads to pulmonary edema. This results from a loss of myocardial fibrils, mitochondrial changes, and cellular degeneration; chronic changes such as fibrosis are common. Cardiac complications may occur early in post-SCT period.

b. *Diagnosis*
   - Signs and symptoms include weight gain, peripheral edema, tachycardia, dyspnea on exertion, orthopnea, rales, and rhonchi.
   - Echocardiogram is used to measure shortening or ejection fractions.

c. *Management:* Patients may continue to deteriorate, as chronic and cumulative damage is usually irreversible. Treatment is limited to supportive measures, including precise fluid management, judicious use of diuretics and inotropic agents, maintaining comfort, and decreasing myocardial oxygen consumption and stress.

7. **Hemorrhagic cystitis** causes significant morbidity for the SCT patient.
   a. *Cystitis* is caused by bladder toxicity from chemotherapy, most often associated with cyclophosphamide. A metabolite produces ulceration of the bladder mucosal tissue. Small vessels in the underlying tissue hemorrhage into the bladder. Viruses of the bladder mucosa may also cause hematuria.
   b. *Diagnosis*
      - Signs and symptoms include red-tinged urine with clots, dysuria or frequency of urination, and symptoms of urethral obstruction from clots such as pain. This can lead to postrenal failure if not corrected.
      - Bladder ultrasound indicates the presence of clots or thickened bladder wall.
   c. *Management*
      - Mild cases respond to aggressive hydration with resolution in 1 to 2 days.
      - Severe cases may require continuous bladder irrigation with a three-way Foley catheter at 500 mL to 3 L/hour to clear developing clots and prevent obstruction. Platelets are used to maintain platelet counts at higher than 20,000/mm^3 for a child who is not bleeding or higher than 50,000/mm^3 for a child who is bleeding. Cystoscopy is used to cauterize the bleeding ulcerative areas; it is usually not a long-term solution because of the diffuse widespread area affected. Instillation of chemicals can be used to stop the bleeding. Continued irrigation is critical as further damage to the bladder may occur if the chemicals are not rinsed from the bladder.
8. **Graft-versus-host disease (GvHD)**
   a. *GvHD* represents engraftment of donor T lymphocytes in the recipient that reject the tissue of the recipient. It predominantly involves the skin, GI tract, and the liver. It is rare for GvHD to occur in syngeneic or autologous transplants. There is increased risk with partially matched allogenic transplants.
   b. *GvHD* is the main cause of morbidity and mortality in allogeneic transplants. It results from histocompatibility differences between the donor cells (graft) and the recipient (host). Donor cells can contain viable immunocompetent T lymphocytes that can recognize the foreign antigens of the host and therefore mount an immunologic response against the host. Recipients with profound cellular immunodeficiency, either congenital or acquired, cannot respond against and reject the donor marrow.
   c. *GvHD* occurs in two forms, acute and chronic, despite HLA-identical donor and recipient transplants and prophylactic immunosuppressive therapy.
   d. *Acute GvHD* occurs within the first 100 days after transplantation with a range in severity from mild and transitory to severe, prolonged, and lethal.

- Signs and symptoms are not always immediately recognized because symptoms may mimic other problems such as infection, VOD, hepatitis, and toxic effects of chemotherapy.
  - *Skin GvHD:* Onset of a maculopapular skin rash initially involving the palms and soles and later progressing centrally may cause intense pruritus and progress to bullous lesions and ulceration. Skin GvHD occurs at or near the time of WBC engraftment.
  - *Gastrointestinal GvHD:* Nausea, vomiting, abdominal cramping, anorexia, paralytic ileus, green and watery, and heme-negative diarrhea. Later heme-positive diarrhea occurs as more of the intestinal mucosa begins to slough. Hypoalbuminemia is noted.
  - *Liver GvHD:* Right upper quadrant pain, hepatomegaly, jaundice, ascites (rare), elevated liver enzymes, and bilirubin occur.
- The degree of organ system involvement is graded from I to IV, describing the severity of illness, prognosis, and response to therapy (Table 8-17).
- Diagnosis is made by biopsy of the skin or rectal or liver tissue.
- *Prophylaxis:* Morbidity and mortality are lessened by prevention rather than treatment of established GvHD. Interventions include selection of histocompatible donors, immunosuppressive therapy, and removal of T cells from the donor marrow before transplantation (associated with a risk of engraftment failure). Irradiation of all blood products before transfusion results in the inactivation of T lymphocytes, whereas adequate platelet and RBC function is maintained. Irradiation should be maintained for 1 year for uncomplicated SCT (return of T-cell immunity).
- *Treatment* of acute GvHD includes corticosteroids, CSA, azathioprine, and antilymphocyte preparations (see Relevant Pharmacology section). Various combinations have not shown consistent impact on reducing GvHD and improving long-term survival because patients continue to die of infections. Mild (grade I) GvHD does not warrant therapy. Treatment of grades II to IV is recommended.
  - Assess early clinical manifestations of GvHD. Distinguish GvHD from other complications such as antibiotic or chemotherapy reactions, irritated bowel, infections, and radiation toxicity.
  - Appropriate skin care will provide comfort and reduce the risk of infection. Oil in the bath water decreases skin dryness and soothes pruritus; if bullae occur, prevent infection and bleeding. Low air-loss beds decrease discomfort of pressure points and may facilitate exudate absorption. Other skin-care products such as hydrogel absorb wound

TABLE 8-17
Clinical Stages of Acute Graft-versus-Host Disease (GvHD)

Stage	Skin	Liver: Bilirubin Level	Gut: Diarrhea Volume
1	Maculopapular rash <25% of body surface area	2–3 mg/mL	7–13 mL/kg/d
2	Maculopapular rash 25%–50% of body surface area	3–6 mg/dL	14–20 mL/kg/d
3	Generalized erythroderma	6–15 mg/dL	21–27 mL/kg/d
4	Desquamation and bullae	>15 mg/dL	>27 mL/kg/d

Data from Cassano WF, Gross S, Graham-Pole J, Rudder S: Graft versus host disease. In Blumer JL: *A practical guide to pediatric intensive care.* St Louis, 1990, Mosby; and *Research protocols for bone marrow transplant.* Memphis, 1995, St Jude Children's Research Hospital.

exudate, provide a physiologically moist environment and promote wound healing and tissue granulation. Provide pain-control measures for the pain associated with skin desquamation.

- Provide measures to resolve the GI tract effects of GvHD. Watch for hypovolemia and shock through strict monitoring of intake and output, daily weights, and assessment of electrolytes. The patient may need to be NPO to reduce further gut activation of the GvHD. Clean the perineal area and soothe irritated skin. Assess for rectal lesions. Hemoccult test all emesis and stool to determine presence of GI tract bleeding.

e. *Chronic GvHD* occurs beyond 100 days up to 2 years. It is disabling and frequently fatal and is more likely to occur if the child has the acute form of GvHD.

- Signs and symptoms affect the same target organs as affected in acute GvHD, but different symptoms occur, including skin lesions, sclerosis, hair loss, dystrophic nails, dysphagia, heartburn, chronic diarrhea, and malabsorption.
- Management involves steroids, CSA, azathioprine, and artificial tears to prevent ocular damage from the associated keratoconjunctivitis.

REFERENCES

Abramson JS, Wheeler JG, Quie PG: The polymorphonuclear phagocytic system. In Stiehm ER, editors: *Immunologic disorders in infants and children,* ed 5. Philadelphia, 2004, W. B. Saunders, pp 68-80.

Algren C, Arnow D: Pediatric variations of nursing interventions. In Hockenberry MJ, editor: *Wong's nursing care of infants and children.* St. Louis, 2003, Mosby, pp 1101-1167.

American Academy of Pediatrics: Report of the Committee on Infectious Diseases. In *The red book,* ed 26. 2003, American Academy of Pediatrics.

American Association of Blood Banks: *Technical manual,* ed 14. Bethesda, Md., 2002, AABB.

American Association of Blood Banks, American Red Cross, Council of Community Blood Centers: *Circulation of information for the use of human blood and blood components, 1994.* Washington, DC, 1994, The Red Cross.

American College of Chest Physicians, Society of Critical Care Medicine Consensus Conference: Definitions for sepsis and organ failure and guidelines for the use of innovative therapies in sepsis. *Crit Care Med* 20(6):864-873, 1992.

American Red Cross: *Blood components, 1994.* Washington, DC, 1994, The Red Cross.

Anderson DC, et al.: Impaired chemotaxigenesis by type III group B streptococci in neonatal sera: relationship to specific anticapsular antibody and abnormalities of serum complement. *Pediatr Res* 17(6):496-502, 1983.

Andrew M, Montgomery RR: Acquired disorders of hemostasis. In Nathan DG, Orkin SH, editors: *Nathan and Oski's hematology of infancy and childhood.* Philadelphia, 1998, W. B. Saunders.

Bellanti J: *Immunology III.* Philadelphia, 1985, W. B. Saunders.

Bellanti JA, Kadlec JV: Host defense mechanisms. In Chernick V, Kernig EL, editors: *Kernig's disorders of the respiratory tract in children,* ed 5. Philadelphia, 1990, W. B. Saunders, pp 182-201.

Berger M, Frank MM: The serum complement system. In Stiehm ER, editor: *Immunologic disorders in infants and children,* ed 3. Philadelphia, 1989, W. B. Saunders, pp 97-115.

Bernini JC, et al.: Beneficial effect of intravenous dexamethasone in children with mild to moderately severe acute chest syndrome complicating sickle cell disease. *Blood* 92(9):3082-3089, 1998.

Bousvaros A, Walker WA: Development and function of the intestinal mucosal barrier. In MacDonald T, editor: *Ontogeny of the immune system of the gut.* Boca Raton, Fla., 1990, CRC Press, pp 2-16.

Centers for Disease Control and Prevention: 1994 revised classification system for human immunodeficiency virus in children less than 13 years of age. *MMWR Morb Mortal Wkly Rep* 143(RR-12):1-10, 1994.

Chakraverty R, et al.: The incidence and cause of coagulopathies in an intensive care population. *Br J Haematol* 93(2): 460-463, 1996.

Christensen RD, Rothstein G: Efficiency of neutrophil migration in the neonate. *Pediatr Res* 14:1147-1149, 1980.

Department of Health and Human Services: *HIV/AIDS surveillance report*. Washington, DC, 2002, CDC.

El Bahir H, Laundy M, Booy R: Diagnosis and treatment of bacterial meningitis. *Arch Dis Child* 88(7):615-620, 2003.

Fischer A, Notarangelo LD: Combined immunodeficiencies. In Stiehm RE, Ochs HD, Winkelstein JA, editors: *Immunologic disorders in infants and children*, ed 5. Philadelphia, 2004, Elsevier Saunders.

Gennery AR, Cant AJ: Diagnosis of severe combined immunodeficiency. *J Clin Pathol* 54(3):191-195, 2001.

Goldman AS, Ham-Pong AJ, Goldblum RM: Host defenses: development and maternal contributions. *Adv Pediatr* 32:71-100, 1985.

Gonzales-Ryan L, et al.: Hematopoietic stem cell transplantation. In Rasco Baggott C, et al., editors: *Nursing care of children and adolescents with cancer.* Philadelphia, 2002, W. B. Saunders.

Grant MJ: Host defenses. In Curley MAQ, Moloney-Harmon PA, editors: *Critical care nursing of infants and children.* Philadelphia, 2001, W. B. Saunders, pp 655-694.

Griffin TC, McIntire D, Buchanan GR: High-dose intravenous methylprednisolone therapy for pain in children and adolescents with sickle cell disease. *N Engl J Med* 330(11):733-737, 1994.

Grossman M: Children with AIDS. In Sande MA, Volberding PA, editors: *The medical management of AIDS.* Philadelphia, 1988, W. B. Saunders, pp 319-329.

Guyton AC, Hall JE, editors: *Textbook of medical physiology*, ed 9. Philadelphia, 2000, Elsevier Science, 2000.

Hacein-Bey-Abina S, Le Deist F, Carlier F: Sustained correction of X-linked severe combined immunodeficiency by ex vivo gene therapy. *N Engl J Med* 346:1185-1186, 2002.

Hacein-Bey-Abina S, von Kalle C, Schmidt M: A serious adverse event after successful gene therapy for X-linked severe combined immunodeficiency. *N Engl J Med* 348: 255-256, 2003.

Hanson C, Shearer WT: AIDS and other acquired immunodeficiency diseases, Part I. In Feigin R, Cherry J, editors: *Textbook of pediatric infectious diseases*, ed 4. Philadelphia, 1998, W. B. Saunders.

Harpin VA, Eutter N: Barrier properties of the newborn infant's skin. *J Pediatr* 102(3): 419-425, 1983.

Hoste E, et al.: Significant increase of activated partial thromboplastin time by heparinization of the radial artery catheter flush solution with a closed arterial catheter system. *Crit Care Med* 30(5): 1030-1034, 2002.

Hughes WT: *Pneumocystis carinii* pneumonia. In Pizzo PA, Wilfert CM, editors: *Pediatric AIDS: the challenge of HIV infection in infants, children and adolescents.* Baltimore, Md, 1994, Williams & Wilkins, pp 405-418.

Hughes WT, Anderson DC: *Pneumocystis carinii* pneumonia. In Feigin R, Cherry J, editors: *Textbook of pediatric infectious diseases*, ed 4. Philadelphia, 1998, W. B. Saunders.

Jacobe SJ, et al.: Outcome of children requiring admission to an intensive care unit after bone marrow transplantation. *Crit Care Med* 31(5):1299-1305, 2003.

Jakubik LD, Thompson M: Care of the child with sickle cell disease: acute complications. *Pediatr Nurs* 26(4):373-379, 2000.

Jenkins TL: Sickle cell anemia in the pediatric intensive care unit: novel approaches for managing life-threatening complications. *AACN Clin Issues* 13(2):154-158, 2002.

Klein RB, et al.: Decreased mononuclear and polymorphonuclear chemotaxis in human newborns, infants, and young children. *Pediatrics* 60(4):467-472, 1977.

Kline NE: Prevention and treatment of infections. In Rasco Baggott C, et al., editors: *Nursing care of children and adolescents with cancer.* Philadelphia, 2002, W. B. Saunders.

Landor M, Rubinstein A: Human immunodeficiency virus infection in children. In Spirer Z, Roifman CM, Branski D, editors: *Pediatric immunology: pediatric and adolescent medicine.* New York, 1993, Karger, pp 102-130.

Laxon CJ, Titler MG: Drawing coagulation studies from arterial lines: an integrative literature review. *Am J Crit Care* 3(1):16-22, 1994.

Leonard M: Diagnostic evaluations and staging procedures. *Nursing care of children and adolescents with cancer.* Philadelphia, 2002, W.B. Saunders.

Levi M, deJonge E, van der Poll T: New treatment for disseminated intravascular coagulation based on current understanding of the pathophysiology. *Ann Med* 36(1):41-49, 2004.

Levy MM, et al.: 2001 SCCM/ESICM/ACCP/ATS/SIS International Sepsis Definition Conference. *Crit Care Med* 31(4):1250-1256, 2003.

Lexi-Comp Online 2004. Retrieved February 1, 2005. At: http://www.cronline.com.

Lexi-Comp Online Laboratory Values 2004. Retrieved February 1, 2005. At: http://www.cronline.com/crlsql/servlet/cronline.

Lott JW, Kenner C: Keeping up with neonatal infection: designer bugs, part II. *MCN* 19(5):264-271, 1994.

Mahon PM: Orthoclone OKT3 and cardiac transplantation: an overview. *Crit Care Nurs* 11(8):42-50, 1991.

Makhoul I, Makhoul H, Claxton D, Rybka W: 2003, April 18. Pure B-cell disorders. *E-Medicine,* Topic 216. Retrieved August 2, 2004, at http://www.emedicine.com/med/topic216.htm

Malloy MB, Perez-Woods RC: Neonatal skin care: prevention of skin breakdown. *Pediatr Nurs* 17(1):41-48, 1991.

Mandell GL, Dolin R, Bennett JE, editors: *Principles and practice of infectious diseases,* ed 6. Philadelphia, 2004, W. B. Saunders.

Manno CS: What's new in transfusion medicine? *Pediatr Clin North Am* 43:793-808, 1996.

Maschmeyer G. Pneumonia in febrile neutropenic patients: radiologic diagnosis. *Curr Opin Oncol* 2001;13(4):229-235.

Masuda K, Kinoshita Y, Kobayashi Y: Heterogeneity of Fc receptor expression in chemotaxis and adherence of neonatal neutrophils. *Pediatr Res* 25(1):6-10, 1989.

Miller D. Immunosuppression in pediatric transplant patients. *Pediatr Nurs* 21(1):21-29, 2001.

Miller ME: Immunocompetence of the newborn. In Chandra RK, editor: *Primary and secondary immunodeficiency disorders.* New York, 1983, Churchill Livingstone, pp 157-164.

Miller ME: The inflammatory and natural defense systems. In Stiehm ER, editor: *Immunologic disorders in infants and children.* ed 2. Philadelphia, 1980, W. B. Saunders, pp 165-180.

Mudge-Grout CL: *Immunologic disorders.* St Louis, 1992, Mosby-Year Book.

Nathan DG, Orkin SH, Oski FA: *Nathan and Oski's hematology of infancy and childhood,* vol 2. Philadelphia, 1998, W. B. Saunders.

Nevins TE: Overview of new immunosuppressive therapies. *Curr Opin Pediatr* 12(2):146-150, 2000.

New York State Department of Health: HIV prophylaxis following occupational exposure. *HIV clinical guidelines for the primary care provider,* ed 3. New York, 2003, New York State Department of Health AIDS Institute.

O'Neill Shigeoka A: 2003, January 21. Severe combined immunodeficiency. *E-Medicine,* Topic 2083. Retrieved February 1, 2005 at: http://www.emedicine.com/ped/topic2083.htm

O'Neill Shigeoka, A: (2002, August 27). T-cell disorders. *E-Medicine,* Topic 2212. Retrieved February 1, 2005, format: http://www.emedicine.com/ped/topic2212.htm.

Oski FA, Brugnara C, Nathan DG: A diagnostic approach to the anemic patient. *Nathan and Oski's hematology of infancy and childhood.* Philadelphia, 1998, W.B. Saunders.

Owusu-Ofuri S, Riddington C: Splenectomy versus conservative management for acute sequestration crises in people with sickle cell disease. *The Cochrane Database of Systematic Reviews* (1): 2004.

Panzarella C, et al.: Management of disease and treatment-related complications. In Rasco Baggott C, et al., editors: *Nursing care of children and adolescents with cancer.* Philadelphia, 2002, W. B. Saunders.

Quigley SM, Whitney DE: Skin integrity. In Curley MAQ, Moloney-Harmon PA, editors: *Critical care nursing of infants and children.* Philadelphia, 2001, W. B. Saunders, pp 511-544.

Riddington C, Wang W: Blood transfusion for preventing stroke in people with sickle cell disease. *The Cochrane Database of Systematic Reviews* (1), 2003.

Risch L, Fischer JE, Herllotz R, Huber AR: Heparin-induced thrombocytopenia in paediatrics: clinical characteristics, therapy and outcomes. *Intens Care Med* 30(8): 1615-1624, 2004.

Scott JP: Hematology. In Behrman RE. Kliegman RM, editors: *Nelson's essentials of pediatrics.* Philadelphia, 2000, W. B. Saunders, pp 605-644.

Sevier NM, Kline NE: Conditions that produce fluid and electrolyte imbalance. In Hockenberry MJ, editor: *Wong's nursing care of infants and children.* St. Louis, 2003, Mosby, pp 1207-1254.

Sindhi R: Sirolimus in pediatric transplant recipients. *Transplant Proc* 35(suppl 3A):113S-114S, 2003.

Tancabelic J, Haun SE: Mangement of coagulopathy with recombinant factor VIIa in a neonate with echovirus type 7. *Pediatr Blood Cancer* 43(2):170-176, 2004.

Tortora GJ, Grabowski SR: *Principles of anatomy and physiology,* ed 10. New York, 2002, Harper Collins College Publishers.

Vilalta R, et al.: Rapamycin use and rapid withdrawal of calcineurin inhibitors in pediatric renal transplantation. *Transplant Proc* 35:703-704, 2003.

Weinberg G: Antiretroviral therapy of human immunodeficiency virus infection. In Mandell GL, Douglas JE, Bennett R, editors: *Principles and practices of infectious diseases,* ed 5. New York, 2000, Churchill Livingstone.

Wethers DL: Sickle cell disease in childhood: Part I. Laboratory diagnosis, pathophysiology and health maintenance. *Am Fam Physician* 62(5):1013-1020, 2000.

Wilkinson JD, Greenwald BM: The acquired immunodeficiency syndrome: impact on the pediatric intensive care unit. *Crit Care Clin* 4(4):831-844, 1988.

The Working Group on Antiretroviral Therapy and Medical Management of HIV Infected Children: Guidelines for the use of antiretroviral agents in pediatric HIV infection, *MMWR* 47(RR-4):1-31, 2004.

CHAPTER

9 Multisystem Issues

Multiple Trauma

Tracy Ann Pasek and Kimberly Ann Etzel

Critically injured children and their families require the expertise of pediatric nurses, intensivists, and other health care professionals for trauma care. The admission to an intensive care unit (ICU) is unplanned and unexpected, causing stress and anxiety. The pediatric intensive care unit (PICU) nurse must have knowledge of development, injury, treatment, and prevention to care for the injured child and family effectively.

EPIDEMIOLOGY AND INCIDENCE

In the United States, traumatic injuries are the third leading cause of death over all ages (MacKenzie and Fowler, 2000). Childhood injury exceeds all other causes of death combined. Death from unintentional (accidental) injury accounts for 65% of all injury deaths for children younger than 19 years of age (Nguyen, 2003).

Overall, the leading causes of fatal childhood injuries are motor-vehicle crashes (MVCs), fire/burns, drowning, falls, and poisoning (Centers for Disease Control and Prevention [CDC], *Childhood Injury Fact Sheet*, 2004). Between 1972 and 1992, MVCs were the leading cause of death for children 1 to 19 years of age, followed by homicide or suicide (predominantly by firearms), and then drowning (Nguyen, 2003). In 2000, MVCs were reported to continue to be a leading cause of pediatric death. Among children 1 to 4 years of age, MVCs, drowning, and fire were the **most** common causes of injury death. MVCs were also the most common cause of injury death among children

5 through 14 years of age, followed by firearm and drowning deaths (Maternal and Child Health Bureau, 2002).

According to the National Highway Traffic Safety Administration (NHTSA) in 2001, MVCs remained the leading cause of death for children of every age from 4 through 14 years (NHTSA, Traffic Safety Facts, 2001). In 2004, the CDC reported that alcohol was involved in about 35% of adolescent-driver fatalities and about 40% of all adolescent drownings (CDC, *Facts on Adolescent Injury*, 2004).

Several factors influence childhood injuries: age and stage of development, gender, behavior, and environment. Developmental milestones also correlate with the mechanism of pediatric injuries.

A. Age and Stage of Development, Gender

Children's abilities to react and respond to others, coordinate, anticipate, and judge the consequences of their actions are factors that change predictably as children's physical, communicative, social, and intellectual abilities develop. The mechanism and outcomes of injuries vary by age (National Pediatric Trauma Registry [NPTR], 1996). Males are more likely than females to die of any type of injury (CDC, *Facts on Adolescent Injury*, 2004). Males are twice as likely to become injured as are females (NPTR, 1996).

B. Mechanisms

Falls are the leading cause of injury and are most common in the infant and toddler groups. Children tend to fall from objects, balconies, windows, and trees. Falls occur most often in homes, followed by school yards and playgrounds (The American College of Surgeons, 1997). The next major mechanism is MVC, followed by pedestrian injury (i.e., when children are struck by motor vehicles) (Table 9-1). Most pediatric injuries occur as a result of blunt trauma; penetrating trauma accounts for only a small portion. Head injuries are the most severe and are responsible for the most deaths (Nguyen, 2003).

C. Environment

Although they constitute a smaller percent of injuries than blunt forces, penetrating injuries in children aged 13 to 18 years have increased in recent years, attributable in large part to the proliferation of handguns and increased urban violence in our society.

In 2003 state and local protection services received approximately 2.9 million referrals for child abuse or neglect, of which 906,000 children were determined to be victims (National Clearing house on Child Abuse and Neglect, 2005). Sixty-three

TABLE 9-1
The Top Five Leading Causes of Injury

Age (years)	0-5	6-10	>10
Mechanism	Fall Motor vehicle Pedestrian Struck* Stab	Falls Pedestrian Bike Motor vehicle Sports	Motor vehicle Falls Bike GSW Sports

Modified from Tepas JJ, Faillace WJ: Pediatric trauma. In Mattox KL, Feliciano DV, Moore EE, editors: *Trauma*, ed 4. New York, 2000, McGraw-Hill Health Professions Division, pp 1075-1098.
*Struck: struck by an object.
GSW, Gun shot wound.

percent of victims experienced neglect. During 2003 it is estimated that 1500 children suffered fatalities related to abuse or neglect. Neglect represented more than one third of the fatalities, with multiple maltreatment and physical abuse following closely.

Child maltreatment resulting from blunt trauma to the head or from shaking is the leading cause of head injury among infants and young children. Infants are at the greatest risk for dying of homicide during the first week of life, and the greatest risk is on the first day of life (CDC, *Childhood Injury Fact Sheet*, 2004). Children younger than 1 year of age account for 44% of child maltreatment fatalities. Male and female victims have similar rates for all types of maltreatment except for child sexual abuse. Child sexual abuse is four times higher among females than among males (Administration on Children, Youth, and Families, 2000).

For every child who dies of an injury, 40 others are hospitalized and 1120 are treated in emergency departments. An estimated 50,000 children acquire permanent disabilities each year from abuse. Thus, pediatric trauma continues to be a major threat to the health and well-being of children. The National Safety Council estimates that approximately $16 billion is spent per year caring for injured children between birth and 16 years of age (Tepas and Faillace, 2000).

INJURY PREVENTION AND FAMILY EDUCATION

In all age groups, prevention is paramount to safety and health. When children are admitted to the PICU, nurses are primary advocates for preventive care and guidance. Using knowledge of development as a foundation, safety education and anticipatory guidance for both parents and children can be incorporated into many nursing interventions and parent teaching (Table 9-2). Although it is difficult to approach the subject of prevention in a critical setting, the opportunity to teach families about how to prevent reoccurring injuries should not be lost.

MECHANISMS OF INJURY

Mechanism of injury can be described as the effect of energy on human tissue. Several mechanisms of injury are responsible for pediatric trauma, including kinetic, thermal, electrical, chemical, and radiant energy. It follows that specific injuries are classified according to the responsible mechanism. Other mechanisms include water submersion, cold exposure, asphyxia, and unintentional injury (see Child Maltreatment section) (Zuspan, 2003).

A. Kinetic Energy

Kinetic energy is the energy of motion. It is the force that is responsible for most traumatic injuries. Kinetic forces cause blunt, crush, shear, acceleration-deceleration, and penetrating injuries.

1. **Blunt-force trauma:** Most pediatric injuries are due to blunt-force trauma, which results in injuries to the solid and hollow organs as well as to the long bones. It also produces crushing, shearing, or tearing of tissue both externally and internally. Some examples of blunt-force trauma are falls, MVCs, lap-belt injuries, and pedestrian versus motor-vehicle accidents. To illustrate the vulnerability of children to multiple trauma, consider a pedestrian versus MVC. Pediatric victims may experience a common phenomenon called *Waddell's triad.* Children are struck higher on the body than adults. The first impact occurs when the bumper strikes the child's legs. The second impact is the child's chest, followed

Text continued on p. 645.

TABLE 9-2
Psychosocial and Developmental Risk Factors: Predispositions for Childhood Injury

Developmental Risk Factors	Mechanisms/Types of Injury	Prevention Strategies and Parent Teaching
INFANT		
Learns to roll, sit, crawl, and walk	Falls (most frequent) • walker-related • rolling from high surfaces • fall from adults' arms	Use safety straps • high chair • stroller • changing table • swing • infant seat Keep doors closed to stairs and laundry chutes Secure window screens
Cries to communicate until language develops	Homicide	Promote parenting skills and coping interventions • support networks • health promotion (balanced diet, adequate sleep)
Depends on others for needs and safety	Drowning Burns/scalding Motor vehicle crashes	Never leave child unattended • bathtub, pool, water sources • walker Test temperature of water before bathing Use safety locks/gates on stairs, doors, and windows Restrain infant in an approved rear-facing infant seat in rear seat
Explores through touch, taste, feelings, and motion	Suffocation Choking Aspiration Poisoning Burns/scalding	Avoid drinking hot liquids, cooking, smoking while holding infant Test temperature of food before feeding and water before bathing Use heat retardant nightwear Keep crib side rails up and lower mattress when infant can sit Keep crib free of toys Keep small objects, inappropriate toys, and household items out of reach Avoid latex balloons Position infant on back for sleep

Continued

TABLE 9-2
Psychosocial and Developmental Risk Factors: Predispositions for Childhood Injury (*cont'd*)

Developmental Risk Factors	Mechanisms/Types of Injury	Prevention Strategies and Parent Teaching
TODDLER		
Explores their body and world	Falls from greater heights than infants	Use safety locks/gates on stairs, doors, and windows
	• windows	Keep crib side rails up and lower mattress when infant can sit
	• porches	Supervise playground activity
	• playground equipment	Keep doors closed and use child protective devices on doorknobs
	Riding toys	Have child wear helmet
Desires increased independence	Choking	Cut food into small pieces
		Avoid foods such as peanuts, hard candy, and popcorn
		Remind toddlers not to run with food/toys in their mouths
Lacks concept of danger	Heat injuries, burns/scalds	Avoid drinking hot liquids, cooking, or smoking while holding child
Lacks comprehension of cause-effect	Chemical burn injuries	Test temperature of food before feeding and water before bathing
	Drowning	Use heat retardant nightwear
		Never leave child unattended in bathtub, pool, water sources
		Avoid latex balloons
		Use electrical outlet covers
		Keep appliances and cords out of reach
		Avoid tablecloths
		Help child avoid dangerous situations by teaching and reinforcing associated risks
		Restrain toddler in an approved car seat in rear seat
PRESCHOOL-AGE		
Desires increased independence	Bike vs. pedestrian accidents	Provide safe riding toys
Learns skills by imitating others	Falls	Avoid permitting child to ride inappropriate things such as tractor, lawn mower, ATV
Develops increased motor skills		Teach street safety by stop/look/listen and buddy system when crossing
Lacks well-developed sense of direction		Teach helmet safety
Lacks well-developed peripheral vision		Use safety locks/gates on stairs, doors and windows
		Supervise playground activity
		Keep doors closed and use child protective devices on doorknobs
		Use electrical outlet covers
		Keep appliances and cords out of reach

Experiences the world through egocentrism, imagination, and fantasy		Help children avoid dangerous situations by teaching and reinforcing associated risks
General age-specific safety	Burns (fire-related most common; overall rare in this age)	Keep pot handles turned inward or toward back of stove Keep matches and lighters out of reach Teach child to stop, drop, and roll Use 3-point restraints or approved car seat of motor vehicle
SCHOOL-AGE		
Well-developed motor skills May lack the cognitive skills to analyze and judge situations accurately Increasing advanced motor skills Learning to ride bicycle	Motor vehicle crashes Falls • balconies • windows • playground equipment • trees Head injuries	Avoid riding inappropriate equipment/toys such as lawn mower or ATV Teach street safety by looking both ways, holding hands, and not crossing the street alone Teach helmet safety Supervise playground activity Teach swimming skills and water safety
Increasing independence Developing relationship with peers		Help children avoid dangerous situations and remind them of potential dangers
General age-specific safety	Burns (fire-related most common; overall rare in this age)	Keep pot handles turned inward Keep matches and lighters out of reach Teach child to stop, drop, and roll Use 3-point restraints in rear seat in motor vehicle
ADOLESCENT		
Increased activity in sports Able to drive motor vehicles	Motor vehicle crashes Spinal cord injuries, head injuries, and long bone fractures	Use 3-point restraints in motor vehicle Encourage adolescents not to use drugs and alcohol before operating a motor vehicle Encourage use of helmets with motorcyles and sports activities
Desires increased independence	Drowning Firearm injuries Homocide/suicide	Validate peer pressure while helping adolescent to live within the limits set by his/her parents Teach swimming skills and water/boat safety

Continued

TABLE 9-2
Psychosocial and Developmental Risk Factors: Predispositions for Childhood Injury (*cont'd*)

Developmental Risk Factors	Mechanisms/Types of Injury	Prevention Strategies and Parent Teaching
Developing relationship with peers Participates in risk-taking behavior and succumbs easily to peer pressure Believes injury will not happen to them and judgment may not be well defined		Teach firearm safety • treat firearms with respect • do not play with firearms • treat all firearms as if they were loaded • use gun locks if gun is in home
ALL AGE GROUPS		
General safety		Teach parents and children that restraint devices are the most effective safety devices in preventing serious injury and death in MVC (American College of Surgeons) Use age-appropriate restraint device and position while in motor vehicle Teach child to treat driveways and parking lots the same as streets Firearm safety • keep firearms in areas secure from children • utilize gun locks if firearms are in home • reinforce gun safety and not to play with guns Teach swimming skills and water safety Restrict exposure/teach safety related to environmental elements such as sun/cold Encourage use of helmet and protective gear for bike riding and appropriate sports
Maintain a safe environment		Increase knowledge related to age-appropriate toys/activities and playground equipment Have smoke detectors/fire ladders and fire extinguishers in home Practice fire and emergency evacuation plans at home at least every 6 months
Safety around animals	Animal bites	Introduce infants to pets slowly and cautiously Teach children pet safety Do not tease animals Do not approach unfamiliar animals Teach injury prevention as part of a healthy lifestyle Health care professionals should help increase parents' awareness of the community programs that can help them with injury prevention and the challenges they may face in keeping their children safe

by the face and head, with the vehicle's hood. Common injuries within this triad include a midshaft femur fracture, abdominal injury, and head injury (Simone, 2003) (see Specific Injury section).

2. **Crush injury**

   A crush injury occurs when compressive strain (energy) is concentrated in one body area. Crush injuries include animal bites or being caught in machinery or equipment (e.g., finger caught in a car door).

   a. Patients who experience *crush injuries* from extreme forces (e.g., high-speed MVC, earthquakes) are at particular risk for the development of rhabdomyolysis and myoglobinuria. Volume depletion from fluid sequestration in damaged tissues and poor fluid intake can lead to acute renal insufficiency.

   b. *Myoglobinuria* is usually associated with rhabdomyolysis, or muscle destruction. The cellular release of myoglobin is often accompanied by an increase of creatine kinase (CK). When excreted into the urine, myoglobin can precipitate, causing tubular obstruction and acute renal insufficiency. Myoglobinuria causes little or no morbidity or mortality except when it is associated with the secondary complications of rhabdomyolysis, including hyperkalemia, hypocalcemia, and acute renal failure (ARF). In patients experiencing myoglobinuria, physical examination reveals generalized muscle weakness, often with painful muscle groups, trauma, or areas of ischemic pressure necrosis where the patient has lain for extended periods. Expect any patient with extensive trauma to have some degree of myoglobinuria (Arnold, 2003; Dunmez, 2003).

   c. *Animal bites* can lead to a localized infection, cellulitis, and, in some instances, surgical intervention. Bites vary from a small puncture wound or laceration to crushing of major arteries, veins, and nerves. Pets are most likely to be involved in animal bites from cats, dogs, ferrets, and other small animals (Walker, 2003).

      - Dog bites may result in a child being admitted to the ICU, depending on the location and severity of the bite. Dog bites are associated with a lower incidence of infection than human bites; however, cat bites or scratches have a higher risk for infection (Hodge and Trecklenburgh, 2000). Bites to the airway region may be severe and require mechanical ventilation and surgery, and underlying injuries such as fractures may also be present. Potential complications include infection (the most common) and rabies (the most serious).
      - Parent concerns are often focused on cosmetic implications for the future and on bleeding (Walker, 2003). The discrepancy between the potential complications and common parental concerns presents teaching opportunities for critical-care nurses.
      - Wound care should include irrigation under pressure and cleansing of the site with benzalkonium chloride to kill rabies. A wound culture should be obtained. The nurse should anticipate radiographic studies and the administration of tetanus toxoid and antibiotics (Walker, 2003).
      - Providing education to the family regarding prevention strategies for the future is crucial. Education should include information about how to approach dogs and other animals, when to avoid approaching them, as well as available community resources for dog-bite education (Chapman et al., 2000).

3. **Shear injury:** Shear injury occurs when forces are applied in opposite directions (the brain within the cranium). When a shear injury is present in the absence of a

significant trauma history and in combination with retinal hemorrhages, inflicted trauma, such as shaken-infant syndrome (SIS), must be ruled out (see Child Maltreatment section).

4. **Acceleration-deceleration injury:** Acceleration-deceleration injuries occur when a body stops suddenly and the internal organs keep moving inside the body, for example, in high-speed MVC. The internal organs and vessels, such as the spinal cord, hepatic artery and vein, and descending thoracic aorta, rupture or tear. This type of injury can occur in a high-speed MVC when the child is thrust against the seat belt.
5. **Penetrating injury**
   a. *Penetrating injuries* occur from firearms, knives, or other objects (Chandy, 2004).
   b. The severity of *knife wounds* is related to the anatomic area inflicted with the knife, the length of the blade, and the angle of penetration (Creel, 1997). An exit wound may or may not be present, and the blade may be impaled. Objects and toys can become missiles that can penetrate a child's body. For example, the young child running with a toy in his or her mouth who subsequently falls can sustain a penetrating injury to the oropharynx. Damage to the internal organs results from kinetic force along the path of the penetrating object (Czerwinski and Maloney-Harmon, 2003).
   c. *Firearm injuries* are the second leading cause of injury and death in the United States. The case fatality rate for children is 17%. The severity of injury appears to be increasing (Nance et al., 2003). Youth firearm injury severity can be measured by the hospital course (e.g., immediate operating room, immediate PICU admission, death) (Snyder et al., 2003). Injuries from low-velocity weapons are generally less destructive than from high-velocity weapons (e.g., semiautomatic weapons) because high-velocity weapons include hydrostatic pressure (Czerwinski and Maloney-Harmon, 2003). Injuries from firearms are related to the type of weapon, the size and caliber of bullet, the muzzle velocity of the projectile, the number of bullets that penetrate the body, bullet trajectory, and the distance from which the firearm was discharged. Dense organs, such as the liver and muscles, sustain greater damage than less dense organs, such as the lungs (Czerwinski and Maloney-Harmon, 2003). The damage to body tissues from a bullet or missile is related to shock waves, cavitation, and pulsation of the cavity (Czerwinski and Maloney-Harmon, 2003).
      - *Gunshot wound (GSW) characteristics:* Gunshot wounds (GSWs) to the head are more fatal than are GSWs to the extremities; GSWs to the head are less common than are GSWs to the extremities (Nance et al., 2003). Outcomes are usually fatal for children who suffer from intracranial firearm injury (Nance et al, 2003). The bullet may course through multiple routes once it is in the body. It may ricochet off bone, resulting in bony fragments. Moreover, the bullet itself may fragment. Fragments of any type will increase the size and severity of the wound (Czerwinski and Maloney-Harmon, 2003). A bullet may tumble or somersault within the body, causing increased damage and greater wound severity. Penetrating forces produce entrance and, most often, exit wounds (Czerwinski and Maloney-Harmon, 2003).
      - *Bullet wounding mechanisms:* Crushing of tissues occurs when the missile initially strikes and creates a permanent cavity. *Yaw* is the deviation of a bullet from a straight path. If the bullet strikes the body at an angle, the angle of yaw is increased and more damage occurs (Czerwinski and

Maloney-Harmon, 2003). Temporary cavitation occurs as a result of the missile losing energy to the surrounding tissues as it enters the body. This cavity can exceed the size of the bullet, and it is achieved within milliseconds of penetration. Cavitation is defined by bullet velocity. It is produced from the effects of combustion (muzzle blast) and is commonly seen with shotgun wounds. Internal explosion of gas and powder results in burns (Czerwinski and Maloney-Harmon, 2003).

- *Risk for injury:* Dense, less elastic tissues (e.g., bone, brain, liver, spleen, fluid-filled organs) can be damaged severely by the formation of a temporary cavity because of the greater amount of energy imparted (Czerwinski and Maloney-Harmon, 2003). Lower-density, elastic tissues (e.g., the lung) are less affected by cavitation because less energy is transferred to the tissue. Examples of fluid-filled organs are the heart and gastrointestinal (GI) tract (Czerwinski and Maloney-Harmon, 2003).
- *Nursing implications and treatment for GSW patients:* Basic principles (the ABCs) of trauma apply to victims of GSWs.
  - The primary survey should also include rapid assessment for the location of entry and exit wounds, if any. The nurse should be aware that GSWs to the neck could cause significant airway complications (e.g., hematoma, and direct injury to the larynx). Anticipation of endotracheal intubation or cricoidthyrotomy for GSWs to the neck is reasonable.
  - Understanding the nature of fatal firearm injuries and the potential treatment options is vital to improving care of the maximally injured pediatric patient (Nance et al, 2003). The cascade of physiologic derangements that often accompany severe injury plays a large part in patient demise; it follows that multiple body regions being affected will increase the likelihood of death (Nance et al., 2003). Most children who arrive at trauma centers alive but subsequently die of nonintracranial fatal firearm injuries die quickly as the result of major vascular and thoracic injuries (Nance et al., 2003).
  - Ultrasound can be useful in localizing a bleeding source in a child with a multicavitary injury, but it can have limitations in the assessment phase for these patients (Nance et al, 2003). "Damage control" for abdominal injuries was introduced more than a decade ago (Nance et al., 2003; Rotondo et al., 1993). This management approach emphasizes an abbreviated initial laparotomy with control of hemorrhage and contamination followed by an ICU course of aggressive resuscitation aimed at restoring metabolic homeostasis (Nance et al., 2003). After this, definitive repair of injuries and abdominal closure 12 to 48 hours after the initial laparotomy are recommended (Nance et al., 2003).
  - Following the primary survey, intravascular access should be established and fluids administered (20 mL/kg). Accurate, precise description of the wound and surrounding landmarks should follow. If the GSW is to the child's head, the nurse should anticipate computed tomography (CT) scan, surgical debridement, and antibiotic therapy postoperatively if complications of infection develop. GSWs to the abdomen can result in immediate peritonitis (e.g., major vascular injuries, hollow organ injuries).
  - Several wound-outcome measures should be assessed throughout the child's PICU course, including the incision color, the surrounding

tissue (degree, color, and pain intensity), and the progression of exudate (type, color, and amount). The nurse should also assess the type of closure materials present (e.g., staples), epithelial resurfacing, and collagen deposition (e.g., healing ridge) (Bates-Jensen and Wethe, 1998).

- Vigilant pulmonary, neurologic, and peripheral vascular assessment is necessary to detect complications such as bullet embolization. If bullet embolization is suspected or confirmed, anticipate surgical debridement and anastomosis of the involved injured major vessels. Wounds that are close to major vessels warrant astute observation for hematoma formation. GSWs to bones are treated as compound fractures that require surgical exploration and debridement.
- It is advisable to start teaching the family as close to the PICU admission as possible. Teaching should include prevention and signs and symptoms of posttraumatic stress disorder (PTSD).

B. Exposure Injuries

1. **Thermal injury:** Thermal injury occurs when the rate of heat absorption is greater than the rate of heat dissipation and results in scalds and flame burns (see Burns).
2. **Electrical injury:** When electricity—either through current or lightning—comes into contact with the body, its electrical energy is converted to heat. The heat causes injury. Most electrical injuries are due to low-voltage alternating current in the home setting (see Burns).
3. **Chemical injury:** When a chemical is applied to the body, it causes injury by either producing heat or denaturing protein (see Burns and Toxicology). An example of chemical injury is an abusive parent who pours bleach on a child's skin.
4. **Radiant burns:** Exposure to the sun or to nuclear or therapeutic radiation can cause radiant burns (see Burns).
5. **Heat and cold exposure injuries**
   a. *Environmental exposure* during extreme cold results in hypothermia and frostbite. Hypothermia begins when a child's temperature is 35°C. Children are at risk for hypothermia because of their large body surface area (BSA)-to-mass ratio and less subcutaneous fat for heat production. Blood loss, alcohol use, and the injuries themselves may be hypothermia-related conditions.
   b. *Frostbite* may accompany hypothermia and multiple-trauma injuries and occurs when ice crystallizes in the body's cells. Frostbite usually affects the fingers, hands, feet, toes, ears, and nose (Barkin, 1999). The severity (degree) of frostbite depends on the environmental temperature and humidity, the duration of exposure, windchill factor, immobility, and tightness of clothing (Barkin, 1999). The American College of Surgeons (1997) defines four categories of frostbite, ranging from partial- to full-thickness tissue freezing: *First-degree* is manifested by pain, hyperemia, and edema of the involved area. *Second-degree* frostbite is a partial-thickness cold injury in which large fluid-filled blisters develop, followed by tissue necrosis. *Third-degree* frostbite causes full-thickness and subcutaneous tissue necrosis, initially characterized by small blisters containing dark fluid. The affected body part is cool, numb, blue or red, and does not blanch. Over the course of days, the affected tissues become necrotic and require debridement. *Fourth-degree* frostbite is full-thickness cold injury extending to the muscle and bone. The body part is

numb, cold, and bloodless with no blisters or edema. Gangrene develops, which may necessitate amputation.

- The focus of frostbite treatment is pain control, reperfusion, infection prevention, and safe manipulation of the affected region. Prevention of future injuries is important and can be accomplished by effective patient and family teaching.
- Administer preemptive intravenous (IV) analgesics for pain associated with rewarming, reperfusion, and manipulation of body part. Combination therapy (pharmacologic and nonpharmacologic interventions) can be useful (see Chapter 1).
- Wash wounds with mild soap and water if they appear clean; consider chlorhexidine gluconate (Hibiclens) if wounds appear or are suspected of being soiled. If a dressing is required, use a gel dressing to provide a pain-free, nonocclusive barrier. Topical silver sulfadiazine (e.g., Silvadene) may be applied to open wounds (Walker, 2003a). Cover gel or silver dressings with a secondary dressing (e.g., sterile gauze wrap). Anticipate administering prophylactic antibiotics and tetanus toxoid. Keep blisters intact unless a decision is made to debride them (Walker, 2003a).
- Avoid applying dry heat. Rewarm deep frostbite rapidly in a water bath at a temperature range of 102°F to 108°F (39°C to 42°C), ideally 104°F (40°C). Prevent mechanical friction by avoiding tissue-to-tissue contact and touching the extremity to the basin during a rewarming bath. Elevate the affected extremity, particularly after rewarming, to treat gross edema (Walker, 2003a).

c. Prolonged environmental exposure to heat may result in heat cramps, heat exhaustion (heat syncope), and heat stroke (Walker, 2003b). Of these, *heat stroke* is a true medical emergency. It is crucial to detect and treat heat cramps before they progress to heat exhaustion and finally heat stroke (Laskowski-Jones, 2000). Heat stroke kills up to 80% of victims who are not treated appropriately (Auerbach et al., 1999). Children are at risk for heat-related emergencies because they acclimate more slowly to exercise in the heat compared with adults *(exertional heat stroke)* (Laskowski-Jones, 2000). Other predisposing risk factors for heat stroke that may be considered unique for the pediatric population include, but are not limited to, dehydration, fatigue, sleep deprivation, fever, muscular exertion, history of seizures, sunburn, and the use of certain drugs (e.g., amphetamines, cocaine) (Auerbach et al., 1999).

- Heat exhaustion occurs in athletes who sweat profusely and experience significant volume depletion. Core body temperatures with heat exhaustion are between 38°C (100.4°F) and 40.5°C (104.9°F). Symptoms include nausea, vomiting, dizziness or syncope, weakness, and mild changes in mental status changes (e.g., confusion, inattention). Treatment consists of vigorous rehydration with IV fluids if mental status or GI problems preclude oral intake. Children experiencing heat exhaustion should be moved to a cooler environment, and measures to cool the body (e.g., ice packs to the neck or axilla, cool towels, fanning) should be used (American Academy of Pediatrics, 2000).
- *Heat stroke* is an acute medical emergency caused by an extreme buildup in body heat with a failure of the body's normal thermoregulatory mechanisms. It manifests with core body temperatures usually exceeding

40.5°C (>104.9°F) and sometimes even exceeding 41.7°C (107.0°F). It is life threatening, with a mortality rate of around 10% despite good medical management. Shock, circulatory abnormalities, disseminated intravascular coagulation (DIC), rhabdomyolysis, arrhythmias, and seizures are prominent features. Treatment involves immediate transport to an emergency medical facility. Rapid cooling, close management of circulation and hydration, and intensive multisystem monitoring and support are essential (Laskowski-Jones, 2000).

C. Drowning, Submersion, and Anoxic Injury

1. **Drowning** is an important and preventable cause of death in childhood (Brenner et al., 2001). **Submersion injury** (drowning and near drowning) is a unique, well-studied, and common cause of asphyxial injury, and it can serve as a model for understanding many of the prognostic, pathophysiologic, and therapeutic aspects of all types of asphyxial injuries in the pediatric population (Ibsen and Koch, 2002). Examples of other asphyxial injuries include inhalation, traumatic asphyxia, apnea, strangulation, suffocation, foreign-body aspiration, and others (Isben and Koch, 2002).
2. The three most important **risk factors** that contribute to drowning and near drowning are (1) the inability to swim or the overestimation of swimming capabilities, (2) risk-taking behavior, and (3) inadequate adult supervision. Sites where childhood drownings occur may be distinguished as domestic (e.g., bathtubs, buckets), artificial pools (e.g., swimming pools, hot tubs), natural freshwater (e.g., ponds, pits), and salt water (Brenner et al., 2001). Most submersion events occur in fresh water (Isben and Koch, 2002).
3. **Pathophysiology**
   a. During the initial minutes after submersion, there is panic and struggle to surface. This is when small amounts of fluid are aspirated into the hypopharynx, triggering laryngospasm. The victim then swallows large volumes of water. In most cases, the initial laryngospasm abates and the victim aspirates large volumes of water. Laryngospasm continues, and there is little aspiration. Vomiting and aspiration of gastric contents may occur with evolving hypoxemia. The hypoxemia causes neuronal injury, and eventual circulatory collapse ensues with coincident myocardial damage, multiple-organ-system dysfunction, and further ischemic brain injury (Isben and Koch, 2002).
   b. Cardiac pathophysiologic changes associated with submersion injury are consistent with hypoxic-ischemic injury (Isben and Koch, 2002). Pulmonary pathophysiologic changes result from initial hypoxemia, increased permeability of the capillary endothelium, surfactant disruption, or aspiration of gastric contents or caustic materials (Isben and Koch, 2002). Sequalae associated with these changes may include acute lung injury or acute respiratory distress syndrome, alveolar collapse, atelectasis, intrapulmonary shunting, and ventilation-perfusion mismatch (Isben and Koch, 2002). Additionally, submersion injury victims will be at increased risk for infection as a result of mechanical ventilation (Isben and Koch, 2002).
4. **Hypothermia**

   Hypothermia is often associated with submersion injuries and is dependent on the temperature of the water (Isben and Koch, 2002). The mammalian "dive reflex" is elicited by contact of the face with cold water and consists of breath-holding, intense peripheral vasoconstriction with bradycardia, decreased cardiac output, and increased mean arterial pressure (MAP). The role of this reflex in human submersion remains unclear (Isben and Koch, 2002).

5. **Recovery and outcome**
   a. Near-drowning victims are likely to have a poor outcome if they (1) spend more than 10 minutes under water (2) do not receive basic life support within 10 minutes of the incident, (3) have a core temperature below 33°C, (4) have a Glasgow Coma Score (GCS) of 5 or lower, (5) have persistent apnea, (6) have an arterial blood pH less than 7.1, and (6) were immersed in water warmer than 10°C (Chandy, 2000).
   b. Prediction of functional neurologic outcome versus death or severe disability becomes more reliable with time as the child is treated and recovery or response to therapy is observed (Isben and Koch, 2002). Neurologic examination within the first 24 to 72 hours of therapy (combined with other imaging and testing procedures) is the best indicator of neurologic outcome (Isben and Koch, 2002). Magnetic resonance spectroscopy rather than CT may be useful in the early evaluation of hypoxic-ischemic injury (Isben and Koch, 2002). Early electroencephalography (EEG) is complicated by the use of sedatives, analgesics, and muscle relaxants consistent with resuscitation and initial treatment. A flat or severely attenuated EEG or burst suppression record is often a poor prognostic indicator, but it is most likely reflective of the initial insult and resuscitation (Isben and Koch, 2002). Similar findings that persist in the absence of such medications are more predictive of a poor neurologic prognosis (Isben and Koch, 2002).
6. **Treatment in the ICU**
   a. One focus of treatment for a near-drowning victim is core rewarming. Methods used for core rewarming include the administration of warmed IV fluids and blood, the introduction of heated oxygen into the lungs using an endotracheal tube, and warm fluid lavage into organs and spaces (e.g., stomach, bladder) (Chandy, 2000). If the heart and lungs do regain normal function following rewarming measures, further attempts at resuscitation are likely to be futile (Chandy, 2000).
   b. The focus of mechanical ventilation after hypoxic-ischemic injury should be preventing ventilator-induced lung injury rather than the degree of ventilation (controlling neurologic outcome with mild or moderate hyperventilation to avoid hypercapnia) (Isben and Koch, 2002).
   c. Fluid resuscitation and inotropic agents may be required to restore adequate tissue perfusion as a result of impaired myocardial contractility, persistent hypoxemia, hypothermia, acidosis, suboptimal intravascular volume, and electrolyte abnormalities (Isben and Koch, 2002). Long-term morbidity and mortality after near drowning are due to hypoxic-ischemic brain injury; neuroresuscitative strategies have included monitoring and management of intracranial pressure (ICP), barbiturates, hypothermia, calcium-channel blockers, free radical scavengers, and others (Isben and Koch, 2002).

HISTORY

A. Trauma Resuscitation

Trauma resuscitation begins immediately after the injury, with first aid initiated by family or bystanders, and continues with the prehospital care providers and emergency department staff. The initial assessment and treatment must be organized and methodical to decrease trauma-related morbidity and mortality.

B. Injury History

1. The **history surrounding the injury** is obtained from family, bystanders, prehospital providers, and the patient (if possible). Pertinent historical information is obtained and relates to three important areas: mechanism of injury, patient history, and the plausibility of the mechanism of injury and patient history. The critical-care nurse plays a pivotal role in assimilating details specific to the mechanism of injury and the presenting injury and complications. The following serves as a guide for the nurse and lists basic information that should be obtained relative to each mechanism of injury.
   a. *Motor-vehicle occupant:* Scene fatalities, use of restraining devices (e.g., car seat, three-point restraints, booster seat, lap belt), front or backseat passenger, ejection from the vehicle, site of impact (e.g., side, rear-end, head-on), motor-vehicle speed, object of collision (e.g., oncoming vehicle, stationary vehicle or object), passenger compartment intrusion, entrapment
   b. *Pedestrian–motor-vehicle crash:* Speed of the vehicle, travel of the patient after the impact, being run over by or pinned under the vehicle, the type of surface on which the patient landed, the point of impact on the patient's body
   c. *Bicycle–motor-vehicle crash:* Speed of the bicycle, speed of the vehicle (if moving), use of a bicycle helmet
   d. *Fall:* The height from which the patient fell, the number of steps, the surface onto which the patient landed, and the area of body that hit the ground first
   e. *Penetrating injury:* The type of weapon used, number of bullets fired, caliber of bullets, firing range, number and location of stab wounds
2. The **following questions** related to the injury history help elicit valuable information to anticipate ICU course and outcome.
   a. *Airway:* Did the child have a choking or vomiting episode? Was assistance needed to maintain the child's airway?
   b. *Breathing:* Did the child stop breathing or have difficulty breathing? If so, for how long did this occur? Was rescue breathing initiated?
   c. *Circulation:* Was blood lost? About how much? Was cardiopulmonary resuscitation (CPR) initiated? How long was it in progress?
   d. *Disability:* Did the child sustain a loss of consciousness? If so, for how long? Was the child easily arousable? Does the child have antegrade (loss of memory after the injury) or retrograde (loss of memory before the injury) amnesia? Does the child recognize family members and familiar objects? Was the child able to wiggle his or her fingers and toes? Did the child appear flaccid? Did the child appear frightened, apprehensive, and anxious?
   e. *Other:* Was any first aid administered? Were any splints or bandages applied? Did the child get up and walk around after the injury, or was the child found in the same position as immediately following the injury?
3. **Additional information** may integrate the mechanisms of injury with the patient's social history. Family and developmental history may be elicited from the following questions:
   a. *Developmental plausibility: Is the mechanism of injury consistent with the injuries seen and the history related to these injuries?* Does the mechanism of injury match the patient's history? That is, if the mechanism of injury in an infant was a fall from a couch (approximately 1 foot high) onto a carpeted floor and the infant is in cardiopulmonary arrest, intentional injury must be suspected (see Child Maltreatment section).

b. *Credibility of witnesses:* Are family members or bystanders changing their stories to match the child's injuries? Are witnesses reluctant to divulge information? For example, the mechanism of injury in a 13-year-old child is a gunshot wound to the chest from a drive-by shooting. It is a warm evening; all the neighbors are outside, and yet no one sees the car or driver. Such witnesses may be afraid to come forward for fear of gang retaliation.
c. *Patient's overall appearance:* How does the child appear overall? Does the child appear well nourished and clean? Is the child's appearance developmentally appropriate? Does the child appear to be the correct size and weight for his or her age? Does the child have any bruises, scars, or other signs of child maltreatment? How is the parent-child relationship? Does the parent or caregiver comfort or scold the child for the injury? Does the parent label the child as "clumsy" or "accident prone"? Does the child go willingly to strangers, or does the child shrink from human touch? (see Child Maltreatment section).

C. Patient Health History

Parents may have been involved in the injury and may be receiving treatment elsewhere (e.g., for an MVC). Family members called to the hospital might not be able to provide information about the patient's health history. Parents or legal guardians must be notified when an injury occurs; however, emergency treatment is not withheld until parental consent is obtained.

The critical-care nurse can use the acronym AMPLE to guide the assessment of the basic past health history:

- *Allergies* to medications
- *Medications* the patient regularly receives (both over-the-counter and prescription)
- *Medical history* or illness as well as special needs (e.g., hearing impairment, use of special devices)
- *Last meal* eaten
- *Events* or environment that led to the injury (obtained in injury history)

INITIAL ASSESSMENT

The initial assessment of the multiply injured child includes the primary and secondary assessments. Children have unique anatomic and physiologic features that make them different from adults; these features should be taken into consideration when conducting the primary and secondary assessments.

A. Primary Assessment

1. In the **primary assessment,** life-threatening injuries are detected and treated. Life-threatening injuries include airway obstruction; open, tension, and bilateral hemopneumothoraces; traumatic arrest; flail chest; cardiac tamponade; and hemorrhagic shock.
2. **Life-saving interventions** are initiated simultaneously with the detection of these injuries and include airway stabilization and restoration of breathing and circulation.
3. **Airway and cervical spine assessment**
   a. *Developmental considerations*
      - Because the young child's airway has a narrow diameter, airway obstruction occurs easily. The tongue is relatively large compared with the oral cavity and can easily obstruct the airway. The larynx is more cephalad

and anterior, and the vocal cords are short and concave (American College of Surgeons, 1997).

- The epiglottis is U-shaped and protrudes into the pharynx. The cricoid cartilage is the narrowest area of the airway in children younger than 10 years of age. The smaller the child, the greater the disproportion between the size of the cranium and the midface, producing a greater propensity for the posterior pharyngeal area to buckle as the relatively larger occiput forces passive flexion of the cervical spine (American College of Surgeons, 1997). If the neck is hyperflexed or hyperextended, airway obstruction results from the laxity of the airway structures. The lower airways are small in diameter, with less supporting cartilage in infants and young children; thus airway obstruction from mucus and edema easily occurs (see also Chapter 2). Children younger than 8 years are susceptible to cervical spine injury because of their larger head size, weak neck musculature, and horizontal facets (Muir and Town, 2003). Furthermore, these young children have lax intraspinal ligaments and capsules, thus increasing their susceptibility to pseudosubluxation of the cervical spine (American College of Surgeons, 1997). Their fulcrum of cervical mobility is high (C2-3) compared with C5-6 and C6-7 in the adult (American College of Surgeons, 1997), which accounts for the fact that C1-3 fractures are the most common cervical fracture in pediatric patients. Therefore, suspected cervical-spine injuries should always be suspected until proven otherwise (Muir and Town, 2003).

b. *Assessment and interventions*

- The airway is assessed for patency. The presence of loose teeth, vomit, and blood is determined. The cervical spine is maintained in neutral alignment, usually by securing the child on a pediatric long board with a cervical immobilization device and a cervical collar. Use a board with an occipital cutout or well. If the long board does not have a cut-out place, 1-inch padding under the child from the buttocks to the shoulders will maintain spinal alignment (Zaritsky et al., 2001). Flexion of the cervical spine must be avoided to prevent airway compromise or aggravation of an existing spinal cord injury. The front of the cervical collar is opened to inspect the neck for jugular vein distention and tracheal deviation and to palpate the carotid pulse and then closed. The cervical collar must fit properly to prevent flexion and extension of the cervical spine. A properly fitting collar has these features: the chin rests securely in the chin holder, the collar does not cover the ears, and the bottom of the collar rests on the upper sternum (Bernardo and Waggoner, 1992).
- Signs and symptoms of spinal cord injury are quickly ascertained, such as numbness, tingling, and inability to wiggle the toes and fingers. Full spinal immobilization is maintained throughout the initial treatment.

4. **Respiratory assessment**

a. *Developmental considerations*

- The chest wall in younger children is cartilaginous, allowing blunt and penetrating energy forces to be easily transmitted to underlying lung and cardiac tissues. Significant chest injury can be present in the absence of rib fractures. Fractures of the first and second ribs are not common in children and indicate significant force when present. An increasing number of fractures correlate with increasing mortality. Similarly, flail segments indicate severe parenchymal injury (e.g., pulmonary contusion) (American College of Surgeons, 1997). The mediastinum is mobile, allowing for increased problems with pneumothoraces.

- Breathing is primarily diaphragmatic until the age of 7 to 8 years. Chest retractions can be observed during respiratory distress. The crying child swallows air, resulting in gastric distention. This distention impedes diaphragmatic movement and respiratory excursion.
- Children have fewer alveoli and therefore less respiratory reserve compared with adults. The work of breathing must be continuously assessed. Breath sounds may be easily transmitted because of the thin chest wall, allowing a false assumption that breath sounds are equal.
- Oxygen consumption is higher in infants compared with that in adults, allowing hypoxemia to occur rapidly (Vernon-Levett, 2003). This higher consumption results in more rapid respiratory rates.

b. *Assessment and interventions*

- Respirations are assessed by observation and inspection. The qualities of respirations are determined by assessing the presence of breath sounds high in the axillae and anterior chest. Unequal bilateral breath sounds may indicate a pneumothorax on the diminished side. Signs of respiratory distress include retractions of the intercostal muscles, nasal flaring, grunting (in infants), adventitious breath sounds, or diminished or absent breath sounds. Rescue breathing with 100% oxygen by bag-valve-mask is initiated in the apneic or bradypneic child.
- The chest is exposed and inspected for any surface trauma, penetrating wounds, paradoxical movements, and flail segments. The rib cage is gently palpated for tenderness, crepitus, and flail segments. The sternum is palpated for tenderness as well.

5. Circulatory assessment

a. *Developmental considerations*

- Children have a higher oxygen requirement and faster metabolic rate, requiring a higher cardiac output per kilogram of body weight (Rupp and Day, 2003). Although the child's circulating blood volume of 80 mL/kg is small, it is larger on a milliliter per kilogram basis compared with an adult's. Even small amounts of blood loss can decrease circulating blood volume and compromise perfusion. Hypotension does not develop until a 20% to 45% blood loss occurs (Rupp and Day, 2003); therefore hypotension is a *late* sign of circulatory compromise in the child. Adequate tissue perfusion is reflected by a capillary refill time of less than 2 seconds (see Chapter 3).
- Tachycardia is the initial response to hypovolemia, and it occurs with decreased oxygen delivery. Tachycardia is usually the first and often the only sign of shock. This increased heart rate increases cardiac output. When this compensatory mechanism fails, tissue hypoxia and hypercapnia occur, leading to bradycardia (Rupp and Day, 2003) and hypotension. Bradycardia and hypotension, therefore, are *late* signs of cardiac failure. Bradycardia and hypotension are both ominous signs of impending respiratory and circulatory collapse.

b. *Assessment and interventions*

- Circulation is assessed by auscultation of heart sounds for their rate, rhythm, and quality. If the pulse is absent or, if peripheral pulses or blood pressure are nonpalpable in the presence of an electrical rhythm (pulseless electrical activity or PEA), chest compressions are immediately initiated. Muffled heart tones, distended veins, and shock (Beck's triad) may indicate cardiac tamponade, which may necessitate pericardiocentesis or open pericardiotomy (American College of Surgeons,

1997). Major external hemorrhage is controlled by application of direct pressure.

- Peripheral circulation is assessed by palpating a radial or brachial pulse, measuring capillary refill (should be less than 2 seconds), and assessing skin color (pink) and temperature (warm). Deviations in peripheral circulation may indicate decreased blood flow to the periphery, which can result in decreased oxygen and substrate delivery to the tissues.

6. **Neurologic assessment**
   a. *Developmental considerations*
      - Infants and children are susceptible to brain injury for a number of reasons. They have a larger head-to-body ratio. The skull is malleable because of its thin cranial bones; so less protection is afforded to the brain tissues. Nerve myelinization is not complete at birth, and this unmyelinated brain tissue is particularly vulnerable to injury, especially shearing forces.
      - Fontanelles and sutures may remain open until approximately 18 to 24 months. Following head injury, the open fontanelles and sutures may help to equalize increased ICP, thus hiding the signs of intracranial injury (see Chapter 4).

   b. *Assessment and interventions*
      - A brief neurologic evaluation establishes the patient's level of consciousness and pupillary size and reactivity. Responsiveness may be more difficult to evaluate in the preverbal child. Alterations in developmentally expected behaviors, such as lack of stranger anxiety in an 8-month-old infant, decreased muscle tone in a 2-month-old infant, or inability to focus and follow objects in a 6-month-old infant, may indicate changes in neurologic functioning. Changes in the child's level of consciousness may indicate decreased oxygenation (pulmonary exchange) or perfusion (hypovolemia), not necessarily brain injury.
      - Throughout the primary assessment, the nurse talks to the child to determine his or her level of consciousness and to provide emotional support. The *AVPU* method of evaluation determines the child's response to stimulation (Liebman, 2003):
        - *A*wake
        - Responsive to *V*erbal stimuli
        - Responsive to *P*ainful stimuli
        - *U*nresponsive
      - The infant should respond by looking around and being wary of strangers. The verbal child should be able to state his or her name and perhaps other information. The child who changes from awake to sleepy to disoriented should be watched closely. The pediatric GCS score (see GCS in Chapter 4) should be obtained to record the best eye, motor, and verbal responses.

7. **Exposure**
   a. *Developmental considerations:* Children have a larger BSA-to-weight ratio compared with adults. This ratio renders them susceptible to convective and conductive heat loss. Infants younger than 6 months of age do not have the neuromuscular maturity to shiver to maintain body heat. *Nonshivering thermogenesis* then occurs, where brown fat is broken down to provide warmth; unfortunately, oxygen consumption increases and decompensation ensues (Walker, 2003b).

   b. *Assessment and interventions:* The child is completely undressed to allow inspection of all injuries. Overhead warming lights and warm ambient temperature should help maintain body temperature within a normal range.

Warm blankets should be applied to respect modesty, prevent convective heat loss, and promote comfort.

B. Secondary Assessment

A complete head-to-toe assessment is conducted to detect and treat all non–life-threatening injuries.

1. The **head** is examined for depressions, lacerations, hematomas, and impaled objects. The anterior and posterior fontanelles in infants are palpated; a tense and bulging fontanelle may indicate increased ICP. The scalp is palpated for lacerations and observed for dirt, glass, and other debris.
2. The **face** is inspected for deformities, lacerations, foreign bodies, and impaled objects. The orbits, facial bones, and mandible are palpated for pain and crepitus. Asymmetric facial movement is observed, which may indicate facial nerve paralysis. Classic Le Fort (facial) fractures, although rare in children, should be suspected in any blunt-force or penetrating facial trauma. Malocclusion is indicative of a fractured mandible. *An example of a combined traumatic finding to the head or face would be a child with a self-inflicted GSW to the mandible who has a palate impaled with a tongue piercing.*
3. The **eyes** are assessed for pupillary reactivity, symmetry, and extraocular movements. Blood in the anterior chamber of the eye *(hyphema)* should be reported immediately because this finding indicates a serious injury. Foreign bodies should be noted, and penetrating objects are stabilized in place with gauze and tape. A ruptured globe is possible if the eye is swollen shut and bruised and a penetrating or direct blunt force was applied during the injury. The presence of tearing should be noted as well. Visual acuity may be easily assessed by asking the young child to point to an object or by having an older child verbalize his or her ability to see. The presence of contact lenses should be ascertained, and the contact lenses should be removed. Periorbital bruising or "raccoon's sign" is indicative of a basilar skull fracture. Scleral hemorrhage may be observed if compression forces were applied at the time of injury.
4. The **ears** are examined for cerebrospinal fluid or bloody drainage. Such drainage can be collected onto a gauze pad; however, the ear is never packed with gauze. Hematotympanum should be noted. Ecchymosis over the mastoid process or "Battle's sign," is indicative of a basilar skull fracture; when ecchymosis over the mastoid process is noted, the skull fracture is more than 12 hours old. Ear lacerations should be covered with gauze soaked in normal saline (NS) until definitive repair is scheduled.
5. The **nose** is examined for cerebrospinal fluid or bloody drainage, deformities, lacerations, or bruising. Drainage can be collected onto a gauze pad, but the nares are not packed with the gauze.
6. The **oral cavity,** including the tongue, mucous membranes, and teeth, are examined for injury. Displaced permanent teeth can be placed in milk or NS and dated; debris should not be removed from the tooth because this material aids in reimplantation. Dental apparatus, such as braces, may have been damaged during the injury and should be assessed by a pediatric dentist or orthodontist.
7. The **neck** examination involves opening the front piece of the cervical collar for inspection of the anterior neck. The neck is assessed for lacerations, swelling, deformities, jugular-vein distention, and impaled objects. The neck is palpated for pain, tenderness, and subcutaneous emphysema. Tracheal positioning is noted; the normal position is midline. Tracheal deviation is noted above the sternal notch in young children. The larynx is palpated for integrity; a fractured

larynx is easier palpated than visualized. The awake child's voice is assessed for hoarseness or changes. A hoarse or "gravelly" voice may also indicate tracheal trauma and the possible need for airway intervention. After the neck is assessed, the collar is secured.

8. The **chest** is reinspected for symmetry, flail segments, open wounds, and impaled objects. The anterior chest is examined for cutaneous lesions that might indicate underlying pulmonary or cardiac injury. The chest is auscultated for the presence of normal and adventitious breath sounds. The anterior rib cage and both clavicles are palpated for pain and tenderness. Pain with inspiration should be noted. The heart sounds are auscultated and should be clear and distinct. The point of maximal impulse (PMI) should be noted.
9. The **abdomen** is observed for distention, bruising, penetrating wounds, and impaled objects. Bowel sounds should be auscultated. The abdomen is then palpated for pain, rigidity, and tenderness. The lower abdomen is palpated for bladder tenderness and distention.
10. The **pelvis** is palpated for tenderness and intactness. Any pain or displacement on palpation is indicative of a pelvic fracture. Femoral pulses are assessed for equality and strength. The bladder is palpated for distention. The genitalia, urinary meatus, perineum, and rectum are inspected for signs of trauma, bleeding, and impaled objects. Blood at the urinary meatus may indicate a urethral tear. The prostate gland is difficult to palpate in the preadolescent boy. A flaccid rectal sphincter is indicative of spinal cord injury. The rectal examination may be deferred in cases of severe rectal trauma when an examination under anesthesia (EUA) or surgical intervention is needed or when a foreign body is lodged in the rectal vault. Priapism may be noted. Anal examinations specific to abuse are difficult to interpret due to a number of variables: (1) the size of the object introduced, (2) the presence of force, (3) use of lubricants, (4) degree of cooperativeness from the victim, (5) the number of episodes of penetration, (6) the time since the last contact (Finkel and DeJong, 2001).
11. The **extremities** are inspected for any deformities, open wounds or fractures, contusions, and impaled objects. Each extremity is palpated for pain, and the peripheral pulses are assessed for equality and amplitude. Skin color and temperature are reassessed as well as capillary refill time. Asking the child to wiggle his or her toes and fingers and asking whether he or she can feel the nurse touching the toes and fingers indicate neurovascular and neuromotor integrity. Hand grasps and foot flexion and extension determine strength and motor-nerve functioning.
12. The **back** examination involves carefully log-rolling the child to inspect the back. To log-roll the child, one person is assigned to keep the child's head midline and execute the move. Additional staff members are needed to roll the child onto his or her side at the surgeon's command. Another person examines the back for any deformities, lacerations, hematomas, impaled objects, or abrasions on the posterior surface and flank. Each vertebra is palpated for stability and the presence of pain. After this examination, the surgeon gives the command to roll the child to the supine position, maintaining in-line cervical stabilization the entire time. The child's motor and neurovascular statuses are assessed immediately before and after the logrolling to assess the presence of spinal cord injury.
13. **Vital signs and pulse oximetry** readings are measured continuously and recorded every 5 minutes until the child is stable and then every 15 minutes for the first hour of treatment. Temperature is measured frequently to evaluate the effectiveness of warming measures and to detect and treat hypothermia. The child's vital signs should be compared with the age-appropriate norms for heart

and respiratory rates and blood pressure ranges. Immediately after the injury, however, the child's physiologic requirements may not fall within age-appropriate ranges. Therefore these parameters should serve as a guide only.

C. Trauma Scoring

After the primary and secondary assessments are completed, a trauma score and a pediatric GCS are assigned. The Trauma Score (TS), an objective method for determining injury severity, can be used as an adjunct with continued reassessment data to help use established guidelines for treatment of trauma patients (Haley, 2003).

Three trauma scores are used in pediatric trauma. The Pediatric Trauma Score (PTS) assesses six parameters important in the outcome of pediatric trauma: size, airway, blood pressure, central nervous system (CNS), fractures, and wounds. The TS assesses respiratory rate and effort, blood pressure, and capillary refill. It also includes the GCS score. The Revised Trauma Score (RTS) comprises the GCS score (see Chapter 4), blood pressure, and respiratory rate. The TS and RTS are adult scores, but they are used in children. Ideally trauma scores are calculated during three phases: in the prehospital setting, on arrival to the emergency department, and 1 hour later.

INITIAL TREATMENT

A. Airway and Cervical Spine

1. In the unconscious child, the **airway initially is opened** and maintained using the jaw thrust maneuver. This maneuver is the safest technique for opening the airway in the child with a suspected cervical spine injury (Liebman, 2003). The head-tilt/chin-lift method is not used in pediatric trauma patients because this method may convert a cervical spine fracture without neurologic injury into a cervical spine fracture with neurologic injury. Because the child's oral cavity is relatively small, the upper airway is easily obstructed by the lax oropharyngeal musculature in the unconscious child.
2. **Foreign material,** such as teeth, vomit, or blood, is cleared from the oral cavity with a tonsillar tip (Yankauer) suction tube. Stimulation of an intact gag reflex must be avoided as gagging, vomiting, and aspiration may result. Blind finger sweeps are not recommended for foreign-body removal in infants and young children because foreign material may be displaced distally and injury to the friable oral mucosa may result.
3. An **oropharyngeal airway** may be placed in unconscious children to maintain airway patency. Oral-airway size must be appropriate because an artificial airway that is too small may push the tongue backward. One that is too large may damage the delicate, soft intraoral tissues, causing bleeding and swelling and further complicating airway management (Liebman, 2003). The oropharyngeal airway is measured from the corner of the mouth to the angle of the jaw (Schermer, 1997). This type of airway is inserted directly using a tongue blade to pull the tongue forward. This airway is *not* rotated 90 degrees as in the adult because damage may occur to the oral tissues. Furthermore, the tongue may be displaced posteriorly into the pharynx, causing an airway obstruction.
4. **Nasopharyngeal airways** are not recommended in pediatric trauma patients. In the child with a head injury, a basilar or cribriform plate fracture may be present. During insertion of a nasopharyngeal airway, entry into the cranial vault may occur.

5. These **basic airway maneuvers** are acceptable for short-term airway control. Endotracheal intubation is preferred for extended periods. The equipment is prepared and cardiorespiratory and pulse oximetry monitors are used. The child's vital signs are closely monitored for cardiac dysrrhythmias, lower oxygen saturation, or bradycardia. During endotracheal intubation, neutral cervical spine alignment is maintained by the surgeon or another skilled practitioner to avoid hyperextension. Endotracheal intubation is best accomplished by rapid-sequence technique by a skilled practitioner.
6. A **combination of medications** is often used during rapid-sequence intubation to prevent increased ICP and to produce adequate states of sedation, analgesia, and paralysis (Vernon-Levett, 2003). Succinylcholine and rocuronium both have a short onset of action. Atropine may be included for children less than 5 years of age and with the use of succinylcholine to prevent bradycardia. The sedatives and anesthetic agents used are based on the condition and stability of the patient. For a normotensive patient, midazolam, etomidate, thiopental, or propofol may be used. For a hypotensive or hypovolemic patient, medications may include etomidate, ketamine, or midazolam (with mild hypotension). If the patient is asthmatic, ketamine or midaozolam can be used. A patient with actual or suspected head injury should receive thiopental, propofol, or etomidate when normotensive and etomidate or low-dose thiopental when hypotensive (Zaritsky et al., 2001). Note that even a single induction dose of etomidate may block the normal stress-induced increase in adrenal cortisol production for 4 to 8 hours or longer in debilitated patients (Lexi-Comp Inc., 2005).
7. An **uncuffed endotracheal tube** is used in children 8 years of age and younger because the cricoid cartilage serves as an effective seal. The orotracheal route is preferred. The endotracheal tube is secured with tape and benzoin or with commercially prepared devices. After intubation, a nasogastric (if a basilar skull fracture is not present) or orogastric tube is inserted and connected to low continuous suction. Young children are aerophagic, and aggressive ventilation may lead to gastric distention (Semonin-Holleran, 1992). The gastric tube is measured from the corner of the mouth, over the ear to the xiphoid process, and marked with tape. Once the tube is properly placed, it is secured with tape. A chest radiograph is taken to confirm the endotracheal tube depth. Indicators of correct airway placement include symmetric chest movement, equal bilateral breath sounds auscultated in all fields and absent over stomach, end-tidal carbon dioxide detection, and condensation in the endotracheal tube. Endotracheal suctioning may be required if copious secretions or oral trauma is present.
8. The **most common complication of endotracheal intubation** is inadvertent intubation of the right main-stem bronchus or dislodgment of the endotracheal tube into the right main-stem bronchus if the patient is positioned for procedures or transported within the facility. When this situation arises, chest expansion may not be equal, and breath sounds are absent or diminished in the left side of the chest. Pulse oximetry readings may be low, and ventilation may be difficult. Prompt recognition of this complication is essential; it is corrected by withdrawing the endotracheal tube until equal breath sounds and equal chest movement are observed. Documentation of endotracheal tube placement at the nose or lip may be valuable.
9. In children where airway patency and control is not possible because of extensive craniofacial injuries, an **emergency tracheostomy or cricothyrotomy** may be required.
10. **Spinal precautions** are maintained during emergency treatment. Spinal precautions include the application of a rigid cervical collar, cervical immobi-

lization device (CID), and an immobilization board. If the child vomits, the child is log-rolled as a unit with the equipment remaining intact, and then suctioning is performed. Anteroposterior, lateral, oblique, and odontoid cervical spine radiographs from C1 through T1 may be obtained to determine the presence of spinal fractures. When obtaining the lateral views, the child's arms are pulled downward by a surgeon or nurse to allow for radiographic visualization of T1. The radiographs are assessed for vertebral symmetry, alignment, and spacing. If the child does not have radiographic evidence of bony spinal abnormalities *and* the child has normal neurologic findings *and* no pain on palpation, the spinal immobilization devices may be removed. Normal neurologic findings include absence of pain with full range of cervical motion, this is often difficult to assess in the presence of distracting injuries or head trauma. An MRI may be needed to evaluate the spine further.

B. Breathing

1. **High-flow oxygen** through a non-rebreather face mask at a flow rate of 10 to 15 L is administered. The face mask fits properly if it is snug and covers the nose and mouth. If the child will not tolerate a face mask and oxygen saturation levels are maintained at 98% to 99%, the oxygen can be administered in a blow-by fashion.
2. **If apnea or shallow breathing occurs,** ineffective respirations are present; in such cases, artificial ventilation is initiated with a bag-valve-mask and 100% high-flow oxygen. If breathing is spontaneous, but effective respirations are not achieved, endotracheal intubation is performed. The chest should rise and fall symmetrically when the bag is squeezed. If the chest does not rise, the face mask and head should be carefully repositioned while maintaining spinal precautions (Liebman, 2003). The bag-valve-mask device should have a bag capacity of at least 450 mL, be self-refilling, and come in pediatric and adult sizes. The pop-off valve should be occluded to allow for the need for higher ventilation pressures (Emergency Cardiac Care Committee and Subcommittees, 1992).
3. A **pulse oximeter** detects the percent of oxygen saturation in the blood and is a useful adjunct for determining adequacy of oxygenation.
4. **Mechanical ventilation** is initiated once proper endotracheal placement and adequate ventilation are achieved. The initial settings include an age-appropriate rate, 100% oxygen, and a low positive end-expiratory pressure (PEEP). The ventilator settings are adjusted according to the child's response to treatment.
5. **Life-threatening thoracic injuries** include tension hemothoraces, pneumothoraces, and pericardial tamponade. All these conditions are rare but must be anticipated. Pneumothoraces are initially treated with rapid needle decompression followed by chest tube placement. Pericardial tamponade is treated with a pericardiocentesis or a pericardial window in the operating room.

C. Circulation

1. **Cardiorespiratory and blood pressure monitors** are employed immediately after the child's arrival at the hospital. The appropriate cuff size should be two-thirds the size of the child's upper arm or thigh.
2. **Intravenous (IV) cannulation** with the largest catheter diameter possible is attempted in the upper, preferably uninjured extremity. Intraosseous access should be considered if IV access cannot be achieved in a reasonable amount of time (Zaritsky et al., 2001). If intraosseous access is unsuccessful, central venous

cannulation or cutdown should be attempted by an experienced physician or surgeon in the antecubital space or via the saphenous system. During IV cannulation, blood is obtained and sent for the following tests, depending on the location of injury. In suspected abdominal trauma, the following are assessed: hemoglobin, hematocrit, and platelet count; electrolytes and glucose; blood urea nitrogen (BUN) and creatinine; amylase, lipase, aspartate aminotransferase (AST; previously serum glutamic-oxaloacetic transaminase [SGOT]) and alanine aminotransferase (ALT; previously serum glutamic-pyruvic transaminase [SGPT). Creatine phosphokinase (CPK) is assessed for a child with suspected cardiac trauma. Type and crossmatch or type and screen are required if operative management is anticipated or blood will be administered. Blood toxicology screening is done for patients with suspected drug or alcohol use (Emergency Cardiac Care Committee and Subcommittees, 1992). The IV crystalloid fluid of choice is lactated Ringer's solution (LR), which is administered at a maintenance rate in the absence of hypovolemic shock. The fluid is warmed if rapid infusion is administered. A stopcock can be connected to the tubing if fluid boluses are anticipated. Overhydration is avoided in children with significant head injury to prevent cerebral edema.

3. In the **tachycardic or hypotensive child,** a 20 mL/kg fluid bolus of crystalloid is administered. If no improvement in heart rate or blood pressure is observed, a second bolus is administered. If no response is apparent, a 10 mL/kg bolus of warm, O-negative blood may be administered rapidly. More than two boluses of fluids may be required.
4. **External hemorrhaging** is controlled with direct pressure to the wound. Elevation of a bleeding extremity, in conjunction with direct pressure, may help to slow the bleeding process. Tourniquet and hemostat applications are controversial and are not used.
5. The application of a **pneumatic antishock garment (PASG)** has limited value in the pediatric population. Its use in children is generally limited to inflation of a leg compartment for splinting of a femur fracture.
6. **Traumatic arrest (empty heart syndrome)** is treated with cardiopulmonary resuscitation and rapid infusion of warmed crystalloid and blood products. Thoracotomy and open cardiac massage are rarely performed for blunt trauma and are usually a last-chance effort to resuscitate the child. Prognosis is poor.

D. Disability and Neurologic Checks

1. **Frequent neurologic checks** are performed to observe for changes in level of consciousness, motor, and sensory function. The pediatric GCS score is helpful to document serial neurologic assessments. Changes in the child's level of consciousness may indicate hypovolemia or increased ICP. Vomiting and irritability are early signs of increased ICP. In infants a bulging fontanelle or an increased head circumference is a *late* sign of increased ICP.
2. **Normoventilation** with 100% oxygen is initiated in the child with a severe head injury to keep the $Paco_2$ between 35 and 45 mm Hg. Hyperventilation is initiated to achieve a $Paco_2$ of approximately 30 mm Hg if signs of a lesion (e.g., epidural) or rapid decompensation are present. A $Paco_2$ less than 28 mm Hg may contribute to brain ischemia.
3. Procedures and treatments are **explained to the child** at a level he or she can understand. Words of praise and comfort go far to help reassure the frightened, injured child.

E. Exposure

1. Passive and active **warming measures** are initiated to prevent conductive and convective heat loss. Passive warming measures include warm blankets and increased ambient room temperature. Active warming measures include the administration of normothermic IV fluids and blood products to help with core warming.
2. **Temperature measurements** are obtained via the oral, rectal, or tympanic routes. Temperature probes on endotracheal tubes, esophageal probes, or urinary bladder thermistors are other options for temperature measurement.

F. Gastrointestinal (GI) and Genitourinary (GU)

1. An **orogastric or nasogastric tube** should be inserted to prevent gastric distention, vomiting, and aspiration. Initial drainage can be tested for the presence of blood. Gastric contrast can be administered through the gastric tube before CT testing.
2. In the absence of trauma or blood at the urinary meatus or suspected urethral trauma, an **indwelling bladder catheter** may be inserted and connected to a urinary drainage bag. If urethral trauma is suspected, a retrograde urethrogram must be performed before insertion of an indwelling bladder catheter. When drug or alcohol use is suspected, urinalysis and toxicology and blood toxicology screen are indicated. In postmenarchal females, urinary chorionic gonadotropin (UCG) testing should be done to rule out pregnancy.
3. A **stool smear** should be tested for occult blood.

G. Musculoskeletal

1. All long-bone fractures are immobilized. The child's neurovascular status is assessed immediately before and after splinting to ensure that an injury has not occurred or been aggravated. Open fractures, lacerations, or wounds require careful evaluation and cleaning.
2. Amputated body parts are wrapped in dry or moistened gauze, sealed in a plastic bag, and then placed in an ice water bath. At no time should the amputated part touch the ice directly, as tissue necrosis may occur. Subspecialists (e.g., plastic surgery and reimplantation specialists) will determine whether reattachment is possible after evaluating the child's amputated parts. Whether the child and family view the amputated part or injured limb is decided on an individual case basis. Younger children may become frightened of the wound, whereas older children may be curious, and their imagined injury may be worse than the reality (see Chapter 1). Tetanus prophylaxis, antibiotics, and analgesic administration are necessary.

ADDITIONAL INTERVENTIONS

A. Diagnostic Testing

1. During any **intrahospital transport**, an experienced nurse and physician attend to the child. Appropriate resuscitation equipment is taken during the transport in case the child's condition deteriorates.
2. **Chest radiographs** are obtained to determine the placement of endotracheal, gastric, and chest tubes. These films also confirm the presence of pneumothoraces or hemopneumothoraces, rib and clavicle fractures, and diaphragm integrity. Abdominal radiographs confirm the placement of gastric tubes and bladder catheters; stomach and intestine intactness can be observed as well. Free air is

noted, and the pelvis is examined for fracture. Skeletal radiographs are obtained according to the suspected injury. Radiographs are obtained in the trauma room with portable x-ray equipment or in the radiology suite. The child's primary nurse should remain with the child during these studies to explain procedures and monitor the child's condition.

3. **CT scanning** is undertaken in children with significant head, face, chest, or hemodynamically stable abdominal trauma. Angiography may be obtained for suspected severe vessel injury from blunt or penetrating trauma.
4. **Peritoneal lavage** is rarely performed to diagnose hemorrhage or visceral perforation in the pediatric population because CT scanning is the procedure of choice, along with assessment of the child's overall appearance and stability (Haley and Schenkel, 2003). Peritoneal lavage may be indicated when a multiply injured child requires immediate operative intervention (e.g., head injury), when CT scan is unavailable, or when CT scan findings are normal but a hollow viscous (bowel) injury is suspected (Simone, 2003). The use of focused abdominal sonography for trauma (FAST) has provided an excellent screening tool for initial assessment of the peritoneum and pericardial spaces. Unfortunately this modality remains very operator dependent. The need for surgical management remains dependent on hemodynamic stability. CT has emerged as the standard for evaluation of children with blunt abdominal trauma (MacKenzie and Fowler, 2000).

B. Pain Assessment

1. Because **critically ill pediatric trauma patients** may be nonverbal (e.g., endotracheally intubated) or preverbal because of cognitive development, a multidimensional assessment scale is helpful for assessing pain. Although self-report remains the recommended method to assess pain intensity, the Faces, Legs, Activity, Cry, and Consolability (FLACC) Scale (see Chapter 1) can be used with children as young as infants. The FLACC Scale can be especially useful when assessing postoperative pain because the scores are determined by observation of specific distress behaviors (Maloney-Harmon and Czerwinski, 2003). The FLACC scale lends itself well to children who have an artificial airway, who have significant cognitive delay, and who are unable to self-report pain because of conditions associated with multiple trauma (e.g., multiple surgical procedures) (Willis et al., 2003). The acronym FLACC denotes the following assessment categories: face (expression, muscle movement), legs (position, movement), activity (body position, movement), cry (degree, quality), and consolability (degree, effective interventions) (Merkel et al., 1997). The Behavioral Pain Assessment Scale is a valid, reliable, and clinically useful tool (Manworren and Hynan, 2003) (see Chapter 1). This scale lends itself well to the trauma population ranging in age from 2 months to at least 7 years, considering the potential communication challenges associated with these children (Manworren and Hynan, 2003). The FLACC may also be suitable for surgical trauma patients (Willis et al., 2003). Critical care nurses may be able to use the FLACC scale to guide analgesic choice (Manworren and Hynan, 2003).
2. **Newborns** experiencing trauma present unique challenges. The following are general principles for the prevention and management of newborn pain. Pain in newborns may be of a diagnostic (e.g. arterial puncture), therapeutic (e.g. chest tube insertion), or surgical nature. If a procedure is painful for adults, it should be considered painful in newborns. Newborns may experience a greater sensitivity to pain and are more susceptible to the long term effects of painful stimulation (Anand, 2001). Hyperalgesia may be a problem for babies who have experienced previous tissue injury, postoperative pain, localized infection, or

inflammation (Anand, 2001). Adequate pain management may be associated with decreased clinical complications and even decreased mortality. Sedatives do not relieve pain and may mask the newborn's pain response (Anand, 2001).

3. A combination of **environmental, behavioral, and pharmacological interventions** can prevent, reduce, and sometimes even eliminate newborn pain (Anand, 2001). An example would be the use of a sucrose pacifier and swaddling (behavioral and environmental management) together with fentanyl citrate (pharmacologic management) for a chest tube insertion procedure (see Chapter 1).

C. Emotional Support

1. The injured child experiences many **painful and frightening events** before, during, and after the injury. Children have fears of parental separation, pain, disfigurement, and mutilation. It is a nursing responsibility to provide comfort and emotional support to the child during this time of crisis.
2. The assignment of a **primary nurse** to the patient helps the child focus on one person. Speaking in a calm, reassuring voice may help the child to gain composure. For the child who receives spinal immobilization, standing at the child's side near the chest level allows the child to see the nurse without attempting to move the head sideways; standing over the child's head may be frightening and intimidating. Holding the child's hand, stroking the hair, and talking calmly and confidently can help the child to gain trust.
3. The awake or unconscious child should receive **age-appropriate explanations** for procedures. The truth should be told about any pain or discomfort that may occur. Coping measures for painful procedures include deep breathing, guided imagery, counting, singing, or other activities. Allowing the child to wiggle a hand or foot gives the child some sense of control. Child-life specialists may be able to enhance the child's repertoire of coping skills during procedures.
4. The **parents or family members** should be permitted to see the child as soon as possible. The nurse can explain to the family what they will see, hear, and smell on entering the child's room. Explain the current plans for the child's treatment to the family in language that they can understand. Encourage the family to touch the child and to ask questions. The family may welcome having a social worker, religious counselor, or other support person. Parental presence during resuscitation is advocated, along with the proper support and understanding that goes with this type of intervention (Thomas, 2003).

SPECIFIC INJURIES

With patients who experience multiple trauma, critical care nurses are faced with the challenge of assessing and managing more than one injury at a time. Additionally, nurses must be alert for the development of complications, which may be enhanced or obscured as a result of associated injuries. It is not uncommon for the nurse to prioritize care for life-threatening injuries (e.g., head trauma) while planning to manage less severe injuries in the future (e.g., orthopedic trauma). For the purpose of discussion, specific body system injuries are briefly addressed in this section with the understanding that these injuries will not be isolated in the multiple trauma patient. Detailed discussions are found in previous chapters of this book.

A. Head Injuries

1. Head injury usually results from **blunt force** inflicted during motor-vehicle crashes, bicycle crashes, falls, or child maltreatment. Mild (GCS 13 to 15) to

moderate (GCS 9 to 12) head injuries are more common than severe (GCS less than 8). Children with severe head injuries typically require admission to the ICU for management of increased ICP (see Chapter 4).

2. Signs of a **mild to moderate head injury** include persistent vomiting, posttraumatic seizure, and loss of consciousness, usually defined as a GCS of 13 to 15 being mild and 9 to 12 as moderate head injury (Parrillo et al., 2003). Most often, children with mild to moderate head injuries are hospitalized if they have any neurologic deficits, seizures, vomiting, severe headache, fever, prolonged loss of consciousness, skull fracture, altered level of consciousness, or suspected child maltreatment (Vernon-Levett, 2003). The evaluation of children with mild to moderate head injuries includes serial neurologic evaluations with measurement of the level of consciousness, pupillary response, motor and sensory response, and vital signs. Changes in the child's level of consciousness indicate increasing ICP, and treatment must be initiated to prevent subsequent deterioration and possible brainstem herniation. A CT scan without contrast may be performed to identify specific blood collection (that can be surgically evacuated), intraparenchymal injuries, and signs of increased ICP evidenced by compressed ventricles.
3. Signs of a **severe head injury** include a decreased level of consciousness, posturing, combative behavior, and abnormal neurologic findings. Children with severe head injuries require airway and ventilatory control, with a rapid neurologic assessment performed before administration of paralytic and sedative agents. Airway control should be obtained in children with a GCS of 8 or lower. Hypoxemia should be avoided. Hypoxia is defined as apnea, cyanosis, a PaO_2 less than 60 to 65 mm Hg, or oxygen saturation lower than 90%. Hypoventilation should also be avoided and is an indication that assisted ventilation is needed. Hyperventilation is not recommended but may be considered in patients who show signs of cerebral herniation or acute neurologic deterioration after correcting hypotension or hypoxemia. Blood pressure should be monitored frequently. Hypotension can be an indication of spinal or neurogenic shock. Hypotension should be identified and corrected as rapidly as possible. In children, pressure below the 5th percentile for age or by clinical signs of shock must be treated with fluid administration to maintain systolic blood pressure in the normal range (Parrillo et al., 2003). Hypotension with or without hypoxia causes significant mortality rates in children compared with rates in adults (Parrillo et al., 2003). The effect of intracranial hypertension or elevated ICP on outcome after severe brain injury appears to be related to both the absolute peak and duration of elevated ICP and cerebral perfusion pressure (CPP) and compliance. Therefore CPP (MAP – ICP = CPP) should be a parameter that is used in the assessment of hypotension and treatment of ICP. A CPP less than 40 Hg is consistently associated with increased mortality (Parrillo et al., 2003). ICP monitoring is appropriate with TBI traumatic brain injury and maintaining a GCS of 8 or lower (Parrillo et al., 2003). Mannitol may be considered in euvolemic patients who show signs of cerebral herniation or acute neurologic deterioration. IV administration of mannitol (1 g/kg) removes fluid from the interstitial spaces. Prophylactic administration of mannitol is not recommended. Mannitol is administered for signs of acute increases in ICP or for increased pressure with ICP at various infusion rates ranging from 0.25 to 1 g/kg. Phenobarbital or phenytoin/fosphenytoin may be administered to prevent seizures. Fosphenytoin offers several advantages over parenteral phenytoin including the ability to administer intramuscularly or IV without a filter, less discomfort at the infusion site, and a lower potential for cardiac

toxicity. However, the cost has been a limiting factor (Holliday et al., 1998). A CT scan without contrast is performed to determine the extent of the injury, followed by operative management as indicated.

4. Ongoing **assessment and goals of treatment** include measures to ensure adequate cerebral oxygen delivery and prevention of secondary brain injury (Vernon-Levett, 2003). These treatment goals include continuation of previously noted emergency treatment: (1) optimal ventilation and oxygenation; (2) maintenance of normal PCO_2; (3) maintenance of normal ICP and monitoring; (4) ventricular drainage of cerebrospinal fluid (CSF); (5) administration of diuretics (mannitol or lasix); (6) promotion of venous drainage with head midline and head of bed elevation; (7) optimization of systemic arterial pressure and cerebral perfusion pressure along with temperature control and prevention and recognition strategies for seizures; (8) therapeutic options based mainly on adult studies including avoidance of hyperthermia and consideration of hypothermia for refractory intracranial hypertension (Parrillo et al., 2003); and finally, (9) monitoring the child for the potential development of diabetes insipidus (DI).

B. Maxillofacial Injuries

1. Children sustain **maxillofacial injuries** from blunt forces, such as pedestrian, MVC, or bicycle injuries. Maxillofacial injuries include trauma to the dentition, mandible, and midface. Maxillofacial injuries are suspected in children who sustain blunt or penetrating forces to the face. The face is observed for bruising, lacerations, open wounds, and impaled objects. The awake child is asked to open and close the mouth; if the child is unable to do so or malocclusion is present, mandibular fracture is suspected. The face is observed for symmetry, and the cranial nerves are assessed for intactness. The nose is palpated for tenderness and observed for bruising, and the nares are observed for bleeding or blood clots. The face is palpated for "step-offs," tenderness, and pain. The maxilla is palpated between two gloved fingers for continuity. Loose and missing teeth are noted, as is the presence of orthodontic appliances or false teeth. Anteroposterior, open mouth, panorex radiographs, and CT scanning may be obtained in the stable child to determine the extent and location of facial injuries.
2. **Dental injuries** occur from direct forces to the face. In very young children, only the temporary (primary) teeth may be involved; however, if the injury displaces or avulses the temporary dentition, the underlying follicles (the location of the developing permanent teeth) may be involved (Chase, 1995). The most serious damage to teeth occurs in the permanent teeth that have a partially developed root (Chase, 1995).
3. **Mandibular fractures** are classified according to their location: condylar, angle, symphysis, dentoalveolar, and body fracture. Intermaxillary fixation is an option for fractures of the mandibular condyles, whereas open reduction and internal fixation of angle and body fractures are conducted (Chase, 1995). Antibiotics are administered to prevent infection. Scrupulous attention to airway management and oral hygiene are imperative. Children may have concerns about their inability to talk, and alternative methods for communication are required. The older child and adolescent may have concerns about his or her appearance and should be reassured that any bruising and edema will subside over time.
4. **Midfacial fractures** are classified using the Le Fort categories. A Le Fort I fracture is horizontal across the maxilla above the alveolar process and horizontal plate of the palatine and palatal process of the maxilla. The Le Fort II fracture involves the orbital floors, lamina papyracea of the ethmoid bone, and separation of the frontal

nasal suture. A Le Fort III fracture involves craniofacial disarticulation where the facial bones are separated from the cranial buttress systems (Seyfer and Hansen, 2000). Le Fort fractures are treated with internal fixation.

5. **Nasal fractures** occur in the bony pyramid, cartilaginous nasal vault, the septum, or all three. A pediatric speculum is inserted into the naris to observe for a septal hematoma; if not detected early, such a hematoma may lead to an abscess and destruction of the nasal cartilage. Treatment may be immediate or delayed, depending on the child's condition. Treatment includes a closed reduction while the young child receives general anesthesia, whereas a topical cocaine application and local anesthetic with IV sedation may be adequate for older children (Seyfer and Hansen, 2000).

C. Spinal Cord Injuries

1. **Spinal cord injuries without radiographic abnormalities**
   a. Spinal cord injuries occur less frequently than injury to other body systems, but there is a lifelong impact on the child and the family. When these injuries do occur, the outcomes are permanent and devastating. Children have relatively large heads, and the laxity of the juvenile spine allows spinal cord injury to occur without bony abnormalities, a phenomenon known as SCIWORA (*s*pinal *c*ord *i*njury *w*ith*o*ut *r*adiographic *a*bnormalities) (Dickman et al., 1993).
   b. *SCIWORA* is defined as the occurrence of a spinal cord injury despite normal plain radiographic studies. In addition, flexion/extension films of the cervical spine and CT scans are also normal. There are wide differences in the reporting of SCIWORA; its incidence ranges from 5% to 70% of all pediatric spinal cord injuries, depending on the study examined. A true incidence is probably close to 20% of all pediatric spinal cord injuries. SCIWORA occurs almost exclusively among younger children, and two thirds of cases occur in patients 8 years or younger. SCIWORA is very uncommon in adolescents and rare among adults. Cervical and thoracic spinal levels are injured with almost equal frequency, and lumbar levels are rarely involved.
   c. SCIWORA is due to the flexibility of the ligaments and elasticity of the immature spine. A young child's vertebral column can withstand elongation without evidence of deformity even with the presence of a spinal cord injury. The infant spine can withstand up to 2 inches of stretch without disruption. In contrast, the spinal cord ruptures only after 1/4 inch of stretching. Mismatching of elasticity response between the spinal column and spinal cord is the major factor contributing to the high incidence of SCIWORA injuries in young children.
   d. In all cases of suspected SCIWORA injury, an MRI should be performed. It is possible that compressive, treatable lesions may be identified that were not seen on plain films. It is important to understand that once a SCIWORA injury is diagnosed, the child is at increased risk for recurrence of this episode. Recurrent injuries are typically more severe than initial injuries and may have permanent sequelae. Many centers maintain patients in external braces, such as a stiff cervical collar for several months, to prevent further injury. In general, once a diagnosis of SCIWORA is made, most practitioners are very conservative in their approach, and some type of external immobilization is usually necessary for at least 1 to 2 months (Brokmeyer, 1999) (see Chapter 4).
2. **Management of spinal injuries**
   a. *Spinal injuries* are always suspected in multiply injured children. Spinal cord injuries can be divided into *partial* and *complete* loss of function at a given level. Partial injuries can be subdivided into several general types. The *anterior*

cord syndrome is characterized by the loss of corticospinal and spinothalmic pathways, with preservation of posterior column function. The *central cord syndrome* results from injury to the centrally located fibers affecting upper motor limb and spinothalmic function. *Brown-Sequard syndrome* commonly results from penetrating spinal cord injuries and causes damage to the ascending spinothalmic fibers and motor pathways. The region of the spine and the forces that cause them classify bony injuries.

b. Complete *spinal immobilization* is maintained until it is clinically determined that a spinal cord injury is not present. Children with high spinal cord injuries must receive airway control and mechanical ventilation, and children with lower cervical injuries are closely observed for worsening of their respiratory status. Children with high spinal cord lesions may require more IV fluid than children with lower spinal cord lesions because spinal shock causes peripheral vasodilatation (warm shock) and relative hypovolemia. Therefore, at a minimum, normal maintenance infusion rates are required. The infusion of vasopressors, such as dopamine or phenylephrine (Neo-Synephrine), may also be indicated. High dose methylprednisolone (30 mg/kg) is administered early in treatment (within 6 to 8 hours of the injury) to be effective. Lateral, anteroposterior, and odontoid radiographs of the cervical spine are obtained, and anteroposterior and lateral views of the thoracic and lumbar spine are obtained as indicated. Flexion-extension radiographs to determine for stability of the bony canal are not performed until it is determined that spinal cord injury is not present. Such flexion-extension tests may be performed in SCIWORA injury once additional diagnostic testing is completed. Serial neurologic assessments are performed to determine whether the injury is worsening.

c. *Unconscious, multiply injured children* remain in complete spinal immobilization until they are awake and able to complete a neurologic examination. Additional diagnostic tests, such as magnetic resonance imaging (MRI) or somatosensory-evoked potentials (SSEPs), may be indicated to determine the presence or extent of the spinal cord injury. Operative management for bony spinal stabilization or other vertebral repair may be indicated in children with vertebral fractures or dislocations. The treatment of spinal and spinal cord injuries can include external immobilization for temporary stabilization (cervical collars and bed rest) or traction (Gardner-Well tongs) to obtain or maintain alignment. Extended external-fixation devices can be applied, such as a halo vest. An MRI may also be effective in evaluating possible spinal cord injuries in the obtunded, unconscious, or intubated patient (Frank et al., 2002).

D. Thoracic Injuries

1. Thoracic injuries in infants and young children usually result from blunt-force trauma incurred in falls. Older children usually sustain thoracic injuries in MVCs as pedestrians or passengers (Kamerling, 2003). Penetrating chest trauma occurs more often in adolescents from violence.
2. Common thoracic injuries and their symptoms and treatments are outlined in Table 9-3 (see also Chapter 2).

E. Abdominal Injuries

1. **Blunt force** is the most common cause of abdominal trauma in children, with subsequent hemorrhaging a cause for traumatic death. More than 90% of serious abdominal injuries are the result of blunt trauma. The costal margins of the child do not extend down as far as those of an adult and provide little protection for the upper abdominal viscera. The compactness of the abdominal contents allows

TABLE 9-3
Clinical Manifestations and Treatment of Thoracic Injuries

Condition	Clinical Manifestations	Treatment
Rib fractures	Pain Crepitus Bruising	Medicate for pain; splinting
Closed pneumothorax	Dyspnea Tachypnea Decreased or absent breath sounds on the affected side Pain Dullness with percussion	Needle thoracostomy; insertion of chest tube
Open pneumothorax	Sucking noise on inspiration Bubbling noise on expiration Dyspnea Tachypnea	Application of an occlusive dressing, taped on three sides
Tension pneumothorax	Dyspnea Jugular vein distention Decreased or absent breath sounds on the affected side Tracheal deviation away from the affected side Decreased or absent chest wall movement Hyperresonance with percussion Possible mediastinal shift away from the affected side	Needle thoracostomy; insertion of a chest tube
Hemothorax	Dyspnea Tachypnea Tachycardia Pallor Restlessness Hypotension Dullness with percussion Decreased or absent breath sounds	Insertion of a chest tube Fluid resuscitation
Pulmonary contusion	Dyspnea	Oxygenation Ventilation
Cardiac contusion	Tachycardia Dysrhythmias Chest pain	Oxygenation Fluid administration Cardiac monitoring
Tracheobronchial rupture	Crepitus Subcutaneous emphysema Pneumomediastinum Pneumopericardium	Intubation Ventilation
Pericardial tamponade	Beck's triad (muffled heart tones, decreased arterial pressure, elevated venous pressure) Agitation Decreased peripheral perfusion Pulsus paradoxus Jugular vein distention	Ventilation Pericardiocentesis Fluid resuscitation Cardiac monitoring Thoracotomy

From Bernardo LM, Trunzo R: Pediatric trauma. In Kitt S, Selfridge-Thomas J, Proehl J, Kaiser J, editors: *Emergency nursing: a physiologic and clinical perspective,* ed 2. Philadelphia, 1995, W.B. Saunders.

kinetic forces to be transmitted to multiple organs. The most commonly injured organ is the spleen, followed by the liver (McSwain, 2000). Injuries also occur to the pancreas and intestinal tract (see Chapter 7).

2. **Signs of abdominal trauma** include tenderness on palpation and abdominal distention, abrasions, or contusions. Hypovolemic shock may be observed if internal hemorrhaging is present. The absence of bowel sounds does not confirm an abdominal injury because an ileus can occur as a result of the child crying, swallowing air, or being frightened (Fabian and Croce, 2000). Although elevations in liver function test (LFT) results may be noted with liver injuries, such elevations are not specific to the liver trauma. Tenderness in the left upper quadrant may be associated with a splenic injury. Pain in the left shoulder may be elicited on abdominal palpation or deep breathing (Kehr's sign). Elevations of serum amylase and lipase levels indicate a possible pancreatic injury, and a tender mass in the epigastric region may also be palpated (Jurkovich, 2000). Free air may be noted on radiographs when injuries occur to the GI tract, whereas CT scan identifies specific injuries to each solid abdominal organ.
3. Most, if not all, **gunshot wounds** to the abdomen require surgical exploration, whereas many **stab wounds** to the abdomen may be selectively (i.e., observed) managed if the surgeon determines that the knife has not penetrated into the abdominal cavity. CT scanning with contrast is indicated in the stable child who sustains blunt abdominal trauma. This diagnostic method is preferred over peritoneal lavage because of its accuracy in detecting the location and extent of abdominal injuries. Such children receive serial hemoglobin and hematocrit testing to determine if internal bleeding is present. Nursing care involves maintaining IV infusions; an NPO (nothing by mouth) status; and close evaluation of the level of consciousness, circulatory status, and abdominal findings (abdominal girth, presence of pain, tenderness, bruising). Although conservative, nonoperative management is usually indicated for most blunt-force injuries, a surgical approach is indicated if hemorrhaging or peritonitis is suspected. The unstable child who does not respond to fluid resuscitation is prepared for transfer to the operating room for operative management.

F. Genitourinary (GU) Tract Injuries

1. GU tract injuries usually result from **blunt-force trauma** (Simone, 2003); however, the incidence of penetrating trauma is on the rise (see Chapter 5).
2. Injuries to the **female genitalia** occur from falls, straddle injuries, and sexual abuse or assault. Because these injuries are not easily observed in the emergency department, they require examination under anesthesia (EUA) in the operating room (Simone, 2003). Testicular trauma results from straddle-type injuries. Most testicular injuries occur in adolescents who are struck in the scrotum while playing sports or during an altercation (Corriere, 1994). Testicular fractures can be diagnosed with ultrasound and are then repaired. Direct forces are the most common causes of penile injuries (e.g., zipper injuries, toilet seat trauma).
3. The child's GU tract system is **more vulnerable to certain injuries** than is the adult's system. Children's kidneys are larger and have less perinephric fat. The rib cage affords less protection to the kidneys. Preexisting abnormalities (e.g., Wilms' tumor, ectopic kidneys, hydronephrosis) can predispose a kidney to injury. Ureteral elasticity and torso mobility allow for ureteral injuries to occur. The bladder is an abdominal organ in the younger child and is less protected when full. A full bladder can rupture between a car's seat belt and the child's vertebral column as a result of a deceleration injury (American Urological Association, 2004). The bladder neck, especially in girls, is less protected. Boys

are more vulnerable to urethral injuries as a result of the length and position of the urethra (Hoover and Belinger, 1987). The tissues of prepubescent girls are smaller and considerably more rigid than those of the adolescent or adult, thus increasing the risk of tearing with either blunt or penetrating trauma. Prepubescent girls also have a thin vesicovaginal septal wall.

4. Symptoms of **renal trauma** include abdominal, back, or flank tenderness; physical signs include localized abrasions, bruises, lacerations, and hematuria. The degree of hematuria does not correlate with the degree of injury; in fact, minor or no hematuria may occur in serious injuries, such as a renal pedicle or parenchymal injury, and gross hematuria may result from a minor renal trauma (Simone, 2003). Renal injury should be suspected when the lower ribs are fractured. Severe GU tract hemorrhaging can lead to hypovolemic shock.
5. **Urinalysis** evaluation is performed to determine the presence of hematuria. The awake, stable child may be able to void spontaneously. The unstable child may require an indwelling bladder catheter for evaluation and output measurement unless catheterization is contraindicated. A retrograde urethral contrast study should be performed before catheterization in suspected urethral injuries (American Urological Association, 2004). Treatment is specific for the location and extent of the injury, ranging from observation and bed rest to surgical exploration.

G. Musculoskeletal Injuries

1. **Musculoskeletal injuries** commonly occur in children and include open and closed fractures, dislocations, nerve injuries, tendon injuries, and amputations. Growing bones are porous, and the periosteum is strong and thick. These features lead to partial fracturing of the bone, such as greenstick fractures, rather than complete fractures. Although the thicker periosteum allows quicker fracture healing, it may impede fracture reduction (Olney and Toby, 1995). The ligaments are strong, allowing for the higher occurrence of fractures versus ligament injury. Children have an epiphyseal growth plate (physis) located at the articulating ends of the bones between the epiphysis and metaphysis (Phelan, 1994). The physis is responsible for longitudinal bone growth, and injury to the growth plate may result in growth disturbance or arrest. Growth generally is completed in boys by 16 years of age and in girls by 14 years of age. Children who sustain injuries near the physis require follow-up to detect limb-length discrepancies and angular deformities (Olney and Toby, 1995). Nerve and tendon injuries occur from crushing forces, such as wringers, lawn mowers, or farm equipment. Amputations occur from knives, bicycle spokes, and crushing injuries from lawn mowers, farm equipment, motor vehicles, and powerboats.
2. **Musculoskeletal trauma** is suspected in the child with point tenderness; soft-tissue swelling or discoloration; limitations in range of motion; loss of function; altered sensory perception; and changes in pulse, temperature, or capillary refill distal to the injury (Liebman, 2003). Musculoskeletal trauma is rarely life threatening, so the priorities of airway, breathing, and circulation are addressed before treating any fractures. Neurovascular status is assessed before and after any intervention, such as splinting, swathing, or dressing. Analgesics should be administered. Radiographs include the joint above and below the injury and comparative views (radiographs of the injured and uninjured extremities).
3. Most **fractures** are simple and nondisplaced, requiring only the application of a cast. A schematic representation of fractures is found in Figure 9-1. The casted extremity is assessed for swelling of the toes or fingers, odor from the cast, and changes in skin color and temperature. If the child complains of sharp pain or numbness, compartment syndrome should be suspected.

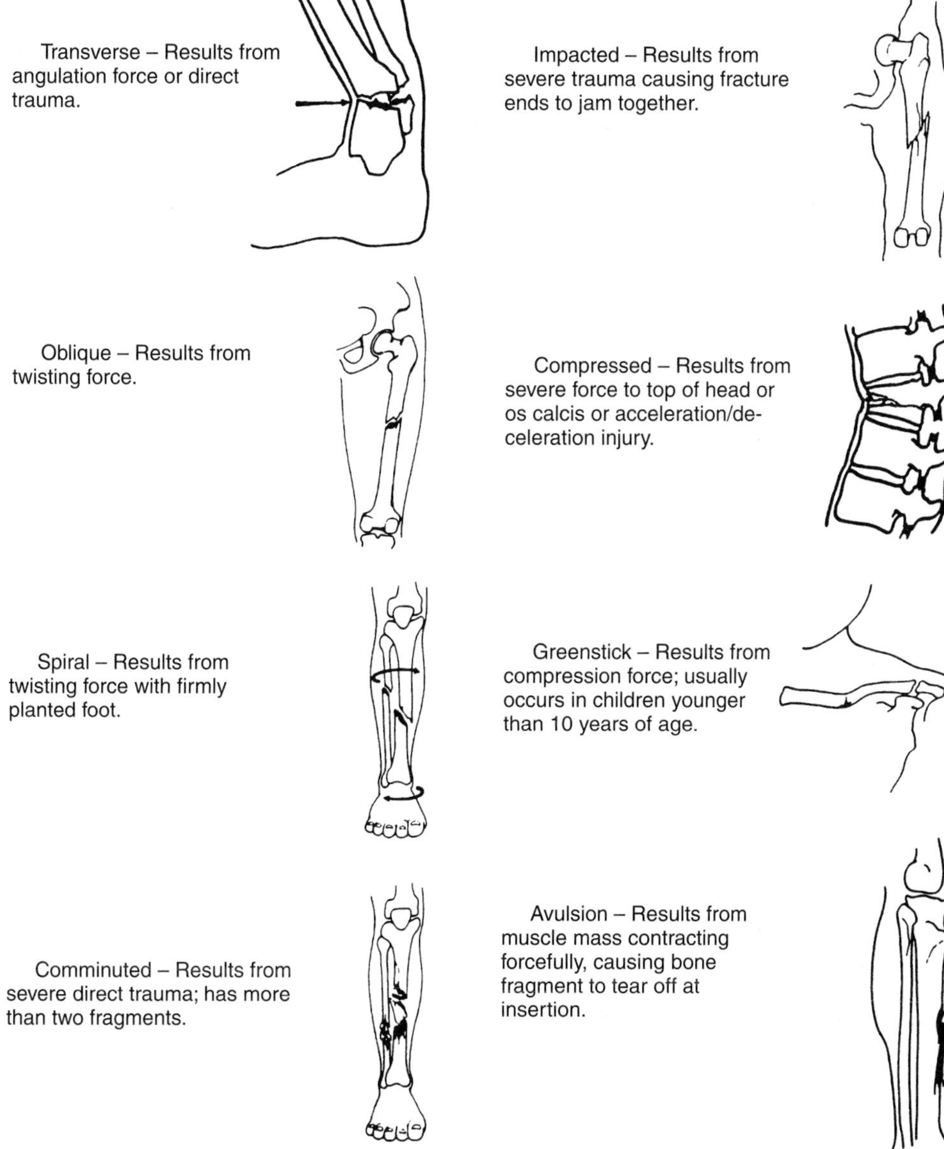

FIGURE 9-1 ■ Types of fractures.

a. *Nondisplaced fractures* may be too edematous to allow casting. In such cases, a splint is applied, and the cast is applied later, when the swelling has resolved. *Displaced fractures* may require a closed reduction, in which the orthopedic specialist and nurse apply manual traction-countertraction to realign the fractured bone. Conscious sedation is administered, using IV analgesics and sedatives such as midazolam, fentanyl, or ketamine. Once the fracture is reduced, the medications are stopped, the cast is applied, and postreduction radiographs are obtained. If the closed reduction was not successful, an open reduction and internal fixation is required.

b. *Open fractures* are divided into three types. *Type I open fractures* are less than 1 cm long, are usually a clean puncture with little soft-tissue involvement (Mason, 2003), and can be treated with casting, provided a window is cut into

TABLE 9-4
Classification of Open Fractures

TYPE I
Wound <1 cm long
Usually moderately clean puncture through which a spike of bone has pierced the skin
Little soft tissue damage
No sign of crushing injury
Fracture usually is simple, transverse, or short oblique with little comminution

TYPE II
Laceration is >1 cm long
No extensive soft tissue damage, flap, or avulsion
Slight or moderate crushing injury
Moderate comminution of fracture
Moderate contamination

TYPE III
Extensive damage to soft tissues, including muscles, skin, and neurovascular structures
High degree of contamination
Great deal of comminution and instability as a result of high-velocity trauma

TYPE IIIA
Soft tissue coverage of bone is adequate despite extensive laceration, flaps, or high-energy trauma
Includes segmental or severely comminuted fractures from high-energy trauma regardless of size of wound

TYPE IIIB
Extensive injury to or loss of soft tissue, with periosteal stripping and exposure of bone
Massive contamination
Severe comminution from high-velocity trauma
After irrigation and debridement, a segment of bone is exposed
Local or free flap is needed for coverage

TYPE IIIC
Any open fracture associated with arterial injury that must be repaired, regardless of degree of soft tissue injury

Mason KJ: Pediatric musculoskeletal trauma. In Moloney-Harmon PA, Czerwinski SJ, editors: *The care of the pediatric trauma patient.* St. Louis, 2003, W.B. Saunders.

the cast to allow for wound visualization and dressing changes. *Type II open fractures* have a laceration larger than 1 cm with slight or moderate crushing and no extensive soft-tissue damage (Mason, 2003). *Type III injuries* have extensive damage to soft tissues, muscle, skin, and neurovascular structures; contamination is present (Mason, 2003). Antibiotics are administered IV; they are also irrigated into the wound. Sterile dressings are applied to open fractures, and tetanus prophylaxis is administered. Debridement is continued every 24 to 48 hours until the wound is clean (Mason, 2003). Types II and III injuries may be treated with external fixation (Table 9-4).

c. *Physeal fractures* are described using the Salter-Harris classification and are outlined in Figure 9-2. Open fractures that involve the growth plate may be treated with smooth K-wires in addition to external fixation (Mason, 2003).
d. *Elbow fractures* occur in children, with supracondylar fractures being the most common. Injury to the brachial artery is most often associated with supracondylar and intercondylar fractures. If a brachial artery injury is

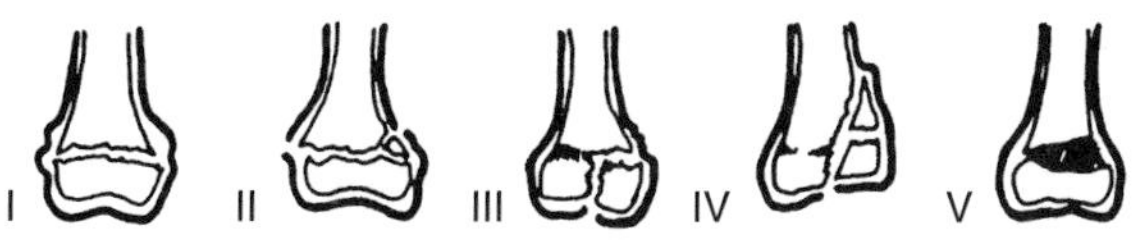

FIGURE 9-2 ■ Salter-Harris classification of physeal injuries.

suspected, an arteriogram must be performed, followed by emergent surgical repair of the vessel (Lewin and Murthy, 2000). If not assessed rapidly and treated properly, complications can result. A complete neurovascular assessment is performed, along with Doppler examination of the arterial blood supply. Unfortunately, compartment syndrome can occur with supracondylar fractures. The consequences of missed compartment syndrome can be devastating, including Volkmann's ischemia or even loss of the limb (Lewin and Murthy, 2000). Operative management for a closed reduction is undertaken. Skeletal or skin traction can be implemented, and closed reduction and percutaneous pinning are options as well (Mason, 2003). Careful ongoing evaluation of the child's neurovascular status is imperative. If the injured arm is the child's dominant one, the child must learn to use the nondominant arm. This learning requires patience, and the child may become frustrated. The prolonged immobilization also plays havoc on the child's development and temperament, and opportunities for creative release of energy are necessary.

e. *Femoral fractures* are common, with about 70% occurring in the midshaft area (Mason, 2003). The injured thigh is swollen, firm, and shortened and may be bruised. The child is unable to move the leg and complains of pain. An anteroposterior radiograph is obtained. Treatment varies according to the child's age. Hip spica casts are applied in infants and toddlers, an intervention that may be performed in the ICU. Most children aged 2 years through 10 years also benefit from the hip spica (Mason, 2003). Spica casting is contraindicated in these children if the shortening is 2 to 3 cm and if there are multiple injuries (Mason, 2003). In cases of shortening, skeletal or skin traction is indicated until early callus formation is observed on radiographs; in multiple injuries, open reduction and external fixation is the treatment of choice (Mason, 2003). Children older than 11 years may receive internal fixation or intermedullary fixation. When skeletal traction is used, pin care is performed on a routine schedule to avoid infection. Signs of pin infection include tenting of the insertion site, redness, and drainage.

- Femur fractures are frequently associated with significant force and therefore can occur in association with head injuries. Spasticity and restlessness are the main challenges for children with moderate to severe head injuries, making femur fracture management complicated. Traction is insufficient to control the fracture fragments, which increases the risk for malunion. Head injury prevents the patient from being able to self-report problems; so skin and compartment assessment is difficult, particularly when early casting was done. Risks associated with traction or casting include malunion, osteomyelitis, skin breakdown, excessive shortening, and rotational deformities (Mason, 2003; Routt, 1998).
- External fixation, IM fixation, and plating are options for stabilizing femur fracture in a head-injured patient. All have distinct advantages. External fixation has the capability to stabilize adjacent joints to prevent excessive soft-tissue movement and contractures (Tolo, 1990). Internal fixation may require supplementary casting and may be useful in older children who are at less danger for growth plate injury (Mason, 2003). Compression plating provides good control of bone fragments, a high rate of union, low risk for

infection, ease of mobilization, and low risk for functionally important limb-length discrepancy (Mason, 2003). Plate removal requires more surgery, and the long scar may have cosmetic disadvantages (Mason, 2003).

- Outcomes and complications of femur fractures in head-injured children are related to ectopic bone formation, particularly around major joints (Hensinger, 1998). Pain and inflammation near a major joint may signal impending ectopic bone formation (Mason, 2003). Physical therapy, pharmacologic management, and additional surgery may be required and subsequently affect recovery.

f. Children with *pelvic fractures* require bed rest. Unstable pelvic fractures may require the application of an external fixation device or, in rare cases, internal fixation may be required. Again, the psychological effects of immobility must be addressed, and options for movement must be given. *Pelvic fractures* are defined as fractures of the bones of the pelvis or a separation of one of the two immobile joints in the pelvis, sacroiliac joint, or symphysis pubis (Mason, 2003). What makes pelvic fractures life-threatening is the close proximity of the orthopedic injury to internal organs and large vessels, the large marrow cavities, and the expansive peritoneal cavity, which can mask bleeding into the abdomen (Mason, 2003). Injuries to the musculoskeletal system, abdomen, and thorax often accompany pelvic fractures as well as multiple contusions and soft-tissue injuries (Mason, 2003).

- Patients with pelvic fracture are at risk for hemorrhage from multiple sources, including osseous, vascular, and visceral structures. Displaced pelvic fractures can injure paravaginal, superior gluteal, and internal iliac arteries, which can compromise the viability of the lower extremity (Mason, 2003).
- Visceral injuries associated with pelvic fracture may be very serious and may involve urologic and neurologic injuries. Specific neurologic injury may include the lumbosacral plexus when sacroiliac disruptions or sacral fractures are incurred (Mason, 2003).
- Another serious complication is infection from contamination of the fracture if it is open and there are communicating or proximal lacerations (Mason, 2003). Emergency pelvic fracture management includes early, immediate immobilization of the pelvis with sand bags, evaluation of associated injuries, and assessment for subtle signs of abdominal bleeding (Mason, 2003). Aggressive replacement of fluid and blood is vital to preventing neurovascular complications to the extremities (Mason, 2003).

H. Nerve injury

Nerve injury is suspected in any crushing trauma. Open wounds near the anatomic location for peripheral nerves should be an indication for nerve involvement (Mason, 2003). Sensory loss is difficult to ascertain in young children; however, two tests can be administered to determine nerve damage. The first test is to observe for a lack of sweating in the affected area using an iodine starch test or a Ninhydrin print test. The second test is the wrinkle test, where the extremity is placed in warm water; if the skin wrinkles, the nerve is intact (Mason, 2003). Nerve injuries are graded from I to V, with grades I through II having the best chances for full recovery. Peripheral nerve injuries tend to heal better in children than in adults; it is believed that the child's brain plasticity assists in nerve regeneration. Children seem to need less formal sensory reeducation following peripheral nerve repair than adults, which may be due to their natural curiosity. The shorter distances required by axons to regenerate before reaching their end-organ may also enhance nerve recovery (Mason, 2003). Moreover, the shorter distances peripheral pain impulses need to travel to reach the cerebral cortex may make up for injury or the degree of nerve myelination.

I. Amputated Digits

1. **Amputated digits or extremities** are classified as *complete* or *incomplete.* Amputated digits or extremities require surgical reimplantation. Such microsurgical techniques are highly specialized and may be available only at level I trauma centers. Before reimplantation, the child's health condition and the condition of the digit or limb must be carefully evaluated. Amputated digits and limbs are carefully wrapped in sterile gauze moistened with NS and placed in a cup or container. The cup or container is then placed in an ice-water bath. The cup is labeled with the child's name, date, and time. An amputated digit cooled according to the aforementioned method can be reimplanted up to 24 hours after the injury (Mason, 2003). The attached body area is assessed for bleeding and neurovascular integrity. The amputated area is carefully wrapped in sterile dressings, and care should be taken to shield the young child's view from the injury. The success of the reimplantation is related to the child's health condition and the viability of the tissues. If the reimplantation is not viable, the child may require prosthesis and subsequent rehabilitation. Unique pain challenges accompany amputation injuries. Emergency management of an incomplete amputation includes controlling bleeding, cleaning the tissue, and cooling the extremity to maximize the tissue viability for reconstruction. Even with viable repairs, rehabilitation may still be required. The child and family should be prepared for the possibility of permanent loss and counseled accordingly.
2. **Neurovascular assessments** include postoperative assessments of arterial and venous circulation. A sign of arterial occlusion is a pale, cool extremity with poor turgor. Brisk bleeding should be noted with a dermal stick and indicates arterial blood flow. A sign of venous occlusion is a cyanotic, cool extremity with tense turgor. The extremity should be elevated unless there are signs of arterial compromise. The patient's room should be warmed to avoid vessel constriction. Postoperative care also includes wound care and dressing changes. The wound may also require further debridements. The patient will receive IV antibiotic therapy (Mason, 2003).

J. Tendon Injuries

Tendon injuries also occur with crush or open injuries, usually in the forearm and hand. The child may not be able to move or wiggle the fingers or refuse to do so because of pain and discomfort. Operative management is necessary to repair tendons. Following tendon repair, the area is assessed for function and neurovascular status; passive flexion exercises are performed with the parents or therapist (Olney and Toby, 1995).

DANGEROUS COMPLICATIONS OF MULTITRAUMA

Dangerous complications of multitrauma include, but are not limited to, rhabdomyolysis, compartment syndrome, fat embolism syndrome (Fort, 2003), and venous thromboembolism (VTE).

A. Rhabdomyolysis

1. **Rhabdomyolysis** is the disintegration of muscle tissue. Injured myocytes release potassium, phosphorous, and thromboplastin. Adenine nucleotides are released and converted to uric acid (Fort, 2003).
2. Several **predisposing trauma-related conditions** are associated with rhabdomyolysis and include crush injuries, electrical shock, severe burns, extended immobility, snake venom, substance abuse (i.e., alcohol, barbiturates,

cocaine, street drug "ecstasy"), tetanus, and reperfusion to damaged cells (as in fasciotomy for compartment syndrome).

3. A classic sign associated with rhabdomyolysis is **dark, reddish brown urine** (Fort, 2003). Laboratory findings reveal that serum CK equals or exceeds a level five times that of normal. Myoglobin is present in the urine. Urine dipstick shows the urine to be heme positive without the presence of red blood cells (RBCs) (Meister and Reddy, 2002). Acute renal insufficiency (elevated BUN and creatinine) is a consequence of severe myoglobinuria wherein the globulin precipitates and blocks the urinary tubules. Myoglobin excretion is facilitated by alkalinization of the urine and increased urine flow. Electrolyte abnormalities may result from rhabdomyolysis, including hyperkalemia and hyperphosphatemia from the damaged muscle cells. Hypocalcemia may develop from the hyperphosphatemia or as a result of calcium deposition in the damaged muscles. Uric acid may be elevated and metabolic acidosis may develop.
4. **Symptoms** associated with rhabdomyolysis include muscle pain, weakness, and cramping. Sinus tachycardia, nausea, vomiting, and fever are other symptoms. Neurologic symptoms of agitation and confusion may be evident. Renal manifestations of rhabdomyolysis may include decreased urine output, potential renal failure, and electrolyte abnormalities. Finally, a patient with this complication may have DIC (Meister and Reddy, 2002).
5. **Nursing implications and treatment:** The nurse caring for a patient with rhabdomyolysis should prepare to normalize electrolyte values; administer IV crystalloids; and administer sodium bicarbonate, insulin, and glucose for hyperkalemia. Administering phosphate-binding antacids and diuretics is part of therapy. In severe instances, the nurse should prepare for Swan Ganz catheter insertion in renal or cardiac disease and anticipate dialysis for irretractable hyperkalemia (Fort, 2003).

B. Compartment Syndrome

1. **Compartment syndrome** is when pressure in the myofascial compartment exceeds capillary perfusion pressure so that blood flow decreases to the tissues within.
2. **Predisposing trauma-related conditions** associated with compartment syndrome include (1) hemorrhage, (2) edema, (3) extravasation, (4) extreme muscle inactivity, (5) external forces (i.e., cast, eschar, tight dressing).
3. **Signs and symptoms** of compartment syndrome include swelling and tenseness along with paresthesia, hypoesthesia, or anesthesia of the affected limb. Complete neuropathy may occur. Other indications of compartment syndrome include warm, shiny skin; loss of pulse (late sign); and, of course, pain.
4. Children who are able to communicate may be able to describe **"loss of two-point discrimination."** This is the inability to distinguish between one or two stimuli (ends of a paperclip) touching the affected extremity.
5. **Nursing implications and treatment:** Nurses have the following responsibilities when treating a patient with compartment syndrome: (1) to keep the affected extremity at the heart level, (2) to perform serial neurovascular examinations at least hourly, (3) to anticipate fasciotomy, and (4) to monitor for the development of rhabdomyolysis.

C. Fat Embolism Syndrome

1. **Fat embolism syndrome (FES)** may be associated with large or multiple bone fractures or intramedullary (bone marrow) manipulation during surgery. FES is a chain of events initiated by the release of fat globules from the bone marrow into the circulation (Fort, 2003). Patients most commonly at risk for trauma-related FES

are those with pelvis, femur, tibia, or rib fractures. Resultant conditions can range from hypoxemia to acute respiratory distress syndrome (ARDS) and DIC (D'Here et al., 1999). The lungs, CNS, and skin are the major organ systems manifesting signs of FES. FES should be considered whenever alveolar-arterial oxygen gradients deteriorate in conjunction with loss of pulmonary compliance and CNS deterioration. As ventilation becomes compromised secondary to decreases in pulmonary compliance, $Paco_2$ levels increase. Hemodynamics deteriorate while pulmonary arterial pressures are increased, often accompanied by decrease in cardiac index (Duke and Rosenberg, 2000).

2. **Nursing implications and treatment:** When caring for a patient at risk for the development of FES, the nurse should move the fractured extremity as little and as carefully as possible before fixation. Arterial blood gases (ABGs), hemoglobin, hematocrit, and platelets should be monitored, and respiratory and neurologic status should be assessed for signs and symptoms of hypoxemia. Fluid and blood therapy may be indicated and, possibly, inatropic support. Treatment of pulmonary dysfunction is supportive (Fort, 2003).

D. Venous Thromboembolism

1. **Risk** for the development of venous thromboemolism (VTE) is related to severe trauma, major vascular injury, central venous catheter placement, and immobilization (Goldhaber and Elliot, 2003a, b). Older age is an increased factor for venous thromboembolism, but it is not clear at what exact age this risk increases substantially. Patients with spinal cord injuries or spinal fractures are at high risk for venous thromboembolism following trauma (Eastern Association for the Surgery of Trauma, 2005).
2. **Nursing implications** for the prevention of VTE: Consider applying sequential compression devices (SCDs) if the patient is at risk and unable to ambulate or perform leg and foot exercises (Cummings and Byrum, 2001). The nurse should avoid applying sequential compression devices when local leg conditions exist that would be compromised by the sleeves (e.g., dermatitis, vein ligation, skin graft, incisions). Ischemic vascular disease, massive edema of legs, pulmonary edema from congestive heart failure (CHF), extreme deformity or contracture of leg, and suspected preexisting VTE are additional contraindications for the use of SCD.
3. **Prevention strategies** that nurses can support include the following: The nurse should assess pedal and posterior tibial pulses every 2 hours for patients at risk. Assessing pulse quality and capillary refill is important. Observe for the presence of cyanotic nail beds, cooler skin temperature, numbness, and tingling. Teach the child and family to report pain and cramping in the lower legs immediately. Removal of SCDs may be necessary in the event of hypotension. The child's family should be taught to avoid massaging the lower legs if they begin to hurt (Crowther and McCourt, 2004).

CHILD MALTREATMENT

A. Definition

1. **Child maltreatment** (child abuse and neglect) is any recent act or failure to act on the part of a caregiver that results in death or serious physical or emotional harm, sexual abuse, or exploitation. This also includes any act or failure to act that presents an imminent risk of serious harm. Child fatalities are the ultimate tragic consequences of maltreatment (Kelley, 2003).

2. **The Child Abuse Prevention and Treatment Act** identifies four major types of maltreatment. *Physical abuse* is the infliction of physical injury to a child. *Child neglect* is failure to provide for a child's basic needs. Child neglect can be physical, educational, or emotional and includes withholding medical treatment. *Sexual abuse* comprises one or some combination of the following activities: fondling a child's genitals, intercourse, incest, rape, sodomy, exhibitionism, and exploitation. **Emotional abuse** involves verbal abuse or mental injury. *Emotional abuse* can be understood in terms of actions or lack thereof that could cause or have caused serious behavioral, cognitive, emotional, or mental disorders (CDC, *Child Maltreatment*, 2004).

B. Etiology and Incidence

1. Numerous **parental and child factors** place a family at risk for child maltreatment (Table 9-5).
2. **Reporting** suspected child maltreatment by nurses and health care professionals is mandated by law. Critical-care nurses who suspect child maltreatment are required to report their suspicions to their local child abuse hotline. Reporters need not have actual knowledge of abuse or neglect (Kelley, 2003). A professional who postpones reporting until all doubt is eliminated probably violates the reporting law. Deliberate failure to report suspected abuse is a crime (Myers, 2002). Reporting is made in good faith, and follow-up by the local child welfare agency is required within a specified period. No litigation can be brought against a nurse for filing a suspected child maltreatment report in good faith. Although it may not seem feasible for a parent to elope from the hospital with a critically ill child, the nurse should consider the need to make arrangements with hospital security in the event this might happen (Kelley, 2003).

C. History of the Injury

1. Child physical abuse is suspected based on the **physical findings and the history** surrounding the injury. The history, in relation to the injury, is what differentiates intentional from unintentional injury.
2. The **history of the injury** should be obtained and well documented. Characteristics of the history that are consistent with child abuse include the following: the history is inconsistent with the injury; the caregiver denies any knowledge of how the injury occurred; the caregiver is reluctant to divulge information or changes the story; the child is developmentally incapable of the injury; there is a delay in seeking treatment; the child has prior hospitalizations or injuries; the caretaker's response is inappropriate to the level of injury; and there is a history of previous placement in foster care or with a child protective agency. All communication is documented using the child's and the caregiver's own words (Kelley, 2003).

D. Physical Abuse

1. **Cutaneous injuries** (e.g., bruises, bite marks, burns) occur from excessive force applied to the child from an adult caretaker and constitute one specific manifestation of physical abuse injury.
2. **Bruises**
   a. Any *bruises* must be evaluated in light of the plausibility of the injury event as stated by the caretaker, the child's health history, the child's level of development, the presence of other injuries, and laboratory data. A cardinal finding is a mismatch with existing injury and the provided history (Kelley, 2003).

TABLE 9-5
Common Indicators of Child Maltreatment

FAMILY BEHAVIORS
Inappropriate parent-child interaction
Extremes of reactions to hospital staff (e.g., hostile, unconcerned)
Unrealistic expectations of the child
Parental denial of any knowledge of how injury occurred
Attribution of blame to sibling for injury
Inappropriate response to severity of injury by parent, such as underreacting or overreacting to child's condition

CHILD BEHAVIORS
Extremes of behaviors (e.g., withdrawn, acting out)
Lack of opposition to painful procedures
Developmental delays
Inappropriate sexual behavior
Somatic complaints (e.g., chronic headaches, sleep disorders, enuresis)
Suicidal behavior and threats
Drug or alcohol abuse

HISTORICAL FINDINGS
Story inconsistent with physical findings or developmental level
Delays in seeking medical treatment
Direct disclosure
Repeat visits to the emergency department

PHYSICAL FINDINGS
Multiple injuries in various stages of healing
Injury type and location inconsistent with child's developmental level
Characteristic pattern reflective of object used to cause injury (e.g., belt marks)
Signs of poor overall care
Genital bleeding or discharge in prepubescent children

RADIOGRAPHIC FINDINGS
Multiple fractures
Cortical metaphyseal fragmentation
Traumatic involucrum*
Skull fractures†
Suture separation

From Czerwinski SJ, Moloney-Harmon PA: Intenational injuries. In Moloney-Harmon PA, Czerwinski SJ, editors: *The care of the pediatric trauma patient.* St. Louis, 2003, W.B. Saunders.
*Not visible radiographically until 7 to 18 days after trauma.
†Evident immediately after trauma.

b. *Bruises* commonly occur in young children as they run and play. Normally, bruises are small, few, and found on the extensor surfaces, such as the shins, elbows, chin, and knees. Bruises indicative of physical abuse are found on the face and head and on areas protected by clothing. Periorbital hematomas are especially suspicious for maltreatment. Bruises found on the chest, abdomen, thighs, buttocks, and back are also suspicious for physical abuse. These bruises are usually in various stages of healing and are numerous. Bruises that have the appearance of an object, such as a belt buckle, hand imprint, or looped electrical cord, are always treated as abuse (Kelley, 2003).

- In infants, bruises may be seen near the mouth, lips, and frenulum resulting from physical forces when the caretaker repeatedly attempts to force-feed a bottle into the infant's mouth. Bruises or rope burns may be found around the neck, wrists, or ankles and indicate that the child was restrained. Blistering and abrasions may be present, which may indicate the child's struggle against the restraints. The restraints can be made of rope, cloth, strap, or chain (Kelley, 2003). In infants and young children, paired oval bruises or pinch marks may be found on the cheeks, arms, earlobes, and other areas from human sources (Kelley, 2003).
- School-age children who have repeatedly been subjected to beatings and bruising prefer to wear long-sleeved and long-legged clothing, even in warm weather, to hide the marks.

3. **Bite Marks**

Bite marks are another cutaneous manifestation that is highly indicative of child abuse. Adult bite marks are differentiated from child bite marks by measuring the maxillary intercanine distance; a distance greater than 3 cm indicates that an adult bit the child (Kelley, 2003).

4. **Burns**

a. Burns occur from scalding liquids and contact with hot objects. Flame burns can be implicated in child abuse, such as in arson. An unintentional scald burn can occur if the young child pulls a crock pot or pot of hot liquid onto himself or herself. The intensity of the burn would be greatest about the head, with the depth of burn tapering off as it reaches the chest. An intentional scald injury has a circumscribed area of injury that is full thickness and depicts the patterned configuration of a heating object (e.g., steam irons, curling irons, car cigarette lighters). Usually no splash pattern is seen with intentional burns (Kelley, 2003).

b. The following sample scenarios will help the critical care nurse differentiate between intentional and nonintentional injury.

In response to a young child who soiled himself during toilet training, the caretaker dunks the child's buttocks into a tub of hot water. The resulting scald injury is isolated to the perineum and buttocks. A donut-shaped scarring to the buttocks may be present if the child's buttocks were held against the tub itself. In contrast, a child who inadvertently fell into a tub would have burns about the head or side of the body (Kelley, 2003).

A curious child may suffer an unintentional hand burn by submerging the hand into a bucket of water. The resulting burn would be irregular, partial thickness in depth, and circumferential, as the pain response causes the child to quickly withdraw the hand. On the other hand, the child who suffers an intentional burn has a body part held in hot water by the caretaker. The resultant burn is circumferential, full thickness, and has a clear line of demarcation at the wrists or ankles. The flexion creases are spared from the burn (Kelley, 2003).

A child with any burn in an unlikely place, such as the soles of the feet, buttocks, or perineum must be treated as an intentional injury and investigated accordingly (Kelley, 2003). ■

5. **Internal organ injuries**
   a. As with cutaneous lesions, the history of an internal organ injury is important to ascertain. Internal organ injuries occur from blunt forces applied to the children as they are struck, kicked, punched, beaten, thrown, or stabbed by caretakers. The manifestations of internal organ injury are the same in both unintentional and intentional trauma. Liver lacerations, splenic rupture, pulmonary and cardiac contusions, as well as brain injury can occur through child maltreatment. Blunt abdominal trauma, the most common type of inflicted abdominal trauma in children, is usually the result of a child's being punched or kicked in the abdomen (Ludwig, 2001). Intra-abdominal hemorrhage may result with few external signs. Visceral injuries rarely produce immediate specific signs or symptoms that lead to prompt identification (Ludwig, 2001). Inflicted abdominal injury should be suspected when there are (1) clear signs of abdominal trauma, (2) unexplained shock, (3) unexplained cardiac arrest, (4) unconsciousness with suspected inflicted head injury, and (5) unexplained unconsciousness (Kelley, 2003). Severe internal injuries might not be immediately detected because of the parent's failure to give an accurate history of trauma and also because little or no external evidence of abdominal trauma is seen at the time of examination (Kelley, 2003). Children who sustain child maltreatment tend to be younger and preverbal, and thus unable to verbalize how the injury occurred (see Table 9-5). These children are usually brought in for treatment because of worsening signs of injury, such as abdominal distention, vomiting, or other vague parental history or complaints.

An 8-year-old boy is admitted for a fractured spleen from repeated punching to his abdomen by his mother's boyfriend. He lies motionless with O_2 delivery by a face tent. Several hours pass without the RN administering pain medication that is ordered PRN (as needed) "because he does not appear to be in pain." On closer inspection, the boy's SVO_2 is in the low 90s and he is rigid and clenching his fists. Chest expansion is shallow with ineffective respirations. The next nurse administers his pain medication routinely. His O_2 requirement decreases and his SpO_2 improves. This nurse suspects the patient did not complain of pain or rate it as high because of the fear of being punched by another adult. ■

   b. Emergent situations are those involving children brought to the hospital for treatment who have unstable vital signs, severe dehydration, or malnutrition with possible progression to shock and life-threatening injuries (Kelley, 2003). When rib fractures are present, a significant force was applied to the chest (usually squeezing), and maltreatment must be suspected and investigated (Kelley, 2003). Treatment for inflicted abdominal and chest trauma is the same as for unintentional injury.

6. **Long-bone fractures**
   a. *Maltreated children* sustain long-bone fractures as their extremities are twisted and pulled by caretakers or from being thrown or beaten. Fracture patterns are consistent with the applied blunt forces and include spiral fracture of long bones (from intentional twisting), rib, skull, nose or facial fractures, and femur fractures in children younger than 1 year of age. Fractures to the sternum, spinous processes, scapulae, and humeral fractures are see in children younger than 3 years and are a result of blunt forces (Kelley, 2003). The young child is brought for treatment because of an inability to use an arm or to bear weight on a leg. The injured extremity appears deformed, painful, and swollen, as in unintentional musculoskeletal trauma.

TABLE 9-6
Diagnostic Tests Associated with Suspected Child Maltreatment

Laboratory Studies	Comments/Rationale
COMPLETE BLOOD COUNT	
Hematocrit, hemoglobin	Rules out shock, anemia
	Rules out organic cause of bruising or bleeding
Coagulation studies	
Prothrombin time, partial thromboplastin time, platelets	Elevated levels may be the first indicator of abdominal injury
	Elevated levels are indicative of extensive soft tissue and muscle injury
SERUM	
Amylase	Rules out sexually transmitted disease; all ages; suspected sexual abuse
Creatine phosphokinase	
Syphilis serology	Rules out pregnancy; all postmenarche girls with history suggesting sexual abuse
Human chorionic gonadotropin	Rules out forced or voluntary ingestions and chemical abuse
Toxicology screen	Rules out renal trauma, dehydration, ingestions, sexual abuse
URINE	
Red blood cells, specific gravity, toxicology screen, culture, pregnancy test, sperm	Culture for gonorrhea, *Chlamydia,* and other sexually transmitted diseases is especially important with suspected sexual abuse
	Microscopic examination for sperm; may be omitted if >72 h since abuse incident or if child has bathed
CULTURES	
Wounds, throat, vaginal, rectal	
VAGINAL SECRETIONS	*Trichomonas,* yeast, or *Gardnerella* infections
Vaginal wet preparation	
Saline and potassium hydroxide with whiff test	
RADIOLOGIC STUDIES	
Skeletal X-ray film: skull, ribs, extremities	Rules out fractures; common findings are multiple fractures
	Detects remote injuries and extremely recent injuries
Bone scans	Important in detecting subtle intracranial and internal abdominal injuries
Ultrasound, computed tomography scan, magnetic resonance imaging	

From Czerwinski SJ, Moloney-Harmon PA: Intentional injuries. In Moloney-Harmon PA, Czerwinski SJ, editors. *The care of the pediatric trauma patient.* St. Louis, 2003, W.B. Saunders.

7. **Head trauma**
   a. *Head trauma* from child abuse is the most common cause of child abuse–related death and can also result in brain damage, psychological dysfunction, and physical impairments (Alexander et al., 2001). Head trauma occurs from blunt forces (impact, shaking), penetrating forces (bullet), and lack of oxygenation (asphyxia). Impact injury occurs when the child is struck by a caretaker's hand or object or the child is thrown against an unyielding surface. Resulting injuries include brain insults, skull fractures, facial fractures, and possible eye and ear injuries. Penetrating injuries occur from bullets, knives, or other

objects projected at the child. Again, direct injuries to the brain, head, and face occur. Asphyxia from gagging or choking to stop the child's crying can lead to ischemia and brain damage (Kelley, 2003).

b. Probably the most well-known form of child abuse is *shaken impact syndrome* (Alexander et al., 2001). This syndrome occurs in children younger than 2 years. The child is held by the chest facing the caretaker, and the chest is compressed during the shaking episode. This shaking may cause grip marks to the chest and arms as well as rib and humerus fractures (Kelley, 2003). Violent shaking leads to subdural hematoma formation, metaphyseal chip fractures, and retinal hemorrhages (Kelley, 2003). High spinal cord injury can occur as well. The shaken infant may display lethargy, poor sucking ability, irritability, rhythmic eye opening and deviation, decerebrate or decorticate posturing, seizures, and alterations in muscle tone and responsiveness to voice, touch, or pain. The child presents for treatment either seizing, in cardiac arrest, or with a history of a seizure. The definitive finding in shaken impact syndrome is the presence of retinal hemorrhages; therefore careful ocular examinations are imperative in any young child with a vague history who has seizures or cardiac arrest.

8. *Diagnostic tests* for child maltreatment are summarized in Table 9-6.
9. **Treatment** is initiated based on the extent of the injuries. Surface bruises are photographed, and these photographs are placed in the child's medical record. The child protective agency is contacted. The caretaker or parent is informed of the suspicion of child maltreatment, whose reactions may range from relief to anger. It is best to have this information given to the family by the physician with a nurse or social worker in attendance. The hospital's security officers may need to be nearby in the event the family reacts violently. Abused children may be placed in foster care, and legal action may be taken against the family.
10. In the ICU, abused children may die of their injuries. Because the nurse is in the position to support both the child and family, it may be very difficult to support suspected perpetrators who inflicted the life-threatening injuries. Furthermore, if the child dies of the injuries, homicide charges may be filed. Nurses who care for such children may need support from other resources within the hospital.

E. Sexual Abuse

1. **Sexual abuse** is often defined as the involvement of children or adolescents in sexual activities they do not understand, to which they cannot give informed consent, or that violate sexual taboos (Finkel and DeJong, 2001). Sexual abuse includes exhibitionism; digital or object penetration of the rectum or vagina; sexual touching; vaginal penile or rectal penile penetration; pornography; and prostitution (Kelley, 2003; Reece, 2000). Like physical abuse, sexual abuse involves a host of family, child, and societal factors. Incest, for example, is allowed to continue in families who do not protect their children or who fail to have appropriate caretakers available. Children may be groomed by a perpetrator for increasing sexual involvement over a period of time. The relationship is kept secret and involves threats of harm or special favors. This may be confusing to the child because the activity may "feel good." Children do not know or understand the precise physical act of intercourse. It must be taught (Kelley, 2003). The child feels guilty and betrayed as he or she continues in the relationship. If the child does come forward, the child's story may be discounted, allowing the abuse to continue.
2. **Sexual abuse** happens to both genders, to children of all ages, and to children in every socioeconomic strata. Poverty, drug abuse, alcoholism, an unhappy family life, and living in a family without one or both natural parents may make the child vulnerable to this abuse (Finkel and DeJong, 1994).

3. **Sexual assault (rape)** occurs in children and adolescents and is the forcible act of intercourse. Young children who are victims of sexual abuse tend to act out sexually with their peers, siblings, and adults. They exhibit precocity in sexual remarks or questions that demonstrate their increased awareness of sexual behavior, and frequent and compulsive masturbation may be present (Kelley, 2003). Extreme fears, self-esteem disturbance, and lack of control are nursing diagnoses associated with sexual abuse (Kelley, 2003). These children become obsessed with cleanliness to remove blood or secretions and to avoid "feeling dirty." They have a preoccupation with genital references and may even draw them, a finding that is uncommon in children without sexual abuse. Adolescents may become runaways, develop suicidal thoughts, and engage in prostitution (Kelley, 2003).
4. **Assessment and treatment:** The child with suspected sexual abuse may be brought in for treatment by a caretaker. The caretaker may state that abuse is known, or the caretaker may state that the child has a vaginal or penile discharge or dysuria. Herpetic lesions to the mouth may be another complaint for treatment. Sexual abuse should be suspected in pregnant, young adolescents (10 years to 14 years of age), especially if the pregnancy is concealed, or with vaginal or penile discharge, foreign bodies, sexually transmitted diseases, or rectal or vaginal pain (Kelley, 2003).
5. **The sexually abused or assaulted child must undergo a physical examination and interview.** Experienced professionals in the care of these children must conduct these examinations to avoid contamination of evidence and to allow the child to tell the story only once. The *physical examination* may be deferred in the child with sexual abuse if the last episode occurred more than 72 hours before presentation (Kelley, 2003). If the sexual abuse or assault occurred within 72 hours, the physical examination can be initiated.
6. The **physical examination** may be done with a parent or caretaker present, provided that person is not the perpetrator. One nurse or rape crisis counselor assumes the role of support person, while another nurse assists with obtaining and labeling the specimens. The child can be placed on an adult's lap in the frog-leg position or assume a knee-chest position on the examination table. The left lateral decubitus position allows for examination of the rectum. If at any point the child does not cooperate with the examination and becomes upset and fearful, the examination is stopped. An examination under anesthesia is then performed. The child is never restrained or forced to comply with the examination. Secondary abuse is caused by a physical examination that is so overzealous that it assumes a rape-like quality in the mind of the child (Ludwig, 2000). The external genitalia are examined, and cultures for syphilis, gonorrhea, and chlamydia are obtained. Any lacerations, bruising, and bleeding are noted. A Wood's lamp is also used to observe for semen; a wet prep for sperm or semen detection is also obtained. In the adolescent female victim, a bimanual pelvic examination is indicated. In young females, a pediatric ear speculum may be used to visualize the cervix and cultures are again obtained. The rectal area is examined for bruising, bleeding, or tearing, and cultures are obtained. In the male child, similar cultures of the meatus and rectum are obtained, and both areas are observed for bruising, lacerations, or tearing.
7. All **evidence** is obtained carefully and is secured in an assault kit that is usually provided by the local law enforcement agency. Such kits have prelabeled envelopes for specimen collection. Aside from the cultures, other specimens include a saliva sample, pubic hairs, a comb used to comb the hairs, fingernail scrapings, and blood specimens for Venereal Disease Research Laboratory (VDRL), human immunodeficiency virus (HIV), hepatitis B, and human

chorionic gonadotropin (HCG). Postmenarchal females are usually given the option to take a high dose of oral contraceptives to prevent pregnancy. Pharyngeal cultures are also obtained. The specimens are then sealed, and the collecting nurse's name is written on the outside of the collection box. The box is then hand delivered to the hospital police for safe keeping; then everyone must sign for the box, or it is handed directly to the law enforcement agent, who signs for the box. This chain of evidence avoids potential evidence mishandling or tampering, either of which may jeopardize the legal process. The child's clothes are also obtained and placed in paper bags and given to law enforcement. Follow-up is completed through the hospital, rape crisis center, or regular health care professional.

8. The examining professional carefully **documents** all the physical findings; the nurse documents the chain of evidence and the child's reaction to the examination. The sexually abused or assaulted child is interviewed by a trained professional. The parent or caretaker and child are interviewed separately. The child is not asked any leading questions and is simply asked to talk about what happened. The child may use puppets or dolls to demonstrate what occurred; using paper and crayons for drawing allows the nonverbal or preverbal child to depict the situation. The child is told that he or she did the right thing by coming forward with the story and that the child did not do anything wrong (Kelley, 2003).

F. Neglect

1. **Neglect** is the most prevalent type of child maltreatment; it involves omitting the child's basic needs, including food, shelter, clothing, health care, and a safe environment (Kelley, 2003). Neglect may go undetected when it is associated with poverty. Other factors that may be associated with neglect include parental substance abuse, low self-esteem, social isolation, reliance on physical punishment for discipline, depression, and lack of knowledge regarding growth and development (Kelley, 2003).
2. Neglected children may be brought for **treatment** by law enforcement authorities that respond to a complaint from a neighbor. Although it is unlikely that a child will enter the ICU for neglect alone, signs of neglect should be observed for in children who are admitted for possible child maltreatment, ingestions, or drug overdoses.

G. Psychological Maltreatment (Emotional Abuse)

Emotional abuse usually occurs with other maltreatment forms. In such instances, the caretakers or parents do not provide a nurturing environment. These caretakers berate, belittle, degrade, terrorize, isolate, and reject their children (Kelley, 2003). Signs of emotional abuse include sleep and feeding disorders, hyperactivity, developmental delays, and excessively passive or aggressive behavior. Again, although admission to the ICU is not usually warranted for emotional abuse, these behaviors may be observed in children who are in the ICU for other reasons. Such behaviors should be brought to the attention of the physician and social worker so that investigations into the child's home life can be conducted.

H. Munchausen Syndrome by Proxy (MSBP)

1. **Munchausen syndrome by proxy (MSBP)** is defined by the American Professional Society on the Abuse of Children as a form of child abuse. The child is a victim of maltreatment in which an adult (often the biologic mother) falsifies physical or psychological (or both) signs and symptoms in the child, causing this child to be regarded as ill or impaired (Thomas, 2003). Characteristically, MSBP

is hidden, difficult to detect, and often undiagnosed (Thomas, 2003). The perpetrator gains support of the health care team through skilled deceit, leading professionals to believe she is a devoted, loving mother. The perpetrator "doctor shops" and "hospital jumps" so that tracking the child's true medical history is virtually impossible.

2. Perpetrators usually have the following **commonalities**: (1) feeling unwanted as children; (2) hating their children because of feelings of jealousy over their happy childhood; (3) the medical staff's acceptance motivated them to continue harming their children (Hughes and Corbo-Richert, 1999); (4) suffering some loss through maternal rejection; (5) suffering a lack of maternal attention or love during infancy (Karlin, 1995).
3. MSBP is a **family disorder**. Marital discord is often present. The father may rarely visit his child and may be oblivious to his partner's behavior. Siblings may have complicated medical histories. There may be a history of unexplained SIDS of a sibling. More than one SIDS death is reason for a high index of suspicion (Fulton, 2000).
4. **Countless methods of abuse** may mark this disorder. They include but are not limited to the following: (1) falsifying signs and symptoms (e.g., apnea, cardiac arrest, GI bleeding); (2) poisoning (e.g., insulin, table salt, fingernail polish remover); (3) contamination of blood, urine, or stool samples to feign a false result; (4) injection of urine, stool, saliva or blood in IV access ports; (5) intentional suffocation; (6) blowing air in the gastric tube; (7) application of caustic substances to the skin; (8) withdrawal of blood from the IV line to cause anemia; (9) adding blood to the diaper to feign a GI bleed; (10) pouring chocolate milk (or similar substance) over the child and linen to resemble vomit; (11) excessive compassion toward the child when caregivers are present and ignoring the child when caregivers are not present (Thomas, 2003).
5. Critical care nurses must be knowledgeable of the medicolegal implications surrounding **documentation**. Documentation should describe details of the actual observation of the mother's behavior, including interaction with the child, staff, physician, and spouse. Pertinent quotations should be documented, including precise recording of the patient's condition with and without the suspected perpetrator present (Thomas, 2003). Examples of effective documentation in MSBP might include an exerpt like the following:

1155: Mother not at bedside. Vital signs (VS) stable. BP 110/60, HR 112.
1205: Mother at bedside; stood near dopamine and epinephrine infusions. BP 60/35, HR 38.
1206: Intensivist notified and patient hand-bagged; CPR started. Mother left room.
1207: VS stable and return to normal.
1220: Mother makes trip to the gift shop; asks RNs if they want a soda.
1400: Father wakes mother from nap in parents' lounge; Father told RNs he knew nothing about his child being that sick. Mother and father have a loud argument.
1600: Mother returns from a fast-food restaurant and returns to the bedside.
1605: Nurse finds brown "emesis" all over the bed linen.

Toxicology

Rose Ann Gould Soloway

Most poison exposures in children are managed safely at home with the guidance of the poison center. However, critical-care nurses must recognize; consult with the poison center about; and treat those exposures that are most likely to cause serious injury, illness, or death and therefore those most likely to require treatment in an intensive care unit (ICU).

DEFINITIONS

A. Poisoning Versus Overdose

The term *poison* is often used to refer to nonpharmaceutical substances, and *overdose* is used for pharmaceuticals; however, any substance that enters the body and causes harm is a poison, and therefore the term *poisoning* is used in this section to describe the consequences of any exposure resulting in injury, illness, or death.

B. Poison Exposure

Poison exposure means some type of inappropriate contact with a potentially harmful substance. Such exposure can be through ingestion, inhalation, ocular or dermal contact, or parenteral injection.

C. Routes of Exposure

The manner in which a potentially toxic substance enters the body can influence the time of onset, intensity, and duration of toxic effects. Statistically, most poisonings occur by ingestion. However, never overlook the importance of other routes of exposure, for example, inhalation and dermal routes for organophosphate insecticides; inhalation, nasal, and parenteral routes for drugs of abuse; ocular, dermal, oral, and inhalation for caustic chemicals; inhalation for gases, fumes, and vapors; and parenteral for envenomations. Except for chemical exposures whose effects are confined to the site of exposure, the effects of a poison exposure are determined by the degree of absorption of the substance into the bloodstream, the extent of metabolism to a less toxic or more toxic substance, distribution to target organs, and ultimate elimination from the body.

D. Acute Versus Chronic Exposure

Most poison exposures in children are the result of acute ingestion. Chronic overdoses, or an acute overdose of a drug also taken for a long period, are possible for children who require therapeutic drugs for medical conditions. Chronic exposures are also possible for those abusing drugs, for victims of child abuse, and for victims of Munchausen syndrome by proxy. Kinetics, toxic blood levels, and clinical manifestations of poisoning may differ with acute and chronic administration of a drug.

ROLE OF THE POISON CENTER

The poison center is the source of expert clinical toxicology information. Twenty-four hours a day, 7 days a week, the physicians, nurses, and pharmacists at the poison center can assist in a number of ways:

- Providing expert advice about poisoning by drugs (legal, illegal, foreign, veterinary), household products, industrial chemicals, hazardous materials, environmental toxins, chemical warfare agents, drugs to treat exposure to biological warfare agents, snakes, spiders, plants, mushrooms, and pill identification.
- Determining whether a complex of symptoms could be caused by poisoning.

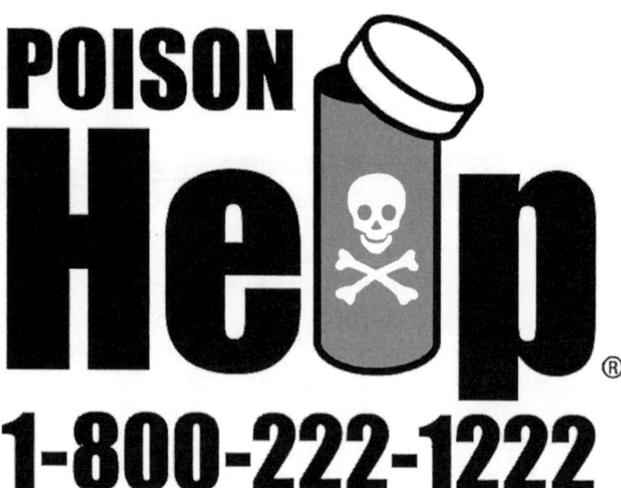

FIGURE 9-3 ■ The new nationwide phone number for poison centers automatically connects callers with the local poison center.

- Locating sources for unusual antidotes (e.g., botulinum antitoxin, exotic snake antivenins), treatments, and laboratory studies.
- Conducting clinical and epidemiologic research.

Each patient becomes an anonymous part of a national database, which collectively identifies actual and in some cases previously unsuspected hazards. These data are uploaded by your local poison center in real time to the American Association of Poison Control Centers Toxic Exposure Surveillance System as part of syndromic surveillance for public health threats. Data also are used to reformulate or repackage products or to require removal of products from the market. The Joint Commission on Accreditation of Healthcare Organizations requires that the poison center phone number be posted in every health care facility. Phone stickers and posters are available from the poison center serving each area.

All U.S. poison centers share the same phone number, 1-800-222-1222 (Figure 9-3). Calls are routed automatically to the local poison center according to the area code and telephone exchange.

EPIDEMIOLOGY AND ETIOLOGY

A. Epidemiology

1. The most comprehensive source of information about poison exposures in the United States is the Annual Report of the American Association of Poison Control Centers Toxic Exposure Surveillance System, published each September in *The American Journal of Emergency Medicine* and on the Web at www.aapcc.org. It allows differentiation between common but relatively benign poison exposures and those with serious consequences.
2. In 2003 there were 2,395,582 poison exposures reported to 64 poison centers in the United States. More than 92% of these exposures occurred in a residence. In 74.5% of reported cases, the poison exposures were managed over the telephone without the patient's needing to seek hands-on medical care. A summary of the number of pediatric exposures and fatalities is in Table 9-7 (Watson, 2003).
3. The most common poison exposures in children during 2003 are listed in Table 9-8, and Table 9-9 lists those substances associated with the largest number of fatalities in all ages. This section focuses on the most dangerous poison exposures, rather than the most common.

TABLE 9-7
Number of Pediatric Poison Exposures, 2003

Age	No. of Exposures	Percent of All Exposures	No. of Fatalities	Percent of All Fatalities
Under 6	1,245,584	52.0	34	3.1
6-12	158,316	6.6	7	0.6
13-19	171,823	7.2	65	5.9

Watson WA, Litovitz TL, Klein-Schwartz et al.: 2003 Annual report of the American Association of Poison Control Centers Toxic Exposure Surveillance System. *Am J Emerg Med* 22(5):335-404, 2004.

TABLE 9-8
Most Common Poison Exposures in Children, 2003

Under Age 6 Years	Age 6-19 Years
Cosmetics and personal care products	Analgesics
Cleaning substances	Cough and cold preparations
Analgesics	Antidepressants
Foreign bodies	Foreign bodies
Topical medicines	Bites and envenomations
Cough and cold preparations	Cosmetics and personal care products
Plants	Cleaning substances
Pesticides	Sedatives/hypnotics/antipsychotics
Vitamins	Stimulants and street drugs
Antimicrobials	Antihistamines

Watson WA, Litovitz TL, Klein-Schwartz et al.: 2003 Annual report of the American Association of Poison Control Centers Toxic Exposure Surveillance System. *Am J Emerg Med* 22(5):335-404, 2004.

TABLE 9-9
The 10 Most Common Causes of Poison-Related Fatalities, All Ages, 2003

Analgesics
Sedatives, hypnotics, and antipsychotic drugs
Antidepressants
Stimulants and street drugs (most, but not all, deaths were associated with illegal drugs)
Cardiovascular drugs
Alcohols
Anticonvulsants
Antihistamines
Gases and fumes
Muscle relaxants

Watson WA, Litovitz TL, Klein-Schwartz et al.: 2003 Annual report of the American Association of Poison Control Centers Toxic Exposure Surveillance System. *Am J Emerg Med* 22(5): 335-404, 2004.

B. Risk Factors

All ages are vulnerable to iatrogenic poisonings (e.g., incorrect drugs or routes of administration in a health care setting); environmental poisons (e.g., carbon monoxide, pesticides, contaminated water); inadvertent ingestion of poisonous substances that were transferred into food containers such as baby bottles, milk containers, and soft drink bottles; and idiosyncratic reactions. Children of any age may be victims of child abuse or Munchausen syndrome by proxy. In addition, there are some age-related physiologic and behavioral factors that may predispose to, exacerbate, or mitigate poison exposures.

1. **Infants** are poisoned when parents misread or disregard medication labels, when potentially harmful substances are left within an infant's grasp, or when older siblings "feed" or "help with" infants. Immature gastrointestinal (GI) tract flora predispose infants to infant botulism from ingestion of honey and to methemoglobinemia from the ingestion of foods or well water high in nitrites. Immature nervous systems exacerbate the risk of poisoning by any central nervous system (CNS) toxin. Rapid respiratory and metabolic rates increase the risk of carbon monoxide poisoning. Immature hepatic and renal systems may or may not increase the risk of poison exposures, depending on the specific mechanisms for metabolism and excretion. An infant's small body weight increases the potential for danger if an infant is envenomated by snakes or spiders.
2. **Toddlers** are poisoned when potentially poisonous substances are left within reach. As consequences of normal growth and development, children grab or climb to reach anything that seems attractive, put everything in their hands into their mouths, and imitate adult behavior, including the taking of medicines. Children are unable to distinguish medicines and household products from benign look-alikes such as candy and soft drinks. Physiologically, toddlers face the same risks as infants in terms of the nervous, hepatic, and renal systems, respiratory and metabolic rate, and body weight.
3. **School-age children** may not be able to read or may misinterpret label instructions on products and medicines, succumb to "dares" of classmates, and may not be able to predict the consequences of their actions. Because of wide variability in normal growth and development, it is difficult generally to predict the physiologic effects of many poison exposures.
4. **Preteens and teenagers** may misinterpret label instructions on products and medicines, succumb to "dares" of classmates, explore more widely outside the home and school environment, abuse drugs, or attempt suicide. Teenagers may be exposed to chemicals on the job. After about age 10, children metabolize acetaminophen in the adult fashion (i.e., generate increased amounts of the hepatotoxic metabolite). As they near the upper end of the teenage range, physiologic responses approach, then equal, expected adult responses.

MANAGEMENT OF PATIENTS WITH POISON EXPOSURES

A. History

1. Usually the basic information is known: Children spill things, brag about taking medicine or "helping mommy," or act guilty about having done something "forbidden."
2. In the absence of history, a high index of suspicion is required to determine whether a poison exposure has occurred. Suspect a poison exposure when there is a sudden onset of illness; unexplained symptoms, findings, or laboratory values; an unusual complex of symptoms; exposure to a fire (carbon monoxide, cyanide); or psychiatric treatment in the child, a family member, or caretaker and therefore access to psychotropic drugs. In older children who are trauma victims, suspect drug or alcohol use as a precipitating factor. Also, previously undiagnosed medical conditions (e.g., glucose-6-phosphate dehydrogenase [G6PD] deficiency)

may predispose to poisoning by some agents (naphthalene mothballs, dapsone), and the poison center can help identify such conditions.

3. To determine whether a poison exposure may have occurred, ask about medicines and products in the home; whether there have been visitors in the home or the child has visited elsewhere; if herbal medicines, home remedies, or foreign preparations have been used or are available; or if the child has been breast-feeding. To assess environmental factors, ask whether anyone else is ill, for example, or whether there have been any home improvement projects or new appliances installed.
4. In addition to ascertaining the nature of any symptoms, determine when they started and in what order they occurred. This information can provide valuable clues in determining what the poison is or whether the available history is accurate.

B. Assessment

1. **Clinical assessment** in cases of poison exposure is no different from physical assessment for any other medical emergency. Characteristic complexes of symptoms, physical findings, and laboratory findings may assist with assessment of exposure to unknown poisons (Table 9-10).
2. The need for **laboratory assessment** depends on whether the poison is known; if so, what the poison is; whether knowledge of test results will affect medical care, prognosis, or disposition of the patient; and, in some cases, whether there are medicolegal considerations.
   a. For many poisonings with *anticipated systemic effects*, baseline electrolytes; renal and hepatic functions; respiratory, cardiovascular, and hematologic parameters; and arterial blood gas (ABG) analyses are necessary.
   b. For some poisons, *quantitative measurement* in urine or serum determines whether treatment is needed. Examples include acetaminophen, aspirin, lead, ethylene glycol, and methanol.
   c. In other cases, *laboratory studies* may confirm the presence of particular substances but do not alter patient care (e.g., tricyclic antidepressants).
   d. At other times, *laboratory values* cannot be returned in time to influence patient care (e.g., cyanide).
   e. In some cases, the *time* between exposure and collection of the laboratory specimen influences the interpretation of laboratory results (e.g., acetaminophen, aspirin, carbon monoxide).
   f. When a poisoning is suspected but not known, a *comprehensive toxicology screen* may be helpful in identifying the agent. How "comprehensive" such a screen is varies from facility to facility; it is essential to know what was tested for before declaring such a screening result to be negative.
   g. It is usual, and desirable, to "treat the patient, not the laboratory." When caring for a poisoned patient, the exact opposite is sometimes necessary to prevent devastating consequences. In some common, potentially fatal poisonings, *metabolites* are responsible for toxic effects, and ideally the patient would be treated before toxic metabolites are generated and while the patient is still asymptomatic. In cases of acetaminophen, ethylene glycol, and methanol poisoning, laboratory studies do guide therapy.

C. Interventions

1. **Prevention of absorption:** Decontamination is the initial step. This may refer to removal from contaminated air, irrigation of exposed eyes and skin, or GI tract decontamination.

TABLE 9-10
Toxicologic Syndromes (Toxidromes)

Toxin	Vital Signs	Mental Status	Signs and Symptoms	Clinical Findings
Acetaminophen	Normal (early)	Normal	Anorexia, nausea, vomiting	RUQ tenderness, jaundice (late)
Amphetamines	Hypertension, tachycardia, tachypnea, hyperthermia	Agitation	Hyperalertness, panic, anxiety, diaphoresis	Mydriasis, hyperactive peristaltism, diaphoresis
Antihistamines	Hypotension, hypertension, tachycardia, hyperthermia	Altered (agitation, lethargy to coma), hallucinations	Blurred vision, dry mouth, inability to urinate	Dry mucous membranes, mydriasis, flush, diminished peristaltism, urinary retention
Arsenic (acute)	Hypotension, tachycardia	Alert to coma	Abdominal pain, vomiting, diarrhea, dysphagia	Dehydration
Barbiturates	Hypotension, bradypnea, hypothermia	Altered (lethargy to coma)	Slurred speech, ataxia	Dysconjugate gaze, bullae, hyporeflexia
Beta adrenergic antagonists	Hypotension, bradycardia	Altered (lethargy to coma)	Dizziness	Cyanosis, seizures
Botulism	Bradypnea	Normal unless hypoxia	Blurred vision, diplopia, dysphagia, sore or dry throat, constipation	Ophthalmoplegia, mydriasis, ptosis, cranial nerve abnormalities, descending paralysis
Calcium channel blockers	Hypotension, bradycardia	Altered (lethargy, confusion)	Nausea	
Carbamazepine	Hypotension, tachycardia, bradypnea, hypothermia	Altered (lethargy to coma)	Hallucinations, extrapyramidal movements, seizures	Mydriasis, nystagmus
Carbon monoxide	Often normal	Altered (lethargy to coma)	Headache, dizziness, nausea, vomiting	Seizures
Clonidine	Hypotension, hypertension, bradycardia, bradypnea	Altered (lethargy to coma)	Dizziness, confusion	Miosis
Cocaine	Hypertension, tachycardia, tachypnea, hyperthermia	Altered (anxiety, agitation, delirium)	Hallucinations, paranoia, panic, anxiety, restlessness	Mydriasis, nystagmus
Cyclic antidepressants	Hypotension, tachycardia	Altered (lethargy to coma)	Confusion, dizziness, dry mouth, inability to urinate	Mydriasis, dry mucous membranes, distended bladder, flush, seizures

TABLE 9-10
Toxicologic Syndromes (Toxidromes) (*cont'd*)

Toxin	Vital Signs	Mental Status	Signs and Symptoms	Clinical Findings
Digitalis	Hypotension, bradycardia	Normal or altered	Nausea, vomiting, anorexia	None
Disulfiram/ethanol	Hypotension, tachycardia	Normal	Nausea, vomiting, headache, vertigo	Flush, diaphoresis
Ethylene glycol	Tachypnea	Altered (lethargy to coma)	Abdominal pain	Slurred speech, ataxia
Iron	Hypotension, tachycardia	Normal or lethargy	Nausea, vomiting, diarrhea, abdominal pain, hematemesis	
Isoniazid	Often normal	Normal or altered (lethargy to coma)	Nausea, vomiting	Status epilepticus
Isopropanol	Hypotension, tachycardia, bradypnea	Altered (lethargy to coma)	Nausea, vomiting	Hyporeflexia, ataxia, odor of acetone on breath
Lead	Hypertension	Altered (lethargy to coma)	Irritability, abdominal pain (colic), nausea, vomiting, constipation	Peripheral neuropathy, seizures, gingival pigmentation
Lithium	Hypotension (late)	Altered (lethargy to coma)	Diarrhea, tremor, nausea	Weakness, tremor, ataxia, myoclonus, seizures
Mercury	Hypotension (late)	Altered (psychiatric disturbances)	Salivation, diarrhea, abdominal pain	Stomatitis, ataxia, tremor
Methanol	Hypotension, tachypnea	Altered (lethargy to coma)	Blurred vision, blindness, abdominal pain	Hyperemic disks, mydriasis
Opioids	Hypotension, bradycardia, bradypnea, hypothermia	Altered (lethargy to coma)	Slurred speech, ataxia	Miosis, decreased peristaltism
Organic phosphorous compounds, carbamates	Hypotension/ hypertension, bradycardia/ tachycardia, bradypnea/ tachypnea	Altered (lethargy to coma)	Diarrhea, abdominal pain, blurred vision, vomiting	Salivation, diaphoresis, lacrimation, urination, bronchorrhea, defecation, miosis, fasciculations, seizures
Phencyclidine	hypertension, tachycardia, hyperthermia	Altered (agitation, lethargy to coma)	Hallucinations	Miosis, diaphoresis, myoclonus, blank stare, nystagmus, seizures

Continued

TABLE 9-10
Toxicologic Syndromes (Toxidromes) (*cont'd*)

Toxin	Vital Signs	Mental Status	Signs and Symptoms	Clinical Findings
Phenothiazines	Hypotension, tachycardia, hypothermia or hyperthermia	Altered (lethargy to coma)	Dizziness, dry mouth, inability to urinate	Miosis or mydriasis, decreased bowel sounds, dystonia
Salicylates	Hypotension, tachycardia, tachypnea, hyperthermia	Altered (agitation, lethargy to coma)	Tinnitus, nausea, vomiting, hyperpnea	Diaphoresis, congestive heart failure
Sedative-hypnotics	Hypotension, bradypnea, hypothermia	Altered (lethargy to coma)	Slurred speech, ataxia	Hyporeflexia, bullae
Theophylline	Hypotension, tachycardia, tachypnea, hyperthermia	Altered (agitation)	Nausea, vomiting, diaphoresis, anxiety	Diaphoresis, tremor, seizures, dysrhythmias

Goldfrank LR, Flomenbaum NE, Lewin NA et al.: Goldfrank's toxicologic emergencies, ed 7. New York, 2002, McGraw-Hill, pp 257-258.
RUQ, Right upper quadrant.

a. *Ocular exposure* is treated by copious irrigation, at least 15 to 20 minutes for acidic substances and 30 minutes for alkaline substances, with subsequent reevaluation. One measure of the efficacy of irrigation is when a pH strip gently touched to the cul-de-sac indicates a neutral pH. Ocular irrigation in children is difficult at best, and the best method is the one that can be initiated quickly and then maintained. Ocular irrigation in teens can be performed as in adults, with an irrigation device.

b. *Dermal exposure* is also treated by copious irrigation for the times specified previously. For older children, a shower is ideal. Protect staff from exposure to harmful substances, initiate irrigation, and remove and bag contaminated clothing.

c. *GI tract decontamination* may include gastric emptying with ipecac syrup, gastric lavage, or whole-bowel irrigation, adsorbing remaining ingested substances with activated charcoal, and then hastening evacuation of the charcoal complex with a cathartic agent.

- *Ipecac syrup* was once used to induce vomiting. Now, the American Academy of Pediatrics no longer recommends the stocking or use of ipecac syrup to treat poisoning, even at home.
- *Gastric lavage* is difficult at best in young children. The efficacy of gastric lavage is limited by the respective sizes of the child, the tube, and the tablets. It is sometimes used in patients with life-threatening overdoses who present shortly after ingestion.
    - Secure the airway and warm normal saline (NS) for instillation. The largest possible orogastric tube should be used, usually a 16- to 32-gauge French. Instill 50 to 100 mL of warm NS at a time, and then allow it to remain in the stomach for a few minutes and drain by gravity. Repeat until lavage fluid is clear. Activated charcoal and a cathartic can be administered before the lavage tube is withdrawn.

  - Gastric lavage is contraindicated for ingestions of caustic substances and hydrocarbons. However, careful lavage with a soft tube is sometimes used within 1 hour of an acid ingestion.
- *Whole-bowel irrigation* is sometimes used to treat poisonings when the amount of substance ingested is extremely dangerous or potentially fatal and when there are no effective treatments. Examples include iron, some sustained-release drugs such as calcium-channel blockers, and sometimes ingested packets of illegal drugs such as cocaine and heroin. The general procedure is the same as for bowel preparations. Secure the airway if necessary, and administer a polyethylene glycol-electrolyte solution until the rectal effluent is clear. The dose is 0.5 L/hour for young children and 1 to 2 L/hour for older children and adults.
- *Activated charcoal* is processed so that each molecule contains multiple binding sites. Activated charcoal adsorbs, or binds to, most clinically important drugs and poisons. This prevents absorption from the GI tract into the bloodstream. Activated charcoal does not adsorb metals (e.g., iron, lithium), caustic substances, ethanol, or many pesticides. When these substances are ingested, activated charcoal may still be indicated because of co-ingestants.
  - The usual dose of activated charcoal is 0.5 to 1 g/kg for young children, 25 to 50 g for older children, and 50 g per dose for teenagers and adults.
  - Activated charcoal should not be mixed with ice cream, syrups, or other items intended to improve palatability. The charcoal adsorbs many of these agents and would therefore be less effective.
  - Single doses of activated charcoal are indicated for most serious poison exposures because it decreases the amount of toxic substance available for absorption into the bloodstream.
  - Multiple doses of activated charcoal (every 2 to 6 hours) are useful in lowering toxic blood levels and shortening the course of poisoning from some substances that undergo enterohepatic or enterogastric recirculation. Some drugs are partially metabolized in the liver, and then active drug is secreted into bile and deposited in the small bowel. Subsequent doses of activated charcoal adsorb the drug as this occurs. This is true regardless of the route of exposure. *Intestinal dialysis* takes advantage of concentration gradients. As drug is adsorbed to charcoal in the GI tract, previously absorbed, unmetabolized drug moves from receptor sites and intracellular spaces into the GI tract. As this occurs, it too is adsorbed by subsequent doses of activated charcoal. Among the drugs for which multiple doses of activated charcoal are indicated are digoxin, carbamazepine, theophylline, phenobarbital, and amitriptyline (American Academy of Clinical Toxicology, 1999).
  - *Cautions:* To prevent a charcoal impaction, always check for active bowel sounds before administering a dose of charcoal. When multiple doses of activated charcoal are given, cathartics are occasionally recommended. If so, it is essential that a cathartic be administered no more than once, or occasionally twice, per day to prevent electrolyte imbalance and dehydration. Errors have occurred when charcoal suspension in sorbitol has been mistakenly administered instead of charcoal in an aqueous suspension. It is also essential that the patient have active bowel sounds. Always check before administering the next dose of charcoal.

- *Cathartics:* If cathartics are used at all to treat a poisoning, sorbitol and magnesium citrate are the most common.
  - *Sorbitol* may be combined with charcoal or administered afterward. It should be administered no more than once per day. The dose is 1 to 2 g/kg.
  - *Magnesium citrate* may be combined with charcoal or administered afterward. It should be administered no more than once per day. The dose is 4 mL/kg.

2. **Enhancement of elimination:** The means and possibility of enhancing elimination depend on a substance's volume of distribution and usual elimination.
   a. *Ion trapping* is useful for some drugs that are more rapidly eliminated in an alkaline environment; examples include salicylates and phenobarbital. In these cases, administering sodium bicarbonate to alkalinize the urine enhances excretion. (Some drugs are more easily eliminated by acidifying the urine, but this is not recommended; precipitation of myoglobin and renal failure may occur.)
   b. *Extracorporeal measures* to enhance elimination of toxins may be useful in certain dangerous poisonings by substances that can be retrieved from the vascular compartment. Depending on the child's age, hemodialysis can be used for salicylates, lithium, methanol, and ethylene glycol, among others; hemoperfusion may be used for theophylline; and exchange transfusion is sometimes used to treat "gray baby syndrome" induced by chloramphenicol.

D. Administration of Antidotes

Few pharmacologic antidotes are available. Most poisonings are treated by decontamination followed by symptomatic and supportive care. If a specific antidote is indicated, it is described as part of the treatment for poisonings considered in the following.

E. Provision of Supportive Care

Provision of symptomatic and supportive care for poisoning ranges from such simple measures as fluids and positioning for hypotension to invasive measures to support cardiovascular, respiratory, and hematologic functioning. Descriptions of individual poisons indicate whether one particular drug (e.g., antiarrhythmic, anticonvulsant, vasopressor) is preferred. Increasing or recurrent symptoms may be expected with some poisonings and occur unexpectedly in others. See Table 9-11 for possible reasons.

TABLE 9-11
Causes of Increasing or Recurring Symptoms and Drug Levels

Incomplete gastrointestinal decontamination: virtually any solid dosage form
Drug concretion or bezoar. Examples: aspirin, iron, meprobamate
Enterohepatic recirculation. Examples: amitriptyline, digoxin, phencyclidine
Ingestion of anticholinergic drug, or drug with anticholinergic properties. Examples: antihistamines, atropine, tricyclic antidepressants, glutethimide
Exposure to especially lipid-soluble substances. Examples: some organophosphate insecticides, anesthetic agents, ethchlorvynol
Incorrect or incomplete history
Incorrect laboratory values
Re-exposure in the hospital

F. Prevention of Future Episodes

Circumstances contributing to iatrogenic poisonings must be considered. For young children, age and development specific poison-prevention teaching may be required. Suspicions of abuse require legal and social service involvement. Drug abuse prevention and treatment programs and psychiatric intervention may be required for older children and teens.

POISONINGS BY PHARMACEUTICAL AGENTS

A. Acetaminophen

Acetaminophen is found in hundreds of prescription and nonprescription analgesics, both alone and in combination with other analgesics, including opioids; in combination with antihistamines in over-the-counter sleeping preparations; and in combination with decongestants, antihistamines, antitussives, expectorants, and analgesics in products to treat coughs, colds, and allergies. Most preparations are oral, but the drug also is available as rectal suppositories.

1. Acetaminophen is rapidly absorbed from the **GI tract**, but food or co-ingestants may delay peak absorption until about 4 hours after ingestion.
2. Acetaminophen is metabolized in the **liver**. After about the age of 10 years, approximately 5% to 10% of the drug is metabolized by a hepatotoxic metabolite that is normally detoxified by the enzyme glutathione. In overdose, the body's glutathione stores are depleted, causing the liver damage characteristic of acetaminophen overdose. In children younger than 10 years, a different metabolic pathway may be followed, presumably providing some degree of hepatic protection. This relative protection is not entirely reliable, and infants and young children can also die of hepatic injury after acute or chronic acetaminophen overdose. There is some renal metabolism of acetaminophen; therefore renal injury, although not as common as hepatic injury, is possible.
3. The **toxic dose** of acetaminophen is related to body weight (or ideal body weight in the case of markedly obese individuals); ingestions of unknown amounts or greater than 150 mg/kg require laboratory assessment of absorbed acetaminophen to predict toxicity.
4. Because the toxic effects of acetaminophen overdose are due to metabolites, **symptoms** of toxicity are delayed. Only rarely, after massive overdose, does a patient develop mental status changes, significant GI tract symptoms, and acidosis within hours after ingestion. Often there are no symptoms of overdose for 6 to 14 hours after ingestion. The earliest symptoms are nausea and vomiting. Within 24 to 48 hours after ingestion, hepatic enzymes rise. The patient may experience increasing GI tract symptoms and right upper quadrant pain, or the patient may feel relatively well. Within 72 to 96 hours after an untreated, severe overdose, hepatic encephalopathy with coagulopathies and hyperglycemia may ensue, followed rapidly by hepatic failure and death.
5. **Assessment**
   a. *History* should include the name of the drug; the amount ingested; the time of ingestion; and whether ingestion was acute, chronic, or both; the type, onset, duration, or absence of symptoms; and whether there were co-ingestants.
   b. *Draw* a serum acetaminophen level at least 4 hours after ingestion. Also draw baseline hepatic, renal, and hematologic studies if the level is toxic or if ingestion was large or chronic by history or occurred more than 8 to 12 hours earlier.

6. **Treatment** of acetaminophen poisoning is straightforward and successful if the antidote administration is initiated within 8 to 12 hours after ingestion. Later administration has some utility. The specific antidote is *N*-acetylcysteine (NAC), which serves as a glutathione precursor and substitute to prevent *N*-acetyl-*p*-benzoquinoneimine-induced hepatocellular injury. Indications for NAC include a toxic acetaminophen level in blood drawn 4 hours or more after ingestion and toxic ingestion by history or suspicion when laboratory results cannot be returned by 8 hours after ingestion. The entire course of therapy must be administered to every patient with an acute ingestion and a toxic acetaminophen level, even if the plasma acetaminophen level becomes negative. NAC is being used to treat effects of the toxic metabolite, not the parent compound.
   a. *Oral NAC*
      - The loading dose is NAC 140 mg/kg administered orally (PO), followed by 70 mg/kg every 4 hours for 17 doses, for a total of 18 doses over 72 hours. Dilute the drug 3-to-1 in juice or a beverage palatable to the patient. In an alert patient, offer the diluted drug over ice in a covered container.
      - Administration of PO NAC is often complicated by vomiting induced by the poisoning and NAC itself. If a dose of NAC is vomited within 1 hour of administration, the dose must be repeated. If an antiemetic is required, use ondansetron or another antiemetic that does not require hepatic metabolism. If necessary for successful NAC administration, a duodenal tube may be passed with fluoroscopic placement.
   b. *IV NAC* was approved by the U.S. Food and Drug Administration (FDA) in January 2004 under the brand name Acetadote.
      - The loading dose is 150 mg/kg, diluted in 200 mL of 5% dextrose, over 15 minutes; 50 mg/kg, diluted in 500 mL of 5% dextrose, is infused over 4 hours. Finally, 100 mg/kg in 1 L of 5% dextrose is infused over 16 hours (Dart and Jones, 2004). Fluid and electrolyte imbalance is a concern for small children; call the poison center for additional dosing information.
   c. *Other treatment* includes daily monitoring of hepatic enzymes and symptomatic and supportive care.
7. **Special considerations** include the need for a high index of suspicion. Acetaminophen poisoning is perfectly treatable if recognized early but potentially fatal if untreated. Those who recover and have no clinical or laboratory evidence of hepatic injury are not expected to experience sequelae. Those who develop liver failure from this poisoning may undergo successful liver transplantation.

B. Anesthetics for Topical Use

Anesthetics for topical use contain benzocaine, dibucaine, and lidocaine. They are found in prescription and nonprescription remedies, including teething lotions, first-aid creams, and drugs infiltrated into wounds before suturing. Children have died rapidly after ingestion of dibucaine.

1. Children experience the **rapid onset** of dysrhythmias, seizures, and methemoglobinemia after ingestion or absorption of these drugs. As little as several milligrams is sufficient for toxic effects to occur.
2. **Suspect methemoglobinemia** in patients who are cyanotic and do not respond to oxygen. Tentative diagnosis can be made by inspection of the blood. A drop of the patient's blood on a piece of filter paper appears brown next to a drop of "normal" blood. Laboratory confirmation reports a percent of methemoglobin, the amount of normal hemoglobin that has been converted to methemoglobin and therefore cannot transport oxygen.

3. **Specific treatment** for methemoglobinemia is the IV administration of methylene blue. Treatment for other toxic manifestations is symptomatic and supportive.

C. Antidepressants

Serotonin reuptake inhibitors (SRI) have become more widely prescribed than tricyclic antidepressants (TCA) and other cyclic antidepressants because there are fewer dangerous effects in overdose and fewer unpleasant side effects for patients. Poison center data support the widespread availability and lower toxicity of SRIs compared with TCAs. In 2003, TCAs alone or formulated with other drugs accounted for 12,710 calls to poison centers and were associated with 93 fatalities and life-threatening effects in 1,373 cases. The corresponding numbers for SRIs were 55,977 exposures, with 106 fatalities and life-threatening effects in 1730 cases.

1. **Tricyclic antidepressants** include amitriptyline, clomipramine, desipramine, doxepin, imipramine, nortriptyline, and others, both singly and in combination with other psychotropic agents. There are no approved therapeutic indications and no safe doses for these drugs in very young children, who may have access to drugs belonging to an older sibling or other family member. Imipramine is used in the treatment of nocturnal enuresis in older children. The tricyclic antidepressants may be used to treat depression in preteens and teenagers, although treatment with selective SRIs is now more common.
   a. In general, these drugs are *rapidly absorbed*. In large ingestions, sufficient drug may be absorbed for its anticholinergic properties to inhibit gastric motility; therefore significant amounts of unabsorbed drug may remain within the GI tract. These drugs are widely distributed and highly protein bound.
   b. *Tricyclic antidepressants* have several effects: anticholinergic, responsible for the dry mouth and hallucinations that sometimes accompany overdose; delayed uptake of norepinephrine, accounting for these drugs' therapeutic utility and for some CNS and cardiac effects of overdose; membrane-depressant effects on the heart, resulting in conduction delays and dysrhythmias; and α-adrenergic blocking properties. Early hypertension may precede the significant hypotension characteristic of this poisoning.
   c. The **toxic dose** cannot be predicted with certainty. Any amount is potentially dangerous for infants, toddlers, and young children. For teenagers and adults, the toxic amount is variable. Ambulance transport, GI tract decontamination, and at least 6 hours of emergency department evaluation are required for all ingestions in young children and ingestions larger than a therapeutic dose in older children. A patient who develops any clinical signs of toxicity within the 6-hour observation period requires admission to a monitored bed until the patient has been asymptomatic for 24 hours.
   d. A **classic presentation** of tricyclic antidepressant poisoning includes the rapid onset of grand mal seizures and coma, perhaps within 30 minutes of ingestion; hypotension; metabolic acidosis; and numerous dysrhythmias, especially ventricular dysrhythmias and conduction delays. Common electrocardiogram (ECG) findings are numerous and include prolonged PR and QRS intervals.
   e. When **assessing the patient,** anticipate the need for intubation if the patient is still conscious. The most useful laboratory study is ABG analysis. Symptomatic patients are likely to develop acidosis that is resistant to correction. Laboratory measurements of drug and metabolite levels correlate loosely with expected toxicity but are not necessary for patient care because they are not used to determine treatment.

f. **Treatment** includes GI tract decontamination, maintaining serum pH between 7.45 and 7.55, cardiac monitoring, and treatment of hypotension, seizures, and dysrhythmias.
   - Administer activated charcoal every 4 hours until the patient is asymptomatic; check for the presence of bowel sounds before each charcoal dose.
   - Sodium bicarbonate is the drug of choice to treat tricyclic antidepressant poisoning. Although hyperventilation is sometimes used to correct acidosis, sodium bicarbonate is preferred because it appears to have therapeutic effects in addition to the correction of acidosis.
   - Lidocaine, magnesium sulfate, or overdrive pacing may be indicated for dysrhythmias unresponsive to a normalized pH. Diazepam may be used for seizures.
   - Hypotension must be treated aggressively and may require invasive support if fluids, positioning, and norepinephrine are ineffective.

g. **Amoxapine** is a cyclic antidepressant that causes few cardiovascular effects after overdose, but it is often associated with status epilepticus. An overdose of amoxapine requires aggressive seizure control, often including intubation and muscular paralysis.

2. **Serotonin uptake inhibitors** include citalopram (Celexa), fluoxetine (Prozac), fluvoxamine (Luvox), paroxetine (Paxil), and sertraline (Zoloft).
   a. *Effects* of single-drug overdoses tend to be mild, including drowsiness and GI effects. Citalopram especially is associated with a greater incidence of seizures and cardiac effects, including QTc prolongation. Treatment includes GI decontamination and symptomatic and supportive care.
   b. *Serotonin syndrome* is potentially life threatening. It may occur idiosyncratically, after large overdoses, or especially with an overdose of more than one drug.
      - As a result of excess serotonin accumulation in the CNS, patients may experience autonomic and neuromuscular effects, including fever, tachycardia, and muscle rigidity. Ascending neuromuscular effects may lead to respiratory compromise.
      - Treatment includes respiratory support, aggressive external cooling, and treatment of muscular rigidity as needed, with measures ranging from benzodiazepines to muscular paralysis.
   c. Because patients are often prescribed more than one drug, those with a *history* of having overdosed on an SRI should be assessed for co-ingestion of other drugs, including other antidepressants.

D. Benzodiazepines

Benzodiazepines are used as adjuncts to anesthesia and as anticonvulsants. Young children may have access to these drugs if these are being taken therapeutically by family members. They may also be abused or self-administered in suicide attempts. In general, overdoses of these drugs can be successfully treated with respiratory support and, sometimes, the antidote flumazenil. (Flumazenil effectively reverses respiratory depression associated with benzodiazepine overdose, but there are contraindications [see later discussion]). Combining a benzodiazepine with ethanol or another CNS depressant significantly increases toxicity, however.

1. Commonly used **benzodiazepines** include alprazolam, oxazepam, lorazepam, diazepam, and chlordiazepoxide. Midazolam is used as an adjunct to anesthesia.
2. Benzodiazepines act by enhancing the effects of **γ-aminobutyric acid (GABA)**, an inhibitory neurotransmitter in the brain. The many types of drugs within the

class make it impossible to generalize about absorption and elimination. Some of those prescribed for therapeutic use in the outpatient setting (e.g., diazepam) have a long half-life; therefore significant and prolonged respiratory depression should be anticipated in someone who abused the drug or took a large quantity.

3. **Effects of overdose** include respiratory and CNS depression. In an uncomplicated overdose, there are no specific drug-related laboratory values of use. In a potential mixed overdose, determination of co-ingestants is important.
4. **Flumazenil** is the specific antidote. A test dose may be used to help determine whether respiratory depression is caused by a benzodiazepine overdose, although it should not be used to maintain wakefulness. Caution must be used to avoid precipitating withdrawal in a patient who is dependent on a benzodiazepine. Flumazenil should never be used if the patient has also overdosed on a tricyclic antidepressant because an increased risk of seizures has been associated with this use. Likewise flumazenil should not be used if the patient is known to have a seizure disorder.
5. **Treatment** includes symptomatic and supportive care. If the patient is habituated to the drug, withdrawal symptoms may occur. A protocol to prevent acute withdrawal and accomplish gradual withdrawal must be implemented.

E. Calcium-Channel Blockers

Calcium-channel blockers include amlodopine, diltiazem, nicardipine, nifedipine, verapamil, and others, in regular and sustained-release preparations. As indications for their use in cardiovascular disease and other conditions have increased, poison exposures and fatalities in children have also increased. No antidote or universally effective treatment exists. Aggressive GI tract decontamination and vigorous supportive care are required.

1. **Calcium-channel blockers** are easily absorbed from the GI tract. Elimination rates vary but can be prolonged for days after an overdose.
2. Most simply stated, **calcium** is required for cellular contraction. These drugs, therapeutically and in overdose, slow the influx of calcium through calcium channels into the intracellular space of cardiac nodal tissue, myocardial tissue, and vascular (especially arteriolar) tissue. The result is conduction delays, diminished cardiac output, and hypotension.
3. The **toxic dose** is variable but small. A single nifedipine tablet was thought to be responsible for the death of a 12-month-old child. The ingestion of any amount of any of these drugs should be considered potentially fatal in a child.
4. **Physical assessment** must be comprehensive. There are multiple mechanisms for hypotension (decreased cardiac output, diminished peripheral vascular resistance), hypoxia and apnea (bradydysrhythmias, heart block, decreased cardiac output), and metabolic acidosis (hypoperfusion, hypoxia). Also common are CNS depression, seizures, possibly hypoxic seizures, headache, and flushing, perhaps as a result of vasodilation, and hyperglycemia (calcium-channel blockers inhibit insulin release). Electrolyte monitoring, ABG analysis, and continuous assessment of respiratory and cardiovascular status are needed.
5. **Treatment** begins with aggressive GI tract decontamination. Although gastric lavage or charcoal-cathartic administration may be part of emergency department treatment, consider whole-bowel irrigation for ingestion of multiple tablets or sustained-release preparations. IV calcium chloride or calcium gluconate is indicated, although it is not usually effective. In a patient with stable electrolyte and acid-base status, calcium chloride is preferred because it contains a higher concentration of calcium. (Extravasation of calcium chloride can cause tissue necrosis, so placement and patency of peripheral IV lines must be checked

before each administration by this route.) Glucagon may be used to increase the heart rate and conduction velocity, although it too is not always effective. Insulin plus dextrose has been used to stabilize blood pressure in patients refractory to other treatments. Otherwise, treatment is symptomatic and supportive.

6. **Serum calcium levels** especially must be monitored closely while treatment continues. No absolute change in the quantity of the patient's calcium stores occurs; there is a change in the distribution of calcium stores.

F. Chloroquine

Chloroquine is used to treat malaria and rarely for other medical conditions, such as rheumatoid arthritis. It is rapidly absorbed and has a narrow therapeutic margin. Exposures are unintentional in children, suicidal in adults, and a result of therapeutic error in all ages (i.e., taking the drug daily rather than weekly, as indicated). Overdoses are infrequent, but hypotension, seizures, cardiorespiratory collapse, and death can occur within 30 to 60 minutes after ingestion. There is no antidote.

1. The **toxic dose** of chloroquine overlaps the therapeutic dose. Children have died after ingestion of less than 1 g.
2. If a patient survives to reach the ICU, **treatment** includes activated charcoal (and possibly a cathartic), if not already administered, and vigorous symptomatic and supportive respiratory, cardiac, and neurologic care. Epinephrine and diazepam are the drugs of choice for cardiac effects and seizures. Close monitoring of electrolytes is necessary. Patients are often hypokalemic.

G. Digoxin

Digoxin overdoses in the pediatric population are usually acute, although chronic intoxication may occur. Children may have access to their own drugs or those of family members. Pediatric therapeutic doses must be carefully calculated and measured, and blood levels must be carefully monitored. Some plants contain cardiac glycosides with digitalis-like effects if ingested, including foxglove *(Digitalis purpurea)* and oleander *(Nerium oleander)*. Poisoning by these plants is treated as for digitalis poisoning.

1. Digitalis usually is absorbed rapidly and excreted renally.
2. The **toxic effects** of digitalis are exacerbations of therapeutic effects. Digitalis interferes with the Na^+-K^+-ATPase pump, found in smooth muscle and abundantly in cardiac tissue. Therapeutically this maintains the correct proportions of intracellular and interstitial sodium, potassium, and calcium necessary for cellular contraction and nodal conduction. When the Na^+-K^+-ATPase pump is poisoned by toxic concentrations of digitalis, intracellular calcium levels rise, intracellular potassium is depleted, and serum potassium levels become markedly elevated. (However, when digitalis is administered for a long period in conjunction with diuretics, patients may present with hypokalemia.) Any and every dysrhythmia can result. Atrial dysrhythmias, bradycardia, and heart block are most common, along with ventricular irritability and hypotension.
3. A **toxic dose** can be estimated by history, but there is no substitute for laboratory evaluation of serum levels and careful evaluation of the patient. The therapeutic range is 0.5 to 2 ng/mL, but toxicity can occur within this range.
4. **Clinical effects of acute overdose** are GI and cardiovascular: nausea, vomiting, hypotension, bradycardia, and dysrhythmias. In chronic overdose, visual changes are also described, especially yellow or green "halos" or "hazes." Laboratory evaluation of electrolytes, especially potassium, and renal function is needed, along with the serum digitalis level. Continuous cardiac monitoring is essential.

5. **Treatment of digitalis overdose** includes prevention of absorption, intensive monitoring, administration of the antidote, and symptomatic and supportive care.
   a. *GI tract decontamination* is indicated, with administration of multiple doses of activated charcoal to enhance clearance of digitoxin.
   b. *Usual measures* are indicated to treat bradycardia and other dysrhythmias, hypotension, and hyperkalemia.
   c. *Administration of the antidote,* digoxin immune Fab, quickly reverses severe hyperkalemia and life-threatening dysrhythmias. IV administration of 40 mg of digoxin immune Fab fragments (1 vial) binds 0.6 mg of digitalis. The poison center can help to make other dose determinations if the amount of ingested digitalis is not available. Patients in renal failure may need dialysis to remove the digoxin immune Fab complex.
   d. If the *antidote is not available,* standard but aggressive treatment is needed to treat hyperkalemia (insulin, glucose, and sodium bicarbonate), support blood pressure, and treat dysrhythmias. Patients in renal failure require dialysis to remove digitalis.
   e. *Monitoring serum digoxin levels* can be confusing after antidote administration, as some laboratory methods measure and report a concentration that includes both free digitalis and that bound to Fab. It is necessary to know whether reported digitalis levels are of free digitalis only. (This is especially important for patients treated therapeutically with digitalis who must remain digitalized.)

H. Diphenoxylate and Atropine

Diphenoxylate-atropine combinations (e.g., Lomotil) are used to treat diarrhea in adults. There is no safe amount of this drug for young children. The combination of powerful opioid and anticholinergic effects is the reason for both its therapeutic usefulness in adults and its danger in children.

1. The **anticholinergic effects** of atropine cause this drug to be retained in the GI tract for prolonged periods. The onset of opioid effects can be delayed for as long as 24 hours after ingestion.
2. Every child who ingests any amount of this drug must be **monitored** in an ICU for 24 hours.
3. **Treatment** includes GI tract decontamination, symptomatic and supportive care, and careful monitoring for the onset of CNS and respiratory depression induced by diphenoxylate, the opioid component of this drug. Naloxone is effective for symptoms of opioid overdose.

I. Oral Hypoglycemic Agents

Oral hypoglycemic agents, including glyburide and glipizide, can cause the delayed onset of significant hypoglycemia in children, even in single-tablet ingestions. Every young child who swallows even one of these pills requires GI tract decontamination and admission, with frequent serum glucose determinations, for 24 hours. If hypoglycemia occurs, treat with IV glucose. Glucagon may be ineffective because small children have little stored glycogen. Octreotide may be administered to stabilize serum glucose.

J. Imidazoline Derivatives

Imidazoline derivatives are available to children in the form of clonidine, an antihypertensive, and such ocular and nasal vasoconstrictors as tetrahydrozoline, naphazoline, and oxymetazoline. All are α_2-agonists with mixed central and peripheral effects. A single tablet of clonidine, inadvertent application of even a used clonidine patch, or just several drops of the other drugs can cause the onset of coma, respiratory depression, and hypotension within 30 minutes of ingestion (or topical application for liquid vasoconstrictors and decongestants). GI tract decontamination is indicated for solid dosage forms. Symptomatic and supportive care is required for 24 to 36 hours, and recovery is expected.

K. Iron

Iron in the form of adult-strength supplements and prenatal vitamins with iron is a dangerous overdose in children younger than 6 years of age. Prescription-strength preparations may contain 60 to 65 mg of elemental iron per tablet, although some contain more than 100 mg of elemental iron. Fatalities in children from iron poisoning have declined because over-the-counter preparations now usually contain less than 30 mg of elemental iron per tablet. Iron supplements are sometimes used in suicide attempts by others, especially pregnant teenagers. (Overdoses of children's chewable multiple vitamins with iron may cause iron toxicity, but they have not been associated with iron-related fatalities in children.) The use of deferoxamine, a specific antidote, is important but may be limited in serious iron poisoning because of side effects, especially hypotension.

1. In **overdose,** iron causes significant corrosive injury to the GI tract. Absorption of iron is thus enhanced. Circulating free iron injures blood vessels and damages hepatocytes. As iron is metabolized, free hydrogen is released; in concert with other events, this produces metabolic acidosis.
2. **Mild symptoms** may occur with ingestion of more than 20 mg/kg of essential iron. **Significant toxicity or death** is possible with ingestions of more than 60 mg/kg; this amount of iron can be ingested by a 10-kg child who swallows just 10 typical prescription-strength adult preparations. The amount of essential iron in each iron salt varies; the potential risk is calculated by determining the iron salt and the amount of essential iron in each preparation, the number of pills missing, and the child's body weight. Actual risk is determined by serum iron levels and the presence or absence of symptoms.
3. The **course of severe iron poisoning** is described in steps, although individual patients may not follow this outline precisely:
   - **a.** *Phase I,* about 30 minutes to 2 hours after ingestion, includes GI tract symptoms, possibly severe, including hemorrhagic gastritis, vomiting, hematemesis, diarrhea, lethargy, and pallor.
   - **b.** *Phase II,* about 2 to 10 or 12 hours after ingestion, is a latent phase during which the patient is asymptomatic. The systemic insults described previously occur during this asymptomatic phase, and the patient abruptly enters phase III.
   - **c.** *Phase III,* about 12 to about 48 hours after ingestion, involves a rapid onset of cardiovascular collapse. Hypotension, increasing lethargy and coma, seizures, pulmonary edema, hepatorenal failure with coagulopathies, and hypoglycemia occur. Death may occur rapidly or after days or weeks of complications, including intestinal necrosis.
   - **d.** In *phase IV,* about 6 weeks after exposure, patients who survive the acute episode may require surgery for severe pyloric scarring.
4. **Assessment** of these patients includes careful evaluation of physical findings and laboratory results. Determine the nature of any symptoms and the time of onset compared with the time of ingestion.
   - **a.** *Initial laboratory studies* include serum iron level drawn 2 hours or longer after ingestion, complete blood count (CBC), and electrolytes. Patients with more than mild GI tract symptoms also require ABG analysis, determination

of electrolyte status, and baseline hepatic and renal function studies. Typing and crossmatch are indicated if there is frank bleeding or guaiac-positive stools.

b. *Iron tablets* (not pediatric chewable vitamins with iron) are radiopaque. An abdominal flat plate may permit counting of tablets in the child's GI tract. (A flat plate demonstrating negative findings cannot be used to rule out iron ingestion.)

5. **Treatment** of the iron-poisoned child includes GI tract decontamination, chelation with deferoxamine, and symptomatic and supportive care.
   a. *GI tract decontamination* may include gastric lavage or whole-bowel irrigation. If an abdominal x-ray examination demonstrates iron pills in the intestinal tract, whole-bowel irrigation is called for until the appropriate number of pills is counted in the rectal effluent or until a repeat radiographic examination documents that the pills have been removed. Iron is not adsorbed to activated charcoal.
   b. *Chelation* is indicated if the serum iron level is greater than 350 mcg/dL in the presence of symptoms, or if the serum iron is greater than 500 mcg/dL. Deferoxamine is administered IV. (Although the drug may be administered intramuscularly, this is inappropriate for the iron-poisoned child who is likely to be hypovolemic and hypotensive.) The usual dose of deferoxamine is 15 mg/kg per hour. Higher doses are sometimes used but may be associated with hypotension. "Vin rosé" colored urine, if it occurs, is a marker for elimination of deferoxamine-iron chelate, but this does not always appear and is not always reliable. Serum iron levels are more accurate.
   c. *Serum iron levels* must be repeated until it is certain that levels are dropping and that there is not a concretion, or clump, of iron tablets being slowly absorbed from the GI tract.
   d. *Symptomatic and supportive care* is otherwise required, but such measures must be aggressive to stop GI tract bleeding, treat hypovolemia and hypotension, and treat coagulopathies and other consequences of hepatic failure.
   e. Two special dangers are associated with *iron poisoning*. Parents and health care providers alike often think of iron as "just" a vitamin and are ignorant of the fact that quite small amounts of this essential element can cause fatalities in children. The asymptomatic latent phase of iron poisoning fools parents and health care providers who misinterpret the absence of symptoms as absence of risk.

L. Isoniazid

Isoniazid (INH) is used to treat tuberculosis. Young children may have access to the drug, and it is used in suicide attempts by teenagers.

1. **Isoniazid**, given therapeutically or taken in overdose, depletes the body of pyridoxine (vitamin B_6). Pyridoxine is a cofactor in numerous enzymatic reactions, including those responsible for the generation of GABA. GABA is an inhibitory neurotransmitter in the CNS; depletion of GABA leads to seizures.
2. An **overdose** of INH precipitates the onset of grand mal seizures, perhaps within 30 minutes of ingestion, and the subsequent development of severe acidosis.
3. The only effective **treatment** for INH-induced seizures is IV pyridoxine. If the dose of INH is known, the dose of pyridoxine is a milligram-per-milligram equivalent. If the dose is unknown, pyridoxine, 5 g IV, should be administered. Diazepam is an effective adjunct, as it enhances the action of GABA, but it cannot assist with synthesis of GABA and is not a substitute for pyridoxine.

4. Once seizures are controlled, **GI tract decontamination** can be carried out. Acidosis often corrects itself once seizures are controlled, but it is amenable to the usual therapies. Treatment otherwise is symptomatic and supportive.

M. Opioids

Opioids are found in a variety of prescription preparations and street drugs. Because the ICU nurse is familiar with the administration of opioid analgesics and antitussives, this section simply emphasizes a few points related to overdose.

1. The **classic triad of symptoms** (miosis, respiratory depression, and coma) may be masked by concomitant administration of other drugs. Abusers of stimulant drugs such as cocaine and amphetamines frequently use an opioid or other depressant simultaneously. Opioids may be abused inadvertently when drug dealers substitute them for or combine them with other drugs.
2. Young children can be **markedly sensitive** to some opioids. Dangerous situations may occur when both parents administer a codeine-containing antitussive.
3. Some opioids are associated with **clinically significant differences:**
   a. *Meperidine (Demerol)* use or abuse is not necessarily associated with pinpoint pupils. Also, normeperidine, the first metabolite of meperidine, is a CNS stimulant; chronic use or abuse is therefore associated with seizures.
   b. *Propoxyphene (Darvon)* and pentazocine (Talwin) may require up to 10 mg of naloxone to reverse the respiratory depression they induce, much higher than the usual naloxone dose.
   c. *Methadone* has a half-life of about 24 hours, much longer than other opioids, and requires sustained doses of naloxone, by IV drip, to prevent respiratory depression until the methadone is eliminated. (Nalmefene hydrochloride, a newer opioid antagonist, has a longer half-life than naloxone, but its use in children has not yet been evaluated.)
4. **Dermal patches and oral lozenges containing fentanyl,** even if they were used and discarded, are a significant risk to children who access them, for example, by retrieving them from a trash can. Discarded fentanyl patches contain sufficient residual drug to seriously poison a child who chews on one, swallows one, or applies one to the skin.

N. Salicylate Poisoning

Salicylate poisoning is most often due to aspirin. However, most fatal salicylate poisonings in children may occur from ingestion of methyl salicylate, a rapidly-absorbed liquid also known as oil of wintergreen, and from GI tract preparations containing bismuth subsalicylate. Older children and teenagers take aspirin in suicide attempts. (Although chronic salicylate poisoning may occur in people on therapeutic doses, such doses are rarely used in children.)

1. **Aspirin** is rapidly absorbed. In therapeutic doses, it has a small volume of distribution and much is bound to serum proteins. It undergoes hepatic metabolism and renal excretion. With chronic administration, receptors are saturated and free salicylate accumulates rapidly.
2. The **actions of salicylate in overdose** are complex and interdependent. Stimulation of the central respiratory drive causes respiratory alkalosis and metabolic acidosis. Interference with carbohydrate and lipid metabolism generates organic acids. Increased metabolic demands result in hypoglycemia, both in the serum and the CNS. Uncoupling of oxidative phosphorylation leads to hyperthermia. Direct CNS toxicity can cause tremor, agitation, seizures, and coma. Sequence and exact clinical effects depend on size, timing, and acuity of

ingestion and the age and health of the patient. A careful evaluation of each patient's status and history is essential.

3. **Acute toxicity** generally correlates with ingested dose. Greater than 150 mg/kg by history may be associated with mild toxicity, greater than 300 mg/kg with greater toxicity, and greater than 500 mg/kg with fatality. More specific determination is based on a serum salicylate level drawn 6 or more hours after ingestion.
4. In the **absence of history**, suspect salicylate poisoning in a patient who presents with tachypnea, tachycardia, hyperthermia, diaphoresis, mental status changes, respiratory alkalosis, metabolic acidosis, or mixed acid-base abnormalities. If present, tinnitus is an important clue, as is frank or occult GI tract bleeding.
5. **Treatment** includes GI decontamination, followed by multiple doses of activated charcoal administered every 4 hours with a cathartic once in 24 hours. Hydration is essential but must be controlled to avoid precipitating pulmonary edema. Potassium supplementation is often needed. Administer sufficient amounts of sodium bicarbonate to correct acidosis and achieve a urine pH of about 8; this enhances renal excretion of salicylate. Hemodialysis is indicated for salicylate levels above about 100 mg/dL in acute ingestions (lower in patients with chronic ingestions) and seriously symptomatic patients. Otherwise, treatment must be aggressive but is symptomatic and supportive.
6. **Special considerations**
   a. *Aspirin tablets* may clump together in the stomach, forming concretions that may be slowly absorbed over a prolonged period. If a large ingestion is suspected, it is essential to measure serial salicylate levels to avert the delayed onset of fatal effects. Ingestion of sustained-release forms of aspirin also can cause the delayed onset of symptoms. Again, it is essential to monitor serial salicylate levels.
   b. Because the *time between ingestion and death* from salicylate poisoning can often be measured in just hours, a high index of suspicion and aggressive management are essential to prevent serious CNS effects and fatalities.

O. Sympathomimetics

Sympathomimetic drugs are represented by both legal and illegal agents in the pediatric age group: cocaine is a legal, useful topical vasoconstrictor and a widely abused street drug; amphetamines are used as weight control agents, to treat hyperactivity disorders, and as the street drug "speed"; legal decongestants and appetite suppressants are sold as "street speed" or amphetamine look-alikes. Ephedra, even if it is not available legally, can be obtained via the Internet. Children are poisoned by ingesting appetite suppressants or an overdose of cough, cold, or allergy preparations containing decongestants and by swallowing available street drugs. Teenagers are poisoned by taking overdoses of appetite suppressants, by abusing street drugs, or by attempting to avoid arrest by swallowing illicit drugs. Hallucinogenic amphetamines (MDMA, MDA, "Ecstasy," "Adam," "Eve") are abused as "party drugs" or "rave drugs." The intended use, route of administration, and duration of action of these drugs may differ, but the acute clinical effects are indistinguishable, and treatment of acute effects is essentially the same. (Discussion of the numerous known medical consequences of cocaine and amphetamine abuse is beyond the scope of this review.)

1. The **toxic dose** is variable and may be idiosyncratic. In street drugs, the actual amount of drug, as opposed to adulterants, is unknown.
2. **Clinical effects** are as expected for any sympathomimetic agent: tachycardia, hypertension, diaphoresis, mydriasis, agitation and tremulousness, and central

vasoconstriction, including cardiac, cerebral, and visceral. In significant poisoning, ventricular dysrhythmias, seizures, hyperthermia, and coma may develop. The hallucinations sought by users of "party" or "rave" drugs are accompanied by other sympathomimetic effects, especially extreme hyperthermia.

3. **Clinical assessment and laboratory evaluation** are straightforward. When possible, identification of the drug involved helps to predict the duration of effects: a few hours for cocaine unless complicated by cardiac, cerebral, or other events caused by vasoconstriction, hyperthermia, or seizures; 18 to 24 hours for amphetamines, with the same caveat; variable for the other drugs and dependent to some extent on whether they are sustained-release preparations. Although radiographic examinations are not generally indicated in poisoning by sympathomimetic drugs, in the case of swallowed illegal drugs, they may help to visualize the number and location of the packets.
4. **Treatment** of these poisonings includes GI tract decontamination where indicated and then symptomatic and supportive care. A single dose of activated charcoal with a cathartic is indicated unless drug packets (e.g., vials, condoms, balloons, foil) have been swallowed. In these cases, multiple doses of activated charcoal may be indicated until the packets pass.

POISONING BY NONPHARMACEUTICAL AGENTS

A. Carbon Monoxide

Carbon monoxide is a colorless, odorless, tasteless, nonirritating gas—a product of incomplete combustion. The most common residential sources are house fires, exhaust from automobiles and gas-powered equipment, furnaces, space heaters, wood- and coal-burning stoves and fireplaces, and gas ovens and hot water heaters. Methylene chloride, found in paint strippers, is metabolized to carbon monoxide after ingestion, inhalation, or dermal absorption.

1. Carbon monoxide has an **affinity for hemoglobin** 200 times greater than that of oxygen. Besides displacing oxygen at hemoglobin receptor sites, it inhibits the release of oxygen from hemoglobin. Therefore inadequate amounts of oxygen are circulating, and that which is circulating is less available to tissues.
2. The **effects of carbon monoxide poisoning** are related to hypoxemia; the greater the amount of carboxyhemoglobin, the more severe the symptoms. Direct cellular toxicity also occurs. A carboxyhemoglobin level of about 10% may be associated with headache, nausea, and lethargy. As the carboxyhemoglobin level increases, GI tract and CNS symptoms increase. At a level of 50% the patient is unconscious, and victims of carbon monoxide exposure die at levels of about 70% or greater. Symptoms of chronic carbon monoxide exposure (e.g., due to malfunctioning furnaces or clogged chimneys) are often mistaken for a viral or flulike illness.
3. **Evaluating** victims of carbon monoxide poisoning requires close attention to symptoms experienced at any time since exposure, not just at the time of evaluation. The carboxyhemoglobin level at the time of presentation may have declined markedly since the patient was exposed. After an acute exposure to carbon monoxide, those who have lost consciousness, even if they are now awake, and fetuses are at greatest risk.
4. The **initial treatment** for carbon monoxide poisoning is 100% oxygen. Hyperbaric oxygen is indicated for those who were or are unconscious, pregnant women, those who remain symptomatic after oxygen administration, and those with recurrent symptoms.

5. **Other treatment** is symptomatic and supportive.
6. **Special considerations**
   a. Children and household pets are at greatest risk for carbon monoxide poisoning because of their rapid respiratory and metabolic rates. When a family is poisoned by carbon monoxide, children are generally more seriously ill.
   b. *Aggressive treatment* is required because long-term neuropsychiatric sequelae have been documented in adults with carbon monoxide exposure. Because of the difficulty or impossibility of conducting and interpreting such tests in children, long-term sequelae are postulated but not documented.
   c. Consider carbon monoxide poisoning in any family or gathering in which a number of people become ill with GI tract and CNS complaints.
   d. Unless the source of carbon monoxide is known (e.g., a suicide attempt with automobile exhaust, house fire) or remedied (e.g., repair of a faulty furnace), patients and their families must not return to a possibly contaminated environment.
   e. Encourage the installation of carbon monoxide alarms.

B. Caustic Substances

Caustic substances are those that can cause chemical burns. Young children are injured by unintentional contact with household substances, whereas older children may ingest these substances in suicide attempts. Occasionally children are exposed when they attempt unsupervised experiments. Strongly acidic and alkaline substances can cause chemical burns. Although the sources and mechanisms of injury are different, treatment and nursing care for both are essentially the same. The single exception is hydrofluoric acid, which is considered separately.

1. **Sources**
   a. *Acids* such as sulfuric acid, hydrochloric acid, and muriatic acid (dilute hydrochloric acid) are found in homes in toilet-bowl cleaners, swimming pool chemicals, metal cleaners, and concrete and masonry cleaners. These products tend to be liquids and usually are associated with greater injury to the stomach than to the esophagus after ingestion.
   b. *Alkaline substances* are liquids or solids found in wet cement, drain openers, oven cleaners, laundry detergent, and automatic dishwasher detergent. Examples include sodium hydroxide, potassium hydroxide, calcium hydroxide, sodium carbonate, and some phosphates. Children who bite into ammonia capsules are likely to develop an alkaline burn to the tip of the tongue.
2. **Mechanism of injury**
   a. *Acids* precipitate proteins and dehydrate tissues; exposure causes vascular thrombosis and the rapid formation of eschar. This hard crust helps to limit further penetration of acid into tissue. In general, serious injury is associated with exposure to products with a pH lower than 2.
   b. *Alkaline substances* cause vascular thrombosis and liquefaction necrosis. They disrupt cell walls and combine with lipids, which accounts for the soapy appearance of tissue and provides no protection whatsoever from further penetration of the chemical into tissue. In general, serious injury is associated with products with a pH higher than 12.
3. The **degree of injury** is determined by several factors. In addition to pH, the physical form of the substance may influence toxicity: liquid products transit the oropharynx and esophagus quickly and may cause the greatest injury to the stomach. However, a very viscous liquid may cause significantly greater injury.

Solids and crystals are associated with injury to the lips, mouth, oropharynx, and esophagus. Duration of contact with tissue also influences the extent of injury. The presence of food and liquid in the stomach minimizes the amount and duration of contact between the caustic substance and the gastric mucosa.

4. **Ocular and dermal exposure** to caustic substances requires copious irrigation with saline or water, as indicated earlier in this chapter. If there are any symptoms after irrigation, ocular exposures to caustic substances require ophthalmologic consultation. After initial irrigation, dermal exposures to caustic substances are treated as thermal burns of similar degree.
5. After **ingestion of a caustic product**, there is no strict correlation between the presence or absence of symptoms (including pain) and presence, location, or degree of injury.
   a. *Mild effects* of inflammation and irritation, similar to a first-degree thermal burn, require only symptomatic and supportive care.
   b. *Partial- or full-thickness injuries* are the equivalent of second- and third-degree thermal injuries. With ingestion of an acid (generally a liquid), there is risk of gastric perforation within about 3 days of ingestion. Otherwise, the risk of perforation is greatest during the granulation phase, perhaps up to 2 weeks. Then the development of scar tissue and esophageal stricture commences.
   c. *Initial pain* may be oral, substernal, or epigastric.
6. **Assessment** of the patient includes visual inspection of exposed tissue, evaluation of acid-base and fluid and electrolyte status, determination of hemoglobin and hematocrit, and perhaps radiographic examinations to determine the presence or absence of free air.
7. **Treatment**
   a. *Dilution* with a small volume of water helps to minimize contact between the caustic substance and tissue. Large volumes are not indicated because that would increase the risk of vomiting, causing esophageal reinjury and the possibility of aspiration.
   b. *Observe for respiratory distress.* Soft-tissue swelling and aspiration of caustic material can contribute to respiratory difficulty. If significant edema is present, oral or nasotracheal intubation is dangerous, and a tracheotomy or cricothyrotomy is needed.
   c. *Observe for signs of fluid and electrolyte imbalance* to evaluate loss of fluids or third-spacing of fluids.
   d. *Observe for acidosis* if the patient has ingested a large quantity of an acid, as may occur in a suicide attempt. Although direct injury is generally confined to points of contact with the chemical, acidosis is one possible systemic manifestation associated with acid ingestion.
   e. *Esophagoscopy and endoscopy* may be indicated. If the initial injury is thought to be severe or if circumferential burns are found on esophagoscopy, additional surgical procedures may be indicated. Gastrostomy may be performed to remove necrotic tissue; place a string or stent in the esophagus, or place a gastric feeding tube. Esophagectomy and colonic interposition (removing the esophagus and replacing it with a length of the patient's own colon) may also be performed.
   f. The *use of steroids* is controversial and depends on the preference and experience of individual gastroenterologist and surgeon. Steroids may decrease the formation of restrictive scar tissue after circumferential burns but may also weaken tissue and predispose the patient to infection.
   g. *Antibiotics* are prescribed for patients taking steroids and for patients with specific indications.

h. Observe the patient for signs of *perforation and sepsis.* Perforation may be accompanied by abdominal distention and a change in the amount or character of the patient's pain.
i. *Analgesics* are indicated.
j. Patients must remain *NPO (taking nothing by mouth)* until esophagoscopy is performed.

8. **Special considerations**
a. Until the patient is *decontaminated,* health care providers must avoid contact with caustic material.
b. If the patient has sustained a *serious injury,* psychosocial considerations for the patient and the family come to the forefront. Ocular and dermal exposures may cause significant disfigurement, and ocular exposures may result in permanent blindness. Ingestion with significant injury means that the patient may require permanent tracheostomy or gastrostomy or both, major surgery and follow-up for esophagectomy and colonic interposition, or regular esophageal dilation for many years to come. Also, the risk of developing cancer at the site of the injury, although delayed for decades, is greater than in the general population.

9. **Hydrofluoric acid** is different from other acids, and indeed from other caustic agents, in that it is absorbed dermally, even through intact skin, and can cause both local and systemic effects. It is used industrially to etch glass and computer chips, as a cleaning agent for metals and air-conditioning units, and as a rust remover. Products with low (but potentially dangerous) concentrations of hydrofluoric acid are sold for home use as rust removers and metal brighteners. Hydrofluoric acid is toxic by all routes of exposure, but dermal exposure is the most common and is discussed here.
a. In *concentrations above 50%,* hydrofluoric acid causes immediate local tissue injury along with significant pain. In concentrations between 20% and 50%, the onset of local injury and pain can be delayed for 8 hours or longer. In concentrations lower than 20%, the effects of exposure may not be evident for 24 hours.
b. *Hydrofluoric acid* is absorbed through the skin and precipitates both calcium and magnesium. The result is intense pain at the site of the exposure. With significant exposure, systemic hypocalcemia, hypomagnesemia, hyperkalemia, and possibly fatal ventricular dysrhythmias are present.
c. *Initial treatment* is copious irrigation with running water, even in the absence of local effects. With exposure to the hands, subungual concentrations of hydrofluoric acid may be difficult to remove and often necessitate removal or splitting of the nails or injection of calcium (discussed later).
d. *Local pain* is treated with a calcium gluconate gel, prepared by mixing 3.5 g of calcium gluconate powder in 5 oz of water-soluble gel (Seamens, 2001), and is applied to painful areas until the pain subsides. When pain recurs, additional gel is applied. The patient should apply the gel liberally at home if pain recurs and return for further care if the gel ceases to be effective.
e. *More serious exposures* may be treated with subcutaneous, intravenous (IV), or intra-arterial infusions of calcium gluconate. Even minimal dermal exposure to high concentrations of hydrofluoric acid may cause systemic hypocalcemia. These patients must be admitted to monitored beds, and serial calcium levels must be closely monitored until it is certain the patient is out of danger.

C. Cyanide

Cyanide is thought of as a fast-acting lethal poison, but in some circumstances a slower onset of symptoms is possible. Treatment involves supportive care and the rapid administration of amyl nitrite, sodium nitrite, and sodium thiosulfate, packaged as a cyanide antidote kit.

1. There are many **potential sources** of cyanide poisoning. Victims of fires may develop cyanide poisoning along with carbon monoxide poisoning. A number of plant seeds (apples, peaches, plums, pears, nectarines, and cherries) contain amygdalin, which generates hydrogen cyanide after ingestion. Laetrile, an ineffective treatment for cancer, is derived from apricot kernels and has caused death from cyanide poisoning. Cyanide is a metabolite of nitroprusside; rapid or prolonged treatment can cause symptoms of cyanide poisoning. (Cyanide and thiocyanate levels should be monitored.) Nonoccupational cyanide poisoning in adults and teenagers is likely to result from suicidal ingestion of laboratory or photographic chemicals. Children have died rapidly after swallowing professional jewelry-cleaning solutions containing cyanide. Acetonitrile, which is metabolized to cyanide, is found in liquids used to dissolve artificial fingernail glue; delayed onset of symptoms and death have occurred when this product was swallowed.
2. Cyanide interferes with the **action of cytochrome oxidase** and therefore with aerobic metabolism and cellular utilization of oxygen. Other enzyme systems are affected as well.
3. The **toxic dose** depends on the form of the chemical and route of administration. Small amounts of cyanide salts can cause rapid loss of consciousness and death. Substances that are metabolized to cyanide (e.g., amygdalin glycosides, acetonitrile, nitroprusside) have a delayed onset of action, and the toxic dose is variable.
4. **Clinical effects** are related to hypoxia and typically progress within minutes from dizziness and headache to coma and death. Acidosis and hypotension are prominent. Patients with lesser exposures and those exposed to substances that must be metabolized have a less precipitous onset of symptoms.
5. **ABGs** must be followed closely. Cyanide can be measured in serum, but levels cannot be returned in time to be useful for acutely poisoned patients.
6. **Antidotal treatment** is with a three-part cyanide antidote kit. First, methemoglobin is induced with nitrites; cyanmethemoglobin is formed as cyanide is thus removed from cytochrome oxidase. Administration of sodium thiosulfate results in the formation of relatively nontoxic thiocyanate.
   a. *Amyl nitrite ampules* are broken, placed in a cloth, and held in front of the patient's mouth for 15 of 30 seconds, then repeated. This permits the formation of about 5% methemoglobin. This step may be skipped in favor of immediate administration of IV sodium nitrite.
   b. *Sodium nitrite* induces the formation of additional methemoglobin. The desired level of methemoglobin is 20% up to no more than 40%. In children, the amount of sodium nitrite is calculated according to body weight and titrated to actual hemoglobin levels. Doses must be carefully calculated because inducing too high a level of methemoglobinemia worsens hypoxia. **High levels cannot be treated with methylene blue because to do so would liberate free cyanide.**
   c. Administration of *sodium thiosulfate* results in the formation of thiocyanate, which is eliminated renally.
   d. *Treatment* also includes respiratory support and symptomatic and supportive care.
7. **Special considerations**
   a. Too high a level of *methemoglobin* can itself be fatal. Pediatric doses of nitrites must be carefully calculated, and methemoglobin levels must be monitored.
   b. *Brain-dead victims* of cyanide poisoning may be considered as organ donors.

D. Envenomations

Envenomations by snakes and spiders will not be considered in depth in this book. Always consult the poison center when treating a patient with a snake or spider bite. All venoms are extremely complex mixtures; any bite resulting in symptoms indicates a poisoning with the potential for serious multisystemic effects. Children are at greater risk than adults because of their small body size in relationship to the amount of venom injected.

1. The **venom of the Crotalidae** (rattlesnakes, copperheads, and cottonmouths [water moccasins]) can cause the rapid onset of life-threatening effects, although this is not expected with bites of copperheads and cottonmouths. Action at numerous venom receptors results in hypotension, increased capillary permeability resulting in local ecchymosis and edema, pulmonary edema, local tissue injury, myocardial injury, and bleeding and clotting disorders. Local wound care and intensive supportive care are both essential. Definitive antidotal treatment is the administration of antivenin; Fab antivenin (CroFab) is derived from sheep and has superseded equine polyvalent crotalid antivenin as the treatment for crotalid envenomations. There is no substitute for administration of sufficient quantities of antivenin in a patient poisoned by a rattlesnake. Common treatment errors include withholding antivenin in a patient with a life- or limb-threatening envenomation for fear of allergic reactions and performing fasciotomy in lieu of administering sufficient antivenin in patients with peripheral edema.
2. The **venom of the Elapidae** (the coral snakes) can cause fatal poisoning by its neuromuscular effects, specifically, respiratory muscle paralysis. Onset of symptoms is delayed for 6 to 8 hours after envenomation. Fortunately, such fatalities are extremely rare. Treatment includes the administration of antivenin and respiratory support.
3. The **venom of the black widow spider** *(Latrodectus mactans)* also can cause paralysis of respiratory muscles, although this is not usual. More common effects are immediate, intense pain at the site of the bite (which can be identified by two tiny fang marks, about 0.5 cm [$^1/_4$ in] apart); muscle weakness, ataxia, and ptosis, especially in children; and intensely painful muscle contractions, across the abdomen for lower-extremity bites and across the back and shoulders for upper-extremity bites. Treatment includes administration of analgesics and a benzodiazepine. Antivenin is available, but its use is usually required only for severe systemic effects.

E. Ethanol

Ethanol is found in alcoholic beverages, mouthwash, and cosmetics such as perfumes, tonics, and hair spray. It is used therapeutically as the antidote for ethylene glycol and methanol poisoning when fomepizole is not available. Young children are poisoned unintentionally or by adults who give them alcoholic beverages. Preteens and teenagers may indulge in binge drinking and may be alcohol dependent. In these cases, they are as vulnerable as adults to atrial dysrhythmias following binges and to medical and behavioral consequences of alcoholism.

1. **Ethanol** is rapidly absorbed and widely distributed. It is well known as a CNS depressant. In children, ethanol's hypoglycemic effects are significant; the immature liver does not maintain sufficient glycogen stores to counteract ethanol-induced hypoglycemia.
2. **Symptoms** related to ethanol-induced CNS depression are lethargy, ataxia, respiratory depression, hypothermia, and coma. These effects may begin within an hour of ingestion, followed within a few hours by hypoglycemic seizures, coma, and death. Metabolic acidosis may be present in large ingestions.

3. **Toxicity** may occur with an ethanol ingestion of 1 g/kg. This may be roughly estimated as the amount of alcoholic product ingested multiplied by the percent of ethanol in the product divided by the body weight of the patient (in kilograms). A fatal dose in children is approximately 3 g/kg; the fatal dose in teenagers and adults is widely variable.
4. **Physical assessment** is straightforward. Laboratory studies required include serum ethanol level, electrolytes, glucose, and ABG analysis.
5. **Treatment:** Gastric emptying is not useful longer than 1 hour after ingestion. Activated charcoal does not adsorb ethanol. Careful monitoring and correction of serum glucose are essential. Other treatment is symptomatic and supportive. Ethanol is removed by hemodialysis, which may be indicated for serious or potentially fatal ingestions.
6. **Special consideration:** Even preteens and young teenagers may be alcohol dependent. Be alert for signs of impending withdrawal: tremors, agitation, hallucinations, and seizures. Benzodiazepines are usually indicated for initial management of alcohol withdrawal.

F. Ethylene Glycol

Ethylene glycol is the ingredient in automobile antifreeze, the most common source of glycol poisoning in the pediatric population. Unintentional ingestions are the norm in young children, whereas adolescents drink antifreeze in suicide attempts or as an ethanol surrogate. This is a dangerous poisoning because ethylene glycol is sweet but extremely toxic in small amounts. Effects are due to metabolites and are therefore delayed. Parents or victims mistakenly may believe that absence of early symptoms indicates absence of toxicity.

1. **Ethylene glycol** is rapidly absorbed from the GI tract and is widely distributed. During the several steps in its metabolism, glycolic acid, lactic acid, and a number of other organic acids are generated, leading to the metabolic acidosis characteristic of this poisoning. Oxalic acid precipitates with calcium, leading to the deposition of calcium oxalate crystals in soft tissue (including the kidney) and renal failure.
2. The **toxic dose** is variable but small; the potential fatal dose is 1 to 1.5 mL/kg.
3. **Toxic effects** are delayed for as long as 12 to 24 hours; early effects resemble alcoholic inebriation. As the poisoning progresses, nonspecific symptoms of lethargy and GI tract complaints evolve into ataxia, seizures, coma, and renal failure. In the absence of specific history, ethylene glycol poisoning should be suspected in any patient who presents with or develops both coma and metabolic acidosis.
4. A **serum ethylene glycol level** is most useful but is not always easily obtained. The presence or absence of an anion gap metabolic acidosis is more easily ascertained and is extremely useful. ABG analysis is required. A few hours after ingestion, the urine can be examined for the presence of calcium oxalate crystals. A serum ethanol level should be drawn in anticipation of antidotal therapy with ethanol if fomepizole is not available.
5. **Treatment** includes prevention of absorption (if possible), prevention of metabolism to toxic metabolites, and enhanced elimination.
   a. *Gastric emptying* is useful only within 1 hour of ingestion.
   b. *Specific antidotes* to ethylene glycol poisoning are the alcohol dehydrogenase inhibitors fomepizole and ethanol. The goal of antidotal treatment with fomepizole or ethanol is to prevent metabolism of ethylene glycol into toxic components until ethylene glycol can be eliminated renally or by hemodialysis. Either antidote is administered until the serum ethylene glycol level is less than 20 mg/dL. Dosing of both is altered by concurrent hemodialysis.

- Fomepizole is administered IV every 12 hours. The loading dose is 15 mg/kg; maintenance dose is 10 mg/kg for four doses, followed by 15 mg/kg until therapy is no longer needed (Dart, 2004).
- The initial dose of ethanol is calculated according to age, whether ethanol is already present, and whether the patient is habituated to ethanol. Subsequent doses are titrated to the serum ethanol level, which should be maintained at 100 mg/dL. To prevent ethanol-induced hypoglycemia, serum glucose must be carefully monitored and corrected if necessary.

c. *Hemodialysis* is indicated if the ethylene glycol level is greater than 50 mg/dL.

d. *Serial ethylene glycol levels* should be determined until they are less than 10 mg/dL. Metabolism of ethylene glycol to nontoxic metabolites is enhanced by administration of pyridoxine and thiamine.

e. *Renal function and acidosis* must be aggressively monitored and corrected.

6. Special considerations: A high index of suspicion is necessary because ethylene glycol is toxic in extremely small quantities and because the most effective time to initiate treatment is before metabolism and symptoms occur. Aggressive treatment is necessary, not only to prevent renal damage and death but to minimize the risks of peripheral nervous system damage in survivors.

G. Methanol

Methanol is the ingredient in windshield-washer solution. It also is found in gas-line additives, fuel for chafing dishes and model airplanes, and deicing compounds. It is extremely toxic in small amounts, has a sweet taste, and, in the case of windshield washer solutions, resembles blue soft drinks, especially when transferred to beverage containers. It is also used as an ethanol surrogate and in suicides. The metabolites of methanol are responsible for its toxicity.

1. **Methanol** is rapidly absorbed from the GI tract. It is metabolized briefly to formaldehyde, then to formic acid. Generation of organic acids accounts for metabolic acidosis, and generation of formic acid accounts for optic nerve damage.
2. The **toxic dose** is variable but small, with permanent blindness associated with an ingestion of perhaps 10 mL of methanol and fatality associated with just a few milliliters more.
3. Because **toxicity** is due to metabolites, there may be no symptoms for 10 to 24 hours. The early nonspecific symptoms include inebriation, GI tract complaints, and lethargy. As formic acid is generated, ocular complaints begin. They have been described variously as double vision, dim vision like being in a snowstorm, and actual blindness. The patient progresses to seizures and coma.
4. Because the area of **physical assessment** requiring unusual attention is examination of the optic disc for hyperemia and the retina for edema, ophthalmologic consultation should be secured promptly. Determination of ethanol levels is ideal but often difficult to obtain. Presence or absence of an anion gap metabolic acidosis is critical information, as is measurement of ABGs. An ethanol level should be determined in anticipation of antidotal therapy with ethanol.
5. **Treatment** includes prevention of absorption (if possible), prevention of metabolism to toxic metabolites, and enhanced elimination.

   a. *Gastric emptying* is useful only within 1 hour of ingestion.

   b. *Specific antidotes* to methanol poisoning are the alcohol dehydrogenase inhibitors fomepizole and ethanol. The goal of antidotal treatment with fomepizole or ethanol is to prevent metabolism of methanol into toxic components until methanol can be eliminated renally or by hemodialysis. Either antidote is administered until the serum methanol level is less than 20 mg/dL. Dosing of both is altered by concurrent hemodialysis.

- Fomepizole is administered IV every 12 hours. The loading dose is 15 mg/kg; maintenance dose is 10 mg/kg for four doses, followed by 15 mg/kg until therapy is no longer needed (Dart, 2004).
- The initial dose of ethanol is calculated according to age, whether ethanol is already present, and whether the patient is habituated to ethanol. Subsequent doses are titrated to the serum ethanol level, which should be maintained at 100 mg/dL. To prevent ethanol-induced hypoglycemia, serum glucose must be carefully monitored and corrected if necessary.

c. *Hemodialysis* is indicated if the methanol level is greater than 50 mg/dL.

d. *Serial methanol levels* should be determined until they are less than 10 mg/dL. Eventual metabolism of methanol to carbon dioxide and water is enhanced by administration of folate if the patient is already symptomatic. If the patient is still asymptomatic, leucovorin may be given instead.

e. *Ocular status* must be monitored. Acidosis must be aggressively monitored and corrected. Other treatment is symptomatic and supportive.

6. **Special considerations:** A high index of suspicion is necessary because methanol is toxic in extremely small quantities and because the most effective time to initiate treatment is before metabolism occurs. Aggressive treatment is necessary, not only to prevent blindness and death but to minimize risks of peripheral nervous system damage in survivors.

H. Hydrocarbons

Hydrocarbons may be categorized in many ways: by chemical composition, intended purpose, volatility, and toxic effects. Some hydrocarbons are of particular danger to the pulmonary tract if aspirated, although not usually damaging to the GI tract if ingested. These include gasoline, kerosene, lamp oil, mineral spirits, mineral seal oil, and other substances used as fuels, lighter fluids, lubricants, and polishes.

1. When **ingested,** these liquids may be irritating and cause nausea, diarrhea, and eructation. However, they are not absorbed from the GI tract and are not expected to cause systemic effects.
2. **Aspiration** of any amount of hydrocarbon is dangerous; when it occurs, pneumonitis is likely. Depending on the exact substance and its viscosity, expected effects include airway irritation, pulmonary edema, disruption of surfactant, and impaired oxygen exchange. The victim experiences hypoxia, cyanosis, and perhaps alveolar collapse. Chest radiographic findings may range from isolated basilar infiltrates to "whiting out," especially after aspiration of such low-viscosity hydrocarbons as charcoal lighter fluid. Bacterial pneumonia may follow.
3. **Relevant history** includes a history of coughing or choking after ingestion of a hydrocarbon; in these cases, aspiration is likely, and the victim must be assessed in a health care facility. Physical assessment should focus on pulmonary findings and CNS abnormalities secondary to hypoxia. Laboratory studies are necessary to determine the status of oxygenation. A chest radiograph should be taken quickly if the patient is severely symptomatic on arrival at the health care facility; otherwise, it should be deferred until 2 hours after exposure to permit detection of changes.
4. **Treatment** of patients with hydrocarbon aspiration may need to be aggressive but is symptomatic and supportive. In general, steroids are not indicated, and antibiotics are indicated only if bacterial pneumonia develops.

I. Mushrooms

Mushrooms of many varieties can be poisonous and even fatal when ingested by the unwary. Children may eat wild mushrooms unintentionally, as they do many other things. More dangerous is the situation where an adult identifies wild mushrooms incorrectly and then cooks and serves them. In these cases, much more of the material is ingested; also, there could be multiple victims. Mycologists divide mushrooms into numerous species; toxicologists divide them into several groups based on symptoms. The poison center can help you narrow the group of mushroom (thus treatment) on the basis of symptoms and can identify a mycologist for positive identification of wild mushrooms and their spores. (Any available mushroom specimen must be wrapped in waxed paper or a dry paper bag and stored safely until it can be transported for identification or until it can be determined that specific identification is not necessary.) There are a few situations in which mushroom ingestion precipitates an ICU admission.

1. In the United States, there are **two types** of mushrooms that are inherently sufficiently toxic to cause fatalities. Both are differentiated by the delayed onset of GI tract symptoms. Sometimes people do not associate nausea, vomiting, and diarrhea with mushrooms eaten hours or even the day before.
   a. *Amanita phalloides, A. verna,* and *A. virosa* are hepatotoxic. The onset of significant GI tract symptoms occurs 8 or more hours after ingestion. Death from hepatic and renal failure may occur in about 5 days. There are no antidotes and no universally effective treatments. If ingestion is recognized early enough, GI tract decontamination is necessary. Hemodialysis may remove hepatotoxic metabolites.
   b. *Gyromitra esculenta* is sometimes mistaken for the edible morel, with hepatotoxic consequences. Vigorous GI tract decontamination is required if the ingestion is recognized early enough. Ingestion of *Gyromitra* species results in monomethylhydrazine poisoning, similar to isoniazid (INH). Treatment is as for INH poisoning, including pyridoxine 25 mg/kg.
2. **Other toxic mushrooms** in the United States cause the rapid onset of GI tract and perhaps other symptoms, typically within 30 minutes to 2 hours. Numerous mushrooms can cause cholinergic, anticholinergic, or hallucinogenic effects. Treatment includes GI tract decontamination and then symptomatic and supportive care. Numerous mushrooms can cause the rapid onset of GI tract symptoms with associated fluid and electrolyte imbalances. Treatment may include GI tract decontamination and then symptomatic and supportive care with an emphasis on monitoring and replacing fluids and electrolytes.

J. Organophosphate Insecticides

Organophosphate insecticides are absorbed via ingestion, inhalation, and dermal contact. Highly toxic organophosphates such as sarin, tabun, and soman were developed as nerve gas agents for warfare and terrorist events; less toxic organophosphates include malathion, dursban, and diazinon, which are used in household settings. Children can be exposed by household exterminations (e.g., for fleas and termites), garden applications, and exposure to agricultural sprays and adolescents by occupational exposure and in suicide attempts.

1. Organophosphate insecticides are **acetylcholinesterase inhibitors.** By binding to acetylcholinesterase, organophosphate insecticides prevent acetylcholine from being hydrolyzed to choline and acetic acid. There is continued stimulation of acetylcholine receptors in the CNS and at muscarinic and nicotinic sites in the autonomic nervous system. Expected effects of exposure thus are referable to the CNS and to the autonomic nervous system. Onset of symptoms is variable: rapid for nerve gas agents and "typical" household pesticides, delayed and prolonged for extremely fat-soluble agents and for those that must first be metabolized to toxic agents (e.g., fenthion).

a. *Muscarinic symptoms* can be remembered by the mnemonic *sludge: s*alivation, *l*acrimation, *u*rination, *d*efecation, *g*astrointestinal effects (e.g., nausea), and *e*yes (e.g., pinpoint pupils).
b. *Nicotinic effects* can be remembered by the mnemonic *mtwthf: m*ydriasis, muscle twitching, and cramps; *t*achycardia; *w*eakness; *(t)h*ypertension; and *f*asciculations.
c. *CNS effects* include tremor, agitation, confusion, ataxia, lethargy, seizures, and coma.

2. The **greatest threat** to the patient is respiratory distress, both from bronchorrhea and from weakness or even paralysis of the respiratory muscles. The greatest threat to the health care provider is poisoning by being exposed to a patient who has not been decontaminated.
3. **Physical assessment** of the patient must necessarily be thorough because acetylcholinesterase inhibition has broad and diverse systemic effects. The specific laboratory study required is measurement of red blood cell (RBC) cholinesterase. (Often the more easily measured plasma cholinesterase level is measured, but this test is not as useful because it can be affected by many things other than organophosphate insecticide poisoning.) The range of normal varies, but a significant decrease from the expected normal is indicative of cholinesterase inhibition and organophosphate insecticide poisoning.
4. A patient with dermal exposure must be **decontaminated.** Protect staff with impermeable gowns and gloves to minimize or prevent dermal exposure, remove and isolate contaminated clothing, and wash the patient thoroughly (twice with copious amounts of soap and water). Even the vomitus of patients who have ingested these compounds can be hazardous to staff members.
5. **Atropine** is administered to occupy muscarinic receptors and alleviate muscarinic effects. The necessary dose is titrated to symptoms, especially bronchorrhea. The pediatric dose is 0.05 mg/kg, repeated every 5 to 10 minutes until bronchial secretions are controlled; atropine by IV drip may be required for hours or days, depending on the amount of insecticide absorbed and its duration of effects.
6. **Pralidoxime (2-PAM)** is administered to cleave the organophosphate-acetylcholinesterase bond before it "ages," or becomes permanent within 24 hours after exposure. It is used in severe organophosphate insecticide poisoning and may be administered concurrently with atropine. Like atropine, it is administered until the patient remains asymptomatic.
7. Otherwise, **care** is symptomatic and supportive, with aggressive respiratory care.
8. **Special considerations:** Patients are often undertreated because health care providers are reluctant to administer the necessarily high and prolonged doses of atropine or pralidoxime. Permanent neurologic effects have been associated with exposure to some organophosphate insecticides. Young children are especially susceptible to the effects of these insecticides.
9. **Carbamate insecticides** have the same acute toxic effects as organophosphate insecticides. However, pralidoxime is not indicated for poisoning by carbamate insecticides, which do not form permanent bonds with acetylcholinesterase.

PSYCHOSOCIAL CONSIDERATIONS

Parents often feel guilty about a poisoning episode. Although it is objectively true that most such incidents can be anticipated and avoided, the reality is that young children are extremely curious and move very fast. Even the most vigilant parents must blink their eyes, turn their backs, tend to another child, or experience a momentary lapse in concentration. Most parents realize what they could have done differently to prevent the poisoning. It probably is most productive for health care providers to focus on what parents did right: recognized a dangerous situation; sought emergency assistance; cooperated with health care providers who attempted to elicit a history, identify the drug or product, and reconstruct the scenario; and provided support to the poisoned child and other family members during recovery. This can be followed by specific poison prevention information, which can be obtained from the poison center.

For older children or teens whose poisoning represented self-destructive or sociopathic behavior, psychiatric or social service consults are required.

If there is any suspicion of child abuse or Munchausen by proxy, there may be legal requirements to be fulfilled in addition to the need for psychiatric and social services referrals for the parents.

Septic Shock

Michelle A. Dragotta, Barbara A. Woodruff, and Debra M. Bills

A. Developmental Anatomy and Physiology

1. **Immunity** of the young child is not equal to that of the developmentally mature host. Several aspects of the infant and young child's first, second, and third lines of defense are immature (see the developmental distinctions noted in Chapter 8). The healthy infant and young child are not immunocompromised; rather, they are immunologically *inexperienced.*
2. **Cardiac output regulation:** See Chapter 3 on maturational differences in cardiac output and its associated components (heart rate, stroke volume, preload, contractility, and afterload). Changes in the child's cardiac output (CO) accompany the child's growth and development. CO is greatest at birth (200 mL/kg per minute) and then decreases throughout childhood to adolescence (100 mL/kg per minute) (Hazinski, 1999). This decrease is related to two events (Alyn and Baker, 1992): (1) a decrease in fetal hemoglobin and (2) an increase in adult hemoglobin and less oxygen requirements secondary to a changing surface area. In the young child, CO is directly proportional to heart rate (Hazinski, 1999).
3. **Oxygen consumption:** Oxygen consumption is the volume of oxygen consumed by the tissues per unit of time. Oxygen consumption is the product of the CO and the amount of oxygen extracted from each milliliter of blood, expressed as mL/kg per minute. Changes in the child's oxygen consumption accompany the child's growth and development. As with CO, oxygen consumption decreases throughout childhood. Normal values in the fetus are 8 mL/kg per minute (Alyn and Baker, 1992); in the infant, 10 to 14 mL/kg per minute; and in the child, 5 to 8 mL/kg per minute (Hazinski, 1999).

B. Etiology

1. Children have a **predisposition** to sepsis and septic shock as a result of environmental and genetic factors; this predisposition may be associated with immune dysfunction (Carcillo, 2003).
2. All microorganisms potentially can lead to **septic shock,** including bacteria, viruses, fungi, rickettsiae, spirochetes, protozoa, mycoplasmas, *Chlamydia* organisms, and parasites.

3. **Causative microorganisms** often vary with the following factors:
   a. *Patient's age:* Watson (2003) and colleagues have shown that age is the most significant influence in the epidemiology of severe sepsis. Table 9-12 illustrates the occurrence and case fatality of certain pathogens Watson's group found in relation to the age of the child with severe sepsis (Watson et al., 2003).
   b. *Immunocompetence:* In immunocompromised patients, the usual source is the patient's endogenous flora. In immunocompetent patients, the usual source is exogenous flora, with some evidence that patients may benefit from protective isolation against intensive care unit (ICU) acquired microorganisms (Maki, 1995).
   c. *Location:* In hospital-acquired *(nosocomial)* infection, the etiologic organism is usually specific to the individual unit and institution and geographic region. Community-acquired infection compromises a significant proportion of infections in the pediatric intensive care unit (PICU). In one study the PICU had nearly twice as many community-acquired infections as the adult medical-surgical ICU (Brown, 1985).
   d. *Site of infection:* Patients with invasive monitoring devices, mechanical ventilation, and invasive catheters are more likely to fall victim to nosocomial infections (Urrea, 2003). It has been reported that bacterial, urinary tract, and respiratory tract infections are more frequently related to these infections (Raymond, 2000; Richards 1999; Stover, 2001).

C. Epidemiology

1. **Incidence**
   a. Watson and colleagues (2003) reported that *sepsis* accounts for 42,000 cases a year, with 4400 associated deaths in the United States per year. In 1995, 7% of all deaths in children were caused by severe sepsis (National Center for Health Statistics, 2002). This number represents 2275 more deaths than pediatric patients who died of cancer (National Cancer Institute, 1999).

TABLE 9-12
Occurrence and Case Fatality of Select Pathogens Among Children with Severe Sepsis by Age

	Less than 1 Year (n = 4643)		1-10 Years (n = 2724)		11-19 Years (n = 2308)	
Organism	**Cases %**	**Case fatality %**	**Cases %**	**Case fatality %**	**Cases %**	**Case fatality %**
Meningococcus	0.3	20.0	8	10.4	2.3	15.1
H. Influenza	1.6	4.2	2.4	1.6	1.9	6.8
Pseudomonas	3.6	14.6	7.7	12.4	6.9	9.4
Staphylococcus (all types)	22.7	8.6	11.2	7.9	14.4	7.8
Staphylococcus aureus	2.3	5.7	2.9	0	3.5	3.8
Streptococcus (all types)	12.1	10.2	9.8	13.9	6.9	8.8
Pneumococcus	1.7	12.8	4.0	19.1	2.0	6.4
Group A Strep	0.3	0	0.7	5.0	0.2	0
Group B Strep	3.1	7.6	0.1	50.0	0.8	5.6
Fungus	10.0	10.8	13.3	16.8	10.4	11.6

Reprinted with permission from Watson RS et al: The epidemiology of severe sepsis in children in the United States. *Am J Respir Crit Care Med* 167:698, 2003.

b. The burden of *sepsis* continues despite advances in medical care (Watson et al., 2003). The annual estimated cost of sepsis is between $1.97 billion to $4 billion dollars (Carcillo, 2003; Watson et al., 2003). Chronic illness is a major predisposing factor of sepsis (Watson et al., 2003). Watson and colleagues (2003) showed that infants have more underlying etiologies related to neurologic and cardiovascular disease, whereas children usually have etiologies of cancer and immunodeficiency disorders (Watson et al., 2003).

2. **Risk factors**
   a. *Susceptible patients* are those with extremes in age (neonates and children younger than 3 years of age), noncompliance with immunization schedules, malnourishment or failure to thrive, chronic illness, malignancy, immunosuppressive therapy (e.g., malignancy, transplant recipient), primary immunodeficiency, asplenia, acquired immunodeficiency syndrome (AIDS), and congenital heart disease.
   b. *Aggressive microorganisms* have changing resistance patterns.
   c. Several factors increase the *risk of infection* in children who are in the PICU. These include invasive procedures, immunosuppression, and the physiologic immunodeficiency related to the age of the child (Urrea, 2003).

D. Pathophysiology

1. **Septic shock** has been defined by Carcillo as "infection with hypothermia or hyperthermia, tachycardia (may be absent with hypothermia), and altered mental status in the presence of a least one, but usually more than one, of the following: decreased peripheral pulses compared with central pulses, capillary refill prolonged for more than 2 seconds *(cold shock)* or flash capillary refill *(warm shock)*, mottled or cool extremities *(cold shock)*, and decreased urine output (less than 1 cm^3/kg)" (Carcillo, 2003).
2. All surfaces of the body exposed in any way to the external environment serve as the **first line of defense.** When the microorganism breeches any of these barriers, it gains access to the body's internal environment.
3. The **inflammatory-immune response,** the **second line of defense,** is then triggered in an effort to eliminate or neutralize the microorganism and its toxins, contain the microorganism invasion, prevent access to the body's systemic environment (i.e., bloodstream), and promote rapid healing of involved tissues.
4. When the microorganism overwhelms the **second line of defense,** it invades the body's tissues, and the microorganism and its toxins are released systemically into the blood stream (Natanson et al., 2001).
   a. With systemic release of the microorganism and its toxins, there is an activation and release of various mediators and cytokines, referred to as a *system inflammatory response syndrome* (SIRS). SIRS is the body's systemic inflammatory-immune and hormonal response to severe injury or illness originating from a variety of sources, such as infection, hemorrhage, trauma, pancreatitis, and thermal injuries (American College of Chest Physicians [AACP] and Society for Critical Care Medicine [SCCM], 1992). SIRS is not dependent on an infection. The presence of SIRS accompanied by an infectious process is referred to as *sepsis* (ACCP and SCCM, 1992). Sepsis represents a continuum of clinical states in which the patient displays varying degrees of severity, specifically with regard to hypoperfusion, organ dysfunction(s), and hypotension (Table 9-13).
   b. Two factors that influence the *morbidity and mortality of SIRS* are the ability to treat the underlying disease of the patient and whether or not multiple-organ dysfunction syndrome is present (Kaplan, 2001).

TABLE 9-13
Related Pathogenesis of Systemic Inflammatory Response System (SIRS), Sepsis, Septic Shock, and Multiple Organ Dysfunction Syndrome (MODS)

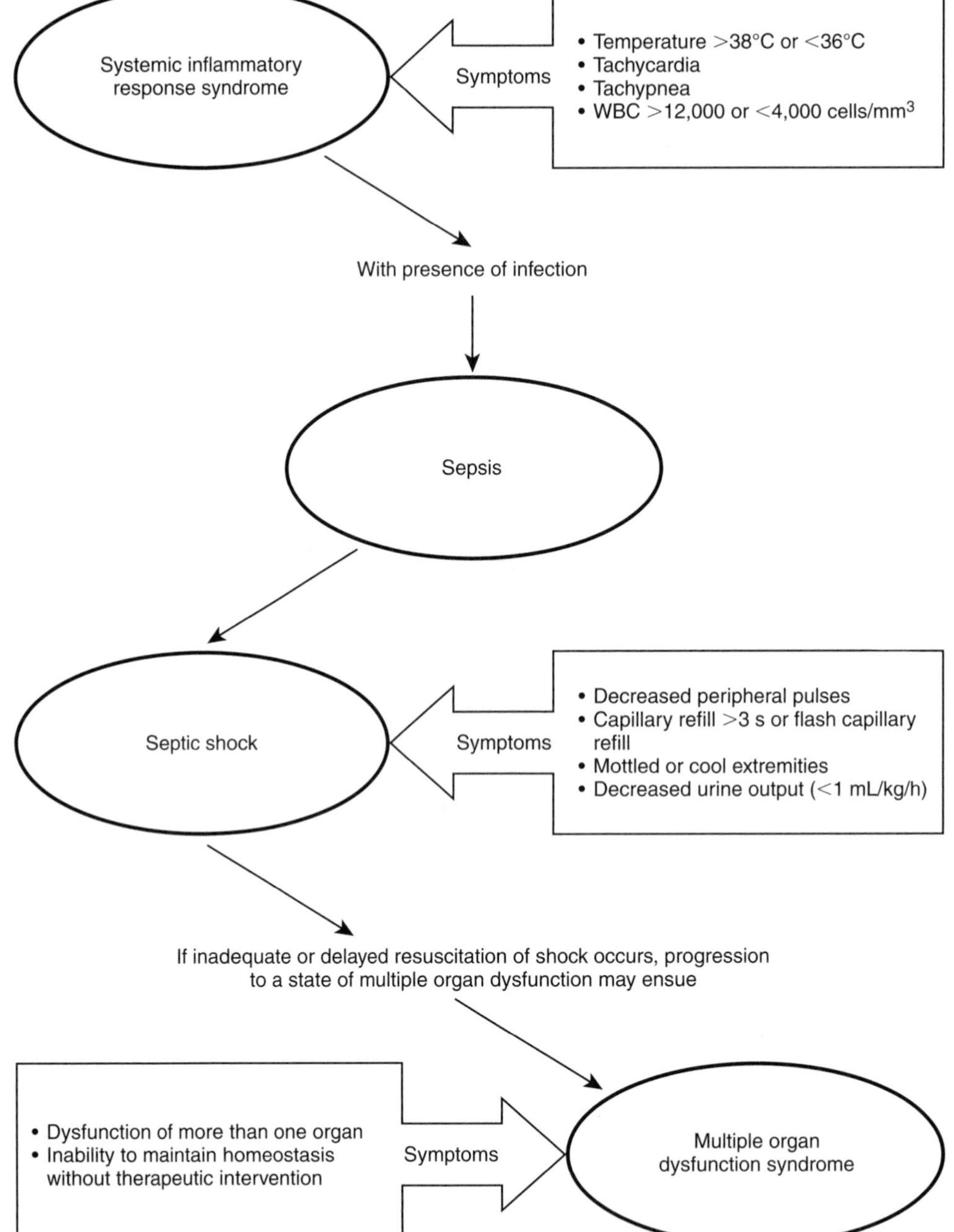

Modified from the American College of Chest Physician/Society of Critical Care Medicine Consensus Conference: Definitions for sepsis and organ failure and guidelines for the use of innovative therapies in sepsis. *Crit Care Med 20:864-874, 1992.*

c. *Mechanisms* within the inflammatory response and SIRS are the same, the differences being in the extent and magnitude of the response. Events or mechanisms of the inflammatory response serve protective functions, whereas SIRS causes deleterious outcomes.

5. The **activation and release of various mediators** result from two sources: exogenous and endogenous.
   a. *Exogenous* mediators are released by the invading microorganism. Microorganism mediators include, but are not limited to, endotoxin (released from gram-negative bacteria), exotoxin (released from gram-positive bacteria), and mannan (released from fungal cell walls).
      - *Endotoxin,* a lipopolysaccharide that is an integral part of the outer membrane of all gram-negative bacteria, is the most commonly studied toxin in sepsis. Endotoxin is shed as bacteria multiply or die. The core lipid A chain of the lipopolysaccharide is identical in every gram-negative organism. Antibodies for the core lipid A have been developed and have been investigated in several clinical studies. Results of these studies have failed to support conclusively their use in the treatment of septic shock (Natanson et al, 2001). Endotoxin administration to normal adult human volunteers (Suffredini et al., 1989) and animals (Natanson et al., 1989) results in cardiovascular changes similar to those seen with sepsis.
      - Endotoxin levels have been correlated to the incidence of lactic acidosis, adult respiratory distress syndrome (ARDS), renal insufficiency, and myocardial dysfunction in adults (Danner et al., 1991) and the severity of disease and outcomes in children (Brandtzaeg et al., 1989; Mertsola et al., 1991).

   b. *Endogenous mediators* are synthesized or activated by the host in response to an insult or invading microorganism *(exogenous mediators).* Endogenous mediators play an important role in the *normal* inflammatory-immune response, but an exaggerated activation results in life-threatening events, such as cardiovascular instability (Natanson et al., 2001).

   c. *Exogenous mediators* (e.g., endotoxin) initiate an amplified, exaggerated activation of a myriad of host physiologic processes (Carcillo, 2003).
      - Plasma enzyme cascade activation (Baldwin, 2002) involves complement (see Chapter 8 for background information), which in SIRS results in excessive inflammation and excessive cellular activation with associated mediator release; coagulopathy, which in SIRS results in excessive intravascular coagulation with endothelial damage, microvascular obstruction, and altered tissue perfusion; fibrinolysis, which in SIRS results in hemorrhage; and kallikrein-kinin (bradykinin) acting to enhance margination of neutrophils, which in SIRS results in massive vasodilation, increased capillary permeability, excessive inflammation, excessive cellular activation with associated mediator release, and bronchoconstriction.
      - Cellular responses induce recruitment of all types of white blood cells (WBCs), platelets, mast cells, fibroblasts, and endothelial cells to participate (Baldwin, 2002).
      - Several types of *biochemical mediators* are released as a result of exaggerated recruitment and activation of the aforementioned cells:
         - Cytokines are hormone-like substances that serve as physiologic communicators between cells participating in the inflammatory-immune response (see Table 8-4). These include interleukins, interferons, tumor necrosis factor (TNF), and colony-stimulating factors (CSFs).

- Lipid mediators are arachidonic acid metabolites (prostaglandins, leukotrienes, and thromboxane) and platelet-activating factor (PAF). Arachidonic acid is a normal constituent of cell membranes that is released from the walls of injured WBCs and metabolized through two pathways (lipoxygenase and cyclooxygenase); it results in lipid mediators. The lipoxygenase pathway results in the formation of thromboxane, prostacyclin, and prostaglandin, subsequently affecting vascular tone and permeability. The cyclo-oxygenase pathway results in the formation of leukotrienes, subsequently causing vascular and airway constriction and increased capillary permeability. PAF is produced by endothelial cells, WBCs, and others and normally participates in the activation of platelets and other cells in inflammation and coagulation. In SIRS, PAF triggers exaggerated mediator release, subsequently resulting in hemodynamic changes, endothelial damage, and excessive coagulation (Baldwin, 2002).
- Toxic oxygen metabolites (oxygen-derived free radicals) are produced by numerous sources, including xanthine oxidase systems, activated phagocytes, mitochondria, and arachidonic acid pathways. Normally the metabolites are produced in small amounts during oxidative metabolism in a localized area and metabolized through numerous innate enzyme systems or membrane antioxidants (Baldwin, 2002) and have bactericidal activity. In SIRS the metabolites damage cell membranes of endothelial cells and other tissues, which results in increased permeability, edema, and exaggerated inflammation. Toxic oxygen metabolites are thought to play a significant role in organ damage seen during septic shock (Baldwin, 2002).
- Proteolytic enzymes *(proteases)* are produced by numerous phagocytic cells, such as neutrophils and macrophages. The enzymes assist the phagocyte in the digestion of bacteria and other foreign material, participate in wound healing, and serve as enzymatic catalysts for the enzyme cascades (e.g., complement, coagulation, fibrinolysis, and kallikrein-kinin) (Baldwin, 2002). In SIRS, proteolytic enzymes cause vascular and tissue damage, increased permeability, and edema.
- Nitric oxide is thought to be an endothelium-derived relaxant factor that serves as a potent modulator of vascular tone and permeability.
- Nitric oxide causes several different effects when systemic inflammation occurs. They include excessive vasodilation, vasopressin hyposensitivity, decreased cardiac contractility, and impaired tissue perfusion (Deich, 2002; Vallet, 2002).

d. Three of the most influential mediators of gram-negative septic shock include *endotoxin, TNF, and interleukin-1 (IL-1)* (Baldwin, 2002). TNF is produced by monocytes and macrophages. It results in enhanced inflammatory-immune responses and promotes the adhesion of neutrophils to endothelial cells and the release of other mediators. Clinical manifestations include body temperature changes, tachypnea, alveolar thickening, tachycardia, increased vascular permeability, hypotension, metabolic acidosis, and altered blood distribution to organs, such as the kidney and gut (Baldwin, 2002). IL-1 is produced by lymphocytes, macrophages, and endothelial cells and is released in response to TNF. It results in many of the same findings as TNF as well as further release of TNF, PAF, and other mediators, such as IL-2 (Baldwin, 2002). Many of the clonic manifestations of IL-1 and TNF overlap, and actions of TNF and IL-1 are synergistic (Baldwin, 2002).

6. The **mechanisms** of each of the mediators vary, *but* the overall result of the exaggerated release of exogenous and endogenous mediators includes a distributive shock state characterized by maldistribution of blood volume, cardiac dysfunction, imbalance of oxygen supply and demand, and metabolic alterations (Figure 9-4).

a. *Maldistribution of blood volume* results from neuroendocrine activation, including the release of catecholamines, glucagon, glucocorticoids, aldosterone, renin, and angiotensin (Baldwin, 2002). Release of catecholamines results in vasoconstriction and redistribution of blood flow. Biochemical-mediator release results in reduced peripheral resistance or increased peripheral vasodilation, leading to blood pooling in the peripheral vasculature and increased microvascular permeability, leading in turn to leakage of interstitial fluid from the vascular space. Direct endothelial damage also leads to increased microvascular permeability. Coagulation activation leads to decreased blood flow and microthrombi formation secondary to increased platelet aggregation and increased margination and chemotaxis of neutrophils (Figure 9-5).

b. *Cardiac dysfunction:* There is inconclusive evidence of decreased coronary artery blood flow as the cause of cardiac dysfunction in sepsis and septic shock (Baldwin, 2002). Alterations in the responsiveness of the sympathetic nervous system result in changes in contractility, cardiac output, and cardiac index, which are normally enhanced through the sympathetic nervous system stimulation of myocardial β-adrenergic receptors. In early sepsis, there is enhanced β-adrenergic stimulation. Later in the continuum, the myocardium becomes less sensitive to circulating catecholamines, and contractility declines (Baldwin, 2002). Ceneviva (1998) and colleagues have shown that children more often demonstrate decreased cardiac output with a decrease in left ventricular function.

- Mediator release is thought to be the culprit for cardiac dysfunction in sepsis and septic shock. Myocardial depressant factor is thought to be released by the pancreas during hypoperfusion and ischemia. Endotoxin's mechanism of action on the myocardium is unclear but is thought to be either a direct effect or an indirect effect through the stimulation of other mediators that reduce cardiac contractility (Baldwin, 2002). Many other mediators (e.g., IL-2, thromboxane, prostaglandin, leukotriene, TNF) continue to be investigated with respect to their effects on various aspects of hemodynamics, including cardiac contractility (Baldwin, 2002). The hemodynamic profile characterized by low systemic vascular resistance (SVR) and profound tachycardia contributes to diminished coronary artery perfusion and further cardiac dysfunction (Carcillo, 1993).

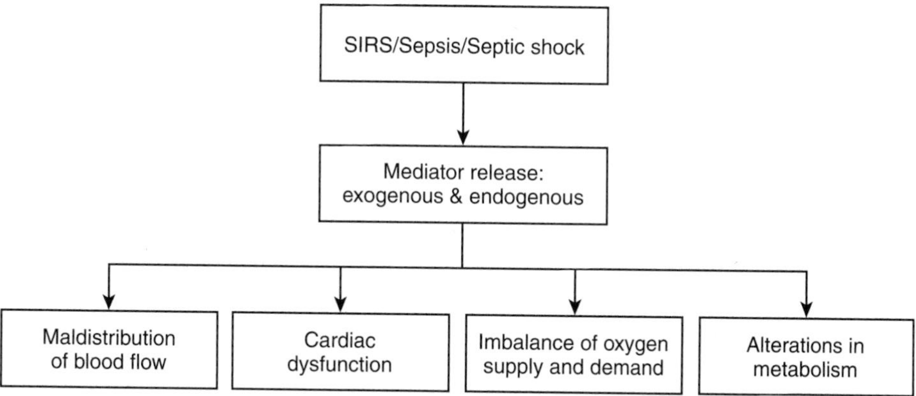

FIGURE 9-4 ■ Outcomes of mediator release in systemic inflammatory response syndrome (SIRS), sepsis, and septic shock.

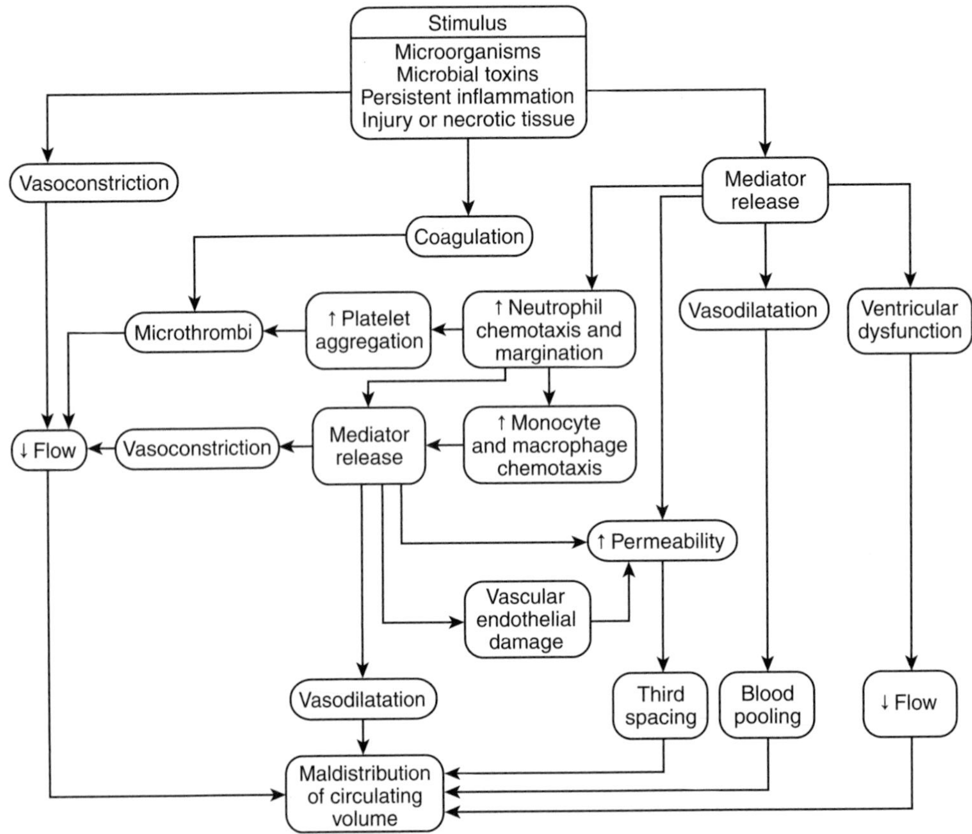

FIGURE 9-5 ■ Processes leading to maldistribution of circulating volume. (From Robins EV: Maldistribution of circulating volume. In Huddleston VB, editor: *Multisystem organ failure: pathophysiology and clinical implications*, ed 2. St. Louis, 1996, Mosby-Year Book.)

c. *Imbalance of oxygen supply and demand*

- Hypoxemia is usually the result of respiratory failure and pulmonary edema secondary to mediator release and increased permeability (Hazinski et al., 1999). Maldistribution of blood flow exacerbates hypoxemia and may lead to ventilation perfusion abnormalities and intrapulmonary shunting. Imbalance of oxygen supply and demand with SIRS and septic shock is due to the decrease in the maximum oxygen delivery secondary to myocardial dysfunction and the decrease in the tissue's ability to extract the oxygen.
- In normal circumstances, with healthy tissues and normal or increased oxygen transport, oxygen consumption is maintained at a constant. In other words, oxygen consumption is independent of oxygen transport. More oxygen is normally delivered to the tissues than is normally consumed. Delivering more oxygen does not change the amount consumed by the tissues (Baldwin, 2002). As oxygen availability to the tissues decreases, consumption is initially maintained by increasing the oxygen extraction ratio. When oxygen availability falls to a critical level, oxygen consumption falls (Figure 9-6).
- The relationship between oxygen transport and oxygen consumption is altered in clinical conditions such as sepsis, ARDS, and multiple-organ dysfunction syndrome (MODS) (Baldwin, 2002). Oxygen consumption is dependent on oxygen transport. The amount consumed is related to the amount delivered and is referred to as *supply dependency* or *pathologic supply*

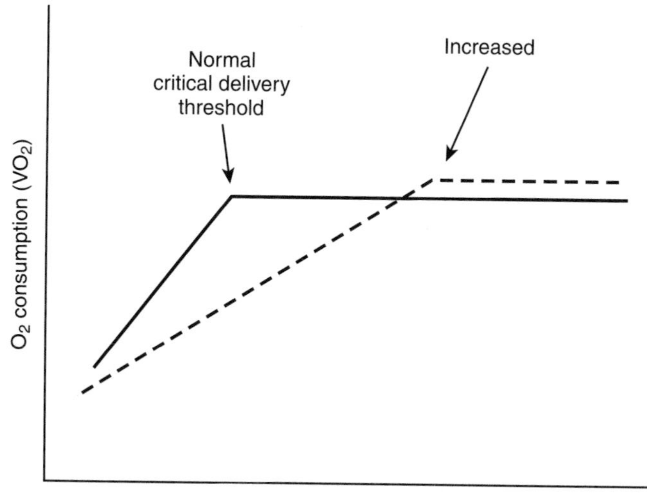

FIGURE 9-6 ■ Relationship between oxygen delivery and oxygen consumption. (From Schumaker PT and Samuel RW: Oxygen delivery and uptake by peripheral tissues. *Crit Care Clin* 5:259, 1989.)

dependency. The cause of supply-dependent oxygen consumption in sepsis is through cellular defect (some evidence of impaired oxidative metabolism), maldistribution of blood flow at the microcirculatory level, or impaired oxygen diffusion (Baldwin, 2002).

- The outcome is inadequate tissue perfusion. Adenosine triphosphate (ATP) is generated through increased glycolysis, which results in the by-product pyruvate and subsequently lactate and causes metabolic acidosis (Baldwin, 2002). If tissue demand is greater than supply, cellular injury occurs.

d. *Alteration in metabolism* (Baldwin, 2002)

- Initially, metabolic alterations serve as compensatory mechanisms aimed at meeting the body's increased needs (Baldwin, 2002). These alterations result from neurohormonal responses primarily mediated by the sympathetic nervous system and initially characterized by hypermetabolism (an increase in resting energy expenditure, an increase in cardiac output, and an increase in oxygen consumption and carbon dioxide production), hyperglycemia, and hypercatabolism. Particular attention should be paid to patients with purpura fulminans or chronic steroid use for signs of adrenal insufficiency (Dichter and Curley, 2001). Carcillo (1997), states, "Any patient whose perfusion and blood pressure is unresponsive to vigorous volume resuscitation and vasoactive support should be evaluated for adrenal insufficiency."
- Inadequate substrate metabolism occurs. In carbohydrate metabolism, glycogen stores are depleted, usually in less than 12 hours. The liver initiates gluconeogenesis, whereas glucose utilization by cells decreases, glucose transport into the cells decreases, and serum glucose concentration increases. In lipid metabolism, catecholamine and decreased insulin lead to catabolism of triglycerides to free fatty acids and ketones for energy (from adipose tissue) with the potential for lipemia or hypertriglyceridemia. In protein metabolism, amino acids are needed for gluconeogenesis. The primary sites of amino acids include skeletal muscle, connective tissue, and unstimulated gut. Therefore autocannibalism occurs with rapid loss of skeletal muscle to provide amino acids. In combination with decreased protein synthesis, there is an eventual deficiency of amino acids.

7. Compensatory responses to shock are mechanisms to increase tissue perfusion and prevent cellular, tissue, and vital organ injury in the presence of all shock states. Most compensatory mechanisms are dependent on various "sensing" mechanisms to recognize changes in the cardiac output or arterial blood pressure.

a. *Compensatory mechanisms* are sequentially stimulated in an effort to maintain perfusion.
   - *Stretch receptors* (in the right atrium and pulmonary artery) sense volume changes, either from decreased circulating volume or in the case of septic shock from increased venous capacitance. Stimulation of these receptors results in an increase in sympathetic discharge to the medullary vasomotor center.
   - Baroreceptors within the renal juxtaglomerular apparatus are stimulated by reduced renal afferent arteriolar pressure. The reduction in pressure causes activation of the renin-angiotensin-aldosterone system, which results in vasoconstriction of arterioles (and, to a lesser extent, veins), increased renal tubular reabsorption of sodium and water, and stimulation of the adrenal cortex. The stimulation of the adrenal cortex increases the production of aldosterone, causing retention of renal sodium, thus expanding extracellular fluid volume (Hazinski and Jenkins, 2002). A drop in mean arterial pressure (MAP) or pulse pressure close to physiologic range results in the decreased stretching of arterial baroreceptors (in aortic arch, carotid bodies, and splanchnic vessels) and loss of their inhibitory effect on the vasomotor center *(baroreceptor reflex)*. Sympathetic vasomotor stimulation causes norepinephrine release from nerve endings and widespread vasoconstriction. Once MAP falls below 80 mm Hg for the aortic arch and 60 mm Hg for the carotid bodies, the activity of these baroreceptors is eliminated (Kumar and Parrillo, 2001).
   - Norepinephrine-epinephrine vasoconstrictor reflex: Sympathetic vasomotor stimulation causes stimulation of the adrenal medulla and the release of epinephrine primarily, although some norepinephrine is secreted as well. This reflex accentuates and prolongs vasoconstrictive effects throughout the body, including constriction of afferent and efferent arterioles of the kidney resulting in decreased glomerular filtration, decreased urine output, and increased sodium retention (Hazinski and Jenkins, 2002).
   - Vascular chemoreceptors are sensitive to changes in PO_2, PCO_2, and decreased pH (increased hydrogen ion concentration) and are activated when the blood pressure is less than approximately 80 mm Hg. On activation sympathetic tone increases substantially. The chemoreceptors have a limited role during normal physiologic homeostasis but an active role during shock (Kumar and Parrillo, 2001).
   - CNS ischemia reflex serves as the most powerful stimulus to sympathetic tone in severe shock (Kumar and Parillo, 2001). Medullary chemoreceptors are sensitive to increased carbon dioxide associated with decreased cerebral perfusion and to blood pressure lower than 60 mm Hg (Kumar and Parillo, 2001).

CLINICAL ASSESSMENT

A. History

1. **Chief complaint:** The history is guided by the child's chief complaint. The chief complaint is noted in the patient's or the primary caretaker's own words.
2. **History of the present illness** includes the date and mode of onset, course, duration, influencing factors, and exposure to infectious agents including

contact with infectious persons, animal (domestic or wild) bites, ingestion of contaminated food or water, and foreign travel. Signs and symptoms to be noted include the following:

a. *General:* Fatigue, change in level of activity, chills, fever, weight loss, change in feeding, night sweats, malaise
b. *Mental status:* Confusion, restlessness, syncope, irritability, somnolence
c. *Skin:* Rash, petechiae, pallor, mottling, lesions, ulcers, rhinitis
d. *Lymph nodes:* Enlargement (adenopathy), tenderness
e. *Respiratory:* Tachypnea, respiratory tract infection, respiratory distress, dyspnea, orthopnea, cough, hemoptysis, sputum, chest pain
f. *Cardiovascular:* Tachycardia, flushed skin
g. *Abdomen:* Anorexia, altered bowel sounds, diarrhea, constipation, melena, vomiting, hematemesis, protuberant abdomen (not age appropriate), abdominal pain, masses, hepatosplenomegaly
h. *Genitourinary tract:* Hematuria, number of voids or diapers per day

3. **Medical history**
   a. Aspects that *alter* the child's resistance to infection include recent injury, diet and nutrition, immunization history, and birth history.
   b. Aspects that *increase* the child's risk of infection include prolonged antibiotic therapy, previous surgeries (e.g., thymectomy, splenectomy), liver or spleen disorders (functional splenectomy), metabolic and immune disorders (diabetes mellitus, renal disease, primary immunodeficiency, and allergies or hypersensitivities), malignancy, and transplantation.
   c. *Previous infections,* including childhood infectious diseases, should be noted.
4. **Family history** should note familial diseases that may increase the child's risk of infection.
5. **Medication history** should include those that increase the child's risk of infection. Also consider any dietary supplements the child is taking.
6. **Social-cultural history and habits** include psychosocial history, environmental exposures such as radiation (either inadvertent exposure or radiation therapies [total or localized]) or chemical (inadvertent exposure to benzene, lead, etc.), and recent travel.

B. Nursing Examination of the Patient

1. **Inspection** includes level of consciousness, level of activity, general appearance, and respiratory rate, rhythm, and effort. Skin and mucous membranes should be examined for color and consistency, the presence of lesions, and the presence of generalized or localized edema, which is usually periorbital or sacral. Pedal edema may occur after the child begins to walk. Characteristics of fontanelles and jugular venous distention are noted to assess hydration status. Precordial activity (sometimes referred to as *sternal bulging*) is noted and is due to hypertrophy of the right ventricle, causing the lower end of the sternum and ribs to project forward. Although the point of maximal intensity (PMI) may be visible in some children, especially those who are thin, a prominent or heaving precordium may be an indication of cardiac dysfunction.
2. **Palpation**
   a. *Skin and mucous membranes* are palpated for moisture, texture, refill, and temperature (note any demarcation in temperature from distal to proximal extremities and extremities versus the trunk). With cardiac dysfunction, blood is circulated at an insufficient rate, and compensatory vasoconstriction occurs in the extremities to shunt blood toward vital organs. Normal capillary refill is less than or equal to 2 seconds. The presence and intensity of peripheral

pulses are noted. Also note proximal versus distal pulse quality because it is reflective of perfusion status.

b. The level at which the *normal liver border* may be palpable is related to age. In the infant, the liver is normally felt up to 3 cm below the right costal margin; in the 1-year-old child, up to 2 cm below the right costal margin; and in the 4- to 5-year-old child, up to 1 cm below the right costal margin. The presence of hepatomegaly may indicate cardiac dysfunction, tumor, or hepatitis. An enlarged liver may also indicate fluid overload because the liver may act as a sponge and become engorged when central venous pressure (CVP) increases.

3. **Auscultation:** The presence and quality of breath sounds are noted. Respiratory rate and heart rate should be evaluated within the context of the child's age, clinical condition, and other external factors, such as fever. Apical heart rate and rhythm are auscultated. In the infant and young child, cardiac output is directly proportional to heart rate because stroke volume is small (Hazinski, 1999). Blood pressure is a late sign of decompensation but is still obtained. Blood pressure should be evaluated in the context of the child's age, clinical condition, and other parameters reflective of perfusion.
4. **Phases and clinical manifestations of septic shock** (Table 9-14).
5. **Stages** may be identified in the clinical progression of septic shock in *some* children (Baldwin, 2002). During the hyperdynamic compensated phase, blood pressure is maintained. In the later, hyperdynamic uncompensated phase, blood pressure begins to fall. The hypodynamic state essentially appears congruent to cardiogenic shock.
6. **Correlating clinical findings with ACCP and SCCM proposed terminology (2001)**
   a. *Infection* is a microbial phenomenon characterized by an inflammatory response to the presence of microorganisms or the invasion of normally sterile host tissue by those organisms.
   b. *Bacteremia* is the presence of viable bacteria in the blood.
   c. *SIRS* is the acute development of two or more of the following (ACCP and SCCM, 1992) (see Table 9-13):
      - Fever (greater than 38°C) or hypothermia (lower than 36°C)
      - Tachycardia (age related)
      - Tachypnea (age related)
      - Leukocytosis (WBC >12,000/mm^3), leukopenia (WBC <4,000/mm^3), or greater than 10% bands
   d. *Sepsis* is the systemic response to infection; it is diagnosed by the presence of SIRS associated with an infectious process and characterized by two or more of the aforementioned findings for SIRS. Documented bacteremia is not necessary for the diagnosis of sepsis. The International Sepsis Definitions Conference in 2001 agreed that the definition of severe sepsis would remain intact (Carcillo, 2003).
   e. *Severe sepsis* is defined as, "Sepsis and organ failure determined by various organ failure scores" (Carcillo, 2003).
   f. *Septic shock* is defined as "infection with hypothermia or hyperthermia, tachycardia (may be absent with hypothermia), and altered mental status, in the presence of at least one, but usually more than one, of the following: decreased peripheral pulses compared with central pulses, capillary refill prolonged for more than 2 seconds (cold shock) or flash capillary refill (warm shock), mottled or cool extremities (cold shock), and decreased urine output (below 1 cm^3/kg)" (Carcillo, 2003).
   g. *MODS* is defined as failure of more than one organ (Carcillo, 2003).

TABLE 9-14
Phases and Clinical Manifestations of Septic Shock

Organ System	Sepsis	Hyperdynamic Septic Shock*	Hypodynamic Septic Shock†
Central nervous system	Change in activity Change in feeding Change in response	Clouded sensorium Irritability Disorientation Lethargy	Disorientation Lethargy Obtundation
Cardiovascular	Sinus tachycardia Bounding pulses	Sinus tachycardia Bounding pulses Warm, dry, flushed skin Widened pulse pressure ± Diminished perfusion ± Mottled extremities ↑↓ Capillary refill Generalized edema Relative hypovolemia Progressive hypotension	Sinus tachycardia Weak, thready pulse Dysrhythmias Narrowed pulse pressure Diminished perfusion ↓ Mottled extremities ↓ Capillary refill Generalized edema Hypotension
Pulmonary	Tachypnea	Tachypnea Progressive hypoxemia	Pulmonary edema
Metabolic	Fever or hypothermia Respiratory alkalosis	Fever or hypothermia Hyperglycemia or hypoglycemia Progressive metabolic acidosis	Fever or hypothermia Hyperglycemia or hypoglycemia Severe metabolic acidosis
Hematology/ immunology	Leukocytosis/leukopenia ↑ Immature neutrophils (bands)	Leukocytosis/leukopenia ↑ Immature neutrophils (bands)	Leukocytosis/leukopenia
Renal		↓ Urine output	↓ Urine output

Data from Carcillo JA: Management of pediatric septic shock. In Holbrook PR, editor: *Textbook of pediatric critical care,* Philadelphia, 1993, WB Saunders, pp 114-142; Robbins EV: Maldistribution of circulating blood volume. In Huddleston VB, editor: *Multisystem organ failure: pathophysiology and clinical implications,* St. Louis, 1992, Mosby, pp 85-108; Rosenthal-Dichter C: Septic shock. In Slota MC, editor: *Core curriculum for pediatric critical care nursing,* Philadelphia, 1998, WB Saunders, p 638.

*Hyperdynamic septic shock is characterized by increased cardiovascular findings and seemingly "good" perfusion; the body's demands are still not adequately met.

†Hypodynamic septic shock may be accompanied by signs and symptoms of deteriorating organ dysfunction(s).

C. Invasive and Noninvasive Diagnostic Studies

1. Laboratory

a. *Serum hematologic studies* include the following:

- CBC
- WBC count (Chapter 8): Total WBC count is generally considered normal at 5000 to 10,000/mm^3 but is age specific. Leukocytosis occurs in all forms of shock as a result of the demargination of neutrophils (Kumar and Parrillo, 2001). Leukopenia occurs in late septic shock *or* in infants and young children who are less able to replace neutrophils repeatedly in the face of an overwhelming infection. The WBC differential measures the five subcategories of circulating WBCs and is reported as a percentage. Neutropenia may be seen. An increased percentage (more than 10%) of bands (immature neutrophils) is seen when there is an increased demand for or decreased supply of neutrophils in the presence of an overwhelming infection (a shift

to the left). A lymphocyte count of less than 1000 for longer than 7 days may be seen (Carcillo, 2003). Absolute granulocyte or neutrophil counts (AGC or ANC) may be low. An ANC lower than $1000/mm^3$ carries a moderate risk for infection, and an ANC lower than $500/mm^3$ carries a high risk for infection.

- Hemoglobin is variably affected. Usually with the extravasation of intravascular water there is erythrocytosis.
- Platelet count increases acutely but may be followed by thrombocytopenia with progressive septic shock.
- Other serum tests of inflammation that may be helpful include erythrocyte sedimentation rate (ESR) and C-reactive protein, which are elevated secondary to an infectious process.

b. *ABG analysis* (Baldwin, 2002): Respiratory alkalosis occurs early in the course of septic shock. Initial respiratory alkalosis occurs as a compensatory mechanism to reduce carbon dioxide in the presence of increasing lactic acidosis from decreased perfusion. As septic shock progresses and respiratory reserves fail, metabolic acidosis develops. The body is unable to compensate for the increasing acid buildup. An anion gap acidosis is present because of the elevated levels of lactic acid.

c. *Routine chemistries:* Electrolytes, sodium, potassium, chloride, and bicarbonate are required to assess an anion gap. Blood urea nitrogen (BUN) and creatinine levels initially appear normal. Lactate should be followed serially because it is a marker of tissue oxygen debt and supply-dependent oxygen consumption. It is a late marker of tissue hypoperfusion but one of the few available means of estimating tissue oxygenation. Arterial lactate levels greater than 2 mEq/L are associated with increased mortality in the adult population.

d. *Blood cultures* may identify causative microorganism. Aerobic and anaerobic cultures are usually obtained. Obtaining blood cultures is a *simultaneous* priority with administering broad-spectrum antibiotic coverage. Attempt to obtain blood cultures before the administration of antibiotics, but *never "hold" antibiotic administration to obtain blood cultures.*

- The timing of culture results is dependent on the type of microorganism and the stage of the illness (Grimes, 1991). Results from cultures for common microorganisms such as streptococci, staphylococci, and *Enterobacter* are available in 24 to 48 hours. Results from a pneumococcal culture are available in 3 to 4 days.
- Results from blood cultures may be negative. Some microorganisms, such as *Mycobacterium tuberculosis,* shed intermittently, causing negative results from cultures. This is common in patients with active tuberculosis (Grimes, 1991). In these instances, serial cultures may be required. Some patients, especially those who have received antibiotics, may also yield negative results from blood cultures. Only 50% of the patients with clinical signs of sepsis will have an organism isolated (Hazinski, 1999).

e. *Other specimens and cultures*

- Sputum specimens from the lower respiratory tract versus oropharyngeal secretions may be helpful.
- Fecal cultures are used to find organisms that are not a part of the normal bowel flora or to determine normal flora that become pathogenic (e.g., *Clostridium difficile, Escherichia coli*).
- Urine specimens with bacterial counts of less than 10,000/mL of urine are considered free of infection. Bacterial levels between 10,000 to 100,000/mL in urine cultures are inconclusive and require a second specimen. Bacterial

counts greater than 100,000/mL of urine represent a definitive urinary tract infection.

- Cerebrospinal fluid: Lumbar puncture may be needed to evaluate spinal fluid (Hazinski and Jenkins, 2002). Gram stains are particularly useful with cerebrospinal fluid infections for the purpose of selecting antibiotics.

2. **Radiologic:** *Routine chest radiograph* is useful for ruling out pneumonia as the source of infection. Radiographic studies of other areas of the body are indicated by the child's history and physical examination.
3. **Invasive hemodynamic monitoring**
   a. All patients with suspected shock should have an indwelling *arterial catheter* to monitor blood pressure serially. Blood pressure assessment via manual sphygmomanometer or automatic noninvasive oscillometric techniques may be inaccurate in patients in shock secondary to marked peripheral vasoconstriction.
   b. *CVP* is most often used to manage the child with uncomplicated septic shock to trend intravascular volume status and response to therapy.
   c. A *pulmonary artery catheter* is helpful in managing the child in florid septic shock. It provides continuous monitoring of cardiac filling pressures (CVP and pulmonary artery wedge pressure [PAWP]), an estimate of left ventricular end-diastolic pressure [LVEDP] and volume [LVEDV]), cardiac flow (cardiac output per cardiac index [CO/CI]), cardiac contractility (stroke volume, stroke volume index, stroke work index), and afterload (SVR, systemic vascular resistance index [SVRI]). It also allows for withdrawal of blood from the pulmonary artery catheter to determine oxygen consumption: pulmonary artery oxygen content and mixed venous oxygen saturation (Svo_2).
4. **Hemodynamic parameters** accompany various shock states (Table 9-15).

D. Nursing and Collaborative Diagnoses

- ❖ Fluid-volume deficit related to relative hypovolemia, vasodilation, capillary permeability, decreased intake, and potential inadequate fluid resuscitation
- ❖ Alteration in tissue perfusion related to maldistribution of blood flow secondary to systemic inflammatory response, capillary permeability, vasodilation, vasoconstriction, and microvascular thrombi
- ❖ Inadequate CO resulting from increased energy expenditures and myocardial dysfunction secondary to mediator release and acidosis
- ❖ Impaired gas exchange related to vasoconstriction, increased capillary permeability, and alterations in pulmonary endothelial cells
- ❖ Hyperthermia or hypothermia related to infectious process, mediator release, and increased basal metabolic rate
- ❖ Alteration in nutrition, less than body requirements, related to hypermetabolism secondary to mediator release and inadequate nutritional support

E. Goals and Desired Patient Outcomes

1. **Prevention and early recognition** of children with sepsis or septic shock
2. Early, accurate, and complete **administration of antibiotics**
3. Early and aggressive **fluid resuscitation** until improved perfusion is observed as evidenced by improved mental status, diminished tachycardia, capillary refill of less than 2 seconds, warm extremities, strong pulses, increased urine output, and restoration and maintenance of normal blood pressure (Carcillo, 2002).
4. Restoration of **optimal balance of oxygen supply and demand** and thus **tissue perfusion** as indicated by arterial oxygen saturation of 92% or higher, hemoglobin concentration of 10 g/dL or greater, CI between 3.3 and 6 L per min/m^2 body

TABLE 9-15
Hemodynamic and Oxygenation Profile Changes in Shock

Parameter	Norms	Hypovolemic	Cardiogenic	Septic: Early	Septic: Late
Heart rate (beats/min)	Newborn–3 mo: 85–205 3 mo–2 yr: 100–190 2–10 yr: 60–140 >10 yr: 60–100	↑	↑	↑	↑
MAP	>60 mm Hg	Compensated-normal then decompensated-decreased	Compensated-normal then decompensated-decreased	Compensated-normal then decompensated-decreased	Compensated-normal then decompensated-decreased
CI	2.5–5.5 L/min/M^2	↓	↓	↑ then ↓	↑ then ↓
RAP/PAWP	2–6 mm Hg/6–12 mm Hg	↓	↑	↓ then ↑	↓ then ↑
PVRI	PVRI = Mean PA – PCWP/CI × 80 Norm: 80 – 240 dyne-sec/cm^5/M^2	Normal or ↑	Normal or ↑	Normal or ↑	Normal or ↑
SVRI	SVRI = MAP – RAP/CI × 80 Norm: 800 – 1600 dyne-sec/cm^5/M^2	↑	↑	↓ then ↑	↓ then ↑
Do_2	Do_2 = Cao_2 × CI × 10 Norm: 620 ± 50 mL/min/M^2	↓	↓	↑ then ↓	↑ then ↓
Vo_2	Vo_2 = arterial Do_2 – venous Do_2 Norm: 120–200 mL/min/M^2	↑ then ↓	↑ then ↓	↑ then ↓	↑ then ↓
OER	$Cao_2 - C\bar{v}o_2/Cao_2 \times 100$ Norm: 25 ± 2%	↑ then ↓	↑ then ↓	Normal/↑ then ↓	Normal/↑ then ↓
Svo_2	Norm: 75% (60%–80%)	↓ then ↑	↓ then ↑	Normal/↓ then ↑	Normal/↓ then ↑

Modified from Dichter CH, Curley MAQ: Shock. In Curley MAQ, Maloney-Harmon PA: *Critical care nursing of infants and children,* ed 2. Philadelphia, 2001, W.B. Saunders, p 932.

CI, cardiac index; *MAP*, mean arterial blood pressure; *PAWP*, pulmonary artery wedge pressure; *PVRI*, pulmonary vascular resistance index; *RAP*, right atrial pressure; *SVRI*, systemic vascular resistance index; *Do_2*, oxygen delivery; *Vo_2*, oxygen consumption; *OER*, O_2 extraction ratio.

surface area (BSA), oxygen delivery (DO_2) between 500 and 600 mL/min/m^2, normal oxygen consumption ($\dot{V}O_2$); infants, oxygen 10 to 14 mL/kg per minute; in children, oxygen 7 to 11 mL/kg per minute), superior vena cava oxygen saturation (SVC O_2) greater than 70%, and normalization of serum lactate of less than 2 mEq/L.

5. Early **nutritional support**
6. Minimization of the risk and extent of **organ dysfunction**

F. Patient Care Management

1. Recognize that **each specific intervention** has a place in the overall treatment perspective (Bone, 1993; Natanson et al., 1995). Essential treatment *must* include both *definitive treatment,* including identification, localization, and eradication of the source of infection with antibiotic administration, and *advanced life support treatment,* including oxygenation, ventilation, and circulation with fluid and inotropic administration. *Controversial treatments* are those with conflicting results or undetermined efficacy such as steroids for nonfluid refractory-catecholamine resistant shock and morphine antagonists. *Futuristic treatments* are those currently under investigation or scheduled for investigation in the future such as passive immunization and monoclonal antibody administration. Controversial and futuristic treatments often fall into one of two approaches, which include either neutralizing microbiologic toxins or modulating host inflammatory-immune responses.
2. **Identify those patients at risk** for the development of sepsis or septic shock. Early recognition of sepsis or septic shock can be challenging because either may be subtle and insidious, especially in younger patients such as neonates and infants and patients undergoing treatments or interventions that alter inflammatory-immune response, including glucocorticoid administration. The *classic presentation of fever, tachycardia,* and *vasodilation* with warm, flushed skin is seen in most children with innocuous viral and bacterial infection (tachypnea accompanies a respiratory source of infection) but also in children whose infection progresses to septic shock (Carcillo, 2002). Monitor ongoing changes in the patient or the patient's response(s), such as behavior, temperature patterns (e.g., fever), and WBC count.
3. **Initial resuscitation**
   a. *Assessment of airway, breathing, and circulation (ABCs):* Rapid cardiopulmonary assessment, proposed by the American Heart Association Pediatric Advanced Life Support (PALS) Program (Table 9-16), includes a primary survey of life-threatening conditions followed by a secondary survey. About 80% of children with septic shock require intubation and mechanical ventilatory support within 24 hours of admission (Carcillo et al., 2002). Obtain vascular access using PALS guidelines (Hazinski, 2002). Central access and two intravenous (IV) access lines are preferred. Once the ABCs are ensured, the child should receive, as required, antibiotic administration, volume resuscitation, and vasoactive agents.
   b. *Antibiotic administration:* Blood culture specimens should be obtained before the administration of antibiotics, but antibiotics should never be withheld to obtain a culture. *Administering antibiotics and obtaining cultures are a concomitant priority.* With the emergence of many resistant organisms, antibiotics may be given in accordance with regional resistant/sensitivity patterns.
   c. *Volume resuscitation:* In a child with septic shock, an aggressive approach is taken: 20 mL/kg fluid bolus with subsequent boluses of 20 mL/kg to a total of 60 mL/kg in the first 10 minutes of resuscitation (Carcillo, 2003). Boluses are

TABLE 9-16
Rapid Cardiopulmonary Assessment of a Healthy and Decompensating Child

Assessment Parameter	Healthy Child	Decompensating Child
AIRWAY PATENCY	Able to maintain independently	Maintainable with interventions such as head positioning, suctioning, adjuncts; unmaintainable requiring intubation
BREATHING		
Respiratory rate	Within age-appropriate limits*	Tachypnea or bradypnea as compared to age-appropriate limits* *Note:* Warning parameter: >60 breaths/min
Chest movement (presence)	Chest rise and fall with each respiration	Minimal to no chest movement with respiratory effort
Chest movement (quality)	Silent and effortless respirations; chest rise concomitant with abdomen with each breath	Evidence of labored respirations with retractions; asynchronous movement between chest and abdomen with respirations
Air movement (presence)	Air exchange bilaterally in all lobes	Despite movement of chest, minimal or no air exchange is noted on auscultation
Air movement (quality)	Breath sounds of normal intensity and duration per auscultation assessment	Nasal flaring, grunting, stridor, or wheezing
CIRCULATION		
Heart rate (presence)	Apical beat within age-appropriate limits*	Absent heart rate, bradycardia or tachycardia as compared to age-approriate limits* *Note:* Warning parameters: Infant: <80 bpm Child <5y: >180 bpm Child >5y: >150 bpm
Heart rate (quality)	Heart rate regular with a normal sinus rhythm	Irregular, slow, or very rapid rate; common dysrhythmias include supraventricular tachycardia, bradyarrhythmias, and asystole
Skin	Warm, pink extremities with capillary refill ≤2 s; peripheral pulses present bilaterally with normal intensity	Pallor, cyanotic, or mottled skin; cool extremities; capillary refill time >2 s; peripheral pulses weak or absent; central pulses weak
Cerebral perfusion	Alert to and interested in surroundings; recognizes parents; responsive to fear and pain; normal muscle tone	Irritable, lethargic, obtunded or comatose; minimal or no reaction to pain; loose muscle tone (e.g., floppy)

■ **TABLE 9-16**
■ ■ **Rapid Cardiopulmonary Assessment of a Healthy and Decompensating Child (*cont'd*)**

Assessment Parameter	Healthy Child	Decompensating Child
Blood pressure	Within age-appropriate limits*	A fall in blood pressure from age-appropriate limits, a *late sign of decompensation* *Note:* A fall of 10 mm Hg systolic pressure is significant. Lower systolic blood pressure limit: infant ≤1 mo: 60 mm Hg; infant ≤1 y: 70 mm Hg; child >1 y; 70+ mm Hg (2 × age in y)

Modified from Moloney-Harmon P, Rosenthal CH; Nursing care modifications for the child in the adult ICU. In Stillwell S, editor: *Critical care nursing reference book.* St Louis, 1992, Mosby-Year Book.

*All vital signs are interpreted within the context of age, clinical condition, and other external factors, such as the presence of fever.

preceded and followed by systematic and repeated assessments of clinical parameters of perfusion and are administered until perfusion improves. *Some children require more than 200 mL/kg of fluid within the first hour of presentation.* Fluid boluses for volume resuscitation should be administered via IV push and within 20 minutes of presentation (Carcillo, 2003). Early intervention to reversing the shock state is associated with successful resuscitation (Han et al., 2003). The type of fluid initially is isotonic crystalloid fluid (lactated Ringer's [LR] or 0.9% NaCl).

d. *Vasoactive agents* (Table 9-17): If volume resuscitation fails to restore perfusion or severe hypotension is present, vasoactive agents are indicated. A mixed α- and β-adrenergic agent, such as dopamine (5 mcg/kg per minute), is usually initiated. If blood pressure remains inadequate, dopamine is increased to β-adrenergic concentrations (10 mcg/kg per minute). If blood pressure continues to be decreased, inotropic agents are added. In the presence of hypotension, the drug of choice is epinephrine. For the current parameters in treating the pediatric septic shock patient, refer to Figure 9-7.
   - *Note:* Protocols should be used *only* as guides to therapy. Vasoactive support should be evaluated using consistent clinical criteria rather than numeric values only.

4. Cardiovascular management

a. *Support and optimize cardiac output:* CO may be within the normal range or increased at times in the continuum of septic shock, but it is still inadequate to meet the body's demands. Normal or increased CO is often accompanied by low blood pressure and SVR, thus affecting perfusion and oxygen transport. Recommendations for each of the constituents of cardiac output serve *only* as a guideline. Each patient should be evaluated individually with regard to age, clinical context (including the changing continuum of septic shock), and total hemodynamic profile.

b. *Increase preload with early, aggressive fluid therapy* (isotonic crystalloids first and colloids later): Volume administration is used to treat hypoperfusion, hypotension, and decreased preload due to increased capillary permeability, vasodilation, and maldistribution of blood flow. In the absence of rales or

TABLE 9-17
Inotropic and Vasoactive Agents Used in the Treatment of Septic Shock

Drug	Site of Action	Dose (mcg/kg/min)	Primary Effect*	Secondary Effect
Dopamine	Dopaminergic	2–5	Increase renal perfusion	Dysrhythmias
	Dopaminergic and β_1	2-10	Inotropy Chronotropy Increase renal perfusion	
	α	10–20	Vasoconstriction	
Norepinephrine	$\alpha > \beta$	1-2	Vasoconstriction Inotropy	>MVO_2 Dysrhythmias <Renal BF
Epinephrine	α and β	0.05–1.5	Vasoconstriction Inotropy Chronotropy	>MVO_2 Dysrhythmias <Renal BF
Dobutamine	β_1	5–20	Inotropy	Tachycardia Dysrhythmias Vasodilation Hypotension
Sodium nitroprusside		0.5–10 (light-sensitive)	Vasodilation (balanced)	<PVR >V/Q mismatch Cyanide toxicity
Nitroglycerin		0.2–20	Vasolidation (venous)	<PVR >ICP
Amrinone		5–10 (load with up to 3 mg/kg over 20 min)	Inotropy Vasodilation	Dysrhythmias <PVR Thrombocytopenia
Milrinone		0.25–0.75 (load with 75 mcg/kg over 20 min)	Inotropy Vasodilation Improves diastolic function	Dysrhythmias <PVR

*Difficult to predict the dose-response effect. Management requires individual titration at the bedside.
MVO_2, myocardial oxygen consumption; *BF*, blood flow; *PVR*, pulmonary vascular resistance; *V/Q*, ventilation/perfusion; *ICP*, intracranial pressure.

hepatomegaly, aggressive fluid resuscitation should be initiated with successive 20 mL/kg boluses of an isotonic crystalloid solution (i.e., normal saline). It is important to check the liver edge between boluses. These boluses should be administered every 10 minutes until the patient receives up to 60 mL/kg of fluid or shock is resolved (Han et al., 2003). A recent study by Rivers and colleagues found that early aggressive volume resuscitation in patients with severe sepsis and septic shock improved the likelihood of survival (Hotchkiss, 2003). Monitor the response to volume administration through repeated, systematic assessment of clinical parameters (see Table 9-16). Serial measurements of cardiac filling pressures (CVP, pulmonary capillary wedge pressure [PCWP]) and ventricular performance (CO/CI, SVR) are useful in monitoring recommended CVPs of 5 to 8 mm Hg or PAWPs of 12 to 15 mm Hg.

c. *Maximize contractility:* The left ventricular ejection fraction (LVEF) and overall contractility are significantly lowered in septic shock. The increased

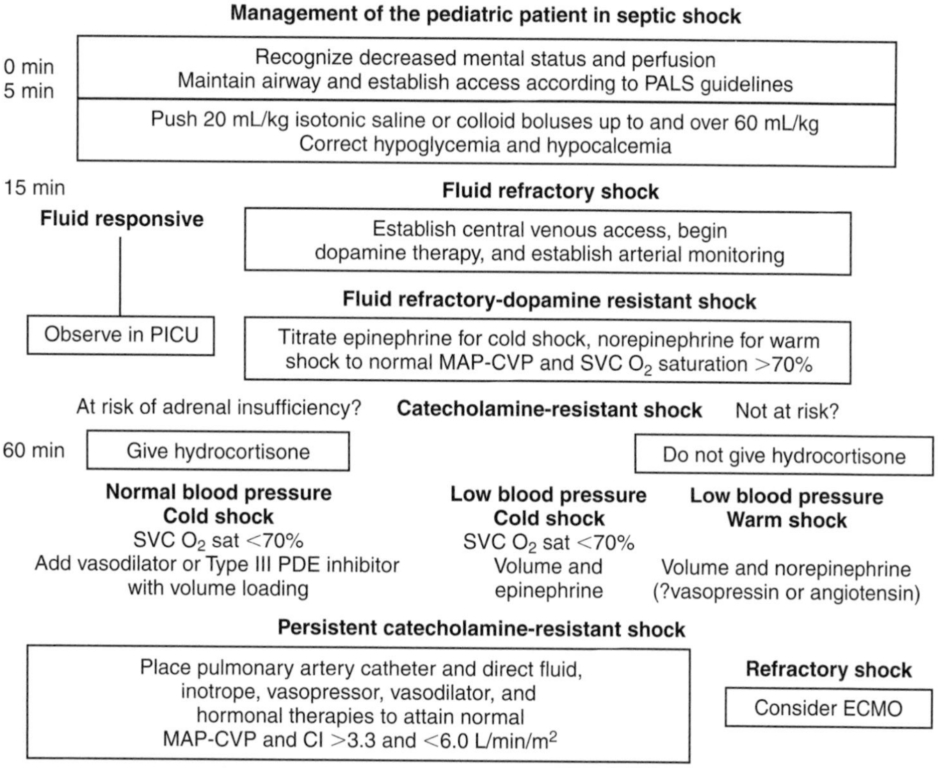

FIGURE 9-7 ■ American College of Critical Care Medicine clinical practice parameters for hemodynamic support of pediatric and neonatal patients with septic shock. *CI*, cardiac index; *ECMO*, extracorporeal membrane oxygenation; *MAP-CVP*, mean arterial pressure-central venous pressure; *PDE*, phosphodiesterase; *SVC O_2*, superior vena cava oxygen saturation.

(From Carcillo JA, Fields AI, and task force members: Clinical practice parameters for hemodynamic support of pediatric and neonatal patients in septic shock. *Crit Care Med* 30(6):1-13, 2002.)

CO is due to an increase in heart rate and ventricular dilation (Dichter and Curley, 2001). Inotropic agents may be indicated for improvement of contractility (see Table 9-17).

d. *Manipulate afterload* (SVR): Persistent hypotension may occur even in the presence of aggressive volume administration and is often related to mediator release and vasodilation rather than low CO/CI. Vasopressors may be indicated, and larger doses may be required over time because of continuing mediator release, capillary leakage, and decreased responsiveness of α- and β-adrenergic receptors. Hypodynamic shock is characterized by increased SVR, low CO/CI, and high LVEDP. Direct-acting vasodilators (e.g., nitroprusside, nitroglycerin) as well as inodilators (e.g., amrinone, milrinone) may be indicated (Dichter and Curley, 2001). The goal for vasodilation therapy is to reduce afterload while increasing contractility, CO/CI, and tissue perfusion. Manipulation of afterload most often occurs in combination with an inotropic agent. The inotropic agent maintains the blood pressure and enhances contractility, whereas the vasodilator reduces the afterload and cardiac filling pressures.

e. *Support and optimize heart rate:* Various inotropic and vasoactive agents may result in tachyarrhythmias and worsen the clinical and hemodynamic picture. Tachycardia may be significant because two thirds of coronary artery perfusion occurs during diastole and is determined primarily by aortic diastolic pressure and duration of diastole. Tachydysrhythmias will need to be managed aggressively (Dichter and Curley, 2001).

5. **Respiratory management**
   a. The *goal of respiratory management is to balance oxygen delivery with the individual patient's tissue oxygenation requirements* rather than normalizing hemodynamic parameters and laboratory values to age-appropriate values (Curly, 2001).
   b. *Assess and maximize tissue oxygenation* (see Chapter 2). Support airway and ventilation. Position the child to support maximal airway patency. Provide supplemental oxygen. Anticipate intubation because most children with septic shock require intubation and mechanical ventilation.
   c. *Assess tissue oxygenation* using parameters such as ABG analysis, oxygen saturation, and oxygen content. Normal PaO_2 is 80 to 100 mm Hg on room air. With supplemental oxygen, the lower limit of the normal PaO_2 expected for a given FiO_2 is estimated by multiplying the FiO_2 by 5. Hypoxemia is present if the hemoglobin saturation is less than 90%. *Oxygen content* (CaO_2) is the quantity of oxygen in each 100 mL of blood and includes both the amount dissolved in the plasma and carried in the hemoglobin. Normal oxygen content is 18 to 20 mL/dL of blood.

$$CaO_2 = [\text{Hgb (g/dL)} \times 1.36 \text{ mL } O_2/\text{g Hgb} \times SaO_2] + (0.003 \times PaO_2)$$

   d. *Assess oxygen utilization* using the parameters of oxygen delivery and oxygen consumption.
      - *Oxygen transport or delivery* (DO_2) is the volume of oxygen delivered to the tissues each minute and reflects the quantity of oxygen available to the tissues.

$$DO_2 \text{ (mL/min/m}^2) = CI \times \text{Arterial } O_2 \text{ content}$$

      - *Oxygen consumption* ($\dot{V}O_2$) is the amount of oxygen consumed by the tissues per minute and reflects an overall index of total body metabolism. VO_2 in infants and children, which ranges from 5 to 14 mL O_2/kg per minute, can be measured, estimated, or calculated:

$$\dot{V}O_2 = CO \times [(SaO_2 - S\bar{v}O_2) \times (\text{Hgb concentration} \times 1.36 \text{ mL/g})] \times 10$$

      - *Oxygen extraction ratio* is determined by dividing oxygen consumption by oxygen transport or delivery with the normal value, around 20% to 25%.

$$O_2 \text{ Extraction ratio} = \frac{\dot{V}O_2}{\dot{D}O_2} = \frac{CaO_2 - CvO_2}{CaO_2}$$

      - *Mixed venous oxygen saturation ($S\bar{v}O_2$)* is a continuous reflection of the balance between oxygen supply and oxygen demand, with the normal range between 70% and 80%.
   e. *Optimize oxygen delivery:* See Chapter 2.
   f. *Minimize oxygen demand:* It is beneficial to limit the patient's metabolic demands, especially patients with little or no metabolic reserve. Interventions include reducing pain, agitation, and fear. It is also important to provide adequate ventilation and sedation to decrease the patient's work of breathing. For each degree Celsius, the metabolic demands change by 13%. Therefore it is important

to decrease both heat and cold stress (Dichter and Curley, 2001). Avoid reducing fever below 37°C, as this will shift the oxyhemoglobin curve to the left, thereby decreasing the oxygen delivery to the tissues (Curly, 2001).

6. **Minimize iatrogenic complications**
   a. Barotrauma can be prevented by using the lowest possible peak pressure that will allow for adequate ventilation (Awad, 2003).
   b. *Minimize the risk of and assess for further cardiac dysfunction* by monitoring electrolytes and watching for tachyarrhythmias secondary to vasoactive and inotropic agents or electrolyte imbalance.
   c. *Minimize the risk of and assess for aspiration* by placing a nasogastric tube, ensuring the tube's patency and function, and elevating the head of the bed 30 degrees if tolerated.
   d. *Minimize the risk of and assess for renal toxicity* by optimizing tissue perfusion and judiciously using medications that are toxic to the kidneys.
7. **Supportive and investigational therapies**
   a. *The best management is prevention:* Proper handwashing is the single most effective means of preventing nosocomial infections. Good handwashing is essential. Not surprisingly, research has shown that the hands of health care workers are the primary mode of spreading nosocomial infections (Trampuz and Widmer, 2004). All personnel should wash their hands before and after every patient contact. However, compliance to handwashing recommendations is low, rarely exceeding 40% (Trampuz and Widmer, 2004). A study by Slota and colleagues (Slota et al., 2001) demonstrated that compliance with handwashing was associated with a reduction in nosocomial infections and that gown and glove isolation appeared to have an additional protective effect on children who had undergone solid organ transplantation. Patients with severe neutropenia or high-dose corticosteroid therapy are at risk for infection from endogenous microorganisms and airborne fungi (e.g., *Aspergillus*). The risk of *Aspergillus* infection is directly related to counts of airborne fungi. Outbreaks of fungemias are usually linked to building construction or dysfunction in air-control systems. Placement of patients in positive pressure rooms with spore-free high-efficiency particulate air (HEPA)-filtered air reduces this risk.
   b. The *gastrointestinal (GI) tract normally serves as an effective barrier* by preventing contents of the bowel from entering the body and by preventing body contents from leaking into the intestinal lumen (Winkelstein, 1999). Gram-negative bacteria, normally present within the intestinal lumen, are isolated from the body's internal environment by GI tract mucosa impermeability to gram-negative bacteria, GI tract lymphoid tissue preventing invasion of gram-negative bacteria, and anaerobic bacteria (commensal bacteria) preventing overgrowth of gram-negative bacteria (Hazinski, 1999).
      - *Gastrointestinal hypoperfusion* caused by sepsis may also disrupt the patient's gut barrier function. This may lead to translocation, which is the movement of bacteria across the mucosal barrier and into the bloodstream (Dichter and Curley, 2001). Enteral feedings may limit bacteria overgrowth (Dichter and Curley, 2001). Compromised host defenses (first, second, or third line of defense) that increase the risk for translocation include changes in GI tract pH, thermal or traumatic injury, radiation therapy, immunosuppression, nutritional compromise, and liver dysfunction (altered Kupffer's cell function). Alteration in normal GI tract flora (through viral or bacterial infection, reduction or impairment of motility, or antibiotic administration) and alteration in gut membrane permeability (related to decreased perfusion [e.g., shock] or GI tract mucosal injury) also increase the risk for translocation.

- *Assess for evidence of GI tract compromise.* Note the amount and consistency of diarrhea, guaiac-positive stools (or more obvious GI tract bleeding), and bacterial counts; stool cultures may indicate bacterial overgrowth. Increases in gastric output may be caused by numerous factors but may serve as an early indicator of GI tract compromise. Abdominal distention is also an early indicator of GI tract compromise. Mucosal pH can be measured indirectly via a balloon-tipped catheter (gastric tonometry). Normal pH reflects adequate perfusion, whereas an acidotic pH reflects tissue hypoxia. Ileus is a late sign of GI tract compromise.
- *Supportive GI tract therapies* include stress ulcer prophylaxis. Sepsis may cause gastrointestinal hypoperfusion. This in turn can lead to ulceration of the stomach and intestines, thereby increasing the risk of bleeding. The administration of histamine (H_2)-receptor antagonists may control gastric acidity and prevent gastric bleeding (Dichter and Curley, 2001).
- *Selective digestive decontamination (SDD)* may be used in patients who are at risk from translocation of bacteria across the mucosal barrier into the bloodstream (Pearson, 2002). Many advocates of SDD work in adult ICUs where the presence of nosocomial pneumonia is not only more common but also has a far greater significance than in the PICU (Pearson, 2002). No significant evidence is available to support SDD in the PICU (Pearson, 2002).

c. *Nutritional support* should be provided via the enteral route. The gut mucosa will atrophy quickly in the absence of enteral nutrients. The gut mucosal barrier can be preserved by the initiation of early enteral nutrition (Awad, 2003).

- Enteral feedings enriched with glutamine are vital in the preservation of gut mucosal integrity (Awad, 2003). Some advantages exist to using the enteral route over the parenteral route. Studies in animals have shown that the enteral nutrition route will be maintain mucosal integrity, decrease bacterial translocation, and maintain the immunologic function of the GI tract (Awad, 2003).

d. *CSFs:* Neutrophils are important to help eradicate pathogens, and yet they also cause excessive release of oxidants and proteases, which may cause injury to organs. Several randomized trials of G-CSF (granulocyte colony-stimulating factor) in patients with pneumonia have been completed. Findings show that although the WBC increased to 70,000 mm^3, there were no negative effects on lung function. The study further showed that there was no increase in survival as well as no decrease in the number of ICU days or decrease in organ function (Hotchkiss, 2003) (see Chapter 8).

e. *Prophylactic antibiotics:* Penicillin prophylaxis is recommended for patients with splenic dysfunction (sickle cell anemia) or who have had a splenectomy to prevent pneumococcal infection. Rifampin prophylaxis is recommended for those who have had close contact with *Haemophilus influenzae* or meningococcal disease.

f. *Vaccines:* Changes in the immunization program have the potential to significantly affect the incidence of community-acquired sepsis. The hepatitis B vaccine is currently given at birth. The American Academy of Pediatrics (2000) advises that all children be immunized again hepatitis B virus (HBV) before age 12 years. *H. influenza* type-B vaccine can be administered at 2 months of age. Meningococcal vaccine is recommended for high-risk patients. MMR (measles, mumps, rubella) booster vaccines are advised because of continued outbreaks of measles in vaccinated school-age children (Wong, 2001).

G. Relevant Pharmacology

1. **Inotropic and vasoactive agents:** see Table 9-17.
2. **Ibuprofen** is a cyclo-oxygenase inhibitor that can block arachidonic acid metabolism through the cyclo-oxygenase pathway.
3. **Drotrecogin alfa (Xigris):** Drotrecogin alfa (activated protein C) works to regulate the coagulatory and inflammatory responses seen in sepsis. It is an anticoagulant and is the first anti-inflammatory agent proven to be effective in sepsis (Hotchkiss, 2003). The use of activated protein C has demonstrated a greater survival in adult patients with both septic shock and severe sepsis (Patel et al., 2003). Barton and colleagues performed a preliminary analysis regarding the safety, pharmacokinetics, and pharmacodynamics of activated protein C in pediatric patients with severe sepsis (Barton et al., 2004). Currently, a large phase 3 randomized study is being conducted to determine the safety and efficacy in children (Barton et al., 2004).
4. **Hydrocortisone:** A study by Han and colleagues demonstrated that the use of hydrocortisone is associated with greater shock reversal in pediatric patients (Han et al., 2003). The use of hydrocortisone is a newer treatment modality and is being investigated widely. The results of another study showed high-dose hydrocortisone (50 mg/kg IV bolus followed by a 50 mg/kg infusion over 24 hours) in Dengue shock syndrome demonstrated significant benefits (Han et al., 2003). The empiric treatment of hydrocortisone in pediatric patients with purpura fulminans, catecholamine-resistant shock, or other risk factors for adrenal insufficiency is recommended in the ACCM-PALS guidelines. The use of hydrocortisone in pediatric patients is worthwhile because stress doses of the drug appear to lessen the potential effects of SIRS in sepsis.

COMPLICATIONS OF SEPTIC SHOCK

A. Implications for Other Systems

Given the complexity of the immune system, it is not surprising that a systemic inflammatory response and septic shock influence many body organs and systems. Because many body systems are affected, organ-specific dysfunction may result. Complications of septic shock include ARDS (see Chapter 2), disseminated intravascular coagulation (DIC; see Chapter 8), acute renal failure (see Chapter 5), and MODS.

B. Multiple-Organ Dysfunction Syndrome (MODS)

MODS is the cause of 97% of all deaths occurring in the PICU (Dichter and Curley, 2001). MODS and associated severe sepsis are the main cause of death in the ICU (Awad, 2003). Severe sepsis can potentially lead to the progressive deterioration of multiple organ systems of MODS (Awad, 2003). The criteria for pediatric patients with MODS are detailed in Table 9-18.

1. **Frequency** of specific organ involvement in children experiencing MODS:
   - a. *Respiratory system* (88%)
   - b. *Cardiovascular* (44%)
   - c. *Neurologic* (24%)
   - d. *Hematologic* (7%)
   - e. *Renal* (5%)
2. The **mortality** associated with MODS is related to the number of organ systems involved in the dysfunction process. A recent study found that as the number of

TABLE 9-18
Criteria for Pediatric Patients with MODS

Organ System	Criteria
Respiratory	RR >90/min Pa_{O_2} <40 mm Hg (in absence of cyanotic heart disease) Pa_{CO_2} >65 mm Hg Pa_{O_2}/Fi_{O_2} <200 mm Hg Mechanical ventilation (>24 h if postoperative) Tracheal intubation for airway obstruction
Cardiovascular	Systolic BP <40 mm Hg (infant <12 months) Systolic BP <50 mm Hg (children >12 months) HR <50 bpm or >220 bpm (infant <12 months) HR <40 bpm or >200 bpm (infants >12 months) Cardiac arrest Continous vasoactive drug infusion to maintain blood pressure
Neurologic	Glasgow coma scale <5 Fixed and dilated pupils Persistent (>20 min) intracranial pressure (>20 mm Hg or requiring therapeutic intervention)
Hematologic	Hemoglobin <5 g/dL WBC count <3000 cells/mm^3 Platelets <20,000/mm^3 Disseminated intravascular coagulation (PT >20 s or PTT >60 s in presence of positive FSP assay)
Renal	BUN >100 mg/dL Serum creatinine >2 mg/dL Dialysis
Gastrointestional	Blood transfusion >20 mL/kg in 24 hours because of gastrointestinal hemorrhage
Hepatic	Total bilirubin >5 mg/dL and SGOT or LDH more than twice normal value (without evidence of hemolysis) Hepatic encephalopathy > grade II

Modified from Dichter CH, Curley MAQ: Shock. In Curley MAQ, Moloney-Harmon PA, editors: *Critical care nursing of infants and children,* ed 2. Philadelphia, 2001, W.B. Saunders, pp 921-945; and Goh A et al.: Sepsis, severe sepsis and septic shock in pediatric multiple organ dysfunction syndrome. *J Paediatr Child Health* 35(5):488-492, October 1999.

BP, Blood pressure; *bpm,* beats per minute; *BUN,* blood urea nitrogen; *HR,* heart rate; *LDH,* luteinizing hormone; *PT,* prothrombin time; *PTT,* partial thromboplastin time; *SGOT,* serum glutamic oxaloacetic transaminase; *WBC,* white blood cell count.

dysfunctional organs increased from two to five, mortality increased accordingly, from 54% to 100% (Awad, 2003).

3. A study by Goh and colleagues (1999) found that children with a larger number of **simultaneous organ dysfunctions** develop more severe categories of sepsis. They also found that as organ dysfunction increased, so did mortality. In addition, the mean admission PRISM II (pediatric risk of mortality score) increased with worsening stages of sepsis (Goh et al., 1999).
4. **Sepsis** is not as strongly associated with MODS in children as in the adult population. Although sepsis is an important cause of MODS, it may not significantly increase mortality in children compared with adults (Goh et al., 1999).

Burns

Mary Jaco, Christine Owens Lane, Paula Dickerson, and Mary D. Gordon

Burns in the pediatric patient introduce diagnostic and therapeutic difficulties related to correct estimation of burn size and depth, fluid resuscitation and maintenance, airway management, vascular access, and thermal maintenance. Children present with age-related limitations of physiologic reserve, making it difficult for them to respond to an extensive burn injury. Recognition of the physiologic and psychosocial needs of children is paramount to providing optimal burn care.

A. Incidence

1. The incidence of burn injury in the United States has declined significantly over the years. As of the 1990s, reportable burn injuries are estimated at more than 1 million per year, almost half from previous surveys (ABA Burn Fact Sheet, 2000).
2. Children ages 4 and younger are at the greatest risk to suffer burn-related injuries, with an injury rate more than twice that of children aged 5 to 14 years (National SAFE KIDS Campaign, 2004).
3. Scald burns are the most common type of burn injury in children, followed by flame, and contact with hot solids. Chemical and electrical burns are relatively rare (Figure 9-8) (Purdue et al., 2002).
4. Nationally, about 10% of child abuse cases involve burning (Ruth et al., 2003).

MECHANISMS OF INJURY

A. Dimensions of Cellular Injury

1. The **local burn wound** is the result of heat necrosis of cells and results in coagulation necrosis of tissue that has both breadth and depth, that is, surface area and depth or degree.
2. The **extent** of cellular destruction depends on the intensity of the heat, the duration of exposure, and the tissue involved. When absorption of heat energy exceeds the ability of the tissue to dissipate the absorbed heat, cellular injury will result in varying depths.
3. The **pathology** of a cutaneous injury can be viewed in two ways:

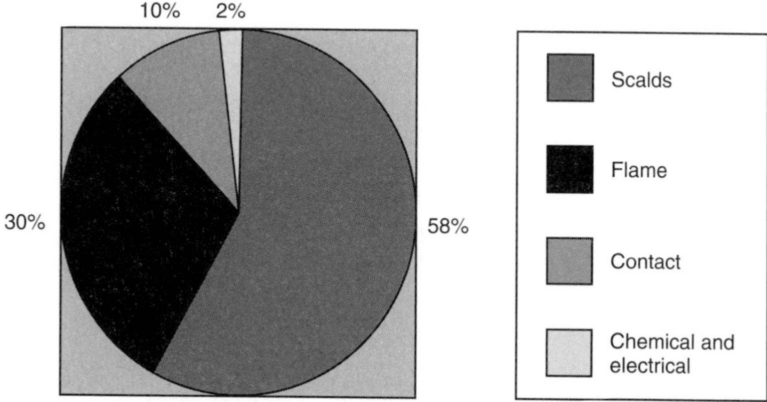

FIGURE 9-8 ■ Etiology of burn injuries in children 1 to 4 years old.

a. *Functional classification:* Classification of the burn injury based on functional changes considers the extent and depth of the burn and defines more precisely the pathology (Figure 9-9).
   - The zone of hyperemia is the most superficial area. It is considered viable tissue and recovers in a matter of days. The injury is analogous to the erythema in first-degree burns (i.e., sunburn).
   - The zone of stasis is less superficial and central to the zone of hyperemia. It is caused by vascular damage and the inflammatory response, resulting in compromised tissue perfusion. Over the ensuing 2 to 3 days after the burn, part or all the zone of stasis may evolve into a deeper injury. If resuscitation promptly restores compromised tissue blood flow, this tissue typically survives.
   - The zone of coagulation is the area having the most intimate contact with the heat source and therefore the most damage. Because it is characterized by cellular death, coagulation necrosis is the result of most burn injury.

b. *Descriptive classification:* A descriptive classification is based on the destruction of the skin layers. This classification indicates which layer of skin has been injured and uses the familiar terminology of first-, second-, third- and fourth-degree burns (Figure 9-10).

B. Thermal Injury

1. Thermal injuries result from direct heat, exposure to caustic chemicals, or contact with an electrical current. Radiation burns are rare.
2. Thermal injuries may be further subdivided into flame, flash burns, scalds, and contact burns.

C. Scald Injury

1. Scald injuries are caused by hot liquids, such as water, grease, and tar.
2. Characteristically in immersion scalds, the underlying burn tissue initially appears red and dry. The red discoloration under these circumstances is due to hemoglobin fixed in the tissues. Immersion scald burns in children are usually full-thickness burns (Advanced Burn Life Support Course, 2001).

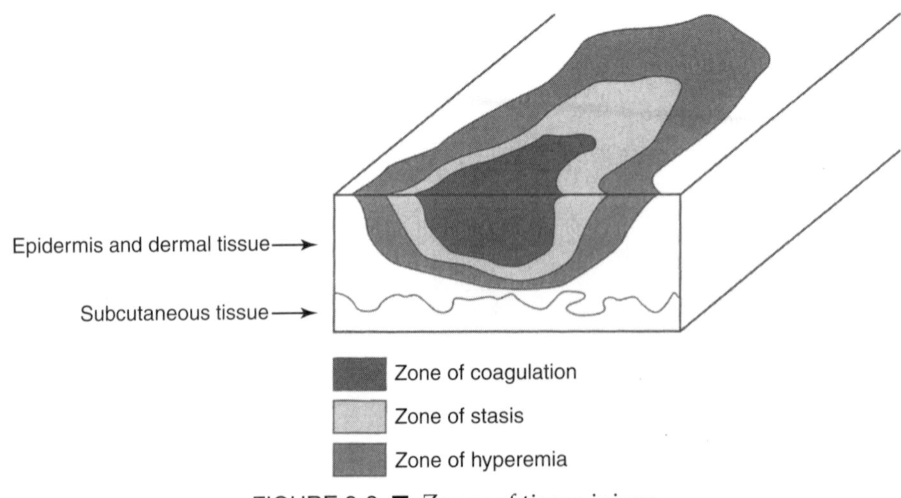

FIGURE 9-9 ■ Zones of tissue injury.

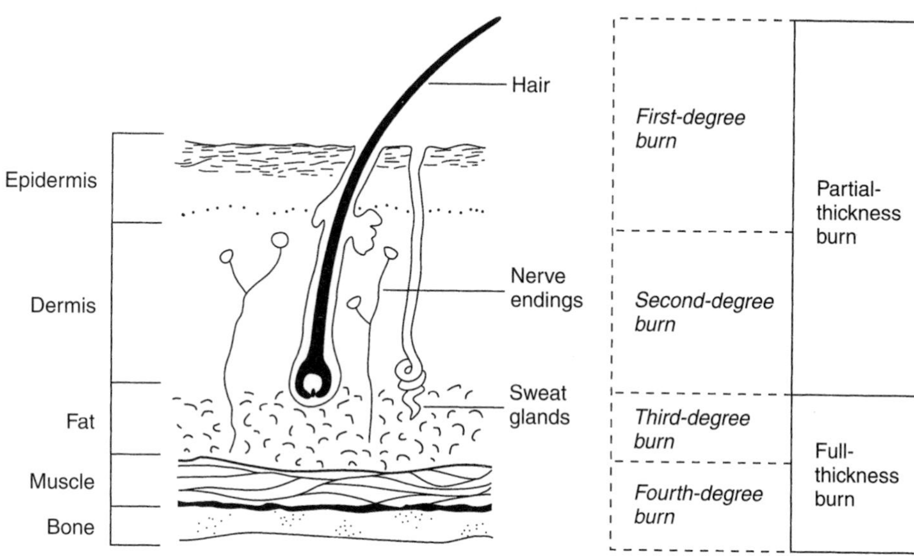

FIGURE 9-10 ■ Schematic cross-sectional representation of the skin

D. Electrical Injury

1. **Electrical injuries** from contact with high-voltage electricity are caused by the following mechanisms: The electrical current passes through the skin, causing cutaneous and deep tissue injury both locally and distant from the contact sites and often producing extensive underlying tissue (muscle or bone) damage. Contact points are often dry, circumscribed, and depressed. Deep tissue damage may result in extensive subfascial edema and tissue necrosis. A fasciotomy may be indicated to reduce pressure within the muscle compartment, thus maintaining blood flow to injured muscles.
2. **Associated complications** may include the following:
   a. *Neurologic complications* (secondary to the electrical current itself) may include cerebral complaints such as loss of consciousness, headaches, seizures, decreased memory, emotional liability, or learning impairment and peripheral complaints such as sensorimotor loss, paresthesias, paralysis, or paresis.
   b. *Renal complications* may include acute tubular necrosis and acute renal failure related to hemochromogens (myoglobinuria and hemoglobinuria) released following muscle necrosis.
   c. *Cardiac arrhythmia and arrest* can occur when the current disrupts the heart's conduction system.
   d. *Skeletal injuries* (i.e., fractures, spinal cord injuries) may be related to powerful tetanic contractions by the muscle or a fall from a height after contact with high-voltage electrical current.
   e. The electrical current arcs external to the body, causing cutaneous injury. Heat may cause ignition of clothing and environmental objects. If clothing is ignited, a large surface area may sustain deep soft-tissue burns resulting from the very high temperature. There may be no actual current damage. These wounds are the *flash-flame type.*

E. Chemical Injury

1. **Chemical burns** occur when the victim comes in direct contact with caustic chemicals, such as acids, alkalies, or petroleum-based products. Severity

is related to the agent, its concentration, its volume, and the duration of contact.

a. *Prompt measures* to remove the chemical ensure the most optimal result. Delay in treatment permits continued tissue damage. Search for a neutralizing agent wastes valuable time, but more important is that the increased heat of the neutralizing reaction may cause further tissue damage (Advanced Burn Life Support Course, 2001).
b. *Initial treatment* consists of removing all the patient's clothing, brushing the skin if the caustic agent is a powder, and irrigating the involved area with copious amounts of tap water or placing the patient in a shower. Irrigation should continue from the time of the injury through evaluation in the hospital. Alkalies may require longer irrigation because they have a high binding affinity with the tissue and thus are more difficult to remove. Alkalies frequently cause greater damage than the acidic compounds.
c. *Chemical injury* to the eye deserves special attention because of the potential for permanent damage to the cornea. The eye should be flushed immediately and continuously until an ophthalmologic consultation is obtained. Irrigate with NS or a balanced salt solution. Tap water can be used if NS is not available.
d. Besides irrigation, *specific treatment modalities* for chemical agents (i.e., hydrofluoric acid, phenol, phosphorus) can be determined by contacting a regional poison-control facility, the hazardous materials division of the fire department, or the chemical manufacturer.

F. Contact Injury

Contact burns are caused by hot, solid objects. Severity is related to size and length of time the object is in contact with skin.

EMERGENT PHASE: INITIAL ASSESSMENT AND MANAGEMENT

The **emergent phase** (1 to 3 days after the burn) begins with the initial hemodynamic response to thermal injury and lasts until capillary integrity is restored and fluid replacement is completed.

A. Care at the Scene of Accident

1. **First aid**
   a. The most important first-aid treatment is *minimizing* the burn wound depth and extent, which is accomplished by eliminating the source of the injury and stopping the burning process (Merz et al., 2003).
   b. After the burning agent is eliminated, *cover* the burns with clean, dry linen. Measures to conserve body heat are essential for all burn victims, particularly for the infant and young child. Wet compresses may be applied to small wounds but not to large injuries. Water increases body heat loss through the wound, a principal concern in small children. Wet dressings also promote hypothermia, which may accentuate the shock state, causing a further decrease in tissue perfusion, cardiac output, and perfusion to vital organs. Ice or ice water should never be used directly on the skin because of the potential for cold injury or for conversion of a lesser burn to a deeper injury (due to vasoconstriction) (Purdue et al., 2002).

2. **Rapid primary and secondary assessment**
   a. At the accident scene the primary and secondary assessments are performed as later described but in a *more rapid manner*. The priority quickly becomes to expediently transport the patient to a hospital.
   b. Burn patients are considered *multiple trauma victims* and must be assessed for other traumatic injuries in addition to the burn, especially if the burn is the result of a motor-vehicle crash or an explosion of some kind. Any coexisting trauma must be evaluated and treated during the primary and secondary surveys.

B. Care in the Emergency Department

1. **Primary assessment**
   a. *Assess the airway and breathing.*
      - Airway management for the burn patient should be managed as for any trauma victim, including performing basic life support measures if indicated, providing 100% FiO_2 via face mask, assessing respirations for adequacy of rate and depth, and assessing for bilateral breath sounds.
      - Special considerations: The upper airway is susceptible to edema and obstruction as a result of exposure to heat and smoke. Because of relatively small airways in children, upper-airway obstruction may occur early and rapidly. Circumferential full-thickness burns to the neck or chest may restrict ventilation.
      - Upper-airway obstruction or lower-airway compromise should be identified and treated accordingly and may require endotracheal intubation and mechanical ventilation.

   b. *Assess circulation.*
      - Determine the extent and depth of the burn. Children with burns covering 10% or more of their total body surface area (TBSA) require circulatory volume support.
      - Establish intravenous (IV) access for fluid resuscitation if indicated. Place two peripheral large-bore IV catheters, appropriate for the size of the child. The peripheral percutaneous route is the method of choice for immediate initial access; if the only accessible veins have overlying burned skin, do not hesitate to use them (Advanced Burn Life Support Course, 2001; Advanced Trauma Life Support Course, 1997). Unless indicated by other associated injuries, first-responders need not start an IV line if the primary hospital or burn center is less than an hour away from the scene of injury (Purdue et al., 2002). Cannulation of small veins may be difficult in any infant or child but even more so in a child with severe vasoconstriction. Maintaining venous access is a major priority. All IV catheters should be sutured. Adhesive tape is ineffective in securing IV catheters to burned tissue and may compromise blood flow in edematous extremities if applied circumferentially.
      - Evaluate skin color, sensation, and capillary refill. Circumferential third-degree burns of the extremities may impair circulation as a result of edema formation. Maintain continuous elevation of the burned extremities.
      - Monitor arterial pulses hourly for 24 to 48 hours on all extremities with deep burns, circumferential burns, or electrical burns. Use an ultrasonic flow device if pulses are not palpable. Escharotomies should be performed at the earliest sign of circulatory compromise (i.e., decreased pulse, complaints of deep aching muscle pain).
      - Insert a urinary catheter to monitor the effectiveness of fluid resuscitation.

c. *Assess neurologic status.*
   - Use the Glasgow Coma Scale (GCS) with a modified verbal score for children younger than 4 years of age (Advanced Trauma Life Support Course, 1997). Typically, the burn victim is initially alert and oriented (Advanced Burn Life Support Course, 2001). For a decreased level of consciousness, consider an associated injury, substance abuse, hypoxia, or preexisting medical condition.

d. *Expose and examine.*
   - Remove all clothing so the extent and severity of injury can be examined. In the case of chemical burns, the clothing could be contaminated and cause further injury. Clothing should not be discarded if there is a suspicion of criminal activity because it might be used as evidence.
   - Remove all jewelry on burned extremities; jewelry might create a tourniquet effect, restricting blood flow.

2. **Secondary assessment**

a. *Obtain a history of the burn injury.* Initial management and definitive care are guided by the mechanism, duration, severity, and time of the injury. As much information as possible should be obtained regarding the incident:
   - Cause of burn?
   - Did the injury occur in a closed space?
   - Time of injury?
   - Were harmful chemicals involved?
   - Were others involved?
   - Assess for intentional injury (possible child abuse; Table 9-19).

b. *Obtain medical history.* Underlying medical conditions frequently complicate burn management and prolong recovery. Determine the presence of preexisting disease or associated illness; medications, alcohol, or drugs; allergies or sensitivities; recent exposure to communicable diseases (i.e., varicella, tuberculosis); status of tetanus immunization (burn wounds are tetanus-prone wounds and immunizations should be consistent with the recommendations of the American College of Surgeons); and status of other immunizations. Tetanus prophylaxis, although important, can be delayed up to 72 hours to establish the patient's immunization status (Advanced Burn Life Support Course, 2001). This status, however, must be documented so as not to be overlooked. As an aid to gaining necessary information, the mnemonic "AMPLE" can be used:
   A = Allergy
   M = Medications
   P = Previous illness
   L = Last meal/fluids
   E = Events related to the injury

c. *Complete physical examination.* This includes a complete head-to-toe examination and assessment to evaluate more fully any and all injuries or abnormalities, including the burn injury. The severity of a burn injury and its morbidity and mortality are determined by the type of burn; size, depth, and anatomic location of the wound; the patient's age; and any preexisting illness or associated trauma.
   - The **extent of a burn** is calculated as a percentage of TBSA. Various methods are available to determine the extent of burn surface area.
     - In the **rule of ones or hand rule,** the palm of an individual's hand represents approximately 1% of the TBSA. Therefore, using the victim's hand as a guideline, the extent of a small burn or one with an irregular outline or distribution can easily be estimated.

■ **TABLE 9-19**
■ ■ **Etiology and Characteristic Patterns of Intentional and Unintentional Burn Injuries in Children**

Type of Burn	Etiology	Unintentional Characteristic Wound Pattern	Intentional Characteristic Wound Pattern
SCALDS			
SPILL/SPLASH Occur when a hot liquid falls from above victim or when a hot liquid is thrown or poured on victim	***hot liquids*** water tea coffee soup grease	• "arrowhead" appearance • irregular margins • nonuniform depth • the liquid cools as it flows downward producing a deeper burn in the topmost area with the depth becoming progressively more shallow and narrower as the fluid flows downward	• essentially the same as unintentional
IMMERSION Occurs when the victim falls into a container of hot liquid or when victim is placed in container of hot liquid	usually water hot tap water boiling water	• splash marks • varying depth of burn • indistinct borders between burned and nonburned skin • multiple areas of burn as the patient struggles to get out of the hot liquid	• absence of splash marks • burn depth is uniform • unvaried appearance • well demarcated "waterline" burn vs. nonburn margins • bilateral symmetrical burns of the extremities, a "stocking & glove" distribution • burns of the buttocks and/or perineum • sparing of the flexor creases in both the groin and popliteal spaces • usually full-thickness
FLAME BURNS	fire		• extreme depth of injury and relatively circumscribed areas compared to unintentional burns
CONTACT BURNS	hot solids	• usually one sided • lack of apparent pattern caused by patient movement	• faithfully depicts the outline of the hot object (e.g., grate/grill pattern • uniform in all directions

- The **rule of nines** measures the percentage of burn surface area by dividing the body into multiples of nine. In the infant or child, the rule is adjusted because the child's head has a larger proportional percentage of the TBSA.
- The **Berkow** (Figure 9-11) or **Lund and Browder chart** allows for a more accurate assessment that takes into account differences in BSA related to age and divides the body into smaller areas (e.g., foot, lower leg, thigh).
- Other methods use a standard **height and weight nomogram** to calculate the body surface area burned in square meters (m^2).

Parkland Memorial Hospital
Dallas, Texas

Burn Record
To be completed on admission

Name____________________

Age________ Date of Birth____________

Admit Date____________________

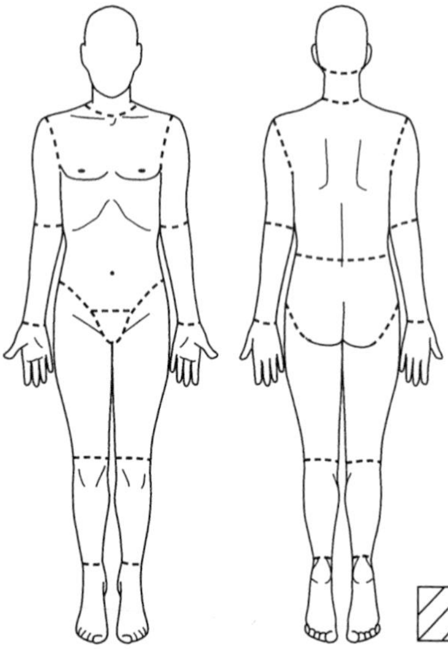

Date of Burn________ Time of Burn________

Weight (kg)________ Height________

2°______ + 3°______ = ______%

First 8 hrs

Second 8 hrs

Third 8 hrs

Albumin

Maintenance

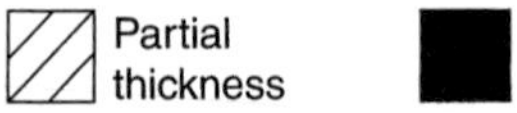

Partial thickness

Full thickness

Percent Surface Area Burned (Berkow Formula)

Area	**1 y**	**1–4 y**	**5–9 y**	**10–14 y**	**15 y**	**Adult**	**2°**	**3°**
Head	19	17	13	11	9	7		
Neck	2	2	2	2	2	2		
Ant trunk	13	13	13	13	13	13		
Post trunk	13	13	13	13	13	13		
R buttock	2½	2½	2½	2½	2½	2½		
L buttock	2½	2½	2½	2½	2½	2½		
Genitalia	1	1	1	1	1	1		
RU arm	4	4	4	4	4	4		
LU arm	4	4	4	4	4	4		
RL arm	3	3	3	3	3	3		
LL arm	3	3	3	3	3	3		
R hand	2½	2½	2½	2½	2½	2½		
L hand	2½	2½	2½	2½	2½	2½		
R thigh	5½	6½	8	8½	9	9½		
L thigh	5½	6½	8	8½	9	9½		
R leg	5	5	5½	6	6½	7		
L leg	5	5	5½	6	6½	7		
R foot	3½	3½	3½	3½	3½	3½		
L foot	3½	3½	3½	3½	3½	3½		
						Total		

FIGURE 9-11 ■ Berkow formula burn record.

TABLE 9-20
Depth and Degree of Burn

Depth	Degree	Characteristics
Superficial	***First***	Local pain and erythema Dry; without blisters Heals in 3–5 days Example: sunburn
Partial thickness Superficial partial thickness	***Second***	Appears red to pale ivory Moist or with blisters Very painful Heals in 14–28 days with variable amount of scarring Caused by flash burns, scalds, or brief contact with hot objects
Deep partial thickness		Mottled; areas of waxy white injury Dry surface May be clinically indistinguishable from full-thickness burn Heals spontaneously in about 15–40 days unless infection converts it to full-thickness injury
Full thickness	***Third***	Elasticity of dermis is destroyed Appears white, cherry red, brown, or black Appears dry, hard or leathery Painless May require escharotomies if circumferential Caused by flame burns, chemical, electrical, or prolonged contact with source of heat
	Fourth	Involves the fat, fascia, muscle, or bone Seen in electrical and deep thermal burns

- Depth of burn
  - Descriptive classification: See Table 9-20 and Figure 9-10.
  - Burns may be more severe (deeper) than they initially appear in the very young (and elderly) because of their thin skin.
  - Depth of injury is often very difficult to estimate accurately in the first 24 hours after the burn; wounds must be reevaluated on a daily basis to provide a more accurate determination of depth.
- Type of burn
  - Identify the type of burn: Although appropriate initial interventions often occur before arrival at the emergency department, never assume this step has been completed (i.e., chemical burns).

d. *Obtain baseline diagnostic studies.* Baseline laboratory studies are essential to evaluate the patient's subsequent progress. Evaluate arterial blood gases (ABGs) and carboxyhemoglobin (if indicated), hematocrit and hemoglobin, electrolytes, albumin, urinalysis, blood urea nitrogen (BUN), chest radiographic examination, and 12-lead electrocardiogram (ECG) with electrical injury, ectopy, or history of underlying cardiovascular disease.

e. *Initial wound care.* Wound care is not considered a component of emergency care except in chemical burns, in which immediate removal of the agent is essential (see Chemical Burns). Substantial wound care, such as excessive manual debridement or application of topical antimicrobials (in the field or

TABLE 9-21
American Burn Association: Burn Center Referral Criteria

A burn unit may treat adults or children or both. Burn injuries that should be referred to a burn unit include the following:

1. Partial thickness burns greater than 10% total body surface area (TBSA)
2. Burns that involve the face, hands, feet, genitalia, perineum, or major joints
3. Third-degree burns in any age group
4. Electrical burns including lightning injury
5. Chemical burns
6. Inhalation injury
7. Burn injury in patients with preexisting medical disorders that could complicate management, prolong recovery, or affect mortality
8. Any patients with burns and concomitant trauma (such as fractures) in which the burn injury poses the greatest risk of morbidity or mortality. In such cases, if the trauma poses the greater immediate risk, the patient may be stabilized initially in a trauma center before being transferred to a burn unit. Physician judgement will be necessary in such situations and should be in concert with the regional medical control plan and triage protocols.
9. Burned children in hospitals without qualified personnel or equipment for the care of children
10. Burn injury in patients who will require special social, emotional, or long-term rehabilitative intervention

From Guidelines for the operations of burn units. In Resources for optimal care of the injured patient: 1999, Committee on Trauma, American College of Surgeons.

primary hospital), is not necessary if the patient will be transferred to a burn care facility.

f. Patients must *have nothing by mouth (NPO)* until they have been seen and evaluated in a hospital and, if necessary, transported to a burn center. A nasogastric tube should be inserted in all patients with a burn size of over 20% body surface area, as they are susceptible to gastric dilatation due to a paralytic ileus, and in all patients who are intubated (Advanced Burn Life Support Course, 2001).

C. Stabilization and Transport

1. Patients with burn injuries who meet the **ABA Criteria for Burn Center Referral** (Table 9-21) should be assessed, stabilized, and promptly transferred. This may be directly from the accident scene to the burn center, or patients may first require transportation to the closest hospital, depending on their condition and the traveling distance necessary.
2. The burn victim must be appropriately **stabilized** following the principles outlined in the primary and secondary surveys.
3. **Documentation** should include the circumstances of injury, including any first-hand accounts, which can be vitally important in the case of suspected child abuse. All resuscitative measures and all medications given must also be documented.
4. **Communication and collaboration** between the referring facility and the burn center are extremely important in ascertaining that the patient's medical needs are met, the most appropriate form of transportation is used, and the patient is safely transported.

D. Systemic Responses: Assessment and Care

An extensive burn affects all organ systems and is manifested by a biphasic pattern of early hypofunction (i.e., decreased cardiac output, increased capillary permeability) followed by hyperfunction (i.e., hypermetabolism). The events, magnitude, and duration of the systemic manifestations of burn shock are proportional to the extent of burn injury and plateau at approximately 50% to 60% burn surface area. Although the exact etiology of burn shock is not totally understood, characteristic fluid volume shifts and hemodynamic changes that accompany burn shock have been identified.

1. **Cardiovascular response**
   a. The *initial response* to a large burn injury is characterized by a decrease in cardiac output and increased peripheral vascular resistance. An uncharacterized factor present in circulation following massive burns has been implicated for this characteristic myocardial depression. The increased peripheral vascular resistance develops as an initial physiologic response to hypovolemia, decreased cardiac output, and the release of vasoactive mediators from the stress response following injury.
   b. *Cardiac output* returns to normal 24 to 36 hours after the burn (Merz et al., 2003). Peripheral vascular resistance returns to normal as cardiac output improves. As cardiac output improves, it exceeds normal values as the characteristic hyperdynamic state develops. Tachycardia develops as a physiologic response to hypovolemia, decreased cardiac output, and elevated catecholamine levels.
   c. *Microvasculature changes* in the cell wall result in the disruption of normal capillary barriers separating the intravascular and interstitial compartments, resulting in free exchange of fluid and plasma. This increased permeability permits essentially all elements of the vascular space, except red blood cells (RBCs) and platelets, to escape, creating a relative hypovolemia. The fluid requirement necessary to restore and maintain tissue perfusion is directly related to the burn size. Capillary leak and edema following small burns are localized to the burn wound. Injury greater than 30% burn surface area produces not only localized burn wound edema but a systemic capillary permeability and general body edema. The rate of progression of tissue edema is dependent on the adequacy and volume of fluid resuscitation. The maximal amount of edema occurs 8 to 12 hours after injury in small burns but up to 24 hours after injury in large burns (Rutan, 1998). Capillary integrity is restored approximately 18 to 24 hours post burn. Large burns may take up to 30 hours to regain capillary integrity.
2. **Pulmonary response:** In large burns without an inhalation injury, early alterations in pulmonary function occur indirectly through the release of inflammatory mediators (i.e., thromboxane) and intravascular hypoproteinemia resulting in a transient hydrostatic pulmonary edema with a mild derangement in oxygenation. A decrease in lung compliance may be related to chest wall edema, circumferential burns to the chest wall, smoke inhalation injury, preexisting lung disease, or fluid-volume overload.
3. **Hematologic response**
   a. Within several hours of injury, as *edema* forms, the fluid shift and intravascular volume deficit result in hemoconcentration (Rutan, 1998). The hematocrit increases secondary to loss of circulating plasma volume. Blood viscosity also increases.
   b. The characteristic *anemia* associated with burn injuries has multiple causes. Only about 10% of the RBC mass is lost to hemolysis during the burning process or by the extravasation of RBCs into the wound (Rutan, 1998). Heat-injured RBCs have a shortened half-life and increased clearance. The ongoing post-burn RBC hemolysis has been attributed to the release of inflammatory mediators (i.e., oxygen radicals, lipid peroxides). Although the exact nature is

not known, there is an impaired production of new RBCs by the bone marrow with a shortened RBC lifespan. Additionally, there is an ongoing effective blood loss related to daily wound care and multiple surgical procedures.

c. Initially there is a *depression in serum clotting factors* with a concomitant rise in fibrinogen degradation products, followed by a post-resuscitation rise in increased levels of coagulation components. Platelet alterations include an increase in adhesiveness and shortened survival time.

4. **Gastrointestinal response:** Decreased gastrointestinal (GI) tract activity, caused by decreased tissue perfusion, is the by-product of hypovolemia and the neuroendocrine responses to injury. These responses cause an increased risk for the development of a burn-stress related ulceration (Curling's), and the incidence of ulceration has been greatly reduced by the routine use of antacid or histamine (H_2) antagonist therapy. With adequate fluid resuscitation, GI tract activity returns to normal within 24 to 48 hours.
5. **Renal response:** With decreased intravascular volume there is a decrease in renal plasma flow and glomerular filtration rate (GFR), resulting in low urine output (Merz et al., 2003). If fluid resuscitation is inadequate or if resuscitation is delayed, oliguria ensues leading to acute renal failure. As the capillary integrity is restored, interstitial fluids are pulled back into the intravascular compartment, and diuresis occurs.
6. **Metabolic response:** With increased catecholamine and glucagon production, there is a mobilization of hepatic glycogen stores, coupled with a relative decrease in insulin production that commonly results in high serum glucose levels in the early post-burn period. Within 24 to 48 hours after the burn, there is an increase in metabolism directly related to the severity of the injury. This hypermetabolic state is characterized by increases in oxygen consumption and heat production, with an increase in both core and skin temperatures. Severe injury accelerates nitrogen flow. Both protein synthesis and breakdown are increased. In patients not meeting nutritional goals, breakdown rates exceed synthesis, resulting in a negative nitrogen balance. As capillary integrity is restored, electrolyte replacement therapy becomes an ongoing process and continues until wound closure is achieved. As the wounds heal, either spontaneously or by skin grafting, the metabolic rate gradually returns to normal levels. The decrease in metabolic requirements is a gradual process. In children with large burns, metabolic requirements remain higher even after the burn wound is fully mature (Saffle and Hildreth, 2002).
7. **Immune and inflammatory response:** Although the exact mechanisms of the immunologic and inflammatory response are not known, characteristic pathophysiologic activities are being recognized as a result of the burn injury. Alteration in the skin's protective function provides opportunity for invasion of microorganisms and primes the defensive mechanisms of the inflammatory and immune systems. It is hypothesized that a massive systemic inflammatory response is caused by the local trauma of a burn. It appears that a burn is a mediator-induced injury; although the local effects occur immediately, the systemic response to the mediators produced within a burn progresses and peaks 5 to 7 days after the injury. It is unclear whether the immunosuppression after a burn injury is the result of biochemical substances (i.e., oxidants, histamine, prostaglandins, arachidonic acid metabolites) liberated from the burn itself, or are produced in response to the burn. Additionally, the immunosuppressive effects of anesthetic agents, surgical procedures, multiple transfusions, and the use of systemic antibiotics emphasize post-burn immunologic abnormalities during the clinical course of burn therapy.

8. **Hypothermia:** Children are more prone to the development of hypothermia secondary to their increased BSA–to-mass ratio. Because of the increased BSA-to-mass ratio, children have greater evaporative water loss and greater heat loss from evaporation and convection. Hypothermia remains a major problem until the wounds have been skin grafted or healed. Hypothermia alone, without any injuries, can cause apnea, progressive metabolic acidosis, and ventricular arrhythmias.

E. Concomitant Injuries: Assessment and Care

1. Inhalation injury

a. An *inhalation injury* may be the most important determinant of mortality in burn patients, having a greater effect than either TBSA burn or age. Inhalation injury exists in approximately 10% to 20% of hospitalized burn patients (Guy and Peck, 1999). More than 50% of burn-center mortalities are attributed to the pulmonary complications of inhalation injury. Advances in fluid resuscitation, metabolic support, and wound management have increased the survival rate of burn patients, but little progress has been made in the survival rate of the burn patient with inhalation injury. Respiratory failure, during the first few hours to days after a burn injury, can be caused by asphyxia, upper airway obstruction, or chemical injury to the airway. The resulting injury can occur alone or in combination with a cutaneous injury.

b. *Classification of injury*

- **Acute asphyxia**: Related to hypoxia and carbon monoxide excess.
  - The process of combustion involves consumption of oxygen; therefore air inspired by fire victims has considerably lower than normal oxygen concentration, particularly when the fire occurs in a closed space. In a fire, as oxygen is consumed during combustion, carbon monoxide is released because it is a basic by-product of incomplete combustion (Cioffi, 1998).
  - Carbon monoxide causes toxicity by three mechanisms: the formation of carboxyhemoglobin, shifting the oxygen-hemoglobin dissociation curve to the left, and binding to other heme-containing proteins, namely cytochrome enzymes and myoglobin. Carbon monoxide is a colorless, tasteless, odorless, nonirritating gas with an affinity for hemoglobin 200 times greater than that of oxygen. As carbon monoxide is transported across the alveolar membrane, it preferentially binds with hemoglobin, in place of oxygen, to form carboxyhemoglobin. Carbon monoxide impedes the dissociation of oxygen from hemoglobin, shifting the oxygen-hemoglobin dissociation curve to the left, thereby impairing oxygen unloading at the tissue level. The result is a major impairment in oxygen delivery. Ninety-seven percent of oxygen is carried to the tissues on hemoglobin. Carboxyhemoglobin also interacts with the myoglobin of cardiac muscle and the cytochrome system, further interfering with oxygen utilization. In victims with preexisting coronary disease, hypoxia of the myocardium may precipitate angina, dysrhythmias, or cardiac arrest. Cerebral hypoxia may lead to cerebral edema. Even if victims recover, neurologic symptoms may persist if the damage is severe (Cioffi, 1998; Guy and Peck, 1999).
  - Tachypnea and cyanosis may be absent because the partial pressure of oxygen in arterial blood ($Pa{O_2}$) as perceived by the peripheral chemoreceptors (the carotid body and aortic arch) is normal. The peripheral chemoreceptors controlling respiratory drive respond to changes in the $Pa{O_2}$, and not to changes in the arterial oxygen saturation ($Sa{O_2}$), even in the presence of high carboxyhemoglobin levels. Standard pulse oximeters

TABLE 9-22
Carboxyhemaglobin Level and Associated Signs and Symptoms

Carboxyhemaglobin Level (%)	Symptoms
0-5	Normal value
<15	Often found in smokers
15-20	Headache, mild dyspnea, confusion
20-40	Disorientation, fatigue, nausea, syncope
>50	Coma, seizures, respiratory failure, death

are unable to distinguish between hemoglobin molecules saturated with oxygen (oxyhemoglobin) and those saturated with carboxyhemoglobin, producing a false elevation in oxygen saturation in victims with significant carbon monoxide toxicity (Advance Burn Life Support, 2001).

- Carbon monoxide toxicity is evaluated by measuring the arterial carboxyhemoglobin level. Elevated levels of carboxyhemoglobin serve as indirect evidence for exposure to combustion products. Multiple signs and symptoms have been associated with carboxyhemoglobin levels (Table 9-22). A low carboxyhemoglobin level does not indicate minimal exposure. Administration of 90% to 100% O_2 displaces some, if not all, the carboxyhemoglobin before arrival to the emergency department or before an ABG analysis can be performed. Carbon monoxide has a constant half-life and is reduced by 50% in 4 hours at room air, and in less than 1 hour if an oxygen concentration of 100% is used (Monafo, 1996).

- Airway injury related to edema or obstruction
  - Heat injury, from inhaling hot air, is limited to the upper airways (above the glottis) and may cause sufficient edema to produce mechanical obstruction (Purdue et al., 2002). Direct thermal injury to the lower tracheobronchial tree and alveoli is rare because of the protective reflex closure of the glottis and the heat-dissipating capacity of the upper airway. Mucosal damage may result from both the heat and the chemical components of smoke. Mechanical obstruction of the airway is not limited to those with inhalation injury. The edema that accompanies scalds or even grease burns to the face and neck can be associated with enough edema to cause external airway compromise.
- Airway injury related to smoke inhalation
  - Airway injury due to smoke is essentially a chemical injury caused by inhalation of the by-products of combustion and is related to the composition (i.e., benzene from plastics) and duration of the inhaled smoke. When the toxic material is inhaled, it adheres to the mucous membranes, producing a chemical burn to the tracheobronchial mucosa or as far down as the particles descend into the lung. Diagnosing the severity of the injury may be based more on the clinical course of the disease process than on initial physical findings. Generally, admission chest radiographic examinations underestimate the severity of lung damage because the injury is usually initially confined to the airways (Advanced Burn Life Support, 2001).

c. *Clinical assessment* (Table 9-23): The onset of symptoms is unpredictable, and a patient with possible inhalation injury must be observed closely. Many patients demonstrate minimal symptoms early after injury, and only when airway

TABLE 9-23
Clinical Assessment: Inhalation Injury

History	Initial Physical Findings	Initial Diagnostic Findings
"Closed space" injury Exposure to noxious gases or smoke Duration of exposure Unconsciousness CPR Alcohol or drug abuse Underlying disease Others involved Accidental or intentional	Burns: Chest, face, neck, head Edema: Face, neck, head Singed: Nasal or facial hair, eyebrows Soot: Mouth, pharynx, naris Ulcerations: Mouth, pharynx Carbonaceous sputum Tachypnea Dyspnea or stridor Cyanosis Bronchorrhea Hoarseness Wheezing, crackles, rhonchi Retractions Nasal flaring CNS signs and symptoms: With decreased level of conciousness assess for: Hypoxemia Hypovolemia Elevated carboxyhemaglobin	ABG: Within normal limits or hypoxemia and acidosis Carboxyhemaglobin: Within normal limits or increased Chest x-ray examination: Admission usually clear Bronchoscopy: Mucosal edema or sloughing Erythema Ulceration Carbonaceous material

edema develops do symptoms become evident. Because of relatively small airways, upper-airway obstruction in the pediatric patient may occur early and rapid. Securing the endotracheal tube is a particular problem in the presence of burn injury. Facial edema—coupled with wounds, secretions, and topical creams—increases the difficulty of securing and maintaining proper tube placement (Purdue et al., 2002).

2. **Additional trauma:** Assess for associated injuries: The burn is often the most obvious injury, but other trauma or life-threatening injuries may be present in approximately 5% to 10% of burn patients (i.e., fractures, soft-tissue injury, head injury, thoracic trauma, abdominal injury). The burn injury may be compounded with blunt trauma from explosions, motor-vehicle crashes, jumping to escape further injury, or falling from a height. Associated injuries should be identified and appropriately managed in the same manner as for any trauma patient.

F. Fluid Resuscitation

1. **Initiating fluid therapy**
   a. *Fluid resuscitation* should be initiated in infants with burns covering 10% or more of their TBSA and in older children with burns 15% or more of their TBSA (Herndon, 2002).
   b. The primary goal of *fluid resuscitation* is first to restore volume and then to maintain intravascular volume at a level ensuring adequate tissue perfusion to vital organs. It is a balance, avoiding organ ischemia as well as preserving heat-injured but viable tissues while avoiding the complications of inadequate or excessive therapy.
   c. In children, *resuscitation therapy* must be more exact, owing to limited physiologic reserves (especially those younger than 3 years of age).

d. Because of the *greater surface area* in relation to body mass, proportionately children require more fluid for burn resuscitation than an adult with a similar size burn. Thus provision for daily maintenance fluids in addition to the fluid requirements dictated by burn size must be emphasized (Herndon, 2002; Morehouse, 1992).

e. The *volume infused* should be continually titrated to avoid both under-resuscitation and over-resuscitation. Constant reevaluation of the patient's clinical course is essential.

f. *Venous access* for infants and children must be established early in post-burn period. IV cannulation of central vessels can be difficult as well as risky, and thus the use of femoral or saphenous veins may be necessary. Another option is intraosseous fluid administration for children less than 8 years of age.

2. **Fluid resuscitation formulas:** The quantity of fluid to be given is based on the extent of burn surface area and the patient's weight.

   a. Numerous effective formulas have been developed for calculating fluid resuscitation for burn patients. All use both an electrolyte solution and a colloid, and all include large volumes of sodium as the primary volume expander. They differ in the amounts of free water and the time of administration post-burn.

   b. Most formulas advocate the use of crystalloid solutions, commonly Ringer's lactate, because of its similar composition to the intravascular fluid being lost into the burn wound. Young children have relatively small glycogen stores; thus hypoglycemia may occur. It may be necessary to provide dextrose-containing fluids during resuscitation. However, avoid a rapid infusion of hypotonic fluid in a young child because it may cause a rapid sodium shift causing cerebral edema, seizures, brainstem herniation, and death.

   c. Ultimately any formula used for fluid replacement is only a starting point and serves only as guide to clinical resuscitation. Indications for altered fluid resuscitation requirements include inhalation injury, associated trauma, delay in starting resuscitation fluids, extensive depth and surface area burn, deep circumferential burns, high-voltage electrical injury, extensive muscle damage, preexisting medical conditions, and extreme age groups (neonate and infant).

   d. An example of calculating fluid replacement using the *Parkland formula (Baxter formula):*

      - The volume calculated by the resuscitation formula is administered over the first 24 hours following injury. The Parkland formula is

      4 mL of Ringer's lactate × % TBSA burn × weight in kg = 24-hour fluid-volume

      - Calculations are based on the time of injury, not the time of the patient's arrival at the hospital.
      - One half of the calculated volume is given over the first 8 hours post-burn, and the remainder is given over the next 16 hours. The rationale for administering proportionately more fluid during the first 8 hours post-burn is to compensate for the plasma loss; because most of the loss is resolved within 12 hours, the subsequent 16 hours generally call for less fluid.

   e. *Weigh* the patient on admission to permit accurate determination of fluid replacement needs.

   f. *Calculate* basal fluid needs for normal daily maintenance requirements (Table 9-24). Recommended maintenance fluid is 5% dextrose in ½ normal saline.

   g. *Calculate* fluid replacement based on burn size (Table 9-25).

TABLE 9-24
Calculation of Maintenance Fluids in Children Based on Child's Body Weight

Child's Weight		Daily Fluid Requirements
Up to 10 kg		100 mL/kg/24 h
11 to 20 kg		1000 mL for the first 10 kg
	plus	50 mL/kg for each kg over 10 kg
21 to 30 kg		1500 mL for the first 20 kg
	plus	25 mL/kg for each kg over 20 kg
31 to 40 kg		1750 mL for the first 30 kg
	plus	10 mL/kg for each kg over 30 kg

TABLE 9-25
Example of Calculating Fluid Resuscitation in Children

Parkland Burn Resuscitation Formula
First 24 Hours Postburn

4 mL Ringers Lactate* × weight in kg × % burn surface area

Give half of the calculated amount in the first 8 h postburn and the remaining amount over the next 16 h; plus daily maintenance volume as needed to maintain appropriate urine output.

Example: 10 kg child with 50% burn surface area:

4 mL × 10 kg × 50% burn surface area = 2000 mL RL* over 24 h

First	8 hours = 1000 mL RL
Second	8 hours = 500 mL RL
Third	8 hours = 500 mL RL

Second 24 Hours Postburn

Albumin 25%	0.1mL × weight in kg × % burn surface area
D5 W†	1mL × weight in kg × % burn surface area Plus daily maintenance volume as needed to maintain appropriate urine output

*Titrate RL and D5RL based on serum glucose levels.
†D51/4NS for infants and small children.

h. An example of calculating fluid replacement using the *Shriners Hospital Galveston formula:*

- The volume calculated by the resuscitation formula is administered during the first 24 hours following injury.
- Twenty-four-hour calculations are based on the time of injury, not the time of the patient's arrival at the hospital.
- The volume requirements are calculated based on m^2 body surface area (BSA) and m^2 body surface area burned (TBSA). Body surface area (m^2) is calculated from height and weight values using a standard nomogram.
- The formula calculates fluid for the first 24 hours after injury:

$$5000\ \text{mL/m}^2\ \text{BSA burn} + 2000\ \text{mL/m}^2\ \text{BSA} = \text{total fluid resuscitation}$$

The fluid administered is Ringer's lactate or 5% dextrose in Ringer's lactate. Colloids may be given later in the first 24 hours to raise plasma volume if needed.

3. **Monitoring fluid resuscitation**
   a. *Adequate resuscitation* is reflected by the following:
      - Normal mentation: Mental clarity can be assessed with the GCS; also recognition of parent is expected.
      - Stable vital signs: Assessment of vital signs can be challenging in the younger population of patients but should include the following parameters: pulse rate, blood pressure, distal extremity color, capillary refill, body temperature, serum base deficit, and oxygen saturations.
      - Adequate urine output: 1 mL/kg hourly in children who weigh less than 30 kg and 30 to 50 mL hourly for children who weigh more than 30 kg (Warden, 2002). Using urine output as an indirect measurement of cardiac output has been found to be a generally reliable guide to adequacy of resuscitation, as maintenance of renal blood flow can be taken to reflect adequate perfusion to other organs as well (Morehouse, 1992).
   b. Place an *indwelling bladder catheter* for accurate urinary output measurements and document hourly for all age groups. Begin at the rate calculated for burn resuscitation and adjust as necessary to achieve adequate urine output.
   c. *During resuscitation,* fluid rates are adjusted hourly ($^1/_2$ hourly in infants) to achieve appropriate urine output.
   d. A *decreased urine output* is most frequently the result of inadequate fluid administration, but always check the Foley catheter for obstruction.
   e. *Serum glucose:* Monitor serum glucose levels every 1 to 2 hours.
      - Infants are at risk for hypoglycemia because of limited glycogen reserves that may become rapidly depleted when stressed, as in trauma (or sepsis) (Hazinski, 1999). In the early post-burn period, blood glucose levels may drop rapidly rather than increase as with older children or adults.
      - Titrating Ringer's lactate and D5 Ringer's lactate together during the first 24 hours post-burn may be necessary to avoid either hypoglycemia or hyperglycemia.
   f. *Assess and treat glycosuria* because it will be difficult to assess accurately resuscitation and perfusion if an osmotic diuresis occurs, which further depletes the intravascular volume (Warden, 2002).
   g. *Serum and urine electrolytes* should be within normal range, and there should be absence of metabolic acidosis. Low hemoglobin and hematocrit levels on admission may signal the need for further evaluation.
   h. *Cool and clammy extremities,* delayed capillary refill, and mental numbness are clinical warning signs of shock.
   i. Remember, *small changes in vital signs* may reflect much greater hemodynamic changes in the child compared with the adult.
4. **Consequences of inadequate fluid resuscitation**
   a. *Delayed treatment* or too little resuscitation volume can cause acute renal necrosis, acute renal failure, conversion of partial-thickness wound to full-thickness wound, or formation of stress ulcers in the GI tract.
   b. *Over-resuscitation* can cause pulmonary edema and related complications, excessive wound edema, and compartment syndrome.
5. **Fluid management after resuscitation (second 24 hours post-burn)**
   a. As *capillary integrity* is restored, the plasma volume deficit is replaced with colloid-containing fluids in an attempt to replace the protein loss, restore plasma oncotic pressure, and minimize the volume requirements during the second 24 hours post-burn.

b. *Post-resuscitation urine output* and replacement of evaporative water loss are maintained by infusion of 5% dextrose in ½ normal saline based on daily basal fluid requirements (see Table 9-24).
c. *Very young children,* especially infants, are more sensitive to acute changes in serum sodium concentrations; the use of hypotonic solutions may lead to severe hyponatremia.
d. *Rapid shifts in serum sodium concentrations* may produce cerebral edema, intracranial bleeding, or seizures (Hazinski, 1999).
e. Thus the *use of salt-containing solutions* in combination with 5% dextrose (i.e., D5 ½ NS, D5 ¼ NS) should be used in infants and very young children.

6. **Fluid management after 48 hours:** Following the initial 48 hours, there is a gradual reabsorption of edema fluid, and diuresis occurs. Fluid administration during this time is based on need using electrolyte status and nutritional requirements. Intake and output and daily weights are closely monitored to help maintain fluid and electrolyte balance during this post-burn period.

G. Wound Assessment and Care

The potential for wound infection is one of the major problems in patients who sustain a thermal injury. The scope and importance of wound care and daily wound assessment cannot be overemphasized. Particular attention is aimed at methods and techniques to prevent infection, facilitate wound healing, promote patient comfort, maintain optimal function, and minimize deformities. Assessment and documentation of wound appearance are as much a part of wound care as the dressing change itself. Any signs of infection, such as odor, drainage, and cellulitis, must be noted so as to care appropriately for the patient. Wound care begins in the emergent phase and continues through the acute and rehabilitative phases. It is performed on admission to the burn center and subsequently performed twice daily.

1. **Wound cleansing**
   a. The *burn wound* is cleansed by performing hydrotherapy, also known as "tanking" or "tubbing." Various cleansing agents can be used, including diluted chlorhexidine gluconate, diluted povidone-iodine, and for smaller wounds a nonperfumed mild soap. Hydrotherapy can take different forms, depending on the child's age, condition, and extent of burn.
      - Spray hydrotherapy is the use of a showerhead to allow water to run intermittently or continuously over the burn wounds. The spray loosens and softens eschar (burn-injured tissue), aids in debridement, and rinses extraneous material from the wounds. It also helps prevent cross contamination of wounds. Spray hydrotherapy is commonly done on patients with more extensive wounds or limited mobility (Carrougher, 1998).
      - Immersion hydrotherapy can be used for patients with smaller burns in a less acute stage of injury. Soaking, again, can aid in debridement of loose eschar, removal of adherent dressings, and assisting patients in participation in range-of-motion exercises (Carrougher, 1998).
      - Showering can be used for older children who are ambulatory and able to participate more fully in their own wound care. Encouraging the child to help remove dressings can often help in decreasing pain and anxiety.
      - If the patient's condition is critical and these procedures cannot be performed, the wounds must be cleaned by bed bath. The utmost care must be taken in this circumstance so as not to cross contaminate wounds.

   b. Generally, *hydrotherapy* should be limited to 20 to 30 minutes for patients with acute burns to avoid heat loss, pain, and stress. There is also the potential for excessive sodium loss through the burn wound (water is hypotonic) (Carrougher, 1998).

2. **Wound debridement**
   a. *Debridement* involves the removal of necrotic tissue, foreign material, and cellular debris from the wound bed, which may be accomplished during hydrotherapy, as part of routine dressing changes, or during surgical procedures. The three types of debridement of the wound are mechanical, chemical, and surgical debridement.
      - Mechanical debridement is the removal of burn eschar as fragments of the necrotic tissue are sloughed naturally during the wound healing process. This is accomplished by cleaning the wound with coarse mesh gauze, the application and removal of gauze dressings, hydrotherapy, irrigation, and the use of scissors and forceps to gently lift and trim loose necrotic tissue. Wet to dry dressings may also be used to debride exudative wounds; however, every effort must be made to avoid injury to newly formed tissue when using this method.
      - Chemical or enzymatic debridement is accomplished by the use of commercially made topical preparations that cause rapid lysis of necrotic tissue. Enzymatic debridement agents should be applied only within the area of the wound and should be discontinued once the eschar has been removed and granulation tissue is present. Comparatively, because of the natural process of infection, bacteria and inflammation hasten the separation of devitalized tissue. However, infection also destroys epidermal appendages and in effect deepens the wound. Eschar generally starts to separate from the wound bed 2 to 3 weeks following injury as a result of the natural proteolytic action of enzymes released from subeschar bacteria and the patient's leukocytes.
      - Surgical debridement is accomplished by excision of the burn wound. Two methods of surgical debridement are tangential and full-thickness excision.
         - *Tangential excision* involves the shaving away of thin layers of eschar until the viable dermal tissues are reached.
         - *Full-thickness excision* involves the removal of nonviable tissue at the level of viable tissue, usually down to subcutaneous fat or fascia.
3. **Topical preparations for burn wounds**
   a. The moist, protein-rich avascular eschar provides an excellent culture medium for microorganisms. Within 1 week after the injury, bacteria are consistently present on any remaining eschar. Additionally, the thermal thrombosis that renders the eschar avascular prevents easy penetration by parenteral antibiotics and impedes delivery of the cellular components of the host defense system to the microorganisms. Consequently, parenteral antibiotics exert little effect on the rapid colonization of the burn wound.
   b. A better understanding of the pathogenesis of burn-wound infection has led to the development of effective topical antimicrobial agents. The development of topical antimicrobials has reduced the use of prophylactic systemic antibiotics in the treatment of burn patients. Topical antimicrobials can temporarily control but not eradicate bacterial growth in necrotic or ischemic tissue, but the potential for invasive burn wound infection in any burn-injured patient remains. Patients with extensive burns in whom timely excision and grafting cannot be accomplished are those in which burn wound infection occurs with the greatest frequency (Sheridan, 2003).

TABLE 9-26
Topical Antimicrobial Agents

Agent	Advantages	Disadvantages
1% Silver sulfadiazene silvadene, SSD, thermazene	Broad spectrum antimicrobial activity Painless upon application Readily available Minimal sensitivity May be used with open or closed dressing technique Most commonly used topical agent Moderate eschar penetration	Transient leukopenia
Mafenide acetate cream (sulfamylon)	Penetrates through burn eschar and cartilage Effective gram-negative coverage	Painful upon application May cause metabolic acidosis (alternating sulfamylon and silvadene application may diminish this effect)
Bacitracin	Effective against gram-positive organisms Low toxicity	Limited effect against gram-negative organisms Limited ability to penetrate eschar
0.5% silver nitrate solution	Excellent antibacterial spectrum	Requires dressing Messy May cause electrolyte imbalances (hyponatremia and hypochloremia)

c. Factors affecting the choice of an antimicrobial agent include the depth, extent, and location of the burn; wound culture results; and current status of the wound (i.e., eschar intact, autograft).

d. Advantages and disadvantages of specific topical agents are listed in Table 9-26.

4. **Special care areas**

a. The skin around the eye is very delicate; so this area should be washed gently and debridement avoided. Any eschar in this area should be allowed to remain until it separates naturally. To decrease the risk of chemical conjunctivitis, the nurse must avoid any cleansing agent used on the face from entering the eye. Similarly, if silver sulfadiazine is used on the face, the eye area should be avoided.

b. Injury to the nose can lead to tissue and cartilage loss; so cleansing should be gentle and debridement avoided, leaving eschar to separate naturally. Mafenide acetate cream is often used on deep burns of the nose because of the ability to penetrate the underlying cartilage. The patient with nasogastric or nasotracheal tubes should be closely monitored for pressure necrosis, and nasal tubes should be supported or padded to avoid pressure.

c. The lips are very delicate and should be gently washed with water or normal saline-soaked gauze. Topical antimicrobial ointments such as Bacitracin are used, rather than creams, and are reapplied as needed to prevent the lips from drying and cracking.

d. Pressure on the ears should be avoided to prevent pressure necrosis and chondritis. Pillows are avoided in patients with burns to the ears for this reason. Also, cloth ties used to secure endotracheal or nasogastric tubes should be positioned to prevent contact with the ear, thus avoiding pressure necrosis and chondritis. The topical of choice for deep burns to the nose is mafenide acetate.

e. To avoid the development of web-space contractures, fingers and toes are wrapped separately with individual gauze wraps.

f. Thorough cleansing of the perineum is required because of the increased risk of infection. The perineum should be cleansed and topical agents reapplied after urination or defecation.

g. Dressings over exposed muscle, tendon, or bone must be kept moist to prevent desiccation. This can be accomplished by using normal saline or an antimicrobial solution and rewetting the dressing every 4 hours. Alternatively, a moisture retentive dressing, such as Second Skin, may be used.

5. **Early burn wound excision:** Surgical excision of the eschar covering the burn wound begins as soon as the injured child has completed fluid resuscitation and is hemodynamically stable (Merz et al., 2003). Early burn wound excision and skin grafting have been shown to contribute to reduced morbidity and mortality in the burn patient by reducing the incidence of infection and sepsis, promoting more rapid healing and reducing scarring (Gordon and Marvin, 2002; Sheridan, 2003). Some burn centers serially excise a maximum of 20% TBSA during each operation, whereas other burn centers excise the complete wound during the initial operation (Merz et al., 2003; Muller, 2002).

6. **Temporary wound coverage:** Temporary wound closure is often necessary in children who are severely burned and have minimal donor sites. Temporary wound closure is also necessary in children who are delayed admissions and have heavily colonized burn wound eschar. The benefits of temporary coverage include the provision of a barrier to infection; a decrease in the loss of fluid, electrolytes, and protein through the wound; and a decrease in the child's pain. Adherence of biological or synthetic dressings also indicates that wound conditions are favorable for autografting. These dressings are also sometimes used to cover partial-thickness burns to enhance healing and reduce pain (Sheridan, 2003).

a. *Homograft or allograft* is a biological dressing and is a skin graft from another human (i.e., cadaver skin). These grafts "take," meaning that they become vascularized by anastomosis of the blood vessels between the wound and the biological graft. Eventually, usually in 1 to 3 weeks, rejection occurs, and ultimately the homograft is removed and the wound is covered with autograft.

b. *Heterograft or xenograft* is a layer of skin from a different species, usually porcine (pig) skin. True vascularization does not occur; however, blood vessels from the wound do grow into the interstices of the biological graft; so when it is removed, easily controlled capillary bleeding occurs.

c. *Synthetic dressings* are a combination of biologic and synthetic materials. One such dressing is Biobrane, which is a biosynthetic dressing composed of a nylon fabric bonded to a semipermeable silicone rubber membrane, with collagen peptides coated to both layers. The silicone rubber membrane helps to prevent fluid loss. The collagen peptides bind with fibrin to provide primary adherence during the first 24 to 48 hours. The nylon provides flexibility and a media for the ingrowth of tissue, providing secondary adherence after 48 hours. In addition to the aforementioned uses for temporary wound dressings, Biobrane is also often used to cover fresh donor sites (Carrougher, 1998).

7. **Autograft:** Permanent wound closure is accomplished with autograft (i.e., a layer of unburned skin removed from the body of the patient). Autograft promotes final wound closure, reduces the amount of scarring, and provides better functional repair.
   a. *Split-thickness autograft* comprises the epidermis and a partial layer of the dermis and is harvested using a dermatome to obtain uniform thickness. Thinner grafts are used on patients with extensive burns to allow for more rapid reharvesting of donor sites.
   b. *Full-thickness graft* is one in which a segment of full dermis and epidermis in transplanted. Primary closure of this site must be done by suture repair or a split-thickness graft. For this reason the use of full-thickness grafts is limited to the repair of small burns.
   c. *Sheet grafts* are used, whenever possible, when the wound location has cosmetic or functional importance (i.e. face, neck, hands, feet).
   d. *Meshed autograft* is indicated for patients with extensive burns because the meshing allows for the maximum coverage of wounds while using limited donor sites. Meshed grafts are usually expanded up to four times their normal size but can be meshed up to nine times their size. For example, the expansion ratio of a 2:1 mesh allows coverage of a wound twice the size of the initial donor site. Meshed grafts also allow for blood, plasma, and wound exudate to escape from the wound bed through the interstices, thus preventing interference with graft vascularization. Unfortunately, with meshed graft, the mesh pattern is often visible after healing (Merz et al., 2003).
   e. *Cultured epithelial autograft* (CEA) is a process by which skin is "grown" in a commercial laboratory using the patient's own keratinocytes and fibroblasts. A skin biopsy is taken from an area of unburned skin and the initial 3-inch square epidermal grafts are supplied in approximately 2 to 3 weeks, with additional grafts being subsequently available. The grafts are applied to the excised wound bed, often using a dermal substitute, such as allograft dermis. This method of grafting is expensive and the grafts are often fragile; hence the use of CEA is usually limited to patients with massive burn injuries and minimal available donor site (Sheridan, 2003).
8. **Donor sites:** Donor sites are often selected for cosmetic reasons but may be limited by the extent of the burn wound. After removal of the autograft skin, a newly created partial-thickness wound is established. Donor sites are usually covered with fine mesh gauze or a synthetic wound covering. The dressing is trimmed as it separates from the healing wound until the donor site is completely healed and none of the dressing remains. With proper care, multiple skin grafts can be harvested from the same site; however, the quality of the grafts diminishes with successive harvests. The head is the most common donor site area on a child.
9. **Preventing graft loss:** Postoperatively, grafts are immediately at risk for failure from infection, bleeding, and mechanical forces such as shearing and friction. The surgical dressing must be monitored for bleeding, odor, and drainage. If any of these are present, the dressing may be removed for further inspection because infection or excessive bleeding can disrupt the graft's viability. The nurse must use the utmost care when moving or lifting the patient so as not to disrupt the fragile graft (Gordon and Marvin, 2002). Various methods are used to protect grafts in vulnerable areas; for example, surgeons may place a

synthetic dressing over autograft on a patient's back because of the increased risk of graft loss.

H. Child Abuse Protection Support

1. **Assessment**
   a. All *pediatric burns* should be assessed for the possibility of child abuse or neglect as a contributing factor. Burns fall within a continuum from accidental to intentional. Neglect that contributes to a burn injury must be considered under the child abuse category.
   b. The *initial assessment* includes documenting the characteristics of the wound (see Table 9-19). The assessment also includes documenting caretaker explanations of child's injuries that are improbable or inconsistent, allege self-injury, blame other children, or exhibit an unexplained delay in seeking treatment (12 hours or more).
2. **Reporting**
   a. *Remember* that the purpose of reporting a suspicious injury is to prevent further harm.
   b. *Inform* physicians of observations indicative of abuse or neglect. Provide all assessment data that could potentially indicate abuse or neglect to the hospital social or psychological services, the physicians, and proper authorities.
3. **Therapeutic interventions**
   a. Be up front with the *family* about reporting the injury to officials. The nurse must be honest and nonavoidant.
   b. Allow the *child* to talk about the cause of the burn injury. Let the child set the pace; do not force them to describe the event. Include other health care providers as needed.

ACUTE PHASE: ASSESSMENT AND MANAGEMENT

The **acute phase** (3 days to weeks after the burn) begins with the onset of diuresis of edema fluid mobilized from the interstitial space and continues through closure of the burn wound.

A. Pulmonary Care

1. **Assess and document** breath sounds, chest excursion, respiratory rate, rhythm, and depth every 2 hours. Turn the patient, and encourage the patient to cough and deep breathe every 2 hours. Administer humidified oxygen therapy as ordered. Elevate the head of the bed 30 to 45 degrees if not contraindicated. Monitor oxygen saturation hourly, and evaluate ABGs as needed. Suction secretions every 1 to 2 hours as needed. Assess and document pulmonary function after suctioning.
2. **Monitor** for indications of impending airway obstruction (i.e., stridor, wheezing, rales, hoarseness, tachypnea, use of accessory muscles for breathing, oxygen desaturation, head bobbing, nasal flaring). Prepare for possible endotracheal intubation and mechanical ventilation. Because children have relatively small airways, upper-airway obstruction may occur early and rapidly.
3. **Observe** for erythema or blistering around the nose and mouth, soot in the sputum, or tracheal tissue in pulmonary secretions. During the acute phase, the burn tissue separates from the airway, causing difficult ventilation obstruction due to the debris.

B. Metabolic and Nutritional Support

1. Burn injury is one of the greatest insults the body can sustain, and it requires **caloric and protein levels** exceeding those of any other traumatic injury (Mayes and Gottschlich, 2001). Increased metabolic requirements of severe burns make nutritional management a requirement. Energy expenditure in the pediatric patient may reach 2 $^1/_2$ times normal.
2. Providing **aggressive nutritional support** to patients with major burns to meet energy requirements, replace protein losses, promote wound healing, and strengthen the immune system is a primary goal of burn therapy. Children normally require greater caloric and protein requirements per kilogram of body weight than an adult. For the pediatric burn patient, the nutritional demands required by the hypermetabolic state of the burn injury superimposed on those for growth may result in a compromise in growth with little net weight gain for the duration of the recovery period (Saffle and Hildreth, 2002). Determine nutritional goals by using one of the various formulas for estimating the energy requirements in pediatric burn patients.
3. **Indirect calorimetry** can also be used to calculate the metabolic requirements of the patient. It can also detect significant underfeeding or overfeeding. The respiratory quotient (RQ) is calculated as the ratio of oxygen consumption to CO_2 production (Vo_2/Vco_2). Starvation is indicated by an RQ of 0.7 or less, normal metabolism produces an RQ of 0.75 to 0.90, and overfeeding results in an RQ of 1.0 or greater (Saffle and Hildreth, 2002).
4. For patients with functioning GI tracts, nutrition provided by the **enteral route** is preferred because it supports the absorptive mechanism of the GI tract and preserves mucosal integrity, which may in turn minimize bacterial translocation from the GI tract (Gottschlich and Jenkins, 1998; Saffle and Hildreth, 2002). For young children with less than 15% TBSA or older children with less than 25% TBSA, oral intake is generally acceptable (Mayes and Gottschlich, 2001). Initiating enteral tube feedings within 24 hours after larger injuries can improve nitrogen balance and nutritional support (Saffle and Hildreth, 2002). Children who are unable to consume the required amount of calories to meet their nutritional goals need enteral tube feedings. Assess gastric residuals every 1 to 2 hours with enteral tube feedings, and assess GI tract function every 4 hours. Note the presence of abdominal distention and diarrhea.
   a. *Assess electrolyte status* every 8 to 12 hours. Weigh the patient daily and maintain strict input and output. The patient's weight should remain within 10% of the patient's usual preburn weight (dry weight).
   b. *Administer antacids* or H_2 blockers as ordered. Assess for GI tract bleeding every 2 to 4 hours.
   c. *Avoid any disruptions of feeding.* Enteral feedings can continue preoperatively, intraoperatively, and postoperatively without increased risk of aspiration. By avoiding disruptions in feeding, it is easier to meet the patient's nutritional goals.
   d. *Enteral feeding* can often times cause diarrhea. The causes include high glucose loads, medications, infectious causes, and contaminated feeds. Treatment ranges from medications, fiber-containing enteral feedings, altering the formula, reducing the infusion rate, or holding the feeding for a day or 2 (Gottschlich and Jenkins, 1998; Saffle and Hildreth, 2002). Check stool culture and culture tube feedings at the end of the hang time. Be aware of the warm environment in the patient's room and the hang time of

the tube feeds. Monitor the process, policies, and protocols for nursing practice.

e. *Parenteral nutrition* is necessary for those unable to meet nutritional goals through the enteral route.

C. Burn Wound Sepsis

1. Although **infection** remains the most common cause of morbidity and mortality in burn patients, the infected site is now more often the lung rather than the burn wound. The use of topical antimicrobial agents and early excision of burn wounds, coupled with early wound closure, have reduced the incidence of serious wound infections that cause mortality.
2. The definition of **burn wound sepsis** is microorganisms exceeding 10^5 per gram of tissue with tissue invasion of subjacent unburned tissue.
   a. *Assessment* of the burn wounds for signs of infection is a daily nursing responsibility. The wound should be completely exposed for a clear assessment. The nurse should monitor and document wound condition and care. Early signs of infection that the nurse should monitor for include cellulitis, odor, increase in wound pain, a change in wound exudates or wound appearance, and loss of previously healed skin grafts (Carrougher, 1998). In addition, the nurse should observe for hemorrhagic and vesicular or necrotic areas in the burn wound. Gray, dark brown, or black spots could indicate burn-wound infection (Heggers et al., 2002).
   b. *Obtain* routine cultures of sputum, urine, and the wound; these cultures must be free of contamination from the normal flora and placed in a sterile container with the appropriate media for transport. Document the use of antimicrobials, both topical and systemic, when sending cultures to the laboratory (Heggers et al., 2002).
3. **Infection control strategies** must be in place to decrease the chance of complications associated with sepsis.
   a. *Administer* tetanus toxoid prophylaxis.
   b. Continually *monitor* temperature with Foley thermistor or soft rectal probe. The expected temperature should be 37.2° to 38.3°C (99° to 101°F) rectally.
   c. *Use* aseptic technique during all aspects of patient care. Use sterile technique when performing invasive procedures. Change invasive lines every 3 days and tubing according to unit policy.
   d. Daily *clean* all equipment around the bedside, including the bed, with a germicidal solution.

D. Septic Shock

1. The **definition** of septic shock is the presence of sepsis with hypotension, despite adequate fluid resuscitation, along with the presence of perfusion abnormalities that may include, but are not limited to, lactic acidosis, oliguria, or an acute alteration in mental status. Patients who are receiving inotropic or vasopressor agents may not be hypotensive at the time perfusion abnormalities are measured.
2. **Cardinal signs** of sepsis: Clinical manifestations may vary based on age.
   a. *Hyperventilation*
   b. *Thrombocytopenia* (<50,000 platelets/mm^3)
   c. *Hyperglycemia*
   d. *Disorientation*
   e. *Hypothermia*
   f. *Intolerance of enteral feedings* (high residuals)

g. *Decreased urine output*
h. *Change in sensorium*

3. **Management of septic shock**
   a. *Initial fluid resuscitation* should begin as soon as shock is recognized. Aggressive fluid resuscitation with crystalloids or colloids must start immediately. Fluid boluses of 20 mL/kg over 5 to 10 minutes are given while monitoring for effectiveness (heart rate, urine output, capillary refill, and loss of consciousness). Vasopressors should only be considered for use after the patient has received adequate fluid resuscitation. Within the first 6 hours of resuscitation, maximizing cardiovascular function and oxygen delivery is the goal (Dellinger et al., 2004). Young infants may need to be intubated early because of low functional residual capacity.
   b. *Antibiotic treatment* should be started within the first hour of resuscitation. Appropriate cultures should be obtained before the antimicrobial therapy is initiated. Reassess the antibiotic treatment after 48 to 72 hours to identify a narrower spectrum of therapy.
   c. *Nutritional support* during sepsis is crucial to the patient's outcome. During sepsis, enteral feeding may be complicated by delayed gastric emptying and diarrhea (Chang and Peck, 2001). If enteral feedings are not tolerated, total parenteral nutrition (TPN) may be considered.
   d. The *therapeutic endpoints* are capillary refill of less than 2 seconds, normal pulses with no differential between peripheral and central pulses, warm extremities, urine output greater than or equal to 1 mL/kg per hour, normal mental status, decreased lactate and increased base deficit, and mixed venous oxygen saturation greater than 70%. (Dellinger et al., 2004).

E. Pain and Anxiety Assessment and Management

1. **Pain assessment**
   a. The *burn injury* itself is the source of continuous (background) pain. Loss of the epidermal and partial loss of the dermal layer leave nerve endings exposed, creating a painful wound. This type of pain begins from the time of injury until wound healing.
   b. *Acute pain,* or procedural pain, is associated with the multiple procedures required during the clinical course of the burn injury, such as dressing changes, surgical excision and grafting (donor sites, contracture release), daily physical therapy, and ambulation.
   c. *Pain scales* are useful to quantify painful episodes and to evaluate whether pain management is effective. Table 9-27 contains pain assessment scales suitable for the pediatric burn patient.
2. **Pain management**
   a. If *pain is not well managed* during the initial acute phase, severe anxiety may develop and pain management may be difficult to achieve.
   b. *Background pain* can be managed by oral medications, including acetaminophen, nonsteroidal anti-inflammatory drugs (NSAIDS), or opioids (Marvin, 1998). These medications should be administered on a routine basis to maintain a therapeutic blood level (Senecal, 1999).
   c. *Procedural pain* is generally managed by IV medications, primarily morphine. Patients without venous access may have oral analgesic agents; ibuprofen and acetaminophen with codeine, oral morphine, or a fentanyl oralet may be administered 30 to 60 minutes before a painful procedure (Senecal, 1999). Closely monitor the patient for procedural pain after administration of opioids; when the stimulus is removed, the patient could begin to appear

TABLE 9-27
Recommended Pain Measurement Tools for Burned Patients

Infants and Toddlers	CHEOPS 40 The Observer Pain Scale
Preschoolers	Faces Pain Rating Scale Oucher Pediactric Pain Questionnaire CHEOPS
School-age children	Faces Pain Rating Scale Visual analog Numeric scale Pediactric Pain Questionnaire Procedure Behavior Checklist
Adolescents	Visual analog Numeric scales Adjective scales McGill Questionnaire

Meyer et al: Management of pain and other discomforts in burned patients. In Herndon D, editor. *Total burn care*, ed 2. London, 2002, Saunders.

oversedated. Also monitor acetaminophen blood levels because if levels are high, liver damage can result.

d. After *fluid resuscitation* has been started and the patient is physiologically stable, begin administering small incremental IV doses of opioids for procedural and breakthrough pain.

e. A *PCA (patient-controlled analgesia)* pump is useful for children over the age of 5 years who are able to follow directions (Gordon and Marvin, 2002).

f. *Moderate or deep sedation* may be required to manage the more painful procedures. Combining opioids and benzodiazepines are useful in treating pain; however, meticulous assessment and monitoring of the patient are essential. Medications should be delivered based on the patient's age, weight, and response. Continuous oxygen saturation monitoring is essential and emergency airway equipment must be available at all times. Personnel qualified to monitor sedation must be present at all times (Krauss et al., 2000; Senecal, 1999).

g. During *sepsis*, medication for pain should be minimized to avoid overdosing (Marvin, 1998).

h. When appropriate, *develop strategies* to give the patient some control over painful encounters. Allow the family to help when appropriate.

i. Several *nonpharmacologic adjunctive approaches* to pain management work well for the pediatric burn patient, including distraction, imagery, relaxation, music, hypnosis, and positive reinforcement (Senecal, 1999).

3. Fear assessment

a. The *psychological response* of fear and anxiety is caused by multiple factors, including fear of the unknown; separation from parents, family, and friends for extended periods; multiple invasive procedures during hospitalization; inability to communicate with patients receiving mechanical ventilation and chemical paralyzation; altered sleep patterns and increased activities during the day and night; unfamiliar surroundings, equipment, and people; and pain. Anxiety may also develop as a result of the traumatic nature of the burn injury.

   b. The *"fear thermometer"* (Silverman anad Kurtines, 1996) is a tool to assess anxiety in the pediatric population. The following script is useful when working with the patient: When you are having your skin cleaned in the bath, how ________ (e.g., anxious, afraid, frightened, nervous) are you feeling? (Robert, 2000).

4. **Interventions to relieve anxiety**
   a. *Anxiolytics* are usually a helpful adjunct to opioids to reduce anxiety associated with a procedure. The most common medication is benzodiazipine.
      - Lorazepam: IV or PO dose is 0.03 mg/kg/dose every 4 hours
      - Taper lorazepam dose for patients taking a benzodiazipine for more than 5 days.
      - Reduce dose by 50% every second day (Robert, 2000).

   b. *Reduce the patient's anxiety level* by explaining procedures and talking to the patient while performing nursing interventions.
   c. *Allow frequent visiting* for families. Encourage the family to bring items from home to remind the child of family life before the injury. Organize care into routines similar to home (i.e., a time to sleep, eat, play, dressing changes, visitors).
5. **Itch assessment:** The severe itching of burn scars and wounds is another symptom that must be addressed and managed. Scratching the wounds leads to breakdown in the skin and, potentially, infection. The nurse may use an assessment tool such as the 1–10 Visual Analog Scale (Field et al., 2000) or the Itch Man Scale to rate the intensity of itching (Meyer et al., 2002).
6. **Itch management**
   a. *Dry, scaly healed skin* is more susceptible to itch. Skin-moistening shampoos should be used daily, followed by moisturizing lotion applied three to four times a day to healed skin.
   b. *Medications* that can be used for treatment include diphenhydramine 1.25 mg/kg every 6 hours, hydroxyzine 0.5 mg/kg every 6 hours, and cyproheptadine 0.1 mg/kg every 6 hours. Each medication would be added to the treatment regimen in this order until the itch is controlled (Meyer et al., 2002).

F. Pressure-Sore Prevention Strategies

1. Many **risk factors** are unique to the burn patient that contribute to an increased risk of pressure-sore development.
   a. The initial hypovolemic and burn shock episode shunts blood away from the skin and to the vital organs.
   b. As fluid resuscitation is delivered, massive edema begins to develop in both burned and unburned body areas. The weight of the extremities can be profound at this stage of edema formation.
   c. Fluids "weep" from the burn wounds, providing a constantly moist environment for burned and unburned skin.
   d. Septic shock episodes may occur periodically during the post-burn course, which will shunt blood away from the skin.
   e. The larger the burn wound, the more repeated trips to the operating room, the longer the cumulative anesthesia time, and the cumulative number of postoperative immobilization days.
   f. The risk of pressure-sore development increases each time Ace wraps or splints are applied to burned extremities.
   g. The increased metabolic rate, caused by the burn injury, can create rapid nutritional deficiencies.

h. Management of pain and anxiety is a balancing act. The patient with pain and anxiety will attempt not to move in an effort to reduce the painful stimuli. However, if too much medication is given, the patient will lose the natural tendency to move or change positions. Background pain must be managed, allowing for natural movement by the patient.

2. The heightened awareness of the increased risk of pressure sores in the burn patient population is important because prevention strategies must be implemented on the day of admission and continued until discharge in order for prevention to be successful. The most current prevention strategies are listed in the *Guideline for Prevention and Management of Pressure Ulcers.*

G. Physical and Occupational Therapy

1. The initiation of a **rehabilitation program** is crucial for the patient sustaining a burn injury. The aim of a rehabilitation program is to restore function and prevent deformities (Serghiou et al., 2002; Ward, 1998).
2. **Positioning** focuses on the prevention of contractures and deformity development. The nurse working with the burn therapist must pay attention to the depth and location of burns and appropriately position the head, extremities, and body so that wound healing is promoted.
3. **Splinting** aids in achieving optimal positioning while protecting joints with deep burns and fresh skin grafts. The nurse must be aware of the splints, assess for proper placement, and recognize potential problems associated with the splinting, such as pressure sores.
4. The **goals of exercise** are to reduce edema, maintain functional joint motion, stretch scar tissue, and return the patient to the optimal level of function (Serghiou et al., 2002). Initially, postoperative exercise must not be done to grafted areas. However, as soon as possible, the exercises must begin. It may take only 1 to 4 days for a burn scar contracture to develop (Ward, 1998). Active exercises can start on admission and continue throughout the rehabilitation continuum of care. Passive exercises are done with patients who are not able to complete active exercises at that time. Gentle, slow stretching results in blanching of the burn scar.
5. **Early ambulation and performance of age-appropriate activities of daily living** (ADLs) are crucial in the recovery process of the patient with a burn injury and aid in producing optimal functional outcomes.

H. Social and Cultural Assessment and Care

1. Several factors complicate the **psychosocial sequelae** of the burn-injured child. Circumstances surrounding the accident generate feelings of guilt, helplessness, despair, and anger from families. Disfigurement is frequently associated with a burn injury, and severe, lengthy episodes of pain are common. Risks of numerous medical and surgical complications increase during hospitalization. Because of the rollercoaster ride of good days and bad days, progress is made very slowly. Hospitalizations are lengthy, and even longer periods of rehabilitation follow discharge. Burn care may precipitate a financial disaster for the family. Because burn care requires a team approach, there are many people, procedures, and tasks the child must become familiar with each day.
2. Fear of **body image** changes: Fear of not being accepted by their friends and of being different and wondering how people in general will treat them is common in burn patients. The fear usually occurs as the time for discharge approaches. Planning for discharge begins on admission to the ICU. Encourage burn-injured

patients to vent their concerns. Psychological counseling for patient and family is helpful. School reentry programs facilitate a successful return to school.

3. **Anger, depression, and withdrawal** are common sequelae of burn injury and require intervention through education and psychological support. The goal is to assist the child in developing positive coping skills.
4. **Financial concerns** are real because the expense of burn care is enormous. Provide for early social work involvement to facilitate financial assistance for the family if needed.

I. Patient and Family Education

1. Provide the patient and family with frequent opportunities for **education** about the burn injury and care regimens required for optimal recovery. Support the family to be involved in ADLs, and develop a partnership with the parents. Develop a trusting relationship with the patient and family. Provide honest but positive information.
2. Promote **restful periods** for the patient during the day and night, and promote a quiet environment.
3. The **rehabilitative phase** begins on admission to the ICU and comprises prevention of functional deficits and psychosocial support. As wounds heal, correction of functional deficits begins with ongoing psychosocial support.

Disaster Preparedness

Nancy Blake

In the past decade, terrorism has unfortunately become an increasingly real threat to the citizens of the United States. *Terrorism* by definition is the unlawful use of force or violence against persons or property to intimidate civilians or to coerce a government or a civilian population in the furtherance of political and social objectives (www.bioterrorism.slv-edu, 2002). Because the scale of a terrorist attack can be often widespread, this type of disaster can be overwhelming to a nation's health care system.

A report to the Congressional Committee from the United States General Accounting Office (GAO) regarding hospital preparedness for a bioterrorist incident was published in August 2003. This report stated that although most urban hospitals nationwide reported participating in basic planning and coordination of activities for bioterrorism response, they did not have the medical equipment, especially ventilators, needed to handle the number of patients who would likely require medical attention as the result of a bioterrorism incident. Four of five hospitals reported having a written emergency response plan that addresses bioterrorism; however, many hospitals lacked key resources, such as laboratories. Many reported being involved in state or local planning and had conducted some training of staff members; however, few had actually conducted drills to prepare for a bioterrorist attack. Most hospitals admitted a lack of preparedness, particularly in terms of having adequate resources to handle a large influx of patients (GAO Report, 2003).

PEDIATRIC PREPAREDNESS

1. Besides being generally unprepared to deal with a large-scale attack, most hospitals are specifically unprepared to care for pediatric patients. State and

federal plans historically have not included provisions for pediatric patients, although that is changing. Children have unique needs for which adult models cannot be adapted easily. In February 2003, a National Consensus Conference was convened to address pediatric preparedness for disasters and terrorism. The conference was funded by grants from the Agency for Healthcare Research and Quality (AHRQ) and the Emergency Medical Services for Children Program (EMSC) of the Maternal Child Health Bureau and sponsored by the Program for Pediatric Preparedness of the National Center for Disaster Preparedness, Mailman School of Public Health, Columbia University, the Children's Health Fund, and the Children's Hospital at Montefiore (Pediatric Disaster Consensus Conference, 2003).

2. Several special pediatric considerations in terrorism and disaster preparedness were identified:
   a. Children are more vulnerable to chemical agents that are absorbed through the skin or inhaled.
   b. Children are especially susceptible to dehydration and shock from a biological attack.
   c. Children cannot be decontaminated in adult decontamination units.
   d. Children require different dosages, antibiotics, and antidotes to many agents.
   e. Children are more susceptible to the effects of radiation exposure and require responses that are different from those required by adults.
   f. Because they have unique psychosocial vulnerabilities, children require special management plans in the event of mass casualties and evacuation.
   g. Emergency responders, medical professionals, and children's health care institutions require special expertise and training to ensure optimal care of those exposed to chemical, biological, or nuclear agents.
   h. Children's developmental ability and cognitive levels may impede their ability to escape danger.
   i. Emergency medical services (EMS) and medical and hospital staff may not have pediatric training, equipment, or facilities (Pediatric Disaster Consensus Conference, 2003).
3. Before the Pediatric Disaster Consensus Conference, a group was commissioned by the Secretary of Health and Human Services, National Advisory Committee on Children and Terrorism, that made recommendations related to the needs of children in a disaster. That group was commissioned to make recommendations regarding the following:
   a. The preparedness of the health care system to respond to terrorism as it relates to children.
   b. Changes to the health care and EMS protocols necessary to meet the special needs of children.
   c. Changes, if necessary, to the National Strategic Stockpile under Section 121 of the Public Health Security and Bioterrorism Preparedness and Response Act of 2002 to meet the emergency health security of children (National Advisory Committee, 2003).
4. The following recommendations were made by the National Advisory Committee on Children and Terrorism:
   a. All planning and training mechanisms must specifically include elements that focus on the needs of infants, children, and adolescents.
   b. Direct attention will be addressed to settings where children normally gather.
   c. Coordination and integration response efforts must be made at all levels of government.
   d. In event of an incident, priority will be given to returning children to their normal routine (National Advisory Committee, 2003).

5. The needs of pediatric patients are now being addressed at many levels by many government agencies, including the National Center for Disaster Preparedness and the Emergency Medical Services for Children Program.

TYPES OF TERRORISM

Terrorism exists in a variety of forms:

- Violence, explosions, and hijackings
- Nuclear or radiologic attacks
- Chemical attacks
- Biological attacks

A. Violence, Explosions, and Hijackings

1. The United States has an **organized trauma system** to deal with small-scale violence or explosions but is not prepared for large-scale attacks. Given the current political climate, it is important that we be prepared to deal with large-scale emergencies. In the past, attacks within the United States, including the Oklahoma City bombing, the Columbine High School shootings, and the shootings at the Jewish Community Center in Granada Hills, California, have overwhelmed emergency departments and pediatric critical care centers.
2. **Mass casualty incidents (MCIs)** require that patients be assessed and triaged quickly but comprehensively. An MCI is characterized by an influx of large numbers of casualties that exceed the capabilities of local emergency and medical personnel. Nurses perform the primary and secondary survey, as with any other trauma patient. Tables 9-28 and 9-29 list the assessment components of the pediatric trauma patient.
3. As patients go through triage, they are sent to the appropriate level of care. The **JUMPStart triage model** is a model that can be used to triage pediatric patients during mass casualty events. (More information about this triage model can be obtained by visiting www.jumpstarttriage.com.)
4. In **preparing for MCIs,** it is important to have the appropriate size and amount of emergency medication, supplies, and equipment. Many new documents related to mass casualty incidents in pediatrics have been published, but much more work needs to be done to handle large-scale disasters involving pediatric patients. One crucial step is to ensure that pediatric patients can be placed in a pediatric intensive care unit (PICU) as quickly as possible and that the PICU nurses know how to treat victims of weapons of mass destruction.
5. **Trauma injuries** would result from some type of blast injury, given that explosions and bombings are often the weapons of choice for terrorists. Such injuries can result from either primary or secondary blasts.
   a. *Primary blast injuries* are the result of sudden changes in atmospheric pressure caused by an explosion. The following are examples of primary blast injuries:
      - Ear injuries (e.g., perforated eardrums)
      - Pulmonary injuries, including hemorrhagic contusion and hemopneumothorax
      - Gastrointestinal hemorrhage, bowel perforation or rupture

   b. *Secondary blast injury* occurs when victims are struck by flying objects and debris.
   c. *Tertiary blast injuries* occur when the body is hurled through the air and struck by another object.

TABLE 9-28
Primary Survey of the Pediatric Trauma Patient

Component	Actions
Airway	Assess for patency; look for loose teeth, vomitus, or other obstruction; note position of head. Suspect cervical spine injury with multiple trauma; maintain neutral alignment during assessment; evaluate effectiveness of cervical collar, cervical immobilization device, or other equipment used to immobilize the spine. Open cervical collar to evaluate neck for jugular vein distention and tracheal deviation.
Breathing	Auscultate breath sounds in the axillae for presence and equality. Assess chest for contusions, penetrating wounds, abrasions, or paradoxic movement.
Circulation	Assess apical pulse for rate, rhythm, and quality; compare apical and peripheral pulses for quality and equality. Evaluate capillary refill; normal is less than 2 seconds. Check skin color and temperature. Assess level of consciousness; check for orientation to person, place, and time in the older child.
Disability	In a younger child, assess alertness, ability to interact with environment, and ability to follow commands. Is the child easily consoled and interested in the environment? Does the child recognize a familiar object and respond when you speak to him or her? Check pupils for size, shape, reactivity, and equality. Note open wounds or uncontrolled bleeding.
Expose	Remove clothing to allow visual inspection of entire body.

B. Nuclear/Radiologic Attacks

1. The threat of **nuclear attack** was more of an issue before the end of the Cold War. Radiation accidents/attacks can arise from problems with nuclear reactors, industrial sources, and medical sources. It is important that clinicians understand how such an attack can occur and how to treat patients affected by it. Medical consequences depend on the type of device used. A radiologic or nuclear attack occurs in one of five ways:
   a. *Simple radiological device (SRD):* A deliberate act of spreading radioactive material without the use of an explosive device, such as putting a high-activity radioactive isotope in a public place, exposing numerous individuals to various levels of radiation.
   b. *Radiologic dispersal device (RDD):* A type of device formed by combining an explosive agent with radioactive materials that might have been stolen. The initial explosion kills or injures those closest to the bomb, and radioactive substances remain to expose and contaminate survivors and possibly emergency responders.
   c. *Nuclear reactor sabotage:* This type of incident is uncommon because of sophisticated shielding but could occur with an attack on a nuclear reactor.
   d. *Improvised nuclear device (IND):* An IND is a device designed to cause a nuclear detonation; it is a radiologic dispersal device. Because it is difficult to detonate such a weapon correctly, this type of incident is uncommon; a high level of sophistication is required to engineer it, but a stolen device would generate high levels of radiation.
   e. *Nuclear weapon* (American College of Radiology, 2002)

TABLE 9-29
Secondary Survey of the Pediatric Trauma Patient

Component	Actions
Head, eye, ear, nose	Assess scalp for lacerations or open wounds; palpate for stepoff defects, depressions, hematomas, and pain. Reassess pupils for size, reactivity, equality, and extraocular movements; ask the child if he or she can see. Assess ears and nose for rhinorrhea or otorrhea. Observe for racoon eyes (bruising around the eyes) or Battle's sign (bruising over the mastoid process). Palpate forehead, orbits, maxilla, and mandible for crepitus, deformities, stepoff defect, pain, and stability; evaluate malocclusion by asking child to open and close mouth; note open wounds. Inspect for loose, broken, or chipped teeth as well as oral lacerations. Check orthodontic appliances for stability. Evaluate facial symmetry by asking child to smile, grimace, and open and close mouth. Do not remove impaled objects or foreign objects.
Neck	Open cervical collar and reassess anterior neck for jugular vein distention and tracheal deviation; note bruising, edema, open wounds, pain, and crepitus. Check for hoarseness or changes in voice by asking child to speak.
Chest	Obtain respiratory rate; reassess breath sounds in anterior lobes for equality. Palpate chest wall and sternum for pain, tenderness, and crepitus. Observe inspiration and expiration for symmetry or paradoxic movement; note use of accessory muscles. Reasses apical heart rate for rate, rhythm, and clarity.
Abdomen/pelvis/ genitourinary	Observe abdomen for bruising and distention; auscultate bowel sounds briefly in all four quadrants; palpate abdomen gently for tenderness; assess pelvis for tenderness and stability. Palpate bladder for distention and tenderness; check urinary meatus for signs of injury or bleeding; note priapism and genital trauma such as lacerations or foreign body. Have rectal sphincter tone assessed, usually by physician.
Musculoskeletal	Assess extremities for deformities, swelling, lacerations, or other injuries. Palpate distal pulses for equality, rate, and rhythm; compare to central pulses. Ask child to wiggle toes and fingers; evaluate strength through hand grips and foot flexion/extension.
Back	Logroll as a unit to inspect back; maintain spinal alignment during examination; observe for bruising and open wounds; palpate each vertebral body for tenderness, pain, deformity, and stability; assess flank area for bruising and tenderness.

2. There are **two categories of radiation incidents:**
   - **a.** *External exposure,* which is irradiation from a source that is either distant or close to the body. External irradiation can be divided into *whole-body* exposure or *local* exposure.
   - **b.** *Contamination,* defined as unwanted radioactive material in or on the body (ACR, 2002).
3. **Response is based on the type of incident.** Most external exposures result in irradiation of the victim. A person exposed to external radiation does not become

radioactive and poses no hazard to nearby individuals. Once the victim is removed from the source of radiation, the irradiation ceases.

4. **Contamination incidents** require a different approach. Caregivers and support personnel must be careful not to spread the contamination to uncontaminated parts of the victim's body, to themselves, or to the surrounding area. Internal contamination can result from inhalation, ingestion, direct absorption through the skin, or penetration of radioactive materials through open wounds (Yu, 2003). Treatment of serious or significant medical conditions should always take precedence over radiologic assessment or decontamination of the patient.
5. **Treatment** of patients of a radiologic attack involve the following priorities:
    a. *Treat and stabilize life-threatening injuries.* A radiologic assessment should be performed by an individual with radiologic health training. Radiologic measurements can be done using a Geiger counter.
    b. *Prevent and minimize internal contamination.* Time is critical to prevent radioactive uptake. Potassium iodide (KI) is administered to prevent radioiodine from accumulating in the thyroid gland. The pediatric dose of KI is listed in Table 9-30. KI should be given within 2 hours of contamination.
    c. *Assess internal contamination and decontamination.* Patients who are contaminated but not seriously injured should be decontaminated before they are treated.
    d. *Contain contamination and decontamination.*
    e. *Minimize external contamination to medical personnel.* Staff should wear personal protective clothing and, if the area is highly contaminated, respirators should be worn.
    f. *Assess internal contamination* (concurrent with the preceding).
    g. *Assess local radiation injuries and burns and flush if they are contaminated.*
    h. *Follow-up* on patients with significant whole-body irradiation or internal contamination.
    i. *Counsel* the patient and his or her family about the potential for long-term risks and effects (Linnemann, 2001).

C. Chemical Attacks

1. **Chemical warfare agents** are hazardous chemicals that have been designed for use by the military to irritate, incapacitate, injure, or kill during wartime (Los Angeles County, 2003). The most recent attacks were the Sarin gas attacks in Japan in the mid 1990s in which few deaths resulted, but the influx of contaminated patients to medical facilities was overwhelming to the medical

TABLE 9-30
Guidelines for KI Dose Administration

Patient/Age	Exposure, GY (RAD)	KI Dose* (MG)
>40 years of age	>5 (500)	130
18-40 years of age	0.1 (10)	130
12-17 years of age	0.05 (5)	65
4-11 years of age	0.05 (5)	65
1 month-3 years of age	0.05 (5)	32
Birth-1 month of age	0.05 (5)	16
Pregnant or lactating women	0.05 (5)	130

This table was created from recommendations developed at the Consensus Conference and in part is based on reviewed reference materials from the American Academy of Pediatrics, Centers for Disease Control, and FDA.
*Children/adolescents weighing more than 70 kg should receive the adult dose (130 mg).

system. Chemical attacks may be combined with explosions and blast attacks. These are sometimes called "dirty bombs." To have chemical contamination associated with explosions, victims will be in close proximity of the explosion or blast attack.

2. Many **nerve agents** are transported on a daily basis by truck or rail cars in the United States. Potentially tear gas, which is sold in stores, could be used in an attack. Chemicals can be absorbed through the eyes, skin, airways, or a combination of these routes.
3. The following are types of **chemical agents:**
   a. *Nerve agents* are the most toxic of all weaponized military agents. They can cause sudden loss of consciousness, seizures, apnea, and death. The diagnosis is usually made on clinical signs and symptoms. Nerve agents inhibit cholinesterase. Examples of these agents are tabun, sarin, saman, and VX.
   b. *Vesicants* cause blistering. The most common vesicants are sulfur, mustard, and lewisite. Mustard and lewisite cause injury to the eyes, skin, airways, and some internal organs.
   c. *Cyanide* is a chemical agent that is widely used in the United States. Terrorists may use it in confined spaces such as subway cars, shopping centers, convention centers, and small buildings. Shortly after inhalation, victims often become anxious and start to hyperventilate. Convulsions, asystole, and death also can occur. Antidotes should be administered immediately.
   d. *Pulmonary intoxicants* can cause severe life-threatening lung injury after inhalation. The effects are generally delayed for several hours. Examples are phosgene and chlorine. An example of this type of accident occurred at the Union Carbide plant in 1984 in Bhopal, India, which was due to an industrial accident (not to a terrorist attack). These intoxicants are irritating to the eyes and respiratory tract and can cause severe pulmonary edema of a noncardiac nature.
   e. *Riot-control agents* stimulate the lacrimal glands to produce tears and cause eye, nose, mouth, skin, and respiratory tract irritation. These are routinely used by police to control an out-of-control crowd or individual. The effect is immediate and lasts about 30 minutes. Examples of these agents are CN (Mace 7), OC (Oleoresin capsicum or Pepper Spray), and Adamsite or CS (tear gas) (Los Angeles County, 2003).
   f. *Antidotes* for the above agents are listed in Table 9-31.
4. **Decontamination Standards**
   a. Staff needs to be trained to *decontaminate* patients appropriately, and the staff should have the appropriate personal protective equipment (PPE). Hospitals should have the equipment required to decontaminate victims.
   b. *Decontamination shelters* should have the following:
      - A water connection compatible with the facility's water lines
      - The ability to collect and contain large quantities of water
      - Something to mix with the water to remove the chemicals
      - Adequate lighting
      - Connection to electricity, whether plugged into the hospital or into a generator
      - A conveyor system for nonambulatory patients
      - Allowance for patient privacy
      - Room for two or three personnel, preferably non–health care providers
      - Room for families in pediatric facilities. Parents may also require decontamination. Parents can also help with decontaminating their children (Hudson et al., 2003).

TABLE 9-31
Antidote Therapy for Chemical Weapons Attacks

Chemical	Antidote	Decontamination (including removal of clothing)	Other
Nerve Agent	Atropine, 2-PAMCl	Soap and water	Diazepam (Valium)
Sulfur Mustard	None, supportive	Soap and water	Delayed onset, delayed bullae, pulmonary care
Lewisite	BAL, supportive	Soap and water	Acute onset, treat acidosis, volume depletion, pseudomembranes
Cyanide	Methemoglobin, amyl nitrite, sodium nitrite, sodium thiosulfate	Soap and water	Bicarbonate, O_2, fluids, treat acidosis, sudden loss of consciousness
Phosgene	None, supportive	Soap and water	IVF, monitor volume, O_2, early intubation, steroids, watch for pulmonary edema
PFIB	None, supportive		Monitor O_2, watch for pulmonary edema
Ammonia	None, supportive	Irrigate eyes–water only Soap and water	Milk, bronchodilators, Silvadene, GI endoscopy, watch for mediastinitis, liquefaction necrosis
Chlorine	None, supportive	Irrigate eyes–water only Soap and water	Bronchodilators, steroids, intubation, bronchoscopy
CN (mace)	None	Irrigate eyes–water only Soap and water	Remove foreign body from eye, watch for bronchospasm
CS (tear gas)	None	Irrigate eyes–water only Soap and water	
Oleoresin capsicum	None	Irrigate eyes–water only Soap and water	From chili pepper, dermatitis, eye injury

c. *Special considerations* must be made when decontaminating children. Because children might not be at a developmental level to understand what is going on, they may be uncooperative, even combative. Children are lower to the ground and so might be exposed to more of the contaminant; in addition, their large surface-to-volume ratio places them at higher risk of absorption and exposure to the contaminant. Because of their size, a smaller dose may be lethal, so it is important to get them decontaminated as quickly as possible. Children are at a higher risk of thermoregulation and must be placed in a neutral thermal environment and out of the extreme heat or cold. It is important to keep the family unit together if possible so that parents can keep smaller children safe. If parents are not available, appropriate arrangements for supervision must be made.

d. A diagram of a *decontamination trailer* with all the preceding requirements is illustrated in Figure 9-12.

D. Biological Attacks

Biological warfare is a very real threat. In 1999 the Association of Professionals in Infection Control developed a template for hospitals to adopt when dealing with

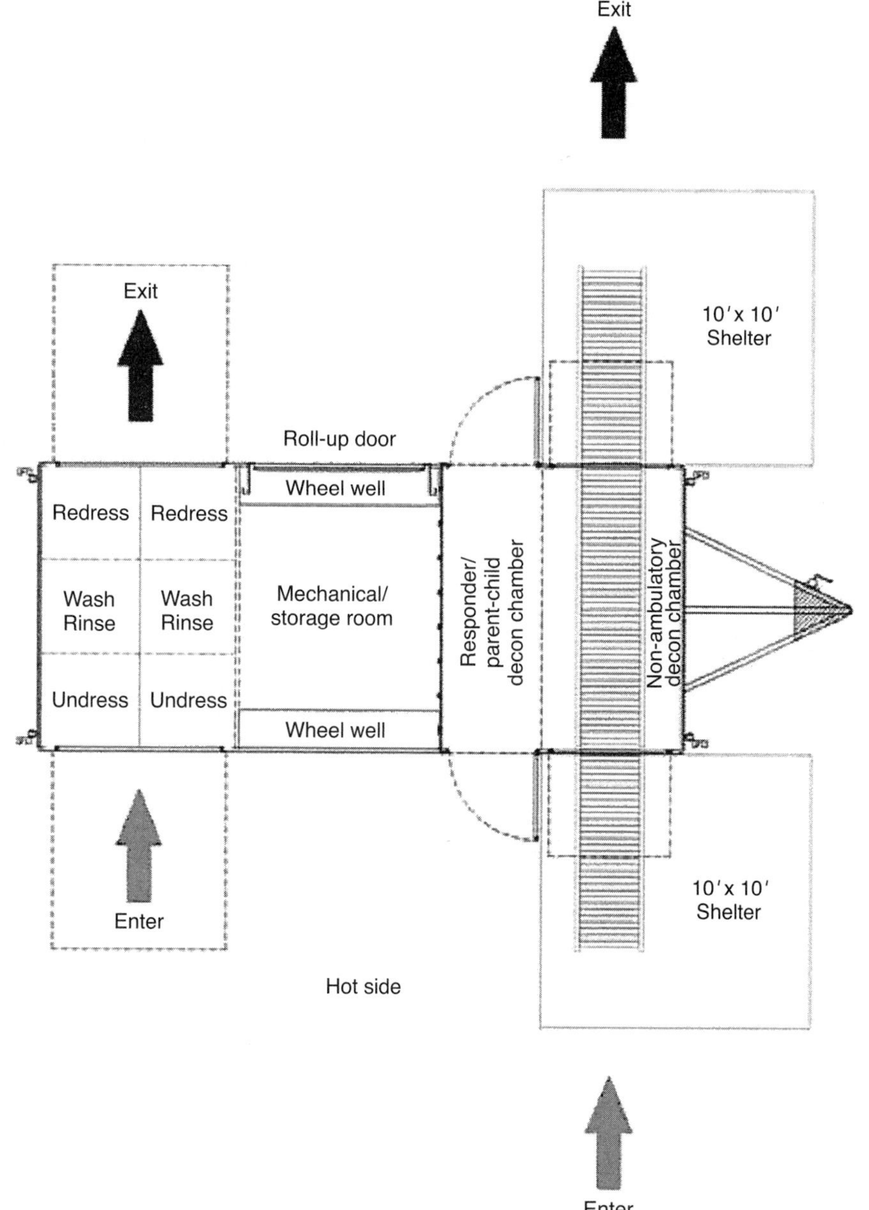

FIGURE 9-12 ■ Decontamination trailer. (Used by permission from Nor E First Response, Inc. MEDecon SCT-19. April 2004. Website: www.nor-e.com/trailers.htm)

bioterrorism; this template is entitled the "Bioterrorism Readiness Plan: A Template for Healthcare Facilities" (APIC, 1999). A biological attack is called *bioterrorism.*

Bioterrorism is defined as the deliberate release of microorganisms (bacteria, viruses, fungi, or toxins) into a community to produce death or disease or to poison humans, animals, or plants (Los Angeles County, 2003). Biological weapons are often called the "poor man's bomb" because they are relatively inexpensive to produce and disseminate. A bioterrorist attack is a real threat, as evidenced by the anthrax attacks in 2001, which resulted in 22 cases of anthrax exposure, five deaths, and a nation on high alert.

1. **Anthrax**
   a. *Etiology*
      - An acute infectious disease caused by *Bacillus anthracis*
      - Some spores viable and infectious in soil for up to 50 years
      - Found most frequently in sheep, goats, and cattle
      - Three types: cutaneous, gastrointestinal, and pulmonary (usually based on the route of exposure)

   b. *Clinical features*
      - Cutaneous
        - Local skin involvement if there is direct contact with spores or bacilli
        - Most often found on head, chest, and forearms
        - Itchy, papular lesion that turns into a vesicle and within 2 to 6 days is black eschar
        - Usually not fatal if treated
      - Pulmonary
        - Nonspecific flulike symptoms
        - 2 to 4 days after initial symptoms, abrupt onset of respiratory failure
        - Hemodynamic collapse
        - Widened mediastinum
        - Dormant in early prodomal stage; high mortality rate after respiratory symptoms
      - Gastrointestinal
        - Abdominal pain, nausea, vomiting, and fever following ingestion of contaminated food, usually meat
        - Bloody diarrhea, hematemesis
        - Positive culture after 2 to 3 days
        - Usually fatal after progression to sepsis
        - Less common form

   c. *Mode of transmission (route of exposure)*
      - Inhalation of spores
      - Cutaneous contact
      - Ingestion of contaminated food
      - Not communicable person-to-person

   d. *Incubation period*
      - 2 to 60 days for pulmonary
      - 1 to 7 days for cutaneous and gastrointestinal modes

   e. *Treatment/therapy* (Table 9-32)

2. **Smallpox:** Smallpox disease was declared eradicated by the World Health Organization (WHO) in 1980 (Los Angeles County, 2003). A smallpox vaccine was available in 2003 for health care workers, but it was not widely used because of issues related to the exclusion criteria and some issues with cardiac problems after receipt of the vaccine. Smallpox is a strong bioterrorism threat because it has a high morbidity in an otherwise normal population.
   a. *Etiology*
      - Acute viral illness caused by the variola virus
      - Airborne transmission
      - One case is a public emergency

   b. *Clinical features* (Figure 9-13)
      - Acute viral symptoms such as influenza
      - Skin lesions appear quickly, progressing from macules to papules to vesicles

TABLE 9-32
Recommended Therapy and Prophylaxis of Anthrax in Children

Form of Anthrax	Category of Treatment (Therapy or Prophylaxis)	Agent and Dosage
Inhalational	Therapy[a] Patients who are clinically stable after 14 days can be switched to a single oral agent (ciprofloxacin or doxycycline) to complete a 60-day course[b] of therapy.	Ciprofloxacin[c] 10-15 mg/kg IV every 12 h (max 400 mg/dose) ***or*** Doxycycline 2.2 mg/kg IV (max 100mg) every 12 h ***and*** Clindamycin[d] 10-15 mg/kg IV every 8 h ***and*** Penicillin G[e] 400-600k mcg/kg/d IV divided every 4 h
Inhalational	Postexposure prophylaxis (60-day course[b])	Ciprofloxacin[f] 10-15 mg/kg PO (max 500 mg/dose every 12 h ***or*** Doxycycline 2.2 mg/kg (max 100 mg) PO every 12 h
Cutaneous, endemic	Therapy[g]	Penicillin V 40-80 mg/kg/d PO divided every 6 h ***or*** Amoxicillin 40-80 mg/kg/d PO divided every 8 h ***or*** Ciprofloxacin 10-15 mg/kg PO (max 1 gm/day) every 12 h ***or*** Doxycyline 2.2 mg/kg PO (max 100 gm) every 12 h
Cutaneous (in setting of terrorism)	Therapy[g]	Ciprofloxacin 10-15 mg/kg PO (max 1 gm/day) every 12 h ***or*** Doxycyline 2.2 mg/kg PO (max 100 gm) every 12 h
Gastrointestinal	Therapy[a]	Same as for inhalational

This table was created from recommendations developed at the Consensus Conference and in part is based on reviewed reference materials from the AAP, CDC, FDA, and Infectious Disease Society of America.

[a] In a mass casuality setting, in which resources are severely limited, oral therapy may need to be substituted for the preferred parenteral option. This may be most acceptable for ciprofloxacin because it is rapidly and well absorbed from the gastriontestinal tract with no substantial loss from first pass effect.

[b] Children may be switched to oral amoxicillin (40-80 mg/kg/d divided every 8 h) to complete a 60-day course (assuming the organism is sensitive). It is recommended that the first 14 days of therapy or postexposure prophylaxis, however, include ciprofloxacin and/or doxycycline regardless of age. A three-dose series of vaccine may permit shortening of the antibiotic course to 30 days.

[c] Levofloxacin or ofloxacin may be acceptable alternatives to ciprofloxacin.

[d] Rifampin or clarithromycin may be acceptable alternatives to clindamycin as drugs that the target bacterial protein synthesis. If ciprofloxacin or another quinolone is used, doxycycline may be used as a second agent because it also targets protein synthesis.

[e] Ampicillin, imipenem, meropenem, or chloramphenicol may be acceptable alternatives to penicillin as drugs with good CNS penetration.

[f] According to most experts ciprofloxacin is the preferred agent for PO prophylaxis.

[g] Ten days of therapy may be adequate for endemic cutaneous disease. However, a full 60-day course is recommended in the setting of terrorism because of the possibility of concomitant inhalation exposure.

- By day 2 to 4, nonspecific flulike symptoms, fever, myalgias
- Rash scabs over in 1 to 2 weeks

c. *Mode of transmission (route of exposure)*
- Large and small respiratory droplets
- Patient-to-patient transmission is likely
- Patients are more infectious if they are coughing
- Infectious at the onset of rash until scabs separate (approximately 3 weeks)

d. *Incubation period*
- 7 to 17 days
- Average, 12 days

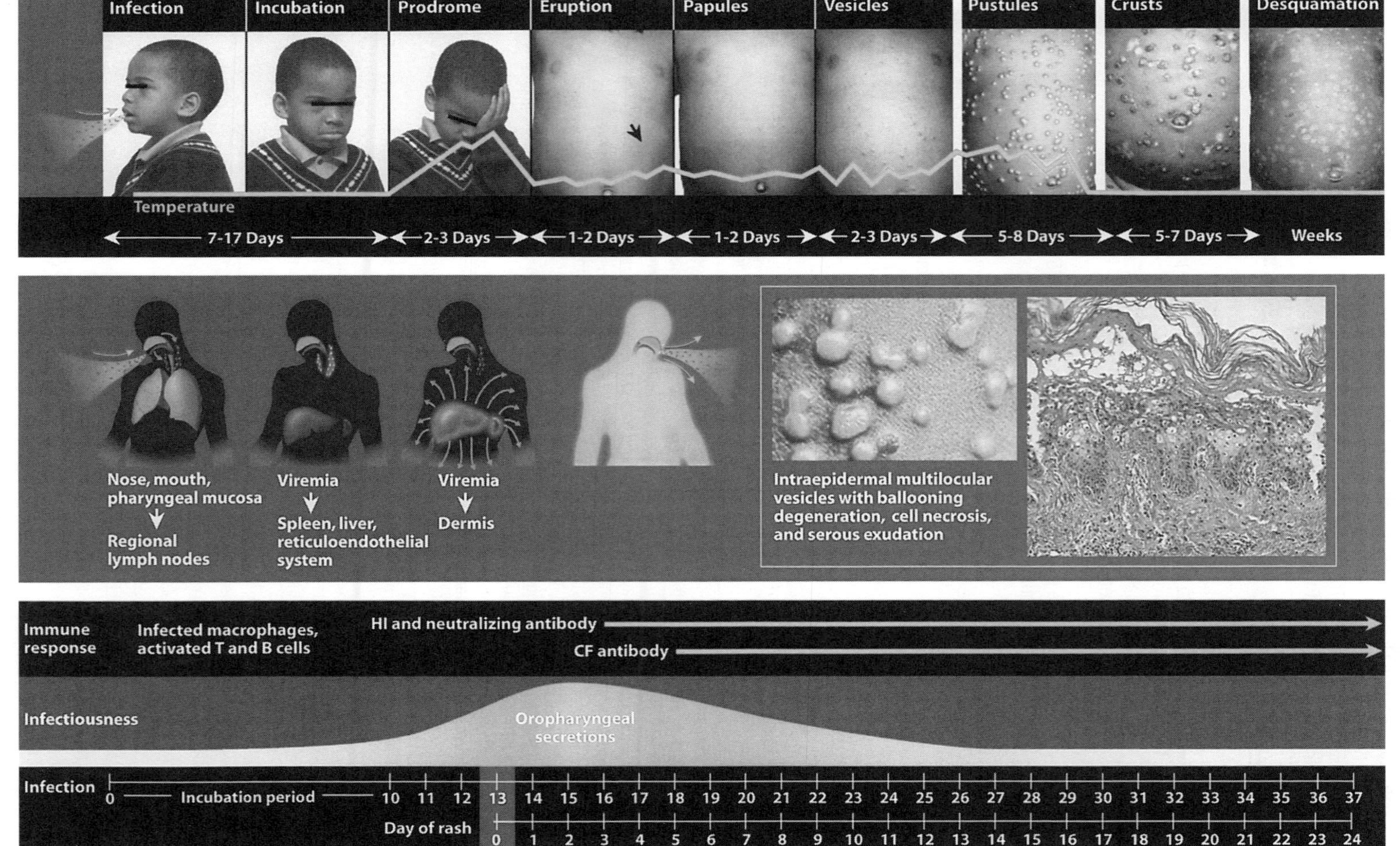

FIGURE 9-13 ■ Clinical manifestations and pathogenesis of smallpox and the immune response.

e. *Treatment* (Table 9-33)
- Vaccine is available
- Vaccine can be given up to 3 days after exposure and still be effective
- After 3 days can try variola immune globulin (VIG)
- Negative isolation is required (Los Angeles County, 2003)

3. Plague

a. *Etiology*
- Acute bacterial disease caused by the gram-negative bacillus *Yersenia pestis*
- Usually transmitted by infected fleas
- Can be airborne, causing pneumonic plague
- Naturally occurring in rodents

b. *Clinical features of pneumonic plague*
- Fever, cough, chest pain
- Hemoptysis
- Mucopurulent or watery sputum with gram-negative rods on Gram stain
- Bronchopneumonia on x-ray

c. *Mode of transmission (route of exposure)*
- Infected rodent to humans by infected fleas
- Bioterrorism-related outbreaks likely in the event of aerosol dispersion
- Person-to-person spread is possible via large aerosol droplets

d. *Incubation period*
- 2 to 8 days if due to flea-borne transmission
- 1 to 2 days if pulmonary exposure has occurred
- Droplet precautions until the patient has completed 72 hours of antimicrobial therapy
- Special air handling is not necessary

e. *Treatment* (see Table 9-33)

4. Tularemia

a. *Etiology*
- Caused by the bacteria *Francisella tularensis,* which typically is the cause in animals (rabbit, deer)
- Almost all exposed will be infected

b. *Clinical features*
- 2 to 10 days after exposure: fever, chills, headache, muscle pain, nonproductive cough, pneumonia
- If ingested, regional lymphadenopathy will occur

c. *Mode of transmission (route of exposure)*
- Humans can be infected from handling infected animals or from diseased fleas, ticks, or mosquitoes
- Can also be spread by aerosol
- Not transmitted person to person

d. *Incubation period:* 2 to 14 days after exposure

e. *Treatment* (see Table 9-33)

5. Botulism

a. *Etiology*
- Caused by *Clostridium botulinum*
- Food-borne cause is most common
- Can be airborne

b. *Clinical features*
- Gastrointestinal symptoms
- Drooping eyelids, jaw clench, difficulty swallowing or speaking
- Descending paralysis

- Blurred vision
- No sensory deficits

c. *Mode of transmission (route of exposure)*
- Usually in food
- Can be aerosolized
- Not transmitted from person to person

d. *Incubation period*
- Ingestion: 12 to 36 hours
- Aerosolized: 24 to 72 hours

e. *Treatment* (see Table 9-33)

6. **Viral hemorrhagic fevers**

a. *Etiology*
- Diverse group of organisms, such as Ebola virus and yellow fever
- Animal or insect hosts
- Humans infected from a bite from an infected animal or insect
- Can be released from an aerosol

b. *Clinical manifestations*
- Vary according to virus
- Usually a nonspecific illness, lasting less than a week, with high fever, headache and systematic illness followed by flushing, maculopapular rash and conjunctival infection, progressing to diffuse hemorrhagic disease and multiorgan system failure
- Severe illness may lead to disseminated intravascular coagulation (DIC), shock, seizures, and even death
- Mortality varies from 10% to 90%

c. *Mode of transmission* (route of exposure)
- Some of these fevers can be transmitted person to person
- Infected flea or animal bite
- Can be aerosolized

d. *Incubation period:* 2 to 22 days

e. *Treatment* (see Table 9-33)

PSYCHOLOGICAL EFFECTS

Since the disasters of September 11, 2001, much research has been done related to the psychological effects of children resulting from such events Blaschke et al (2003) name three specific mental health factors unique to pediatrics:

- Response is dependent on cognitive, physical, emotional, or social development.
- Response is influenced by the emotional state of the caregivers.
- Fear or discomfort may cause children to struggle against their providers (Blaschke et al., 2003).

Reactions and symptoms of these events vary in children. If they are directly affected by the events, they will experience more obvious symptoms. Some initial symptoms may be hyperventilation, tachycardia, and other symptoms related to fear and paranoia. If left untreated, these symptoms can lead to depression, poor appetite, and weight loss, and children sometimes regress into an earlier stage of growth and development. For example, children who are potty trained may start to wet the bed. They may also have nightmares.

After a major disaster, children are more fearful of what comes next, that the event will recur, that someone they love will be killed or injured, or that they will be left alone. Nurses can help to alleviate these fears by intervening as they do with other

■ TABLE 9-33

■ ■ Recommended Therapy and Prophylaxis in Children for Additional Select Diseases Associated with Bioterrorism

Disease	Therapy or Prophylaxis	Treatment, Agent, and Dosage[a]
Smallpox	Therapy	Supportive care
	Prophylaxis	Vaccination may be effective if given within the first several days after exposure
Plague	Therapy	Gentamicin 2.5 mg/kg IV every 8 h ***or***
		Streptomycin 15 mg/kg IM every 12 h (max 2 gm/day, although only available for compassionate usage and in limited supply, is a preferred agent) ***or***
	Prophylaxis	Doxycyline 2.2 mg/kg PO every 12 h ***or***
		Ciprofloxacin[c] 20 mg/kg PO every 12 h
Tularemia	Therapy	Same as for plague
Botulism	Therapy	Supportive care, antitoxin may halt progession of symptoms but is unlikely to reverse them
Viral hemorrhagic fevers	Therapy	Supportive care, ribavirin may be beneficial in select cases[d]
Brucellosis	Therapy[e]	TMP/SMX 30 mg/kg PO every 12 h **and** Rifampin 15 mg/kg every 24 h ***or*** Gentamicin 7.5 mg/kg IM for the first 5 d

This table was created from recommendations developed at the Consensus Conference and in part is based on reviewed reference materials from the AAP, CDC, and Infectious Disease Society of America

[a] In a mass casuality setting, parenteral therapy might not be possible. In such cases, oral therapy (with analogous agents) may need to be used.

[b] Concentration should be maintained between 5 and 20 mcg/mL; some experts have recommended that chloramphenicol be used to treat patients with plague meningitis, since chloramphenicol penetrates the blood-brain barrier. Use in children younger than 2 years may be associated with adverse reactions but might be warranted for serious infections.

[c] Other fluoroquinolones (levofloxacin, ofloxacin) may be acceptable substitutes for ciprofloxacin; however, they are not approved for use in children.

[d] Ribavirin is recommended for Arenavirus, Bunyavirus and may be indicated for a viral hemorrhagic fever of an unknown etiology, although not FDA approved for these indications. For intravenous therapy use a loading dose: 30 kg IV once (maximum dose, 2 gm), then 16 mg/kg IV every 6 h for 4 days (maximum dose, 1 g) and then 8 mg/kg IV every 8 h for 6 days (maximum dose, 500 mg). In a mass casuality setting it may be necessary to use oral therapy. For oral therapy use a loading dose of 30 mg/kg PO once then 15 mg/kg/day PO in 2 divided doses for 10 days.

[e] For children younger than 8 years. For children older than 8 years, adult regimens are recommended. Oral drugs should be given for 6 weeks. Gentamicin, if used, should be given for the first 5 days of a 6-week course of TMP/SMX (trimethoprim/sulfamethoxazole).

traumatic events. They can answer questions and encourage family-centered care. Nurses need to assess the children's growth and developmental levels and treat them accordingly. Nurses also need to assess the psychological symptoms and determine whether the symptoms are severe or out of the ordinary; in the latter situation, social workers or the appropriate mental health members should be notified and allowed to intervene. The Red Cross has numerous resources for health care team members called "Helping Children Cope with Disaster."

CONCLUSION

When an terrorist attack occurs, regardless of the exact type, the impact—biological, chemical, or radiologic—will be overwhelming to the health care system. The potential impact of large numbers of critically ill patients is a real concern, but the overwhelming impact of the additional "worried well" patients can shut down a health care system. It is important that all health care workers have some understanding of the potential of a terrorist attack and how to care for themselves and others during this type of disaster. It is also important that hospitals be prepared to deal with MCIs and that they are aware of their need for "surge capacity," specifically, the ability to increase the census and care for more patients in a disaster.

The need for psychological treatment for the effects of bioterrorism cannot be minimized. Even patients with no physical effects may go the hospital to be checked for illness or injury. Initial triage of psychological symptoms is important in the elimination or minimization of long-term psychological effects.

Depending on the environment and area of the world where nurses are practicing, they may experience terrorist incidents more frequently; all nurses, however, need to be knowledgeable about dealing effectively with these issues. They also need to be aware of how care needs differ for adult patients and pediatric patients.

Initial Stabilization and Transport

Bradley A. Kuch and Carol A. Singleton

Pediatric critical care transport is a highly specialized area of medicine in which the critically ill infant or child is stabilized and transported to a facility specializing in his or her care. The need for patient transport is indicated by the specific elements of care that cannot be provided by the referring institution. These may include diagnostic procedures, airway management, mechanical ventilation, or extracorporeal membrane oxygenation (ECMO). Transferring patients to a facility specializing in this type of care is often complicated by the severity of illness of pediatric patients and the increased risk of mortality found in the transport setting. These children require more interventions (e.g., endotracheal intubation, inotropic support) and continuous cardiovascular monitoring (both invasive and noninvasive), which warrants a crew with an in-depth understanding of pediatric disease pathology and care. For example, it has been demonstrated that identification and rapid stabilization of the pediatric patients with septic shock decrease morbidity and mortality rates in the transport setting (Han et al., 2003). In an effort to provide the same level of care found in the pediatric critical care unit (PICU), the pediatric critical care specialty transport team was created.

In 1991, Pollack et al set the precedent for specialized care by establishing evidence showing an associated decrease in morbidity and mortality in patients who were treated for respiratory failure and head trauma in tertiary care centers versus nontertiary centers (Pollack, 1991). A more recent investigation found that nonspecialized emergency medical services (EMS) personnel underutilized basic therapies such as oxygen administration during the transport of pediatric patients with respiratory illness (Scribano et al., 2000). McCloskey and colleagues demonstrated a decrease in morbidity events in patients who were transported by pediatric critical care specialty teams when compared with adult teams (McCloskey and Orr, 1999).

In 1990 the American Academy of Pediatrics (AAP) recognized this area of medicine as an integral part of the pediatric emergency care system and ultimately granted it section status (Woodward et al., 2002). As the support for pediatric specialty care teams grows, so does the need for education and a complete understanding of the principles associated with the safe effective transport of the critically ill child (Warren et al., 2004).

A. Principles and Philosophy of Pediatric Interfacility Transport

1. **Goals of the critical care transport team**
   a. To provide an *extension of the critical care unit* (i.e., skills, equipment) to the referring facilities (Day et al., 1991)
   b. To provide *timely and safe transportation* to a pediatric critical care center without an increase in morbidity or mortality
   c. To provide the *highest quality of care* for critically ill infants and children who require interfacility transport
2. **Trauma versus critical care**
   a. *Scoop and run:* This term is given to the concept of transport, in which a patient is taken to a facility within the "golden hour." The "golden hour" is often described as the period immediately following a traumatic injury where intervention is critical for patient survival. The "golden hour" philosophy has never been validated and was developed in an era when prehospital personnel did not provide advanced airway management. Therefore patients were at increased risk for adverse events, including death, during transport.
      - Nonspecialty care teams have adopted the "scoop and run" philosophy of patient transport as the standard of practice in the trauma setting. One reason for this is that there is little triage by a coordinating physician at the time of a trauma call. Most calls received are from local emergency medical service (EMS) personnel at the scene; thus all calls are considered critical and deserve immediate transport to a trauma care center.
      - A clinical situation in which scoop and run would be appropriate would be a patient who had uncontrollable bleeding or a significant head injury for which the immediate lifesaving intervention would be an emergent trip to the operating room.
      - Time is critical in regard to the time of arrival to the scene or referring facility by a team who can provide critical care interventions.
   b. *Stay and resuscitate* suggests that certain aspects of resuscitation must be delivered as quickly as possible (McCloskey, 1995). The initial resuscitation of any patient starts with the ABCs (*airway, breathing, and circulation*) and must be delivered at either the accident scene or the referring institution.
      - Han and colleagues demonstrated a 96% survival rate in patients with septic shock who received early resuscitative interventions from community hospital physicians leading to shock reversal versus only 63% in those whose shock was not reversed (Han et al., 2003).
      - This approach to transport care is supported by the American Heart Association Pediatric Advance Life Support concept for treating shock and respiratory failure.
3. **Legal issues**
   a. *COBRA/EMTALA:* The Consolidated Omnibus Budget Reconciliation Act (COBRA) passed in 1985 was intended to prevent patients with unstable medical conditions from being transferred without treatment from the initial hospital (Warren et al., 2004). The statute is also titled the Emergency Medical Treatment and Active Labor Act (EMTALA) and more accurately describes the statute. Under EMTALA, physicians are obligated to stabilize patients with identified emergency conditions. They also may transfer a stabilized patient who requires a higher level of care. Responsibilities of the referring physicians and hospitals include, but are not limited to, the following:
      - Providing all medical treatment within its capacity
      - Identify a receiving hospital that will accept and provide qualified personnel to treat the patient's clinical needs

- Qualified personnel, with appropriate equipment, must accompany the patient.

b. The decision of who is best qualified to assist the referring hospital in the safe *transport* of the neonatal or pediatric patient is most often made by the common consent of the referring doctor and the transport team.

4. **Patient family issues:** The transport team's role in the area of family support has continued to undergo many changes. Previously most teams rarely allowed family members to travel with the patient and team. The psychological impact on families in acute or worsening medical conditions (see Chapter 1) has been considered in several studies. These studies support the value of parental presence in decreasing stress in both the patient as well as the parent. Woodward has stated that "allowing the presence of family members helps minimize the family's fear of being left to wonder what is happening to their child" (Woodward and Flaegler, 2000). The concept of parental presence is becoming incorporated into many transport systems.

   a. In 2000 Woodward and colleagues conducted a survey of parents whose children were transported via ambulance to a large regional children's hospital. They found that allowing the parent to accompany the child during transport was a positive experience that did not hinder intratransport medical care (Woodward and Flaegler, 2000).

   b. In the incidence of neonatal transports, the possibility of parental presence is impacted by the inpatient status of the mother. Some programs address the issue of bonding while decreasing parental stress by using a toy or doll made of Dutch wool called a *Snoedel* (Children's Hospital of Pittsburgh). The Snoedel is left with the mother or family to hold against their skin and then bring to the hospital during their first visit. The wool absorbs the parent's scent, thus offering comfort to the baby during parental absence.

   c. The transport team is the first specialized group of caretakers involved in the child's care. Transport team members are key participants in a child's definitive medical care. Involving parents in the process benefits the family, patient, and transport system (Woodward and Flaegler, 2000).

B. Transport Physiology

The care of critically ill or injured patients during air medical transport is a complex, ever-changing situation that requires a firm knowledge of flight physiology and an understanding of a few fundamental laws of physics. These include atmospheric composition, basic gas laws, and transport-related stresses that affect both the patient and transport team.

1. **Atmospheric composition** is an important physical property of which an understanding is essential for building the foundation of the flight physiology. The atmosphere is composed of seven basic gases: nitrogen (78%), oxygen (21%), argon (0.94%), carbon dioxide (0.03%), hydrogen (0.01%), neon (0.0018%), and helium (0.00015%). The percentage of each gas in the atmosphere remains constant up to approximately 70,000 feet above sea level. Each gas is responsible for a percentage of the total atmosphere that corresponds to its partial pressure.

2. **Gas laws:** A complete understanding of gas laws as they relate to temperature, pressure, and volume is crucial for the safe, effective transport of a patient via either a helicopter or fixed-wing aircraft (Blumen and Rinnert, 1995; Nehrenz, 1997).

   a. *Boyle's law* states that "at a constant temperature, the volume of a given gas is inversely proportional to the pressure. . . ."

$$P_1 V_1 = P_2 V_2$$

In other words, a known volume of gas will expand as the pressure that surrounds it decreases. Boyle's gas law affects any enclosed gas-filled space whether inside or outside the body cavity.

Example: An intubated 13-year-old trauma patient is being transported via a fixed-wing aircraft to a level 1 trauma center. As the aircraft lifts off and climbs to 8000 feet above sea level, the endotracheal tube cuff will increase in size, causing more pressure on the trachea walls. When the aircraft starts to descend for landing, the cuff will decrease to its size prior to landing, thus decreasing the pressure that was previously on the tracheal walls. ■

b. *Dalton's law* describes the *partial pressure* of various gases, the effect that altitude has on them, and states "the total pressure of a gas mixture equals the sum of the individual (partial) pressures of all the gases in the mixtures. . . ."

$$P = P_1 + P_2 + P_3 + P_4$$

Another illustration of Dalton's law is as follows: Each gas present in a gas mixture exerts a partial pressure that equals the fractional volume of gas multiplied by the total pressure (Table 9-34).

Example: What is the partial pressure of oxygen being delivered to a patient being mechanically ventilated at 2000 feet above sea level (706 torr) with 50% oxygen? ■

Partial pressure = barometric pressure × gas concentration
Partial pressure = 706 torr × 50% oxygen
Partial pressure = 353 torr

c. *Charles' law* states that "when pressure is constant, the volume of a gas is very nearly proportional to its absolute temperature. . . ."

$$\frac{V_1}{V_2} = \frac{T_1}{T_2}$$

Charles' law explains the direct relationship between volume and temperature; as the temperature of a gas increases, so does the volume of that gas.

TABLE 9-34
Level of Inspired Oxygen Related to Altitude

Altitude (ft)	Barometric Pressure (mm Hg)	Inspired Oxygen Tension (mm Hg)
0	760	149
1000	733	143
2000	707	138
3000	681	133
4000	656	127
5000	632	122
6000	609	117
8000	564	108
10000	523	99

Example: You are transporting a 50 kg patient who is septic and receiving a 1 L bolus of fluid using large-bore tubing and a pressure bag. As you leave the building and assess your patient during the frigid 15°F winter day, you notice a drop in pressure on the manometer (pressure bag) and the volume stops running. You promptly add more air to the bag to ensure that the bolus continues to run. As you add gaseous volume to the pressure bag, you are witnessing Charles' law at work. The decrease in temperature causes a direct decrease in gaseous volume in the bag. ■

d. *Guy-Lussac's Law* states, "When a volume of gas is constant, the pressure of this gas is directly proportional to the absolute temperature for a constant volume of gas."

$$\frac{P_1}{T_1} = \frac{P_2}{T_2}$$

In simpler words, Guy-Lussac's law illustrates the direct relationship between pressure and temperature.

Example: While completing the morning checks when the aircraft was in the heated hanger (74°F), the pressure of oxygen was 1800 psi. Later that morning, the pilot moves the aircraft outside (32°F) so that the maintenance crew can clean the hanger. Before the first flight, you check the oxygen level once more and discover a pressure of 1550 psi. The change in pressure is explained by Guy-Lussac's law of temperature and pressure. As the temperature decreases, so will the pressure. ■

e. *Henry's law* states that "a quantity of gas dissolved in a liquid is proportional to the partial pressure of the gas in contact with that liquid...." In other words, the partial pressure of a gas above the liquid equals the quantity of gas dissolved in the liquid.

Example: You are transporting a 15-year-old scuba diver who is suffering from decompression sickness after a rapid ascent from a depth of 90 feet. The cause of this illness is the rapid ascent from an environment with a high pressure (i.e., a depth of 90 feet) to an area of relatively low pressure (sea level), causing a release of gas bubbles from the blood. If the teen would have slowly ascended from the depth allowing time for the gas-liquid interface to equilibrate, the situation could have been completely avoided. ■

3. **Transport related stresses** can be placed into two distinct but related categories: environmental and self-imposed. Temperature, hypoxia, dehydration, noise, and vibration are stresses imposed by the environment. Self-imposed stresses can easily be remembered by the acronym DEATH; the components include ***d***rugs, **e**xhaustion (fatigue), ***a***lcohol, ***t***obacco, and ***h***ypoglycemia (Holleran, 1996). In combination with the environmental factors, the self-imposed stresses can magnify the physical and mental fatigue, leading to errors in judgment and decreasing the level of performance. To limit these factors, the transport team must have a solid understanding of the principles of transport-related stresses and the physiologic effects they have on both the patient and crew.
   a. *Hypoxia* is described as the relative state of oxygen deficiency that tissues experience from a decreased oxygen supply. Hypoxia is one of the most important stresses that may be encountered during the air medical transport and is found within four physiologic categories (Table 9-35).
   - *Hypoxic hypoxia* is the oxygen deficiency that is present at the alveolar level. The transfer of gas from the alveolus to the arterial system is compromised, resulting in a low partial pressure of oxygen in the blood.

TABLE 9-35
Clinical Effects and Treatment of Hypoxia

Systems	Signs and Symptoms	Treatment
Cardiovascular	Tachycardia Arrhythmias Hypertension Hypotension *(late)* Bradycardia	1. Identify which type of hypoxia is present: - Hypoxic - Hyperemic - Stagnant - Histotoxic
Pulmonary	Hyperventilation Dyspnea Tachypnea Cyanosis *(late)*	2. Deliver supplemental oxygen - Depending on the severity, a FiO_2 of 1.0 may be required. - An increase may be needed in spontaneously breathing and mechanically ventilated patients alike 3. Patient monitoring - Heart rate/rhythm - Respiratory rate - Blood pressure - End tidal CO_2 - Ventilator parameters
Neurologic	Seizures Restlessness Euphoria Belligerence Unconsciousness	4. Monitor equipment - Indwelling catheters and tubes - Mechanical ventilator - Invasive pressure monitoring equipment 5. Descend - Increase the partial pressure of oxygen by descending to a lower altitude

- *Hyperemic hypoxia* or *anemic hypoxia* occurs when the oxygen carrying capacity of the blood is decreased, resulting in a limited oxygen delivery to the tissues.
- *Stagnant hypoxia* is defined as the lack of adequate blood flow to the body or a specific area of the body. Stagnant hypoxia results from clinical situations with low cardiac output as a component of its pathophysiology.
- *Histotoxic hypoxia* (*cellular/tissue poisoning*) refers to the clinical situations that affect the cell's ability to metabolize molecular oxygen. A patient may have a normal arterial partial pressure of oxygen (PaO_2), but their tissue is unable to use it because of the cellular metabolic dysfunction.

b. *Changing barometric pressure* is the primary cause for many physical symptoms that the flight crew may experience. As an aircraft climbs, the barometric pressure decreases and in turn the gases within the body cavity expand. The expansion may cause complications such as *barotitis media, barosinusitis, and barodontalgia.*

- *The gastrointestinal (GI) system* can hold a significant amount of gas *(methane)*, which is a by-product of normal digestion. As the aircraft climbs, the volume of the gas in the GI tract expands (Boyle's law of volume and pressure), causing discomfort and pain. The patient may release the expanded gas by either belching or flatus (Holleran, 1996). Nasogastric tubes should be vented, allowing excess gas to escape.

c. *Thermal regulation:* The transport environment exposes both the patient and crew to a wide range of temperatures. Prolonged exposure to this environment has been found to have negative physiologic effects. These effects include increased oxygen consumption, vasoconstriction or vasodilation, an increased susceptibility of motion sickness, disorientation, and an increased metabolic rate (Blumen and Rinnert, 1995; Holleran, 1996).

d. *Humidity:* As altitude increases, the level of humidity in the ambient atmosphere decreases. The crew must be aware of the effects that this environmental change will have on both the patient and fellow team members. These effects include dry eyes, chapped lips, thickening of pulmonary secretions, and sore throat. Increasing fluid intake via the oral (crew) or intravenous (IV) routes (patient) will aid in replenishing the fluid lost during flight (McCloskey et al., 1995).

e. *Noise and vibration* are common occurrences in the transport setting, dependent on the mode of transportation: ambulance, fixed-wing aircraft (airplane), or rotor-wing aircraft (helicopter). Noise and vibration may or may not affect patients. Some might experience anxiety, which can be exhibited by an increase in heart rate, blood pressure, or combativeness. Noise presents the crew with the added difficulty of patient assessment. It makes the use of a stethoscope for auscultation of breath sound virtually impossible (Hunt et al., 1991).

f. *Fatigue* is the end product of all contributing stresses on transport personnel. It has been linked to judgment errors, narrowed attention span, limited response, and possibly the cause of several fatal accidents (Blumen and Rinnert, 1995; Holleran, 1996).

C. Transport Equipment

The equipment routinely carried by the transport team should be able to provide ongoing intensive care until the team safely arrives at the receiving institution. The American Academy of Pediatric Task Force on Interhospital Transport recommends the following guidelines for transport equipment (AAP Task Force on Intrahospital Transport 1999). The equipment will do the following:

- Provide the capability for **life support** in the transport setting
- Be **lightweight** (*loadable by two persons*), portable, and self-contained, with a battery life twice the expected transport duration
- Be **durable** enough to withstand altitude and thermal changes, acute decompression vibration (*4-G decelerative forces*), and repeated use
- Have **AC/DC** capabilities
- Have **no electromagnetic field interference**
- Be able to **fit** through standard hospital doors and into transport vehicles and be easily secured to prevent shifting while en route
- **Supplies and medications** carried should be sufficient to maintain ongoing critical care during the transport

D. Team Configuration

The composition of a critical care transport team varies from institution to institution. At present the guidelines for training transport team personnel are designed and implemented by the program director. The goal is for team members to have the clinical skills and expertise needed to deliver the level of care found in the critical care area of the receiving hospital.

1. **Configuration models** that currently exist include RN (registered nurse)/RT (respiratory therapist), RN/RN, RN/EMT-P (paramedic), RN/MD, RN/RT/MD, CRNP (certified registered nurse practioneer)/RN, and CRNP/RT. A program may choose a constant configuration or change based on patient acuity (Table 9-36).

TABLE 9-36
Examples of RN/RT Team Configuration as Related to Clinical Situation

Type of Patient	Staff to Accompany and Remain with Patient
Stable with one IV	RN/RCP team
Stable with arterial line	RN/RCP team
On mechanical ventilator	RN/RCP team
Vasoactive drips/MV	RN/RCP team
ECMO referral	RN/RCP/transport MD
Sepsis shock w/o access	RN/RCP/transport MD

Note: Application of this specific triage strategy to other pediatric referral centers may be limited.
ECMO, Extracorporeal membrane oxygenation; *IV,* intravenous; *MD,* medical doctor; *MV,* mechanical ventilation; *RCP,* respiratory care practitioner; *RN,* registered nurse.

2. The **Transport Section** of the AAP recommends that an RN be a member (most likely the team leader) of the team during every transport (AAP Task Force on Interhospital Transport, 1999). The task force states that the rationale behind this is "that an RN is the most likely to offer the level of education, versatility, and licensing requirements."

E. Advanced Skills Training

It has become common practice in pediatric transport systems to use an RN/RT or RN/RN team without the addition of a physician after a period of specialized training. These individuals are expected to identify and manage problems that might and often do occur during transport. Frequently the team is expected to intervene on arrival to a referring hospital where staff either is uncomfortable or lacks the skill to perform a specific procedure. The AAP Section on Transport medicine has published specific guidelines that address appropriate training procedures and other team-related issues (AAP Task Force on Interhospital Transport, 1999).

1. Many programs require **experience** in the emergency department (ED) or critical care areas, which serves as a foundation for the development of advanced skills.
2. Many, if not most, programs require staff to have successfully completed one or more **advanced life support courses** (Advanced Cardiac Life Support [ACLS], Pediatric Advanced Life Support [PALS], Neonatal Resuscitation Program [NRP]). In general, advanced skill training focuses on (but is not limited to) interventional skills, such as advanced airway management, needle thoracostomy, cannulation of umbilical vessels, and placing intraosseous catheters.
3. Individual programs develop **training sessions** that not only address technical skills, but a didactic component, including core topics such as pathophysiology, diagnosis, assessment, therapy, and complications for each disease entity.
4. Following initial training, **credentialing** may occur within the medical structure of the institution. Ongoing competency assessment programs are expected by the AAP (AAP Task Force on Interhospital Transport, 1999).
5. **Commission on Accreditation of Medical Transport Systems (CAMTS)** is a voluntary accreditation service focused around patient care and safety in the transport environment. CAMTS certification verifies that a transport program meets current standards, which are based on medical research, ground transport, and aviation developments.

INITIAL STABILIZATION OF THE NEONATAL OR PEDIATRIC PATIENT

A. Principles and Practice

The initial stabilization of any infant or child starts at the referring facility before the request for transport. This responsibility is federally mandated by EMTALA and COBRA laws. Patient assessment and therapeutic intervention should be based on the procurement of a patent airway, ensuring effective ventilation, and stabilizing circulation. These assessments and interventions are outlined in the American Heart Association's Pediatric Advanced Life Support course (Zaritsky et al., 2002).

1. The transport team's **resuscitative efforts** should be focused on stabilizing the patient before transport. The "routine" delivery of intensive care to the critically ill child is complicated by numerous environmental factors during transport including the following:
   a. *Cramped surroundings* cause restricted access to the patient due to seatbelts of both the patient and the team members.
   b. *Limited access* to all equipment and limited ability to carry anything but essential equipment are issues.
   c. *Low light conditions,* constant vibration, and/or noise produced by engines may decrease the ability to hear alarms and assess the patient. It may also affect readings of various monitoring devices. The combination of vibration, electronic distortion, and background sound challenges even the most technically advanced equipment.
   d. *Constant movement* of the vehicle increases the risk of accidental extubation.
   e. *Low temperatures* present a significant challenge to team members as they deliver care and also attempt to maintain adequate body temperatures.

B. Transport Population

The pediatric transport patient population differs greatly from that of the adult patient population. Figure 9-14 shows the diagnostic categories of 4905 patients transported by five pediatric specialty care teams from different regions around the United States.

C. Initial Call and Triage

The initial call may be triaged by a command physician who collects patient information and gives recommendation for stabilization. Stabilization begins at the time of the call. An outline of the components for effective information gathering and therapeutic considerations are presented in Table 9-37.

D. Patient Assessment

1. **Airway:** Assessment of the pediatric airway includes airway patency, maintaining an airway, and airway protection. Rapid assessment of these areas will determine the next intervention. It may be as simple as repositioning the child's head (not recommended in patients with questionable cervical spine injury) or as complex as endotracheal intubation. The decision can be made based on the presence or absence of the following:
   a. *Patent airway (ventilation/CO_2):* Obstruction of the upper airway can be easily identified by the absence of audible or palpable airflow, upper airway stridor, or asynchronous chest and abdominal motion. If any of the aforementioned symptoms are present, the upper airway should be visually inspected. In this situation, the patient may possibly require repositioning of the head,

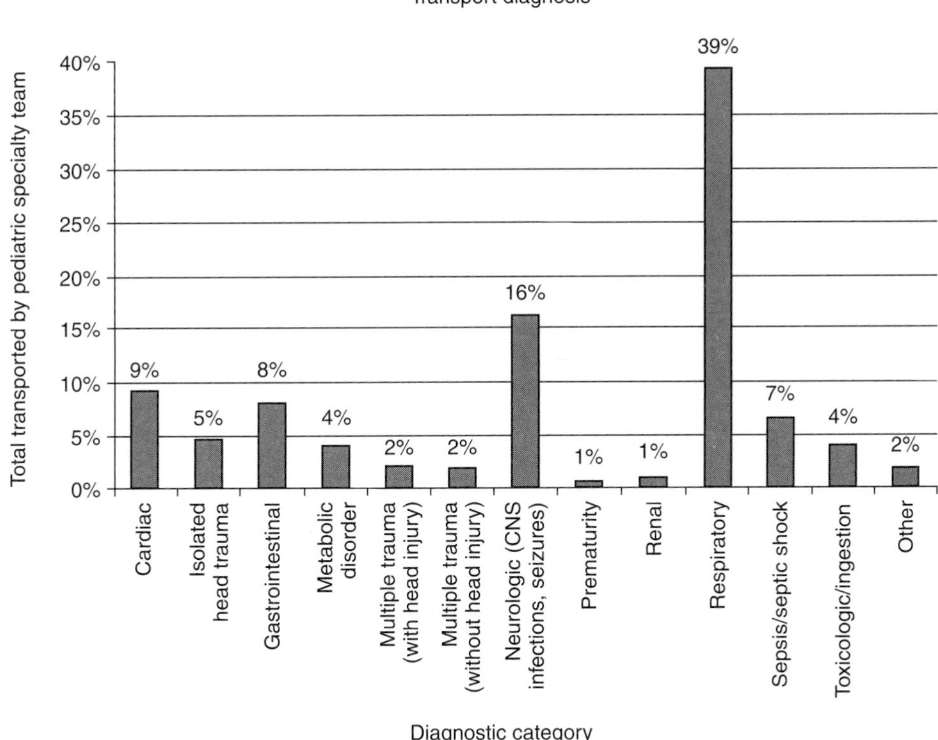

FIGURE 9-14 ■ Database of five regional pediatric specialty care teams.

suctioning of the oral pharynx, or placement of a nasal pharyngeal airway to ensure a patent pathway for respiration to occur.

b. *Maintaining an airway:* Patients with an altered level of consciousness or neuromuscular weakness may be unable to maintain their own airway. Presentation can include limited airflow (decreased breath sounds), "snoring respirations," an inability to control secretions, or obstructive apneas. These patients are at risk for pulmonary insufficiency, leading to hypoxia, hypercarbia, and respiratory acidosis.

c. *Protective airway reflexes (cough and gag):* Assessment of the upper airway reflexes are performed by using a soft-suction catheter to elicit a cough or gag. The presence of this protective reflex will illustrate that the infant or child can protect his or her own airway in case of emesis during transport.

2. **Breathing *(oxygenation/O_2)***: The initial step in the assessment of breathing is a visual inspection of the patient. Identifying the patient's position (i.e., tripod position in epiglottitis), respiratory pattern and rate, level of distress, and behavior (obtunded or anxiousness) will provide the clinician with an immediate assessment of the severity of the situation.

   a. *Respiratory rate:* An accurate respiratory rate should be obtained before interacting with the patient; interaction with a stranger often causes anxiety in the young child, leading to an elevated respiratory rate.

      - *Tachypnea* in a child can be a caused by pain, anxiety, shock, respiratory distress, metabolic acidosis (i.e., diabetic ketoacidosis), and increased body temperature. Identifying the exact cause is often difficult but may be assisted by the use of pulse oximetry, blood gas analysis, or measurement of the patient's temperature.

TABLE 9-37
Information Outline for Initial Transport Triage Call

Initial Call
(Stabilization Begins at the Time of Call)

I. Report should include a brief but concise past medical history as well as a history of the present illness:
- Present Condition
- Vital signs (ABCs = *airway, breathing, circulation*)
  - Patent airway
  - Respiratory rate
  - Heart rate
  - Blood pressure
  - Perfusion
- Neurologic assessment
  - Level of consciousness (LOC)
  - Glasgow Coma Scale (GCS)
  - Presence of seizure activity
- Lab data
  - Blood glucose level
  - Complete blood count (CBC)
  - Electrolytes
  - Cultures
- Radiologic interpretations

II. Treatment recommendations from the transport physician may include, but are not limited to, the following:
- Fluid resuscitation
- Inotropic support
- Aerosolized medication recommendation
- Anticonvulsant therapy
- Antibiotics

III. Decision regarding mode of transportation and team composition:
- Patient condition
- Safety
- Distance
- Accordance with the referring physician recommendation on the patient's medical necessity
  - EMTALA laws
  - Ultimately responsibility falls on the referring physician

- *Bradypnea* is uncommon; it may be caused by a head injury, hypothermia, medications such as narcotics, or impending respiratory failure.
- *Apnea* is common in the premature infant population and can lead to cyanosis and bradycardia. It can be an ominous sign in an older infant and should be closely monitored. If apnea continues, treatment is recommended to ensure a positive neurologic outcome. The causes of apnea may be serious in nature and have been implicated as the first sign in the progression of life-threatening critical illness.

b. *Pattern:* Respiratory pattern should be assessed along with the respiratory rate. Assessment should include the depth of each breath, the inspiratory and expiratory time (i.e., prolonged expiratory phase), and the presence of an increased work of breathing (WOB).
- Increased WOB (respiratory distress) is explained with greater detail in Chapter 2.

- The following clinical findings are signs and symptoms of respiratory distress: grunting, nasal flaring, retractions, paradoxical respiration, and tachypnea.
  - Oxygen is the drug of choice in most cases involving patients who present with signs of an increased WOB. It is important to obtain the patient's normal arterial saturation level, especially with a history of cardiac disease (see Chapter 3).
- **Breathing patterns** can aid in distinguishing the underlying cause of the clinical manifestations with which a particular patient presents:
  - *Periodic breathing* is defined by the periodic pause in the respiratory cycle lasting less than 10 seconds without an associated cyanosis or bradycardia. This pattern is found in premature and newborn infants (Weintraub et al., 2001).
  - *Kussmaul breathing* is a deep, continuous breathing pattern commonly observed in patients with diabetic ketoacidosis (DKA). This breathing pattern causes hyperventilation, which partially compensates for profound metabolic acidosis.
  - *Cheyne-Stokes breathing* is commonly found in patients with neurologic injury. It also has been associated with congestive heart failure in the adult population.

c. *Breath sounds:* Auscultation of the chest in all lobular regions should be performed to determine whether any adventitious breath sounds are present. Proper assessment of the breath sounds should include documentation of the amplitude of the sound produced, timing of the sound (i.e., early, late), and the quality of air movement respiration. Some of the most commonly used terms to describe adventitious breath sounds include wheezes, crackles or rales, rhonchi, and stridor. Chapter 2 describes in more detail the clinical assessment of pulmonary function.

d. *Skin color:* Assessment of skin color should focus on identifying the presence of cyanosis. It may be found either centrally (lips) or peripherally (nail beds). The first line of treatment should be the administration of supplemental oxygen. The causes of cyanosis can be pulmonary and nonpulmonary (see Chapter 2).

3. **Circulation/peripheral perfusion:** Assessment of circulation and peripheral perfusion can be done simultaneously during the initial patient survey. The assessment should include heart rate, central versus peripheral pulses, capillary refill time, level of consciousness, and urine output. Early identification and reversal of children with decreased poor perfusion limit the adverse outcomes associated with uncompensated shock and multiorgan dysfunction syndrome (MODS).

a. *Heart rate* is evaluated for rate, rhythm, strength, and the presence of a murmur. Chapter 3 covers in detail the clinical assessment of cardiovascular function.

b. *Central and peripheral pulses* are compared by evaluating the pressure differences and the quality between the central (i.e., femoral, carotid, axillary) and the peripheral pulses (i.e., radial, dorsalis pedis, posterior tibial).
- Narrowed pulse pressure is indicative of circulatory compromise.
- "Thready" pulse can occur as a result of a narrowing pulse pressure.
- "Wide pulse" pressures or "bounding pulses" are commonly found in early septic shock.

c. *Capillary refill* is assessed by applying pressure to an extremity and observing the time it takes for the blanched area to reperfuse. Less than 2 seconds is considered normal, whereas a capillary refill time greater than 2 seconds may indicate poor perfusion and may require medical intervention. *Flash* or *brisk capillary refill* is present when the blanched area reperfuses in less than 1 second and is considered "warm shock" (Carcillo, 2003).

- Other indicators of poor skin perfusion include pallor, mottling, peripheral cyanosis, and cold extremities.

d. *Altered level of consciousness* is often found as an early sign of shock because of inadequate cerebral perfusion (Carcillo, 2003). See Chapter 4 for a detailed review of age-specific neurologic assessments.

e. *Urine output* is an indicator of renal perfusion and is considered inadequate when it is less than 1 mL/kg per hour (Carcillo, 2003). Low urine output may be present before any other sign of decreased perfusion.

f. *Liver size* should be assessed in any patient with signs of decreased cardiac output or respiratory distress of unknown etiology. The liver edge in a healthy child should be palpated less than 3 cm below the right costal margin (see Chapter 3). If the is liver enlarged, the patient may be in cardiogenic shock (Carcillo and Fields, 2002; McCloskey et al., 1995).

4. Neurologic: A brief neurologic evaluation should be part of the ongoing assessment, together with the ABCs. Focus should be directed to several areas:

a. *Level of consciousness (LOC):*

- Age-appropriate behavior: One can expect a child to be crying or frightened; however, irritability may be an early sign of neurologic deterioration.
- Alertness, level of activity, and quality of cry are all easily assessed at the time of transport.
- Ominous signs of neurodeterioration include a child's failure to respond to parents or not crying during a noxious stimulus, such as starting an IV. Urgent medical intervention and support are warranted.
- Use of the Glasgow Coma Scale (GCS) (see Chapter 4) or AVPU (alert, voice response, pain response, unresponsive) scale provides a brief ongoing method of evaluation of LOC.

b. *Pupillary response*

- Observe for size, equality, and reactivity.
- Responses may indicate increased intracranial pressure (ICP), inadequate oxygenation, hypothermia, or ischemic encephalopathy.
- Pupillary changes may be a result of pharmacologic intervention.

c. *Seizure activity*

- Seizures are a common occurrence in transport.
- Woodward and colleagues stated that "the etiologies of seizures and treatments required can be varied and complex. Familiarity with seizure etiologies and treatment options will allow one to manage the event effectively in the short run, while safely transporting the patient for definitive evaluation and therapy" (Woodward et al., 1999).
- Comprehensive review of seizures, classification, and defining characteristics is covered in Chapter 4.

d. *Signs of increased ICP:*

- Irritability progressing to lethargy
- Decreased ability to follow commands
- Changes in response to painful stimuli
- Pupillary changes, decreasing response to light
- LOC and GCS can be used to evaluate neurologic changes.

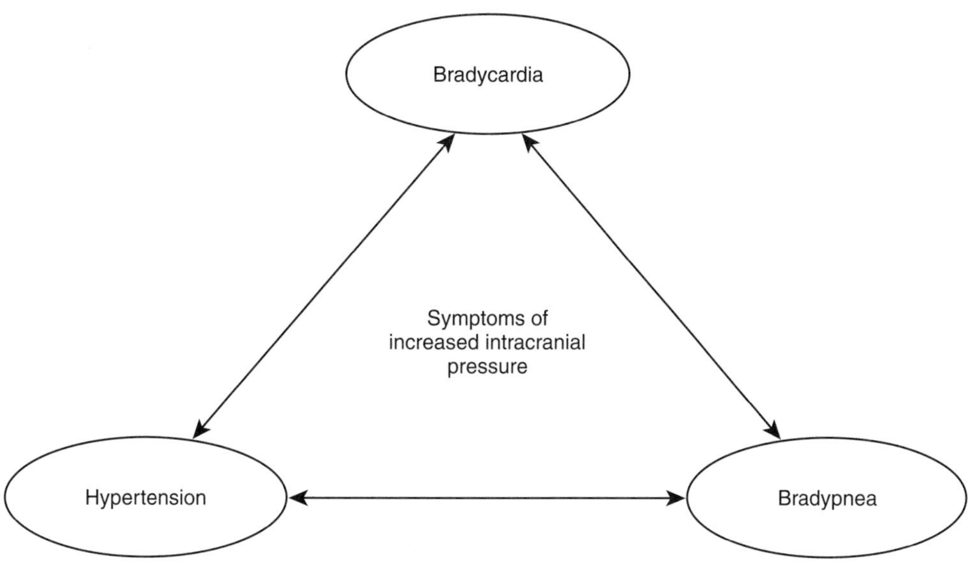

FIGURE 9-15 ■ Cushing's triad.

- Ongoing evaluation and intervention can avert later signs of increased ICP (Figure 9-15).

5. **GI assessment:** Clinical assessment should be focused on four main areas (see Chapter 7):
   - **a.** *Inspection* for abdominal distention, masses, obvious loops of bowel
   - **b.** *Auscultation* for the presence or absence of bowel sounds
   - **c.** *Palpation* to note presence of guarding or pain
   - **d.** *Percussion*
   - **e.** *Review* of recent GI losses
6. **Head-to-toe assessment**
   - **a.** *Brief* head-to-toe assessment should be made in all patients.
   - **b.** *Special areas of focus* may be included based the on reason for call as well as team's initial assessment. This may include abdominal survey or observing the skin for rashes or bruises.

E. Airway Management

The single most important intervention during the initial stabilization of any patient is establishment of a functional patent airway. Understanding the clinical indications and techniques used during the stabilization of the pediatric airway is focused around the basic anatomic difference found between the pediatric and adult patient (see Chapter 2). Some of the more common airway interventions used in the pediatric population include nasal pharyngeal airways, oropharyngeal airways, laryngeal mask airways (LMA), and endotracheal intubation. Each of these techniques has relative indications and contraindications that provide the practitioner with a useful means of deciding which maneuver is needed to ensure a safe, effective airway (Table 9-38).

1. **Nasal pharyngeal airways** (NPA, nasal trumpet) are used in the semiconscious patient with intact airway reflexes (*cough and gag*) to relieve the obstruction created by posterior pharynx. The appropriate-sized NPA is found by measuring the distance from the nares to the tragus for length and using the largest diameter that passes through the nasal passage without traumatizing the mucosa. Always remember the following:

TABLE 9-38
The Indications and Contraindications of Various Airway Adjuncts

Airway Adjuncts	Indications	Contraindications	Clinical Limitations
Nasopharyngeal	Upper-airway obstruction in the semiconscious patient Airway obstruction caused by a clinched jaw (*clonus*)	Coagulopathies Cerebral spinal fluid leaks Basilar skull fractures	No protection against aspiration Risk of laryngospasm Difficult to find pediatric sizes
Oropharyngeal	Upper-airway obstruction caused by the posterior displacement of the tongue against the pharyngeal wall As an adjunct until endotracheal intubation	Coagulopathies Functional gag reflex Consciousness	No protection against aspiration Trauma to lips and teeth Risk of laryngospasm
Laryngeal mask airway (LMA)	Airway in an unconscious patient without protective airway reflexes Difficult airway situation Respiratory failure	High pressures required to effectively ventilate Full stomach Intact airway reflexes	Limited use in patients requiring high ventilatory pressures No protection against aspiration Correct placement of the LMA is difficult to maintain when moving a patient
Endotracheal intubation	Respiratory failure Upper airway obstruction Hemodynamic instability (*shock*) Loss of protective airway reflexes (*cough and gag*) Suspected increased intracranial pressure	Intubation is often indicated by the failure or limitations of the prementioned adjuncts. Therefore the need for endotracheal intubation has only technical contraindications	Requires highly trained clinicians to perform Demands an advanced knowledge of the pediatric airway and the pharmacologic agents used during intubation

a. *Lubricate* the exterior of the tube with a water-soluble lubricant.
b. If the *airway is too large*, it may cause blanching of the exterior nares.
c. It may cause *laryngospasm, nasal ulceration, or bleeding*.

2. **Oropharyngeal airways** (OPAs, oral airway) are used to relieve the obstruction created by the base of the tongue and the posterior portion of the oropharynx, thus providing a patent pathway for ventilation to occur. Sizing of the oral airway is done by aligning the selected airway on the side of the face with the flange just outside the teeth and the tip at the angle of the mandible. Use of the OPA provides no protection against aspiration of blood, stomach contents, or other material in a patient with an altered LOC. In the pediatric transport setting, patients that tolerate an oral airway may require endotracheal intubation before transfer to protect against aspiration. Important issues to remember when caring for a patient with an oropharyngeal airway include the following:
   a. A *tongue depressor* should be used to displace the tongue downward, which facilitates placement of the oral airway.

b. If the *oral airway is too small,* it may "push" the tongue into the posterior pharynx, exacerbating the airway obstruction.
c. If the *oral airway is too large,* the distal end may force the epiglottis into the entrance of the airway, causing obstruction.
d. This type of airway is not well tolerated in patients with *intact airway reflexes.*
e. Oral airway does not protect against *aspiration.*

3. **Laryngeal mask airway** (LMA) is an airway adjunct often used in the operating room as the primary method of securing an artificial airway. It consists of a tube with a large balloon or mask at the end that seals the hypopharynx. Placement of the LMA is relatively simple and is accomplished by blindly advancing it into the pharynx until resistance is met. The balloon is then inflated and ventilation is assessed. In 2001 the American Heart Association recognized the LMA as an acceptable alternative to endotracheal intubation in unresponsive patients when performed by health care providers trained in its use. Important facts about the LMA include the following:
   a. It has *relative ease of placement* (Pennant and Walker, 1992).
   b. It is *contraindicated* in conscious patients with intact gag reflex (Zaritsky et al., 2002).
   c. *Sedation or neuromuscular blockade* may be required to prevent coughing or gagging during placement (Martin et al., 1999; Tung, 2005).
   d. It does not protect against *aspiration* (Martin et al., 1999; Tung, 2005; Zaritsky et al., 2002).
   e. It has limited use in patients who require *high ventilatory pressures* (Martin et al., 1999).
   f. *Correct placement* of the LMA is difficult to maintain when moving a patient.
   g. An LMA is an acceptable method of *initial airway stabilization;* an endotracheal tube is the recommended method of airway management during transport (Warren et al., 2004).
4. **Oral endotracheal intubation** (OETI), when performed by the skilled practitioner, is considered the airway adjunct of choice in the patient with respiratory failure. Endotracheal intubation can be complicated by a number of undesirable factors that can lead to catastrophic pulmonary and neurologic complications. These factors include prolonged hypoventilation leading to decreased cardiopulmonary reserve, increased ICP, hemodynamic instability (shock), and the potential of a full stomach. The successful endotracheal intubation is defined by the limitation of the adverse effects that may occur as a result of airway manipulation in the critically ill patient. To limit these effects, many pediatric emergency care systems have adopted the technique of rapid sequence intubation (RSI) for all patients requiring OETI (Sagarin et al., 2002). RSI is a systematic approach to OETI, which has a 3- to 5-minute period of breathing 100% oxygen, the simultaneous administration of an induction agent and neuromuscular blockade, and when intubating conditions are present, a proper sized endotracheal tube is passed into the trachea (Figure 9-16). It has been associated with higher success rate and lower rate of serious adverse effects (Sagarin et al., 2002). When assisting with the endotracheal intubation of the pediatric patient, the practitioner should remember a few important points:
   a. Always *gather* the equipment first. Intubation equipment includes a high FiO_2 delivery appliance, functional proper-sized resuscitation bag (BVM), proper-sized laryngoscope blades with functional bulbs and handle, endotracheal tubes (one proper size and one size smaller), and a stylet, monitoring equipment, suction and suction equipment, clinically indicated drugs for

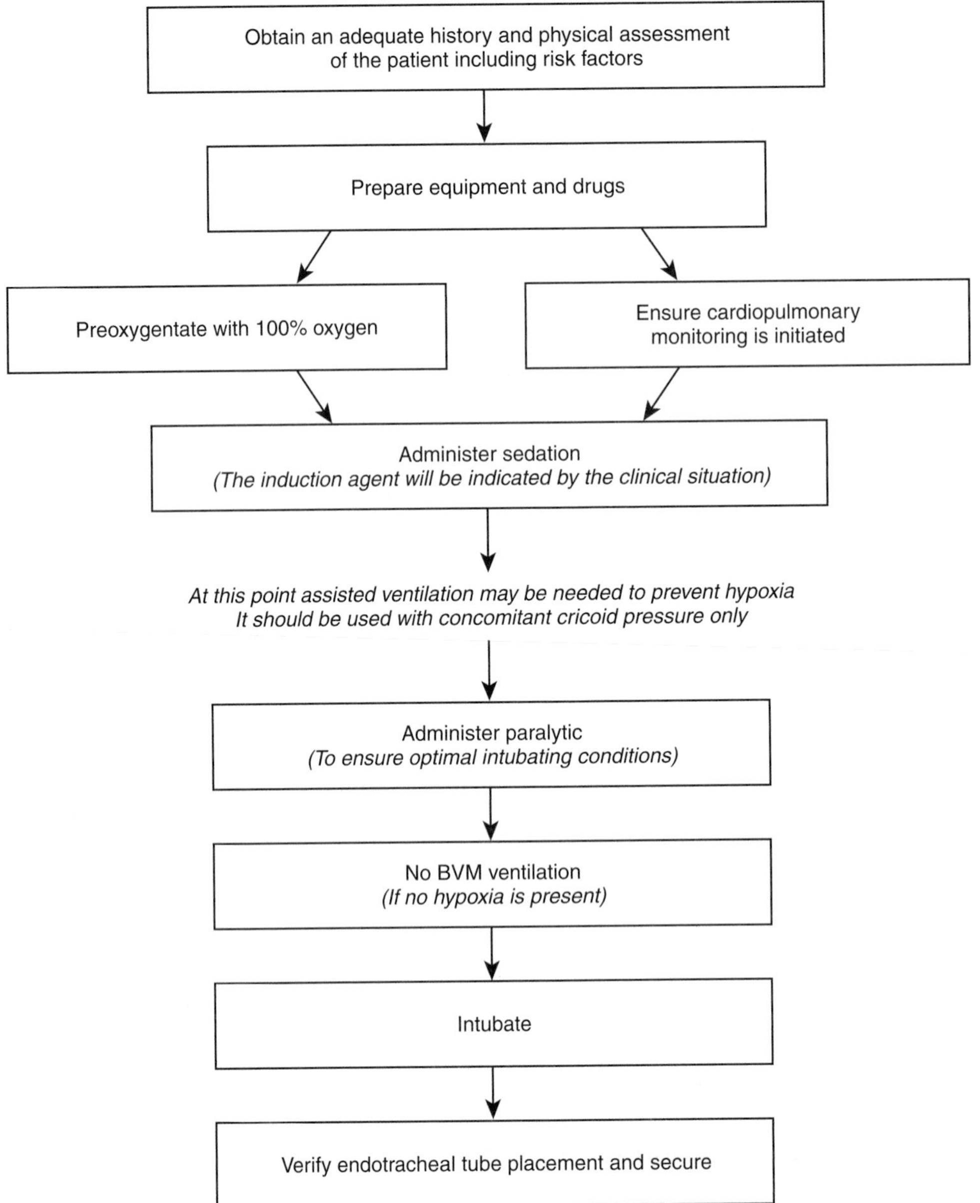

FIGURE 9-16 ■ Steps for rapid-sequence intubation.

induction and paralysis, a device to secure the endotracheal tube (ETT), and an end-tidal carbon dioxide detection device (for secondary confirmation).

b. Use *sedation* first, then neuromuscular blockade second.

c. Always *confirm* ETT placement by multiple methods. Equal bilateral breath sounds, no air entry into the stomach (epigastric region), end-tidal carbon dioxide detection, effective chest rise, oxygen saturation (Spo_2), and condensation in the ETT tube are effective ways to identify an appropriately placed ETT.

F. Vascular Access

1. **Establishing** peripheral vascular (PIV) access before transport is essential.
2. In the presence of **cardiovascular collapse,** PIV access may be difficult. PALS guidelines advocate that peripheral access be obtained rapidly. The term *rapidly*

is defined by the patient's acuity rather than by a 90-second time frame as previously published.

3. If PIV access cannot be obtained, **intraosseous (I/O) vascular access** in the proximal tibia or distal femur should be initiated. Updated 2001 guidelines now state that I/O access can be used in children older than 6 years of age.
4. **Central venous access** is not advocated as a first choice. However, it may be attempted by qualified personnel after initial access is obtained.
5. In the neonatal population, **umbilical venous access** is the preferred means of access, and it is easily located and cannulated by trained health care practitioners.

G. Fluid Resuscitation

The rapid administration of isotonic fluid is imperative for the reversal of dehydration and the treatment of low cardiac output states such as shock. The recommended crystalloid solutions are normal saline (0.9% NSS), and lactated Ringer's (Carcillo, 2003; Carcillo et al., 2002). Colloids (5% albumin) may also be used as an initial resuscitation fluid; the evidence is inconclusive, however (Carcillo, 2002; Lighthall and Pearl, 2003).

1. **Fluid administration** should be given as a rapid IV bolus of either 10 mL/kg in the neonatal population or 20 mL/kg in the pediatric population over 10 minutes (Figure 9-17) and repeated as needed.
2. After each bolus, the patient should be **reassessed**. The assessment must include heart rate, blood pressure, urine output, capillary refill, and LOC (Carcillo and Fields, 2002).
3. **Initial fluid resuscitation** may require 40 to 60 mL/kg. Recent guidelines from the American College of Critical Care Medicine recommend the initiation of vasopressor support in the patient with septic shock who does not respond to total 60 mL/kg of volume (Carcillo and Fields, 2002).
   a. *Indications* for the administration of isotonic IV in the neonatal population include a capillary refill time longer than 2 seconds, sustained tachycardia, tachypnea, hypotension, mottled or cyanotic appearance, cool skin temperature, dehydration, or narrowed pulse pressure (High and Yeatman, 2000).
   b. *Pediatric patients* who require fluid resuscitation may present with delayed capillary refill longer than 2 seconds, sustained tachycardia, tachypnea, hypotension, mottled or cyanotic appearance, cool skin temperature, dehydration, or narrowed pulse pressure (High and Yeatman, 2000).

H. Vasoactive Drug Support

Inotropic agents are useful in the treatment of shock (cardiogenic or distributive) or in any condition that myocardial function is impaired. ACCM-PALS guidelines call for rapid, stepwise execution of therapeutic interventions with the goal to restore normal blood pressure and perfusion within 1 hour of patient presentation (Han et al., 2003). Institution of these guidelines should be recommended by the command physician (Figure 9-18). Han and colleagues demonstrated that the early reversal of shock using therapeutic interventions consistent with the ACCM-PALS guidelines is associated with improved outcome when initiated by the community physician (Han et al., 2003).

1. **Inotropic agents** work through α- and β-adrenergic receptors. The hemodynamic impact of catecholamine infusions may be blunted by inadequate fluid resuscitation in shock states (Han et al., 2003).
2. **Dobutamine** may be administered to improve capillary refill in normotensive patients by improving cardiac output.
3. Hypotensive patients commonly require **epinephrine or dopamine**. Epinephrine may be more effective because children and infants commonly have an age-

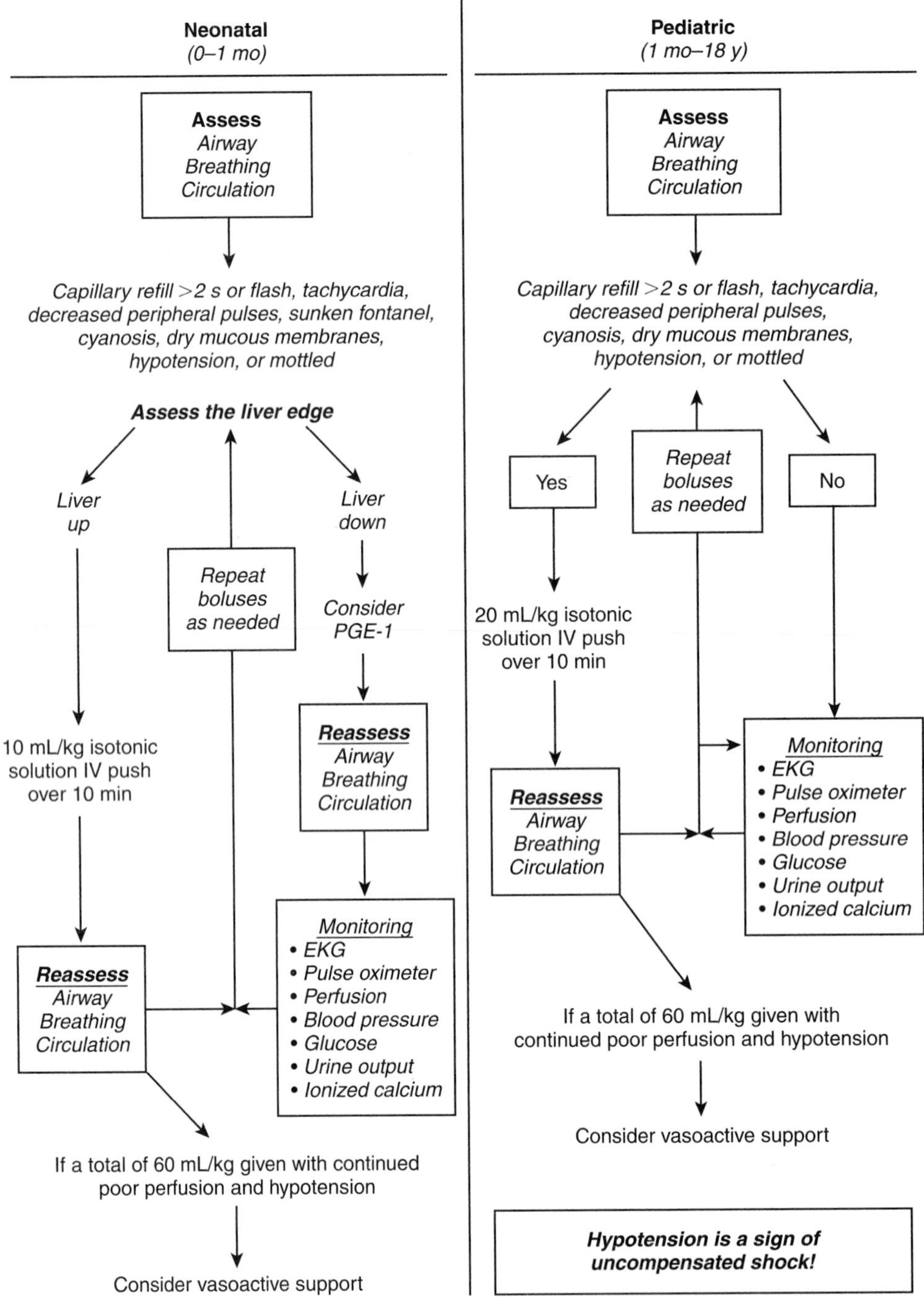

FIGURE 9-17 ■ Pathway for the initial fluid resuscitation.

specific insensibility to dopamine (Han et al., 2003). For patients in shock, intrinsic norepinephrine stores are often depleted, making dopamine an ineffective agent.

4. In warm shock, **norepinephrine** is commonly used (Carcillo, 2003).
5. **Detailed review** of agents, along with dosages, is found in Chapter 3 and in the Shock section of this chapter.

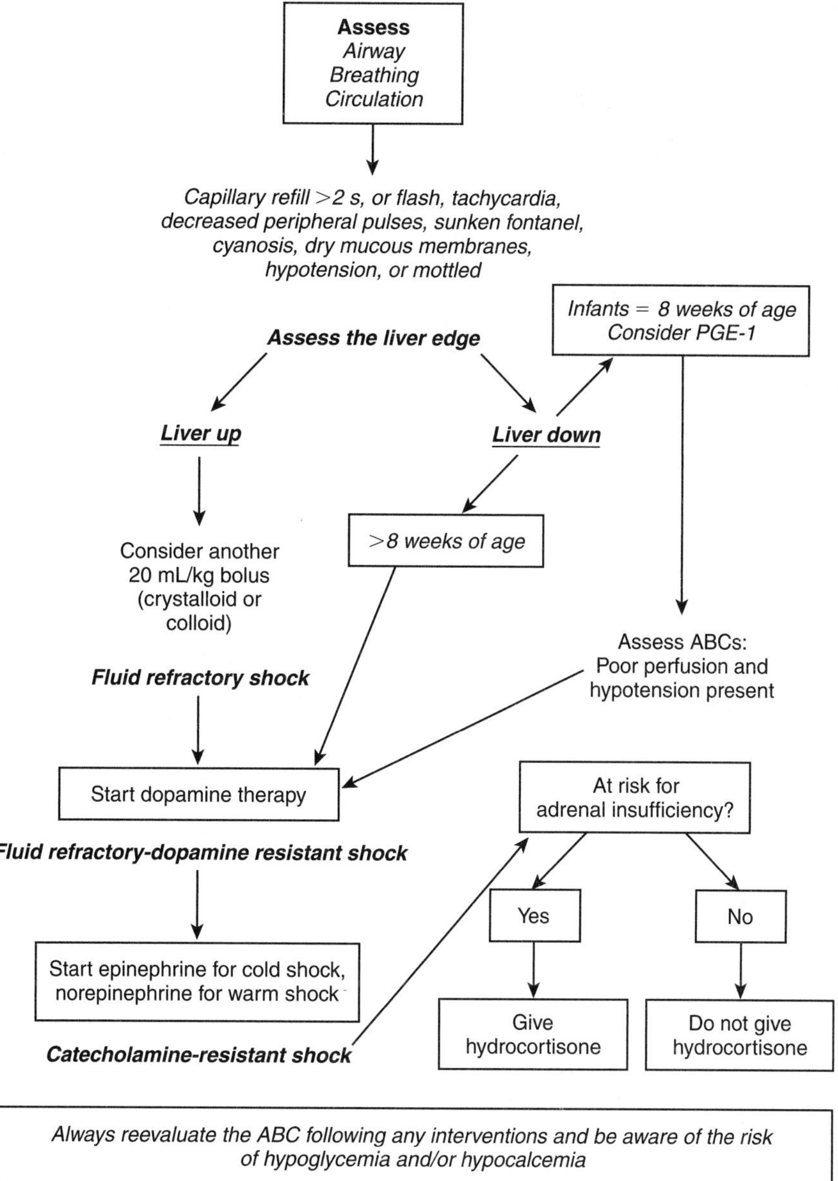

FIGURE 9-18 ■ Vasoactive support.

6. In the transport setting, **inotropes** may be administered through a peripheral vein or I/O in the absence of central venous access. The greatest effects and safety are attained via central access and should be obtained as soon as possible.

I. Glucose

Hypoglycemia can result quickly as the critically ill child depletes his or her glycogen stores. Losek demonstrated that 18% of children requiring resuscitative interventions were found to be hypoglycemic with an associated increase in mortality (Losek, 2000). Early identification of hyperglycemia or hypoglycemia can easily be accomplished with a bedside rapid glucose testing system.

1. **Hypoglycemia:** The presentation of hypoglycemia in the neonate may include seizures, altered LOC, jitteriness, apnea, irregular respirations, hypothermia,

and hypotonia. In the infant or child, it may present as coma, anxiety, headache, weakness, abdominal pain, and seizures (Schacher and Silfin, 2003). If a patient presents with a history of poor feeding or any of the associated symptoms mentioned herein, a serum or whole-blood sample is used to rule out hypoglycemia as an underlying cause. If hypoglycemia is present, a 200 mg/kg bolus of glucose should be administered (Figure 9-19).

a. *Causes of hypoglycemia* include the following:
   - **Ingestions:** Salicylates, alcohol, hypoglycemic agents, β-adrenergic blocking agents, and propranolol
   - **Infection:** Gram-negative sepsis, septic shock
   - **Endocrine disorders:** Insulin-dependent diabetes mellitus (IDDM), growth hormone deficiencies, hypothyroidism, and Addison disease. The most common complication in children with IDDM is hypoglycemia (Bhatia and Wolfsdorf, 1991).
   - **Other:** Congestive heart failure, respiratory failure, and idiopathic ketotic hypoglycemia

b. *Complications of hypoglycemia* include coma, seizures, aspiration pneumonia, and hypoxia due to the patient's inability to maintain his or her own airway (Jaimovich, 2002). Rapid identification and management of a patient with neurologic compromise will limit risk of these untoward events.

2. **Hyperglycemia/diabetic ketoacidosis (DKA):** See Chapter 6 for etiology, pathophysiology, and definitive treatment of DKA, the leading cause of morbidity and mortality in children with insulin-dependant diabetes mellitus (type 1). Death is most commonly associated (57% to 87%) with the occurrence of cerebral edema (Dunger et al., 2004). A child who presents with a long duration of symptoms, signs of circulatory compromise, altered LOC, who is under the age of 5 years, or who is a patient with "new-onset" DKA is associated with the

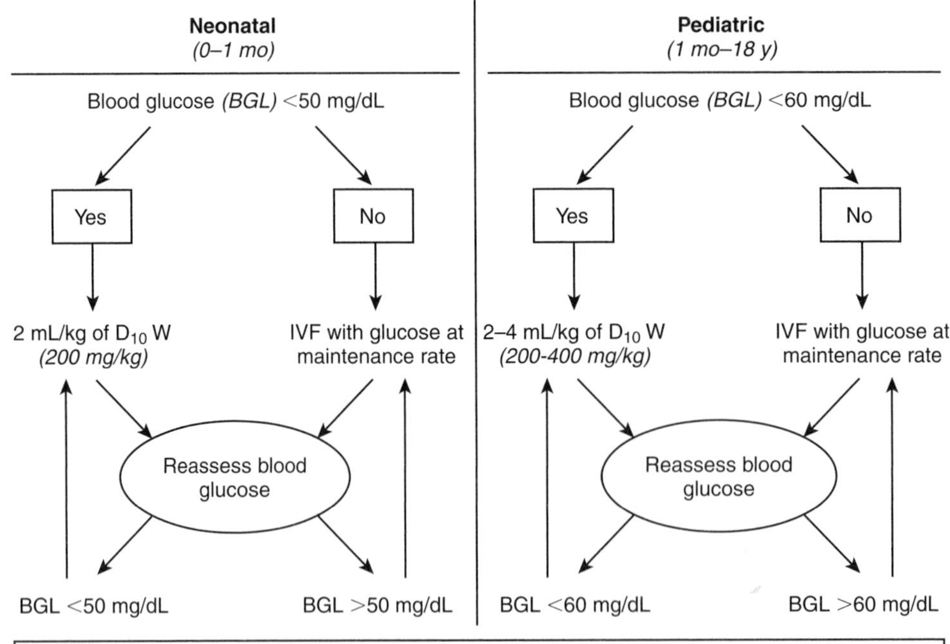

FIGURE 9-19 ■ Transport management of hypoglycemia via peripheral access.

highest risk of cerebral edema and should be managed in a PICU (White, 2003). In the transport setting, the initial treatment is focus on the reversal of hypovolemic shock secondary to the severe dehydration, which is a major component of this disease process (Figure 9-20).

a. *Causes of hyperglycemia* include the following:

- Type 1: Insulin-dependent diabetes mellitus (IDDM) is an autoimmune disease that is most commonly found in infants and children. Type 1 is associated with DKA.

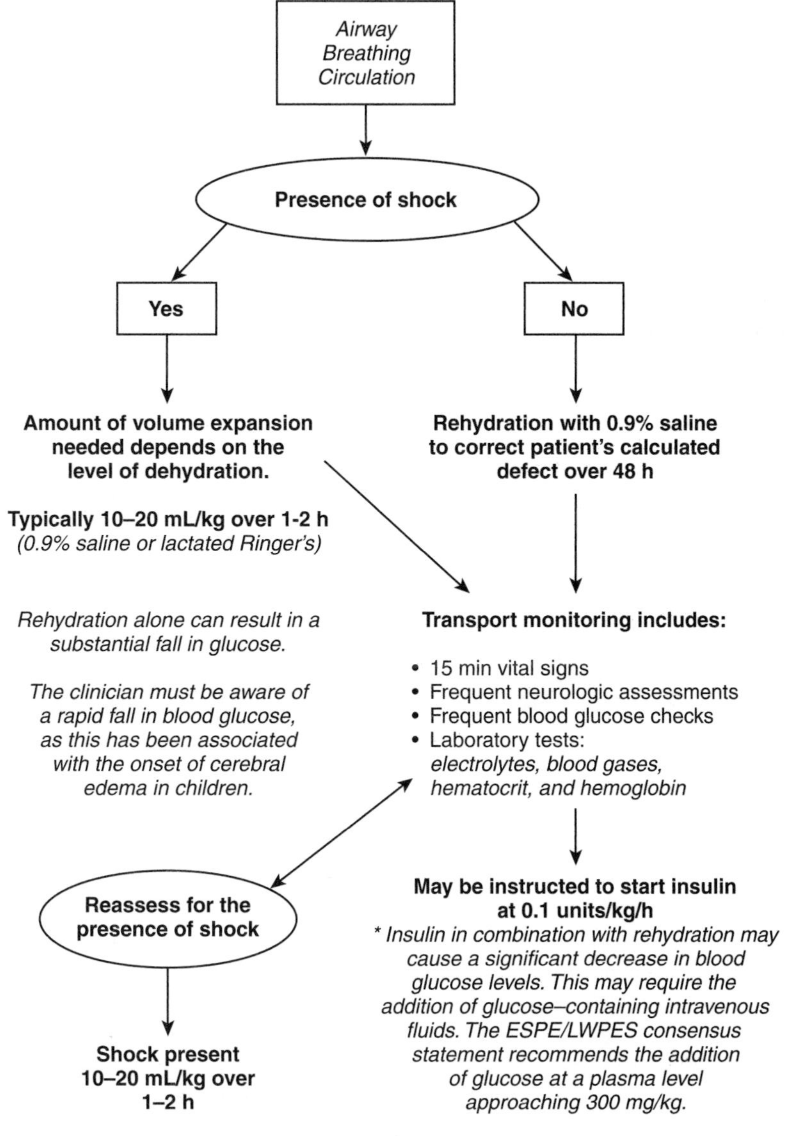

The figure is merely an example of the initial stabilization of a pediatric patient with diabetic ketoacidosis. The dosages and specific treatment regimens can be found in the *ESPE/LWPES consensus statement on diabetic ketoacidosis in children and adolescents (Dunger 2004).*

FIGURE 9-20 ■ Initial stabilization of a patient with diabetic ketoacidosis.

- Type 2: Non–insulin-dependent diabetes mellitus (NIDDM) is most often found in adults and is related to insulin resistance.

b. *Associated complications* of hyperglycemia/DKA include cerebral edema (*most common*), heart disease, myocardial infarction, adult respiratory distress syndrome, thrombosis, aspiration pneumonia, pulmonary embolism, and rhabdomyolysis (White, 2003).

J. Respiratory Care

Respiratory distress may be caused by a variety of pulmonary and nonpulmonary pathologies (see Chapter 2). Nonpulmonary causes include sepsis, congenital cardiac disease, and shock. Pulmonary pathophysiology can be divided into two distinct areas of origin:

- Upper airway, including croup, epiglottitis, foreign-body aspiration, tracheal malacia, subglottic stenosis (*acquired and congenital*), and vocal cord paralysis
- Disorders affecting the lower airway and the lung parenchyma, including asthma, bronchiolitis, bronchomalacia, pneumonia, acute respiratory distress syndrome (ARDS), hyaline membrane disease (*neonatal RDS*), and aspiration.

Patient assessment should be aimed at identifying the origin of respiratory distress.

1. **Supplemental oxygen delivery** in the pediatric transport setting requires knowledge of the basic principles of oxygen therapy as well as the baseline arterial saturation for patients with congenital heart disease (AARC Guidelines, 2002). A concise report of the patient's medical history should reveal the presence of any underlying cyanotic heart disease.
   a. The previously healthy child who demonstrates signs of *respiratory distress*, hypoxia, cyanosis, and shock should be administered supplemental oxygen as the first step.
   b. The *proper device* for oxygen delivery is based on the patient's age, size, fraction of inspired oxygen (FiO_2) needed, and inspiratory flow rate (Table 2-11).
2. **Aerosolized medications** have become the treatment of choice in the pediatric patient presenting with an increased work of breathing (WOB) secondary to acute reversible airway obstruction. Medications are indicated, depending on the origin of the airway obstruction (i.e., upper versus lower airway). Table 9-39 includes a synopsis of commonly used pharmacologic agents for the acute treatment of airway obstruction. Clinicians must assess known drug allergies or past adverse drug reactions.
   a. Selection of a delivery method is based on the severity of illness and the duration of treatment needed to electively reverse acute airway obstruction. Both small-volume *(intermittent)* and large-volume (*continuous*) nebulizers can be used to administered medications via a mask, oxyhood (*infant*), or an artificial airway (Bower et al., 1995).
   - **Small-volume nebulizer** can be used to deliver intermittent drug aerosol treatments for either acute exacerbation of or the daily therapeutic delivery of maintenance medications. In the emergency treatment of bronchospasm, this type of nebulizer can be used to deliver multiple single-dose treatments as needed.
     - Robertson and colleagues describe the safe and effective use of multiple nebulized low-dose albuterol (0.15 mg/kg initially followed by 0.05 mg/kg) treatments in pediatric patients with acute asthma when given every 20 minutes for a total of six treatments (Robertson et al., 1985).

TABLE 9-39
Medications for the Acute Treatment of Airway Obstruction

Pharmacologic Agent	Mode of Action	Indications	Contraindications	Complications
Racemic epinephrine *(Vaponephrine)*	Equal α and β adrenergic stimulation Causes both vasoconstriction and bronchodilation	Bronchospasm Upper airway inflammation	Hypersensitivity to epinephrine or other components of the drug suspension Cardiac arrhythmias	Bronchospasm Palpitations Cough Muscle tremors Nervousness Tachycardia
Albuterol sulfate *(Ventolin, Proventil)*	β_2-adrenergic stimulation Little β_1 receptor activity	Bronchospasm	Hypersensitivity to albuterol or other components of the drug suspension Congestive heart failure Hypertension	Bronchospasm Palpitations Cough Muscle tremors Nervousness Tachycardia
Levalbuterol *(Xopenex)*	Single isomer β_2-agonist	Bronchospasm	Hypersensitivity to albuterol or other components of the drug suspension	Tachycardia Hypertension Anxiety Headache Chest Pain Nausea
Ipratropium bromide *(Atrovent)*	Anticholinergic agent that causes bronchodilation by parasympathetetic pathways	Used in conjunction with β_2-agonist for the treatment of bronchospasm	Hypersensitivity to ipratropium or other components of the drug suspension	Dry mouth Blurred vision Nausea Palpitations Cough Bronchospasm

- Multiple doses of ipratropium bromide (Atrovent) added to frequent high doses of nebulized albuterol might aid in the treatment of severe bronchospasm (Schuh et al., 1995).
- *Nebulized racemic epinephrine* (Vaponephrine) has become a common treatment for children with upper-airway obstruction secondary to croup (Klassen, 1999). It also has been found to be effective in the treatment of bronchiolitis. Its positive effect in infants with bronchiolitis has been demonstrated by improvement in clinical scores and a decrease in airway resistance (Bertrand et al., 2001; Numa et al., 2001).

- **Large-volume nebulizers** are used to deliver aerosolized medications continuously over an extended period. Its use has been associated with a more rapid clinical improvement in children with severe status asthmaticus compared with intermittent delivery of the same drug concentration in the PICU (Papo, 1995).

3. **Adjunctive therapies**
   a. Glucocorticoids in conjunction with aerosolized medication have been found to be beneficial in the treatment of acute upper-airway and lower-airway obstruction alike. They may be administered either by mouth (PO), intramuscularly (IM), IV, or by nebulization (Klassen, 1999; Volovitz and Nussinovitch, 2002). The effect of glucocorticoids is not immediate; thus the

initial treatment of these patients should focus on stabilizing the airway, breathing, and circulation.

- **Dexamethasone** (Decadron) is most commonly used to treat upper-airway inflammation. Strong evidence has been published, demonstrating a more rapid clinical improvement, shortened hospital stays, and a significant reduction in the rate of endotracheal intubation in patients who receive dexamethsone versus those who do not (Klassen, 1999).
- **Methylprednisolone** (Solu-Medrol), when given as an initial bolus of 2 mg/kg followed by 1 mg/kg every 6 hours, improves clinical index scores, facilitates recovery from bronchospasm, and decreases the rate of relapse in children with status asthmaticus (Younger et al., 1987).
- **Budesonide** (Pulmicort) has been proven an effective alternative to oral steroids as maintenance therapy in asthma. Nebulization of budesonide results in a high percent of the drug being deposited in the upper airway. With this in mind, Klassen and colleagues investigated its use in the treatment of children with croup and found a more rapid clinical improvement, a lower rate of hospitalization, and shorter stays in the emergency department compared with use of a placebo (Klassen et al., 1994).

b. IV medications may be indicated in the patient with refractory bronchospasm and impending respiratory failure. Their use must include continuous cardiopulmonary monitoring and frequent clinical assessments to monitor respiratory and neurologic status.

- **Terbutaline** is the IV β-agonist of choice in the United States. It is most commonly used in patients who do not respond to continuous nebulized treatment and is initiated as an initial loading dose of 5 to 10 mcg/kg over 5 minutes. Recommended dosages for continuous infusion of terbutaline are 0.1 to 6.0 mcg/kg per minute (Heinrich et al., 2001; Stephanopoulos et al., 1998).
  - Adverse reactions to terbutaline include arrhythmias, tachycardia, hypertension, hypotension, nausea, and palpitations.
- **Magnesium sulfate** administration via either a single bolus or continuous infusion may be beneficial in the treatment of refractory bronchospasm (Bloch et al., 1995; Ciarallo and Fields, 1996; Okayama et al., 1987). Boluses are most commonly given in doses between 25 and 75 mg/kg over 20 minutes (Heinrich et al., 2001). Glover and colleagues describe the safety of continuous infusions at a rate of 25 mg/kg per hour in children who weigh less than 30 kg and 20 mg/kg per hour in children who weigh more than 30 kg (Glover et al., 2002).
  - Adverse reactions to intravenous magnesium sulfate include nausea, flushing, somnolence, vision changes, and muscle weakness (Glover et al., 2002). The most severe effects occur at a concentration of greater than 12 mg/dL and include respiratory depression and arrhythmias (DeNicola et al., 1994).

4. Mechanical ventilation

a. *Indications:* The noise, vibration, poor lighting, and lack of assistive personnel make advanced airway procedures extremely difficult while in the transport vehicle. For this reason, the indications for the initiation of mechanical ventilation in the transport setting tend to be more aggressive and include, but are not limited to, cardiac or respiratory arrest, combativeness (safety), airway obstruction, impaired control of ventilation, impending respiratory failure, inadequate gas exchange, fluid refractory shock, or circulatory failure (McCloskey and Orr, 1995).

b. *Ensuring effective ventilation* in the mechanically ventilated patient is an essential skill in the transport setting. The movement associated with transport as well as multiple patient transfers add to the increased risk of ETT displacement.

- A rapid visual inspection of the child's chest should reveal a gentle symmetrical rise and fall with each mechanical breath. The unilateral rise of a patient's chest may be the first sign of either a mainstem intubation or a pneumothorax. If this occurs the clinician should perform a physical assessment of the patient. A radiograph or illumination of the chest may also aid in the identification of a pneumothorax.
- Auscultation of the patient's chest and abdomen should be done post intubation as part of initial airway assessment. If they have already been intubated by the referring hospital the team should assess the patient's breaths sounds immediately upon arrival.
- A disposable end-tidal carbon dioxide (CO_2) detector is a useful tool for identifying whether the ETT is in the trachea. The CO_2 detector is placed on the 15-mm flange of the ETT while it is in the trachea, and then the patient is given a manual breath. The presence of exhaled CO_2 will result in a color change inside the CO_2 detector. PALS guidelines recommend giving six artificial breaths before assessing color change on the CO_2 detector (Zaritsky et al., 2002). If there is no color change when the CO_2 detector is in place, the ETT is in the esophagus, the patient has little or no pulmonary perfusion, or the ETT is completely occluded.
- Use of continuous end-tidal CO_2 monitoring may aid in identifying changes in mechanical ventilation during transport. Its usefulness has been demonstrated in identifying esophageal intubations, displacement of the artificial airway, and adjunctive in monitoring mechanically ventilated pediatric patients in an environment with excessive noise (Bhende et al., 1995). The use of end-tidal CO_2 monitors should not replace the use of blood gas analysis.

c. *Trouble shooting:* Use of the DOPE algorithm (Table 9-40) may aid in identifying situations that might cause acute patient decompensation during mechanical ventilation (Zaritsky et al., 2002).

d. *Humidity:* Inadequate humidification in the patient with an artificial airway can cause damage to tracheal epithelium, reduce motility of cilia, and result in excessive mucus production and plugging (Barhart and Czervinske, 1995). A heat and moisture exchanger (HME) is a lightweight hygroscopic condenser that adds humidity by retaining moisture from patient's exhaled gas.

- HME may add resistance to the airway, thus increasing the WOB in the spontaneously breathing patient.
- HME should be used with caution in patients with excessive pulmonary secretions because there have been reports of ETTs becoming completely obstructed with thickened mucus (Barhart and Czervinske, 1995).
- It is important to ensure the proper-sized HME for the patient because this may add a significant amount of dead space to the ventilation circuit, elevating the patient's $PaCO_2$. If the HME is too small, it will add resistance to the ventilation system.

K. Thermoregulation

The maintenance of normothermia in the transport setting is complex because of the constant changing physical environment and the increased risk of ineffective thermoregulation of the critically ill child.

TABLE 9-40
Algorithm for Trouble Shooting a Mechanically Ventilated Patient in Respiratory Distress

D.O.P.E.
D = Displacement of the airway
O = Obstruction of the airway
P = Pneumothorax
E = Equipment failure

Data from AHA PALS Handbook.

TABLE 9-41
Normal Neonatal and Infant Temperature Values

Temperature Site	Celsius (°C)	Fahrenheit (°F)
Skin	36-36.5	96.8-97.7
Axillary	36.5-37.0	97.7-98.6
Rectal	36.5-37.0	97.7-98.8

Information from McCloskey KA, Orr RA, editors: *Pediatric transport medicine.* St Louis, 1995, Mosby.

1. **Hypothermia**
   a. The neonatal or infant population is at a greater risk for hypothermia because they have a limited nutritional reserve, a large surface area-to-body ratio, extremely low birth weight, and increased metabolic demands (McCloskey and Orr, 1995). These risks are especially elevated in the infant who is unconscious, sedated, or immobilized (Curley and Moloney-Harmon, 2001). The following should be considered in the stabilization of the hypothermic infants:
   - Ensure that the infant is completely dry and remove any wet clothing or linen.
   - Place a stocking cap on the infant's head or swaddle the infant in a blanket.
   - Transport the infant (i.e., one who weighs less than 10 lbs) in a double-walled incubator. A heat shield, insulated incubator cover, or a heating mattress/pack may be needed to maintain a stable thermal environment within the incubator.
   - Monitor both skin and axillary temperatures throughout transport (Table 9-41). Skin temperature is monitored by placing a skin-temperature probe directly onto the infant's abdomen (McCloskey and Orr, 1995).

   b. Pediatric hypothermia may be caused by environmental exposure, infection, shock, surgery, traumatic brain injury, congenital nervous system malformation, and medications such as vasopressor, sedatives, or anesthetics (Curley and Moloney-Harmon, 2001). The following will aid in the reversal of hypothermia in the pediatric patient:
   - Remove all wet clothing and linens.
   - Cover the patient in warm blankets, and use a radiant insulated blanket to prevent continued heat loss during transport.
   - Resuscitation of a patient in cardiopulmonary arrest should continue until the patient's core temperature reaches 30°C.

c. Hypothermia impairs both myocardial function and vascular tone, which may lead to profound hemodynamic collapse. Profound hypotension may occur from the rewarming process secondary to the peripheral vasodilation (Curley and Moloney-Harmon, 2001).

2. **Hyperthermia**

a. Clinical hyperthermia is a state of sustained elevated body temperature greater than 37.8°C orally or 38.8°C rectally. As in hypothermia, the causes of hyperthermia are either internal or environmental in nature. Internal causes include fever (*most common*), malignant hyperthermia, traumatic brain injury, central nervous system malformation medications (*phenytoin, histamine blockers, and antibiotics*), or heat-related illnesses (Curley and Moloney-Harmon, 2001). Environmental causes include exposure to extreme elevated ambient temperatures and accidental overheating. Treatment of hyperthermia may include, but is not limited, to the following:

- Antipyretic therapy such as aspirin, acetaminophen, and ibuprofen effectively "reset the hypothalamic set-point" to normal limits (Curley and Moloney-Harmon, 2001).
- Aspirin has been associated with gastritis, GI bleeding, diminished platelet function, and Reye syndrome (Curley and Moloney-Harmon, 2001).
- The use of external cooling may aid in controlling elevated body temperature in the transport setting.
- When fever is associated with suspected bacteremia, treatment will include antibiotics (Curley and Moloney-Harmon, 2001).

CONCLUSION

The goal of any pediatric transport system is to provide an extension of the critical care unit to the referring facilities, ensure a timely and safe transport to a pediatric critical care center without an increase in morbidity or mortality, and to provide the highest quality of care for critically ill infants and children who require interfacility transport. The first step in this process is the initial stabilization, which must begin at the referring facility before the request for transfer. Stabilization begins with a thorough assessment of the child's airway, breathing, and circulation. Once identified, airway compromise, ineffective respiration, stabilization of circulation, and correction of hypoglycemia must be treated without delay. Using the American Heart Association's Pediatric Life Support (PALS) course guidelines may be beneficial in both assessing and treating the critically ill child. The second step is the transfer to a facility specializing in pediatric care. This transfer is often complicated by the severity of illness and the innate increased risk of mortality found in the transport setting. Children needing medical transport often require more advanced procedures such as endotracheal intubation, inotropic support, and continuous cardiovascular monitoring (invasive and noninvasive), which warrants a crew with an in-depth understanding of pediatric disease pathology and advanced care.

REFERENCES

Multiple Trauma

Administration on Children, Youth, and Families, U.S. Department of Health and Human Services: *Child Maltreatment 2000*. Washington, DC, 2000, U.S. Government Printing Office. Available at http://www.acf.hhs.gov/programs/cb/publications/cm00/outcover.htm. Accessed November 1, 2002.

Alexander RC, Levitt CJ, Smith WL: Abusive head trauma. In Reece RM, Ludwig S, editors: *Child abuse: medical diagnosis and management,* ed 2. Philadelphia, 2001, Lippincott, Williams & Wilkins, pp 47-80.

American College of Surgeons Committee on Trauma: *Advanced trauma life support,* ed 6. Chicago, 1997, American College of Surgeons, p 293.

American Urological Association: *Pediatric considerations: reconstruction and trauma-bladder trauma.* Available at http://urologyhealth.org/pediatric/index.cfm?cat=10&topic=36. Accessed February 8, 2004.

Anand KJS: Consensus statement for the prevention and management of pain in the newborn. *Arch Pediatr Adolesc Med* 155:173-180, 2001.

Arnold WC: Myoglobinuria. Available at http://www.emedicine.com/ped/topic1535.htm. Accessed February 22, 2005. Updated 2003.

Auerbach PS, Donner HJ, Weiss EA: *Field guide to wilderness medicine.* St Louis, 1999, Mosby.

Barkin RM: Hypothermia and frostbite. In Barkin RM, Rosen P, editors: *Emergency pediatrics,* ed 5. St Louis, 1999, Mosby, pp 335-341.

Bates-Jensen G, Wethe J: Acute surgical wound management. In Sussman C, Bates-Jensen B, editors: *Wound care: a collaborative practice manual for physical therapists and nurses.* Gaithersburg, Md, 1998, Aspen Publishers, p. 230.

Bernardo L, Waggoner T: Pediatric trauma. In Sheehy S, editor: *Emergency nursing: principles and practice,* ed 3. St Louis, 1992, Mosby, pp 683-690.

Brenner RA, Trumble AC, Smith GS et al: Where children drown: United States, 1995. *Pediatrics* 108(1): 85-89, 2001.

Brinker D: Pain management. In Maloney-Harmon PA, Czerwinsk SJ, editors: *Nursing care of the pediatric trauma patient,* Philadelphia, 2003, W. B. Saunders, pp 118-137.

Brinker MD, Joosten KFM, Liem O, et al: Adrenal insufficiency in meningococcal sepsis: bio-available cortisol levels and impact of interleukine-6 levels and intubation with etomidate on adrenal function and mortality. *J Clin Endocrinol Metab* June 28, 2005.

Brokmeyer D: *Pediatric spinal cord and spinal column trauma.* The American Association of Neurological Surgeons/Congress of Neurological Surgeons, 1999. Available at http://www.neurosurgery.org/sections/pediatric/Ped_spine.html. Accessed February 8, 2004.

Centers for Disease Control and Prevention, National Center for Injury Prevention and Control (CDC): *Childhood injury fact sheet.* Available at http://www.cdc.gov/ncipc/factsheets/childh.htm. Accessed February 6, 2004.

Centers for Disease Control and Prevention, National Center for Injury Prevention and Control (CDC): *Child maltreatment.* Available at http://www.cdc.gov/ncipc/factsheets/cmfacts.htm. Accessed February 4, 2004.

Centers for Disease Control and Prevention, National Center for Injury Prevention and Control (CDC): *Facts on adolescent injury.* Available at http://www.cdc.gov/ncipc/factsheets/adoles.htm. Accessed February 4, 2004.

Centers for Disease Control and Prevention, National Center for Injury Prevention and Control (CDC): *Injury fact sheet.* Available at http://www.cdc.gov/ncipc/cmprfact.htm. Accessed February 4, 2004.

Chandy D: *Drowning and near-drowning: prevention and treatment.* Available at http://www.thedoctorwillseeyounow.com/articles/other/drown_7. Accessed February 8, 2004.

Chapman S, Cornwall J, Righetti J, et al: Preventing dog bites in children: randomized controlled trial of an education intervention. *BMJ* 320(7248):1512-1513, 2000.

Chase D: Maxillofacial injuries. In Buntain W, editor: *Management of pediatric trauma.* Philadelphia, 1995, W. B. Saunders, pp. 201-218.

Conway A: Developmental and psychosocial considerations. In Thomas DO, Bernardo LM, Herman B, editors: *Core curriculum for pediatric emergency nursing.* Sudbury, Mass, 2003, Jones and Bartlett Publishers, pp 34-48.

Corriere J: Urinary tract injuries. In Ford EG, Andrassy RJ, editors: *Pediatric trauma.* Philadelphia, 1994, W. B. Saunders, 223-243.

Creel J: Mechanisms of injury due to motion. In Campbell J, editor: *Basic trauma life support: advanced prehospital care,* ed 3. Englewood Cliffs, NJ, 1997, Prentice Hall, pp 1-20.

Crowther M, McCourt K: Get the edge on deep vein thrombosis. *Nurs Manage* 35(1):21-29, 2004.

Cumings C, Byrum D: The beat goes on: cardiac pacers—how to use them, what to know about them. *Am J Nurs* 101(suppl): 9-12, 2001.

Czerwinski SJ, Moloney-Harmon PA: Intentional injuries. In Moloney-Harmon PA, Czerwinski SJ, editors: *The care of the pediatric trauma patient*. St Louis, 2003, W. B. Saunders, pp 152-159.

D'Heere M, Houghton D, Ginzburg E: Fat embolism syndrome. *J Trauma Nurs* 6(3):73-76, 1999.

Dickman CA, Zabranski JM, Rekate HL, et al: Spinal cord injuries in children without radiographic abnormalities. *West J Med* 158:67, 1993.

Duke JC, Rosenberg SG: Anesthesia. In Mattox KL, Feliciano DV, Moore EE, editors: *Trauma,* ed 4. New York, 2000, McGraw-Hill Health Professionals Division, pp 311-348.

Dunmez, O: *Crush syndrome*. Available at http:www.uninet.edu/cin2003/conf/donmez/donmez.html. Accessed February 3, 2006.

Eastern Association for the Surgery of Trauma: *Trauma guidelines*. Available at http://www.east.org. Accessed February 22, 2005.

Emergency Cardiac Care Committee and Subcommittees, American Heart Association: Guidelines for cardiopulmonary resuscitation and emergency cardiac care. *JAMA* 268(16):2262-2275, 1992.

Fabian TC, Croce MA: Abdominal trauma, including indications for celiotomy. In Mattox KL, Feliciano DV, Moore EE, editors: *Trauma,* ed 4. New York, 2000, McGraw-Hill Health Professionals Division, pp 583-602.

Finkel MA, DeJong AR: Medical findings in child sexual abuse. In Reece RM, Ludwig S, editors: *Child abuse medical diagnosis and management,* ed 2. Philadelphia, 2001, Lippincott, Williams & Wilkins, pp. 207-286.

Fort CW: How to combat 3 deadly trauma complications. *Nursing* 33(5): 58-63, 2003.

Frank JB, Lim CK, Flynn JM: The efficiency of magnetic resonance imaging in pediatric cervical spine clearance. *Spine* 27(11):1176-1179, 2002.

Fulton D: Early recognition of Munchausen syndrome by proxy. *Crit Care Nurs Quart* 23(2):35-42, 2000.

Goldhaber SZ, Elliot CG: Acute pulmonary embolism: part I: epidemiology, pathophysiology, and diagnosis. *Circulation* 108(22):2726-2729, 2003a.

Goldhaber SZ, Elliot CG: Acute pulmonary embolism: part II: risk stratification, treatment, and prevention. *Circulation* 108(23):2834-2838, 2003b.

Haley K: Initial trauma assessment and intervention. In Thomas DO, Bernardo LM, Herman B, editors: *Core curriculum for pediatric emergency nursing*. Sudbury, Mass, 2003, Jones and Bartlett Publishers, pp 409-421.

Haley K, Schenkel K: Thoracic trauma. In Thomas DO, Bernardo LM, Herman B, editors: *Core curriculum for pediatric emergency nursing*. Sudbury, Mass, 2003, Jones and Bartlett Publishers, pp 445-449.

Hensinger RN: Complications of fractures in children. In Green NE, Swiontkowski MF, editors: *Skeletal trauma in children,* ed 2, vol 3. Philadelphia, 1998, Saunders, pp 121-147.

Holliday SM, Benfield P, Plosker GL: Fosphenytoin. *Pharmacoeconomics* 14(6): 685-690, 1998.

Hodge D, Trecklenburgh FW: Bites and stings. In Fleisher GR, Ludwig S, editors: *Textbook of pediatric emergency medicine,* ed 4. Philadelphia, 2000, Lippincott, Williams & Wilkins, pp 979-998.

Hoover D, Belinger M: Genitourinary trauma. In Ehrlich F, Heldrich F, Tepas J, editors: *Pediatric emergency medicine*. Rockville, Md, 1987, Aspen Publishers, pp 307-313.

Hughes LM, Corbo-Richert B: Munchausen syndrome by proxy: literature review and implications for critical care nurses. *Crit Care Nurse* 19:71-77, 1999.

Isben LM, Koch T: Submersion and asphyxial injury. *Crit Care Med* 30(11 suppl):S402-S408, 2002.

Jurkovich GJ: The duodenum and pancreas. In Mattox KL, Feliciano DV, Moore EE, editors: *Trauma,* ed 4. New York, 2000, McGraw-Hill Health Professionals Division, pp 735-762.

Kamerling SN: Thoracic injury. In Moloney-Harmon PA, Czerwinski SJ, editors: *The care of the pediatric trauma patient.* St Louis, 2003, W. B. Saunders, pp 207-226.

Karlin NJ: Munchausen syndrome by proxy. *Brattleboro Retreat Psychiatry Review*, 1995, pp 1-7. Available at http://www.brateretreat.org/btpr/v4nl.html. Accessed October 12, 1999.

Kelley SJ: Child abuse and neglect. In Thomas DO, Bernardo LM, Herman B, editors: *Core curriculum for pediatric emergency nursing.* Sudbury, Mass, 2003, Jones and Bartlett, pp 573-584.

Laskowski-Jones L: Responding to summer emergencies. *Dimens Crit Care Nurs* 19(4):2-12, 2000.

Laskowski-Jones L: Responding to winter emergencies. *Dimens Crit Care Nurs* 18(6):13-20, 1999.

Lewin JD, Murthy V: Humeral diaphysis of midshaft fractures. In Hoppenfeld S, Murthy VL, editors: *Treatment and rehabilitation of fractures.* Philadelphia, 2000, Lippincott, Williams & Wilkins, pp 22-190.

Lexi-Comp Formulex. Hudson, Ohio, 2005, Lexi-Comp.

Liebman MA: Initial resuscitation of the pediatric trauma victim. In Moloney-Harmon PA, Czerwinski SJ, editors: *The care of the pediatric trauma patient.* St Louis, 2000, W. B. Saunders, pp 62-70.

Ludwig S: Visceral injury manifestations of child abuse. In Reece RM, Ludwig S, editors: *Child abuse: medical diagnosis and management,* ed 2. Philadelphia, 2001, Lippincott, Williams & Wilkins, pp 157-175.

Ludwig S: Child abuse. In Fleisher GR, Ludwig S, editors: *Textbook of pediatric emergency medicine,* ed 4. Philadelphia, 2000, Lippincott, Williams & Wilkins, pp 1669-1704.

MacKenzie EJ, Fowler CJ: Epidemiology. In Mattox KL, Feliciano DV, Moore EE, editors: *Trauma,* ed 4. New York, 2000, McGraw-Hill Health Professionals Division, pp 21-40.

Manworren RCB, Hynan LS: Clinical validation of FLACC: preverbal patient pain scale. *Pediatr Nurs* 29(2):140-146, 2003.

Mason KJ: Pediatric musculoskeletal trauma. In Moloney-Harmon PA, Czerwinski SJ, editors: *The care of the pediatric trauma patient.* St Louis, 2003, W. B. Saunders, pp 248-275.

McSwain NE: Kinematics of trauma. In Mattox KL, Feliciano DV, Moore EE, editors: *Trauma,* ed 4. New York, 2000, McGraw-Hill Health Professionals Division, pp 127-151.

Maternal and Child Health Bureau: *Child health USA 2002.* Available at http://www.mchb.hrsa.gov\chusa02\main_pages\page_03.htm. Accessed February 18, 2004.

Meister J, Reddy K: Rhabdomyolysis: an overview. *Am J Nurs* 102(2):75-79, 2002.

Merkel SI, Voepel-Lewis T, Shayevitz JR, et al: The FLACC: a behavioral scale for scoring postoperative pain in young children. *Pediatr Nurs* 23:292-297, 1997.

Muir R, Town DA: Spinal cord injury. In Moloney-Harmon PA, Czerwinski SJ, editors: *The care of the pediatric trauma patient.* St Louis, 2003, W. B. Saunders, pp 248-275.

Munchausen Syndrome by Proxy Survivors Network. Available at http://www.mbpsnetwork.com/. Accessed March 10, 2004.

Myers JEB: The legal system and child protection. In Myers JEB, Berliner L, Briere J et al., editors: *The APSAC handbook on child maltreatment,* ed 2. Thousand Oaks, Calif, 2000, Sage Publications, pp 305-327.

Nance ML, Branas CC, Stafford PW et al: Nonintracranial fatal firearm injuries in children: implications for treatment. *J Trauma Inj Infect Crit Care* 55(4):631-635, 2004.

National Clearinghouse on Child Abuse and Neglect Information: *Child maltreatment 2003: summary of key findings.* Washington, DC, 2005, HHS. Available at http://nccanch.acf.hhs.gov/pubs/factsheets/canstats.cfm. Accessed February 2, 2006.

National Highway Traffic Safety Administration: *Traffic safety facts 2001.* Available at http://www.nhtsa.dot.gov. Accessed February 18, 2004.

Nguyen TD: *Considerations in pediatric trauma.* Available at http://www.emedicine.com/med/topic3223.htm. Last updated October 2, 2003. Accessed January 31, 2004.

Olney B, Toby E: Musculoskeletal injuries. In Buntain W, editor: *Management of pediatric trauma.* Philadelphia, 1995, W. B. Saunders, pp 394-427.

Parrillo JE, et al: Guidelines for the acute medical management of severe traumatic brain injury in infants, children, and adolescents. *Crit Care Med* 31(6 suppl): 417-486, 2003.

Phelan A: Musculoskeletal trauma. In Kelley SJ, editor: *Pediatric emergency nursing,* ed 2. Norwalk, Conn, 1994, Appleton & Lange, pp 323-334.

Reece RM: Preface. In Reece RM, editor: *Treatment of child abuse.* Baltimore, Md, 2000, Johns Hopkins University Press, pp xiii-xvi.

Routt MLC: Fractures of the femoral shaft. In Green NE, Swiontkowski MF, editors: *Skeletal trauma in children,* ed 2. Philadelphia, 1998, W. B. Saunders, pp 405-429.

Rotondo MF, Schwab CW, McGonigal MD: Damage control: an approach for improved survival in exsanguinating penetrating abdominal injury. *J Trauma* 35:375-383, 1993.

Rupp LA, Day MW: Children are different: pediatric differences and the impact on trauma. In Moloney-Harmon PA, Czerwinski SJ, editors: *The care of the pediatric trauma patient.* St Louis, 2003, W. B. Saunders, pp 35-61.

Semonin-Holleran R: Trauma in childhood. In Neff J, Kidd P, editors: *Trauma nursing: the art and science.* St Louis, 1992, Mosby, pp 527-553.

Seyfer AE, Hansen JE: Facial trauma. In Mattox KL, Feliciano DV, Moore EE, editors: *Trauma,* ed 4. New York, 2000, McGraw-Hill Health Professionals Division, pp 415-435.

Simone S: Abdominal genitourinary injury. In Moloney-Harmon PA, Czerwinski SJ, editors: *The care of the pediatric trauma patient.* St Louis, 2003, W. B. Saunders, pp 189-205.

Schermer, CR: *Injuries due to falls from heights.* Subcommittee on Injury Prevention and Control. Chicago, October 17, 2002, American College of Surgeons Trauma Program. Available at http://www.facs.org/trauma/falls.html. Accessed February 3, 2006.

Snyder AK, Chen LE, Foglia RP et al: An analysis of pediatric gunshot wounds treated at a level I pediatric trauma center. *J Trauma Inj Infect Crit Care* 54(6):102-106, 2003.

Tepas JJ, Faillace WJ: Pediatric trauma. In Mattox KL, Feliciano DV, Moore EE, editors: *Trauma,* ed 4. New York, 2000, McGraw-Hill Health Professionals Division, pp 1075-1098.

Thomas K: Munchausen syndrome by proxy: identification and diagnosis. *J Pediatr Nurs* 18(3):174-180, 2003.

Tolo VT: External fixation in multiply injured children. *Orthop Clin North Am* 21:393-400, 1990.

Tuffs-New England Medical Center: National Pediatric Trauma Registry Fact Sheet (NPTR): fact sheet 2, October 1993. Available at http://www.nptr.org/rehab/factshee.htm. Accessed February 18, 2004.

U.S. Department of Health and Human Services Administration for Children and Families. *Child maltreatment 2003: reports from the states to the National Child Abuse and Neglect data systems. National statistics on child abuse and neglect 2005.* Available at www.acf.hhs.gov/programs/cb/publications/cmreports.htm.

Vernon-Levett P: Traumatic brain injury in children. In Moloney-Harmon PA, Czerwinski SJ, editors: *The care of the pediatric trauma patient.* St Louis, 2003, W. B. Saunders, pp 171-188.

Walker JH: Bites and stings. In Thomas DO, Bernardo LM, Herman B, editors: *Core curriculum for pediatric emergency nursing.* Sudbury, Mass, 2003, Jones and Bartlett, pp 513-520.

Walker JH: Cold-related emergencies. In Thomas DO, Bernardo LM, Herman B, editors: *Core curriculum for pediatric emergency nursing.* Sudbury, Mass, 2003a, Jones and Bartlett Publishers, pp 507-512.

Walker JH: Heat-related emergencies. In Thomas DO, Bernardo LM, Herman B, editors: *Core curriculum for pediatric emergency nursing.* Sudbury, Mass, 2003b, Jones and Bartlett, pp 503-506.

Willis MHW, Merkel SI, Voepel-Lewis T, et al: FLACC behavioral pain assessment scale: a comparison with the child's self-report. *Pediatr Nurs* 29(3):195-198, 2003.

Zaritsky AL, Nadjarbu VM, Berg RA, et al: *Instructor's manual: pediatric advanced life support.* Dallas, 2001, American Heart Association, pp 264-293.

Zuspan SJ: Mechanism of injury. In Moloney-Harmon PA, Czerwinski SJ, editors: *The care of the pediatric trauma patient.* St Louis, 2003, W. B. Saunders, pp 53-61.

Toxicology

American Academy of Clinical Toxicology, European Association of Poison Centres and Clinical Toxicologists: Position statement and practice guidelines on the use of multi-dose activated charcoal for the treatment of acute poisoning. *J Toxicol Clin Toxicol* 37:731, 1999.

Behrman RE et al., editors: *Nelson textbook of pediatrics,* ed 16. Philadelphia, 2000, W. B. Saunders.

Dart RC et al: *Medical toxicology,* ed 3. Philadelphia, 2004, Lippincott Williams & Wilkins.

Ford MD et al: *Clinical toxicology.* Philadelphia, 2001, W. B. Saunders.

Goldfrank LR et al: *Goldfrank's toxicologic emergencies,* ed 7. New York, 2002, McGraw-Hill, pp 1255-1266.

Lampe KF, McCann MA: *AMA handbook of poisonous and injurious plants.* Chicago, 1985, American Medical Association.

Spoerke DG, Rumack BH: *Handbook of mushroom poisoning: diagnosis and treatment.* Boca Raton, Fla, 1994, CRC Press.

Watson WA, Litovitz TL, Klein-Schwartz W et al: 2003 Annual report of the American Association of Poison Control Centers Toxic Exposure Surveillance System. *Am J Emerg Med* 22:335-404, 2004.

Septic Shock

American College of Chest Physicians (ACCP) and Society for Critical Care Medicine (SCCM): Consensus conference: definitions for sepsis and organ failure and guidelines for the use of innovative therapies in sepsis. *Crit Care Med* 20(6):864-874, 1992.

Alyn IB, Baker LK: Cardiovascular anatomy and physiology of the fetus, neonate, infant, child, and adolescent. *J Cardiovasc Nurs* 6(3):1-11, 1992.

Awad S: State-of-the-art therapy for severe sepsis and multisystem organ dysfunction. *Am J Surg* 186(5A):23S-30S, 2003.

Baldwin KM: Shock, multiple organ dysfunction syndrome, and burns in adults. In McCance KL, Huether SE, editors: *Pathophysiology: the biologic basis for disease in adults and children,* ed 4. St Louis, 2002, Mosby, pp 1483-1512.

Barton P, et al: Safety, pharmacokinetics, and pharmacology of drotrecogin alfa (activated) in children with severe sepsis. *Pediatrics* 113(1):7-17, 2004.

Bone RC: Sepsis, the systemic inflammatory response syndrome, and multiple organ dysfunction syndrome: recent advances. *Sepsis and septic shock: current issues and recent development—abstract brochure.* Anaheim, Calif, 1993, National Teaching Institute, AACN.

Brandtzaeg P, Kierulf P, Gaustad P, et al: Plasma endotoxin as a predictor of multiple organ failure and death in systemic meningococcal disease. *J Infect Dis* 159:195-204, 1989.

Brown RB, Hosmer D, Chen HC, et al: A comparison of infections in different ICUs within the same hospital. *Crit Care Med* 13:472-476, 1985.

Cancer incidence and survival among children and adolescents: United States SEER program 1975-1995. Bethesda, Md: National Cancer Institute, SEER Program, 1999. NIH Pub. No. 99-4649.

Carcillo JA: Management of pediatric septic shock. In Holbrook PR, editor: *Textbook of pediatric critical care.* Philadelphia, 1993, W. B. Saunders, pp 114-142.

Carcillo JA: Pediatric septic shock and multiple organ failure. *Crit Care Clin* 19:413-440, 2003.

Carcillo JA, Cunnion RE: Septic shock. *Crit Care Clin* 13:553-574, 1997.

Carcillo JA, Fields AI: Clinical practice parameters for hemodynamic support of pediatric and neonatal patients in septic shock. *Crit Care Med* 30(6):1365-1574, 2002.

Ceneviva G, et al: Hemodynamic support in fluid-refractory pediatric septic shock. *Pediatrics* 102(2):e19, 1998.

Curley MAQ, Thompson JE: Oxygenation and ventilation. In Curley MAQ, Moloney-Harmon PA, editors: *Critical care nursing of infants and children,* ed 2. Philadelphia, 2001, W. B. Saunders, pp 233-307.

Danner RL, Elin RJ, Hosseini JM, et al: Endotoxemia in humans. *Chest* 99:169, 1991.

Deich E, Vincent JL, Windsor A. *Sepsis and multiple organ dysfunction: a multidisciplinary approach.* London, 2002, W. B. Sanders.

Dichter CH, Curley MAQ: Shock. In Curley MAQ, Moloney-Harmon PA, editors: *Critical care nursing of infants and children,* ed 2. Philadelphia, 2001, W. B. Saunders, pp 921-945.

Goh A, et al: Sepsis, severe sepsis, and septic shock in pediatric multiple organ dysfunction syndrome. *J Paediatr Child Health* 35(5):488-492, 1999.

Grimes DE: *Infectious diseases.* St Louis, 1991, Mosby.

Han Y, et al: Early reversal of pediatric-neonatal septic shock by community physicians is associated with improved outcome. *Pediatrics* 112(4):793-799, 2003.

Hazinski MF: *Manual of pediatric critical care.* St Louis, 1999, Mosby, pp 85-288.

Hazinski MF, editor: *Textbook of pediatric advanced life support.* Dallas, 2002, American Heart Association.

Hazinski MF, Jenkins ME: Shock, multiple organ dysfunction syndrome, and burns in children. In McCance KL, Huether SE, editors: *Pathophysiology: the biologic basis for disease in adults and children,* ed 4. St Louis, 2002, Mosby, pp 1513-1539.

Hotchkiss R, Karl I: Medical progress: the pathophysiology and treatment of sepsis. *N Engl J Med* 348(2):138-150, 2003.

Kaplan L: *Systemic inflammatory response syndrome.* Available at http://emedicine.com/MED/topic2227.htm. Last updated October 11, 2001. Accessed February 18, 2004.

Kumar A, Parrillo JE: Shock: classification, pathophysiology, and approach to management. In Parrillo JE, Bone RC, editors: *Critical care medicine: principles of diagnosis and management,* ed 2. St Louis, 2001, Mosby, pp 371-420.

Maki DG: Nosocomial infection in the intensive care unit. In Parrillo JE, Bone RC, editors: *Critical care medicine: principles of diagnosis and management.* St Louis, 1995, Mosby, pp 893-954.

Mertsola J, Kennedy WA, Waagner D, et al: Endotoxin concentration in cerebrospinal fluid correlate with clinical severity and neurologic outcome of *Haemophilus influenzae* type b meningitis. *Am J Dis Child* 145:1099-1103, 1991.

Natanson C, Eichenholz PW, Danner RL, et al: Endotoxin and tumor necrosis factor challenges in dogs stimulate the cardiovascular profile of human septic shock. *J Exp Med* 169:823, 1989.

Natanson C, Hoffman WD, Parrillo JE: Septic shock and multiple organ failure. In Parillo JE, Bone RC, editors: *Critical care medicine: principles of diagnosis and management.* St Louis, 1995, Mosby, pp 355-374.

Natanson C, Hoffman WD, Parrillo JE: Septic shock and multiple organ failure. In Parrillo JE, Bone RC, editors: *Critical care medicine: principles of diagnosis and management,* ed 2, St Louis, 2001, Mosby, pp 437-452.

National Center for Health Statistics: Deaths from 282 selected causes. Available at http://www.cdc.gov/nchs/datawh/statab/unpubd/mortabs/gmwkiii.htm. Last updated June 14, 2002. Accessed July 10, 2002.

Parillo JE, Dellinger RP: Shock: classification, pathophysiology, and approach to management. In Parillo JE, Kumar A, editors: *Critical care medicine,* ed 2. St Louis, 2001, Mosby, pp 371-420.

Patel G, et al: New treatment strategies for severe sepsis and septic shock. *Curr Opin Crit Care* 9:390-396, 2003.

Pearson G: *Handbook of paediatric intensive care.* Philadelphia, 2002, W. B. Saunders, pp 276-277.

Raymond J, Aujard Y, the European Study Group: Nosocomial infections in pediatric patients: a European, multicenter prospective study. *Infect Control Hosp Epidemiol* 21:260-263, 2000.

Richards MJ, Edwards JR, Culver DH, Gaynes RP: Nosocomial infections in pediatric intensive care units in the United States. *Pediatrics* 103:39-45, 1999.

Slota M, et al: The role of gown and glove isolation and strict handwashing in the reduction of nosocomial infection in children with solid organ transplantation. *Crit Care Med* 29(2):405-412, 2001.

Stover BH, Shulman ST, Bratcher DF, et al: Nosocomial infection rates in US children's hospitals' neonatal and pediatric intensive care units. *Am J Infect Control* 29:152-157, 2001.

Suffredini AF, Fromm RE, Parker MM, et al: The cardiovascular response of normal humans to the administration of endotoxin. *N Engl J Med* 321:280, 1989.

Trampuz A, Widmer A: Hand hygiene: a frequently missed life-saving opportunity during patient care. *Mayo Clin Proc* 79:109-116, 2004.

Urrea M, Pons M, Serra M, et al: Prospective incidence study of nosocomial infections in a pediatric intensive care unit. *Pediatr Infect Dis J* 22:490-494, 2003.

Vallet B: Endothelial cell dysfunction and abnormal tissue perfusion. *Crit Care Med* 30:S229-S234, 2002.

Watson RS, Carcillo JA, Linde-Zwirble WT, et al: The epidemiology of severe sepsis in children in the United States. *Am J Respir Crit Care Med* 167:695-701, 2003.

Winkelstein ML: The child with gastrointestinal dysfunction. In Wong DL, editor: *Whaley and Wong's nursing care of infants and children,* ed 6. St Louis, 1999, Mosby, pp 1533-1580.

Wong D: *Wong's essentials of pediatric nursing,* ed 6. St Louis, 2001, Mosby, pp 360-362.

Burns

American Burn Association (ABA): *Burn incidence and treatment in the US: 2000 fact sheet.* Chicago, 2000, ABA.

American Burn Association (ABA): *Advanced burn life support course: provider's manual.* Chicago, 2001, ABA.

American College of Surgeons Committee on Trauma: *Advanced trauma life support course,* ed 6. Chicago, 1997, American College of Surgeons.

Carrougher G: Burn wound assessment and topical treatment. In Carrougher G, editor: *Burn care and therapy.* St Louis, 1998, Mosby.

Chang YH, Peck MD: Nutrition in sepsis and infection. In Holcombe BV, Gottschlich MM, editors: *The science and practice of nutrition support.* Dubuque, Iowa, 2001, Kendal/Hunt.

Cioffi WG: Inhalation injury. In Carrougher GJ, editor: *Burn care and therapy.* St Louis, 1998, Mosby.

Dellinger RP, Carlet JM, Masur H et al: Surviving sepsis: campaign guidelines for management of severe sepsis and septic shock. *Crit Care Med* 32(3):858-871, 2004.

Field T, Peck M, Hernandez-Reif M et al: Postburn itching, pain, and psychological symptoms are reduced with massage therapy. *J Burn Care Rehabil* 21:189-193, 2000.

Gordon M, Marvin J: Burn nursing. In Herndon D, editor: *Total burn care,* ed 2. London, 2002, W. B. Saunders.

Gottschlich MM, Jenkins ME: Metabolic consequences and nutritional needs. In Carrougher GJ, editor: *Burn care and therapy.* St Louis, 1998, Mosby.

Guy JS, Peck MD: Smoke inhalation injury: pulmonary complications. Medscape 1999. Available at http://www.medscape.com/viewarticle/408744.

Heggers JP, Hawkins H, Edgar P et al: Treatment of infection in burns. In Herndon D, editor: *Total burn care,* ed 2. London, 2002, W. B. Saunders.

Krauss B, Green S: Primary care: sedation and analgesia for procedures in children. *N Engl J Med* 343(13):938-945, 2000.

Marvin JA: Management of pain and anxiety. In Carrougher GJ, editor: *Burn care and therapy.* St Louis, 1998, Mosby.

Mayes T, Gottschlich M: Burns and wound healing. In Holcombe BV, Gottschlich M, editors: *The science and practice of nutrition support.* Dubuque, Iowa, 2001, Kendal/Hunt.

Merz J, Schrand C, Mertens D et al: Wound care of the pediatric burn patient. *AACN Clin Issues* 14(4):429-441, 2003.

Meyer WJ, Marvin JA, Patterson DR et al: Management of pain and other discomforts in burned patients. In Herndon D, editor: *Total burn care,* ed 2. London, 2002, W. B. Saunders.

Monofo WW: Initial management of burns. *N Engl J Med Curr Concepts* 335:1581-1585, 1996.

Muller M, Herndon D: Operative wound management. In Herndon D, editor: *Total burn care,* ed 2. London, 2002, W. B. Saunders.

National SAFE KIDS Campaign (NSKC): *Burn injury fact sheet.* Washington, DC, 2004, NSKC.

Purdue GF, Hunt JL, Burris AM: Pediatric burn care. *Clin Pediatr Emerg Med* 3:76-82, 2002.

Robert R, Blakeney P, Herndon DN: Abuse, neglect, and fire setting: when burn injury involves reporting to a safety officer. In Herndon D, editor: *Total burn care,* ed 2. London, 2002, W. B. Saunders.

Robert R, Blakeney P, Villarreal C et al: Anxiety: current practices in assessment and treatment of anxiety in burn patients. *Burns* 26:549-552, 2000.

Rutan RL: Physiologic response to cutaneous burn injury. In Carrougher GJ, editor: *Burn care and therapy.* St Louis, 1998, Mosby.

Ruth GD, Smith S, Bronson M et al: Outcomes related to burn-related child abuse: a case series. *J Burn Care Rehabil* 24(5):318-321, 2003.

Saffle JR, Hildreth M: Metabolic support of the burned patient. In Herndon D, editor: *Total burn care,* ed 2. London, 2002, W. B. Saunders.

Senecal SJ: Pain management of wound care. *Nurs Clin North Am* 34(4):847-860, 1999.

Serghiou MA, Evans EB, Ott S et al: Comprehensive rehabilitation of the burned patient. In Herndon D, editor: *Total burn care,* ed 2. London, 2002, W. B. Saunders.

Sheridan RL: Results of technical and organizational progress. *JAMA Contempo Updates* 290(6):719-722, 2003.

Silverman W, Kurtines W: *Anxiety and phobic disorders: a pragmatic approach.* New York, 1996, Plenum Press.

Warden G: Fluid resuscitation and early management. In Herndon D, editor: *Total burn care,* ed 2. London, 2002, W. B. Saunders.

Weber JM: Epidemiology of infections and strategies for control. In Carrougher GJ, editor: *Burn care and therapy.* St Louis, 1998, Mosby.

Disaster Preparedness

AAP: *Disaster preparedness to meet children's needs.* Available at www.aap.org/terrorism. Accessed September 2004.

AAP Committee on Environmental Health: Chemical terrorism and its impact on children: a subjective review. *Pediatrics* 105(3):662-670, 2000.

American Academy of Pediatrics: Chemical-biological terrorism and its impact on children: a subject review. *Am Acad Pediatr* 105(3):662-670, 2000.

American College of Radiology: ACR Disaster Planning Task Force—2002: *Disaster preparedness for radiology: professional response to radiological terrorism,* Version 2.0. Reston, Va, 2002, American College of Radiology.

Association for Professionals in Infection Control (APIC) Bioterrorism Taskforce and CDC Hospital Infectious Program Bioterrorism Working Group: *Bioterrorism readiness plan: a template for healthcare facilities,* Washington, DC, 1999, APIC.

Bernardo LM, Kapsen P: Pediatric implications in bioterrorism: education for healthcare providers. *DMR (Disaster Management and Response)* I(2):52-54, 2003.

Blaschke G, Palfrey J, Lynch J: Advocating for children during uncertain times. *Pediatr Ann* 32(4):271-274, 2003.

Bradley B, Greshan L, Sidelinger D, Harstein B: Pediatric health professional and public health response. *Pediatr Ann* 32(2):87-94, 2003.

Burklow T, Yu C, Madsen J: Industrial chemicals: terrorism weapons of opportunity. *Pediatr Ann* 32(4):230-234, 2003.

Children's Hospital: *Hospitals rethink disaster plans after September 11.* Available at www.childrenshospital.net/nachri/news/terrorism.html. Accessed September 1, 2004.

Christopher GW, Cieslak T, Pavlin JA, Eitzen EM Jr: Biological warfare: a historical perspective. *JAMA* 278:412-422, 1997.

Cieslak T, Henretig F: Ring-a-ring-a-roses: bioterrorism and its particular relevance to pediatrics. *Pediatrics* 15: 107-111, 2003a.

Cieslak T, Henretig F: Bioterrorism. *Pediatr Ann* 32(3):154-165, 2003b.

Davidhizer R, Shearer R: Helping children cope with public disasters. *Am J Nurs* 102:26-33, 2002.

Department of Health and Human Services, Office of Inspector General State of California: *Review of public health preparedness and response for bioterrorism program funds.* A-09-02-1007, Sacramento, Calif, August 2003, The Department.

Ferguson S: Preparing for disasters: enhancing the role of pediatric nurses in wartime. *J Pediatr Nurs* 17(4):307-308, 2002.

Fulton GL: *Controversies in preparation and response for children in the face of terrorism or disaster.* Available at www.ems-c.org/disasters/framedisasters.htm. Accessed September 2003.

Government Accounting Office (GAO): *Report to the congressional committees. Hospital preparedness: most urban hospitals have emergency plans, but lack certain capacities for bioterrorism response.* GAO-03-924, Washington, DC, 2003, GAO.

Hanze D: How to help children and adolescents deal with the threat of terrorism. *JSPN* 7(1):42-44, 2002.

Hudson T, Reilly K, Dulagh J: Considerations for chemical decontamination shelters. *DMR* 4:110-113, 2003.

Linnemann RE: *Managing radiation medical emergencies.* Philadephia, 2001, Radiation Management Consultants.

Los Angeles County EMSA and Public Health: *Terrorism agent information and treatment guidelines for clinicians and hospitals,* June 2003.

Los Angeles County Department of EMS Agency. *Medical management of CBRNE,* Los Angeles, 2000, The Agency.

Maloney-Harmon P, Czerwinski S: *Nursing care of the pediatric trauma patient.* St Louis, 2003, W. B. Saunders.

National Advisory Committee on Children and Terrorism Recommendations to the Secretary, June 2003.

National Center for Disaster Preparedness: Pediatric preparedness for disasters and terrorism: a national consensus conference executive summary 2003. Columbia University, National Center for Disaster Preparedness.

Newberry L, editor: *Sheehy's emergency nursing: principles and practice,* ed 5. St Louis, 2003, Mosby.

Rotenberg J: Diagnosis and management of nerve agent exposure. *Pediatr Ann* 32(4):242-250, 2003a.

Rotenberg J: Cyanide as a weapon of terror. *Pediatr Ann* 32(4):236-240, 2003b.

Rotenberg J, Burklow T, Selancho J: Weapons of mass destruction: the decontamination of children. *Pediatr Ann* 32(2):98-105, 2003.

Tasota F, Henker R, Hoffman L: Anthrax as a biological weapon: an old disease that poses a new threat. *Crit Care Nurse* 22(5):21-35, 2002.

U.S. Department of Justice: *Emergency response guidebook for weapons of mass destruction incidents,* Washington, DC, 2001, The Department.

Veenema TG, editor: *Disaster nursing and emergency preparedness for chemical, biological and radiologic terrorism and other hazards.* New York, 2003, Springer.

Waeckerle JF: Domestic preparedness for events involving weapons of mass destruction. *JAMA* 283(2):252-254, 2000.

Wheeler D, Poss WB: Mass casualty management in a changing world. *Pediatr Ann* 32(2):98-105, 2003.

Yu C: Medical response to radiation-related terrorism. *Pediatr Ann* 32(3):169-176, 2003.

Yu C, Burklow T, Madsen J: Vesicant agents and children. *Pediatr Ann* 32(4):254-257, 2003.

Initial Stabilization and Transport

AAP Task Force on Intrahospital Transport: *Guidelines for air and ground transport of neonatal and pediatric patients,* ed 2. Elk Grove Village, Ill, 1999, American Academy of Pediatrics.

Barhart SL, Czervinske MP: *Perinatal and pediatric respiratory care.* Philadelphia, 1995, W. B. Saunders.

Bertrand P et al: Efficacy of nebulized epinephrine versus salbutamol in hospitalized infants with bronchiolitis. *Pediatr Pulmonol* 31:284-288, 2001.

Bhatia V, Wolfsdorf JL: Severe hypoglycemia in youth with insulin-dependant diabetes mellitus: frequency and causative factors. *Pediatrics* 88:1187-1193, 1991.

Bhende MS et al: Evaluation of a portable infrared end-tidal carbon dioxide monitor during pediatric interhospital transport. *Pediatrics* 95(6):875-878, 1995.

Bloch H et al: Intravenous magnesium sulfate as an adjunct in the treatment of acute asthma. *Chest* 107:1578-1581, 1995.

Blumen IJ, Rinnert KJ: Altitude physiology and the stresses of flight. *Air Med J* 14: 87-100, 1995.

Bower LK et al: Selection of an aerosol delivery device for neonatal and pediatric patients. *Respir Care* 40(12):1325-1335, 1995.

Carcillo JA: Pediatric septic shock and multiple organ failure. *Crit Care Clin* 19:413-440, 2003.

Carcillo JA, Fields AI: Clinical practice parameters for hemodynamic support of pediatric and neonatal patients in septic shock. *Crit Care Med* 30:1365-1378, 2002.

Ciarallo L, Sauer AH, Shannon MW: Intravenous magnesium therapy for moderate to severe pediatric asthma: results of a randomized, placebo-controlled trial. *J Pediatr* 129:809-814, 1996.

Cowley RS: An economical and proved helicopter program for transporting the emergency critically ill and injured patients. *J Trauma* 13:1029, 1973.

Curley MAQ, Moloney-Harmon P: *Critical care nursing of infants and children,* ed 2. Philadelphia, 2001, W. B. Saunders.

Day S et al: Pediatric interhospital critical care transport: consensus of a national leadership conference. *Pediatrics* 88: 696-704, 1991.

DeNicola LK et al: Treatment of critical severe status asthmaticus in children. *Pediatr Clin North Am* 41:1293-1324, 1994.

Dunger DB et al: ESPE/LWPES consensus statement on diabetic ketoacidosis in children and adolescents. *Arch Dis Child* 89:188-194, 2004.

Glover ML, Machado C, Totapally BR: Magnesium sulfate administered via continuous intravenous infusion in pediatric patients with refractory wheezing. *J Crit Care* 17:255-258, 2002.

Han YY et al: Early reversal of pediatric-neonatal septic shock by community physicians is associated with improved outcome. *Pediatrics* 112(4):793-799, 2003.

Heinrich WA et al: Status asthmaticus in children. *Chest* 119:1913-1929, 2001.

High K, Yeatman J: Transport considerations for the pediatric trauma patient. *J Emerg Nurse* 26:346-351, 2000.

Holleran RS: *Flight nursing principle and practice,* ed 2. St Louis, 1996, Mosby.

Hunt RC et al: Inability to assess breath sounds during air medical transport by helicopter. *JAMA* 265(15):1982-1984, 1991.

Jaimovich DG, Vidyasagar D: *Handbook of pediatric and neonatal transport medicine,* ed 2. Philadelphia, 2002, Hanley & Belfus.

Klassen TP et al: Nebulized budesonide for children with mild-to-moderate croup. *N Engl J Med* 331:285-289, 1994.

Klassen TP: Croup, a current perspective. *Pediatr Clin North Am* 46:1167-1178, 1999.

Lighthall GK, Pearl RG: Volume resuscitation in the critically ill: choosing the best solution. *J Crit Ill* 18:252-260, 2003.

Losek JD: Hypoglycemia and the ABC's (sugar) of pediatric resuscitation. *Ann Emerg Med* 35:43-46, 2000.

Martin SE, Ochsner MG, Jarman RH: The LMA: a viable alternative for securing the airway. *Air Med J* 18:89-92, 1999.

McCloskey KA, Orr RA: *Pediatric transport medicine.* St Louis, 1995, Mosby.

McCloskey KA, et al: Pediatric specialty care teams are associated with reduced morbidity during interfacility transport. *Pediatrics* 104(suppl):687, 1999.

Myers TR: AARC guidelines: neonatal and pediatric O_2 delivery. *Respir Care* 47(6):707-716, 2002.

Nehrenz G: *Internet J Aeromedical Transportation* 1(1), 1997. Available at http://www.ispub.com/journals/IJAMT/VOL1N1/altox.htm.

Numa AH, Williams GD, Dakin CJ: The effect of nebulized epinephrine on respiratory mechanics and gas exchange in bronchiolitis. *Am J Respir Crit Care Med* 164:86-91, 2001.

Okayama H et al: Bronchodilating effect of intravenous magnesium sulfate in bronchial asthma. *JAMA* 257:1076-1078, 1987.

Pennant JH, Walker MB: Comparison of the endotracheal tube and laryngeal mask in airway management by paramedical personnel. *Anesth Analg* 74(4):531-534, 1992.

Papo MC, Frank J, Thompson AE: A prospective, randomized study of continuous versus intermittent nebulized albuterol for severe status asthmaticus in children. *Crit Care Med* 21(10): 1479-1486, 1995.

Pollack MM: Improving outcomes from tertiary pediatric intensive care: a statewide comparison of tertiary and nontertiary care facilities. *Crit Care Med* 19:150-159, 1991.

Robertson CF et al: Response to frequent low doses of nebulized salbutamol in acute asthma. *J Pediatr* 106:672-674, 1985.

Sagarin MJ, Chiang V, Sakles JC: Rapid sequence intubation for pediatric emergency airway management. *Pediatr Emerg Care* 18:417-422, 2002.

Scribano PV et al: Use of out-of-hospital intervention for the pediatric patient in an urban emergency medical service system. *Acad Emerg Med* 7:745-750, 2000.

Schachner H, Silfin M: Endocrine emergencies. In Crain EF, Gershel JC, editors: *Clinical manual of emergency pediatric,* ed 4. New York, 2003, McGraw-Hill.

Schuh S et al: Efficacy of frequent nebulized ipratropium bromide added to frequent high-dose albuterol therapy in severe childhood asthma. *J Pediatr* 126(4):636-645, 1995.

Stephanopoulos DE et al: Continuous intravenous terbutaline for pediatric status asthmaticus. *Crit Care Med* 26: 1744-1748, 1998.

Tung BJ: The pediatric rescue airway. *Air Med J* 24(2):55-58, 2005.

Venkataraman ST, Rubenstein JS, Orr RA: Interhospital transport: a pediatric perspective. *Crit Care Clin* 8(3):515-523, 1992.

Volovitz B, Nussinovitch M: Management of children with severe asthma exacerbation in the emergency department. *Pediatr Drugs* 4(3):141-148, 2002.

Warren J et al: Guidelines for the inter- and intrahospital transport of the critically ill patient. *Crit Care Med* 32:256-262, 2004.

Weintraub Z et al: The morphology of periodic breathing in infants and adults. *Respir Physiol* 127(2-3):173-184, 2001.

White NH: Management of diabetic ketoacidosis. *Rev Endocr Metab Disord* 4(4):343-353, 2003.

Woodward GA, Chun TH, Miles DK: It's not just a seizure: etiology, management, and transport of the seizure patient. *Pediatr Emerg Care* 15:147-155, 1999.

Woodward GA, Fleegler EW: Should parents accompany pediatric interfacility ground ambulance transport? The parent's perspective. *Pediatr Emerg Care* 16:383-390, 2000.

Woodward GA, et al: The state of pediatric interfacility transport: consensus of the second National Pediatric and Neonatal Interfacility Transport Medicine Leadership Conference. *Pediatr Emerg Care* 18: 38-43, 2002.

Younger RE et al: Intravenous methylprednisolone efficacy in status asthmaticus of children. *Pediatrics* 80:225-230, 1987.

Zaritsky AL et al., editors: *Pediatric advanced life support provider manual.* Dallas, 2002, American Heart Association.

Appendix: Case Studies

Each of the system-based chapters in this book presented an overview of developmental anatomy and physiology and the pathophysiology involved in various conditions commonly encountered in children hospitalized in pediatric critical care units. To facilitate analysis of clinical signs and symptoms and problem solving related to patient care, the following case studies are presented for further review of selected patient problems.

CASE STUDY A: CARDIOVASCULAR SYSTEM—HYPOPLASTIC LEFT HEART SYNDROME (HLHS)

David, a 19-day-old, 4-kg male born to a 17-year-old gravida 1, para 1 mother, was discharged on day 2 of life. Examination at discharge was without detectable pathology. Two days before presentation, David was noted to be eating poorly. One day before, he was lethargic. The morning of presentation he was difficult to arouse, refused to eat, had marked respiratory effort, and was pale.

In the emergency room, initial vital signs were heart rate (HR) of 60 bpm, respiratory rate (RR) of 90/min with marked retractions, flaring, and grunting, right arm blood pressure of 40/19, and afebrile. The infant was immediately sedated, paralyzed, intubated, and placed on mechanical support with an Fio_2 of 100%. Initial arterial gases were Sao_2 65%, Po_2 30 mm Hg, Pco_2 38 mm Hg, pH 6.9, and base deficit (BD) -15. Femoral central venous access was placed. Following the infusion of albumin, initiation of dopamine and dobutamine drips, and repeated administration of bicarbonate, the saturation remained at 70%, blood pressure was 45/20, and the HR was 200 bpm (sinus tachycardia). Prostaglandin E_1 infusion was initiated, and in 10 minutes, saturation rose to 80%, pH was 7.30, and BD was -5. Blood pressure rose to 60/35, and the infant began producing urine.

Echocardiogram examination revealed mitral and aortic atresia, a hypoplastic aortic arch, severe coarctation, a diminutive nonapex-forming left ventricle, and a restrictive patent ductus arteriosus (PDA) with bidirectional flow. ■

1. What physiologic event precipitated the initial patient decompensation?
   a. Aspiration of gastric contents
   b. Physiologic closure of the PDA
   c. Delayed closure of the PFO
   d. Excess perfusion to the extremities

   Answer: b. Physiologic closure of the PDA decreases perfusion to the aorta below the area of obstruction with acidosis and shock resulting. When the ductus is open, all four limb pressures will be equal because perfusion is maintained distally, depending on the location of the coarctation. In severe low output, all pressures will be diminished because of poor distal perfusion. With normal perfusion, a closed ductus results in a blood pressure differential between upper and lower extremities.

Four days later, with normal kidney and liver function and a normal cranial ultrasound, a Norwood operation with a 3.5-mm Blalock-Taussig (BT) shunt was performed without incident. Initial blood gases and vital signs in the ICU were Sao_2 86%, Po_2 48 mm Hg, Pco_2 26 mm Hg, pH 7, BD -19, HR 195 bpm in junctional rhythm, and blood pressure 50/30 on Fio_2 of 80%. Urine output was scant, extremities cool, and pulses not palpable. The infant was on dopamine, fentanyl, and epinephrine drips. ■

2. Which of the following statements regarding the relationship between the oxygen saturation, heart rate, blood pressure, and blood gases is *not* correct?
   - **a.** Saturations are high, thus most of the cardiac output is being directed to the lungs (pulmonary overcirculation), resulting in hypotension, tachycardia, and acidosis.
   - **b.** Junctional rhythm is most likely a response to the acidosis, low cardiac output, or swelling in the region of the SA node related to surgery.
   - **c.** A higher Fio_2 is required to decrease pulmonary vasodilation.
   - **d.** Bicarbonate can be used to treat the metabolic acidosis, and a decreased ventilatory rate may achieve a slight relative respiratory acidosis.

   Answer: c. Higher Fio_2 can be detrimental, leading to most of the cardiac output being directed to the lungs, resulting in hypotension, tachycardia, and acidosis. Oxygen should be weaned rapidly to 21% to 30% to decrease pulmonary vasodilation. A hypoxic gas mixture may be required. Afterload-reducing agents may decrease SVR and restore a QP:QS ratio of 1:1. Junctional rhythm is most likely a response to the acidosis, low cardiac output, or surgical edema. Bicarbonate can be used to treat the metabolic acidosis, and the ventilatory rate can be decreased to achieve a slight relative respiratory acidosis.

3. What are the treatment options for junctional tachycardia?
   - **a.** Pacing
   - **b.** Antiarrhythmics
   - **c.** Treatment of underlying conditions
   - **d.** All of the above

   Answer: d. Junctional tachycardia (JT) often results from low cardiac output, catecholamine release, fever, or exogenous pressors and can be detrimental to cardiac output in infants. JT can be treated with pacing, antiarrhythmics, or treatment of underlying conditions. It would be difficult to effectively override an HR in the 190s with pacing. Also, it is important to decrease the metabolic rate through cooling, paralyzation, and sedation.

Chest tube output was 40 ml/hr for the first 3 hours after surgery and has stopped. The baby remains oliguric, hypotensive, tachycardic, and acidotic. ■

4. What are the potential causes of this hemodynamic state?
   - **a.** The infant may be dry intravascularly, requiring volume resuscitation.
   - **b.** The acute bleeding may have resulted in a clot formation in the atrium or chest tube itself, which may be causing tamponade.
   - **c.** Acute tubular necrosis is a common postop occurrence.
   - **d.** A and B

   Answer: d. The infant may be dry intravascularly, requiring volume resuscitation, or acute bleeding may have resulted in clot formation in the atrium or chest tube itself, which may cause cardiac tamponade. If so, a chest x-ray study would demonstrate a widened mediastinum. An echogram may show fluid, a clot behind the heart, or an underfilled ventricle. Pulsus paradoxus may be present. If cardiac output is severely compromised or bleeding is ongoing, the chest needs to be opened to evacuate the clot or blood, possibly at the bedside. A return to the operating room may be necessary. Other supportive measures include volume and calcium replacement and treatment of acidosis.

The infant survives and is being prepared for discharge. His parents tell you they wish to have more children. They want to know why this happened and what the risks are for future pregnancies. In preparation for discharge, you are reviewing current health needs and the need for future surgery. ■

5. Which of the following statements is correct in counseling this family in regard to risk, infant nutrition, caloric need, and growth and development?
   a. A family history is necessary to evaluate for other congenital heart diseases (CHD) since the risk is higher in families with more than one child with CHD.
   b. Growth is usually normal or exceeds normal after the initial surgery.
   c. Development is usually severely delayed.
   d. Nutritional demands are often less than requirements for the general population.
   Answer: a. A family history will help to evaluate the potential risk for subsequent pregnancies. In hypoplastic left heart syndrome (HLHS) the actual recurrence risk may be higher than the quoted increased risk of 2% to 4%. A genetic evaluation may be desired. Growth will be slower than normal. Development is often within the expected range, although there may be some lags in gross motor skills with severe cyanosis or failure. Caloric demands are greater than requirements for the general pediatric population, and with cardiac failure, requirements of 130 kcal/kg per day or higher may be required. In some cases, reflux occurs. Feeding tubes and PT/OT may be required to provide adequate nutrition. Ongoing monitoring of SaO_2 is also standard in some centers. Parents need to learn that the child can still overcirculate and should not be stressed with activities or feeds.

6. What is the benefit of the second-stage repair?
   a. Increases volume through increased systemic-to-pulmonary shunting
   b. Increases ventricular pressure to enable high saturations
   c. Reduces the pressure and volume overload on the ventricle by removing the systemic-to-pulmonary shunt
   d. None of the above
   Answer: c. Second-stage repair reduces the pressure and volume overload on the ventricle by removing the systemic-to-pulmonary shunt, which would become relatively smaller anyway. This procedure may increase energy and growth but may not significantly increase saturation. It does provide for stable saturation until the final procedure, however, so that the infant can no longer overcirculate.

Long-term problems associated with the Fontan procedure include ventricular dysfunction (sometimes requiring transplant), protein-losing enteropathy, dysrhythmias, recurrent effusions and ascites, arteriovenous malformations (more common after the second stage), and exercise limitations.

CASE STUDY B: MULTISYSTEM ISSUES—TOXICOLOGY

A 3-year-old boy was found with an open bottle of his mother's prenatal vitamins with iron. The color of the tablet coating is seen inside the child's mouth. Twenty-five tablets are unaccounted for.

1. Following ingestion of iron, gastrointestinal (GI) decontamination may include all of the following, *except:*
   a. Ipecac syrup
   b. Gastric lavage
   c. Activated charcoal
   d. Whole bowel irrigation

   Answer: c. Activated charcoal does not bind iron. Inducing emesis with ipecac syrup may be helpful if the child has not vomited and is performed early after ingestion (but is not recommended as home therapy). Gastric lavage is helpful in removing pills and pill fragments if performed soon after ingestion. Whole bowel irrigation is the standard of care to remove large amounts of ingested iron.

2. For the next several hours, it is important to observe this child for the development of any of the following, *except:*
   a. GI bleeding
   b. Coma
   c. Acute tubular necrosis
   d. Metabolic acidosis
   e. Coagulopathies

   Answer: c. In overdose, iron causes significant corrosive injury to the GI tract. Circulating free iron injures blood vessels and damages hepatocytes and can cause GI bleeding. As iron is metabolized, free hydrogen is released and in concert with other events produces metabolic acidosis. Symptoms of severe toxicity include coma, cardiovascular collapse, seizures, hepatic failure, and coagulopathies.

3. The child experienced vomiting, diarrhea, and abdominal pain for about 3 hours and then gradually fell into an undisturbed sleep. The most likely explanation is:
   a. The iron tablets have been eliminated from the GI tract and the child is out of danger.
   b. The child is now in the asymptomatic latent phase, during which iron is being absorbed and metabolized.
   c. Since the child's symptoms are not characteristic of iron poisoning, he probably has a GI virus or food poisoning.
   d. These symptoms are characteristic of an allergic reaction to vitamin supplements and were precipitated by the large amount of vitamins in these adult-strength supplements.

   Answer: b. The asymptomatic latent phase occurs between 2 and 12 hours after ingestion. Systemic insults occur during this phase, then the child abruptly enters the third phase with a rapid onset of cardiovascular collapse.

4. The most effective definitive therapy for acute iron intoxication is:
   a. Deferoxamine
   b. Volume expanders
   c. Hemodialysis
   d. Resin hemoperfusion
   e. Exchange transfusion

   Answer: a. Deferoxamine is an iron-chelating agent (it binds iron) and is administered as an intravenous infusion.

CASE STUDY C: MULTISYSTEM ISSUES—TRAUMA

Suzy, a 5-year-old girl, was hit by a car while crossing the street. Paramedics arrived at the scene within 10 minutes of the accident. She was found to have labored, irregular breathing and a heart rate of 50 bpm. She was intubated immediately, and hyperventilation was initiated. On arrival at the emergency department she was manually ventilated and cardiac compressions were in progress. She was stabilized following a brief resuscitation period. Rapid neurologic assessment revealed enlarged but reactive pupils, fluid draining from the left ear, bruising over the left mastoid bone, and decorticate posturing. She was given a bolus of mannitol (Osmitrol) and furosemide (Lasix) and sent to radiology for a CT scan. Head CT results revealed a skull fracture, small cerebral laceration, and diffuse cerebral swelling. She was taken to the operating room for a ventricular intracranial pressure (ICP) catheter followed by admission to the pediatric intensive care unit (PICU). ■

1. Based on the clinical examination, Suzy most likely has which of the following types of skull fractures?
   a. Growing skull fracture
   b. Basilar skull fracture
   c. Right frontal bone skull fracture
   d. Depressed skull fracture
   Answer: b. Basilar fractures present with specific symptoms related to a break in the basilar portion of the skull bones. Battle's sign represents postauricular hematoma and swelling from damage to the sigmoid sinus temporal bone. Rhinorrhea represents cerebrospinal fluid (CSF) leakage into the middle ear cavity with drainage through the eustachian tube. Otorrhea represents CSF leakage from the ear canal related to a tear of the dura mater.

2. In most patients the most effective way to acutely lower ICP is by:
   a. Administering furosemide
   b. Hyperventilation
   c. Hyperoxygenation
   d. Administering a barbiturate
   Answer: b. Although intervention needs to be individualized for each patient, a lower $PaCO_2$ causes the pH to increase (decreased hydrogen ion concentration) and decreases cerebral tissue acidosis. Precapillary arterioles constrict in response to decreased hydrogen concentration. Cerebral blood flow, cerebral blood volume, and ICP decrease. Hyperventilation may be used as a rescue intervention or when herniation is imminent to reduce ICP, but other interventions are necessary to maintain adequate perfusion pressure.

On the second day of admission, Suzy's ICP acutely increased to 55 mm Hg and remained elevated for 6 minutes and then returned to its baseline. During this period, the mean arterial blood pressure was 90 mm Hg, the right pupil was dilated and fixed, and she had decerebrate posturing. ■

3. Suzy's waveform is best described as:
   a. C wave
   b. P1 wave
   c. A wave
   d. B wave
   Answer: c. A waves (plateau) are spontaneous, rapid, irregular increases in ICP to 50 to 100 mm Hg lasting 5 to 20 minutes. A waves are frequently associated with dilated pupil(s), vomiting, abnormal posturing, decreased level of consciousness, widened pulse pressure, dysrhythmias, and decreased

respirations. They represent impaired cerebral blood flow and occur most often with decreases in blood pressure associated with hypovolemia.

4. Which of the following nursing interventions is indicated at this time?
   a. Elevate the head of bed 45 degrees
   b. Administer lidocaine
   c. Administer oxygen
   d. Open the ventriculostomy drain
   Answer: d. CSF drainage will promote displacement of excess cerebral volume. CSF drainage by clamping and unclamping of the drainage device is controlled by physician order.

5. During the acute period of ICP elevation, Suzy's cerebral perfusion pressure (CPP) was:
   a. 15 mm Hg
   b. 90 mm Hg
   c. 35 mm Hg
   d. 40 mm Hg
   Answer: c. CPP calculation: CPP = MAP (mean arterial pressure) – ICP
   Normally CPP is greater than 50 mm Hg in the child and greater than 60 mm Hg in the adolescent.

6. If a child with a closed head injury develops polyuria, hypernatremia, and serum hyperosmolality, the nurse suspects:
   a. Diabetes mellitus (DM)
   b. Diabetes insipidus (DI)
   c. Syndrome of inappropriate antidiuretic hormone (SIADH)
   d. Thyrotoxicosis
   Answer: b. Diabetes insipidus (DI) can result from head trauma. It is a clinical condition characterized by a decrease in urine concentration, resulting in excessive diuresis, urine osmolality less than 200 mOsm/kg, specific gravity (SG) less than 1.005, serum sodium greater than 145 mmol/L, serum osmolality greater than 300 mOsm/kg, tachycardia, and dehydration. This may be an ominous sign in head trauma.

7. Suzy's ICP is stabilized by the fourth day. Follow-up CT demonstrated blood in the subarachnoid space. Suzy is most at risk for which of the following complications?
   a. Obstructive hydrocephalus
   b. Epidural hematoma
   c. Blindness
   d. Motor paralysis
   Answer: a. Blood in the subarachnoid space will result in decreased reabsorption of CSF, which leads to ventricular dilation.

CASE STUDY D: GASTROINTESTINAL SYSTEM—LIVER FAILURE

A 10-month-old girl, Sara, is admitted to the PICU with acute mental status changes. One of Sara's siblings died of suspected liver failure. Sara's laboratory studies include the following results: total bilirubin 5.2 mg/dL, aspartate aminotransferase (AST) 4268 IU/L, ammonia

220 mcmol/L, albumin 3.2 g/dL, platelets 180,000/mm^3, white blood cell count (WBC) 8.2 × 10^9/L, and prothrombin time (PT) 33 seconds. She is on 0.5 L of oxygen per nasal cannula, is lethargic, and does not respond to stimuli. ■

1. Which of the following assessment findings would you observe?
   a. Jaundice
   b. Petechiae
   c. Erythematous diffuse rash
   d. Cyanosis
   Answer: a. An accumulation of yellow pigment in the skin and other tissues, jaundice is evident when total bilirubin is greater than 3 mg/dL. Kernicterus is the presence of yellow pigment in the basal ganglia of the brain seen in the neonatal period with an elevated indirect hyperbilirubinemia. Dark-colored urine and pale-colored stool may occur.

2. Which of the following blood products would best treat Sara's coagulopathy?
   a. Platelets
   b. Packed red blood cells
   c. Fresh frozen plasma (FFP)
   d. 25% albumin
   Answer: c. Coagulopathy in liver disease is related to the liver's abnormal production of prothrombin and other clotting factors and its ineffective removal of activated clotting factors. FFP contains the necessary clotting factors.

3. The rationale for administering lactulose (Cephulac) enemas is to:
   a. Promote ammonia excretion
   b. Provide supplemental glucose
   c. Promote intestinal reabsorption of ammonia
   d. Prevent intestinal bacterial translocation
   Answer: a. A diseased liver may be unable to remove toxic metabolites (such as ammonia) normally formed during the degradation of proteins, amino acids, and blood. Ammonia accumulation may contribute to the encephalopathy that occurs. Lactulose acidifies colonic flora and promotes ammonia elimination.

4. The family consents to a liver biopsy to assist with the child's diagnosis. The postbiopsy interventions by the nurse caring for Sara would include:
   a. Left-side-lying positioning, vital signs taken every 15 minutes for 1 hour, monitoring of gastric pH
   b. Prone positioning, vital signs taken hourly for 1 hour, monitoring of serial hematocrits
   c. Right-side-lying positioning, vital signs taken every 15 minutes for 1 hour, monitoring of serial hematocrits
   d. Left-side-lying positioning, vital signs taken every 15 minutes for 1 hour, monitoring of gastric pH
   Answer: c. Nursing interventions include right-side-lying position to apply pressure to the biopsy site, vital signs taken every 15 minutes for 1 hour to monitor for bleeding and hypotension, and monitoring of serial hematocrits to assess for bleeding.

5. Sara's change in neurologic status can be attributed to:
   a. Jaundice
   b. Esophageal varices

c. Asterixis
d. Hepatic encephalopathy
Answer: d. Hepatic encephalopathy is the leading cause of morbidity and mortality in patients with liver failure. The etiology of hepatic encephalopathy is not known.

CASE STUDY E: NEUROLOGIC SYSTEM—HEAD INJURY

Mary, a 9-year-old girl, fell 20 feet from a tree house. Upon impact, she lost consciousness for approximately 2 minutes. When the paramedics arrived, she was conscious with a Glasgow Coma Score (GCS) of 14. She was breathing spontaneously 26 bpm, heart rate was 110 bpm, and blood pressure was 110/72. The cervical spine was immobilized and the patient was transferred to the emergency department.

In the emergency department, Mary had periods of irritability alternating with unresponsiveness and apnea. The GCS decreased to 8. She was intubated and two peripheral intravenous lines were started. A 20 mL/kg bolus of normal saline was given. The patient was immediately transferred to radiology for a CT scan. The CT scan revealed a biconvex-shaped (lenticular) hyperdense area with a midline shift. ■

1. The CT scan report best describes which of the following?
   a. Subdural hematoma
   b. Epidural hematoma
   c. Diffuse cerebral swelling
   d. Intracranial hematoma
   Answer: b. The CT scan demonstrated an epidural hematoma as a biconvex-shaped (lenticular) hyperdense area. If the clot is large, there is usually a midline shift.

2. What is the treatment of choice for this patient?
   a. Return the patient to the emergency department and continue to assess neurologic status
   b. Transfer the patient to the pediatric intensive care unit (PICU) for more extensive monitoring
   c. Remain in the radiology department for CT scans of the abdomen and chest
   d. Transfer the patient to the operating room for immediate evacuation of the clot
   Answer: d. The patient must be transferred to the OR to evacuate the clot. Epidural hematomas can expand rapidly because of their usual arterial source. Intracranial pressure can increase quickly with brain herniation and cerebral ischemia.

Several hours later, the patient is in the PICU. She remains intubated and ventilated, has arterial pressure, central venous pressure, ICP, and $Pbto_2$ monitoring. The arterial pressure is 110/65 mm Hg, MAP is 80 mm Hg, ICP is 18 mm Hg, $Pbto_2$ is 24 mm Hg, HR is 122. ■

3. What is the cerebral perfusion pressure?
   a. 56 mm Hg
   b. 30 mm Hg
   c. 62 mm Hg
   d. 130 mm Hg
   Answer: c. CPP calculation: CPP = MAP (mean arterial pressure) – ICP

4. Which of the following sets of patient parameters has the worst prognosis?
   a. ICP 15 mm Hg, CPP 50 mm Hg, $Pbto_2$ 30 mm Hg
   b. ICP 25 mm Hg, CPP 65 mm Hg, $Pbto_2$ 22 mm Hg
   c. ICP 10 mm Hg, CPP 80 mm Hg, $Pbto_2$ 40 mm Hg
   d. ICP 12 mm Hg, CPP 40 mm Hg, $Pbto_2$ 15 mm Hg

   Answer: d. The abnormally low CPP and $Pbto_2$ represent cerebral ischemia. A $Pbto_2$ less than 15 is associated with high mortality.

5. On day 2, Mary's CPP is 40 mm Hg, ICP is 25 mm Hg, and $Pbto_2$ is 15 mm Hg. Which of the following are first-line interventions to improve the patient's condition?
   a. Increase MAP with fluids and vasopressors
   b. Hyperventilate to achieve a $Paco_2$ of 30 mm Hg
   c. Start a pentobarbital infusion
   d. Administer phenytoin

   Answer: a. Initial management is directed at correcting hypotension and improving cerebral blood flow to prevent cerebral ischemia. Fluids and vasopressors are used to improve CBF, CPP, and MAP. Hyperventilation is only used when conventional therapies have been exhausted and $Pbto_2$ monitoring is available to assess brain oxygenation. Pentobarbital coma is used for refractory intracranial hypertension (i.e., all other therapies have failed to control ICP). Phenytoin may be prophylactically prescribed to prevent early-onset seizures.

Despite fluids, vasopressors, sedation, paralysis, and mannitol, Mary's ICP remains less than 25 mm Hg, CPP is less than 50 mm Hg, and $Pbto_2$ is less than 20 mm Hg. A decision is made to start a pentobarbital infusion. ■

6. Which of the following neurodiagnostic tests or monitoring is used to evaluate burst suppression?
   a. CT scan
   b. EEG
   c. Cranial ultrasound
   d. Sjo_2 monitoring

   Answer: b. Continuous EEG monitoring is used to evaluate burst suppression.

7. Which of the following infusions is commonly used with a pentobarbital infusion?
   a. Dopamine
   b. Vecuronium
   c. Mannitol
   d. Morphine

   Answer: a. Hypotension is a common side effect of pentobarbital, and vasopressors such as dopamine are commonly used to support circulation.

CASE STUDY F: NEUROLOGIC AND ENDOCRINE SYSTEMS—BRAIN TUMOR/DI

Tanya, a 5-year-old girl, was admitted to the PICU following craniotomy for excision of a suprasellar tumor. Approximately 12 hours after admission the following were noted: decreased level of consciousness, tachycardia, hypotension, and a urine output of 15 mL/kg per hour with a specific gravity (SG) of 1.003. Laboratory studies revealed serum sodium 160 mmol/L, serum osmolality 340 mOsm/kg, and urine sodium 20 mmol/d. The diagnosis of diabetes insipidus (DI) was made. Initial treatment consisted of urine replacement (ml/ml) with half normal saline (NS). Twenty-four hours later her level of consciousness improved, urine output remained at 10 to 15 mL/kg per hour with a low SG, serum sodium was 150 mmol/L, and serum osmolality was 305 mOsm/kg.

Desmopressin (DDAVP) 5 mcg/kg intranasally was begun. Within 2 hours her urine output had dropped to 3 mL/kg per hour with an SG of 1.010. IV replacement of urinary losses was discontinued, and maintenance fluids were continued. Urine output and SG were monitored every hour. When urine output exceeded 2 mL/kg per hour and SG fell below 1.010, another intranasal dose of desmopressin was administered. Two days later the IV was discontinued, and the DI was managed with twice daily doses of desmopressin and ad lib oral intake. ■

1. This child would require fluid and electrolyte correction over a period of 48 hours to prevent which of the following?
   a. Cerebral dehydration and hemorrhage
   b. Cerebral edema and herniation
   c. Cerebral hemorrhage and edema
   d. Cerebral dehydration and herniation

   Answer: b. Slow correction of a hyperosmolar state is necessary to prevent cerebral edema and possible herniation. A rapid decrease in serum osmolality causes water to move into the cells (which were previously at equilibrium with the serum osmolality), precipitating cellular swelling.

2. The cardiovascular signs and symptoms of DI are primarily due to:
   a. Decreased preload
   b. Decreased afterload
   c. Decreased contractility
   d. Decreased conduction

   Answer: a. Intravascular volume loss is secondary to the absence of ADH with unchecked free water loss by the kidney. Treatment with exogenous ADH increases water reabsorption by the kidney, maintaining blood volume.

3. Desmopressin is the synthetic form of which of the following?
   a. ADH
   b. Renin
   c. Aldosterone
   d. Insulin

   Answer: a. Desmopressin is a form of ADH replacement therapy for the treatment of DI. The primary pathophysiologic abnormality in DI is ADH deficiency.

CASE STUDY G: HEMATOLOGY/ONCOLOGY—BONE MARROW TRANSPLANT (BMT) AND SHOCK

Rob, a 13-year-old boy with a history of leukemia, received a bone marrow transplant 80 days ago. He was admitted to the intensive care unit in septic shock. ■

1. Which of the following indicate an attempt by the kidneys to compensate for the changes in the child's condition?
   a. Increased serum bicarbonate, vasoconstriction of arterioles, secretion of renin
   b. Decreased serum bicarbonate, vasoconstriction of arterioles, secretion of renin

c. Increased sodium excretion, vasodilation of arterioles, secretion of renin
d. Increased sodium reabsorption, vasodilation of arterioles, secretion of renin
Answer: a. In an effort to correct acidosis, the kidney increases the bicarbonate in the serum to increase uptake of the hydrogen ions. The arterioles constrict to compensate for decreased perfusion and decreased renal blood flow. The kidneys release renin in response to sympathetic stimulation. Renin is converted to angiotensin I, which is converted to angiotensin II, which causes vasoconstriction and secretion of aldosterone. To maintain adequate volume, sodium reabsorption is increased.

2. On day 2, Rob's blood urea nitrogen (BUN) increased to 75 mg/dL, and the creatinine remained at 2.4 mg/dL. The increase in BUN may be an indication of worsening acute renal failure (ARF) and acute tubular necrosis (ATN).
a. True
b. False
Answer: b. An increase in BUN without an increase in creatinine is most likely an indication of dehydration, decreased renal perfusion, or high catabolic state. An indication of ATN would be a rising BUN *and* creatinine level.

3. Rob gained 5 kg during the first 24 hours. This weight gain was largely the result of volume given during the fluid resuscitation. Rob received regular doses of furosemide (Lasix). After several days of high-dose diuretics, Rob's urine output increased to 7 mL/kg per hour, and his weight decreased. The team began to notice a rising serum phosphorus level. This was most likely the result of:
a. Dehydration
b. Muscle wasting
c. Hypocalcemia
d. Hyperkalemia
Answer: c. Alterations in calcium balance are often related to the use of loop diuretics, which block tubular reabsorption of calcium and may cause hypocalcemia. As serum calcium decreases, phosphorus increases. Since the mechanism for excretion of phosphate is primarily generated by the kidneys, patients in renal failure are at high risk for hyperphosphatemia.

4. Rob's serum phosphorus level remained greater than 9 mg/dL despite calcium administration. Options for further treatment of the hyperphosphatemia should include:
a. Hemodialysis or continuous renal replacement therapy (CRRT)
b. Increasing the dose of furosemide
c. Administration of magnesium
d. Administration of epogen
Answer: a. Hemodialysis or CRRT may be required to decrease phosphate levels. Increasing the dose of furosemide may lead to further hypocalcemia and resultant hyperphosphatemia. The administration of magnesium will not decrease the serum phosphate level. Epogen is used to induce erythropoiesis.

CASE STUDY H: MULTISYSTEM ISSUES—BURNS

Angie, an 18-month-old toddler, lives with her mother and 10-year-old sister. At noon Angie pulled the electrical cord to a crockpot of boiling beans, spilling the contents over her face, trunk, and arms. At 12:30 PM Angie's mother brought her to the emergency department. Angie is crying and restless. Angie's temperature is 36.5° C (rectal), HR is 110 bpm and regular, BP is 100/80, respirations are 30/min and nonlabored. Angie weighs 11 kg. ■

1. Most pediatric burn injuries occur in:
   a. Newborns
   b. Infants and toddlers
   c. School-age children
   d. Adolescents
   Answer: b. Most burns occur in the very active and curious age group of infants and toddlers. Among small children, scalds are the predominant burn injury.

2. The extent of cellular destruction within the burn wound depends on:
   a. Duration of exposure
   b. Intensity of the heat
   c. Tissue involved
   d. All of the above
   Answer: d. Duration of exposure, intensity of heat, and the tissue involved all determine the extent of destruction. When absorption of heat energy exceeds the ability of the tissue to dissipate the absorbed heat, cellular injury in varying depths results.

3. A burn injury in which the entire integument is destroyed can be described as a:
   a. First-degree burn
   b. Second-degree burn
   c. Third-degree burn
   d. Fourth-degree burn
   Answer: c. First- and second-degree burns are partial-thickness burns. A third-degree burn destroys all the layers of skin. Fourth-degree burns involve fat, fascia, muscle, and bone as well.

4. The initial hemodynamic response to a large burn injury includes:
   a. Increase in cardiac output and decrease in peripheral vascular resistance
   b. Increase in cardiac output and peripheral vascular resistance
   c. Decrease in cardiac output and increase in peripheral vascular resistance
   d. Decrease in cardiac output and peripheral vascular resistance
   Answer: c. A large full-thickness burn causes significant fluid losses and resultant hypovolemia. Cardiac output falls and peripheral vascular resistance increases in response to the hypovolemia and the release of vasoactive mediators from the stress response following injury. Cardiac output returns to normal 18 to 24 hours after the burn, and peripheral vascular resistance returns to normal after cardiac output improves.

Angie has mostly large fluid-filled blisters on her trunk and arms. The blisters on her face have ruptured, and the underlying tissue is wet and pink. With the burn record the extent and depth of Angie's burn is calculated to be 21%. ■

5. In the first 8 hours the amount calculated for burn fluid resuscitation (using Table 9-26) is:
   a. 924 mL
   b. 462 mL
   c. 223 mL
   Answer: b. 4 mL × 11 kg × 21% × 2 = 462 mL

6. The amount calculated for maintenance fluid requirements per 24 hours (using Table 9-25) is:
   a. 1000 mL
   b. 1050 mL
   c. No daily maintenance fluids needed
   Answer: b. 1050 mL per 24 hours.

7. To determine the adequacy of fluid resuscitation, the minimum desired urine output for Angie would be:
   a. 30 mL/hr
   b. Three wet diapers per shift
   c. 11 mL/hr
   d. 5 mL/hr
   Answer: c. Minimum urine output is 1 mL/kg per hour.

8. In the emergent period of care the primary cause of shock related to the burn injury is:
   a. Cardiogenic
   b. Hypovolemic
   c. Neurogenic
   d. Septic
   Answer: b. The first and primary goal is fluid resuscitation aimed at restoring and then maintaining intravascular volume at a level adequate for tissue perfusion to vital organs. Septic and cardiogenic shock may occur later.

9. With a large burn the patient may experience a decrease in lung compliance related to:
   a. Fluid volume overload
   b. Restrictive burns to the chest
   c. Smoke inhalation injury
   d. All of the above
   Answer: d. A decrease in lung compliance may be related to chest wall edema, circumferential burns to the chest wall, smoke inhalation injury, preexisting lung disease, or fluid volume overload.

10. Immediate initial treatment of a chemical burn includes:
    a. Removing all patient clothing and locating a neutralizing agent
    b. Removing all patient clothing, brushing a powdered chemical from the skin, and locating a neutralizing agent
    c. Removing all patient clothing, brushing a powdered chemical from the skin, and administering copious irrigation of the wound with tap water
    Answer: c. Prompt measures to remove the chemical from contact with the skin prevent continued tissue damage. Searching for a neutralizing agent wastes valuable time. In some cases the increased heat of the neutralizing reaction may further damage tissue.

11. The one best initial treatment for a burn-injured patient with suspected carbon monoxide toxicity is:
    a. Fresh air
    b. Administration of 100% O_2
    c. Hyperbaric oxygenation
    d. Mechanical ventilation

Answer: b. Administration of 100% O_2 will displace some if not all the carboxyhemoglobin before the patient's arrival at the emergency department. Carbon monoxide has a constant half-life and is reduced by 50% in 4 hours at room air, in less than 1 hour in 100% O_2, and in 30 minutes when hyperbaric oxygenation is used.

12. In an assessment of suspected child abuse, the physical examination documentation should include:
- **a.** Thorough description of all injuries
- **b.** Characteristic patterns of intentional injury, such as "stocking and glove" distribution
- **c.** Bruising or injuries in varying stages of healing
- **d.** Evaluation of the consistency of the injury with the described history
- **e.** All of the above

Answer: e. All of these assessments are important in determining intentional injury. Deliberate injury by burning is often an unrecognized and unappreciated component of thermal injury. The evaluating team must be aware of the possibility of abuse in any child who incurs a burn injury, especially in children less than 2 years of age.

13. The preferred route of drug administration in the early postburn period is:
- **a.** Intramuscular (IM)
- **b.** Intravenous (IV)
- **c.** Subcutaneous (SC)

Answer: b. In the early postburn period, changes in fluid volume and circulation prevent the use of the IM or SC route for some drugs because absorption by these routes may be erratic.

CASE STUDY I: NEUROLOGIC SYSTEM—INFECTIOUS DISEASE

Jennifer, a 6-year-old girl, is admitted to the PICU following a history of fever and rash for 2 days. On admission to the emergency department, she was manually ventilated with a bag-valve-mask device. Her heart rate and blood pressure were normal, and her temperature was 39°C. Neurologically she responded appropriately to pain, and her pupils were equal and reacted to light (PERL). Her trunk had a fine petechial rash. She rapidly deteriorated in the emergency department, requiring advanced life support. Routine laboratory tests, chest x-ray film, and lumbar puncture (CSF analysis) were obtained before admission to the unit. The tentative diagnosis was bacterial meningitis. ■

1. On the basis of the clinical examination, the pathogen most likely responsible for her meningitis is:
- **a.** *Haemophilus influenzae* type B
- **b.** *Neisseria meningitidis*
- **c.** *Escherichia coli*
- **d.** Enterovirus

Answer: b. Petechial rash may occur with *N. meningitidis. N. meningitidis* is a prominent organism causing bacterial meningitis in children over 2 months of age.

2. Jennifer has a positive Brudzinski sign, which is best described as:
- **a.** Extension of upper and lower extremities

b. Pupil constriction with neck flexion
c. Back pain and resistance after passive extension of the lower legs
d. Flexion of hip and knees after passive flexion of the neck
Answer: d. Brudzinski sign is the flexion of the hips and knees after passive flexion of the neck. Bacterial meningitis is also characterized by nuchal rigidity (stiff neck), Kernig's sign (back pain and resistance with passive extension of the lower legs), photophobia (abnormal intolerance of light), fever, vomiting, lethargy, headache, and alteration in consciousness.

3. Which of the following interventions has highest priority?
a. Ordering a kinetic bed to prevent skin breakdown
b. Administering intravenous broad-spectrum antibiotics
c. Transferring to radiology for a CT scan
d. Assisting with insertion of an ICP catheter
Answer: b. Antimicrobial therapy is the mainstay of bacterial meningitis treatment. Chemoprophylaxis is also given to close contacts of patients with *N. meningitidis* and *H. influenzae.*

4. Typical CSF characteristics following bacterial meningitis include:
a. Elevated WBC, decreased glucose, elevated protein, positive Gram stain
b. Normal WBC, normal glucose, elevated protein, positive Gram stain
c. Elevated WBC, increased glucose, decreased protein, positive Gram stain
d. Decreased WBC, increased glucose, increased protein, negative Gram stain
Answer: a. Elevated WBC (polymorphonuclear cells predominate; may be normal in neonates), decreased glucose (should be compared to serum glucose; may be normal in neonates), elevated protein (normal 10 to 30 mg/dL in children; 20 to 170 mg/dL in neonates), and positive Gram stain. In addition, the organism culture will be positive, and the fluid is usually turbid or cloudy.

5. Jennifer develops a urine output of 0.3 mL/kg per hour. Laboratory studies reveal serum sodium of 125 mmol/L; serum osmolality of 256 mOsm/kg; urine specific gravity (SG) of 1.025; urine sodium of 45 mmol/d, and urine osmolality of 600 mOsm/kg. What would the appropriate therapeutic intervention be?
a. Fluid bolus of normal saline
b. Furosemide IV
c. Fluid restriction
d. Observation
Answer: c. SIADH is associated with meningitis. Symptoms include a serum osmolality of less than 280 mOsm/kg, urine osmolality elevated inappropriately in relation to serum osmolality, serum sodium less than 135 mmol/L, urine sodium greater than 30 mmol/d, and urine SG greater than 1.020. Usually, fluid restriction to insensible losses is sufficient to decrease blood volume and increase serum sodium. Serum sodium should be normalized over 24 to 48 hours to prevent neurologic sequelae.

CASE STUDY J: RESPIRATORY SYSTEM—RSV

James, a 2-month-old boy with a large ventricular septal defect (VSD), is admitted to the emergency department for symptoms of respiratory distress. He has a history of 3 days of low-grade fever, coughing, and congestion and a 3-year-old sibling with an upper respiratory tract infection. The parents note that he has eaten poorly for the last 24 hours and has had only 2 wet diapers. Admission temperature is 38.2° C, HR is 194 bpm, RR is 90/min, blood pressure is 68/50, and Sa_{O_2} is 84%. James is dusky with mottled extremities and is irritable, retracting, and grunting. Audible wheezing and crackling is noted on auscultation. Admitting diagnosis is probable respiratory syncytial virus (RSV) bronchiolitis.

When James's respiratory condition continues to deteriorate in the PICU, endotracheal intubation and mechanical ventilation are required. Intravenous fluids are initiated. James is then noted to be resting comfortably with an HR of 152 bpm, BP 80/62, RR of 36/min on synchronized intermittent mandatory ventilation (SIMV) with an Sa_{O_2} of 98% on Fi_{O_2} of 40%, and normal arterial blood gases. ■

1. Which diagnostic test is most definitive for RSV bronchiolitis?
   a. Chest x-ray
   b. Pulse oximetry
   c. Fluorescent antibody test
   d. Arterial blood gas analysis
   Answer: c. Rapid fluorescent antibody test for RSV may be used to test nasopharyngeal secretions. Direct isolation of the virus is possible through nasopharyngeal washing but may require 2 weeks for positive culture results. The diagnosis is based primarily on clinical observations. Chest radiography may demonstrate hyperinflation, atelectasis, and peribronchial thickening in about half of infected patients.

2. Which of the following is the best measure to prevent the spread of RSV?
   a. Restriction of visiting
   b. Good hand washing
   c. Strict gown and glove isolation
   d. Transfer to a rehabilitation facility
   Answer: b. Good hand washing is required to prevent spread of the virus to other patients and families, particularly high-risk patients. Patients at high risk for RSV infection include immunosuppressed patients and children with congenital heart disease, bronchopulmonary dysplasia (BPD), cystic fibrosis, prematurity, and other chronic illnesses.

3. Medications often used during endotracheal intubation of infants and children include:
   a. Steroids and NSAIDs
   b. Barbiturates, antiemetics, and neuromuscular blockers
   c. Benzodiazepines, neuromuscular blockers, and steroids
   d. Neuromuscular blockers, sedatives, and anticholinergics
   Answer: d. A neuromuscular blocker such as succinylcholine (depolarizing agent) or vecuronium (nondepolarizing agent) is administered to relax the airway. A sedative and narcotic are administered to decrease anxiety and pain. An anticholinergic agent (such as atropine) may be administered to decrease secretions and prevent bradycardia and bronchospasm.

4. Which of the following statements concerning airway pressures in children who are mechanically ventilated is *not* correct?
   a. The greater the lung compliance, the higher the peak inspiratory pressure (PIP) will be.
   b. Positive end expiratory pressure (PEEP) tends to "stent" open the airways, which might otherwise collapse at end expiration.

c. Continuous positive airway pressure (CPAP) provides positive airway pressure sustained throughout spontaneous respiratory cycles.
d. Mean airway pressure is influenced by a variety of mechanisms, including tidal volume, PEEP, and PIP.
Answer: a. Compliance is the relationship of volume to pressure within a closed space. Lung compliance is determined by the elasticity of lung tissue and the presence of surfactant in the alveoli. Therefore, greater compliance will enable *lower* PIPs.

5. Which of the following statements concerning ventilator modes in children is true?
   a. Intermittent mandatory ventilation (IMV) does not allow the patient to breath spontaneously.
   b. SIMV incorporates a sensor that recognizes spontaneous breaths and retimes delivery of the next ventilator breath.
   c. During pressure support ventilation (PSV), a lower pressure limit will provide greater support for the patient.
   d. The trigger is the mechanism that terminates inspiration.
   Answer: b. SIMV incorporates a sensor that recognizes spontaneous breaths and retimes delivery of the next ventilator breath. The spontaneous breaths are not regulated by the preset parameters. IMV delivers a preset number of breaths at preset parameters, but the patient *can* breathe spontaneously from the circuit. PSV allows the patient to breathe spontaneously, triggering ventilator support with a pressure sensor. When spontaneous effort is sensed, gas flow is delivered until the airway pressure reaches a preset minimum limit. The higher the pressure limit, the greater the support for the patient. The trigger is the mechanism that *initiates* inspiration.

6. The nurse caring for James notes a sudden decrease in Sao_2 from 98% to 82%. What is the first priority for nursing interventions?
   a. Administer a sedative agent
   b. Increase the Fio_2 and ventilator rate
   c. Reposition the endotracheal tube
   d. Assess the patency of the endotracheal tube
   Answer: d. Assessment of the patency of the endotracheal tube should be done first. Auscultate the chest to assess for presence and equality of breath sounds. Repositioning the tube may be required if breath sounds are diminished on one side of the chest either through auscultation or radiographic examination. This is frequently the result of the tube migrating into the right main stem bronchus. Endotracheal tube suctioning may be required if auscultation reveals increased secretions or a blocked tube. If atelectasis or edema of the small airways has progressed, increased Fio_2 or increased ventilatory support may be required. Sedative agents should not be administered until all other potential causes of hypoxemia have been ruled out.

7. Evaluate the following arterial blood gases: pH 7.42, Po_2 92 mm Hg, Pco_2 42 mm Hg, base deficit (BD) -1.
   a. Metabolic alkalosis
   b. Within normal limits
   c. Metabolic acidosis
   d. Respiratory alkalosis
   Answer: b. The values are within normal limits.

8. Evaluate the following arterial blood gases: pH 7.28, Po_2 74 mm Hg, Pco_2 59 mm Hg, Hco_3 24 mEq/L, BE 0.
   a. Compensated metabolic acidosis
   b. Uncompensated metabolic alkalosis
   c. Compensated respiratory alkalosis
   d. Uncompensated respiratory acidosis
   Answer: d. If there were evidence of renal compensation, Hco_3 would be elevated above 26 mEq/L and BE would be elevated above +2.

9. The concept of permissive hypercarbia is a strategy that allows:
   a. A higher Pco_2 with normal oxygenation, pH greater than 7.15, and no evidence of cerebral dysfunction
   b. A higher Pco_2 with a minimum Po_2 of 50 mm Hg, pH greater than 7, and a normal mental status
   c. A respiratory alkalosis with Po_2 in the normal range
   d. A respiratory acidosis with Pco_2 ranging from 80 to 100 mm Hg
   Answer: a. Permissive hypercarbia is a strategy for guiding ventilator manipulations that allow hypercarbia to exist with normal oxygenation, pH greater than 7.15, Pco_2 between 45 and 80 mm Hg, and no evidence of cerebral dysfunction. Over time, physiologic compensation normalizes the pH. The benefit is that it allows minimal volume ventilation, which reduces the risk of lung injury.

CASE STUDY K: RENAL SYSTEM—DEHYDRATION

Janet, a 6-month-old infant, has been admitted to the emergency room with a temperature of 38.9° C and a history of cold and flu symptoms over the last 24 hours. The infant is lethargic. Heart rate is 190 bpm. Respiratory rate is 50/min. Blood pressure is 80/45. The infant has a sunken fontanelle and has not had a wet diaper in more than 18 hours. ■

1. Which signs and symptoms would indicate dehydration?
   a. Urine output less than 0.5 mL/kg per hour, decreased urine sodium content, urine osmolarity less than 300 mOsm/L
   b. Urine output less than 0.5 mL/kg per hour, decreased urine sodium content, urine osmolarity greater than 500 mOsm/L
   c. Urine output greater than 1 mL/kg per hour, increased urine sodium content, urine osmolarity greater than 500 mOsm/L
   d. Urine output greater than 1 mL/kg per hour, decreased urine sodium content, urine osmolarity less than 300 mOsm/L
   Answer: b. In the event of decreased fluid balance the kidneys attempt to compensate by increasing sodium reabsorption, which decreases sodium excretion and decreases urine output. As a result, urine osmolarity increases.

2. The most important priority for this patient is to:
   a. Obtain blood cultures
   b. Place a Foley catheter
   c. Obtain vascular access
   d. Intubate and start mechanical ventilation
   Answer: c. Obtaining vascular access to begin fluid replacement and restore adequate circulation would be the first priority. Establishing an airway and breathing are always the first priorities in resuscitation; however, the history

of this child did not indicate the need to assist airway or breathing. It would be important to obtain necessary tests; however, this would come after adequate vascular access has been established.

3. Normal urine output for an infant would be expected to be greater than or equal to:
   a. 0.5 mL/kg per hour
   b. 1 mL/kg per hour
   c. 3 to 5 mL/kg per hour
   d. 5 mL/kg per hour
   Answer: b. An infant's normal urine output is between 1 and 3 mL/kg per hour. A child would be expected to have a urine output greater than or equal to 1 to 2 mL/kg per hour.

4. Water is conserved or eliminated by the kidneys in response to which of the following?
   a. Urine sodium concentration
   b. Serum potassium concentration
   c. Level of ADH
   d. Presence of aldosterone
   Answer: c. Vasopressin, or ADH, plays a role in water balance. The hypothalamus regulates the release of ADH from the posterior pituitary based on the osmolarity of the intravascular and extracellular fluids. The release of ADH causes water reabsorption in the distal tubules and collecting ducts, resulting in increased urine concentration.

CASE STUDY L: ENDOCRINE SYSTEM—DIABETIC KETOACIDOSIS (DKA)

A child presents to the PICU with lethargy, polyuria, serum glucose of 550 mg/dL, a blood pH of 7.25, glycosuria, and ketonuria. ■

1. Hyperglycemia is present in the child with uncontrolled diabetic ketoacidosis (DKA) due to:
   a. Decreased tissue utilization of glucose and increased counterregulatory hormones
   b. Increased counterregulatory hormones and increased tissue utilization of glucose
   c. Increased tissue utilization of glucose and decreased counterregulatory hormones
   d. Decreased counterregulatory hormones and decreased tissue use of glucose
   Answer: a. In the absence of insulin, stored substrates are mobilized and cellular uptake of glucose is inhibited. An increase in counterregulatory hormones contributes to increased glucose production and hyperglycemia.

2. Appropriate therapeutic intervention would be:
   a. Continuous infusion of regular insulin
   b. NPH insulin IV bolus followed by continuous infusion of regular insulin
   c. Regular insulin SC followed by maintenance IV fluids
   d. NPH insulin SC followed by maintenance IV fluids
   Answer: a. Continuous infusion of regular insulin would be an appropriate intervention. Volume expansion is administered as boluses of normal saline during the first 1 to 2 hours. IV fluid rate is determined based on fluid deficit,

maintenance requirements, and any ongoing fluid losses. Dextrose 5% is added to IV fluids when the blood glucose falls below 250 mg/dL.

3. What is the appropriate intervention for serum glucose of 240 with ongoing acidosis?
   a. Decrease insulin and continue to follow glucose
   b. Give a bolus of dextrose
   c. Add 5% or 10% dextrose to IV fluids and continue insulin infusion
   d. Add 5% or 10% dextrose to IV fluids and decrease insulin infusion
   Answer: c. Insulin is needed to suppress ketogenesis and lipolysis and resolve the ketoacidosis.

4. What occurs with the potassium level in DKA with the initiation of insulin?
   a. Nothing
   b. The potassium is low and stays low until the glucose is normal
   c. The potassium is elevated or normal but remains unchanged with insulin administration
   d. The potassium is normal or elevated but decreases with insulin administration
   Answer: d. In acidosis, potassium shifts from the intracellular space into the extracellular space. Insulin and correction of the acidosis shifts the potassium intracellular.

5. Match laboratory data and signs and symptoms of SIADH versus DI.
   a. ______ Inappropriate secretion of antidiuretic hormone
   b. ______ Hypernatremia
   c. ______ Low serum sodium and low serum osmolality
   d. ______ Deficiency of antidiuretic hormone
   e. ______ Serum hyperosmolality
   f. ______ Treatment: fluid restriction
   g. ______ Polydipsia
   h. ______ Treatment: vasopressin or DDAVP
   i. ______ Low urine output in the absence of hypovolemia
   j. ______ Dehydration is a complication
   Answer: SIADH: a, c, f, i; DI: b, d, e, g, h, j

CASE STUDY M: MULTISYSTEM ISSUES—TOXICOLOGY

A 15-year-old girl was found unconscious; a bottle of her mother's amitriptyline was found next to her. She had a grand mal seizure in the ambulance en route to the emergency department. ■

1. Toxicity of tricyclic antidepressants significantly contributes to which effects?
   a. Drooling and respiratory distress
   b. Agitation and restlessness
   c. Prolonged, accelerated hypertension
   d. Dysrhythmias
   Answer: d. Tricyclic antidepressants have the following effects: anticholinergic, resulting in dry mouth, early hypertension and hallucinations; delayed uptake of norepinephrine, resulting in some CNS and cardiac effects; membrane depressant effects on the heart, resulting in numerous dysrhythmias, especially ventricular dysrhythmias and conduction delays; and α-adrenergic blockade, resulting in the hypotension characteristic of this poisoning.

2. The single most important drug in the management of tricyclic antidepressant overdose is:
   a. Dopamine
   b. Glucagon
   c. Lidocaine
   d. Phenytoin
   e. Sodium bicarbonate

   Answer: e. Symptomatic patients are likely to develop acidosis that is resistant to correction. Although hyperventilation is sometimes used to induce respiratory alkalosis, sodium bicarbonate is more effective in treating acidosis and cardiac dysrhythmias.

3. In cases of intentional drug overdose it is especially important to obtain laboratory evaluation of which potential coingestant?
   a. Acetaminophen
   b. Ethanol
   c. Heroin
   d. Salicylates

   Answer: a. Acetaminophen is readily available in the home and is contained in more than 100 products.

4. Following a tricyclic antidepressant overdose, death is usually due to:
   a. Cardiac dysrhythmias
   b. Disrupted neurotransmission in the central nervous system
   c. Hepatotoxicity
   d. Profound hypotension
   e. Refractory seizures

   Answer: a. Cardiac dysrhythmias can occur following antidepressant overdose. The toxic dose cannot be predicted with certainty. Any amount is potentially dangerous in children. At least 6 hours of emergency department evaluation is required for all ingestions in young children and for ingestions larger than the therapeutic dose in older children. Patients who become symptomatic in the 6-hour observation period require admission to a monitored bed until they have been asymptomatic for 24 hours. With intentional overdoses, psych consults are warranted.

CASE STUDY N: MULTISYSTEM ISSUES—TRANSPORT AND SHOCK

A 2-month-old girl was admitted to a local hospital with a 2-day history of wheezing, tachypnea, and other symptoms consistent with an upper respiratory tract infection. The patient tested positive for respiratory syncytial virus (RSV). The patient was placed on oxygen via face tent, given racemic epinephrine aerosols every 6 hours, Xopenex (levalbuterol HCl) aerosols every 8 hours, and Decadron (dexamethasone) IV every 6 hours. The patient had no other past medical history.

The pediatric specialty transport team was called when the patient became more tachypneic, tachycardic, and stopped taking oral fluids. The referring physician gave the following vital signs: temperature 97.9°F, heart rate 180, respiratory rate of 76, and Spo_2 95% on 40% oxygen. An arterial blood gas revealed pH 7.32, Pco_2 45, Po_2 85, and Hco_3 level of 21. Electrolytes and the patient's H and H all were within normal limits. The patient's weight was 5.15 kg. The patient was started on maintenance IV fluids and given lorazepam (Ativan) for agitation. ■

1. The transport team's initial recommendations to the referring physician should include:
   a. Place the patient in 100% oxygen, administer 20 mL/kg of normal saline, obtain a chest X-ray, and have equipment available for intubation if required for patient decompensation.
   b. Place the patient in a cool mist tent and monitor vital signs closely.
   c. Place the infant in parent's arms with blow-by oxygen, allowing her to take a bottle as desired.
   d. Repeat dose of lorazepam for agitation and sustained tachycardia.
   Answer: a. First step in the treatment of respiratory distress is the administration of oxygen. It can be delivered via an oxyhood, nasal cannula, or properly fitting mask. The patient is tachycardic with a heart rate of 180 beats per minute. The cause for this may be the multiple doses of racemic epinephrine, or the patient may be hypovolemic secondary to an increased respiratory rate and lack of PO intake. No evidence of poor perfusion and hypotension (except tachycardia) with reassessment of vital signs is used to determine improvement in the patient's hemodynamic status.

2. The transport team determines that transporting by helicopter is the best mode of transportation for this patient. What are the primary factors leading to this decision?
   a. Time of call is during "rush hour."
   b. Parents request a flight.
   c. Respiratory failure and shock is impending.
   d. Referring hospital is two hours away.
   e. A, C, and D
   Answer: e. This patient is exhibiting signs of impending respiratory failure, therefore requiring the transport team to use the most efficient, expeditious mode of transportation. The patient's status, distance, time of day, and weather are some of the factors that must be assessed in determining the appropriate mode of transport. Early identification and treatment of respiratory failure and shock is essential for decreasing morbidity and mortality rates in this patient population.

Within an hour of the initial call, the team arrived at the bedside to find the patient receiving a racemic epinephrine aerosol, as directed by the transport physician. The patient would awaken with the assessment, cry, and fall back to sleep. Her pupils were 2 mm and reactive bilaterally with a GCS of 10. The fontanel was soft and flat. The patient had no tears with crying. The initial vital signs were as follows: temperature 97.6° F rectal, heart rate 194, blood pressure 70/38, respiratory rate 86, and oxygen saturations 94% on 100% oxygen with aerosol treatment. The patient had copious nasal drainage with moderate subcostal and intercostal retractions. Bilateral breath sounds contained rales with fair to poor aeration. The patient was pale, with a capillary refill of 4 to 5 seconds. Pulses all were palpable. The liver edge was not palpable. The patient received 20 mL/kg of normal saline and was now on maintenance fluid of dextrose 5%, one fourth normal saline at 25 mL/hr. CXR revealed hyperinflation with some patchy areas of consolidation. ■

3. During the initial assessment, the team recognizes the patient has progressed to respiratory failure and intubation is indicated. What important clinical signs would aid the team members in their decision to intubate and ventilate this patient?
   a. HR of 194 bpm and RR of 86 bpm
   b. Spo_2 94% on 100% Fio_2 with moderate retractions

c. Lethargy
d. All of the above
Answer: d. When assessing the need for endotracheal intubation the team should consider cardiovascular, neurologic, and pulmonary status. The combination of these factors will confirm impending respiratory failure and shock. Intubation may assist with the stabilization of the patient's cardiovascular and pulmonary condition.

CASE STUDY O: HEMATOLOGY AND IMMUNOLOGY—SICKLE CELL DISEASE

Quadir is an 18-month-old boy with Hgb SS. He is admitted to the pediatric intensive care unit with anemia, tachycardia, abdominal fullness, splenomegaly, acute left upper quadrant pain, and weakness. ■

1. On the basis of these clinical findings, you suspect that Quadir may have which of the following?
   a. Vaso-occlusive crisis
   b. Splenic sequestration crisis
   c. Aplastic crisis
   d. Acute chest syndrome
   Answer: b. Although many of these clinical findings are seen with vaso-occlusive crisis, aplastic crisis, or acute chest syndrome, the combination of Quadir's age, acute left upper quadrant abdominal pain, and splenomegaly are indicative of splenic sequestration crisis.

2. The first priority in the management of splenic sequestration crisis is recognition and management of:
   a. Respiratory acidosis
   b. Infection
   c. Hypovolemic shock
   d. Severe abdominal pain
   Answer: c. Recognition and management of hypovolemic shock is a first priority. Acute pooling of blood in the splenic sinuses results in an abrupt fall in hemoglobin level. This results in acute splenic enlargement, significant anemia, and, if severe, can progress rapidly to hypovolemic shock and death.

3. Acute management of the critically ill child with severe splenic sequestration crisis includes:
   a. Supplemental oxygen, hydration with isotonic fluids, and repeated exchange transfusions
   b. Hydration with isotonic fluids, serial CBCs, and assessment of splenic size
   c. Supplemental oxygen and repeated transfusion of packed red blood cells
   d. Full or partial splenectomy
   Answer: a. A child with severe splenic sequestration crisis will require supplemental oxygen, hydration with isotonic fluids, and repeated exchange transfusions. A mild crisis may resolve spontaneously.

4. Repeated episodes of acute chest syndrome, another potential complication of sickle cell disease, may lead to all of the following *except*:

a. Pulmonary hypertension
b. Chronic lung injury
c. Pulsus paradoxus
d. Cor pulmonale
Answer: c. Pulsus paradoxus does not result from acute chest syndrome. Repeat episodes lead to pulmonary hypertension, cor pulmonale, and restrictions of vital capacity, which may cause chronic lung injury.

CASE STUDY P: GASTROINTESTINAL SYSTEM—BILIARY ATRESIA

A 3-month-old is admitted to the PICU for respiratory compromise secondary to ascites and hepatosplenomegaly. The child is on oxygen per nasal cannula and is started on aggressive diuretic therapy. ■

1. What is the most likely diagnosis for this infant?
   a. Tylenol overdose
   b. Biliary atresia
   c. Wilson's disease
   d. Hepatocellular carcinoma
   Answer: b. Biliary atresia is a congenital defect that involves the absence of obstruction of the intrahepatic and extrahepatic ducts of the biliary system, resulting in the development of fibrosis and obstruction of bile flow.

2. Which of the following lab values would be elevated?
   a. Platelet count
   b. Ammonia level
   c. Bilirubin level
   d. Blood urea nitrogen level
   Answer: c. Impaired excretion of direct bilirubin into the bile ducts or biliary tract results in increased levels of direct bilirubin with increased amounts absorbed into the blood.

3. What is the etiology of the ascites and hepatosplenomegaly?
   a. Portal hypertension
   b. Hepatic encephalopathy
   c. Jaundice
   d. Coagulopathy
   Answer: a. Portal hypertension can result in ascites and hepatosplenomegaly. The liver becomes firm and enlarged with regeneration and the spleen becomes enlarged due to vascular engorgement. An enlarged spleen and liver, bruising, and petechiae are noted.

4. The child begins to experience bleeding that is thought to be due to esophageal varices. What would be the most likely treatment?
   a. Immediate liver transplantation
   b. Distal splenal-renal shunt
   c. Endoscopic variceal sclerosing
   d. Endoscopic variceal banding
   Answer: c. The sclerosing agent is injected directly into or alongside varices. Assess for complications including ulceration with rebleeding, perforation, and stricture formation.

CASE STUDY Q: MULTISYSTEMS ISSUES—TRAUMA

Thirty-four-month-old Allison arrived at the emergency department (ED) in an ambulance after having been found unresponsive at home. Mother reports that she was "acting differently after hitting her head on a propane tank" early in the day. EMS intubated and boarded the child prior to transport. Your assessment in the ED reveals that the child is unresponsive and flaccid, orally intubated, and manually ventilated with 100% FiO_2. There is no trauma to the head or face and no nasal or ear drainage. Pupils are fixed and dilated. The chest is clear to auscultation with normal heart sounds. Color is pink and skin is warm and well perfused. There is a large ecchymotic area over the left abdomen but no abdominal distention. There is one PIV. She is diagnosed with a subdural hematoma and closed skull fracture. ■

1. What is the first priority for the RN caring for this patient?
   a. Mannitol IV
   b. Lasix IV
   c. Normal saline bolus 20 mg/kg IV
   d. Phosphenytoin IV

   Answer: a. Patient presents with signs of increased ICP (fixed and dilated pupils) and is already intubated and ventilated. Mannitol (Osmitrol) is an osmotic agent that is most effective in treating intracranial hypertension. Mannitol causes an osmotic gradient between the intravascular space and the brain tissue.

2. Allison's vital signs are a heart rate of 123 and blood pressure of 85/53. In addition to respiratory compromise, which of the following vital sign changes would be indicative of Cushing's reflex?
   a. BP 120/90; HR 160
   b. BP 68/32; HR 90
   c. BP 160/50; HR 65
   d. BP 95/60; HR 100

   Answer: c. Cushing's triad is a late sign of profound compromise in brain stem perfusion and impending herniation that consists of increased systolic pressure, bradycardia, and irregular respiratory pattern. The increased systolic pressure produces a widening pulse pressure.

The patient had a craniectomy for evacuation of a subdural hematoma, partial resection of temporal lobe, and placement of an extraventricular drainage (EVD). Upon arrival to the PICU, an ICP reading was unobtainable and the EVD did not drain. Allison received vecuronium and thiopental for transport to CT scan, since she had some spontaneous respiratory effort. Head CT revealed suboptimal placement of the EVD, significant cerebral edema, and uncal herniation. Also, Allison was found to have a grade III liver laceration in the inferior right lobe. Parents arrived to the hospital on the evening of her admission. ■

3. Which of the following serum lab values are most indicative of a grade III liver laceration?
   a. Decreased Hct, elevated ALT, elevated AST
   b. Elevated lipase, elevated ALT, normal BUN
   c. Decreased Hgb, elevated lipase, elevated amylase
   d. Elevated bilirubin, elevated AST, normal Hct

   Answer: a. Due to vascularity of the liver, bleeding is likely with a laceration, resulting in decreased Hct and Hgb. Amylase and lipase enzyme changes are most indicative of pancreatic injury. Hepatic injury results in elevated hepatic enzymes.

Staff caring for Allison have ensured that detailed documentation is in the medical record. The documentation includes the mechanism of injury and other relevant medical history details. ■

4. Which of the following is the most significant factor that should alert the RN that this is potentially a nonaccidental injury?
   a. Allison's diagnoses
   b. Allison's family arrives 12 hours after admission
   c. The discrepancy between the history and injury severity
   d. Allison's age

   Answer: c. The extent of Allison's injuries do not match what one would expect from hitting her head on a propane tank; nothing in the history indicates abdominal trauma. While relevant, the arrival time of the family to the PICU is not the only consideration in nonaccidental trauma suspicion. In this case, it does support the discrepancy between the family report, mechanism, and severity of injury.

Allison's intracranial hypertension worsens, necessitating the addition of pentobarbital and norepinephrine infusions to her therapy. She becomes polyuric and laboratory data is consistent with central diabetes insipidus (DI). Her pupils remain nonreactive. CPPs are between 50 and 70 mm Hg. ■

5. Which of the following signs would indicate possible development of central DI?
   a. Increased CVP; SG greater than 1.005, hyponatremia
   b. Hypertension; serum osmolality greater than 300 mOsm/kg
   c. Hypotension; serum osmolality less than 200 mOsm/kg
   d. Decreased CVP; SG less than 1.005; hypernatremia

   Answer: d. Central DI is associated with extreme water loss in the urine, resulting in dehydration and low specific gravity. A decreased CVP is consistent with dehydration.

6. Which of the following infusions helps to maintain CPP between 50 and 70 mm Hg?
   a. Hypertonic saline
   b. Norepinephrine
   c. Pentobarbital
   d. Vasopressin

   Answer: b. Norepinephrine is an α- and β-adrenergic agent that causes increased contractility and heart rate as well as vasoconstriction, thereby increasing systemic blood pressure. Norepinephrine helps elevate the MAP to maintain a clinically acceptable CPP.

Index

Page numbers followed by *f* indicate figures; *t*, tables; *b*, boxes

F

G

M

N

O

S

W